CO

---

*Leslie Smith contributed to this book in her personal capacity. The views expressed are her own and do not necessarily represent the views of the National Institutes of Health or the United States Government.
†Susan Smith contributed to this book in her personal capacity. The views expressed are her own and do not necessarily represent the views of the National Institutes of Health or the United States Government.

Sole's

Introduction to CRITICAL CARE NURSING

9th EDITION

MARY BETH FLYNN MAKIC, PhD, APRN, CCNS, CCRN, FAAN, FNAP, FCNS
Professor, College of Nursing
University of Colorado Anschutz Medical Campus
Aurora, Colorado;
Research Scientist, Denver Health
Denver, Colorado

LAUREN T. MORATA, DNP, APRN-CNS, CCNS, CPHQ
Director of Quality and Performance Improvement, Clinical Quality
Lakeland Regional Health
Lakeland, Florida

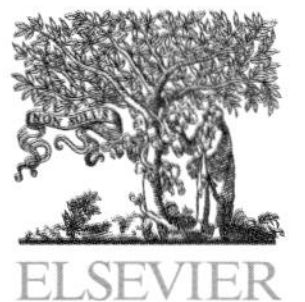

ELSEVIER

Elsevier
3251 Riverport Lane
St. Louis, Missouri 63043

SOLE'S INTRODUCTION TO CRITICAL CARE NURSING, 9TH EDITION ISBN: 978-0-443-11036-8

Previous editions copyrighted 2021, 2017, 2013, 2009, 2005, 2001, 1997, 1993.

Executive Content Strategist: Lee Henderson
Content Development Manager: Danielle Frazier
Senior Content Development Specialist: Maria Broeker
Project Manager: Nayagi Anandan
Design Direction: Patrick Ferguson

Printed in India

Last digit is the print number: 9 8 7 6 5 4 3 2 1

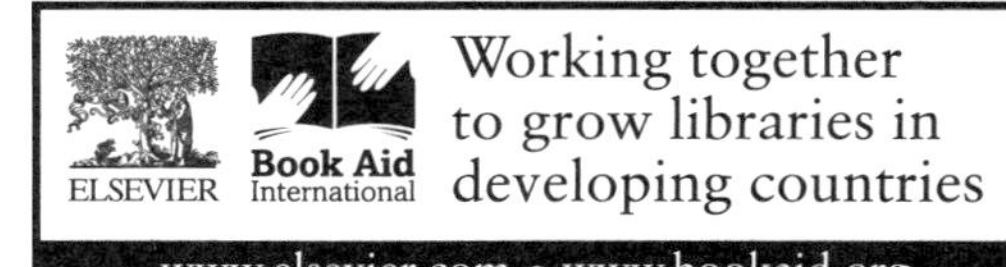

ABOUT THE EDITORS

MARY BETH FLYNN MAKIC

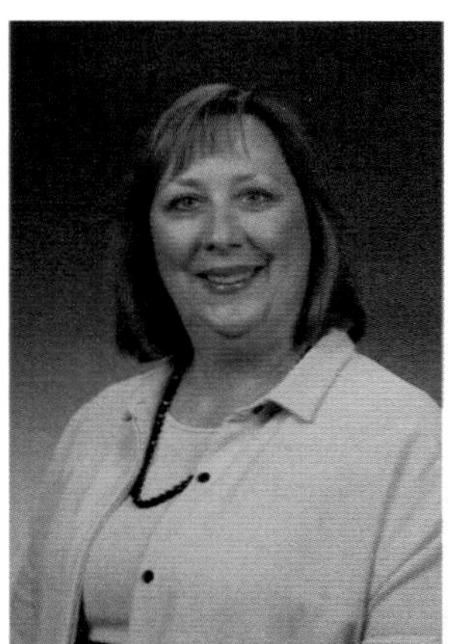

Mary Beth Flynn Makic, PhD, APRN, CCNS, CCRN, FAAN, FNAP, FCNS has more than 30 years of critical care experience in research, evidence-based practice, and clinical education. She is a professor at the University of Colorado Anschutz Medical Campus, College of Nursing and was the program director for the Adult-Gerontology Clinical Nurse Specialist graduate program for 10 years. She is also a research scientist at a level I trauma center in Denver, Colorado. Dr. Makic earned her Bachelor of Science in Nursing from the University of Wisconsin–Madison. She completed her Master of Science at the University of Maryland at Baltimore with a focus on trauma patient populations and the advance practice role of clinical nurse specialist. Her PhD was conferred in 2007 by the University of Colorado Health Sciences Center in Denver, Colorado. She is active in several local and national professional organizations. She also serves on the editorial board of several critical care journals and has published extensively in peer-reviewed journals. Dr. Makic is well known for her passion for improving patient outcomes and nursing through evidence-based practice.

LAUREN T. MORATA

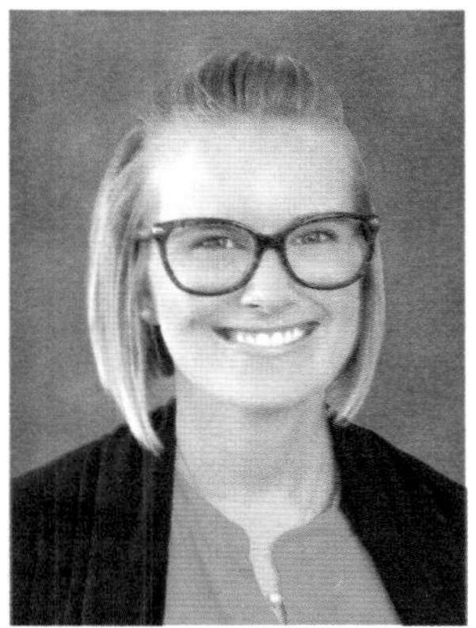

Lauren T. Morata, DNP, APRN-CNS, CCNS, CPHQ has more than a decade of experience as a critical care and trauma nurse and has a passion for evidence-based practice and research. She is the Director of Quality and Performance Improvement at Lakeland Regional Health, where she continues to implement best practices for acute, progressive, and critical care patients. Dr. Morata graduated with a Bachelor of Science in Nursing from the University of Central Florida. She received a Master of Science in Nursing as a clinical nurse specialist from the University of Cincinnati, and a Doctor of Nursing Practice from the University of Central Florida. She has been published in peer-reviewed journals and assisted with the development of the American Association of Critical Care Nurses' Practice Alert on adult prone positioning.

DEDICATION

Since the first edition of this text published in 1991, it was Dr. Mary Lou Sole's mission to provide an easy-to-read text for students, novice nurses, and experienced nurses who want a resource for practice. This book is dedicated to all acute and critical care nurses who care for the lives of our sickest patients at their most vulnerable times. Thank you for all that you do!

MBFM and LTM

To my acute and critical care nursing colleagues, patients, and families, who taught me the importance of excellence in critical care practice. To my parents, sisters, husband, and children, whose unconditional love and support are ever-present and add true meaning to my life.

MBFM

To the acute and critical care clinicians who open this book, I hope the contents within help answer your clinical queries and guide you to provide the best care to your patients. In memory of my father, Tommy Yon, and to my mother, Jackie Yon, both of whom were my first nursing mentors. To my husband and children who provide me with steadfast support and the utmost joy, thank you.

LTM

CONTRIBUTORS AND REVIEWERS

CONTRIBUTORS

Lynelle N. Baba, MS, RN, CCRN, CCNS, FAAN
Clinical Nurse Specialist, Critical Care
University of Kansas Health System
Kansas City, Kansas

Laura Baker, MSN, APRN, ACNPC-AG, CCRN
Nurse Practitioner, Department of Anesthesia & Perioperative Medicine
Medical University of South Carolina
Charleston, South Carolina

Leanne M. Boehm, PhD, RN, ACNS-BC, FCCM, FAAN
Assistant Professor, School of Nursing
Vanderbilt University
Nashville, Tennessee

Amanda Brown, MSN-Ed, RN
Clinical Education Specialist
Critical Care Team
Banner Health
Phoenix, Arizona

Hsin-Mei Chen, PhD, MBA
Assistant Professor, Department of Nursing
Houston Methodist Research Institute;
Manager, Center for Nursing Research, Education and Practice
Houston Methodist Hospital
Houston, Texas

Valerie Danesh, PhD, RN, FCCM, FAAN
Research Scientist, Center for Applied Health Research
Baylor Scott & White Health
Dallas, Texas

Eleanor R. Fitzpatrick, DNP, RN, AGCNS-BC, ACNP-BC, CCRN
Clinical Nurse Specialist, Surgical Intensive Care Unit
Thomas Jefferson University Hospital
Philadelphia, Pennsylvania

Nicole Marie Fontenot, DNP, APRN, ACNP-BC, CCNS, CCRN
Manager of Nursing Science & Academic Outreach
Center for Nursing Research, Education, and Practice
Houston Methodist Academic Institute
Houston, Texas

Shannan K. Hamlin, PhD, RN, AGACNP-BC, CCRN, NE-BC, FCCM
Director, Center for Nursing Research, Education and Practice
Houston Methodist Hospital;
Associate Professor of Nursing
Houston Methodist Institute for Academic Medicine
Houston Methodist Hospital
Houston, Texas

Roberta Kaplow, APRN-CCNS, PhD, AOCNS, CCRN, FAAN
Clinical Nurse Specialist, Nursing
Emory University Hospital
Atlanta, Georgia

Melissa A. Kelley, RN, CPTC
Manager of Recovery Services
LifeLink of Florida
Tampa, Florida

Mary Beth Flynn Makic, PhD, APRN, CCNS, CCRN, FAAN, FNAP, FCNS
Professor, College of Nursing
University of Colorado Anschutz Medical Campus
Aurora, Colorado;
Research Scientist
Denver Health
Denver, Colorado

Lauren T. Morata, DNP, APRN-CNS, CCNS, CPHQ
Director of Quality and Performance Improvement, Clinical Quality
Lakeland Regional Health
Lakeland, Florida

Erica Ochoa, DNP, APRN, FNP-BC, CNRN
Adjunct Professor, Nursing
St. Thomas University
Miami Gardens, Florida;
Adjunct Faculty, Nursing
Arizona College of Nursing
Fort Lauderdale, Florida

Angela D. Pal, PhD, APRN, ACNP-BC, CHSE
Assistant Professor, College of Nursing
University of Colorado Anschutz Medical Campus
Aurora, Colorado

Jan Powers, PhD, RN, CCNS, CCRN, NE-BC, FCCM, FAAN
Director Nursing Research and EBP
Nursing Professional Practice
Parkview Health
Fort Wayne, Indiana

Mamoona Arif Rahu, PhD, MSN, RN, CCRN, TCRN
Trauma Clinical Educator
Department of Trauma Services
Inova Fairfax Medical Campus
Falls Church, Virginia

Catherine D. Robbins, DNP, APRN-BC, CCRN, CNRN
Neurosurgery
Memorial Healthcare System
Hollywood, Florida

Jenny Lynn Sauls, PhD, MSN, RN, CNE
Professor and Director, Nursing
Middle Tennessee State University
Murfreesboro, Tennessee

Sarah E. Schroeder, PhD, ACNP-BC, MSN, RN, AACC
Mechanical Circulatory Support Nurse Practitioner and Program Manager
Department of Mechanical Circulatory Support
Bryan Heart
Lincoln, Nebraska

Maureen A. Seckel, APRN, MSN, ACNS-BC, CCNS, CCRN, FCCM, FCNS, FAAN
Critical Care Clinical Nurse Specialist and Sepsis Coordinator
Consultant
Newark, Delaware

Leslie Smith, DNP, APRN-CNS, AOCNS, BMTCN
National Institutes of Health
Bethesda, Maryland

Susan Smith, DNP, APRN, ACNS-BC
Clinical Nurse Specialist, Critical Care
National Institutes of Health
Bethesda, Maryland

Chelsea Sooy, BSN, RN, CCTC
Director of Quality, Regulatory Affairs and Education
MedStar Georgetown Transplant Institute
MedStar Georgetown University Hospital
Washington, District of Columbia

Linda Staubli, MSN, RN, CCRN, ACCNS-AG
Program Manager, Clinical Quality and Patient Safety
University of Colorado Hospital UC Health
Aurora, Colorado

Sarah Taylor, MSN, RN, ACNS-BC, CBRN
Clinical Nurse Specialist
Trauma Burn Center
University of Michigan Health;
Adjunct Clinical Instructor, School of Nursing
University of Michigan
Ann Arbor, Michigan

Paul Anthony Thurman, PhD, RN, ACNPC, CCNS, CCRN
Nurse Scientist, R Adams Cowley Shock Trauma Center
University of Maryland Medical Center;
Assistant Professor
Adult-Gerontology Acute Care Nurse Practitioner/Adult-Gerontology Clinical Nurse Specialist
University of Maryland School of Nursing
Baltimore, Maryland

Jayne M. Willis, DNP, RN, NEA-BC, CENP
Lecturer, College of Nursing
University of Central Florida
Orlando, Florida

Chris Winkelman, PhD, ACNP-BC, CCRN, CNE, FAANP, FCCM
Associate Professor, Frances Payne Bolton School of Nursing
Lead Faculty, MSN Adult-Gerontology Acute Care Nurse Practitioner Program
Case Western Reserve University
Cleveland, Ohio

REVIEWERS

Manisa Baker, DNP, APRN, CCNS, CCRN
Assistant Professor
Purdue University Northwest
Hammond, Indiana

Linda Bell, MSN, RN
Clinical Practice Specialist-Retired
American Association of Critical-Care Nurses
Aliso Viejo, California

Kimberly Berry, DNP, RN, AGACNP-BC
Critical Care Nurse Practitioner
UCHealth
Aurora, Colorado

Lindsay Boyd, MS, RN
Clinical Nurse Specialist
University of Washington Medical Center
Seattle, Washington

Katharine Courtland, MS, APRN, ACCNS-AG, CCRN
Critical Care Registered Nurse
Emory University Hospital
Atlanta, Georgia

Beverly Copoulos, MSN, CCRN, RN-BC (retired)
Adjunct Faculty–Nursing
Arizona College of Nursing
Tempe, Arizona

Jennifer Downing, MSN, RNC-OB
Adjunct Clinical Instructor
Oklahoma State University-Oklahoma City
Oklahoma City, Oklahoma

Jody Gill-Rocha, MS, BSN, RN
Associate Professor
Mount Carmel College of Nursing
Columbus, Ohio

Kellie Girardot, MSN, RN, AGCNS-BC, TCRN
Trauma Clinical Nurse Specialist
Parkview Regional Medical Center
Fort Wayne, Indiana

Sara Knippa, MS, RN, CCRN, PCCN, ACCNS-AG
Clinical Nurse Specialist, Critical Care
UCHealth
Aurora, Colorado

Laura Madsen, BSN, RN, CCRN, CBRN
Registered Nurse
UCHealth, Burn Center
Aurora, Colorado

Vanessa A. Martinez, DNP, MHA, RN, CPHQ
Senior Director Quality and Safety Improvement
Clinical Quality Consulting
Kaiser Permanente (Kaiser Foundation Hospital and Health Plan)
Oakland, California

Kristi McGuire, EdD, MSN, RN
Assistant Professor of Nursing and BSN Program Director
Nebraska Wesleyan University
Lincoln, Nebraska

Kathleen P. Mierzejewski, MSN, RN
Nursing Instructor
American Institute of Alternative Medicine
Columbus, Ohio

Brianna Moorehead, BSN, RN, CCRN
Clinical Nurse Educator
UCHealth
Aurora, Colorado

Kathy Oman, PhD, RN, FAAN
Professor Emerita, Caritas Coach
University of Colorado College of Nursing
Anschutz Medical Campus
Aurora, Colorado

Jennifer Rechter, MSN, RN-BC, AG-CNS
Clinical Specialist, Medical Intensive Care Unit
Sepsis Coordinator
Parkview Health
Fort Wayne, Indiana

Julie Rials, DNP, APRN-CNP, FNP-BC
Assistant Professor
Oklahoma State University
Oklahoma City, Oklahoma

Rebecca Rich, PharmD, BCCCP, FCCM
Clinical Pharmacy Specialist, Critical Care & Trauma Services
Lakeland Regional Health
Lakeland, Florida

Michael Semanco, PharmD, BCPS, BCCCP
Clinical Pharmacy Specialist–Critical Care & Trauma Services
Lakeland Regional Health Medical Center
Lakeland, Florida

Nicole Seyller, DNP, RN, APN, ACCNS-AG, CCRN, SCRN
Critical Care Clinical Nurse Specialist
UCHealth, Southern Region
Colorado Springs, Colorado

Samuel Simonson, BSN, RN, CCRN
Clinical Nurse Educator
Providence Alaska Medical Center
Anchorage, Alaska

Jenna Sissom, MSN-Ed, RN
Assistant Professor
Lipscomb University
Nashville, Tennessee

Andrea Slivinski, DNP, APRN, ACNS-BC, CEN, CPEN, TCRN
Clinical Nurse Specialist, Trauma
Mission Hospital
Asheville, North Carolina

Amanda Thomson, RN, CCRN, NPD-BC
Nurse Manager
UCHealth
Aurora, Colorado

Rosemary Timmerman, DNP, APRN, CCNS, CCRN-CSC-CMC
Research Scientist Nurse
Providence Alaska Medical Center
Anchorage, Alaska

Tia Wheatley, DNP, RN, AOCNS, AGACNP-BC
Nurse Practitioner & Clinical Nurse Specialist, Hem/Onc & Cell Therapy
Ronald Reagan UCLA Medical Center
Los Angeles, California

Tonka Williams, MHA, MSN, RN, CMSRN
Nursing Director
VCU Medical Center
Richmond, Virginia

John Wood, EdD, MSN, RN
Nursing Instructor (retired)
Graceland University
Independence, Missouri

PREFACE

Acute and critical care nursing deals with human responses to life-threatening health problems. These patients and their families have high levels of acuity and complex physical, emotional, and psychosocial needs. Patients are cared for in critical care units, intermediate care units, outpatient settings, and at home. The critical care nurse is challenged to provide comprehensive care for these patients and their family members. Care of the critically ill patient involves not only the patient's immediate crisis but also consideration of the continuum of care to avoid complications and adverse outcomes.

A solid knowledge foundation in the concepts of critical care nursing is essential for practice. Nurses must also learn the assessment and technical skills associated with management of the critically ill patient.

The goal of this ninth edition of what is now titled *Sole's Introduction to Critical Care Nursing* is to facilitate attainment of this foundation for care of the acutely and critically ill patient. The book continues to provide essential information in an easy-to-learn format. The textbook is targeted to both undergraduate nursing students and experienced nurses who are new to critical care. Both groups have found past editions of the book highly beneficial. In fact, undergraduate students who have taken a critical care course based on this textbook have easily passed critical care courses offered in their first nursing position!

ORGANIZATION

Sole's Introduction to Critical Care Nursing is organized into three parts. **Part I, Fundamental Concepts**, introduces the reader to critical care nursing; psychosocial concepts related to patients, families, and nurses; and legal, ethical, and end-of-life considerations related to high-acuity and critical care nursing practice.

Part II, Tools for the Critical Care Nurse, is a unique feature of this text. Chapters in this section provide vital information on comfort, sedation and delirium, nutrition, recognition of dysrhythmias, hemodynamic monitoring, airway management and mechanical ventilation, management of life-threatening emergencies, and organ donation. These chapters provide current and contemporary information related to the many treatments and technologies that acutely and critically ill patients receive.

The final chapters of the book form **Part III, Nursing Care During Critical Illness**. The nursing process is used as an organizing framework for each chapter. Patient problems with nursing care plans continue to be included so that nurses new to critical care become familiar with interventions common to many critically ill patients. A summary of anatomy and physiology is provided, as are pathophysiology diagrams for common problems seen in critical care. Common pharmacologic interventions are reviewed but are not meant to replace resources that should be accessed within the hospital, clinic, and outpatient practice settings. Multiprofessional collaborations are also presented, as acute and critical care practice requires teamwork to meet the complex needs of patients.

SPECIAL FEATURES

Several features have been incorporated into each chapter to develop clinical reasoning and judgment skills. As the nursing licensure examination has moved to a new model (the Next-Generation NCLEX® Examination) that evaluates nurses' ability to recognize changes in a patient's clinical condition and determine appropriate interventions, practice in translating knowledge into actions is needed. Multiple features within each chapter are designed to develop the nurse's ability to recognize and analyze cues, prioritize hypotheses, generate solutions, take action, and evaluate outcomes. Identification of subtle changes in a patient's condition that require the nurse to develop an evidence-based, person-centered plan of care is necessary to ensure safe delivery of care.

Key features such as Pathophysiology Flow Charts, Clinical and Laboratory Alerts, Pharmacology Tables, and Lifespan and Genetics Boxes facilitate understanding of patient-specific cues that require interventions. Evidence-based practice boxes and clinical exemplars which align with competency-based education pillars in nursing, facilitate understanding of opportunities to generate solutions and implement safe care. The case studies and collaborative plan of care for critically ill patients allow for a deeper understanding of how to apply or translate knowledge into practice to optimize care of acutely and critically ill patients. Knowledge application questions are woven into each chapter, allowing readers to self-evaluate their knowledge. Clinical judgment activities are designed to hone knowledge, critical thinking, and clinical reasoning. Nursing self-care boxes identify strategies to address personal well-being.

Additions and revisions have been made based on reader feedback and current trends.

This edition features a full-color design with updated figures to enhance reader understanding. Many new and revised learning aids appear in this ninth edition to highlight chapter content:

- A **Collaborative Plan of Care for the Critically Ill Patient** is introduced in Chapter 1. It can be individualized to meet specific needs of the patient.
- **Evidence-Based Practice** boxes identify problems in patient care, ask pertinent questions related to the problems, supply evidence addressing the questions, and offer implications for nursing practice. Most of these boxes provide references to systematic reviews and meta-analyses that provide a greater synthesis of the research evidence related to a problem.
- **Clinical Exemplars** present examples that align with the new American Association of College of Nursing domains to include Person-Centered Care; Quality and Safety; Interprofessional Partnership; Information and Healthcare Technologies; Communication; and Diversity, Equity, and Inclusion.
- **Genetics** boxes discuss disorders with a genetic component, including diabetes, Marfan syndrome, and cystic fibrosis.
- **Clinical Alerts** highlight particular concerns, significance, and procedures to help readers understand the potential problems encountered in that setting for selected disorders and disease states.

- **Laboratory Alerts** detail both common and cutting-edge tests and procedures to alert readers to the importance of laboratory results.
- **Lifespan Considerations** alert the reader to the special needs of select populations across the lifespan, such as pregnant patients and older adults, as they relate to critical illness.
- **Transplant Considerations** boxes have been incorporated into several chapters. These boxes include criteria for transplantation, patient management, and strategies for preventing rejection.
- **Case Studies** that are client specific with accompanying questions help readers apply the chapter's content to real-life situations while also testing your clinical judgment skills. Answers for these questions and the **Clinical Judgment Activities** found throughout each chapter are included on the companion Evolve website, which is free to instructors.
- **Nursing Care Plans** describe patient problems, outcomes, nursing interventions, and rationales.
- **Pathophysiology Flow Charts** expand analysis of the course and outcomes of particular injuries and disorders.
- **Pharmacology Tables** reflect the most current and most commonly used critical care medications.
- **Nursing Self-Care** boxes are new to the ninth edition and highlight the importance of the 2020-2030 Future of Nursing report, which states nurses need to address their own personal well-being first to effectively care for others and advance health equity.
- **Key Points** summarize key principles of the chapter.

EVOLVE RESOURCES

We are pleased to offer additional content and learning aids to both instructors and students on our Evolve companion website, which has been customized for the new edition and is available at http://evolve.elsevier.com/Sole/.

For Students. Student resources on the Evolve site include the following:

- **Mastery Questions,** consisting of multiple-choice and multiple-response questions and answer rationales for each chapter.
- **Next-Generation NCLEX® (NGN) Examination–Style Case Studies**
- **Animations and Video Clips,** which feature innovative content from supplemental materials.
- **15 Procedures** from Mosby's Clinical Skills: Critical Care Collection that demonstrate many of the primary procedures important in critical care nursing.

For Instructors. Instructor resources on the Evolve site include the following:

- **TEACH for Nurses Lesson Plans,** which provide the following for each chapter:
  - Objectives and teaching focus.
  - Nursing curriculum standards, concept-based curricula, and mapping to the AACN Essentials, adult CCRN, and PCCN.
  - Teaching and learning activities related to the chapter content.
  - Case study with questions and answers.
- **Answer Keys** to the Clinical Judgment Activities and Case Studies presented in the textbook.
- **PowerPoint slides** for every chapter include lecture notes and audience response questions.
- An electronic **Test Bank** of questions.
- **Next-Generation NCLEX® (NGN) Examination–Style Case Studies**
- An **Image Collection** including all images from the text.

Instructors have access to the student resources as well. Evolve can also be used to do the following:

- Publish your class syllabus, outline, and lecture notes.
- Set up "virtual office hours" and email communication.
- Share important dates and information through the online class calendar.
- Encourage student participation through chat rooms and discussion boards.

Critical care nursing is an exciting and challenging field. Healthcare organizations need critical care nurses who are knowledgeable about basic concepts and research-based practice, technologically competent, and caring toward patients and families. Our hope is that this edition of *Sole's Introduction to Critical Care Nursing* will provide the foundation for critical care nursing practice.

MBFM
LTM

PART I

Fundamental Concepts

1

Overview of Critical Care Nursing

Lauren T. Morata, DNP, APRN-CNS, CCNS, CPHQ
Mary Beth Flynn Makic, PhD, APRN, CCNS, CCRN, FAAN, FNAP, FCNS

INTRODUCTION

Patients in critical care settings have life-threatening conditions requiring constant monitoring and care by a team of multiprofessionals. The nurse/patient ratio is low, sometimes 1:1, to ensure care delivery is timely and response to treatment is continuously assessed. Technology is abundant and readily available to assist in assessing and managing these complex cases and acutely ill patients. Treatments vary but often include mechanical ventilation, multiple invasive lines, hemodynamic monitoring, and administration of many medications and intravenous fluids. Caring for critically ill patients provides ample opportunities to learn new interventions, treatments, and technologies. Many nurses choose to work in critical care settings because they enjoy working in a fast-paced environment that provides frequent, close contact with patients, families, and their multiprofessional colleagues.

CRITICAL CARE NURSING

Definition

Critical care nursing is concerned with physiological and psychological human responses to crisis situation such as trauma, major surgery, or severe complications of illness. The focus of the critical care nurse includes both the patient's and the family's responses to illness and involves prevention as well as attaining the goals of care, whether curative or palliative. Because patients' medical needs have become increasingly complex, critical care nursing encompasses care of both acutely ill and critically ill patients.

Evolution of Critical Care

The specialty of critical care has its roots in the 1950s, when patients with poliomyelitis (i.e., polio) were cared for in specialized units. In the 1960s, recovery rooms were established for the care of patients who had undergone surgery, and coronary care units were instituted for the care of patients with cardiac problems. The patients who received care in these units had improved outcomes. Fig. 1.1 depicts an early cardiac surgical unit.

Critical care nursing evolved as a specialty in the 1970s with the development of general critical care units. Since that time, critical care nursing has become increasingly specialized. Examples of specialized critical care units are cardiovascular, surgical, neurological, trauma, transplant, burn, maternal, pediatric, and neonatal units. Fig. 1.2 shows a modern critical care unit.

Today, critical care nursing practice has expanded beyond the walls of traditional critical care units. For example, critically ill patients are cared for in emergency departments; postanesthesia care units; stepdown, intermediate care, and progressive care units; and interventional cardiology and radiology units. Critical care nurses also provide specialized care during transport of critically ill patients from the field to the acute care hospital and during interfacility transport. With advances in technology, Tele-Critical Care (TCC) has emerged as another setting for critical care nurses. In TCC, patients are monitored remotely by critical care nurses and providers.[1,2] Tele-ICU and ICU telemedicine are terms also used to refer to these remote services. However, the Society of Critical Care Medicine's Tele-ICU Committee recommended the term TCC to replace these existing terms. TCC is not only used in critical care units, but in other parts of the hospital and beyond, such as in disaster scenarios; therefore, the Committee sought a term that better captured the global impact and advances in this critical care service. Implementation of the TCC model has shortened hospital and critical care unit lengths of stay and has reduced mortality.[3] Emerging applications for TCC include the early detection and bundle compliance of sepsis, facilitation of end-of-life discussions, and coordinating patient transfers to the appropriate level of care.[4]

Acute and critical care nurses practice in varied settings to manage and coordinate care for patients who require in-depth assessment, high-intensity therapies and interventions, and continuous nursing vigilance. They also function in various roles and levels, such as staff nurse, educator, advanced practice registered nurse (APRN), and nurse leader. Competencies for critical care nursing practice are listed in Box 1.1.

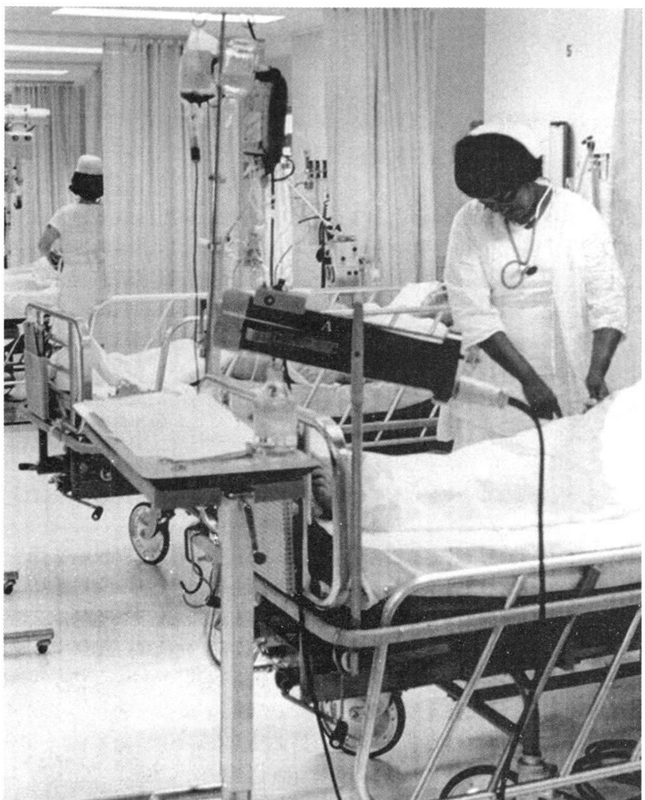

Fig. 1.1 Early cardiac critical care unit circa 1967, called the *cardiac constant care unit*. Note the open-bay concept of care delivery, large cardiac monitor at foot of bed, and absence of multiple pumps. (Reprinted with permission from Cleveland Clinic Center for Medical Arts & Photography © 2011–2019. All rights reserved.)

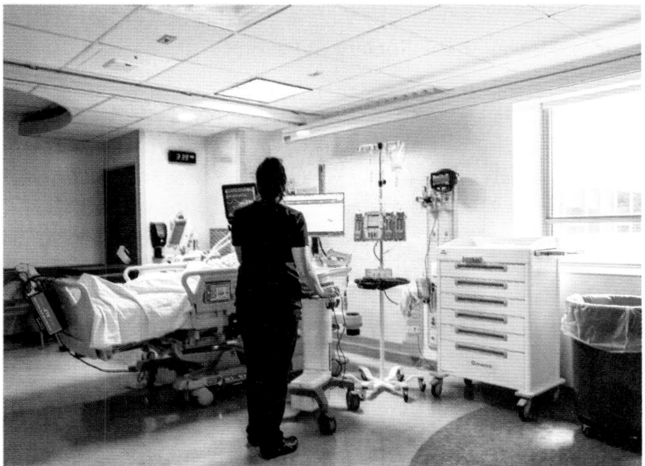

Fig. 1.2 Modern Critical Care Unit. Note the private room and abundance of electronic equipment supporting patient care management. (Courtesy Lakeland Regional Health, Lakeland, Florida.)

CLINICAL JUDGMENT ACTIVITY

Compare perceptions of critical care from the viewpoints of the student, nurse, multiprofessional healthcare team, patient, and family. What are distinguishing similarities and differences in experiences?

BOX 1.1 Synergy Nurse Competencies for Progressive and Critical Care

- Clinical judgment and clinical reasoning skills.
- Advocacy and moral agency in identifying and resolving ethical issues.
- Caring practices that are tailored to the uniqueness of the patient and family.
- Collaboration with patients, family members, and healthcare team members.
- Systems thinking that promotes holistic nursing care.
- Response to diversity.
- Facilitator of learning for patients and family members, team members, and the community.
- Clinical inquiry and innovation to promote the best patient outcome.

Data from The American Association of Critical-Care Nurses. *AACN Synergy Model for Patient Care*. https://www.aacn.org/~/media/aacn-website/nursing-excellence/standards/aacnsynergymodelforpatientcare.pdf?la=en

PROFESSIONAL ORGANIZATIONS

Several professional organizations support critical care practice. These include the American Association of Critical-Care Nurses (AACN) and the Society of Critical Care Medicine (SCCM).

American Association of Critical-Care Nurses

The AACN is a professional organization that was established in 1969 to represent critical care nurses. It is the largest nursing specialty organization in the world, with more than 120,000 members, dedicated to providing knowledge and resources to those caring for acutely and critically ill patients. In addition to the national organization, there are more than 200 chapters in the United States supporting critical care nurses at the local level. The mission of the organization is to drive excellence in acute and critical care for nurses, patients, and families. The vision of the organization supports creating a healthcare system driven by the needs of patients and families in which nurses make their optimal contributions. Values of the organization are the foundation from which it builds the relentless pursuit of excellence and honor principles of integrity, inclusion, transformation, leadership, and relationships.[5]

The benefits of AACN membership include continuing education offerings, educational advancement scholarships, research grants, awards, and several official publications, including *Critical Care Nurse* and *American Journal of Critical Care*. The organization publishes *Practice Alerts*, which present succinct, evidence-based practices to be applied at the bedside. The AACN sponsors the Beacon Award for Excellence, which is given to a unit within a hospital for exceptional care, improved outcomes, and greater satisfaction with care. The organization also pioneered the Clinical Scene Investigator (CSI) Academy to develop bedside nurses as leaders and change agents who improve patient and fiscal outcomes.[6] The AACN website (http://www.aacn.org) provides membership information and a wealth of information related to critical care nursing.

Society of Critical Care Medicine

The SCCM is a multiprofessional society whose mission is to ensure high-quality care for all critically ill patients. The vision of the SCCM is to have care for all critically ill patients provided by an integrated team of professionals directed by an intensivist (provider who has education, training, and board certification in managing critically ill and injured patients). These teams use knowledge, technology, and compassion to provide timely, safe, effective, efficient, and equitable patient care.[7] Membership in the SCCM is open to all providers in critical care, including providers, nurses, respiratory therapists, and pharmacists. The SCCM publishes several journals, including *Critical Care Medicine*. Membership and other information is available online at http://www.sccm.org.

Other Professional Organizations

Several other professional organizations focus on improving care of critically ill patients. Examples include the American College of Chest Physicians (http://www.chestnet.org), the American Thoracic Society (http://www.thoracic.org), and the professional scientific councils of the American Heart Association (http://www.americanheart.org). Nurses can apply for membership in these and other related professional organizations.

> **CHECK YOUR UNDERSTANDING**
> 1. Determine which professional organization's primary focus is to support critical care nursing.
>   A. American Association of Critical-Care Nurses
>   B. American Association of Heart Failure Nurses
>   C. American Nurses Association
>   D. Society of Critical Care Medicine

CERTIFICATION

Critical care nurses are eligible for certification through the AACN. Certification validates knowledge of critical care nursing, promotes professional excellence, and helps nurses maintain a current knowledge base.[8] The AACN Certification Corporation oversees the critical care certification process.

The AACN certification credentials are based on a synergy model of practice, which states that the needs of patients and families influence and drive nurse competencies.[9] (Fig. 1.3 and Box 1.1). Although the synergy model is more than 20 years old, it remains relevant. Each patient and family is unique, with a varying capacity for health and vulnerability to illness. Patients who are more severely compromised have more complex needs, and nursing practice is based on meeting those needs.[10]

Certification at the Bedside

The certifications for nurses in acute and critical care bedside practice are known as *CCRN* and *PCCN*. The CCRN certification is available for nurses who provide care of critically ill adult, pediatric, or neonatal populations. The PCCN certification is for nurses who provide acute care in progressive care, telemetry, and similar units. Once nurses achieve the CCRN or PCCN credential, they may be eligible to sit for additional subspecialty certification in cardiac medicine or cardiac surgery.

Certification for Advanced Practice

Advanced practice certification for critical care nurses is also available. Acute and critical care clinical nurse specialists can seek the ACCNS-AG credential, which is available for those working with adult-gerontology (AG); ACCNS-P, for those working with pediatric; and ACCNS-N, for those working with neonatal populations. Acute care nurse practitioners can become certified as ACNPC-AG.

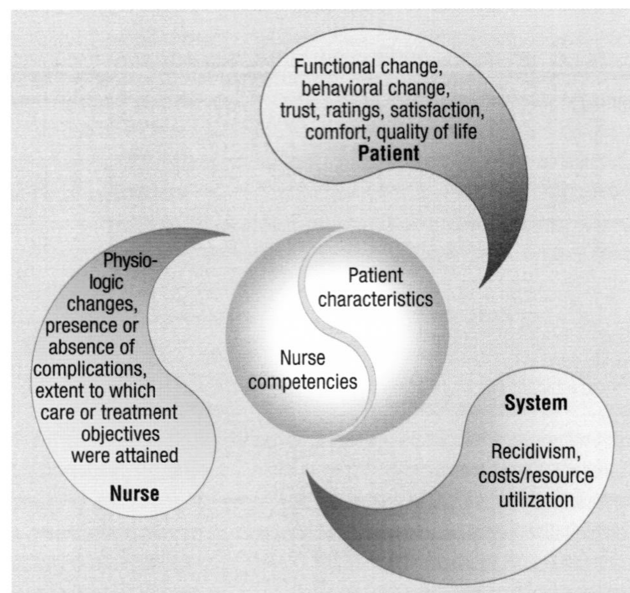

Fig. 1.3 The American Association of Critical-Care Nurses synergy model for patient care. (From Curley M. Patient-nurse synergy: optimizing patients' outcomes. *Am J Crit Care.* 1998;7:69.)

All certifications have eligibility requirements to sit for the examination. Continuing education and ongoing care for acute or critically ill patients are required for recertification.

> **CHECK YOUR UNDERSTANDING**
> 2. A nurse on the unit states, "I don't need to be certified. I've been doing this long enough that it won't bring me any value." Which of the following statements would you use to justify certification?
>   A. "Certification validates the wealth of knowledge and skills you have achieved."
>   B. "The continuing education required to maintain your certification will ensure you use the latest evidence-based practices to effectively care for patients."
>   C. "Patients and their families will know their nurse is a clinical expert when they see you are certified."
>   D. All of the above.

CLINICAL JUDGMENT MEASUREMENT MODEL

The clinical judgment measurement model (CJMM) is used to measure clinical judgment and decision-making. Clinical judgment is an iterative process that requires the individual to apply nursing knowledge to assess the patient, recognize relevant data that informs identification of patient problems and potential complications, and develop and apply potential evidence-based solutions with effective interventions in the delivery of safe care.[11,12] Underlying the model is the nursing process. Elements of the CJMM include:

- Assessment = Recognizing cues
- Diagnosis = Analyzing cues and prioritizing hypothesis
- Planning = Generating solutions
- Implementation = Taking action
- Evaluation = Evaluating outcomes

BOX 1.2 Standards of Professional Performance

The nurse caring for acute and critically ill patients:
- Systematically evaluates the quality and effectiveness of nursing practice.
- Evaluates own practice in relation to professional practice standards, guidelines, statutes, rules, and regulations.
- Acquires and maintains current knowledge and competency in patient care.
- Collaborates with multiprofessional team members, patients, and families to maintain a healthy work environment, effect change and promote optimal outcomes.
- Uses skilled communication to collaborate with the healthcare team to provide care in a safe, healing, humane, and caring environment.
- Acts ethically in all areas of practice.
- Uses clinical inquiry and integrates research findings into practice.
- Considers factors related to safety, effectiveness, cost, and effect in planning and delivering care.
- Provides leadership in the practice setting for the profession.
- Maintains a safe work environment through accountability, implementation of environmental best practices, and health promotion throughout the continuum of care.

Data from Cain C, Miller J. *AACN Scope and Standards for Progressive and Critical Care Nursing Practice.* American Association of Critical-Care Nurses; 2019.

STANDARDS

Standards serve as guidelines for clinical practice. They establish goals for patient care and provide mechanisms for nurses to assess the achievement of goals. Standards of practice delineate the nursing process: assess the patient, analyze and determine nursing diagnosis with expected outcomes, develop a person-centered plan of care, implement interventions, and evaluate progress toward the goals of care. The standards of professional performance (Box 1.2) describe expectations of the acute and critical care nurse.

American Association of Critical-Care Nurses' Competence Framework

The AACN's Competence Framework provides an initial competency for practice approach that validates a core set of knowledge, skills, and abilities (KSAs).[13] The intent is to establish standard entry-level competencies for nurses new to progressive and critical care practice. These KSAs also address a nurse's ability to respond to rapidly changing patient and family needs often encountered within the progressive and critical care practice settings. While each hospital and unit will have specific KSAs, this list is intended to provide a common framework for elements considered essential for the nurse new to acute and critical care practice. Competency requires achievement of core KSAs and the broader set of eight Synergy Nurse Competencies (SNCs).[13] The SNCs encompasses the nurse's ability to assess and perform essential actions required for competent care by the novice nurse. Box 1.1 lists the SNCs. The rapidly changing patient care situations and environment require the nurse to attain competencies in the KSAs and SNCs to respond to the wide range of patient needs effectively.

CRITICAL CARE NURSE CHARACTERISTICS

Essential Practices

Essential nursing practices include monitoring and assessment; reassessment, interpreting information, and problem solving; evaluation of progress towards achieving health outcomes; development of sustainable evidence-based practice; coordination of team activities and the plan of care; patient and family education; and team skill development. The acuteness of a patient's illness makes care the top priority of critical care nurses. A missed detail in care could easily result in an adverse event or even death. Critical care nurses are diligent and highly focused on ensuring optimal outcomes are achieved. They are familiar with the noises, lights, and frequent interruptions. Based on assessment findings, critical care nurses have the knowledge and skills to quickly intervene as indicated. By being proactive and organized, critical care nurses effectively manage complex cases in collaboration with the multiprofessional team. In addition to technical competence, critical care nurses establish relationships with patients and families. Chapter 2, Patient and Family Response to the Critical Care Experience, details the importance of person-centered care in the busy critical care environment.

Challenges of the Profession

Effectively coordinating care of complex cases while meeting the needs of the patients, families, and self, creates a challenging profession, yet one that is incredibly rewarding. Compassion fatigue and moral distress are issues that critical care nurses face because of the fast-paced environment, critical nature of illness, and issues surrounding life and death of patients (See Nursing Self-Care Box).[14-16] Critical care nurses can demonstrate perfectionist tendencies and unrealistic expectations of self, which may further compound high stress levels. Support groups and debriefing conducted by professionals are strategies to help reduce stress, anxiety, and moral distress.

NURSING SELF-CARE BOX

Combating Compassion Fatigue

1. Identification:
   - Physical symptoms: progressive and profound fatigue, aches, sleeplessness, lack of energy
   - Emotional symptoms: withdrawing; isolation; unhappy with career; feelings of failure, incompetence, hopelessness, helplessness, despair
2. Triggers:
   - Staffing shortages
   - Poor social and professional support
   - Overly involved
   - Unable to escape from work
   - Overwhelmed
3. Prevention/Overcoming:
   - Social and professional support
   - Opportunities for professional development
   - Debriefing
   - Mentoring and strong leadership
   - Self-care activities: meditation, exercise, boundary setting, adequate sleep

From Nolte AG, Downing C, Temane A, Hastings-Tolsma M. Compassion fatigue in nurses: a metasynthesis. *J Clin Nurs.* 2017;26(23-24):4364-4378. https://doi.org/10.1111/jocn.13766.[17]

CLINICAL JUDGMENT ACTIVITY

Determine strategies to improve communication and collaboration among the multiprofessional team members in critical care. Self-reflect on skills needed for effective verbal, written, electronic, and text-based communication with the multiprofessional team members.

QUALITY AND SAFETY EMPHASIS

Quality and safety are essential components of patient care. Acute and critically ill patients are at risk for a myriad of harms, which increase morbidity, mortality, length of hospital stay, and costs of care. Application of quality and safety competencies to critical care nursing topics are integrated throughout this text.

Initiatives to Promote Quality and Safety

Nurses and other healthcare professionals have been challenged to reduce medical errors and promote an environment that facilitates safe practices. The Joint Commission has identified *National Patient Safety Goals* to be addressed in hospitals, long-term care facilities, and other agencies that it accredits.[18] Examples are shown in Box 1.3; however, because goals are updated annually, it is important to regularly review The Joint Commission website (http://www.jointcommission.org).

Initiatives to encourage a safe environment are promoted by the government and other national groups, such as the Institute for Healthcare Improvement (IHI). The federal government published a national action plan for reducing healthcare–associated infections.[19] The IHI uses the concept of *bundles* of care to reduce harms, such as infections. Bundles are described as evidence-based best practices that, when implemented as a whole, are intended to improve outcomes; research is being done to evaluate their effectiveness.[20]

Rapid Response Teams. Another strategy to improve patient safety is the implementation of rapid response teams to address changes in patients' conditions. These teams bring critical care expertise to the acute and progressive care bedside for assessment and management of patients whose conditions are deteriorating, providing early intervention and improving outcomes (see Chapter 11, Rapid Response Teams and Code Management).[21] Although most rapid response calls are initiated by healthcare team members, patients and family members are often empowered to activate the team if needed.[22]

BOX 1.3 Examples of Patient Safety Goals

Identify Patients Correctly
- Use at least two methods of patient identification.
- Ensure correct patient identification for blood transfusions.

Improve Communication Among Healthcare Providers
- Ensure the right information is provided to the right clinician.
- Report important results of tests and diagnostic procedures on a timely basis.

Use Medications Safely
- Label all medications and containers, including syringes and medicine cups, at the time of preparation.
- Reduce harm associated with administration of anticoagulants.
- Reconcile medications across the continuum of care.

Use Alarms Safely
- Appropriately manage alarms to reduce alarm fatigue.
- Ensure that alarms are audible and respond to them in a timely manner.

Prevent Infection
- Comply with guidelines for hand hygiene.
- Identify opportunities to improve hand hygiene compliance.

Identify Safety Risks
- Assess patients for suicide risk.
- Reduce the risk of self-harm.

Prevent Mistakes in Surgery and Procedures
- Conduct a preprocedure verification process to ensure that surgery is done on the correct patient and site.
- Mark the correct procedure site on the patient's body.
- Pause before the procedure to ensure that the correct patient, site, and procedure are identified.

Improve Health Care Equity
- Identify health care disparities and establish a written plan to describe ways improve health care equity.

Modified from The Joint Commission. *National Patient Safety Goals.* https://www.jointcommission.org/-/media/tjc/documents/standards/national-patient-safety-goals/2024/hap-npsg-simple-2024-v2.pdf. Published October 4, 2023. Accessed February 8, 2024.

EVIDENCE-BASED PRACTICE

Synthesis of the Evidence

Nurses are encouraged to implement care that is evidence-based and to challenge practices that have "always been done" but are not supported by current, clinical evidence. Evidence-based practice requires a critical review of research and other forms of reliable scientific evidence (i.e., practice guidelines), clinical experience, and consideration of patient preferences. The synthesis of the evidence is used to guide practice interventions. The search for evidence always begins with a review of current, rigorous, high-quality research. Research studies are graded by the rigor of the study methodology and the quality of evidence, and many different rating scales are used. The AACN scale for rating evidence (Table 1.1) is a simple-to-use method for evaluating research studies and other forms of evidence.[23] Meta-analysis of many related research studies is considered to be the highest level of evidence. The Cochrane (https://www.cochrane.org/) and Joanna Briggs Institute, now called JBI, (https://jbi.global/ebp) provide current meta-analysis and evidence summaries on a variety of clinical topics to support evidence-based practice. The next highest level of research findings is derived from randomized controlled trials. Qualitative studies and clinical practice guidelines from national organizations are also important sources of evidence that inform evidence-based practice. Once research studies are critically reviewed and evidence is rated, the findings from the studies are synthesized to elicit practice recommendations. Nurses can get involved in understanding research in many ways, including participating in unit-based journal clubs to critically review studies, rate their quality, and understand how the findings can be used to guide practice.

TABLE 1.1 American Association of Critical-Care Nurses' Levels of Research Evidence

Level	Description
A	Meta-analysis of multiple controlled studies or meta-synthesis of qualitative studies with results that consistently support a specific action, intervention, or treatment
B	Well-designed controlled studies, both randomized and nonrandomized, with results that consistently support a specific action, intervention, or treatment
C	Qualitative, descriptive, or correlational studies; integrative reviews; systematic reviews; or randomized controlled trials with inconsistent results
D	Peer-reviewed professional organizational standards, with clinical studies to support recommendations
E	Theory-based evidence from expert opinion or multiple case reports
M	Manufacturer's recommendation only

From Peterson M, Barnason S, Donnelly B, et al. Choosing the best evidence to guide clinical practice: application of AACN levels of evidence. *Crit Care Nurse*. 2014;34(2):58-68.

Guidelines

Clinical practice guidelines are implemented to ensure that care is appropriate and based on research. Relevant guidelines, such as those guiding nutrition and sedation practices, are discussed throughout the textbook. Many guidelines are available online from national organizations (e.g., SCCM, AHA, Infectious Diseases Society of America [IDSA], etc.), as well as the Agency for Healthcare Research and Quality (AHRQ; https://www.ahrq.gov/research/findings/evidence-based-reports/index.html) and Guideline Central (https://www.guidelinecentral.com/guidelines/).

HEALTHY WORK ENVIRONMENT

The culture of a critical care unit includes shared values, attitudes, and beliefs, which in turn reflect behavioral norms that guide the functional dynamics of staff interactions. Interactions among providers, especially nurses and providers, affect patient safety, clinical outcomes, and the recruitment and retention of nurses.

The AACN initiated a campaign to create work environments that are safe, healing, and humane, as well as respectful of rights and responsibilities and the needs of all people.[24] Essential components of healthy work environments acknowledge the unique contributions of patients, families, nurses, and healthcare team members (Fig. 1.4).[25] Other aspects of a healthy work environment include effective decision-making, appropriate staffing, meaningful recognition, and authentic leadership. Communication and collaboration provide the foundation for achieving a healthy work environment. A healthy work environment promotes nurse retention and job satisfaction.[26]

Communication

Person-centered communication is a strategy to improve communication, quality of care, and mutual trust among patients,

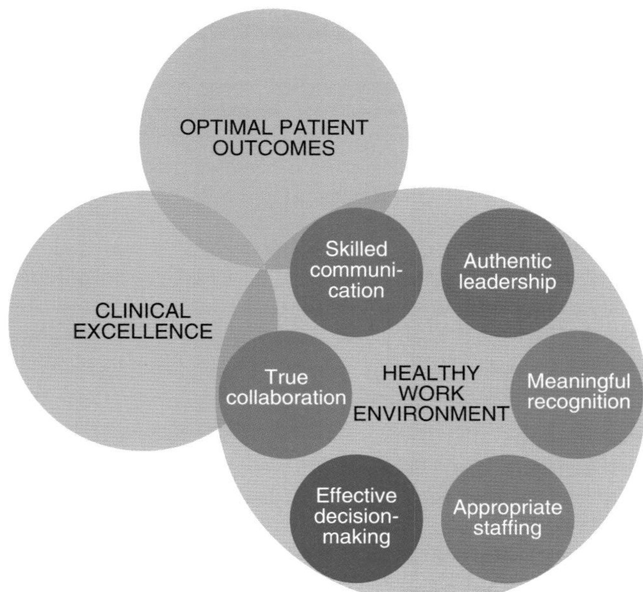

Fig. 1.4 Essential Components of a Healthy Work Environment. Interdependence of healthy work environment, clinical excellence, and optimal patient outcomes. (From American Association of Critical-Care Nurses. AACN standards for establishing and sustaining healthy work environments: a journey to excellence. *Am J Crit Care*. 2005;14[3]:189.)

families, and healthcare professionals.[27] The goal is to elicit more information from patients and to better assess their understanding. Standardized approaches are helpful and are easily learned.[28] Approaches include *Ask-Tell-Ask*, a strategy for encouraging nurses to assess concerns before providing more information, especially when discussing stressful issues with patients and families.[29] *Tell Me More* is a tool that encourages information sharing in challenging situations.

Effective communication is also essential for delivering safe patient care. Many adverse events are directly attributable to faulty communication. Communication breakdowns often occur during *handoff* situations, when patient information is being transferred or exchanged. Common handoff situations include nursing and provider shift reports and patient transfers. Barriers to effective handoffs are noted in Box 1.4. Formal training in handoff communication with both nurses and other team members assists in improving communication and reducing errors, and tools are also available to enhance and evaluate handoffs.[30,31]

The situation, background, assessment, recommendation (SBAR) approach is useful in communication, especially with providers and when conveying information via the phone (Box 1.5).[32] The SBAR technique delivers information in a way that is brief and action oriented. The Clinical Exemplar box illustrates an example of SBAR communication for a patient handoff. Other strategies to improve handoff communication include standardizing processes for the handoff situation, using checklists to prompt and document essential information, and training all personnel in effective communication techniques.

CLINICAL EXEMPLAR

Communication

The *s*ituation, *b*ackground, *a*ssessment, *r*ecommendation (SBAR) report methodology may be particularly helpful in the critical care setting as a method of improving interdepartmental and shift-to-shift information transfer. A sample transfer SBAR report is illustrated.

Situation

My name is (caregiver) Mary Smith, RN, from the (unit) emergency department. I will be transferring (patient name) John Jones, a (age) 34-year-old (sex) man admitted (time/date) 3 hours ago with (diagnosis) diabetic ketoacidosis, to the (receiving department) medical critical care unit. Attending provider is Dr. Michael Miller.

Background

Pertinent history—type 1 diabetes for 20 years; on insulin pump; managed pump failure 24 hours ago inappropriately; renal insufficiency. Summary of episode of care:

- Admitting glucose 648 mg/dL; positive ketones; pH 7.27; PaO_2 90 mm Hg; $PaCO_2$ 20 mm Hg; HCO_3^- 12 mEq/L; K^+ 3.4 mEq/L; BUN 40 mg/dL; creatinine 1.8 mg/dL; admitting weight 65 kg; lethargic
- Received 1 L balanced crystalloid solution (Lactated Ringers) in field. Balanced crystalloid solution (Lactated Ringers) now infusing at 200 mL/h
- Received IV bolus of 6.5 units regular insulin at 1300. Insulin infusion of 100 units regular in 100 mL normal saline infusing at 7.5 units per hour (7.5 mL/h). 1400 repeat glucose 502 mg/dL
- 20 mEq potassium chloride infused in emergency department
- 200 mL urine output last hour—hourly intake and output
- Hemoglobin A1c level 6 weeks ago was 9.2% (outpatient clinical records)

Assessment

- Vital signs: BP 102/60 mmHg; pulse 116 beats/min; respirations 30 breaths/min; temperature 37.5°C
- Intake: 1400 mL; output: 450 mL
- Pain level: 0/10
- Neurological: Lethargic but responsive to stimuli
- Respirations: Deep with acetone odor noted; lungs clear
- Cardiac: S_1/S_2; no murmurs
- Cardiac rhythm: Sinus tachycardia
- Code status: Full
- GI: Abdomen soft/slightly distended; hypoactive bowel sounds
- GU: Voiding frequently; urine concentrated
- Skin: Skin dry with poor turgor; intact
- IV: (Location) right forearm (catheter size) 18 G (condition) no redness/edema
- Assessment: Diabetic ketoacidosis secondary to poorly managed insulin pump failure with gradual improvement of glucose over past 2 hours

Recommendations

- Obtain hourly vital signs
- Repeat glucose, K^+, arterial blood gas due at 1600 today
- Continue balanced crystalloid solution (Lactated Ringers) at 200 mL/h for 4 hours
- IV insulin infusion at 7.5 units (7.5 mL) per hour—bedside glucose monitoring hourly and adjust per protocol
- Monitor urine output hourly
- Contact Dr. Miller with 1600 lab work for further orders
- Refer to diabetes educator and clinical dietitian
- Repeat renal profile in AM

BP, Blood press; *BUN,* blood urea nitrogen; *GI,* gastrointestinal; *GU,* genitourinary; *HCO_3,* bicarbonate; *IV,* intravenous; *K^+,* potassium; *$PaCO_2$,* partial pressure of arterial carbon dioxide; *PaO_2,* partial pressure of arterial oxygen.

BOX 1.4 Barriers to Effective Handoff Communication

- **Physical setting:** background noise, lack of privacy, interruptions.
- **Social setting:** organizational hierarchy and status issues.
- **Language:** differences among people of varying ethnic or cultural backgrounds or geographic areas.
- **Communication medium:** limitations of communication via telephone, email, paper, or computerized records versus face-to-face.

BOX 1.5 SBAR Approach

S—Situation: State what is happening at the present time that has warranted the SBAR communication.
B—Background: Explain circumstances leading up to this situation. Put the situation in context for the reader or listener.
A—Assessment: State what you think is the problem.
R—Recommendation: State your recommendation to correct the problem.

Communication techniques and protocols from other high-risk industries have been implemented in healthcare settings to improve patient safety. Crew resource management (CRM) is a technique that comes from the aviation industry and was developed to promote and improve communication and accountability among team members, a culture of safety, and stress recognition.[33,34]

In a CRM environment, everyone from the captain of the aircraft to the baggage handlers on the ground shares responsibility for safe flight operations. Differences in training are acknowledged, but each member of the team is empowered and has the autonomy to address problems without fear of retaliation or ridicule. Several components of CRM are pertinent to critical care nursing: monitor others' actions by double-checking; verifying, and when necessary, correcting inaccurate or ambiguous information; and situational awareness.[33] If something seems wrong, individuals should trust their "gut instinct" and speak up to correct the situation.[35]

Clear communication is vitally important in the acute and critical care practice environment. Ensuring civil communication, especially during stressful situations, is important for the multiprofessional team and fosters patient safety. The CUS tool (Concerned; Uncomfortable; Safety), developed by the AHRQ predominantly to improve communication within surgical environments, is also effective in other practice settings.[36] The acronym addresses three statements: I am *concerned*; I am *uncomfortable*; this is a patient *safety* issue (https://www.ahrq.gov/hai/tools/ambulatory-surgery/sections/implementation/training-tools/cus-tool.html). Following principles of the CUS tool allows the critical care nurse to voice concerns and place the focus on patient safety.[36]

Collaboration

The ultimate goal of true collaboration in critical care is to create a *culture of safety,* defined as a nonhierarchical culture in which all members have the opportunity and the duty to ensure safe and effective care. Collaboration is founded on mutual respect and the recognition that each discipline involved in patient care brings distinct skills and perspectives to the table.

BOX 1.6 Items to Consider in Daily Multiprofessional Rounds

- Discharge needs
- Greatest safety risk
- Implementation of critical care "bundles"
- Assessment and recommended follow-up
- Cardiac and hemodynamic status
- Volume status
- Neurological status
- Pain, agitation, and delirium
- Pain management needs
- Sedation needs
- Ventilator weaning/extubation plans
- Gastrointestinal status, including bowel management
- Nutrition
- Skin issues
- Chemoprophylaxis: peptic ulcer and venous thromboembolism
- Activity/mobility
- Infection status (culture results/antibiotic stewardship/therapeutic levels of antibiotics)
- Laboratory results
- Radiology test results
- Need for all ordered medications
- Whether central lines and invasive catheters and tubes can be removed
- Whether indwelling urinary catheter can be removed
- Issues that need to be addressed
- Patient/family needs—educational, psychosocial, spiritual
- Code status
- Advance directives
- Parameters for calling the provider
- Treatment goals and strategies to achieve them
- Goals of care align with patient/family wishes
- Plans for discussing care and needs with families

One strategy for collaboration is the implementation of multiprofessional bedside rounds one or two times per day. Intensivist-led rounds and daily goal setting are recommended to address patient care issues and adherence to practice guidelines and bundles of care. Such rounds have the potential to improve communication, collaboration, quality of care, and patient outcomes.[37] Examples of items to be addressed are noted in Box 1.6. It is important to include family members in patient rounds to facilitate communication and involvement. Some teams schedule regular afternoon rounds focused on communication with the family, whereas others include family in routine rounds.

Visualization of goals via standardized data on whiteboards or glass doors of the patient's room is helpful in facilitating communication among the healthcare team and with family members.[38,39]

Conducting morning briefings, or huddles, before interdisciplinary rounds is another strategy to improve communication, collaboration, and patient safety. Suggested content of the morning briefings includes answers to three questions: (1) What happened during the night that the team needs to know (e.g., adverse events, admissions)? (2) Where should rounds begin (e.g., the sickest patient who needs the most attention)? (3) What potential problems have been identified for the day (e.g., staffing, procedures)? [40,41]

CHECK YOUR UNDERSTANDING

3. Determine which strategy is being used when the nurse stops a bedside procedure to assist the provider in donning protective gowns, masks, and hats to reduce infection risk.
   A. Ask-Tell-Ask
   B. Crew resource management
   C. Situation, background, assessment, and recommendation (SBAR)
   D. Teach-back

COLLABORATIVE PLAN OF CARE FOR THE CRITICALLY ILL PATIENT

Critically ill patients have many similarities and needs for patient care. Therefore, a collaborative plan of care for these patients is presented to prevent the need for duplication of many of these common nursing assessments and interventions throughout the textbook. As with any care plan, it must be individualized to the patient because some problems and nursing diagnoses may not be relevant.

COLLABORATIVE PLAN OF CARE

The Critically Ill Patient

Patient Problem

Acute and/or Chronic Pain. Risk factors include underlying physical condition, chronic disorders, and/or treatment.

Desired Outcomes

- Prevention and/or relief of pain.
- Assessment of pain based on a validated pain scale is reduced or at a target level.

Nursing Assessments/Interventions	Rationales
• Assess patient's pain on admission, every 4 hours, and more frequently as needed; using a standardized approach, for example: numeric rating scale for verbal patients; Behavioral Pain Scale (BPS) or Critical-Care Pain Observation Tool (CPOT) for nonverbal patients.	• Establish baseline to assess for changes and responses to treatments and interventions using a standardized approach.
• In collaboration with the team, develop a consistent plan to address the patient's pain; incorporate both pharmacological and nonpharmacological approaches, such as repositioning, music, guided imagery, and animal-assisted therapy.	• Provide a standardized approach to treatment that can be followed by all team members; nonpharmacological approaches can be effective and may reduce the need for and/or dose of medications.
• Explain procedure(s) and expected outcomes.	• Knowledge of expectations may reduce pain associated with procedure(s).

Continued

COLLABORATIVE PLAN OF CARE—cont'd

The Critically Ill Patient

Patient Problem

Anxiety and Decreased Ability to Cope. Risk factors include the stressful critical care environment, sensory overload and deprivation, fear of the unknown, inability to communicate, and many other factors associated with critical illness.

Desired Outcomes

- Prevention and/or relief of anxiety.
- Assessment of agitation based on a validated sedation scale is reduced or at a target level.
- Patient verbalizes reduced fear and anxiety, if able.
- Patient demonstrates positive coping mechanisms.

Nursing Assessments/Interventions	Rationales
• Assess patient's fear and anxiety on admission, every 4 hours, and more frequently as needed; administer sedation per protocol using standardized scales, such as Richmond Agitation-Sedation Scale (RASS) or Sedation-Agitation Scale (SAS).	• Establish a baseline to assess for changes and responses to treatments and interventions; standardized tools facilitate communication, assessment of interventions, and trending.
• In collaboration with the team, develop a consistent plan to address the patient's anxiety; include spiritual support services as requested by the patient and/or family.	• Provide a standardized approach to treatment that can be followed by all team members.
• Communicate with patient; explain procedures; provide calm and reassuring presence; provide information about family and current events.	• Demonstrate concern for the patient; educate about condition. ○ Decreases stress and fear regarding what is occurring beyond their condition and the critical care unit; provides peace of mind regarding their family and loved ones.
• Ask simple questions that can be responded to by nodding, eye blinking, communication boards, speaking devices, and similar strategies; expect frustration.	• Promote effective communication; strategies must be appropriate to culture and physical ability.
• Support family presence; encourage family members to communicate with the patient.	• Promote a sense of well-being.
• Use complementary approaches such as music therapy, guided imagery, and animal-assisted therapy.	• Reduce anxiety.
• Promote regular sleep-wake cycle, daytime activity, and scheduled rest periods; reduce external noise and stimuli as possible.	• Promote rest, healing, and recovery.

Patient Problem

Delirium. Risk factors include critical illness, treatment, and underlying condition.

Desired Outcomes

- Acute confusion is either prevented or decreased.
- No evidence of injury or harm due to delirium.
- Delirium treated properly if diagnosed.

Nursing Assessments/Interventions	Rationales
• Assess delirium using a validated screening tool: Confusion Assessment Method for the ICU (CAM-ICU) or Intensive Care Delirium Screening Checklist (ICDSC).	• Establish a baseline to assess for changes and responses to interventions using a standardized approach.
• Implement the ABCDEF bundle (see http://www.icudelirium.org): ○ Assess for and manage pain. ○ Both awakening and breathing trials for ventilated patients. ○ Choice of sedation and analgesia; incorporate goal-directed sedation. ○ Delirium monitoring and management. ○ Early mobility. ○ Family engagement.	• Prevent delirium using evidence-based interventions; improve cognitive and functional outcomes.
• Speak slowly using simple sentences and nonmedical terminology.	• Promote effective communication with patients with delirium or cognitive impairment.

COLLABORATIVE PLAN OF CARE—cont'd

The Critically Ill Patient

Patient Problem

Decreased Mobility. Risk factors include patient condition and treatment modalities.

Desired Outcomes

- Intact skin and mucous membranes.
- Prevention of loss of muscle mass.
- Stable cardiovascular and pulmonary responses to activity.
- Patient achieves optimum mobility considering illness severity and diagnosis.

Nursing Assessments/Interventions	Rationales
• Collaborate with physical therapist, occupational therapist, and other healthcare team members to determine a treatment plan.	• Develop a treatment plan using experts.
• Ensure that active and passive range of motion (ROM) are done on a regular basis; use commercial ROM devices if available.	• Promote ROM and functional mobility.
• Promote progressive mobility, including out of bed to chair and ambulation as tolerated; assess responses to activity (cardiopulmonary, neurological); use lifting devices and specialized equipment as indicated.	• Maintain muscle mass and ROM; prevent delirium; promote gradual increases in activity while assessing physiological responses; use lift devices to prevent injury to both patient and caregivers.
• Ensure the patient is receiving pharmacological and/or mechanical treatment to prevent venous thromboembolism (VTE).	• Prevent VTE, which is especially common in immobile patients.

Family Problem

Potential for Dysfunctional Family Dynamics. Risk factors include crisis of critical illness, fear of the unknown, inability to effectively communicate with patient, altered family functioning, stress associated with balancing home needs and visitation. (Note: Family includes those self-identified as family members to the patient, including significant others or partners.)

Desired Outcomes

- Family experiences effective communication with the patient and healthcare team.
- Family can identify and discuss dysfunctional behavioral dynamics.
- Effective family coping.
- Reduction of anxiety.
- Able to provide support to patient.

Nursing Assessments/Interventions	Rationales
• Assess family structure; social, environmental, cultural, and spiritual needs; and communication patterns within the family and with the healthcare team.	• Establish a baseline to assess family functioning and response to the patient's illness.
• Identify family spokesperson, create a secure password, and document contact information.	• Establish primary contact for communication; protect patient privacy.
• Establish open, honest communication; provide information; offer support and realistic hope.	• Facilitate communication; meet family's need for information.
• Promote visitation according to patient's condition and family's need for presence. Unrestricted visitation is encouraged.	• Meet common need of family members.
• Assess family's knowledge of the patient's condition, treatment, and prognosis; allow time for questions.	• Identify knowledge deficits and provide opportunities for family education.
• Promote family/significant other's participation in patient care.	• Meet family's need for meaningful contributions to patient care.
• Promote family's communication with the healthcare team, such as participation in multidisciplinary rounds, family rounds, or appointments with key members of the healthcare team.	• Promote open communication and decision-making; reduce family frustration and anxiety of not being able to discuss the patient's condition or understand the plan of care.
• Provide opportunities to discuss the patient's condition and share concerns in a private setting.	• Foster communication in a caring and calm environment.
• Encourage family members to get adequate sleep and rest; provide strategies for communication of changes and updates in conditions should family members go home.	• Promote physical well-being of family members; provide strategies for communication of updates.
• Assess for ineffective coping (i.e., depression, withdrawal, anger, substance use).	• Identify the need for additional communication, support services, intervention, or referral.

Patient Problem

Potential for Pressure Injury. Risk factors include bed rest and physiological alterations associated with critical illness.

Desired Outcomes

- Intact skin and mucous membranes.
- Prevention of pressure injury.

Continued

COLLABORATIVE PLAN OF CARE—cont'd

The Critically Ill Patient

- Patient and family participate in preventive measures.
- Patient and family verbalize understanding of interventions to prevent pressure injury.

Nursing Assessments/Interventions	Rationales
• Assess skin and mucous membranes every shift for alterations and disruption. Pay special attention to bony prominences and areas of pressure associated with devices (e.g., nose, ears); take photos (per hospital policy) of actual and potential skin breakdown.	• Obtain baseline and ongoing assessment of potential skin breakdown or problems in pressure-prone areas; document photos to facilitate assessment.
• Use standardized tools for assessment: Braden or Norton scale.	• Provide a standardized measure for trending skin assessment; score may indicate need for consultation or specialized devices.
• Implement preventive strategies per hospital policy and consultation with wound, ostomy, and continence nurses (WOCNs): mattress overlays, specialized beds, barrier creams, or other strategies.	• Prevent skin breakdown in collaboration with WOCNs.
• Turn and reposition the patient on a regular basis and assess skin during the procedure; prevent shearing when pulling patient up in bed and during turning; use pillows and foam wedges when positioning.	• Relieve pressure and promote circulation; reduce risk for shearing; prevent pressure-related injury associated with positioning.
• Promote adequate nutrition; consult with dietitian and pharmacists to develop nutritional care plan.	• Promote skin integrity and wound healing.
• Prevent and/or treat incontinence. Use external collection devices as appropriate, such as external urinary management devices. Protect skin with barrier cream.	• Reduce risk for skin breakdown associated with incontinence.
• Promote mobility, including out of bed to chair and ambulation as tolerated by the patient; assess skin integrity on return to bed.	• Promote increased circulation and decrease risk for skin breakdown.

Patient Problem

Potential for Insufficient Secretion Removal and Decreased Gas Exchange. Risk factors include disease process/decreased respiratory drive and treatment.

Desired Outcomes

- Airway maintained.
- Decreased work of breathing.
- Oxygen saturation at target level.
- Adequate gas exchange (normal arterial blood gases [ABGs], respiratory rate, lung sounds, level of consciousness).
- Airway free of excessive secretions, edema, or obstruction.
- Lung sounds clear.

Nursing Assessments/Interventions	Rationales
• Assess respiratory rate, depth, and rhythm; monitor ABGs, SpO_2, and $ETCO_2$.	• Assess adequacy of respiration and detect abnormalities.
• Assess for signs of hypoxemia (i.e., restlessness, confusion, agitation, irritability).	• Identify need for treatment to promote oxygenation.
• Auscultate breath sounds.	• Identify adventitious sounds, potentially indicating need for intervention.
• Unless the patient is intubated, encourage coughing and deep breathing on a regular basis; use incentive spirometer and positive expiratory pressure, if indicated.	• Promote alveolar expansion and prevent atelectasis; assess cough ability.
• Suction (nasotracheal or endotracheal) as indicated by patient assessment; hyperoxygenate before suctioning.	• Maintain airway; prevent tissue/mucosal damage from excess suction; provide adequate oxygenation to promote tissue and cerebral perfusion.
• Assess amount, color, and consistency of secretions.	• Identify need for humidification; assess for possible infection.
• Turn and reposition on a regular basis; encourage mobility.	• Prevent atelectasis; promote alveolar function; mobilize secretions.

Patient Problem

Potential for Fluid, Electrolyte, and Acid-Base Imbalances. Risk factors include the disease process, inability to achieve biochemical hemostasis, and critical illness.

Desired Outcomes

- Recognition and early treatment of imbalances.
- Patient is free of musculoskeletal and cardiac changes.
- Patient and family understand the signs and symptoms associated with fluid and electrolyte imbalances.

COLLABORATIVE PLAN OF CARE—cont'd

The Critically Ill Patient

Nursing Assessments/Interventions	Rationales
• Assess for indicators of alterations in fluid, electrolyte, and acid-base balance.	• Use baseline data to assess risks and gauge changes.
• Weigh patient daily.	• Assess changes in fluid status.
• Maintain adequate nutritional intake.	• If nutrition is inadequate, protein stores will be used for energy, resulting in nitrogen balance changes. • Muscle wasting may also increase.
• Administer medications as prescribed (i.e., diuretics, IV fluids, electrolyte replacement).	• Depending on the medication prescribed, the mechanisms may lead to increased fluid, retained fluid, or electrolyte shifts.

Patient Problem

Potential for Impaired Nutrition. Risk factors include "nothing by mouth" status, hypermetabolic state in some disease or illness states, barriers to achieving optimal enteral nutrition, and the need for parenteral nutrition.

Desired Outcomes

- Adequate nutrition to promote resolution of illness, wound healing, and physical strength.
- Maintenance of baseline body weight.
- Nitrogen state is balanced or positive.

Nursing Assessments/Interventions	Rationales
• Obtain baseline height, weight, body mass index (BMI), and laboratory values; assess nutritional risk with standardized tools.	• Use baseline data to assess risks and gauge changes.
• Weigh patient daily.	• Assess changes in caloric intake and fluid status.
• Consult with dietitian, clinical pharmacist, and other team members to generate a nutrition care plan.	• Dietitians and clinical pharmacists are most knowledgeable on strategies to meet nutritional needs of patients.
• Implement guideline-based approaches to nutritional support.	• Develop optimal nutrition plan.
• Assess bowel sounds, abdominal distension, and intake/output on a regular basis.	• Assess for complications such as ileus, impaired nutrition tolerance, fluid overload, diarrhea, and constipation.
• If patient is receiving enteral nutrition, ensure proper tube placement, progress patient to enteral goal as quickly as patient tolerates, keep the head of bed elevated at least 30 degrees, and avoid enteral nutrition interruptions.	• Prevent aspiration associated with improper tube placement, poor absorption, or gastric regurgitation; ensure adequate intake of prescribed nutrition.

Patient Problem

Potential for Decreased Multisystem Tissue Perfusion. Risk factors include decreased cardiac output, cardiac dysrhythmias, hemodynamic instability, treatments such as positive end-expiratory pressure (PEEP), and cardiac abnormalities.

Desired Outcomes

- Adequate cardiac output.
- Oriented to person, time, and place.
- Systolic BP within 20 mm Hg of baseline.
- Mean arterial pressure greater than or equal to 65 mm Hg.
- Heart rate 60 to 100 beats/min.
- Urine output at least 0.5 mL/kg.
- Regular respiratory rate.
- Lung sounds clear.
- Strong peripheral pulses.
- Warm, dry skin.

Nursing Assessments/Interventions	Rationales
• Assess level of consciousness.	• Assess for symptoms of decreased cerebral perfusion.
• Assess heart rate and blood pressure.	• Low cardiac output is associated with abnormally low or high heart rate and manifested by lower blood pressure.
• Assess skin color, moisture, and temperature.	• Assess for perfusion to the periphery manifested by cool, moist skin and possible cyanosis.
• Assess peripheral pulses, including capillary refill.	• Low cardiac output is associated with weak pulses and slow capillary refill.
• Assess urine output hourly.	• Assess for renal perfusion.

Continued

COLLABORATIVE PLAN OF CARE—cont'd

The Critically Ill Patient

Nursing Assessments/Interventions	Rationales
• Assess respiratory rate and lung sounds.	• Assess for impaired perfusion to the lungs.
• Assess for chest pain.	• Decreased perfusion to coronary arteries may result in pain, especially in those with underlying cardiac disease.

Patient Problem

Potential for Infection. Risk factors include invasive devices: ventilator-associated events (VAE), central line–associated bloodstream infections (CLABSI), catheter-associated urinary tract infections (CAUTI), and devices such as traction and intracranial pressure monitoring.

Desired Outcome

- Prevention of infection.

Nursing Assessments/Interventions	Rationales
• Assess for presence of devices that increase the risk for infection.	• Devices interfere with the body's first line of defense.
• Monitor white blood cell (WBC) count.	• Elevation may be associated with infection.
• Assess for signs of infection (depending on device): fever; redness, swelling, pain; color of drainage or secretions.	• Changes often indicate infection.
• Practice meticulous hand hygiene.	• Prevent transmission of organisms.
• Remove devices as soon as they are no longer indicated.	• Decrease risk for infection.
• For the ventilated patient: ○ Elevate head of bed at least 30 degrees. ○ Interrupt sedation and assess for readiness to wean from ventilator daily. ○ Provide oral care daily with toothbrushing. ○ Administer prophylaxis for VTE. ○ Administer prophylaxis for peptic ulcer disease. ○ If available, use an endotracheal tube with port for removal of subglottic secretions. ○ Recommend early tracheostomy during multiprofessional rounds.	• Use evidence-based strategies to reduce infection.
• To prevent CAUTI: ○ Insert indwelling urinary catheter only if indicated. ○ Insertion should be done only by a properly trained individual using strict aseptic technique. ○ Maintain a closed drainage system with unobstructed urine flow. ○ Remove catheter as soon as possible. ○ Consider external urinary management devices. ○ Provide regular perineal and catheter care. ○ Prevent fecal contamination.	• Use evidence-based strategies to reduce infection.
• To prevent CLABSI: ○ Ensure that strict aseptic technique is followed during insertion, including full barrier precautions. ○ Access devices by scrubbing the port or hub with appropriate antiseptic. ○ Perform dressing changes using strict aseptic technique. ○ Change dressings when loose, wet, or soiled. ○ Consider chlorhexidine-impregnated dressings and regular chlorhexidine bathing.	• Use evidence-based strategies to reduce infection.

Patient/Family Problem

Need for Health Teaching (Patient and Family). Risk factors include lack of knowledge about disease process and treatment plan.

Patient/Family Outcomes

- Patient and family verbalize adequate information related to condition and treatment plan.
- Patient and family able to make informed decisions regarding care.

Nursing Assessments/Interventions	Rationales
• Assess patient and family's understanding of condition and treatment plan.	• Establish baseline knowledge and need for instruction.
• Encourage all team members to be involved in patient and family education.	• Provide the expertise of the healthcare team to the patient and family while ensuring direct communication.

COLLABORATIVE PLAN OF CARE—cont'd

The Critically Ill Patient

Nursing Assessments/Interventions	Rationales
• Provide specific, factual information on condition and treatment plan; reinforce teaching after rounds; effectively and consistently communicate the plan of care with members of the healthcare team.	• Provide accurate information to promote continuity of education; facilitate decision-making regarding treatment options.
• Encourage patient and family members to ask questions.	• Ensure accurate information and facilitate understanding of information provided.

BP, blood pressure; *ETCO₂,* end-tidal carbon dioxide; *IV,* intravenous; *SpO₂,* saturation of oxygen in pulsatile blood (by pulse oximetry).
Adapted from Gulanick M, Myers JL. *Nursing Care Plans: Diagnoses, Interventions, and Outcomes.* 10th ed. St. Louis, MO: Elsevier; 2022; Snyder JS, Sump C. *Swearingen's All-in-One Nursing Care Planning Resource.* 6th ed. St. Louis, MO: Elsevier; 2024; Klompas M, Branson R, Cawcutt K, et al. Strategies to prevent ventilator-associated pneumonia, ventilator-associated events, and nonventilator hospital-acquired pneumonia in acute-care hospitals: 2022 update. *Infect Control Hosp Epidemiol.* 2022;43(6):687-713. https://doi.org/10.1017/ice.2022.88; Centers for Disease Control and Prevention. *Healthcare-Associated Infections (HAIs).* https://www.cdc.gov/hai/. Published November 10, 2021; Accessed February 18, 2023.

CLINICAL JUDGMENT ACTIVITY

Compare and contrast strategies for reducing stress and anxiety of critical care nurses.

TRENDS AND ISSUES IN CARE DELIVERY

Aging Population

In developed countries, there is an unprecedented rise in the older adult population, which translates to a higher proportion of older adults in critical care units. Advanced age may increase morbidity and mortality for patients admitted to a critical care unit. Though frailty is often associated with increased age, this does not mean that all older adults are frail. The multiprofessional team must take into consideration the patient's pre-critical care condition, including comorbidities and functional status, as well as the patient's disease process and current acuity.[42]

Healthcare Costs

Healthcare costs continue to escalate while reimbursement rates are reduced. Hospitals are usually reimbursed based on performance and do not receive payment to treat complications that may result from treatment. Evidence-based protocols are being incorporated into order sets to standardize care and reduce complications and associated costs. Readmission rates for certain conditions also affect reimbursement. Both aging and chronic illness increase the likelihood of hospital readmissions. Strategies are being implemented to improve care transitions, especially to the home setting. Collaboration among hospitals, community organizations, caregivers, and patients are essential elements to achieve seamless care among multiple providers and sites. Changing nurse/patient ratios and employing unlicensed assistive personnel are also strategies being implemented to reduce costs. However, outcomes associated with changes in staffing need to be monitored and evaluated to ensure that patient outcomes and patient safety are not compromised.

Healthcare Technology

Technology that assists in patient care continues to grow rapidly. Invasive and noninvasive monitoring systems are used to facilitate patient assessment and to evaluate responses to treatment. Many technological interventions have been introduced to improve patient safety. Point-of-care laboratory testing is done at the bedside to provide immediate values to expedite treatment. Computerized provider order entry and nursing documentation are expected. In many institutions, data from monitoring equipment are automatically downloaded into the electronic health record. Sophisticated computer programs are being developed and tested to analyze physiological data for signs of patient deterioration, such as sepsis, and provide earlier alerts to caregivers. Nurses must become increasingly comfortable with applying the technology, troubleshooting equipment, and evaluating the accuracy of values. The use of technology must be balanced with delivering compassionate care.

As more technological advances become available to sustain and support life, ethical issues have increased. Termination of life support, organ and cell transplantation, and quality of life are just a few issues that nurses must address in everyday practice. Decisions are made regarding applying technology to sustain life or withdrawing technology in futile situations. Nurses must be comfortable addressing ethical issues as they arise in the critical care setting. Increased attention to end-of-life care in the critical care unit is also needed. Palliative care that includes spiritual care is an important intervention that must be embraced by those working in critical care units (see Chapter 3, Ethical and Legal Issues in Critical Care Nursing, and Chapter 4, Palliative and End-of-Life Care).

Using TCC to manage critically ill patients is another emerging trend. Data from monitors and robotics are transferred for evaluation, and the expert conducts an assessment from a distant location.[2] These virtual critical care consultations have improved patient outcomes. Nurses consult with those providing the TCC service based on established protocols and parameters, and then they identify changes in a patient's condition that need to be addressed. These TCC strategies do not replace the high-touch, hands-on care delivered by nurses in the critical care unit, but they assist healthcare workers at remote sites in decision-making and treatment.

CLINICAL JUDGMENT ACTIVITY

Debate the pros and cons of hiring new graduates to work in a critical care unit.

Critical Care Environment

The critical care environment itself is changing. Units are being redesigned with the interests of both patients and nurses in mind. Equipment is becoming more portable, making the transfer of patients for diagnostic testing or to other units easier and safer. In addition, portable equipment can be brought to the bedside for diagnostic testing, preventing the need to transfer unstable patients from the critical care unit. Some institutions have adopted a universal care model, or *acuity-adaptable* rooms. In this setting, patients remain in one unit throughout their hospitalization. The level of nursing care is adjusted to meet the needs of the patient. The universal care model eliminates the need to transfer patients to other units and promotes continuity of care.[43,44]

Critical Care Across the Continuum

Patients are transferred from critical care units much earlier than before. High levels of knowledge and skill are required for nurses who care for patients on progressive care units. Patients are discharged from the hospital often while they are still acutely ill. Nurses must ensure that patients and their family members have the knowledge and skills needed for home care and that adequate resources, such as home healthcare services, are available. Both critical care nurses and APRNs may provide care to these high-acuity patients in the home, often through telehealth technology.

Medications in Critical Care

Implications of the opioid crisis in the critical care setting are widespread. Opioids are commonly administered in the critical care setting. Appropriate prescribing needs to be addressed through education of those ordering medication and collaboration with the critical care pharmacist.[45,46] Patients may have an opioid addiction and require higher doses of routine sedative and pain medications.[47] Given the crisis, more patients with an opioid overdose are being treated in critical care settings.[48]

Medication and fluid shortages are recent issues that affect care delivery and potentially affect patient safety. Most shortages are for medications used in the critical care setting, such as medications used to treat high-acuity conditions and parenteral preparations.[49] During shortages, substitutions are often required, which may be less effective or associated with a greater risk of administration errors and adverse effects.

Antibiotic stewardship in the critical care setting is advocated to reduce the risk for antibiotic resistance. Strategies to promote proper administration of antibiotics include regular audits and feedback, antibiotic time-outs, rapid diagnostic tests, and computerized decision support tools.[50] Regular collaboration with critical care pharmacists is also essential.

Family Presence

Family presence during procedures[51] and open visitation have been standard within hospitals for several years.[52] The presence of family (as defined by the patient) was found to improve communication with the multiprofessional team and foster a sense of trust. Unfortunately, concerns of incivility and violence toward the multiprofessional team and nurses have resulted in more restricted visitation in some settings.[53,54] Welcoming family to support the patient during their hospitalization requires an understanding of the benefits of family presence and visitation as well as recognizing situations that may pose a risk for potential violence and activating hospital resources promptly to de-escalate situations.[54]

Impact of a Pandemic

The severe acute respiratory syndrome coronavirus 2 is the virus that causes Coronavirus disease (COVID-19). The pandemic exposed numerous challenges within the wider healthcare system and had a profound effect on the acute and critical care practice environments. Rapid changes were necessary to address isolation protocols, changes to visitation, limited protective personal equipment, and stressful work environments for the multiprofessional team. The severity and number of individuals with the viral infection overwhelmed healthcare systems and resources. However, the worldwide focus and international collaboration and sharing of information provided numerous resources to guide practice, save lives, and keep clinicians safe. Lessons learned from the COVID-19 pandemic include the importance of open access to resources and the value of TCC.[55] The SCCM and AACN provided just-in-time videos and evolving science-based resources to help guide practice. Acute and critical care nurses played an important role in the fast-paced, dynamically changing challenges associated with the pandemic. Characteristics of critical care nurses fostered delivery of exceptional care to patients despite the profound challenges.[56]

ISSUES RELATED TO THE CRITICAL CARE NURSE

Aging Workforce

Many issues relate to the critical care nurse. Like the population in general, critical care nurses are growing older. To accommodate this growing workforce, hospitals are focusing attention on redesigning the environment with a focus on ergonomics, ease of use, and safety. Innovative staffing models are being developed to continue tapping into the wealth of clinical knowledge and expertise of older nurses who may no longer desire or be able to work full time or 12-hour shifts. Having adequate staffing with paraprofessionals who can assume responsibility for nonnursing tasks is another strategy to facilitate practice.

CLINICAL JUDGMENT ACTIVITY

Envision the critical care unit of the future. Evaluate the environment and how care could be delivered.

Nurses New to Critical Care

Critical care nurses are in demand; therefore, priorities for recruiting, educating, and retaining nurses to work in critical care settings are essential. Many new graduates want to specialize in critical care, yet they are often told that they need to have 1 year of medical-surgical nursing experience. New graduates can be successful in the critical care setting with adequate supervision, orientation, and mentorship.[57] A critical care course, which often includes simulation, assists the nurse in gaining requisite knowledge and skills. Adequate time in orientation, under the guidance of a supportive preceptor to develop and learn the critical care nursing role, facilitates clinical skill acquisition. Starting employment in a progressive or intermediate care unit or applying to critical care nursing fellowships are other strategies for gaining experience prior to working in a high-acuity critical care unit. Many institutions have implemented nurse residency programs to facilitate the transition from the student to staff nurse role.

Psychological Stressors

Bullying and incivility occur in the workforce, especially in high-acuity settings. An environment where these behaviors are tolerated affects nurses, patients, and the organization.[58,59] A healthy work environment that promotes collaboration, respect, decision-making, and communication helps to prevent these behaviors.[60]

Nurses who work in critical care settings are at risk for compassion fatigue, which consists of burnout and secondary traumatic stress. Burnout is a feeling of being ineffective and hopeless when work demands are intense, and traumatic stress stems from exposure to patients with acute illness and trauma.[61] Nurses with less experience are at a higher risk for compassion fatigue.[62] Again, a healthy work environment assists in reducing compassion fatigue in the critical care setting.[61]

CHECK YOUR UNDERSTANDING

4. Determine which of the following is defined by the values of communication, collaboration, and respect:
   A. Burnout
   B. Compassion fatigue
   C. Healthy work environments
   D. Incivility

Critical care nurses must be aware of current and emerging trends that affect their practice and patient care. Involvement in professional organizations, reading professional journals, participating in journal clubs, becoming involved in unit-based nurse practice councils, and attending local and national professional meetings are strategies for nurses to maintain currency in the ever-changing critical care environment.

KEY POINTS

- Critical care nursing encompasses care of both acutely and critically ill patients, prioritizing physiological and psychological responses to crisis of both the patient and family.
- There are several professional organizations with which critical care nurses can engage that provide various resources such as continuing education, grants, awards, and publications that allow for professional advancement.
- Critical care certification is available for bedside and advanced practice nurses, which validates knowledge, promotes professional excellence, and maintains a current knowledge base.
- Standards outline a set of responsibilities nurses are to perform competently. The AACN's Competence Framework is an example of how nurses can achieve such standards through the core set of knowledge, skills, and abilities outlined in the Framework.
- Providing quality and safe care are important aspects of critical care nursing. Several initiatives applicable to all critical care settings can be found through The Joint Commission and IHI.
- Evidence-based care begins with a thorough synthesis of the evidence surrounding the topic or issue of interest, as well as staying up to date on guidelines published by professional organizations.
- A healthy work environment allows nurses to provide high quality and compassionate care and is correlated to improved staffing and retention, a lower incidence of workplace violence, and less moral distress.
- There are a multitude of evolving issues in critical care nursing that continuously change based on the local, national, and global environment. More recent trends include the impact of the aging population, the opioid crisis, medication shortages, the COVID-19 pandemic, workplace violence, and the value of family presence at the bedside.

REFERENCES

1. Subramanian S, Pamplin JC, Hravnak M, et al. Tele-critical care: an update from the society of critical care medicine tele-ICU committee. *Crit Care Med*. 2020;48(4):553–561. https://doi.org/10.1097/CCM.0000000000004190.
2. Udeh C, Udeh B, Rahman N, et al. Telemedicine/virtual ICU: where are we and where are we going? *Methodist Debakey Cardiovasc J*. 2018;14(2):126–133.
3. Panlaqui OM, Broadfield E, Champion R, et al. Outcomes of telemedicine intervention in a regional intensive care unit: a before and after study. *Anaesth Intensive Care*. 2017;45(5):605–610.
4. Deisz R, Rademacher S, Gilger K, et al. Additional telemedicine rounds as a successful performance-improvement strategy for sepsis management: observational multicenter study. *J Med Internet Res*. 2019;21(1):e11161. https://doi.org/10.2196/11161. Published 2019 Jan 15.

5. American Association of Critical-Care Nurses (AACN). *About AACN.* https://www.aacn.org/about-aacn. Published 2019. Accessed February 18, 2023.
6. American Association of Critical-Care Nurses (AACN). *AACN Clinical Scene Investigator (CSI) Academy.* https://www.aacn.org/nursing-excellence/csi-academy?tab=Nurses%20Leading%20Innovation. Published 2019. Accessed February 18, 2023.
7. Society of Critical Care Medicine (SCCM). *About SCCM.* https://www.sccm.org/About-SCCM. Published 2019. Accessed February 18, 2023.
8. American Association of Critical-Care Nurses (AACN). *Value of Certification.* https://www.aacn.org/certification/value-of-certification-resource-center. Published 2019. Accessed February 18, 2023.
9. American Association of Critical-Care Nurses (AACN). *AACN Synergy Model for Patient Care.* https://www.aacn.org/nursing-excellence/aacn-standards/synergy-model. Published 2019. Accessed February 18, 2023.
10. Curley MA. Patient-nurse synergy: optimizing patients' outcomes. *Am J Crit Care.* 1998;7(1):64–72.
11. Tanner CA. Thinking like a nurse: a research-based model of clinical judgment in nursing. *J Nurs Educ.* 20086; 26(6):204-211.
12. Dickison P, Haerling K, Lasater K. Integrating the National Council of State Boards of Nursing clinical judgment model into nursing. *J Nurs Educ.* 2019;58(2):72–78.
13. American Association of Critical Care Nurses. *AACN's Competency Framework for Progressive and Critical Care: Initial Competency 2022.* https://www.aacn.org/education/competence-framework-toolkit. Published 2022. Accessed February 18, 2023.
14. Dodek PM, Norena M, Ayas N, Wong H. Moral distress is associated with general workplace distress in intensive care unit personnel. *J Crit Care.* 2019;50:122–125.
15. Alharbi J, Jackson D, Usher K. Compassion fatigue in critical care nurses. An integrative review of the literature. *Saudi Med J.* 2019;40(11):1087–1097. https://doi.org/10.15537/smj.2019.11.24569.
16. Browning SG. Burnout in critical care nurses. *Crit Care Nurs Clin North Am.* 2019;31(4):527–536. https://doi.org/10.1016/j.cnc.2019.07.008.
17. Nolte AG, Downing C, Temane A, Hastings-Tolsma M. Compassion fatigue in nurses: a metasynthesis. *J Clin Nurs.* 2017;26(23-24):4364–4378. https://doi.org/10.1111/jocn.13766.
18. The Joint Commission. *National Patient Safety Goals.* https://www.jointcommission.org/standards/national-patient-safety-goals/hospital-national-patient-safety-goals/. Published 2022. Accessed August 31, 2022.
19. U.S. Department of Health and Human Services (DHHS). *National Action Plan to Prevent Healthcare-Associated Infections: Road Map to Elimination.* https://health.gov/hcq/prevent-hai-action-plan.asp. Published 2016; Updated September 2021. Accessed February 18, 2023
20. Lavallee JF, Gray TA, Dumville J, et al. The effects of care bundles on patient outcomes: a systematic review and meta-analysis. *Implement Sci.* 2017;12(1):142.
21. Lyons PG, Edelson DP, Churpek MM. Rapid response systems. *Resuscitation.* 2018;128:191–197.
22. McKinney A, Fitzsimons D, Blackwood B, McGaughey J. Patient and family-initiated escalation of care: a qualitative systematic review protocol. *Syst Rev.* 2019;8(1):91. https://doi.org/10.1186/s13643-019-1010-z. Published 2019 Apr 9.
23. Peterson MH, Barnason S, Donnelly B, et al. Choosing the best evidence to guide clinical practice: application of AACN levels of evidence. *Crit Care Nurse.* 2014;34(2):58–68.
24. Barden C. *AACN Standards for Establishing and Sustaining Healthy Work Environments.* 2nd ed. Aliso Viejo, CA: AACN; 2016.
25. Barden C, Distrito C. Toward a healthy work environment. *Health Prog.* 2005;86(6):16–20.
26. Ulrich B, Cassidy L, Barden C, Varn-Davis N, Delgado SA. National nurse work environments - October 2021: a status report. *Crit Care Nurse.* 2022:e1–e18. https://doi.org/10.4037/ccn2022798. [published online ahead of print, 2022 Aug 1].
27. Li J, Wang J, Kong X, et al. Person-centered communication between healthcare professionals and COVID-19-infected older adults in acute care settings: findings from Wuhan, China. *J Gerontol B Psychol Sci Soc Sci.* 2021;76(4):e225–e229. https://doi.org/10.1093/geronb/gbaa190.
28. Hashim MJ. Patient-centered communication: basic skills. *Am Fam Physician.* 2017;95(1):29–34.
29. Shapiro J, Robins L, Galowitz P, et al. Disclosure coaching: an ask-tell-ask model to support clinicians in disclosure conversations. *J Patient Saf.* 2018.
30. Desmedt M, Ulenaers D, Grosemans J, Hellings J, Bergs J. Clinical handover and handoff in healthcare: a systematic review of systematic reviews. *Int J Qual Healthcare.* 2021;33(1):mzaa170. https://doi.org/10.1093/intqhc/mzaa170.
31. Davis J, Roach C, Elliott C, et al. Feedback and assessment tools for handoffs: A systematic review. *J Grad Med Educ.* 2017;9(1):18–32.
32. Müller M, Jürgens J, Redaèlli M, Klingberg K, Hautz WE, Stock S. Impact of the communication and patient hand-off tool SBAR on patient safety: a systematic review. *BMJ Open.* 2018;8(8):e022202. https://doi.org/10.1136/bmjopen-2018-022202. Published 2018 Aug 23.
33. Barton G, Bruce A, Schreiber R. Teaching nurses teamwork: integrative review of competency-based team training in nursing education. *Nurse Educ Pract.* 2018;32:129–137.
34. Haerkens M, Kox M, Noe PM, Van Der Hoeven JG, Pickkers P. Crew resource management in the trauma room: a prospective 3-year cohort study. *Eur J Emerg Med.* 2018;25(4):281–287.
35. Gross B, Rusin L, Kiesewetter J, et al. Crew resource management training in healthcare: a systematic review of intervention design, training conditions and evaluation. *BMJ Open.* 2019;9:e025247. https://doi.org/10.1136/bmjopen-2018-025247.
36. Agency for Healthcare Research and Quality (AHRQ). *Pocket Guide: TeamSTEPPS.* https://www.ahrq.gov/teamstepps/instructor/essentials/pocketguide.html. Published 2014; Updated January 2020. Accessed January 30, 2023.
37. Heip T, Van Hecke A, Malfait S, Van Biesen W, Eeckloo K. The effects of interdisciplinary bedside rounds on patient centeredness, quality of care, and team collaboration: a systematic review. *J Patient Saf.* 2022;18(1):e40–e44. https://doi.org/10.1097/PTS.0000000000000695.
38. Justice LB, Cooper DS, Henderson C, et al. Improving communication during cardiac ICU multidisciplinary rounds through visual display of patient daily goals. *Pediatr Crit Care Med.* 2016;17(7):677–683.
39. Zavalkoff S, Mazaniello-Chezol M, O'Donnell S, et al. Improving transparent team communication with the 'Glass Door' decal communication tool: a mixed methods analysis of family and staff perspectives. *BMJ Open Qual.* 2021;10:e001507. https://doi.org/10.1136/bmjoq-2021-001507.
40. Thompson D, Holzmueller C, Hunt D, et al. A morning briefing: setting the stage for a clinically and operationally good day. *Jt Comm J Qual Patient Saf.* 2005;31(8):476–479.

41. Boscart VM. A communication intervention for nursing staff in chronic care. *J Adv Nurs*. 2009;65(9):1823–1832. https://doi.org/10.1111/j.1365-2648.2009.05035.x.
42. Flaatten H, de Lange DW, Artigas A, et al. The status of intensive care medicine research and a future agenda for very old patients in the ICU. *Intensive Care Med*. 2017;43(9):1319–1328. https://doi.org/10.1007/s00134-017-4718-z.
43. Bonuel N, Cesario S. Review of the literature: acuity-adaptable patient room. *Crit Care Nurs Q*. 2013;36(2):251–271.
44. Kitchens JL, Fulton JS, Maze L. Patient and family description of receiving care in acuity adaptable care model. *J Nurs Manag*. 2018;26(7):874–880.
45. Gross JL, Perate AR, Elkassabany NM. Pain management in trauma in the age of the opioid crisis. *Anesthesiol Clin*. 2019;37(1):79–91.
46. Overton HN, Hanna MN, Bruhn WE, et al. Opioid-prescribing guidelines for common surgical procedures: an expert panel consensus. *J Am Coll Surg*. 2018;227(4):411–418.
47. Goodwin AJ. Critical care outcomes among opioid users: hidden sequelae of a growing crisis? *Crit Care Med*. 2018;46(6):1005–1006.
48. Stevens JP, Wall MJ, Novack L, et al. The critical care crisis of opioid overdoses in the United States. *Ann Am Thorac Soc*. 2017;14(12):1803–1809.
49. Tucker EL, Cao Y, Fox ER, Sweet BV. The drug shortage era: a scoping review of the literature 2001-2019. *Clin Pharmacol Ther*. 2020;108(6):1150–1155. https://doi.org/10.1002/cpt.1934.
50. Pickens CI, Wunderink RG. Principles and practice of antibiotic stewardship in the ICU. *Chest*. 2019;156(1):163–171.
51. Barreto MDS, Peruzzo HE, Garcia-Vivar C, et al. Family presence during cardiopulmonary resuscitation and invasive procedures: a meta-synthesis. *Rev Esc Enferm USP*. 2019;53:e02425.
52. Rosa RG, Falavigna M, da Silva DB, et al. Effect of flexible family visitation on delirium among patients in the intensive care unit: the ICU visits randomized clinical trial. *JAMA*. 2019;322(3):216–228. https://doi.org/10.1001/jama.2019.8766.
53. Bailey RL, Ramanan M, Litton E, et al. Staff perceptions of family access and visitation policies in Australian and New Zealand intensive care units: the WELCOME-ICU survey. *Aust Crit Care*. 2022;35(4):383–390. https://doi.org/10.1016/j.aucc.2021.06.014.
54. Holland KM, Jones C, Vivolo-Kantor AM, et al. Trends in US emergency department visits for mental health, overdose, and violence outcomes before and during the COVID-19 pandemic. *JAMA Psychiatry*. 2021;78(4):372–379. https://doi.org/10.1001/jamapsychiatry.2020.4402.
55. Wei EK, Long T, Katz MH. Nine lessons learned from the COVID-19 pandemic for improving hospital care and health care delivery. *JAMA Intern Med*. 2021;181(9):1161–1163. https://doi.org/10.1001/jamainternmed.2021.4237.
56. Thusini S. Critical care nursing during the COVID-19 pandemic: a story of resilience. *Br J Nurs*. 2020;29(21):1232–1236. https://doi.org/10.12968/bjon.2020.29.21.1232.
57. DeGrande H, Liu F, Greene P, Stankus JA. The experiences of new graduate nurses hired and retained in adult intensive care units. *Intensive Crit Care Nurs*. 2018;49:72–78.
58. Oja KJ. Incivility and professional comportment in critical care nurses. *AACN Adv Crit Care*. 2017;28(4):345–350.
59. Crawford CL, Chu F, Judson LH, et al. An integrative review of nurse-to-nurse incivility, hostility, and workplace violence: a GPS for nurse leaders. *Nurs Adm Q*. 2019;43(2):138–156. https://doi.org/10.1097/NAQ.0000000000000338.
60. Blake N. Building respect and reducing incivility in the workplace: Professional standards and recommendations to improve the work environment for nurses. *AACN Adv Crit Care*. 2016;27(4):368–371.
61. Kelly L, Todd M. Compassion fatigue and the healthy work environment. *AACN Adv Crit Care*. 2017;28(4):351–358.
62. Jakimowicz S, Perry L, Lewis J. Compassion satisfaction and fatigue: A cross-sectional survey of Australian intensive care nurses. *Aust Crit Care*. 2018;31(6):396–405.

2

Patient and Family Response to the Critical Care Experience

Leanne M. Boehm, PhD, RN, ACNS-BC, FCCM
Valerie Danesh, PhD, RN, FCCM, FAAN

INTRODUCTION

Although any hospitalization is stressful, the critical care experience is especially challenging. Critical care presents patients and families with complex issues beyond those directly related to the illness. The personal lives of the patients and those who care about them are affected in many ways. Being in a foreign environment and dealing with an undesirable and often unexpected health problem can result in patients and families experiencing additional trauma, uncertainty, and distress.[1,2] Anxiety, depression, sleep disruption, and acute stress disorder are experienced by many. Family member responses are often manifested in many ways, including concern, fear, nervousness, anger, frustration, anticipatory grief, and impaired problem solving.[3–5] Critical care teams are often so involved with patient care that concerns of families may be neglected. Current practice is evolving toward evidence-based guidelines to deliver family-centered care.[6,7]

Ongoing research into the experiences of critically ill patients and their families consistently supports the premise that critical care nurses must consider the patient and family when providing care.[8–10] Critical care nurses play a unique role in addressing the needs of patients and their families in a complex care environment. For example, advances in life-sustaining procedures and treatments can present ethical considerations in caring for the critically ill, and it is often family members who must evaluate decisions of sustaining life versus the potential loss in quality of life (see Chapter 3, Ethical and Legal Issues in Critical Care Nursing, and Chapter 4, Palliative and End-of-Life Care). Another example is how sociodemographic changes in family structures have altered the traditional definition of what constitutes *family* and *care partner* roles. In these scenarios, critical care nurses may assume an advocacy role in caring for patients and their family members to ensure their needs and wishes are met. The purpose of this chapter is to describe the critical illness experience and its effects on patients and their families.

THE CRITICAL CARE ENVIRONMENT

The *built environment,* or physical layout, of a critical care unit has a subtle yet profound effect on patients, families, and the critical care team. Amid an apparent confusion of wires, tubes, and machinery, a critical care unit is designed for efficient and expeditious life-sustaining interventions. Patients and their family members are cared for in this environment with little or no advance preparation, often causing stress and anxiety. Stress levels can be compounded by unfamiliar and near-constant sensory stimulation from light and noise, loss of privacy, lack of nonclinical physical contact, and emotional and physical pain and trauma. Issues related to the critical care environment include both sensory overload and sensory deprivation.

CLINICAL JUDGMENT ACTIVITY

You are orienting family members to the critical care unit setting for their first visit. The patient sustained traumatic injuries on a hiking trail, and the patient's room environment is similar to that shown in Fig. 2.1. What strategies do you use to introduce the patient's condition and the critical care environment to the family members?

Sensory Stimulation

Many studies have documented the detrimental effects of sensory overload experienced in a typical critical care unit. Lighting and excessive noise can result in adverse outcomes for patients, families, and critical care nurses. Lighting triggers delirium and sleep disruption in critically ill patients.[11] Likewise, the near continuous noise disturbances experienced by critically ill patients prevent them from having the necessary amount and quality of sleep. Individuals entering rooms to assess patients frequently induces sensory disturbance, but is often unavoidable due to acuity of the patient and the need for continuous monitoring.[11] Sensory disturbances can also affect critical care nurses, leading to increased stress, emotional exhaustion, fatigue and burnout, as well as difficult communication and interruptions, which may contribute to medical errors.[12,13]

Conversations, alarms, and staff activities are the main sources of critical care unit noise and major factors contributing to sensory overload. The World Health Organization established guidelines for hospital noise, recommending levels no greater

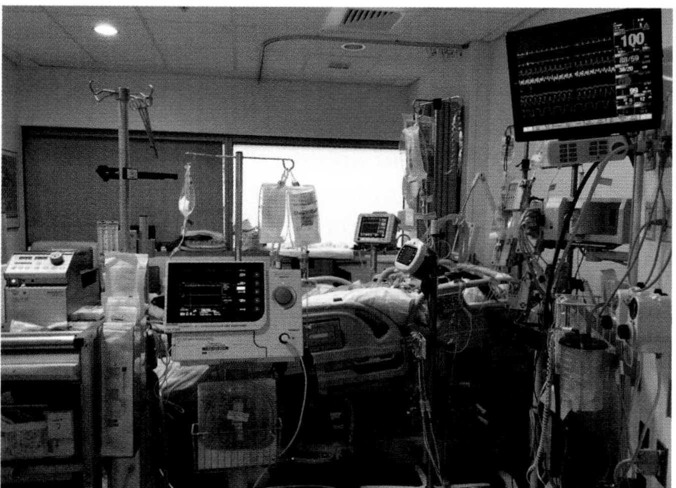

Fig. 2.1 Potential Critical Care Patient Room. If you were the family member and your loved one was this patient, how would you feel when you saw this situation? (Reproduced with permission from Cleveland Clinic Center for Art & Photography© 2019. All rights reserved.)

TABLE 2.1 Noise Levels Associated with Patient Care Devices and Activities

Activity	Sound Level (dB[a])
Call-bell activation	48-63
Oxygen or chest tube bubbling	49-70
Conversations (staff, patients, and family)	59-90
Voice over intercom	60-70
Telephone ringing	60-75
Television (normal volume at 12 feet)	65
Raising or lowering head of bed	68-78
Cardiac monitor	72-77
Infusion pump	73-78
Ventilator sounds	76
Pneumatic tube arrival	88

than 30 dB in daytime and 40 dB at night.[11,14,15] Yet, noise levels in hospitals routinely exceed recommended levels, and efforts to reduce noise have varied success due to the variety and clinical necessity of sound sources. Table 2.1 provides a list of patient care devices and activities with associated sound levels.

Several strategies can be used to reduce noise within the critical care environment: reducing alarm volume when possible, organizing workflow to endorse "quiet time" hours, bundling care to reduce sleep interruptions, closing patient doors, and installing sound-absorbing textiles. Designating a private place behind closed doors for communication with family members also contributes to reducing noise while protecting confidentiality.

Adequate and appropriate exposure to light is a therapeutic modality for the health of both patients and clinicians. Inadequate or poorly placed lighting makes it more difficult to view documents and medication labels and interferes with accurate physical examinations of patients. In addition, the constant artificial lighting present in most critical care units tends to override patients' natural circadian rhythms. Constant artificial lighting has detrimental effects on healthy individuals and has even more of an impact on critically ill patients.[16] Simple measures such as designing patient rooms to take advantage of natural light can reduce depressive symptoms, improve sleep quality, and enhance pain management.

Despite the potential for sensory overload, patients can also experience sensory deprivation in an environment that is very different from their usual surroundings. Sensory deprivation is associated with an increase in perceptual disturbances such as hallucinations, especially in older adults.[14] Nonpharmacologic interventions to provide cognitive stimulation include orienting conversations, encouraging visitation of friends and family, posting family photos within the patient's sight, and tailoring music or television exposure to patient preferences.

Impact of Architectural Design

The design of the critical care unit can affect delivery of care as well as the responses of patients and their families. New hospital construction or renovation of existing facilities provides an opportunity to design hospitals to best meet the needs of patients, families, and clinicians. It is important for members of the critical care team to work with architects and other planners to design a safe and healing environment. Best practices for design of critical care units include private rooms with natural light, views of nature, adequate room for visitors, and noise-reducing features.[11] It is also important when designing or adapting a unit to meet the comfort needs of family members and promote rest should they wish to remain in a patient's room. Physical design of the critical care unit has received much attention over the past 2 decades, resulting in many units that are ideal for clinicians, patients, and their families.[17]

CHECK YOUR UNDERSTANDING

1. A patient is sedated and intubated on arrival to the critical care unit. The family arrives shortly after the patient is admitted. The family members are tearful and appear to be anxious. Which intervention would support the family during this initial visit to the critical care unit?
   A. Encouraging family members to ask questions.
   B. Teaching family members how to perform endotracheal suctioning.
   C. Request that the family wait 1 hour until shift change is complete so that the oncoming nurse can be the point of contact.
   D. Referring family members to the spiritual care team for an initial overview of current status because you need to address urgent changes to the patient's condition.

THE CRITICALLY ILL PATIENT

Many factors influence an individual's response to critical illness, including age and developmental stage, experiences with illness and hospitalization, family relationships and social support, other stressful experiences and coping mechanisms, and personal philosophies about life, death, and spirituality. Patients often remember at least portions of their critical care stay and describe physical experiences like pain, sleep disruption, inactivity, thirst, medical procedures, physical restraints, and difficulty

BOX 2.1 Patients' Recollection of the Critical Care Experience

- Anxiety
- Depression
- Difficulty communicating
- Difficulty sleeping
- Difficulty swallowing
- Fear
- Feelings of dread
- Inability to get comfortable
- Lack of control
- Lack of family or friends
- Loneliness
- Pain
- Physical restraint
- Thirst
- Thoughts of death and dying

swallowing. Memories of psychological experiences may include hallucinations, nightmares, fear, panic, despair, and thoughts of death and dying (Box 2.1).[18] The cumulative effect of these stressors can promote acute anxiety, agitation, and delirium and potentially lead to the development of posttraumatic stress disorder (PTSD), anxiety, and depression in the months to years after critical illness, collectively described as post-intensive care syndrome (PICS).[19–21] Nursing interventions to reduce stress during critical illness can ensure safety, reduce sleep disruption, and minimize noxious sensory overload. Effective strategies are bundling nursing interventions and medical procedures to maximize resting periods and implementation of the **A**ssess, prevent, and manage pain; **B**oth awakening and breathing trials; **C**hoice of sedation; **D**elirium assessment, prevention, and management; **E**arly mobility; and **F**amily engagement and empowerment (ABCDEF) bundle.[22] Chapter 6, Comfort and Sedation, expands on interventions to promote comfort and reduce anxiety.

Orienting

Even if patients are sedated, it is important to remember that many can still hear, understand, and respond emotionally to what is being said. Make every effort to talk to patients and to describe assessments and interventions, regardless of their ability to interact. Reorient patients to the time and place, update them on their progress, and remind them they are safe and have family and people nearby who care about their well-being.

Increase pleasant sensory input by encouraging family members to speak to and touch the patient when not contraindicated by their clinical condition. Reorient the patient every 2 to 4 hours, and address the patient directly to minimize disorientation. Instead of repeatedly questioning the patient (e.g., "Do you know what day it is? Do you know where you are?"), incorporate this content into normal conversation (e.g., "It's 8 o' clock in the morning on the 5th of September. You are still in the critical care unit. Your family will be here to see you in about 10 minutes."). Do not discuss other information or patients, as such information can increase confusion and contribute to sensory overload. Place objects that facilitate orientation, such as a clock or a calendar, within the patient's visual field. Ask family members to bring personal and meaningful items from home to assist in reorienting the patient. These items also humanize the patient and help clinicians recognize that the patient has a unique personality and should be treated accordingly.

Promoting Comfort and Sleep

Promoting rest and sleep are other important nursing interventions. Sleep is frequently interrupted by medication administration, specimen collection (e.g., wound cultures, blood samples), and frequent assessments. During critical illness, patients experience severely altered sleep quality, sleeping an average of 2 to 3 hours in a calendar day and spending more time in light sleep than deep sleep.[7,23] Multiple clinicians are involved in patient care, and interventions are often determined by when staff are available rather than when the timing is ideal for the patient. Bundling nonpharmacological interventions such as removing noxious stimuli, increasing comfort, and promoting day-night cycles are effective ways to promote rest and sleep.[7] Positioning the patient near natural light during the day, reducing light levels in the patient's room at night, and minimizing noise during nighttime hours are strategies to promote day-night cycles. In addition to ensuring adequate patient sleep, sleep promotion is vital for nurses (see Nursing Self-Care Box).

NURSING SELF-CARE BOX

Promoting Sleep Among Nurses

- Alterations in work hours and long work shifts often cause nurses to experience irregular sleep patterns, which may cause both physical and mental health problems.
- Interventions to improve sleep:
  - Aroma inhalation therapy has been found to reduce the impact of sleep disorders, induce deep sleep, and minimize discomfort during sleep.
  - Avoid the use of smartphones and other electronic devices prior to going to sleep.
  - Alcohol and caffeine can disrupt sleep and should be avoided close to bedtime.
  - A hot shower, a period of meditation, or another method of relaxation (e.g., reading) may assist with falling to sleep faster.
  - If sleeping during the day, limit light through the use of blackout shades or an eye mask and reduce noise by using earplugs or white noise.
  - If possible, maintain a consistent sleep-wake cycle on days off.
  - If working the night shift, sleep should either be shifted or split (i.e., sleep for several hours in the morning, then take an extended nap in the afternoon) to ensure wake up occurs close to the start of the next shift.
  - The use of exogenous melatonin may be effective for those with sleep disorders; however, greater research is needed given the inconsistency of dosing and small sample sizes in current studies. Melatonin use should be guided by a sleep specialist.

From Kang J, Noh W, Lee Y. Sleep quality among shift-work nurses: a systematic review and meta-analysis. *Appl Nurs Res.* 2020;52:151227. https://doi.org/10.1016/j.apnr.2019.151227; Lammers-van der Holst HM, Murphy AS, Wise J, Duffy JF. Sleep tips for shift workers in the time of pandemic. *Southwest J Pulm Crit Care.* 2020;20(4):128-130; Carriedo-Diez B, Tosoratto-Venturi JL, Cantón-Manzano C, Wanden-Berghe C, Sanz-Valero J. The effects of the exogenous melatonin on shift work sleep disorder in health personnel: a systematic review. *Int J Environ Res Public Health.* 2022;19(16):10199. https://doi.org/10.3390/ijerph191610199.

Agitation of patients who are critically ill may be caused by pain, discomfort, delirium, and other factors. Critical care nurses are in a position to identify patient stressors and implement interventions to minimize many of them by providing high-quality nursing care, offered with compassion and delivered professionally; explaining procedures or interventions before they are performed; planning care so that the patient has quality time with family members; encouraging shared decision-making; and facilitating communication. Refer to the Collaborative Care Plan found in Chapter 1, Overview of Critical Care Nursing.

CHECK YOUR UNDERSTANDING

2. The family asks the nurse about the patient's sedation and is curious about what the patient may be experiencing. What education could the nurse provide regarding patients who are sedated?
   A. Patients who are sedated are unable to hear, so they do not respond to sounds, and speaking to the patient is not beneficial.
   B. The patient would not be affected by music therapy or familiar voices; therefore, there is no need to play the patient's favorite music or speak to the patient.
   C. The patient may hear, understand, and respond to verbal statements, so continue to speak to and orient the patient.
   D. If the patient hears their loved one's voice, they will become violent and an immediate danger to everyone.

CLINICAL JUDGMENT ACTIVITY

You are in charge of coordinating a family conference to discuss a patient's condition and goals of care. All family members speak Creole and English, with a preference for discussion in Creole. What strategies and resources do you include when planning the family conference?

FAMILY MEMBERS OF THE CRITICALLY ILL PATIENT

Critical care hospitalization is a crisis situation affecting both the patient and the family. Family stress may be detected by the patient, and the patient can suffer as a result. The family is an integral part of the patient's healing process; therefore, critical care nursing interventions must also focus on the family.

Person- and family-centered care recognizes the importance of patients and families collaborating with the critical care team in what is known as *shared decision-making*. This paradigm shift in patient care is widely recognized as an integral part of critical care.[24] Centers for Medicare and Medicaid Services (CMS), the Agency for Healthcare Research and Quality (AHRQ), and many other organizations that are influential in health care acknowledge the importance of person- and family-centered care.[25,26]

The critical care nurse must recognize and acknowledge the importance of care that includes both patients and family members. Families are in a vulnerable state because of the stress they are experiencing in unfamiliar surroundings. For many families, both the hospital and the critical care unit are unfamiliar environments. Most family members have never seen or only rarely visit a critical care unit. The machines and monitors that are commonplace to critical care nurses can be frightening and overwhelming to family members. Fig. 2.1 depicts what a family member sees when entering the room of a critically ill loved one. Imagine your thoughts and feelings if you were to encounter this situation.

CHECK YOUR UNDERSTANDING

3. A patient with a hospitalization 3 months ago involving a critical care stay is following up with their primary care provider. The patient states they are struggling with remembering things that they used to easily recall, such as their children's birthdays. The patient is struggling to complete crossword puzzles, which used to be a mildly challenging hobby. In addition, the patient is suffering from new-onset insomnia and nightmares. Each morning, the patient used to go for a 5-mile jog, but they can barely finish a half mile walk since discharge from the hospital. Determine which condition is affecting the patient based on the assessment findings.
   A. Posttraumatic stress disorder (PTSD)
   B. Critical care unit psychosis
   C. Delirium
   D. Post-intensive care syndrome (PICS)

Family Assessment

Once the patient has been admitted to the critical care unit, a family assessment provides valuable information for plan of care development. Obtain essential information during the admission assessment and gather additional information throughout the hospital stay. Structured tools are available to assess the family but are not consistently used in everyday practice; however, concepts incorporated into tools can guide the nursing assessment. The structural, developmental, and functional categories described in the Calgary Family Assessment Model provide a useful way to gather information about the family.[27] *Structural assessment* is done upon admission, and it identifies immediate family, extended family, and the decision-makers. Other aspects of family structure include ethnicity, race, religion, and spirituality. Designating a spokesperson for primary communication with the family members is beneficial. The *developmental assessment* includes information related to the family's developmental stages and tasks. The *functional assessment* reveals how family members function and behave in relation to one another.

In today's diverse society, it is important to assess the influence of culture and spirituality on both the patient and family. Especially important are beliefs about health and healing, cultural and spiritual practices, personal space and touch preferences, social organization, and the role of the family. Identify the primary language used for verbal and written communication. Use hospital-designated language interpreters when communicating with non-English speakers. Interpreters also serve as cultural guides to facilitate communication and understanding of the critical care experience. A simple approach to cultural and spiritual assessment is to ask three questions that can easily be adapted for most situations: (1) What are your specific religious and spiritual practices? (2) What are your beliefs about illness (and death)? (3) What is most important to you and your family at this time?

An early, proactive approach is advised when assessing a patient's family. Observe the family, interact with them, and note significant facts such as the patient's role, family coping strategies, and socioeconomic issues. The family assessment may reveal whether the family members are angry, feeling guilty, or have unaddressed concerns regarding the patient's condition and care. An illness within the family may also uncover underlying conflicts among family members, especially when family members are estranged or have other unresolved issues. Once an assessment is completed, concisely record the data to identify key information that needs to be shared with all critical care team members caring for the patient.

Family Needs

The most important family needs identified by both family and critical care team members are information and assurance, yet these needs often go unmet. Other commonly identified family needs include proximity, comfort, and support.[28] Globally, many researchers have conducted studies using the Critical Care Family Needs Inventory and identified a predictable set of needs of the family members of critically ill patients: receiving information and assurance, remaining near the patient, being comfortable, having support available, and needing frequent updates on patient status.[29–33] Implementation of family need interventions are effective in reducing family member stress. Addressing family member stress and promoting coping strategies enable the critical care nurse to create a plan of care that assists both patients and their families.

Some family members may be demanding or disruptive or insist on constant vigilance from the nursing staff. These behaviors may reflect a sense of loss of control or memories of an adverse outcome during a previous hospitalization. Recognize these factors as the reason for observed behaviors and determine the best way to communicate and intervene.

Family members often want confirmation that everything is being done for the patient, which may be challenging. Establish a partnership with the family and critical care team built on mutual respect, credibility, competence, and compassion. Nurses can encourage family members to assist in patient assessment (e.g., identify changes) and participate in selected aspects of the patient's care. Depending on institutional policy, it may be possible to enlist family members to help with tasks such as oral care, hygiene, range-of-motion exercises, or repositioning the patient. These activities give family members a sense of purpose and control, reduce distress, and can provide an additional layer of safety when the nurse is unavailable.

Research has been conducted regarding family-centered interventions and their effectiveness in achieving medical treatment goals and improving satisfaction, comprehension, and mental health sequelae.[34] Structured methods for providing family-centered interventions have been developed; however, a single and standardized method to ensure families receive needed care has not been accepted into everyday critical care practice. *The Clinical Practice Guidelines for Support of the Family in the Patient-Centered Intensive Care Unit* were developed by a multiprofessional group of the American College of Critical Care Medicine. The group made 43 recommendations based on the best available evidence. Recommendations that received a grade of C (based on some evidence) or better are listed in Box 2.2.[35] The guidelines remain relevant today.[8,36]

Influences on Patient and Family Responses

Response to critical illness can vary widely and is impacted by a multitude of factors for both the patient and the family. Patients who have survived a prior critical illness generally have less anxiety during subsequent admissions. For other patients, their only prior experience with critical illness may have ended with the death of a family member. This scenario can add considerably to the patient's fears and anxiety. As outlined in the Lifespan Considerations box, older adults often experience an increase in negative outcomes.

LIFESPAN CONSIDERATIONS

Older Adults

- Some older adult patients have a diminished ability to adapt and cope with the major physical and psychosocial stressors of critical illness. This is often the result of multiple losses over the years, including loss of physical function, loss of family members, and loss of resources, such as homes or income.
- Some older adults with chronic illnesses who have endured multiple critical illnesses demonstrate resilience.
- Older adults have a high risk of negative outcomes. Among older adult critical care survivors, health-related quality of life (HRQOL) worsened significantly, and most did not regain their baseline status after 1 year.[37] HRQOL is inversely related to both the severity of the illness and the length of stay.[38]
- Increased mortality, functional decline, and a decrease in HRQOL are common among older critical care survivors, especially after a prolonged length of stay in critical care and among those older than 80 years.[39]

Children and Adolescents

- Assessments for anxiety and depression are relevant for adolescents with close family members receiving care in a critical care setting, irrespective of whether visitation is allowed or restricted.
- New-onset or worsening psychological symptoms of anxiety, depression, and/or PTSD are known concerns for adult family members visiting the critical care unit. Less is known about the psychological risks of allowing children and adolescents to visit or excluding them from visiting adult family members receiving care in the critical care setting. However, based on limited evidence, the effects appear to be positive if the child or adolescent is prepared.[40,41]
- Child Life Specialists, available at some institutions, are professionals educated in the developmental impact of various disease processes and traumatic events on infants, children, and adolescents.[42] These specialists should be consulted as needed to assist with developmentally appropriate preparation for visiting the critical care unit, education regarding the patient's clinical condition, and to provide emotional support.

CLINICAL JUDGMENT ACTIVITY

You are leading a work group responsible for implementing changes to the critical care visitation policy to adopt unrestricted visitation. Several outspoken nurses are highlighting scenarios when unrestricted visitation would interrupt workflow and/or affect nurse satisfaction. What are some of the scenarios you might encounter related to unrestricted visitation policies in the critical care unit, and how would you address them?

BOX 2.2 Evidence-Based Recommendations for Supporting Family Members of Critically Ill Patients

Decision-Making
- Make decisions based on a partnership among the patient, family, and healthcare team.
- Communicate the patient's status and prognosis to family members and explain options for treatment.
- Hold a family conference with the healthcare team within 24 to 48 hours after critical care unit admission and repeat as often as needed.
- Train critical care unit staff in communication, conflict management, and facilitation skills.

Family Coping
- Train critical care unit staff in assessment of family needs, stress, and anxiety levels.
- Assign consistent nursing and provider staff to each patient, if possible.
- Update family members in a language they can understand.
- Provide information to family members in a variety of formats.
- Provide family support using a team effort, including social workers, clergy, nursing and medical staff, and support groups.

Staff Stress
- Keep all healthcare team members informed of treatment goals to ensure that messages given to the family are consistent.
- Develop a mechanism for staff members to request a debriefing to voice concerns regarding the treatment plan, decompress, share feelings, or grieve.

Cultural Support of Family
- If possible, match the provider's culture to that of the patient.
- Educate staff on culturally competent care.

Palliative Care
- Educate staff in palliative care during formal critical care education.

Spiritual and Religious Support
- Assess spiritual needs and incorporate them into the plan of care.
- Educate staff in spiritual and religious issues that facilitate patient assessment.

Family Visitation
- Facilitate open visitation in the adult critical care environment, if possible.
- Determine personalized visitation schedules in collaboration with the patient, family, and nurse; consider the best interest of the patient.
- Provide open visitation in the pediatric critical care unit and neonatal critical care unit 24 hours a day.
- Allow siblings to visit in the pediatric critical care unit and neonatal critical care unit (with parental approval) after participation in a previsit education program.
- Do not restrict pets that are clean and properly immunized from visiting the critical care unit.
- Develop guidelines for animal-assisted therapy.

Family Environment of Care
- Build new critical care units with single-bed rooms to improve patient confidentiality, privacy, and social support.
- Develop signage (e.g., easy-to-follow directions) to reduce stress on visitors.

Family Presence During Rounds
- Allow parents or guardians of children in the critical care unit to participate in rounds.
- Allow adult patients and family members to participate in rounds.

Family Presence During Resuscitation
- Develop a process to allow the presence of family members during cardiopulmonary resuscitation.

Modified from Davidson JE, Powers K, Hedayat KM et al. Clinical practice guidelines for support of the family in the patient-centered intensive care unit: American College of Critical Care Medicine Task Force 2004–2005. *Crit Care Med.* 2007;35(2):605-622.

Communication

Receiving information and feeling safe are predominant, complementary needs of critically ill patients and their family members. Of all the members of the critical care team, nurses spend the most time at the bedside and, as such, are usually the first to hear about any perceived unmet needs of family members. Frequent updates on the patient's condition, anticipated therapies or procedures, and goals of the critical care team are an easy and effective way to allay anxiety while building a relationship of mutual trust. Facilitate communication by providing a simple, honest report of the patient's condition, free of medical jargon. A follow-up assessment to gauge the family's level of understanding helps to tailor the care plan accordingly.

Scheduled rounds between the critical care team and the family assist in maintaining open communication. A predetermined routine for these rounds provides an opportunity for the team to update the family on the patient's condition and answer any questions. It also provides time to identify goals for care and treatment and facilitates shared decision-making. Scheduled family conferences at the bedside or in a conference room, depending on space available and the family's needs, provide a similar opportunity to facilitate communication. If possible, hold a preconference among team members to ensure that consistent messages are delivered during the family conference. Room-based two-way communication boards can also optimize the relay of information by displaying active updates on daily plan of care goals, family questions or concerns for the critical care team, and notes on the patient's likes and dislikes.[43]

Empathetic communication is important during rounds and family conferences. The VALUE mnemonic (Box 2.3) is a useful tool to enhance communication with family members of critically ill patients.[44] The use of structured communication tools

BOX 2.3 Enhancing Communication With Family Members: VALUE Principles

V—Value what the family tells you.
A—Acknowledge family emotions.
L—Listen to the family members.
U—Understand the patient as a person.
E—Elicit (ask) questions of family members.

Data from Lautrette A, Darmon M, Megarbane B et al. A communication strategy and brochure for relatives of patients dying in the ICU. *N Engl J Med.* 2007;356(5):469-478.

have been found to increase understanding of the patient's prognosis and increase agreement on expectations between the family and multiprofessional critical care team while also improving family satisfaction.[45]

Visitation

Visitation practices are important to how patients and families experience critical care. With the exception of pandemic-related constraints,[46] many critical care units have modernized visitation policies by adopting unrestricted visiting hours, which has resulted in family needs being met and a higher satisfaction with the care given.[47,48] Pandemic-related visitation restrictions validated the prevalence of negative effects for patients (e.g., pain, less activity, depressive symptoms), family members (e.g., anxiety, uncertainty, family relational disturbances), and the critical care team (e.g., ethical dilemmas, increased demand for communication and social support), further supporting the need for open visitation.[46]

Some nurses may view family-centered care and open (also referred to as *expanded* or *liberal*) visitation as challenging or stressful; however, administrative support can help nurses to adjust and improve their job satisfaction.[49,50] Reasons cited for opposition to liberal visitation include the presumed increased physiological stress for the patient, family interference with the provision of care, and physical and mental exhaustion of family and friends.[51] An additional concern is that family members will be intrusive, creating burdens for nurses; however, concerns about negative outcomes of unrestricted visitation are unfounded.[52] Contrary to tradition-based practices of restricted visitation, family presence may contribute to the health and well-being of the patient, including improved nutrition intake, increased activities of daily living, and improvements in loneliness, depressive symptoms, agitation, aggression, and satisfaction.[46,53–55] The Clinical Exemplar box illustrates an example of person- and family-centered care.

CLINICAL EXEMPLAR

Person-Centered Care

Ms. K. is a 34-year-old woman with a C7 spinal cord injury that occurred 10 years ago. Her primary caregiver is her 63-year-old mother. Ms. K. has been admitted to the critical care unit with respiratory failure due to pneumonia three times in the past year. The charge nurse reports that Ms. K.'s mother obstructs care and is uncooperative with nursing staff. Ms. K.'s mother requests permission to stay in the patient room overnight throughout the hospitalization because she feels the need to oversee the nursing care. Ms. K's mother describes the hospital-acquired pressure injury (HAPI) with full-thickness skin loss (stage 3) during the last hospitalization. The pressure injury has significantly limited Ms. K.'s activities and is still healing. To address the conflicting concerns related to the privacy of other patients and potential disruptions to care by the nursing staff, the clinical nurse specialist is consulted to develop a plan to both promote family involvement and address nursing concerns. Ms. K.'s mother is permitted to stay overnight, as desired, with the understanding that the nurse may request that she leave the room for brief periods. After several days, the nursing team actively engages Ms. K's mother in nursing tasks (e.g., bathing, turning). As a result of the resolved conflict, the charge nurse proposes a change to unit policy to allow overnight visitors to promote inclusion of family members and care partners in the critical care setting.

Although practice is changing and research is limited, many institutions prohibit visitation by children. The American Association of Critical-Care Nurses (AACN) recommends welcoming children who are supervised by an adult family member.[56] To facilitate child visitation, a unit culture change may be required. Providing children the opportunity to visit a family member in the critical care unit may be traumatic for the child.[41] However, this can be mitigated by appropriately preparing the child (i.e., explaining the environment and the patient's appearance; allowing the child to participate in caregiving; facilitating intimate and private moments).[41] Nurses need to be engaged, and the visiting child needs individual guidance and follow-up.[57] Child Life Specialists are specifically educated and trained to prepare children for these experiences and assist the child in coping with the stress and anxiety of these situations.[42] If available, a Child Life Specialist should be consulted to facilitate and appropriately prepare the child for visiting a family member in the critical care unit. Visitation provides children with an opportunity to learn about their loved one and provides support during times of uncertainty. By allowing the child to visit, the deep bond with their family member is preserved, and the child is given the opportunity to understand the reality of the situation and the patient's condition.[41]

Animal-assisted therapy may also be beneficial to a patient's recovery. Some critical care units have extended visitation to include pet therapy. These institutions have policies that permit the family pet or designated therapy animals to visit the patient.[58,59]

Nurses can assist in promoting policy changes to affect open visitation policies. Unit-based councils and nurse-led research are helpful to create change in visitation policies. A significant benefit of an open visitation policy is its positive effect on the opinions of both patients and families regarding the quality of nursing care. When combined with family support, as demonstrated by the nurses' caring behaviors and interactions, open visitation is influential in shaping the critical care experience for both patients and families.

Family Presence During Resuscitation and Invasive Procedures

In conjunction with open visitation policies, many institutions have implemented policies to allow families to be present during cardiopulmonary resuscitation and invasive procedures. Factors cited for limiting family members' presence include limited space at the bedside, violations of patient confidentiality, not enough clinical staff available to assist family members, increased stress on critical care team members (e.g., performance anxiety, risk for litigation), and increased stress and anxiety for family members; however, these factors have not been substantiated by research. Studies have found that allowing family members to observe resuscitation and invasive procedures has positive effects, and the efforts promote increased knowledge of the patient's condition.[60] Box 2.4 presents the benefits of family presence.

The AACN issues Practice Alerts to guide the critical care community in the implementation of evidence-based policies and procedures. Box 2.5 summarizes the AACN Practice Alert regarding family presence during resuscitation and invasive procedures.

BOX 2.4 Benefits of Family Presence

Being Present Helps Family Members

- Remove doubt about the patient's condition.
- Witness that everything possible is being done.
- Decrease their anxiety and fear about what is happening to their loved one.

Being Present Facilitates Family Members'

- Need to be together with their loved one.
- Need to help and support their loved one.
- Sense of closure and grieving, should death occur.

BOX 2.5 Family Presence During Resuscitation and Invasive Procedures

Expected Practice

- Family members of all patients undergoing resuscitation and invasive procedures should be given the opportunity to be present at the bedside, in accordance with the patient's wishes.
- Prior to the procedure, review responsibilities of the healthcare team with the patient and family in addition to noises or smells that may occur.
- Provide a safe space for the family member that will not interrupt care.
- If possible provide a facilitator to support the family member.
- Re-evaluate the patient's wishes regarding family presence throughout their hospitalization.

Actions for Nursing Practice

- Collaborate with the patient, when possible, to determine who they identify as family.
- Assess the family for safety concerns as well as appropriateness and willingness to be present during procedures/resuscitation.
- Review policies, procedures, and educational programs to include components on topics such as benefits, criteria, contraindications, and role of the family presence facilitator.
- Develop proficiency standards for all staff.
- Develop documentation standards for family presence and debrief with the team as needed.

From American Association of Critical-Care Nurses. *Practice Alert: Facilitating family presence during resuscitation and invasive procedures throughout the lifespan.* https://www.aacn.org/clinical-resources/practice-alerts/facilitating-family-presence-during-resuscitation-and-invasive-procedures-throughout-the-life-span. Published 2023. Accessed February 8, 2024.

CHECK YOUR UNDERSTANDING

4. The family of a critically ill patient has just arrived to the unit. The patient is intubated and sedated for influenza and pneumonia. The family has many questions regarding the patient's condition and prognosis. They are tearful and appear anxious. Which of the following interventions is most likely to address the majority of their needs and minimize their concerns?
   A. Notify the provider of the family's questions.
   B. Share and explain recent laboratory findings with the family.
   C. Coordinate a family conference with the multiprofessional team.
   D. Orient the family to the critical care environment.

DISCHARGE FROM CRITICAL CARE AND QUALITY OF LIFE AFTER CRITICAL CARE

Survivors of critical illness experience many problems, but those cited most are functional disability and weakness, mental health impairments, cognitive dysfunction, and social isolation.[61] Collectively, these symptoms are defined as PICS.[62,63] Focused, multiprofessional postdischarge care, such as outpatient PICS clinics or peer support groups,[64,65] may be necessary to address PICS.

Family members have an increased risk of developing PTSD and caregiver burden after a critical care experience (PICS-family), requiring their own version of personalized follow-up support (e.g., emotional support, home health programs).[66,67] Once home, the demands of follow-up care place an enormous burden on family members, who may be ill-prepared or unwilling to shoulder such a burden. Discharge planning and patient teaching are nursing interventions essential to improving patient and family outcomes. Ongoing family involvement and teaching, beginning at admission and continuing throughout the hospital stay, are crucial interventions. Initiate patient education early and continue it throughout the patient's hospitalization. With the healthcare team, develop a comprehensive discharge plan that includes scheduled follow-up phone calls for ongoing assessment, reevaluation, and support. One technique used to facilitate teaching and learning is the *teach-back method*, in which patients and family members are asked to repeat the information and instructions they have been given.[68,69]

CLINICAL JUDGMENT ACTIVITY

You are caring for a patient whose family members include other medical professionals (i.e., clinical nurse, nurse practitioner, provider). The family is frequently critical of the patient's care and is constantly making suggestions. How do you respond?

CASE STUDY

The patient was involved in a motor vehicle collision. Injuries include a closed head injury, fractures to the left femur, tibia, and fibula, and liver laceration. The patient was unresponsive and hemodynamically unstable upon arrival to the emergency department and was admitted to the critical care unit after a ventriculostomy was placed to reduce and monitor intracranial pressure (ICP). Surgery on the lower extremity fractures is delayed until ICP is controlled. The patient is married with two children (ages 9 and 13). Bandages cover the patient's head and there is a cast to the leg and a ventriculostomy secured through the skull. The patient is sedated, intubated, and dependent on a ventilator.

The patient's significant other is at the bedside and expresses a feeling of "helplessness." Frequently, the significant other is tearful and expresses concern each time a monitoring alarm sounds. The significant other watches the monitors almost constantly and asks what each waveform and number means. The significant other states they want to be able to help in any way possible. According to the significant other, the patient is a hard worker and loves their children very much. A friend who comes to visit tells the significant other to "be strong for the children."

Questions

1. Are the significant other's concerns about the monitor and alarms appropriate? What measures would likely help manage the significant other's concerns?
2. What actions or tasks could be encouraged so the significant other can be more involved in the patient's care?
3. The patient's ICP increases with stimulation, including routine suctioning procedures or when the significant other talks to the patient. Should the significant other be discouraged from talking to the patient? Should visitation be suspended or restricted? Why or why not?
4. Should the patient's children be allowed and/or encouraged to visit? Why or why not?

KEY POINTS

- The critical care environment can cause extreme stress and anxiety for patients and family members due to sensory overload and sensory deprivation.
- Reducing noise and appropriate exposure to light can reduce adverse patient outcomes such as delirium and sleep disruption.
- Distressing physical experiences and memories from the critical care unit can result in PTSD, anxiety, and depression in the months following critical illness.
- Family-centered critical care includes involving family in the patient's healing process (e.g., encouraging them to speak to and touch the patient when not contraindicated).
- Information, assurance, and feeling safe are the most important patient and family-member needs.
- Family presence can contribute to the health and well-being of patients (e.g., improved nutrition intake, reduced depression, increased activities of daily living).
- Allowing family members to observe resuscitation and invasive procedures has positive effects and promotes increased family-member knowledge of the patient's condition.
- Focused, multiprofessional postdischarge care or peer support groups, may be necessary to address the physical, cognitive, mental health, and socioeconomic impairments experienced by patients following discharge after a critical illness (i.e., PICS and PICS-family).

REFERENCES

1. Minton C, Batten L, Huntington A. A multicase study of prolonged critical illness in the intensive care unit: families' experiences. *Intensive Crit Care Nurs.* 2019;50:21–27. https://doi.org/10.1016/j.iccn.2018.08.010.
2. Boehm LM, Jones AC, Selim AA, et al. Delirium-related distress in the ICU: a qualitative meta-synthesis of patient and family perspectives and experiences. *Int J Nurs Stud.* 2021;122:104030. https://doi.org/10.1016/j.ijnurstu.2021.104030.
3. Chang PY, Wang HP, Chang TH, Yu JM, Lee SY. Stress, stress-related symptoms and social support among Taiwanese primary family caregivers in intensive care units. *Intensive Crit Care Nurs.* 2018;49:37–43. https://doi.org/10.1016/j.iccn.2018.05.002.
4. Glick DR, Motta M, Wiegand DL, et al. Anticipatory grief and impaired problem solving among surrogate decision makers of critically ill patients: a cross-sectional study. *Intensive Crit Care Nurs.* 2018;49:1–5. https://doi.org/10.1016/j.iccn.2018.07.006.
5. Turner-Cobb JM, Smith PC, Ramchandani P, Begen FM, Padkin A. The acute psychobiological impact of the intensive care experience on relatives. *Psychol Health Med.* 2016;21(1):20–26. https://doi.org/10.1080/13548506.2014.997763.
6. Davidson JE, Aslakson RA, Long AC, et al. Guidelines for family-centered care in the neonatal, pediatric, and adult ICU. *Crit Care Med.* 2017;45(1):103–128. https://doi.org/10.1097/CCM.0000000000002169.
7. Devlin JW, Skrobik Y, Gelinas C, et al. Clinical practice guidelines for the prevention and management of pain, agitation/sedation, delirium, immobility, and sleep disruption in adult patients in the ICU. *Crit Care Med.* 2018;46(9):e825–e873. https://doi.org/10.1097/CCM.0000000000003299.
8. Coombs M, Puntillo KA, Franck LS, et al. Implementing the SCCM family-centered care guidelines in critical care nursing practice. *AACN Adv Crit Care.* 2017;28(2):138–147. https://doi.org/10.4037/aacnacc2017766.
9. Kleinpell R, Buchman TG, Harmon L, Nielsen M. Promoting patient- and family-centered care in the intensive care unit: a dissemination project. *AACN Adv Crit Care.* 2017;28(2):155–159. https://doi.org/10.4037/aacnacc2017425.
10. McAndrew NS, Jerofke-Owen T, Fortney CA, et al. Systematic review of family engagement interventions in neonatal, paediatric, and adult ICUs. *Nurs Crit Care.* 2022;27(3):296–325. https://doi.org/10.1111/nicc.12564.
11. Bayramzadeh S, Ahmadpour S, Aghaei P. The relationship between sensory stimuli and the physical environment in complex healthcare settings: a systematic literature review. *Intensive Crit Care Nurs.* 2021;67:103111. https://doi.org/10.1016/j.iccn.2021.103111.
12. Blake N. The effect of alarm fatigue on the work environment. *AACN Adv Crit Care.* 2014;25(1):18–19. https://doi.org/10.1097/NCI.0000000000000009.
13. Thomas L, Donohue-Porter P, Fishbein JS. Impact of interruptions, distractions, and cognitive load on procedure failures and medication administration errors. *Journal of Nursing Care Quality.* 2017;32(4):309–317.
14. Berglund B, Lindvall T, Schwela DH, World Health Organization. *Guidelines for Community Noise. World Health Organization's Occupational and Environmental Health Team*; 1999. https://apps.who.int/iris/handle/10665/66217. Accessed February 7, 2023.
15. Horsten S, Reinke L, Absalom A, Tulleken J. Systematic review of the effects of intensive-care-unit noise on sleep of healthy subjects and the critically ill. *Br J Anaesth.* 2018;120(3):443–452.
16. Danielson SJ, Rappaport CA, Loher MK, Gehlbach BK. Looking for light in the din: an examination of the circadian-disrupting properties of a medical intensive care unit. *Intensive Crit Care Nurs.* 2018;46:57–63. https://doi.org/10.1016/j.iccn.2017.12.006.
17. Rashid M. Two decades (1993-2012) of adult intensive care unit design: a comparative study of the physical design features of the best practice examples. *Crit Care Nurs Q.* 2014;37(1):3–32. https://doi.org/10.1097/CNQ.0000000000000002.
18. Topçu S, Ecevit Alpar Ş, Gülseven B, Kebapçı A. Patient experiences in intensive care units: a systematic review. *Patient Exp J.* 2017;4(3):115–127.
19. Rabiee DA, Nikayin DS, Hashem JM, et al. Depressive symptoms after critical illness: a systematic review and meta-analysis. *Crit Care Med.* 2016;44(9):1744–1753. https://doi.org/10.1097/CCM.0000000000001811.
20. Nikayin S, Rabiee A, Hashem MD, et al. Anxiety symptoms in survivors of critical illness: a systematic review and meta-analysis. *General Hospital Psychiatry.* 2016;43:23–29. https://doi.org/10.1016/j.genhosppsych.2016.08.005.
21. Parker AM, Sricharoenchai T, Raparla S, Schneck KW, Bienvenu OJ, Needham DM. Posttraumatic stress disorder in critical illness survivors: a metaanalysis. *Crit Care Med.* 2015;43(5):1121–1129. https://doi.org/10.1097/CCM.0000000000000882.

22. Stollings JL, Devlin JW, Pun BT, et al. Implementing the ABCDEF bundle: top 8 questions asked during the ICU Liberation ABCDEF bundle improvement collaborative. *Crit Care Nurse*. 2019;39(1):36–45. https://doi.org/10.4037/ccn2019981.
23. Romagnoli S, Villa G, Fontanarosa L, et al. Sleep duration and architecture in non-intubated intensive care unit patients: an observational study. *Sleep Med*. 2020;70:79–87. https://doi.org/10.1016/j.sleep.2019.11.1265.
24. Michalsen A, Long AC, DeKeyser Ganz F, et al. Interprofessional shared decision-making in the ICU: a systematic review and recommendations from an expert panel. *Crit Care Med*. 2019;47(9):1258–1266. https://doi.org/10.1097/CCM.0000000000003870.
25. *Guide to Patient and Family Engagement in Hospital Quality and Safety*. U.S Dept. of Health and Human Services' Agency for Healthcare Research and Quality; 2017. https://www.ahrq.gov/patient-safety/patients-families/engagingfamilies/guide.html. Accessed February 7, 2023.
26. Center for Medicaid and Medicare Services. *HCAHPS: Patients' Perspectives of Care Survey*Updated December 1 ; 2021. https://www.cms.gov/Medicare/Quality-Initiatives-Patient-Assessment-Instruments/HospitalQualityInits/HospitalHCAHPS. Accessed February 7, 2023.
27. Shajan Z, Snell D. *Wright & Leahey's Nurses and Families: A Guide to Family Assessment and Intervention*. FA Davis; 2019.
28. Scott P, Thomson P, Shepherd A. Families of patients in ICU: a scoping review of their needs and satisfaction with care. *Nurs Open*. 2019;6(3):698–712. https://doi.org/10.1002/nop2.287.
29. Padilla Fortunatti C, Munro CL. Factors associated with family satisfaction in the adult intensive care unit: a literature review. *Aust Crit Care*. 2022;35(5):604–611. https://doi.org/10.1016/j.aucc.2021.07.006.
30. Chang P-Y, Wang H-P, Chang T-H, Yu J-M, Lee S-Y. Stress, stress-related symptoms and social support among Taiwanese primary family caregivers in intensive care units. *Intensive and Critical Care Nursing*. 2018;49:37–43.
31. Leske JS. Overview of family needs after critical illness: from assessment to intervention. *AACN Clin Issues Crit Care Nurs*. 1991;2(2):220–229. https://doi.org/10.4037/15597768-1991-2006.
32. Leske JS. Needs of adult family members after critical illness: prescriptions for interventions. *Crit Care Nurs Clin North Am*. 1992;4(4):587–596.
33. Mousavi SS, Chaman R, Khosravi A, Mohagheghi P, Mousavi SA, Keramat A. The needs of parents of preterm infants in Iran and a comparison with those in other countries: a systematic review and meta-analysis. *Iran J Pediatr*. 2016;26(5):e4396. https://doi.org/10.5812/ijp.4396.
34. Goldfarb MJ, Bibas L, Bartlett V, Jones H, Khan N. Outcomes of patient- and family-centered care interventions in the ICU: a systematic review and meta-analysis. *Crit Care Med*. 2017;45(10):1751–1761. https://doi.org/10.1097/CCM.0000000000002624.
35. Davidson JE, Powers K, Hedayat KM, et al. Clinical practice guidelines for support of the family in the patient-centered intensive care unit: American College of Critical Care Medicine Task Force 2004-2005. *Crit Care Med*. 2007;35(2):605–622. https://doi.org/10.1097/01.CCM.0000254067.14607.EB.
36. Torbey MT, Brophy GM, Varelas PN, et al. Guidelines for family-centered care in neuro-ICU populations: caveats for routine palliative care. *Crit Care Med*. 2017;45(6):e620–e621. https://doi.org/10.1097/CCM.0000000000002344.
37. Villa P, Pintado MC, Lujan J, et al. Functional status and quality of life in elderly intensive care unit survivors. *J Am Geriatr Soc*. 2016;64(3):536–542. https://doi.org/10.1111/jgs.14031.
38. McKinley S, Fien M, Elliott R, Elliott D. Health-related quality of life and associated factors in intensive care unit survivors 6 months after discharge. *Am J Crit Care*. 2016;25(1):52–58.
39. Heyland DK, Garland A, Bagshaw SM, et al. Recovery after critical illness in patients aged 80 years or older: a multi-center prospective observational cohort study. *Intensive Care Med*. 2015;41(11):1911–1920. https://doi.org/10.1007/s00134-015-4028-2.
40. Ferge JL, Le Terrier C, Banydeen R, et al. Prevalence of anxiety and depression symptomatology in adolescents faced with the hospitalization of a loved one in the ICU. *Crit Care Med*. 2018;46(4):e330–e333. https://doi.org/10.1097/CCM.0000000000002964.
41. Lamiani G, Bonazza F, Del Negro S, Meyer EC. The impact of visiting the Intensive Care Unit on children's and adolescents' psychological well-being: a systematic review. *Intensive Crit Care Nurs*. 2021;65:103036. https://doi.org/10.1016/j.iccn.2021.103036.
42. Association of Child Life Professionals. The child life profession. About Child Life. Accessed February 8, 2023. https://www.childlife.org/the-child-life-profession.
43. Cuenca JA, Manjappachar N, Nates J, et al. Humanizing the intensive care unit experience in a comprehensive cancer center: a patient-and family-centered improvement study. *Palliat Support Care*. 2021:1–7.
44. Lautrette A, Darmon M, Megarbane B, et al. A communication strategy and brochure for relatives of patients dying in the ICU. *N Engl J Med*. 2007;356(5):469–478.
45. Sviri S, Geva D, vanHeerden PV, et al. Implementation of a structured communication tool improves family satisfaction and expectations in the intensive care unit. *J Crit Care*. 2019;51:6–12. https://doi.org/10.1016/j.jcrc.2019.01.011.
46. Hugelius K, Harada N, Marutani M. Consequences of visiting restrictions during the COVID-19 pandemic: an integrative review. *Int J Nurs Stud*. 2021;121:104000. https://doi.org/10.1016/j.ijnurstu.2021.104000.
47. Jacob M, Horton C, Rance-Ashley S, et al. Needs of patients' family members in an intensive care unit with continuous visitation. *Am J Crit Care*. 2016;25(2):118–125. https://doi.org/10.4037/ajcc2016258.
48. Junior APN, Besen BAMP, Robinson CC, Falavigna M, Teixeira C, Rosa RG. Flexible versus restrictive visiting policies in ICUs: a systematic review and meta-analysis. *Crit Care Med*. 2018;46(7):1175–1180.
49. Coats H, Bourget E, Starks H, et al. Nurses' reflections on benefits and challenges of implementing family-centered care in pediatric intensive care units. *Am J Crit Care*. 2018;27(1):52–58. https://doi.org/10.4037/ajcc2018353.
50. Monroe M, Wofford L. Open visitation and nurse job satisfaction: an integrative review. *J Clin Nurs*. 2017;26(23–24):4868–4876. https://doi.org/10.1111/jocn.13919.
51. Riley BH, White J, Graham S, Alexandrov A. Traditional/restrictive vs patient-centered intensive care unit visitation: perceptions of patients' family members, physicians, and nurses. *Am J Crit Care*. 2014;23(4):316–324. https://doi.org/10.4037/ajcc2014980.
52. Trochelman K, Albert N, Spence J, Murray T, Slifcak E. Patients and their families weigh in on evidence-based hospital design. *Crit Care Nurse*. 2012;32(1):e1–e10. https://doi.org/10.4037/ccn2012785.

53. Giuliano K, Giuliano A. Cardiovascular responses to family visitation and nurse-physician rounds. *Heart Lung.* 1992;21(3):290.
54. Hepworth JT, Hendrickson SG, Lopez J. Time series analysis of physiological response during ICU visitation. *West J Nurs Res.* 1994;16(6):704–717. https://doi.org/10.1177/019394599401600608.
55. Moss SJ, Rosgen BK, Lucini F, et al. Psychiatric outcomes in ICU patients with family visitation: a population-based retrospective cohort study. *Chest.* 2022;162(3):578–587. https://doi.org/10.1016/j.chest.2022.02.051.
56. American Association of Critical-Care Nurses. Family presence: visitation in the adult ICU. *Crit Care Nurse.* 2012;32(4):76–78.
57. Knutsson S, Enskar K, Golsater M. Nurses' experiences of what constitutes the encounter with children visiting a sick parent at an adult ICU. *Intensive Crit Care Nurs.* 2017;39:9–17. https://doi.org/10.1016/j.iccn.2016.09.003.
58. Hosey MM, Jaskulski J, Wegener ST, Chlan LL, Needham DM. Animal-assisted intervention in the ICU: a tool for humanization. *Crit Care.* 2018;22(1):22. https://doi.org/10.1186/s13054-018-1946-8.
59. Kramlich D. Complementary health practitioners in the acute and critical care setting: nursing considerations. *Crit Care Nurse.* 2017;37(3):60–65. https://doi.org/10.4037/ccn2017181.
60. Leske JS, McAndrew NS, Brasel KJ, Feetham S. Family presence during resuscitation after trauma. *J Trauma Nurs.* 2017;24(2):85–96. https://doi.org/10.1097/JTN.0000000000000271.
61. Yuan C, Timmins F, Thompson DR. Post-intensive care syndrome: a concept analysis. *Int J Nurs Stud.* 2021;114. https://doi.org/10.1016/j.ijnurstu.2020.103814. 103814-103814.
62. Harvey MA, Davidson JE. Postintensive care syndrome: right care, right now...and later. *Crit Care Med.* 2016;44(2):381–385. https://doi.org/10.1097/CCM.0000000000001531.
63. Marra A, Pandharipande PP, Girard TD, et al. Co-occurrence of post-intensive care syndrome problems among 406 survivors of critical illness. *Crit Care Med.* 2018;46(9):1393–1401. https://doi.org/10.1097/CCM.0000000000003218.
64. Mikkelsen ME, Jackson JC, Hopkins RO, et al. Peer support as a novel strategy to mitigate post-intensive care syndrome. *AACN Adv Crit Care.* 2016;27(2):221–229. https://doi.org/10.4037/aacnacc2016667.
65. Stollings JL, Caylor MM. Postintensive care syndrome and the role of a follow-up clinic. *Am J Health Syst Pharm.* 2015;72(15):1315–1323. https://doi.org/10.2146/ajhp140533.
66. Davidson JE, Jones C, Bienvenu OJ. Family response to critical illness: postintensive care syndrome-family. *Crit Care Med.* 2012;40(2):618–624. https://doi.org/10.1097/CCM.0b013e318236ebf9.
67. Sevin CM, Boehm LM, Hibbert E, et al. Optimizing critical illness recovery: perspectives and solutions from the caregivers of ICU survivors. *Crit Care Explor.* 2021;3(5). https://doi.org/10.1097/CCE.0000000000000420. e0420-e0420.
68. Peter D, Robinson P, Jordan M, Lawrence S, Casey K, Salas-Lopez D. Reducing readmissions using teach-back: enhancing patient and family education. *J Nurs Adm.* 2015;45(1):35–42. https://doi.org/10.1097/NNA.0000000000000155.
69. Ryan-Madonna M, Levin RF, Lauder B. Effectiveness of the teach-back method for improving caregivers' confidence in caring for hospice patients and decreasing hospitalizations. *J Hosp Palliat Nurs.* 2019;21(1):61–70. https://doi.org/10.1097/NJH.0000000000000492.

3

Ethical and Legal Issues in Critical Care Nursing

Jayne M. Willis, DNP, RN, NEA-BC, CENP

INTRODUCTION

Critical care nurses are often confronted with ethical and legal dilemmas related to informed consent, withholding or withdrawing life-sustaining treatment, organ and tissue transplantation, confidentiality, and increasingly, justice in the distribution of healthcare resources. Ethical and legal dilemmas are conflicts that occur when there are equally compelling courses of action and a decision must be made. Many dilemmas are byproducts of advanced medical technologies and therapies developed over the past several decades. Although technology provides substantial benefits to critically ill patients, extensive public and professional debate occurs over the appropriate use of these technologies, especially those that are life-sustaining. One of the primary concerns in critical care is whether a patient's values and beliefs about treatment can be overridden by the technological imperative or the strong tendency to use technology because it is available.

Although many ethical dilemmas are not unique to critical care, they occur more frequently in critical care settings. Therefore, it is crucial that critical care nurses examine the nature and scope of their ethical and legal obligations to patients.

The ethical and legal issues that frequently arise in the nursing care of acute and critically ill patients are examined in this chapter. The discussion includes problems surrounding patients' rights and nurses' obligations, informed consent, and withholding and withdrawing treatment. The elements of ethical decision-making and the involvement of the nurse are discussed, as well as some specific issues with ethical implications.

ETHICAL OBLIGATIONS, NURSE ADVOCACY, AND DECISION-MAKING

Critical care nurses' ethical and legal responsibilities for patient care have increased dramatically since the early 1990s. Evolving case law and current concepts of nurse advocacy and accountability indicate that nurses have substantial ethical and legal obligations to promote and protect the welfare of their patients.

Code of Ethics

The duty to practice ethically and serve as an ethical agent on behalf of patients is an integral part of nurses' professional practice. The nurse's duty is stated in the *Code of Ethics for Nurses With Interpretive Statements,* which was adopted by the American Nurses Association (ANA) in 1976 and revised in 2015 in response to the complexities of modern nursing and in anticipation of healthcare advances. The document describes the moral principles that guide professional nursing practice and serves the following purposes: (1) it delineates the ethical obligations and duties of every individual who enters the profession; (2) it is the profession's nonnegotiable ethical standard; and (3) it is the expression of nursing's own understanding of its commitment to society.[1]

The Code of Ethics consists of nine provision statements. The first three describe fundamental values and commitments of the nurse, the next three describe the boundaries of duty and loyalty, and the final three describe duties beyond individual patient encounters. The interpretive statements of the Code provide specific guidance in applying each provision to current nursing practice. Nurses in all practice areas, including critical care, must be knowledgeable about the provisions of the code and incorporate the basic tenets into their clinical practice.[2] The Code is a powerful tool that shapes and evaluates individual practice and the nursing profession. However, situations may arise in which the Code provides only limited direction. Critical care nurses must remain knowledgeable and abreast of ethical issues and changes in the literature so they may make appropriate decisions when difficult clinical situations arise. Additional ANA position statements related to human rights and ethics are available on the ANA website (https://www.nursingworld.org/practice-policy/nursing-excellence/ethics/).

Ethical Care Obligation

Nurses' ethical obligation to serve as advocates for their patients is derived from the unique nature of the nurse-patient relationship. Critical care nurses assume a significant caregiving role that is characterized by intimate, extended contact with persons who are often the most physiologically and psychologically vulnerable. Nurses also provide support to the patients' families. Critical care nurses have a moral and professional responsibility to act as advocates on the patients' behalf because of their unique relationship with patients and specialized nursing knowledge. Ethical care is a moral orientation that acknowledges individual uniqueness, relationships, and respect for the dynamic nature of life. Core characteristics of ethical care encompass compassion, collaboration, respect, trust, and delivery of dignified care.

CLINICAL JUDGMENT ACTIVITY

You are taking care of Mrs. H., a 90-year-old patient with gastrointestinal bleeding. She has developed numerous complications and requires mechanical ventilation. She is unresponsive to nurses and family members. She has been in the hospital for 2 weeks and requires a transfusion nearly every day to sustain adequate hemoglobin and hematocrit levels. Her prognosis is poor. Before this hospitalization, she lived independently in her own home. Her children tell you they are tired of seeing their mother suffer. How do you respond to the family, and what follow-up do you perform?

Ethical Decision-Making

As reflected in the ANA Code of Ethics, one of the primary ethical obligations of professional nurses is the protection of the patients' basic rights. This obligation requires nurses to recognize ethical dilemmas that actually or potentially threaten patients' rights and to participate in the resolution of those dilemmas.

An ethical dilemma is a difficult problem or situation in which conflicts arise during the process of making morally justifiable decisions. In the critical care setting, ethical principles may have competing priorities. For example, *autonomy* (respect for individual decision-making) may be in direct conflict with *maleficence* (do no harm) or *beneficence* (do good). When these conflicts occur, ethical dilemmas can arise for the healthcare team.[3] In identifying a situation as an ethical dilemma, certain criteria must be met. More than one solution must exist, and there is no clear "right" or "wrong" decision. Each solution must carry equal weight and be ethically defensible. An example of an ethical dilemma is the decision of whether to give the one available critical care bed to a patient with cancer who is experiencing hypotension after chemotherapy or to a patient in the emergency department who has an acute myocardial infarction. The conflicting issue in this example is which patient should be given the bed, based on the moral allocation of limited resources.

Several warning signs can assist the nurse in recognizing an ethical dilemma. If these warning signs occur, the critical care nurse should reassess the situation and determine whether an ethical dilemma exists and what additional actions are needed. Questions to help reassess the situation may include:

- Is the situation emotionally charged?
- Has the patient's condition changed significantly?
- Is there confusion or conflict about the facts?
- Is there increased hesitancy about the right course of action?
- Is the proposed action a deviation from customary practice?
- Is there a perceived need for secrecy around the proposed action?

Arriving at a morally justifiable decision when an ethical dilemma exists can be difficult for patients, families, and health professionals. Critical care nurses must be careful not to impose their own value system on that of the patient. Each patient and family have a set of personal values that are influenced by their environment and culture.

One helpful way to approach ethical decision-making is to use a systematic, structured process, such as the one depicted in Fig. 3.1. This model provides a framework for evaluating the related ethical principles and the potential outcomes, as well as relevant facts concerning the contextual factors and the patient's physiological and personal factors. Using this approach, the patient, family, and healthcare team members evaluate choices and identify the option that promotes the patient's best interests.

Ethical decision-making includes implementing the decision and evaluating the short-term and long-term outcomes. Evaluation provides meaningful feedback about decisions and actions in specific instances, as well as about the effectiveness of the decision-making process. The final stage in the decision-making process is assessing whether the decision in a specific case can be applied to other dilemmas in similar circumstances. In other words, is this decision useful in similar cases? A systematic approach to decision-making does not guarantee that morally justifiable decisions are reached or that the outcome is beneficial to the patient. However, it ensures that all applicable information is considered in the decision.

CHECK YOUR UNDERSTANDING

1. The American Nurses Association (ANA) *Code of Ethics for Nurses With Interpretive Statements* delineates the ethical obligations of every nurse who enters the profession. Which of the following statements are examples of a nurse demonstrating adherence to the code of ethics?
   A. A patient in the critical care unit is asked to participate in a clinical trial on a new medication. The nurse ensures that the patient receives and comprehends information regarding clinical research before they agree to participate.
   B. The nurse participates in the maintenance of their competence and participates in continuing education to remain current in trends in critical care nursing.
   C. The nurse safeguards the patient's right to privacy by sharing relevant patient information only with critical care team members that need that knowledge to carry out patient care duties.
   D. All the above.

CLINICAL JUDGMENT ACTIVITY

You are taking care of Mr. J., a 23-year-old man with a closed head injury. During the night shift, you note a change in the level of consciousness at 3:00 AM. You call the provider, who tells you to watch Mr. J. until rounds the next morning. The provider tells you not to call again. Mr. J.'s neurological status continues to deteriorate. What actions do you take? What is the rationale for your actions?

ETHICAL PRINCIPLES

As reflected in the decision-making model, relevant ethical principles are considered when a moral dilemma exists (Box 3.1). These principles are intended to provide respect and dignity for all persons.

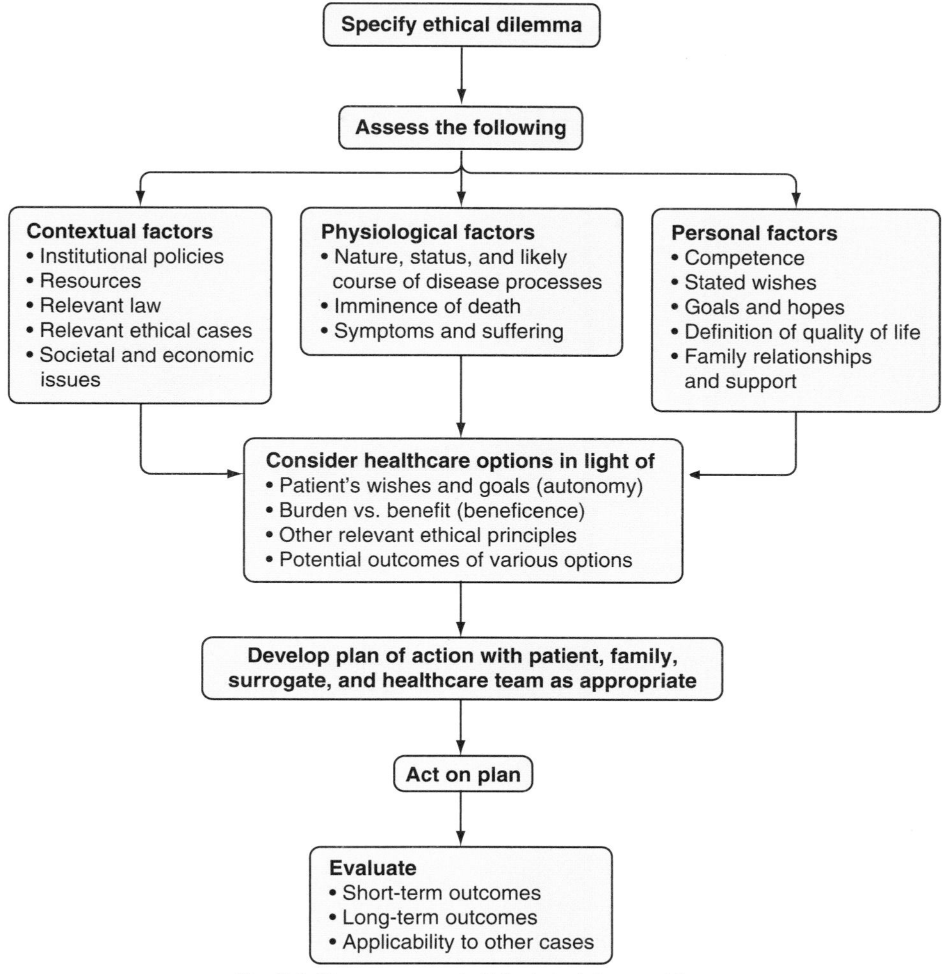

Fig. 3.1 The process of ethical decision-making.

BOX 3.1 Ethical Principles

- **Autonomy:** Respect for the individual and the ability of individuals to make decisions about their own health and future (the basis for the practice of informed consent).
- **Beneficence:** Actions intended to benefit the patients or others.
- **Nonmaleficence:** Actions intended not to harm or bring harm to others.
- **Justice:** Being fair or just to the wider community in terms of the consequences of an action; in health care, justice is described as the fair allocation or distribution of healthcare resources.
- **Veracity:** The obligation to tell the truth.
- **Fidelity:** The moral duty to be faithful to the commitments that one makes to others.
- **Confidentiality:** Respect for an individual's autonomy and the right of individuals to control the information relating to their own health.

Principlism is a widely applied ethical approach based on four fundamental moral principles related to contemporary ethical dilemmas: respect for autonomy, beneficence, nonmaleficence, and justice.[4] The principle of *autonomy* states that all persons should be free to govern their lives to the greatest degree possible. The autonomy principle implies a strong sense of self-determination and an acceptance of responsibility for one's own choices and actions. To respect the autonomy of others means respecting their freedom of choice and allowing them to make their own decisions.

The principle of *beneficence* is the duty to provide benefits to others when in a position to do so and to help balance harm and benefits. In other words, the benefits of an action should outweigh the burdens. A related concept is *non-beneficial treatment*. Care should not be given if it is not beneficial in terms of improving comfort or the medical outcome. The principle of *nonmaleficence* is the explicit duty not to inflict harm on others intentionally.

The principle of *justice* requires that healthcare resources be distributed fairly and equitably among groups of people. The principle of justice is particularly relevant to critical care because most healthcare resources, including technology and pharmaceuticals, are expended in this practice setting.

Other principles are also relevant. The principle of *veracity* states that persons are obligated to tell the truth in their communication with others. The principle of *fidelity* requires that one has a moral duty to be faithful to the commitments made to others. These two principles, along with *confidentiality*, are key to the nurse-patient relationship.

CHECK YOUR UNDERSTANDING

2. A car full of teenagers was in a tragic accident after leaving a football game. Two individuals died at the scene and three were transported to the critical care unit. A friend of the teenagers' calls and asks for information about the three surviving teens. What is the nurse's best response aligned with ethical principles of care?
   A. "I can confirm the individuals are here; however, you'll need to speak to the parents for an update."
   B. "I cannot confirm the individuals are in this hospital; watch the news for updates."
   C. "I'm very sorry, but I need to protect patient confidentiality and I cannot speak to anyone other than direct family members about any patients in the hospital. Please reach out to your friends' parents."
   D. "I can confirm the teenagers are in this hospital and are in critical condition. Have you spoken with law enforcement about the accident to provide essential details about how it happened?"

Creating an Ethical Environment

Critical care nurses and the leadership team focus on nursing initiatives at the unit, service line, and organizational levels to improve quality, patient satisfaction, and nursing retention. The American Association of Critical-Care Nurses' (AACN's) Healthy Work Environment Initiative assists teams to create a positive and fulfilling organizational culture through engagement and empowerment.[5] The program allows nurses to promote, plan, and develop an ethical environment in which to practice.

Addressing ethical problems and participating in ethical decision-making are key to improving the quality of care. Multiprofessional collaboration and collegial working relationships that generate mutual respect are important elements of a successful critical care team.

INCREASING NURSES' INVOLVEMENT IN ETHICAL DECISION-MAKING

Although nurses play a significant role in the care of patients, they often report limited involvement in the formal processes of ethical decision-making. Nurses' perception of this limited involvement may be related to many factors, such as lack of formal education in ethics, lack of institutional mechanisms for review of dilemmas, perceived lack of administrative or peer support for involvement in decision-making, concern about reprisals, and perceived lack of decision-making authority. Research has shown that ethics education has a significant positive influence on moral confidence, moral action, and the use of ethics resources by nurses.[6] If nurses are to fulfill their advocacy obligations to patients, they must become active in the process of ethical decision-making at all levels.

Moral Distress and Moral Resilience

Ethical dilemmas are among the many issues that can lead to *moral distress* for critical care nurses. Moral distress occurs when the nurse knows the ethically appropriate action to take but is unable to act on it or when the nurse acts in a manner contrary to personal and professional values.[7] Moral distress is one of the key issues affecting the workplace environment. Healthy, thriving work environments are eroded when critical care nurses experience unanswered moral distress. The consequences of moral distress are well documented. Nurses with moral distress are sick more often, suffer burnout, and disengage from their work environment, leading to increased turnover and even career changes.[8] Professional nursing and healthcare organizations are addressing the challenges of ethical incongruency by building moral resilience. *Moral resilience* is defined as the ability of nurses to rebalance and resolve ethical incongruency both personally and organizationally when faced with ethical dilemmas.[9] Personal and organizational strategies are needed to assist critical care nurses to address ethical situations in their practice.[10] Box 3.2 lists personal strategies to nurture and grow moral resilience in nursing practice.[10]

BOX 3.2 Critical Care Nurse Strategies to Promote and Sustain Moral Resilience

- Advocate with courage for patients.
- Trust your personal value system.
- Foster your spirituality.
- Show self-confidence in your knowledge.
- Cultivate your own moral compass and practice it.
- Practice reflective review of moral decisions and actions.
- Champion and support colleagues facing ethical dilemmas.
- Foster interpersonal connections during challenging times.
- Seek assistance from colleagues for ethical dilemmas.
- Develop personal care strategies to promote mental health.
- Develop mindfulness practices.
- Build communication skills.
- Know and use organizational resources.
- Embrace mentorship.
- Know and live the ANA Code of Ethics.

Modified from Stutzer K, Bylone M. Building moral resilience. *Crit Care Nurse.* 2018;38(1):77-89; Stutzer K, Rodriguez AM. Moral resilience for critical care nurses. *Crit Care Nurs Clin North Am.* 2020;32(3):383-393. https://doi.org/10.1016/j.cnc.2020.05.002.

Mechanisms to Address Ethical Concerns

A critical element for true collaboration is that healthcare organizations ensure unrestricted access to structured forums such as ethics committees and allow time to resolve disputes among critical participants, including patients, families, and the healthcare team.[5] Actively addressing ethical dilemmas and avoiding moral distress are crucial factors in creating a healthy workplace in which critical care nurses can make optimal contributions to patients and their families.

Institutions should have a formal mechanism in place to address patients' ethical concerns. Bioethics committees are one way to address this need. Typical membership of a bioethics committee includes providers, nurses, chaplains, social workers, and, if available, bioethicists. A multiprofessional committee can serve as an educational and policy-making body and, in some cases, provide ethics consultation on a case-by-case basis. The purpose of ethics consultation is to improve the process and outcomes of patient care by helping to identify, analyze, and resolve ethical problems. This service should be used when the

BOX 3.3 Situations in Which Ethics Consultation May Be Considered

- Disagreement or conflict exists on whether to pursue aggressive life-sustaining treatment, such as cardiopulmonary resuscitation, in a seriously ill patient or to emphasize comfort and palliative care.
- The family demands life-sustaining treatment, such as mechanical ventilation or tube feeding, which the provider and nurses consider futile.
- Competing family members are present and want to make critical decisions on behalf of the patient.
- A seriously ill patient is incapacitated and does not have a surrogate decision-maker or an advance directive.

issues cannot be resolved among the healthcare team, patient, and family. Box 3.3 lists examples of situations in which an ethics consultation may be considered.

Nurses can become more involved with ethical decision-making through participation in institutional ethics committees, multiprofessional ethics forums and roundtables, peer review and quality improvement committees, and institutional research review boards. Nurses can also improve and update their knowledge through formal and continuing education courses on bioethics, as well as through telephone and computerized electronic consultation and reference services. Educational programs and ethics consultation services are available through several ethics and law centers in the United States. Three ethical consultation services are listed in Box 3.4. Additional online educational resources are listed in Box 3.5.

BOX 3.4 Ethics Consultation Services

American Nurses Association Center for Ethics and Human Rights
8515 Georgia Avenue, Suite 400
Silver Spring, MD 20910
http://nursingworld.org/ethics/

Johns Hopkins Berman Institute of Bioethics
Deering Hall
1809 Ashland Avenue
Baltimore, MD 21205
https://bioethics.jhu.edu/

Kennedy Institute of Ethics
Georgetown University
3700 O Street NW
Washington, DC 20057-1212
https://kennedyinstitute.georgetown.edu/

BOX 3.5 Internet Resources for Bioethics

- *American Journal of Bioethics:* http://www.bioethics.net
- American Society for Bioethics and Humanities: http://www.asbh.org
- Department of Medical Ethics & Health Policy – University of Pennsylvania: http://www.bioethics.upenn.edu
- National Institutes of Health Department of Bioethics: http://www.bioethics.nih.gov

Just Culture

The Institute of Medicine report *To Err is Human* was released in 2000 and was the catalyst for a shift in health care from focusing on individuals and blame to considering the system accountable for errors.[11] The term "just culture" was popularized in the patient safety lexicon and outlines the principles for fostering a culture in which frontline staff feels trust and comfort in disclosing errors while maintaining professional accountability.[12] A just culture relies on reporting near misses, errors, and ethical concerns when they occur and does not tolerate conscious disregard of obvious risks to patients, reckless behavior, or gross misconduct. Additionally, it provides a framework to analyze system processes and individual behavior choices to identify opportunities to prevent errors in the future. Just culture is often associated with patient safety, but it can also support healthcare professionals and their mental health by supporting an ethical environment. Critical care nurses need to have the ability to speak up and elevate an ethical issue or an error when encountered. When nurses cannot speak up due to fear of consequences, it can lead to moral distress or patient safety issues. In a 2010 position statement, the American Nurses Association (ANA) advocates for actions that support the just culture concept, citing that it positively impacts the work environment and outcomes.[13]

In 2022, the healthcare community was angered when a former critical care nurse was found guilty of homicide for an unintentional medication error that unfortunately resulted in the death of a patient. The nurse readily disclosed the mistake; however, the nurse was terminated and the nursing license revoked. Admittedly, the nurse in this case bypassed several safety precautions, but it was found that several system issues contributed to the error.[14] The criminal verdict for this unintentional error threatens the just culture philosophy. The ANA released a statement in response to the criminal verdict stating, "This ruling will have a long-lasting negative impact on the profession".[15] The AACN also published a statement saying, "This criminal prosecution and verdict will negatively impact the timely and honest reporting of errors".[16] Human errors by nurses have historically held consequences such as possible reporting to regulatory boards or civil liability. However, the criminalization of this event can undo decades of patient safety work encouraging honest reporting of errors and near misses.

CLINICAL JUDGMENT ACTIVITY

You are caring for Mrs. M., a 68-year-old woman with an acute myocardial infarction. She is in the critical care unit after a successful angioplasty. Her husband brought in her living will, which states that Mrs. M. does not desire resuscitation. Mrs. M. is pain free and alert. As you start your beginning-of-shift assessment, Mrs. M. says, "You know, now that I've made it through the angioplasty, I realize that tubes and machines may not be so bad after all. I haven't made it this far to give up now. If I go into cardiac arrest, I want you to do all that you can for me." What ethical principle is Mrs. M. using? As her nurse, what actions should you take and why?

SELECTED ETHICAL TOPICS IN CRITICAL CARE

Informed Consent

Many complex dilemmas in critical care nursing raise concern of informed consent because patients are experiencing acute, life-threatening illnesses that interfere with their ability to make decisions about treatment or participation in a clinical research study. The doctrine of informed consent is based on the principle of autonomy; competent adults have the right to self-determination or to make decisions regarding their acceptance or rejection of treatment.

Elements of Informed Consent. Three primary elements must be present for a person's consent or decline of medical treatment or research participation to be considered valid: competence, voluntariness, and disclosure of information. Competence (or capacity) refers to a person's ability to understand information regarding a proposed medical or nursing treatment. Competence is a legal term and is determined in court. Healthcare providers evaluate mental capacity. The ability of patients to understand relevant information is an essential prerequisite to their participation in the decision-making process and should be carefully evaluated as part of the informed consent process. Patients providing informed consent should be free from severe pain and depression. Critically ill patients usually do not have the mental capacity to provide informed consent because of the severe nature of their illness or their treatment (e.g., sedation). If the patient is not mentally capable of providing consent, informed consent is obtained from the designated healthcare surrogate or legal authorized representative (proxy). State law governs consent issues, and legal counsel should be consulted for specific questions.

Consent must be given voluntarily, without coercion or fraud, for the consent to be legally binding. This includes freedom from pressure from family members, healthcare providers, and payers. Persons who consent should base their decision on sufficient knowledge. Basic information considered necessary for decision-making includes the following:

- A diagnosis of the patient's specific health problem and condition.
- The nature, duration, and purpose of the proposed treatment or procedures.
- The probable outcome of any medical or nursing intervention.
- The benefits of medical or nursing interventions.
- The potential risks that are generally considered common or hazardous.
- Alternative treatments and their feasibility.
- Short-term and long-term prognoses if the proposed treatment or treatments are not provided.

Informed consent is not a form. It is a *process* that entails the exchange of information between the healthcare provider and the patient or patient's proxy. Frequently, nurses are asked to witness the consent process for procedures and tests. The nurse should serve as an advocate for the patient and ensure that the informed consent process has been completed according to legal standards and institutional policy. Nurses may provide additional patient education to support decision-making, but the process of obtaining informed consent is a provider obligation.

> **CHECK YOUR UNDERSTANDING**
>
> 3. A patient in the critical care unit is being prepped by a provider for an urgent procedure. It becomes apparent to the nurse that the patient does not fully understand the risks and benefits of the procedure. Which of the following describes the role of the nurse in obtaining informed consent? Select all that apply:
>   A. Explain the risks and benefits associated with the procedure.
>   B. Describe the alternatives to the procedure.
>   C. Advocate for the patient by ensuring they are making an informed decision.
>   D. Witness the patient's signature on the consent form after the patient receives and comprehends information regarding the procedure.

Decisions Regarding Life-Sustaining Treatment

Care of persons who are terminally ill or in a persistent vegetative state raises profound questions about the constitutional rights of persons or surrogates to make decisions related to death or life-sustaining care, as well as the rights of the state to intervene in treatment decisions. Table 3.1 reviews three landmark legal cases—Quinlan, Cruzan, and Schiavo—that have influenced legal and ethical precedents in the right-to-die debate. Table 3.2 lists definitions for some terms pertinent to these issues.

The issue of treatment for persons whose quality of life is severely compromised, as in irreversible coma or brain death, is often a result of advanced biomedical technology. Technology frequently sustains life in persons who would have previously died of their illnesses. The widespread use of advanced life-support systems and cardiopulmonary resuscitation (CPR) has changed the nature and context of dying. A "natural death" in the traditional sense is rare; most patients who die in healthcare facilities undergo resuscitation efforts.

The benefits derived from aggressive technological management often outweigh the negative effects, but the use of life-sustaining technologies for persons with severely impaired quality of life, or for those who are terminally ill, has stimulated intensive debate and litigation. Two key issues in this debate are the appropriate use of technology and the ability of the seriously ill person to retain decision-making rights. These issues are based on the ethical principles of beneficence and autonomy.

At the heart of the technology controversy are conflicting beliefs about the morality and legality of allowing persons who are terminally ill or severely debilitated to request the withdrawal or withholding of medical treatment. In these situations, two levels of treatment must be considered: ordinary care and extraordinary care. These levels of care are at two ends of a continuum of potential treatment options. Based on one's beliefs, some therapies fit either category; however, this distinction is still helpful from a legal and ethical perspective. Ordinary care means, in the patient's judgment, the treatment or intervention provides a reasonable hope of benefit and does not place undue burden or expense on the patient, family, or community. Extraordinary care includes those interventions, in the patient's judgment, that do not offer reasonable hope of benefit and are burdensome or expensive to the patient, family, or community.[17]

TABLE 3.1 **Landmark Legal Cases in the Right-to-Die Debate**

Case	Events	Impact
Karen Quinlan	Karen Ann Quinlan was the first modern icon of the right-to-die debate. The 21-year-old Quinlan collapsed at a party after swallowing alcohol and the tranquilizer diazepam (Valium) on April 14, 1975. Doctors saved her life, but she suffered brain damage and lapsed into a "persistent vegetative state." Her family waged a much-publicized legal battle for the right to remove her life-support machinery. They succeeded, but in a final twist, Quinlan kept breathing after the respirator was unplugged. She remained in a coma for almost 10 years in a New Jersey nursing home until her death in 1985.	In finding for the Quinlan family, the courts identified a right to decline life-saving medical treatment under the general right of privacy. According to the court, Quinlan's right to privacy outweighed the state's interest in preserving her life, and her father, as her surrogate, could exercise that right for her.
Nancy Cruzan	Nancy Cruzan became a public figure after a 1983 auto accident left her permanently unconscious and without any higher brain function. She was kept alive only by a feeding tube and steady medical care. Cruzan's family waged a legal battle to have her feeding tube removed. The case went all the way to the U.S. Supreme Court, which ruled that the Cruzans had not provided "clear and convincing evidence" that Nancy Cruzan did not wish to have her life artificially preserved. The Cruzans later presented such evidence to the Missouri courts, which ruled in their favor in late 1990. The Cruzans stopped feeding Nancy in December 1990, and she died later the same month.	The Cruzan case had a significant effect on end-of-life decision-making across the country. After the Cruzan decision, the Patient Self-Determination Act was passed by Congress to allow individuals to make their own decisions about end-of-life care and routine care, should they be unable to make decisions for themselves. The case prompted the development of hospital ethics councils and increased the number of advance directives.
Theresa Schiavo	Theresa Marie "Terri" Schiavo was a Florida woman who sustained brain damage and became dependent on a feeding tube. She collapsed in her home in 1990 and experienced respiratory and cardiac arrest, leading to 15 years of institutionalization and a diagnosis of persistent vegetative state. In 1998 her husband, who was her guardian, petitioned the court to remove her feeding tube. Terri Schiavo's parents opposed the removal, arguing that Terri was conscious. The court determined that Terri would not wish to continue life-prolonging measures. Subsequently a 7-year battle occurred that included involvement by politicians and advocacy groups. Before the court's decision was carried out on March 18, 2005, the Florida legislature and the United States Congress had passed laws to prevent removal of Schiavo's feeding tube. These laws were later overturned by the Supreme Courts of Florida and the United States. On March 31, 2005, after a complex legal history in the courts, Terri Schiavo died at a Florida hospice at the age of 41.	This case received national and international media attention with public debate regarding the moral consequences of withdrawing life support. The movement to challenge the decisions made for Schiavo threatened to destabilize end-of-life law that had developed principally through the cases of Quinlan and Cruzan. Although the Schiavo case had little effect on right-to-die jurisprudence, it illustrated the range of difficulties that can complicate decision-making concerning the termination of treatment in incapacitated persons and the importance of having written advance directives.

Traditionally, extraordinary care includes complex, invasive, and experimental treatments such as resuscitation efforts by CPR or emergency cardiac care, maintenance of life support through invasive means, or renal dialysis. Experimental treatments such as gene therapy are also extraordinary therapies.

Ordinary care involves common, noninvasive, tested treatments such as providing nutrition, hydration, or antibiotic therapy. The noninvasive criterion in the critical care setting does not apply; *ordinary care* is defined as usual and customary for the patient's condition. Maintaining hydration and nutrition through tube feeding is an example of a treatment that falls between ordinary and extraordinary care and is a debatable issue. Therefore, it is important for individuals to document their wishes rather than rely on healthcare team members to assist in the decision-making process related to nutrition and hydration.

The concept of non-beneficial medical treatment is moving to the forefront of the end-of-life debate. Judgment regarding non-beneficial medical treatment in the critical care setting is difficult because it differs greatly among cultures and disciplines. Each goal is then evaluated based on what is achievable or deemed "non-beneficial". The debate over the benefit of specific treatments is essentially a debate on the quality of life and which treatments are worthwhile to assist patients in achieving their goals. The cost of health care and the push toward major healthcare reform is generating public discussion regarding the financial effect of medical treatments at the end-of-life. Discussion on the economics of treatments is as uncomfortable in the United States as is talking about death. This topic has not played a major role in end-of-life decision-making in the past, but experts agree it is becoming more commonly discussed in medical debates.[18]

Cardiopulmonary Resuscitation Decisions. The goals of resuscitation are to preserve life, restore health, relieve suffering, limit disability, and respect the individual's decision, rights, and privacy.[19] Frequently, ethical questions arise about the use of CPR and emergency cardiac care, because such treatment may conflict with a patient's desires or best interests. The critical care nurse should be guided by scientifically proven data, patient preferences, and ethical and cultural norms.

The American Heart Association has developed guidelines to assist practitioners in making the difficult decision to provide or withhold emergency cardiovascular care.[19] The generally accepted position is that resuscitation should cease if the provider determines that efforts are non-beneficial or hopeless. Non-beneficial care constitutes sufficient reason for either withholding or ceasing extraordinary treatments.

TABLE 3.2 Definitions in Critical Care Decision-Making

Concept	Definition
Advance directive	Witnessed written document or oral statement in which instructions are given by a person to express desires related to healthcare decisions. The directive may include, but is not limited to, the designation of a healthcare surrogate, a living will, or an anatomical gift.
Living will	A witnessed written document or oral statement voluntarily executed by a person that expresses the person's instructions concerning life-prolonging procedures.
Medical power of attorney	A patient's legal agent/surrogate whom they trust, such as a family member or friend, to make decisions on their behalf should they become incapacitated.
Healthcare decision	Informed consent, refusal of consent, or withdrawal of consent for health care, unless stated in the advance directive.
Incapacity or incompetent decision	Patient is physically or mentally unable to communicate a willful and knowing healthcare decision.
Informed consent	Consent voluntarily given after a sufficient explanation and disclosure of information.
Proxy	A competent adult who has not been expressly designated to make healthcare decisions for an incapacitated person but is authorized by state statute to make healthcare decisions for the person.
Surrogate	A competent adult designated by a person to make healthcare decisions should that person become incapacitated.
Terminal condition	A condition in which there is no reasonable medical probability of recovery and that can be expected to cause death without treatment.
Persistent vegetative state	A permanent, irreversible unconsciousness condition that demonstrates an absence of voluntary action or cognitive behavior or an inability to communicate or interact purposefully with the environment.
Brain death	Complete and irreversible cessation of brain function.
Clinical death or cardiac death	Irreversible cessation of spontaneous ventilation and circulation.
Life-prolonging procedure	Any medical procedure or treatment, including sustenance and hydration, that sustains, restores, or supplants a spontaneous vital function. Does not include the administration of medications or treatments deemed necessary to provide comfort care or to alleviate pain.
Resuscitation	Intervention with the intent of preserving life, restoring health, or reversing clinical death.
Do not resuscitate (DNR) order	A medical order that prohibits the use of cardiopulmonary resuscitation and emergency cardiac care to reverse signs of clinical death. The DNR order may or may not be specified in patients' advance directives.
Allow natural death	An alternate term with less negative connotations but essentially meaning DNR.
Portable Medical Orders (POLST)	The POLST form is a medical order indicating a patient's wishes regarding treatments that are commonly used in a medical crisis. The POLST complements the advance directive; it is not intended to replace it.

Adapted from The Florida Senate. 2022 Florida Statutes, 765.101. http://www.flsenate.gov/Laws/Statutes/.

Withholding or stopping extraordinary resuscitation efforts is ethically and legally appropriate if patients or surrogates have previously made their preferences known through *advance directives*. It is also acceptable if the provider determines that resuscitation is non-beneficial or has discussed the situation with the patient, family, or surrogate as appropriate and there is the mutual agreement not to resuscitate in the event of cardiopulmonary arrest. For the nurse not to initiate the resuscitation, a *do not resuscitate* (DNR) or "*allow a natural death*" order must be written. Most providers also write supporting documentation regarding the order in the progress notes, such as conversations held with the patient and family members. Additional information is provided in Chapter 4, Palliative and End-of-Life Care.

Family presence during resuscitation and invasive procedures has been a debated topic for the last decade. There is growing evidence that family presence during resuscitation and invasive procedures helps not only families but also the healthcare team.[20] Family presence during resuscitation and invasive procedures is supported by professional organizations, including the Emergency Nurses Association, AACN, and the American Heart Association. Current recommendations are for institutions to establish a process for allowing families who wish to be present to do so. This includes designating a trained clinician or chaplain to support the family throughout the process.

Withholding or Withdrawing Life Support. Withholding life support, withdrawing life support, or both can range from not initiating hemodialysis (withholding) to terminal weaning from mechanical ventilation (withdrawing). Decisions are made based on consideration of all factors in the ethical decision-making model. In all instances of withholding and withdrawing life support, comfort measures are maintained, including management of pain, pulmonary secretions, and other symptoms, as needed.

Most decisions regarding withdrawing and withholding life support are not made in the courts. They are made based on open communication with the patient, family, and surrogate, as appropriate. An ethical decision-making approach is used to decide the best actions to take or not take in the situation. If ethical or legal questions arise, ethics consultation services, ethics committees, and risk managers can provide assistance. The value of clearly stating in writing one's end-of-life issues before becoming critically ill (advance directive) is key to avoiding having treatment given or not given against one's wishes. Equally important is the appointment of a Medical Power of Attorney (MPOA) who knows the patient's wishes, values, and preferences and can make informed end-of-life decisions when the patient cannot (see more discussion in next section).

End-of-Life Issues

Patient Self-Determination Act. In response to public concern about end-of-life decisions and the overall lack of consistent hospital policies, the United States Congress enacted the Patient Self-Determination Act.[21] This Act requires that all healthcare facilities that receive Medicare and Medicaid funding inform their patients about their right to initiate an advance directive and the right to consent to or refuse medical treatment.

Discussions regarding advance directives and end-of-life wishes should be made as early as possible, preferably before death is imminent. The ideal time to discuss advance directives is when a person is relatively healthy, not in the critical care or hospital setting. This allows more time for discussion, processing, and decision-making. Assess patients regarding their perceptions of quality of life and end-of-life wishes in a caring and culturally sensitive way and document the patient's wishes in the medical record. Encourage patients to complete advance directives, including living wills and MPOA, to ensure their wishes will be followed if they are terminally ill or in a persistent vegetative state.

Advance Directives. An *advance directive* is a communication that specifies a person's preference about medical treatment should that person become incapacitated. Several types of advance directives exist, including DNR and allow natural death orders, living wills, healthcare proxies, and other legal documents (Table 3.2). It is important for nurses to know whether a patient has an advance directive and that the directive be followed. To enhance advance directives and ensure common conversation and language, the Portable Medical Orders, more commonly referred to as POLST, have been promoted in many states. The POLST form is a medical order indicating a patient's wishes regarding treatments that are commonly used in a medical crisis. The POLST complements the advance directive and is not intended to replace it. The goal of the POLST is a conversation with an emphasis on advanced care planning, shared decision-making, and ensuring a patient's end-of-life wishes are honored. Not all states participate in the POLST initiative. More information can be found in Chapter 4, Palliative and End-of-Life Care, and at http://www.POLST.org.

The *living will* provides a mechanism by which individuals can authorize the withholding of specific treatments if they become incapacitated. Although living wills provide direction to caregivers, in some states, living wills are not legally binding and are considered advisory. When completing a living will, individuals can add special instructions about end-of-life wishes. Individuals can change their directive at any time.

The MPOA is more protective of patients' interests regarding medical treatment than is the living will. With an MPOA, patients legally designate an agent whom they trust, such as a family member or friend, to make decisions on their behalf should they become incapacitated. The designated person is called the *healthcare surrogate* or proxy. An MPOA allows the surrogate to make decisions whenever the patient is incapacitated, not just at the time of terminal illness. Some legal commentators recommend the joint use of a living will and an MPOA for health care to give added protection to a person's preferences about medical treatment.

Ultimately, if self-determination and informed consent are to have real value, patients or their surrogates must be given an opportunity to consider options and to shape decisions that affect their life or death. Communication and shared decision-making among the patient, family, and healthcare team regarding end-of-life issues are key. Unfortunately, this frequently does not happen before admission to a critical care unit. The critical care nurse must be part of the team that educates the patient and family so they can determine and communicate end-of-life wishes.

Some situations may result in moral distress for the nurse. A nurse who is unable to follow these legal documents because of personal or religious beliefs should request to have the patient reassigned to another nurse. For instance, some advance directives may call for withdrawing life support when certain conditions are met, and this may conflict with the nurse's personal or religious beliefs. Nurses who frequently ask to be reassigned to another patient may need to consider another nursing specialty in which their beliefs do not conflict with advance directives.

The nurse must also be cognizant of the facility's policies regarding advance directives. For example, if a DNR order is on the chart, does it meet all requirements for a legal document per facility policy? Is it signed by the provider? Is the chart notated properly? Is there a healthcare proxy? Are the forms proper? Is there a living will? Is there an identified MPOA? All critical care nurses should review key policies and documents related to DNR and withdrawing and withholding life support, because these situations occur frequently, often during times of crisis decision-making when there is not time to become familiar with policy. Knowledge of institutional policies will facilitate honoring the patients' and families' wishes in a compassionate and caring environment.

Medical Aid in Dying. *Medical aid in dying* (MAiD) is a term used to describe allowing qualified terminally ill patients who have the capacity to make decisions to take a lethal dose of oral medication to end their own lives.[22] Provider-assisted suicide, death with dignity, and assisted death are other terms used to refer to competent patients intentionally choosing the time and circumstances of their death. As of 2023, MAiD is legal in 10 US states and the District of Columbia. Critical care nurses must know the intricacies of the nurse's role in MAiD and differentiate this from the removal of non-beneficial treatments. The key difference between the withdrawal of non-beneficial treatments and MAiD is that MAiD is intended to cause death, whereas withdrawal of non-beneficial treatments and the accompanying sedation are intended to relieve suffering and to allow natural death. It is within the scope of practice for critical care nurses to administer medications to terminally ill patients (or authorized surrogates) who have chosen compassionate extubation. Titrating pain medications and sedatives to ease suffering during removal of the endotracheal tube is not considered euthanasia if the patient stops breathing and is considered ethical and legal in that context. This is an example of the doctrine of double effect, which states that if a planned action has a known, negative adverse effect, it is ethical to act as long as the adverse effect is not the intended goal of the planned action.[23] Administering medications in this context is different from MAiD.

In states where MAiD is legal, the patient must have decision-making capacity and must initiate the process of MAiD. The surrogate is not authorized to make the decision on the patient's behalf, and the nurse cannot administer the prescribed medications with the intent to expedite death. The patient must prepare and self-administer the lethal medications. The ANA adopted a position paper that advocates against nurse involvement in MAiD, citing that these practices are in direct conflict with the Code of Ethics.[24] It is illegal and outside the scope of practice for a nurse to administer medications with the intent to hasten death. Critical care nurses in states where MAiD is legal should be well informed of the state laws and organization's policies in anticipation of patients asking questions about MAiD. Healthcare providers may not start conversations about MAiD and may only respond to questions if the terminally ill patient requests information.

CHECK YOUR UNDERSTANDING

4. The family of a patient who is at the end-of-life has requested pain medication because the patient is grimacing and appears to be in pain. The patient has a do not resuscitate (DNR) status. The nurse assesses the patient and notes the grimacing and an increased heart rate. The patient has orders for IV pain medication, but the nurse is concerned that the medication may affect the patient's breathing and hasten death. What is the appropriate action to take?
   A. Hold the medication and inform the patient's family that giving pain medication can lead to the patient's death and that this would be considered euthanasia.
   B. Inform the patient's family that the patient most likely cannot feel pain because the patient is so close to death.
   C. The patient is suffering; administer the IV pain medication to hasten death.
   D. Administer the IV pain medication as ordered, with the intent to relieve pain.

Ethical Concerns Surrounding Organ and Tissue Transplantation

Organ and tissue transplantation involves numerous and complex ethical issues. The first consideration is given to the rights and privileges of all moral agents involved: the donor, the recipient, the family or surrogate, and all other recipients and donors. Three of the most controversial issues in transplantation are the moral value that should be placed on the human body part, the just distribution of a human body part, and the complex problems inherent in applying the concept of brain death to clinical situations. Additional information on organ donation and transplantation is provided in Chapter 5, Organ Donation.

Ethical Challenges for Nurses in a Disaster or Pandemic

Healthcare events such as natural disasters, mass casualties, and pandemics disrupt the standard of care and pose additional ethical challenges for critical care nurses. Healthcare systems plan for disasters; however, these plans cannot prevent the ethical dilemmas and moral distress that can ensue with events of this enormity. Critical care nurses should familiarize themselves with the ethical foundations for shifting standards of care in these situations to prepare themselves to navigate these challenging times. Three overarching ethical issues during these events include the safety of nurses, patients, colleagues, and families; the allocation of scarce resources; and the changing nature of nurses' relationships with patients and families.[25]

The extraordinary challenges of events such as the coronavirus disease (COVID-19) global pandemic place a tremendous strain on nurses to uphold their ethical obligations to patients, families, and society. Challenges related to the COVID-19 pandemic included scarcity of resources, such as personal protective equipment (PPE), limited family visitation, the potential to ration scarce resources, and severe staffing shortages. The loss of life experienced due to the pandemic compounded by these situations took a toll on the mental health of nurses and exacerbated burnout. The full impact of the pandemic on the nursing workforce is not fully understood yet; however, over half of nurses surveyed indicated they intended to leave or were considering leaving their jobs.[26] The situations that nurses experienced during the pandemic led to an increased awareness of the need for nurses to prioritize self-care practices.

NURSING SELF-CARE

Practices and Resources to Support Resiliency

- Pay attention to your body's signals and care for yourself by taking breaks, eating healthy food, stretching and exercising, and getting quality sleep.
- Include a moment of gratitude on a daily basis and at the beginning of each shift.
- Attend critical incident stress debriefings with your co-workers to address ethical dilemmas or moral distress.
- Engage in activities to build resilience such as journaling and mindfulness.
- Take breaks at work to allow a moment to decompress, especially during challenging shifts.
- Maintain regular exercise.
- Take advantage of available organizational resources, such as the hospital's employee assistance program, ethics committee, and chaplains.
- Learn simple mindfulness exercises that can be used at work and home.
- Do not ignore your feelings and emotions; talk with someone you trust.

Helpful Resources

- American Nurses Association: Resources on self-care and promoting mental health and emotional wellbeing.
  - https://www.healthynursehealthynation.org
- American Association of Critical Care Nurses: Access to a well-being initiative that has a free digital toolkit and virtual support system.
  - https://www.aacn.org/nursing-excellence/well-being-initiative
- National Suicide Prevention Lifeline: This resource is available around the clock by phone at **1-800-273-8255 or "988."**
  - https://988lifeline.org/current-events/the-lifeline-and-988/

Data from Webster L, Wocial LD. Ethics in a pandemic: nurses need to engage in self-care to reduce moral distress. American Nurse Journal. 2020;15(9):18+. https://link.gale.com/apps/doc/A658341793/AONE?u=orla57816&sid=bookmark-AONE&xid=3dff0189[27]; Liu JJW, Ein N, Gervasio J, Battaion M, Reed M, Vickers K. Comprehensive meta-analysis of resilience interventions. *Clin Psychol Rev.* 2020;82:101919. https://doi.org/10.1016/j.cpr.2020.101919.[28]

One specific example of an issue that arose during the recent COVID-19 pandemic was related to vaccinations. The availability of a COVID-19 vaccination with robust efficacy and safety data provided widespread optimism for many clinicians. However, many clinicians experienced frustration and anger when unvaccinated patients or individuals against vaccination presented to the critical care units; they viewed vaccine refusal as an affront to the nurses' hard work and sacrifices. Vaccine refusal is a complex issue that can be affected by multiple factors. Socioeconomic vulnerability, structural racism, and other social determinants of health are some of the factors that influence the vaccination status and beliefs of individuals.[29]

The ANA Code of Ethics can be a resource to help nurses decrease moral distress when they feel compromised due to the inability to practice according to professional values and standards. While the first provision calls on the nurse to practice compassion and respect for every person's inherent dignity, worth, and unique attributes, during disasters and pandemics, nurses shift their focus to an outcome-based framework promoting community and world health (Provision 8). Nurses should take actions that support strategies to avoid entering crisis standards of care; however if the crisis is unavoidable, nurses must work fairly to save the most significant number of lives possible. Provisions 8 and 9 of the Code of Ethics calls on nurses to take a leadership role in public health issues and to collaborate with other health professionals to address health disparities and unjust structures.[1]

CLINICAL JUDGMENT ACTIVITY

Two patients positive for COVID-19 with respiratory failure potentially require mechanical ventilation in the emergency department while waiting on admission to the critical care unit. Only one bed is available, and the unit is short-staffed, requiring the registered nurses to be assigned to more patients than the typical patient load. A nurse is overheard commenting that one of the two patients in the emergency department with COVID-19 has not been vaccinated. What is the critical care nurse's responsibility in caring for individuals who refuse vaccinations that have been demonstrated to be effective in reducing morbidity and mortality? How does the ANA Nursing Code of Ethics provide guidance for the nurse?

Due to their unique relationship with patients and families in vulnerable situations, critical care nurses are frequently confronted with ethical and legal dilemmas. It is imperative that critical care nurses stay abreast of the bioethical and legal issues that may occur in their practice. When nurses apply ethical principles and decision-making processes and utilize available resources to address these dilemmas, they can foster and support optimal outcomes.

CASE STUDY

Mr. W. is a 67-year-old patient in the coronary care unit who has severe heart failure and chronic obstructive pulmonary disease. Mr. W. has been in and out of the hospital for 3 years, requires oxygen therapy at night, and often sleeps in a reclining chair to help with breathing and comfort. He has severe, chronic chest pain, dyspnea, and fatigue. He told his family that he was so tired of being sick and has no joy in life because of his illness. He had a respiratory arrest and was put on the ventilator last night. He awakens after the resuscitation and communicates that he wants the breathing tube to be removed and that he be allowed to die. He is tired of the pain, dyspnea, and overall lack of quality of life. He asks for medication to make him comfortable after the tube is removed. His family agrees with the plan of care.

Mr. W.'s wishes are followed. He is extubated and is given morphine for comfort. Mr. W.'s family members all remain at the bedside, taking turns holding his hand and talking to him.

Questions

1. Apply the ethical decision-making model discussed in this chapter to this case. What are the relevant ethical principles? Are there other areas that must be assessed before proceeding?
2. As the critical care nurse caring for Mr. W., what are your priorities at this point? On what ethical principles are these priorities based?
3. Suppose that you have strong religious beliefs about withdrawal of life support. If you were assigned to Mr. W., what actions should you take?
4. How would an advanced directive assisted Mr. W and his family prior to the patient being intubated? Discuss the benefits of advanced directive for individuals with chronic conditions such as Mr. W.

KEY POINTS

- The Code of Ethics for Nurses, developed by the ANA, establishes ethical standards for nursing professionals.
- In addition to adhering to ethical guidelines from the Code of Ethics, nurses must follow the legal regulations and standards of practice in the state where they practice.
- Ethical dilemmas involve unclear choices that have a range of acceptable options.
- Four frequently used bioethical principles are respect for autonomy, beneficence, nonmaleficence, and justice.
- Nurses must recognize ethical and legal dilemmas in the critical care setting, advocate for patients and families, and activate available resources, as necessary.

REFERENCES

1. American Nurses Association. *Code of Ethics for Nurses with Interpretive Statements*. Silver Spring, MD: American Nurses Association; 2015.
2. Fowler M. *Guide to the Code of Ethics for Nurses: Development, Application and Interpretation*. 2nd ed. Silver Spring, MD: American Nurses Association; 2015.
3. Rainer J, Schneider JK, Lorenz RA. Ethical dilemmas in nursing: an integrative review. *J Clin Nurs*. 2018;27(19–20):3446–3461.
4. Beauchamp T, Childress J. *Principles of Biomedical Ethics*. 8th ed. Oxford, England: Oxford University Press; 2019.
5. American Association of Critical-Care Nurses. *AACN Standards for Establishing and Sustaining Healthy Work Environments: A Journey to Excellence*. 2nd ed. Aliso Vieja, CA: American Association of Critical-Care Nurses; 2016.
6. Grady C, Danis M, Soeken KL, et al. Does ethics education influence the moral action of practicing nurses and social workers? *Am J Bioethics*. 2008;8(4):2–14.
7. McAndrew NS, Leske J, Schroeter K. Moral distress in critical care nursing: the state of the science. *Nurs Ethics*. 2018;25(5):552–570.
8. Lamiani G, Borghi L, Argentero P. When health professionals cannot do the right thing: a systematic review of moral distress and its correlates. *J Health Psychol*. 2017;22(1):51–67.
9. Rushton CH. Cultivating moral resilience. *Am J Nursing*. 2017;117(2):S11–S15.
10. Stutzer K, Bylone M. Building moral resilience. *Crit Care Nurs*. 2018;38(1):77–89.
11. Kohn L, Corrigan J, Donaldson S. *To Err Is Human: Building a Safer Health System*. National Academies Press; 2000.
12. Marx DA. *Patient Safety and the "Just Culture": A Primer for Health Care Executives*. New York, NY: Trustees of Columbia University; 2001.
13. American Nurses Association. *Position Statement Just Culture*; 2010. https://www.nursingworld.org/practice-policy/nursing-excellence/official-position-statements/id/just-culture/.
14. Kelman B. *Vanderbilt Nurse RaDonda Vaught Arrested Reckless Homicide Vecuronium Error*; 2022. https://www.tennessean.com/story/news/health/2020/03/03/vanderbilt-nurse-radonda-vaught-arrested-reckless-homicide-vecuronium-error/4826562002/.
15. American Nurses Association. *Statement in Response to Nurse RaDonda Vaught Conviction*; 2022. https://www.nursingworld.org/news/news-releases/2022-news-releases/statement-in-response-to-the-conviction-of-nurse-radonda-vaught/.
16. American Association of Critical-Care Nurses. *Statement on the Conviction of RaDonda Vaught*; 2022. https://www.aacn.org/newsroom/aacns-statement-on-the-conviction-of-radonda-vaught.
17. National Catholic Bioethics Center. *A Catholic Guide to End-Of-Life Decisions*; 2011.
18. Society of Critical Care Medicine. *Critical Care Ethics: A Practice Guide*. United States: Society of Critical Care Medicine; 2014.
19. American Heart Association. American Heart Association 2020 Guidelines for Cardiopulmonary Resuscitation and Emergency Cardiopulmonary Care. https://cpr.heart.org/en/resuscitation-science/cpr-and-ecc-guidelines.
20. Oczkowski SJW, Ian Mazzetti, Cupido C, Fox-Robichaud AE. Family presence during resuscitation: a Canadian critical care society position paper. *Canadian Respiratory Journal*. 2015;22. https://doi.org/10.1155/2015/532721. Article ID 532721, 5 pages.
21. Public law No. 101-508, 4206, 104 stat. 291 the self-determination act amends the social security act's provisions on Medicare and Medicaid. *Social Security Act*. 1927;42(1990). L U.S.C. 1396.
22. Davidson JE, Hooper FG. Aid in dying: the role of the critical care nurse. *AACN Adv Crit Care*. 2017;28(2):218–222.
23. Wholihan D, Olson E. The doctrine of double effect: a review for the bedside nurse providing end-of-life care. *J Hospice Palliative Nurs*. 2017;19(3):205.
24. American Nurses Association. *American Nurses Association Position Statement: The Nurse's Role when a Patient Requests Aid in Dying*; 2019. https://www.nursingworld.org/~49e869/globalassets/practiceandpolicy/nursing-excellence/ana-position-statements/social-causes-and-health-care/the-nurses-role-when-a-patient-requests-medical-aid-in-dying-web-format.pdf.
25. Morley G, Grady C, McCarthy J, Ulrich CM. Covid-19: ethical challenges for nurses. *Hastings Cent Rep*. 2020;50(3):35–39. https://doi.org/10.1002/hast.1110. Epub 2020 May 14. PMID: 32410225. PMCID: PMC7272859.
26. American Nurses Foundation. Pulse on the Nation's Nurses Survey Series: COVID-19 Two-Year Impact Assessment Survey. https://www.nursingworld.org/~492857/contentassets/872ebb13c63f44f6b11a1bd0c74907c9/covid-19-two-year-impact-assessment-written-report-final.pdf.
27. Webster L, Wocial LD. Ethics in a pandemic: nurses need to engage in self-care to reduce moral distress. *American Nurse Journal*. 2020;15(9). 18+, Available at: https://link.gale.com/apps/doc/A658341793/AONE?u=orla57816&sid=bookmark-AONE&xid=3dff0189.
28. Liu JJW, Ein N, Gervasio J, Battaion M, Reed M, Vickers K. Comprehensive meta-analysis of resilience interventions. *Clin Psychol Rev*. 2020;82:101919. https://doi.org/10.1016/j.cpr.2020.101919.
29. Milliken A, Uveges MK. Nurses' ethical obligations toward unvaccinated individuals. *AACN Advanced Critical Care*. 2022;33(2):220–226. https://doi.org/10.4037/aacnacc2022491.

4

Palliative and End-of-Life Care

Laura Baker, MSN, APRN, ACNPC-AG, CCRN

INTRODUCTION

Advances in critical care technology in the past several decades have vastly improved the ability of healthcare providers to care for critically ill patients, at least in terms of survival rates. Interventions such as extracorporeal membrane oxygenation (ECMO) are increasingly used in the sickest patients, saving many lives but prolonging the dying of others.[1] Left ventricular assist devices (LVADs), once only a bridge to heart transplantation, are now used as "destination" therapy for patients with severe heart failure who are not candidates for transplantation.[2] The appropriate use of these invasive and expensive resources is a matter of much debate, leading to complex ethical issues and decision-making in the care of patients with a critical or chronic illness. Admission to critical care units varies significantly by hospital and region for common medical conditions, demonstrating a lack of agreement on the appropriate intensity of care for many critically ill patients. In 2015, the Institute of Medicine published *Dying in America,* a comprehensive review of the current state of the issue with recommendations for improvement. This important study revealed areas of progress, such as significant increases in healthcare providers' education in end-of-life and palliative care. It also identified significant opportunities for improvement, citing fragmentation of care, increasing healthcare costs, and poor translation of end-of-life education to the bedside.[3] These problems affect the millions of Americans who die every year, the vast majority from progression of long-term illness. In 2022, 3,464,231 resident deaths were recorded in the United States.[3a] Of the 10 leading causes of death, many were chronic processes, including heart and respiratory diseases, cancer, Alzheimer's disease, and complications of diabetes and kidney disease.[4] It can be concluded from this data that more Americans are living with chronic disease prior to their deaths and that many could benefit from palliative care. Early identification of patients appropriate to receive palliative care is warranted to ensure patients receive care consistent with their wishes and to avoid suffering from non-beneficial aggressive care interventions. While earlier models of health care may have suggested adding palliative care once the dying process has begun, newer research and guidelines encourage palliative care concurrent with the active treatment of chronic illness.[5,6]

CRITICAL CARE AT THE END-OF-LIFE

The landmark Study to Understand Prognoses and Preferences for Outcomes and Risks of Treatment (SUPPORT) revealed many disparities between patients' care preferences and actual care received. The most significant findings from the study included a lack of clear communication between patients and healthcare providers, frequent aggressive care, and widespread pain and suffering among inpatients.[7]

Because of the findings from SUPPORT and similar studies, critical care utilization in the final days of life has become an important research focus. When evaluating patients in their last year of life, those admitted to critical care are often older, have multiple comorbidities and generate significantly higher costs when compared to those not admitted to critical care.[8] In addition, patients with chronic conditions are often admitted to critical care for the management of distress symptoms related to their disease process (e.g., dyspnea, pain).[9] Though strides have been made, evidence demonstrates the need for improved communication between healthcare providers and patients regarding disease progression and advanced care planning. Increased national attention on dying in critical care units has stimulated funding for research and development of care guidelines for the dying patient in the critical care setting. Box 4.1 is a compilation of online nursing and research resources to assist with understanding the complexity of caring for the dying patient.

Continuation of Aggressive Care

A large percentage of deaths in the critical care unit are preceded by decisions to withhold or withdraw aggressive support. The percentages vary based on patient population, culture, and unit type.[10,11] Many of these decisions are made by surrogate or proxy decision-makers, because most patients in the critical care unit are unable to make decisions about their own care[12] (see Chapter 3, Ethical and Legal Issues in Critical Care Nursing). Patients, surrogates, and proxies faced with difficult decisions in the critical

BOX 4.1 End-of-Life Online Resources

- Ariadne Labs' Serious Illness Conversation Guide: https://www.ariadnelabs.org/wp-content/uploads/2017/05/SI-CG-2017-04-21_FINAL.pdf
- American Association of Critical-Care Nurses: https://www.aacn.org/clinical-resources/palliative-end-of-life
- Center to Advance Palliative Care: https://www.capc.org/toolkits/integrating-palliative-care-practices-in-the-icu/
- Institute of Medicine, *Dying in America: Improving Quality and Honoring Individual Preferences Near the End-of-Life:* https://nap.nationalacademies.org/catalog/18748/dying-in-america-improving-quality-and-honoring-individual-preferences-near
- National Hospice and Palliative Care Organization: http://www.nhpco.org
- National Library of Medicine: http://www.nlm.nih.gov/medlineplus/endoflifeissues.html
- Northwestern University, Education in Palliative and End-of-life Care Program: https://www.bioethics.northwestern.edu/education/epec.html
- University of Washington, End-of-Life Care Research Program: http://depts.washington.edu/eolcare/
- VitalTalk: https://www.vitaltalk.org/
- 3 Wishes Project: https://3wishesproject.com/

care setting are often experiencing forms of anticipatory grief, depression, and anxiety. As a result, medical information infused with medical jargon may be difficult to comprehend, and decision-making can become impaired.[13–15] Multiple factors influence the continuation of aggressive care in the face of a poor prognosis, including provider differences, provider comfort with difficult conversations, and patient and family beliefs.[16–19] The failure of clinicians, family members, and patients to discuss prognosis, end-of-life issues, and preferences openly and honestly is one of the most significant factors preventing early identification of patients who are unlikely to benefit from aggressive care. As patient advocates, nurses can and must play a key role in ensuring that choices are understood and goals of care are clear.[20] The terms *non-beneficial care, inappropriate care,* and *potentially inappropriate care* have largely replaced *futile care,* with the latter term reserved only for interventions that are not achievable. *Non-beneficial care* is defined as care provided to patients that would result in a quality of life the patient would not want or that is inconsistent with the patient's stated goals of care.[21] The term *inappropriate care* is commonly used and refers to critical care unit interventions with no reasonable expectation of achieving patient survival outside the acute care setting or in situations in which the patient's neurological condition is such that the patient cannot perceive the benefits.[22,23] *Potentially inappropriate care* refers to interventions that have at least some chance of the effect sought by the patient, but clinicians believe that competing ethical considerations justify not providing them (i.e., providing dialysis to a patient with permanent anoxic encephalopathy).[24]

CHECK YOUR UNDERSTANDING

1. A nurse receives a change-of-shift report and assesses that the family may be resistant to a palliative care consult to discuss end-of-life decisions. Which of the following observations may be the reason why aggressive medical care is continued for the patient with a poor prognosis who is unlikely to survive?
   A. Religious and/or cultural beliefs.
   B. Financial or payor status.
   C. Open discussion regarding goals of care for the patient.
   D. Clear communication of prognosis by the multiprofessional healthcare team.

In 2015, five major medical and nursing critical care organizations produced a consensus document based on available evidence, providing guidance to clinicians on how to respond to requests for potentially inappropriate treatment in the critical care unit.[24] A simple, valid assessment tool does not yet exist to accurately predict or determine when an intervention is unlikely to achieve its desired goal, further contributing to conflict at the end-of-life. The identification of the dying patient is often subjective and based on the healthcare providers' opinions and interpretations of diagnostic results and the patient's response to treatment.[25] This makes the determination of the appropriate intensity of care for patients near the end-of-life extremely difficult. While there is no absolute predictor on when and how a patient will die, certain patient characteristics and diagnostic findings have been correlated to an increased likelihood of poor long-term outcomes. These predictors (i.e., critical diagnoses [e.g., cancer; congestive heart failure; chronic lung, renal, or heart disease; stroke], low albumin at admission, length of stay greater than 5 days, multiple organ failure, baseline dementia, residence in a nursing home prior to admission) are important to identify so palliative care services can appropriately be consulted to facilitate goals of care discussions.[26]

Societal values and those of healthcare providers also play a significant role in how end-of-life care in the United States is provided. These values often include a commonly held belief that patients die of distinct illnesses, which implies that such illnesses are potentially curable. Dying is often viewed as failure on the part of the system or providers. The purpose of the healthcare system in the United States is to treat illness, disease, and injury, and this "life-saving" culture often continues to drive aggressive care even when it becomes obvious that the ultimate outcome will be the death of the individual.[3] Fortunately, significant progress has been made in the medical-legal arena in establishing the rights of patients and surrogates to decide for themselves the intensity and duration of care.[27]

CLINICAL JUDGMENT ACTIVITY

The nurse assesses that there is significant disagreement among family members about what course of treatment is best for the patient. What action would be most effective in improving the situation?

Effects on Nurses and the Healthcare Team

Many clinicians experience personal ethical conflicts when providing interventions and aggressive treatment they perceive to be non-beneficial or inappropriate to patients, causing significant moral distress that can lead to burnout.[28–30] Care choices made by patients, surrogates or proxies often differ from those that clinicians might make personally, causing further strain in remaining nonjudgmental in such situations. Recurrent moral distress is often cited as the cause for leaving the profession and a significant cause of job dissatisfaction and stress.[31] Though moral distress is most common and studied among nurses, it is reported in providers and other healthcare providers as well.[32] Interventions to alleviate moral distress through the development of moral resilience include self-care, mindfulness, seeking support from colleagues, ethics education, clarifying goals of care, organizational support, and striving to accept differing values in our patients and families.[33–35]

Patients' dignity is often compromised during a critical care unit stay,[36] and their preferences and wishes may not be elicited by providers in goals of care conferences.[37] Such situations contradict basic nursing ethical principles, causing further moral distress.[20] At times, healthcare providers do not clearly communicate a poor prognosis to patients or the family members, denying them the ability to make informed decisions.[18,38,39] When life support is withdrawn and patients die, caregivers often experience a sense of loss or grief, especially if the patient's stay was prolonged.[40] Customizing interventions aimed at making meaningful end-of-life memories may assist both the family and the healthcare team with the grieving process.[41] Finding a balance between maintaining a professional, healthy distance and being authentic and humane is a difficult task (see Nursing Self-Care box).

NURSING SELF-CARE

The "Sacred Pause" to Prevent Burnout

- Given the frequent exposure to death, critical care nurses are at high risk for burnout if not provided strategies to mitigate the accumulating grief.
- The "Sacred Pause" is an intervention that aims to honor the deceased, recognize the healthcare team, and reduce the risk of burnout.
- The intervention can be initiated by any member of the healthcare team after a death or code event:
  - First, the patient is recognized, and the team is thanked for their efforts.
  - A 45 seconds to 1 minute pause then occurs.
  - After the pause, the team thanks each other and the family, then returns to their work.
- Potential impacts of implementing the "Sacred Pause" are as follows:
  - Bringing closure and helping overcome feelings of grief, disappointment, distress, and failure.
  - Creating feelings of appreciation for the healthcare team's efforts.
  - Instilling and encouraging a sense of teamwork.

Data from Bartels JB. The pause. *Crit Care Nurse.* 2014;34(1):74-75. https://doi.org/10.4037/ccn2014962; Kapoor S, Morgan CK, Siddique MA, Guntupalli KK. "Sacred Pause" in the ICU: evaluation of a ritual and intervention to lower distress and burnout. *Am J Hosp Palliat Care.* 2018;35(10):1337-1341. https://doi.org/10.1177/1049909118768247.

CLINICAL JUDGMENT ACTIVITY

When educating a family about the process of withdrawal of life support, such as mechanical ventilation, the nurse must convey what concepts?

DIMENSIONS OF END-OF-LIFE CARE

Critical care nursing at the end-of-life focuses on five dimensions: (1) alleviation of distressing symptoms (palliative care); (2) communication and conflict resolution; (3) withholding, limiting, or withdrawing therapy; (4) emotional and psychological care of the patient and family; and (5) caregiver organizational support.

Palliative Care

Palliative care, or *palliation,* is the provision of care interventions that are designed to relieve symptoms of illness or injury that negatively affect the quality of life. Common distressing symptoms that may occur with multiple disease states include pain, anxiety, hunger, thirst, dyspnea, increased secretions, diarrhea, nausea, confusion, agitation, and disturbance in sleep patterns.[42,43] The critical care environment tends to exacerbate these symptoms by adding devices (i.e., mechanical ventilation, mechanical circulatory support), by altering sensory stimulation, and through the development of complications associated with both acute and chronic disease processes.[44] Distressing symptoms are common among patients in the critical care unit, and every effort should be made to identify and aggressively treat those symptoms.

Pain management is a major focus of palliative care and begins with proper identification; therefore, frequent nursing assessment is necessary. When assessing pain, the nurse must consider that the expression of pain varies based on individual characteristics. Additionally, throughout the stages of dying, different pain scales may need to be used depending on the patient's ability to communicate.[45] Different nonpharmacological and pharmacological approaches may be necessary to ensure proper pain management. The various pain scales, as well as the medications used to control pain and reduce agitation in the critically ill patient, are discussed in Chapter 6, Comfort and Sedation. When available, complementary and alternative medicine choices can be used with or without traditional treatment regimens to target symptoms such as pain, agitation, anxiety, dyspnea, fatigue, insomnia, nausea, and vomiting. Complementary and alternative medicine is especially helpful when fear of side effects such as increased somnolence is limiting pharmacological management. While generally not curative for symptoms, options such as music, art, acupuncture, acupressure, aromatherapy, Reiki, meditation, and massage therapy can be utilized; research is ongoing in this field.[46,47]

Palliative care is often confused with hospice care, which is reserved for the terminally ill. Palliative care is *not* a substitute for aggressive, life-saving care but rather a complementary supplement to care. In contrast, hospice care is generally reserved for those with a prognosis of 6 months or less to live and is usually *in place of* aggressive life-sustaining or restorative care.[48] There is growing consensus that palliative care should be an integral part of every ill or injured patient's care and should not be reserved only for the dying patient.[49,50] Relief of distressing symptoms should always be provided whenever possible, even when the primary focus of care is life-saving or aggressive treatment. An important part of palliative care consists of "simple" nursing interventions such as frequent repositioning, good hygiene and skin care, and creation of a peaceful environment to the extent possible in the critical care setting. Nurses complete frequent assessments and spend the most time with the patient; therefore, the nurse is the most powerful advocate for appropriate symptom management.

Involving palliative care clinicians in plan of care development avoids critical care unit admissions, reduces length of stay, and decreases healthcare costs for patients with serious or chronic illnesses.[51–53] Additional benefits include improved communication with patients and families, as well as a reduction in distressing symptoms.[54,55] Palliative care may be provided through a consultative model or via an integrative approach, in which palliative care principles are integrated into the daily practice of the multiprofessional team (see Evidence-Based Practice box).

EVIDENCE-BASED PRACTICE

Palliative Care Interventions for Critically Ill Patients

Problem

Integration of palliative care into critical care is advocated to facilitate earlier symptom management, improve communication, identify patient/family goals for care, provide family support and improve end-of-life care. While palliative care services and interventions are advocated in critical care practice settings, the most effective interventions, optimal delivery model, and appropriate outcome measures are unclear.

Clinical Question

In the care of adult patients, which palliative care interventions are most frequently used and what is the impact on outcomes of different palliative care approaches across different countries?

Evidence

PubMed, Embase, Cochrane, CINAHL, and PsycINFO databases were searched using key term variations of "palliative care" and "intensive care" and included randomized controlled trials and observational studies published up to August 2020. A total of 9 randomized trials and 49 cohort studies were included in the systematic review. The methodological quality of the studies varied significantly. Five distinct interventions were identified: (1) communication (24.6%), which involved structured family conferences and informational brochures; (2) ethics consultations (8.8%); (3) education (31.6%), such as didactic sessions, professional development for healthcare clinicians, and simulation; (4) involvement of a palliative care team (49.1%) included screening critical care patients for needs, participating in family conferences, or involvement in multiprofessional rounds; and (5) advanced care planning or goals-of-care discussions (12.3%). Both an integrative model, used in 51.7% of the studies, and a consultative approach, used in 48.5% of the studies, were associated with enhanced palliative care involvement. While functional outcomes for patients were rarely reported, engagement of palliative care service outcomes positively impacted length of stay, decisions around life-sustaining treatments, resuscitation goals, and family communication.

Implications for Nursing

The effectiveness of specific palliative care interventions remains poorly understood, as there are many variations to the most common interventions, delivery modes, and outcomes assessed. However, the most commonly studied intervention was involvement of a palliative care team to assist and support the critical care team in identifying goals of care, facilitating family conferences, or developing palliative care triggers for patients with these unique needs. Based on the systematic review, multiprofessional teams, nurses, patients, and families benefited from the support of a palliative care team member. Nurses should advocate for patients and families to involve a palliative care team member when symptom management and end-of-life care is indicated.

Level of Evidence

C – Systematic Review

Reference

Metaxa V, Anagnostou D, Vlachos S et al. Palliative care interventions in intensive care unit patients [published correction appears in *Intensive Care Med.* 2022;48(4):516]. *Intensive Care Med.* 2021;47(12):1415-1425. https://doi.org/10.1007/s00134-021-06544-6.

CHECK YOUR UNDERSTANDING

2. A nurse is educating a new critical care clinician about palliative care. What key concepts are important to convey during this teaching moment?
   A. Aggressive symptom management.
   B. Improving communication among the healthcare team, patient, and family.
   C. Decreasing patient and family anxiety and distress.
   D. All of the above.

Communication and Conflict Resolution

Clear, ongoing, and honest communication among the members of the healthcare team, the patient, and the family (to include the proxy or surrogate, as appropriate) is a key factor in improving the quality of care for the dying patient in the critical care unit.[25] Unfortunately, communication is also incredibly challenging, in part because of the complex nature of predicting prognosis with accuracy in a critically ill person. Significant differences in perception of the patient's prognosis for recovery have been identified among providers, nurses, and families. The most accurate prognostication occurs when providers and nurses work together, emphasizing the need for a multiprofessional team approach.[56] A shared decision-making model with clinicians, patients, and families collaborating to determine patient prognosis and goals of care is recommended by critical care guidelines.[22] A process-based method for resolving disputes among care teams, patients, and their families has been described and is supported by major nursing and critical care societies.[23,57]

Schedule regular conferences with the patient and family to facilitate communication and identify goals of care. During the conference, make the family feel comfortable talking about death and dying issues, focusing on how the patient would likely choose to proceed in the given situation if able to communicate their wishes. Clarify what the family understands and answer any questions, allowing them to talk about the family member's life and medical history. Provide honest information about the patient's prognosis. Discuss goals for palliative care, emphasizing that patient comfort will be maintained. Use skills of effective communication such as reflection, empathy, and silence. Conclude with a plan and follow-up communication.

Several online resources are available for strengthening the communication skills necessary to facilitate difficult, prognostic, and goal-setting discussions (Box 4.1). This is a skillset that many clinicians spend years researching and improving.

Withholding, Limiting, or Withdrawing Therapy

Most deaths in the critical care unit are preceded by some manner of withholding, withdrawing, or limiting medical treatments, with significant variation among different patient populations.[58,59] Decisions to withdraw, withhold, or limit treatment should be made with participation from the multiprofessional team, family, patient, and proxy or surrogate, as applicable, using a shared decision-making model.[22] Appropriate withdrawal, limiting, or withholding of therapy *does not* constitute medical aid in dying (MAiD) or euthanasia. MAiD involves a provider prescribing a lethal dose of a medication at the request of a competent adult with a terminal illness who intends to use the medication to end their life.[60] Euthanasia occurs when an individual intentionally ends a terminally ill patient's life by administering a lethal dose of medication.[61] MAiD is authorized in only ten states plus the District of Columbia.[62] Euthanasia is illegal throughout the United States and most countries. Minimal moral distress on the part of the healthcare team, patients, and families should result if generally accepted ethical and legal principles are followed during the withdrawal, limiting, or withholding of therapy. Moral distress is further alleviated when conversations regarding wishes surrounding end-of-life and decision-making are made prior to critical illness and captured in the form of advance care planning documents.

A growing number of states have endorsed the use of a standardized end-of-life order set for inpatient or outpatient use, known as Portable Medical Orders or POLST. In 2018, the POLST, which stood for Physician Orders for Life-Sustaining Treatment, became recognized as a word on its own. This change was to promote the importance of the entire healthcare team in end-of-life decision-making and to remove the bias from the phrase "life-sustaining" to liken it to a more neutral document. This form is to be completed through mutual agreement between the provider and patient, proxy, or surrogate. The documentation clearly specifies the kind of care the patient prefers at the end-of-life. POLST has become a strong national movement and represents growing public sentiment in support of having control over personal end-of-life care. As of February 2022, five states in the United States have adopted the National POLST form (Fig. 4.1). Other states have created individualized adaptations unique to their territories. A map available on the POLST website (http://www.polst.org) demonstrates which states either use or are actively working to adopt or adapt a version of the national form.[63]

Regardless of the document used, nurses should advocate for family involvement, open communication, and advanced care planning to facilitate realistic goal setting in critical care. During discussions of withholding, limiting, or withdrawing therapy with a patient, their family, proxy, or surrogate, it is important to emphasize that, while *interventions* may be removed (e.g., mechanical ventilation, mechanical circulatory support, inotropic agents), *care* will remain an ever-constant presence, and the support of the healthcare team will remain unchanged.

CHECK YOUR UNDERSTANDING

3. The nurse is reviewing paperwork brought in by the family. POLST is noted within the paperwork. What would be the appropriate next steps if the patient is sedated and intubated without capacity?
   A. Return the forms to the family, as the POLST is not recognized by the hospital.
   B. Review the documents to evaluate for completeness and assess the patient's wishes per the documentation.
   C. Coordinate a family conference with the multiprofessional team to discuss the POLST.
   D. Both B and C.

Withdrawal Preparation. Preparing patients (if conscious) and families for what will likely occur during the transition to comfort measures is key to alleviating anxiety and undue distress. Anticipate patient symptoms, such as dyspnea during ventilator withdrawal or compassionate extubation, and medicate to alleviate such symptoms, even if high doses of medications are required. Assess pain and agitation using validated tools (see Chapter 6, Comfort and Sedation). Assess the patient's response (e.g., comfort) to determine how much medication is appropriate in a given situation, and titrate therapy as needed to relieve emotional and physical distress. Commonly used medication regimens include opioids, typically morphine sulfate, to manage pain or dyspnea and benzodiazepines for agitation or anxiety.[42,43] Pharmacological management of life-support withdrawal is critical in ensuring a peaceful death for both patient and family (Box 4.2). An actively engaged critical care nurse is vital in ensuring patient comfort and dignity during the withdrawal process.

Ventilator Withdrawal. The most withheld or withdrawn medical intervention in the critical care setting is mechanical ventilation, known as *terminal weaning (TW)* or *terminal extubation (TE)*, also referred to as immediate extubation. TW consist of titrating ventilator support to minimal levels, then either removing the ventilator but not the artificial airway or removing both. TE involves removing the artificial airway and mechanical ventilation without weaning ventilatory support. There is controversy between the two methods, and which type of withdrawal is used is driven by the provider, experience, and patient condition. The impact of each method on patient or family experience warrants further study; however, current research indicates there is no difference in the family's psychological welfare between the two methods.[64]

The response to TW and TE can be assessed with a variety of assessment tools, the patient's self-report, or symptoms (see Clinical Alert box). The critical care nurse should be familiar with the policies and procedures specific to their institution when assessing and documenting the response to TW and TE. When the patient is identified as ready for ventilator withdrawal, prepare the family (if present). If the artificial airway is to be removed, attempt to conceal removal under a towel or covering and have suction ready to manage additional secretions. Excellent practice resources for end-of-life care and ventilator withdrawal are available from a variety of resources (Box 4.1).

Hipaa permits disclosure of polst orders to health care providers as necessary for treatment
Send form with patient whenever transferred or discharged

Medical record # (Optional)

National POLST form: A portable medical order

Health care providers should complete this form only after a conversation with their patient or the patient's representative. The POLST decision-making process is for patients who are at risk for a life-threatening clinical event because they have a serious life-limiting medical condition, which may include advanced frailty (www.polst.org/guidance-appropriate-patients-pdf).

Patient information. **Having a POLST form is always voluntary.**

This is a medical order, not an advance directive. For information about POLST and to understand this document, visit: www.polst.org/form

Patient first name: ______

Middle name/Initial: ______ Preferred name: ______

Last name: ______ Suffix (Jr, Sr, etc): ______

DOB (mm/dd/yyyy): ____/____/____ State where form was completed: ______

Gender: ☐ M ☐ F ☐ X Social security number's last 4 digits (optional): xxx-xx-___ ___ ___ ___

A. Cardiopulmonary resuscitation orders. Follow these orders if patient has no pulse and is not breathing.

Pick 1

☐ **YES CPR: Attempt resuscitation, including mechanical ventilation, defibrillation and cardioversion.** (Requires choosing full treatments in Section B)

☐ **NO CPR: Do not attempt resuscitation.** (May choose any option in Section B)

B. Initial treatment orders. Follow these orders if patient has a pulse and/or is breathing.

Reassess and discuss interventions with patient or patient representative regularly to ensure treatments are meeting patient's care goals. Consider a time-trial of interventions based on goals and specific outcomes.

Pick 1

☐ **Full treatments (required if choose CPR in Section A).** Goal: Attempt to sustain life by all medically effective means. Provide appropriate medical and surgical treatments as indicated to attempt to prolong life, including intensive care.

☐ **Selective treatments.** Goal: Attempt to restore function while avoiding intensive care and resuscitation efforts (ventilator, defibrillation and cardioversion). May use non-invasive positive airway pressure, antibiotics and IV fluids as indicated. Avoid intensive care. Transfer to hospital if treatment needs cannot be met in current location.

☐ **Comfort-focused treatments.** Goal: Maximize comfort through symptom management; allow natural death. Use oxygen, suction and manual treatment of airway obstruction as needed for comfort. Avoid treatments listed in full or select treatments unless consistent with comfort goal. Transfer to hospital **only** if comfort cannot be achieved in current setting.

C. Additional orders or instructions. These orders are in addition to those above (e.g., blood products, dialysis).
[EMS protocols may limit emergency responder ability to act on orders in this section.]

D. Medically assisted nutrition (offer food by mouth if desired by patient, safe and tolerated)

Pick 1

☐ Provide feeding through new or existing surgically-placed tubes
☐ No artificial means of nutrition desired
☐ Trial period for artificial nutrition but no surgically-placed tubes
☐ Not discussed or no decision made (provide standard of care)

E. SIGNATURE: Patient or patient representative (eSigned documents are valid)

I understand this form is voluntary. I have discussed my treatment options and goals of care with my provider. If signing as the patient's representative, the treatments are consistent with the patient's known wishes and in their best interest.

✖ (required)			The most recently completed valid POLST form supersedes all previously completed POLST forms.
If other than patient, print full name:		Authority:	

F. SIGNATURE: Health care provider (eSigned documents are valid) **Verbal orders are acceptable with follow up signature.**

I have discussed this order with the patient or his/her representative. The orders reflect the patient's known wishes, to the best of my knowledge. [Note: Only licensed health care providers authorized by law to sign POLST form in state where completed may sign this order.]

✖ (required)		Date(mm/dd/yyyy): Required / /	Phone #: ( )
Printed full name:			License/Cert. #:
Supervising physician signature:	☐ N/A		License #:

A copied, faxed or electronic version of this form is a legal and valid medical order. This form does not expire. 2019

Fig. 4.1 Portable Medical Orders (POLST), previously referred to as Physician Orders for Life-Sustaining Treatment. (From Portable medical orders for seriously ill or frail individuals. POLST. https://polst.org/. Published October 26, 2022. Accessed November 11, 2022.)

National POLST form – Page 2 *******ATTACH TO PAGE 1*******

Patient full name:

Contact information (optional but helpful)

Patient's emergency contact.(Note: Listing a person here does **not** grant them authority to be a legal representative.Only an advance directive or state law can grant that authority.)

Full name:	☐ Legal representative ☐ Other emergency contact	Phone #: Day: ( ) Night: ( )
Primary care provider name:		Phone: ( )
☐ Patient is enrolled in hospice	Name of agency: Agency phone: ( )	

Form completion information (optional but helpful)

Reviewed patient's advance directive to confirm no conflict with POLST orders: (A POLST form does not replace an advance directive or living will)	☐ Yes; date of the document reviewed:____________ ☐ Conflict exists, notified patient (if patient lacks capacity, noted in chart) ☐ Advance directive not available ☐ No advance directive exists

Check everyone who participated in discussion: ☐ Patient with decision-making capacity ☐ Court appointed guardian ☐ Parent of minor ☐ Legal surrogate / Health care agent ☐ Other: ____________

Professional assisting health care provider w/ form completion (if applicable): Full name:	Date (mm/dd/yyyy): / /	Phone #: ( )

This individual is the patient's: ☐ Social worker ☐ Nurse ☐ Clergy ☐ Other:

Form information and instructions

- **Completing a POLST form:**
  - Provider should document basis for this form in the patient's medical record notes.
  - Patient representative is determined by applicable state law and, in accordance with state law, may be able execute or void this POLST form only if the patient lacks decision-making capacity.
  - Only licensed health care providers authorized to sign POLST forms in their state or D.C. can sign this form. See www.polst.org/state-signature-requirements-pdf for who is authorized in each state and D.C.
  - Original (if available) is given to patient; provider keeps a copy in medical record.
  - Last 4 digits of SSN are optional but can help identify / match a patient to their form.
  - If a translated POLST form is used during conversation, attach the translation to the signed english form.
- **Using a POLST form:**
  - Any incomplete section of POLST creates no presumption about patient's preferences for treatment. Provide standard of care.
  - No defibrillator (including automated external defibrillators) or chest compressions should be used if "No CPR" is chosen.
  - For all options, use medication by any appropriate route, positioning, wound care and other measures to relieve pain and suffering.
- **Reviewing a POLST form:** This form does not expire but should be reviewed whenever the patient:
  (1) is transferred from one care setting or level to another;
  (2) has a substantial change in health status;
  (3) changes primary provider; or
  (4) changes his/her treatment preferences or goals of care.
- **Modifying a POLST form:** This form cannot be modified. If changes are needed, void form and complete a new POLST form.
- **Voiding a POLST form:**
  - **If a patient or patient representative (for patients lacking capacity) wants to void the form:** Destroy paper form and contact patient's health care provider to void orders in patient's medical record (and POLST registry, if applicable). State law may limit patient representative authority to void.
  - **For health care providers:** Destroy patient copy (if possible), note in patient record form is voided and notify registries (if applicable).
- **Additional forms.** Can be obtained by going to www.polst.org/form
- As permitted by law, this form may be added to a secure electronic registry so health care providers can find it.

State specific info	For barcodes/ ID sticker

For more information, visit www.polst.org or email info@polst.org

Copied, faxed or electronic versions of this form are legal and valid. 2019

Fig. 4.1, cont'd

BOX 4.2 Expert Recommendations for Pharmacological Management of Life Support Withdrawal

Key Points

Medications can be used to treat evident symptoms OR in anticipation of symptoms that are not yet present.

Effects of neuromuscular blocking agents should be allowed to wear off prior to withdrawal.

Choice of Opioid and Sedative Medications

Patients who are comfortable on stable doses of an opioid should be continued on that opioid at that dose when starting withdrawal.

Morphine is the opioid of choice to treat pain or dyspnea in an opioid-naive patient.

Fentanyl and hydromorphone are considered safer first-line options for patients with end-stage renal disease (ESRD) and chronic kidney disease (CKD).

Titration of Opioids

Opioids should be titrated to symptoms, with no dose limit.

Opioid-naive patients can be started on bolus doses of 2 mg IV morphine, titrated to effect.

Pain or dyspnea should be treated with a bolus dose of opioid followed by an infusion.

Titration of Sedatives

Sedatives should be used only once pain and dyspnea are treated with opioids.

Combinations of opioids and benzodiazepines can be used during withdrawal.

Sedatives should be titrated to symptoms, with no dose limit.

Benzodiazepine-naive patients can be started on bolus doses of 2 mg IV midazolam, followed by an infusion of 1 mg/h.

Other Medications

Inhaled epinephrine should be used to treat postextubation stridor in conscious patients. This is an important consideration for patients who have been intubated for long periods of time.

Antinauseants should be ordered as needed (PRN) with opioids.

Consider anticholinergic medication (e.g., glycopyrrolate) to prevent upper-airway secretions.

Consider furosemide to prevent congestive heart failure symptoms postextubation.

Adapted from Downar J, Delaney JW, Hawryluck L, Kenny L. Guidelines for the withdrawal of life-sustaining measures. *Intensive Care Med.* 2016;42:1003-1017; Davison SN. Clinical pharmacology considerations in pain management in patients with advanced kidney failure. *Clin J Am Soc Nephrol.* 2019;14(6):917-931. https://doi.org/10.2215/CJN.05180418.

! CLINICAL ALERT

Terminal Weaning or Terminal Extubation

During the process of terminal weaning from ventilatory support or terminal extubation, patients may exhibit symptoms of respiratory distress, such as tachypnea, dyspnea, or use of accessory muscles. These symptoms may suggest a patient will not be comfortably removed from ventilatory support. Titrate pain and sedation medications as needed to relieve such symptoms.

Other Commonly Withheld Therapies. Vasopressors, antibiotics, blood and blood products, dialysis, and nutritional support are other common therapies that may be ethically withheld when goals of treatment shift to palliation instead of cure. Because of the increase in the use of left ventricular assist devices and cardiovascular implantable electronic devices, such as cardioverter-defibrillators, address the deactivation of these devices as appropriate before withdrawing or withholding ventilation or other therapies that may result in cardiac arrest.[58,65]Again, the primary nursing responsibility is to assess and ensure patient comfort during the withdrawal or withholding process.

Palliative Sedation. Palliative sedation (PS) may be used in the setting of end-of-life care where severe symptoms such as delirium, dyspnea, pain, and convulsions are refractory to usual first-line treatment options. The European Association for Palliative Care (EAPC) has defined PS as inducing a state of decreased or absent awareness (unconsciousness) through the monitored use of medications with the intent of relieving the burden of otherwise intractable suffering. PS is to be implemented in a manner that is ethically acceptable to the patient, family, and healthcare providers.[62,66] Medication selection is provider and institution dependent but generally consists of adding medications such as midazolam, propofol, or phenobarbital to the patient's current palliative regimen.[62,67] PS is implemented in collaboration with palliative care specialists and as a multiprofessional approach that takes into consideration the ethical implications. Informed consent should be given, and education should be provided to all involved parties (i.e., patient, family, healthcare team members) regarding the purpose of PS and the anticipated plan. Frequent and close monitoring should be made, as PS is not meant to intentionally cause a patient's death.[68]

Hospice Referral. When it has been determined that aggressive medical care interventions will be withheld or withdrawn, it may be appropriate to initiate a referral to hospice. Hospice is a model of care that emphasizes comfort rather than cure and views dying as a normal human process. It is a philosophy of care rather than a specific place and can be provided in various care settings, as dictated by patient needs.

Hospice care for the critically ill patient is usually provided in an inpatient setting and can include withdrawal of ventilator support or other therapies. For patients who are less dependent on technologies for survival, the dying process may be managed in the patient's home with multiprofessional team support. Referral to hospice may provide a more supportive and tranquil environment for the patient during the dying process. Should such a transfer occur, it is crucial to ensure a smooth transition and good communication among the critical care staff, the receiving hospice provider, the patient, and the family.

Emotional and Psychological Care of the Patient and Family

One of the most challenging aspects of end-of-life care is addressing the emotional and psychological needs of the patient and

CLINICAL EXEMPLAR

Patient-Centered Care

Mr. B is a 74-year-old man with stage IV lung cancer who was hospitalized for respiratory insufficiency requiring bilevel positive airway pressure (BiPAP). His oxygen requirements have significantly increased over the past day, and the team is discussing the need for potential intubation. He is alert, oriented, and able to make his own decisions. While giving his morning medications, the nurse noticed Mr. B was not as positive as he had been on previous shifts. She asks him about things that have cheered him up in the past and he shared that being with family has always helped him to feel joy. He expressed that he was scared to not be able to talk to them anymore if he needed to be intubated but he did not know how much longer he could keep breathing without it because he was feeling tired. During multiprofessional rounds led by the intensivist, the nurse conveyed to the provider Mr. B's discomfort and fear of further decompensation. This communication created the opportunity for shared decision-making and goal setting. With Mrs. B in the room, the provider noted that the BiPAP was not effective and asked, "What are your goals of care: comfort or more aggressive treatment?" Both Mr. and Mrs. B acknowledged that Mr. B would like to be comfortable, spending his final moments with family present and communicating without the presence of the BiPAP mask. A shared decision was made to place Mr. B on high-flow oxygen, and he immediately requested that the remainder of his family be called to visit. Mr. B was able to then spend time sharing memories and talking to his family. By facilitating family participation during multiprofessional rounds, the team was able to effectively address the patient's goals of care; providing dignity and compassion at the end-of-life.

CLINICAL JUDGMENT ACTIVITY

What is palliative care, and how does it apply to patients without a terminal illness?

family (refer to the Collaborative Care Plan found in Chapter 1, Overview of Critical Care Nursing). Needs are as variable as family situations, so carefully assess what the patient's and family's needs *are* instead of making assumptions about what they *ought* to be. Use a nonjudgmental assessment, being keenly aware of the patient's and family's personal feelings or values about the situation. The results of this assessment determine priorities in this dimension of care. Keep in mind that "family" can consist of many different persons in an individual's life. It may include unmarried life partners (same or opposite sex), close friends, and other individuals referred to as "family" who have no legal relationship to the patient.

For some families, spiritual counseling from pastoral care services might be a priority. For others, the need may be for statistics documenting their loved one's chances of survival with a particular diagnosis. One common need among all families is receiving clear, consistent, and accurate information about the patient's condition, what to expect during the withdrawal and dying process (if applicable), and reassurance that the patient will not suffer during the dying process.[69–71] Coordinating the communication process among the patient, family, and healthcare team contributes to building family resilience in the critical care setting and is a key nursing role. Other nursing activities that promote family resilience include managing expectations to ensure a realistic understanding of condition and prognosis, as well as supporting the decision-making process.[71–73] Many institutions have bereavement counselors with extensive training in assisting patients and families through the dying process and its aftermath. Social workers, spiritual care providers, and licensed mental health professionals can frequently assist in meeting the needs of families. Spiritual care providers can be an essential element of end-of-life care, and their presence is valued by nurses, patients, and families.[74]

Maintaining the patient's dignity during the dying process is of the utmost importance. Make time to listen to family accounts of the patient's life before the illness or injury and acknowledge the patient's individuality and humanity. Use a calm manner and voice, maintain a quiet and private environment, and allow unrestricted family presence with the patient before, during, and after the patient's death. Provide items for family comfort, such as tissues, refreshments, and chairs. When no words seem appropriate, maintain a respectful, conscious presence. The patient's death may be a relatively routine part of the critical care nurse's work experience, but family members will likely remember the situation and actions of the healthcare team for many years.

Legacy work is an intervention at the end-of-life that promotes an opportunity for memory sharing, reminiscing, and storytelling among family members and friends while creating tangible and lasting objects. Interventions may include copying the patient's handprint or obtaining a recording of the patient's heart sounds, a rhythm strip, or a voice message. Legacy work is individualized to the patient and can create a positive experience for both the family and the critical care nurse.[75,76] Nursing interventions to support the family at the end-of-life are summarized in Box 4.3.

Caregiver Organizational Support

Providing end-of-life care requires much time, and inadequate staffing patterns may be a barrier to providing optimal care. Nursing leaders should consider the level of care required for this population when staffing to allow nurses

BOX 4.3 Nursing Interventions to Support Care at the End-of-Life

- Assess patient's and family members' understanding of the condition and prognosis to address educational needs.
- Educate family members about what will happen when life support is withdrawn to decrease their fear of the unknown.
- Assure family members that the patient will not suffer.
- Assure family members that the patient will not be abandoned.
- Provide for any needed emotional support and spiritual care resources, such as grief counselors and spiritual care providers.
- Facilitate provider communication with the family.
- Provide for visitation and presence of family and extended family; most family members do not want the patient to die alone.
- Promote memory sharing, storytelling, and the creation of a lasting and tangible object through legacy work.

time to adequately care for the patient at the end-of-life. Should staffing ratios be less than adequate, assistance from colleagues can support the nurse caring for the dying patient and their family.

Other helpful organizational behaviors include bereavement programs for families and assistance or guidance in making funeral arrangements. For situations in which the nurse and the patient or family do not speak the same language, interpreter services are essential to providing excellent end-of-life care. Debriefing or support sessions for staff members may be helpful in easing the stress of caring for dying patients.

Critical care nurses have expressed the need for provider and public education concerning end-of-life issues.[77] Efforts to educate the public on various end-of-life issues are vital to improving care through promotion of advance directives and conversations with loved ones concerning life-support options.[73]

Nurses have also identified the need for professional end-of-life education.[72] The American Association of Critical-Care Nurses (AACN) first developed the *End-of-Life Competency Statements for a Peaceful Death* in 2002, which spurred the improvement of end-of-life education in undergraduate nursing curricula.[74] Training is also available to prepare nurse educators to teach bedside nurses about delivering competent and compassionate care to the dying patient.[75] Empowered nurses and an ethical organizational climate are correlated with lower levels of moral distress.[30] Education can also be provided in an informal setting. Creating committees within a nursing unit focused on identifying areas of practice concerns and creating educational materials can be useful. Naming experienced care team members within the unit as "practice experts" in areas such as communication, symptom management, and final hours can create resources for newer staff learning the practice of palliative care.[76]

Compassion fatigue, known as "secondary traumatic stress," is common in the healthcare field after repeated exposure to the stress of caring for the critically ill and comforting those experiencing loss and grief.[77,78] Classic symptoms of compassion fatigue include: emotional exhaustion, empathy imbalance, difficulty sleeping, anxiety, disassociation, and eventually, burnout.[79] Setting a personal ritual to utilize after a patient death can help empower nurses to reset and continue caring for their patients in times of need.[80]

CULTURALLY COMPETENT AND INCLUSIVE END-OF-LIFE CARE

Many clinicians believe they lack the skills and preparation to guide difficult end-of-life discussions with patients and families of critically ill patients. This discomfort may be magnified when clinicians assist patients and families who are from a culture, religion, or sexual orientation that differs from their own. Cultural influences on care at the end-of-life are highly variable, even by region; therefore, nurses must be sensitive and respectful of these differences to facilitate effective care planning.[81,82]

Research on end-of-life care preferences in various cultural, ethnic, and religious groups has grown rapidly, although it is scarce in smaller cultural groups. Research findings apply to groups in general and *may not apply to individual preferences or situations.* Critical care nurses should become familiar with the values and beliefs of common cultural groups in their practice settings. It is vital for critical care nurses to recognize the influences of their own social, religious, and cultural contexts. There are many ways to be inclusive and embrace diversity, and the following sections provide examples commonly encountered.

Addressing Religious Diversity

Religious doctrine and beliefs profoundly influence patients' and families' choices for end-of-life care.[83] Significant differences in perspective may exist between and *within* many major religious groups, meaning that a "good death" is a definition unique to each individual.[84] Religious practices surrounding the terminally ill and dying may be of paramount importance to patients and their loved ones. Using a validated tool, such as the Religious Beliefs in End-of-Life Medical Care scale, can help to quantify the importance of religion in terms of end-of-life care.[85] It is important to clarify any rituals that may be requested such as arranging Last Rites or pastoral visits to those of the Christian faith, allowing time for meditation for practicing Buddhists, or reciting a declaration of faith and turning the dying to face Mecca as is an Islamic custom.[86,87] Pain management is important to discuss with the patient or family, as some religions have pain modality constraints which may require altering standard palliative order sets.[86]

Creating A Safe Environment

Creating a safe environment for disclosure is important to all patients but especially necessary in the lesbian, gay, bisexual, transgender, queer/questioning (LGBTQ+) population. If a patient feels uncomfortable or fears judgment, lack of disclosure of sexual orientation or gender identification can occur, and the likelihood increases if preferences are not discussed during admission.[88,89] Legal considerations are also necessary for the LGBTQ+ patient and may require involvement of case management services to address advance care directives, establish surrogate decision-makers, and assist with burial rights.[88,89]

When holding conversations with those not fluent in the institution's primary language, use in-person or portable translation services. Adopting an "ask before assume" practice in which assumptions are avoided can help to encourage open discussion and foster patient, family, and provider trust. This in turn creates end-of-life care that is unbiased and patient-preference driven.

CASE STUDY

A 26-year-old Hispanic man sustained severe injuries in a high-speed motorcycle accident, requiring admission to the critical care unit. According to the patient's mother, he had previously been in perfect health, other than having mild asthma as a child. His most significant injuries are a cervical spine fracture and quadriplegia at the C2 level and a devastating traumatic brain injury consisting of a subarachnoid hemorrhage and diffuse axonal injury. He has subsequently developed acute respiratory distress syndrome, requiring high levels of mechanical ventilation support during the first 3 days of his hospitalization. His prognosis for functional recovery from his brain injury is deemed "poor" by the neurosurgeon, and because of his high quadriplegia, he will remain ventilator dependent for life. The patient's family is Cuban, very close-knit, and religious (Catholic), consisting of two sisters, his father and mother, and a grandmother who lives with them. Many of them do not speak English well, including his mother, who is his designated legal surrogate. All are very tearful and devastated by his injuries but remain hopeful that "God will help him recover and move again." His 20-year-old sister, in a private conversation with the nurse, states that her brother had previously told her he would prefer to die if he were ever paralyzed "from the neck down." She is afraid to verbalize these feelings with the rest of the family because she thinks her mother will accuse her of not loving her brother or of wanting to kill him.

Questions

1. What family assessment findings may impact the decision-making process?
2. Based on the assessment details, how does the family's cultural and religious background influence their perspective on this situation?
3. Which assessment findings warrant immediate follow-up? What interventions could the nurse recommend or initiate?
4. What learning needs does this family have? How could these be most appropriately met?
5. What resources would be most helpful to this family at this time? Why?
6. What outcomes would demonstrate the interventions implemented were effective in reducing dysfunctional family dynamics?

KEY POINTS

- The critical care nurse has a vital role in ensuring that patient and family needs for communication, information, support, and comfort are met in a reliable manner.
- Significant moral distress may occur when critical care nurses provide interventions or treatments they perceive to be non-beneficial or inappropriate to patients.
- Nursing self-care is an important step in the management of the critically ill. Preventing burnout can ensure that the critical care nurse is able to continue providing quality care to patients, their families, and friends without emotional and physical consequences.
- Palliative care is an integral part of high-quality, personalized critical care.
- Establishing trust and rapport with patients, families, and surrogates or proxies enables a safe environment for discerning what is most important to individuals at the end-of-life.
- During the withholding, limiting, or withdrawing of therapies, it is imperative that those involved in decision-making for the patient are aware that care and support from the healthcare team will remain unchanged.
- Frequent nursing assessment and collaboration with the multiprofessional team ensures appropriate symptom management at the end-of-life.
- Critical care nurses must simultaneously be aware of the patient's physical needs and their cultural, spiritual, and personal needs at the end-of life.
- Ongoing nursing education on palliative and end-of-life topics is important in ensuring that nurses are empowered to act as patient and family advocates.

REFERENCES

1. Shah M, Patnaik S, Patel B, et al. Trends in mechanical circulatory support use and hospital mortality among patients with acute myocardial infarction and non-infarction related cardiogenic shock in the United States. *Clin Res Cardiol*. 2018;107(4):287–303. https://doi.org/10.1007/s00392-017-1182-2.
2. Michaels A, Cowger J. Patient selection for destination LVAD therapy: predicting success in the short and long term. *Curr Heart Fail Rep*. 2019;16(5):140–149. https://doi.org/10.1007/s11897-019-00434-1.
3. Institute of Medicine. *Committee on approaching death. Dying in America: Improving Quality and Honoring Individual Preferences Near the End of Life*. Washington, DC: National Academies Press; 2014.

3a. Xu JQ, Murphy SL, Kochanek KD, Arias E. *Mortality in the United States, 2021. NCHS Data Brief, no 456*. Hyattsville, MD: National Center for Health Statistics; 2022. https://doi.org./10.15620/cdc:122516.

4. Centers for Disease Control and Prevention. *Number of Deaths for Leading Causes of Death*; 2020. Updated https://www.cdc.gov/nchs/fastats/deaths.htm. Accessed February 11, 2023.
5. Ferrell BR, Temel JS, Temin S, et al. Integration of palliative care into standard oncology care: American society of clinical oncology clinical practice guideline update. *J Clin Oncol*. 2017;35(1):96–112. https://doi.org/10.1200/JCO.2016.70.1474.
6. Quinn KL, Shurrab M, Gitau K, et al. Association of receipt of palliative care interventions with health care use, quality of life, and symptom burden among adults with chronic noncancer illness: a systematic review and meta-analysis. *JAMA*. 2020;324(14):1439–1450. https://doi.org/10.1001/jama.2020.14205.
7. A controlled trial to improve care for seriously ill hospitalized patients. The study to understand prognoses and preferences for outcomes and risks of treatments (SUPPORT). The SUPPORT Principal Investigators. *JAMA*. 1995;274(20):1591–1598. published correction appears in JAMA 1996 Apr 24;275(16):1232.
8. Chaudhuri D, Tanuseputro P, Herritt B, D'Egidio G, Chalifoux M, Kyeremanteng K. Critical care at the end of life: a population-level cohort study of cost and outcomes. *Crit Care*. 2017;21(1):124. https://doi.org/10.1186/s13054-017-1711-4. Published 2017 May 31.

9. Van der Padt-Pruijsten A, Oostergo T, Leys MBL, van der Rijt CCD, van der Heide A. Hospitalisations of patients with cancer in the last stage of life. Reason to improve advance care planning? *Eur J Cancer Care*. 2022;31(6):e13720. https://doi.org/10.1111/ecc.13720.
10. Beil M, van Heerden PV, de Lange DW, et al. Contribution of information about acute and geriatric characteristics to decisions about life-sustaining treatment for old patients in intensive care. *BMC Med Inform Decis Mak*. 2023;23(1):1. https://doi.org/10.1186/s12911-022-02094-z.
11. Lobo SM, De Simoni FHB, Jakob SM, et al. Decision-making on withholding or withdrawing life support in the ICU: a worldwide perspective. *Chest*. 2017;152(2):321–329. https://doi.org/10.1016/j.chest.2017.04.176. [published correction appears in Chest. 2021 Oct;160(4):1576-1577].
12. DeMartino ES, Dudzinski DM, Doyle CK, et al. Who decides when a patient can't? Statutes on alternate decision makers. *N Engl J Med*. 2017;376(15):1478–1482. https://doi.org/10.1056/NEJMms1611497.
13. Petrinec AB, Martin BR. Post-intensive care syndrome symptoms and health-related quality of life in family decision-makers of critically ill patients. *Palliat Support Care*. 2018;16(6):719–724. https://doi.org/10.1017/S1478951517001043.
14. Glick DR, Motta M, Wiegand DL, et al. Anticipatory grief and impaired problem solving among surrogate decision makers of critically ill patients: a cross-sectional study. *Intensive Crit Care Nurs*. 2018;49:1–5. https://doi.org/10.1016/j.iccn.2018.07.006.
15. Li L, Nelson JE, Hanson LC, et al. How surrogate decision-makers for patients with chronic critical illness perceive and carry out their role. *Crit Care Med*. 2018;46(5):699–704. https://doi.org/10.1097/CCM.0000000000003035.
16. Secunda KE, Hart JL. One guideline may not fit all: tailored evidence may improve critical care delivery. *Ann Am Thorac Soc*. 2022;19(8):1273–1274. https://doi.org/10.1513/AnnalsATS.202205-399ED.
17. Yamamoto K, Yonekura Y, Nakayama K. Healthcare providers' perception of advance care planning for patients with critical illnesses in acute-care hospitals: a cross-sectional study. *BMC Palliat Care*. 2022;21(1):7. https://doi.org/10.1186/s12904-021-00900-5.
18. White DB, Ernecoff N, Buddadhumaruk P, et al. Prevalence of and factors related to discordance about prognosis between physicians and surrogate decision makers of critically ill patients. *JAMA*. 2016;315(19):2086–2094.
19. Hoffmann TC, Del Mar C. Clinicians' expectations of the benefits and harms of treatments, screening, and tests: a systematic review. *JAMA Intern Med*. 2017;177(3):407–419. https://doi.org/10.1001/jamainternmed.2016.8254.
20. American Nurses Association. *Code of Ethics with Interpretive Statements*. Silver Spring, MD: American Nurses Association; 2015.
21. Downar J, You JJ, Bagshaw SM, et al. Nonbeneficial treatment Canada: definitions, causes, and potential solutions from the perspective of healthcare practitioners*. *Crit Care Med*. 2015;43(2):270–281. https://doi.org/10.1097/CCM.0000000000000704.
22. Kon AA, Shepard EK, Sederstrom NO, et al. Defining futile and potentially inappropriate interventions: a policy statement from the society of critical care medicine ethics committee. *Crit Care Med*. 2016;44(9):1769–1774. https://doi.org/10.1097/CCM.0000000000001965.
23. Johal HK, Birchley G, Huxtable R. Exploring physician approaches to conflict resolution in end-of-life decisions in the adult intensive care unit: protocol for a systematic review of qualitative research. *BMJ Open*. 2022;12(7):e057387. https://doi.org/10.1136/bmjopen-2021-057387.
24. Bosslet GT, Pope TM, Rubenfeld GD, et al. An official ATS/AACN/ACCP/ESICM/SCCM policy statement: responding to requests for potentially inappropriate treatments in intensive care units. *Am J Respir Crit Care Med*. 2015;191(11):1318–1330. https://doi.org/10.1164/rccm.201505-0924ST.
25. Douglas SL, Daly BJ, Lipson AR. Differences in predictions for survival and expectations for goals of care between physicians and family surrogate decision makers of chronically critically ill adults. *Res Rev J Nurs Health Sci*. 2017;3(3):74–84.
26. Schneider C, Aubert CE, Del Giovane C, et al. Comparison of 6 mortality risk scores for prediction of 1-year mortality risk in older adults with multimorbidity. *JAMA Netw Open*. 2022;5(7):e2223911.
27. Tilse C, Willmott L, Wilson J, Feeney R, White B. Operationalizing legal rights in end-of- life decision-making: a qualitative study. *Palliat Med*. 2021;35(10):1889–1896. https://doi.org/10.1177/02692163211040189.
28. Altaker KW, Howie-Esquivel J, Cataldo JK. Relationships among palliative care, ethical climate, empowerment, and moral distress in intensive care unit nurses. *Am J Crit Care*. 2018;27(4):295–302. https://doi.org/10.4037/ajcc2018252.
29. Henrich NJ, Dodek PM, Gladstone E, et al. Consequences of moral distress in the intensive care unit: a qualitative study. *Am J Crit Care*. 2017;26(4):e48–e57. https://doi.org/10.4037/ajcc2017786.
30. Rodney PA. What we know about moral distress. *Am J Nurs*. 2017;117(2 Suppl 1):S7–S10. https://doi.org/10.1097/01.NAJ.0000512204.85973.04.
31. McAndrew NS, Leske J, Schroeter K. Moral distress in critical care nursing: the state of the science. *Nurs Ethics*. 2018;25(5):552–570. https://doi.org/10.1177/0969733016664975.
32. Henrich NJ, Dodek PM, Gladstone E, et al. Consequences of moral distress in the intensive care unit: a qualitative study. *Am J Crit Care*. 2017;26(4):e48–e57. https://doi.org/10.4037/ajcc2017786.
33. Stutzer K, Rodriguez AM. Moral resilience for critical care nurses. *Crit Care Nurs Clin North Am*. 2020;32(3):383–393. https://doi.org/10.1016/j.cnc.2020.05.002.
34. Rushton CH, Schoonover-Shoffner K, Kennedy MS. A collaborative state of the science initiative: transforming moral distress into moral resilience in nursing. *Am J Nurs*. 2017;117(2 Suppl 1):S2–S6. https://doi.org/10.1097/01.NAJ.0000512203.08844.1d.
35. Rushton CH. Cultivating moral resilience. *Am J Nurs*. 2017;117(2 Suppl 1):S11–S15. https://doi.org/10.1097/01.NAJ.0000512205.93596.00.
36. Douglas SL, Daly BJ, Lipson AR. Differences in predictions for survival and expectations for goals of care between physicians and family surrogate decision makers of chronically critically ill adults. *Res Rev J Nurs Health Sci*. 2017;3(3):74–84.
37. Chiarchiaro J, Ernecoff NC, Scheunemann LP, et al. Physicians rarely elicit critically ill patients' previously expressed treatment preferences in intensive care units. *Am J Respir Crit Care Med*. 2017;196(2):242–245. https://doi.org/10.1164/rccm.201611-2242LE.
38. White DB, Carson S, Anderson W, et al. A multicenter study of the causes and consequences of optimistic expectations about prognosis by surrogate decision-makers in ICUs. *Crit Care Med*. 2019;47(9):1184–1193. https://doi.org/10.1097/CCM.0000000000003807.

39. Kon AA, Davidson JE. Retiring the term futility in value-laden decisions regarding potentially inappropriate medical treatment. *Crit Care Nurse*. 2017;37(1):9–11. https://doi.org/10.4037/ccn2017234.
40. Puente-Fernández D, Lozano-Romero MM, Montoya-Juárez R, Martí-García C, Campos-Calderón C, Hueso-Montoro C. Nursing professionals' attitudes, strategies, and care practices towards death: a systematic review of qualitative studies. *J Nurs Scholarsh*. 2020;52(3):301–310. https://doi.org/10.1111/jnu.12550.
41. Vanstone M, Neville TH, Clarke FJ, et al. Compassionate end-of-life care: mixed-methods multisite evaluation of the 3 wishes project. *Ann Intern Med*. 2020;172(1):1–11. https://doi.org/10.7326/M19-2438.
42. Star A, Boland JW. Updates in palliative care - recent advancements in the pharmacological management of symptoms. *Clin Med*. 2018;18(1):11–16. https://doi.org/10.7861/clinmedicine.18-1-11.
43. Crawford GB, Dzierżanowski T, Hauser K, et al. Care of the adult cancer patient at the end of life: ESMO Clinical Practice Guidelines. *ESMO Open*. 2021;6(4):100225. https://doi.org/10.1016/j.esmoop.2021.100225.
44. Morgan A. Long-term outcomes from critical care. *Surgery (Oxf)*. 2021;39(1):53–57. https://doi.org/10.1016/j.mpsur.2020.11.005.
45. Nordness MF, Hayhurst CJ, Pandharipande P. Current perspectives on the assessment and management of pain in the intensive care unit. *J Pain Res*. 2021;14:1733–1744. https://doi.org/10.2147/JPR.S256406. Published 2021 Jun 14.
46. Zeng YS, Wang C, Ward KE, Hume AL. Complementary and alternative medicine in hospice and palliative care: a systematic review. *J Pain Symptom Manage*. 2018;56(5). https://doi.org/10.1016/j.jpainsymman.2018.07.016. 781-794.e4.
47. Urits I, Schwartz RH, Orhurhu V, et al. A comprehensive review of alternative therapies for the management of chronic pain patients: acupuncture, Tai Chi, osteopathic manipulative medicine, and chiropractic care. *Adv Ther*. 2021;38(1):76–89. https://doi.org/10.1007/s12325-020-01554-0.
48. National Hospice and Palliative Care Organization. Hospice Care. http://www.nhpco.org/about/hospice-care. Accessed February 11, 2023.
49. Gupta N, Gupta R, Gupta A. Rationale for integration of palliative care in the medical intensive care: a narrative literature review. *World J Crit Care Med*. 2022;11(6):342–348. https://doi.org/10.5492/wjccm.v11.i6.342.
50. Zaborowski N, Scheu A, Glowacki N, Lindell M, Battle-Miller K. Early palliative care consults reduce patients' length of stay and overall hospital costs. *Am J Hosp Palliat Care*. 2022;39(11):1268–1273. https://doi.org/10.1177/10499091211067811.
51. Kyeremanteng K, Gagnon LP, Thavorn K, Heyland D, D'Egidio G. The impact of palliative care consultation in the ICU on length of stay: a systematic review and cost evaluation. *J Intensive Care Med*. 2018;33(6):346–353. https://doi.org/10.1177/0885066616664329.
52. Kernick LA, Hogg KJ, Millerick Y, Murtagh FEM, Djahit A, Johnson M. Does advance care planning in addition to usual care reduce hospitalisation for patients with advanced heart failure: a systematic review and narrative synthesis. *Palliat Med*. 2018;32(10):1539–1551. https://doi.org/10.1177/0269216318801162.
53. Effendy C, Yodang Y, Amalia S, Rochmawati E. Barriers and facilitators in the provision of palliative care in adult intensive care units: a scoping review. *Acute Crit Care*. 2022;37(4):516–526. https://doi.org/10.4266/acc.2022.00745.
54. Spijkers AS, Akkermans A, Smets EMA, et al. How doctors manage conflicts with families of critically ill patients during conversations about end-of-life decisions in neonatal, pediatric, and adult intensive care. *Intensive Care Med*. 2022;48(7):910–922. https://doi.org/10.1007/s00134-022-06771-5.
55. Adler K, Schlieper D, Kindgen-Milles D, et al. Integration of palliative care into intensive care: systematic review. *Anaesthesist*. 2017;66(9):660–666. https://doi.org/10.1007/s00101-017-0326-0.
56. Hui D, Hannon BL, Zimmermann C, Bruera E. Improving patient and caregiver outcomes in oncology: team-based, timely, and targeted palliative care. *CA Cancer J Clin*. 2018;68(5):356–376. https://doi.org/10.3322/caac.21490.
57. Mehter HM, McCannon JB, Clark JA, Wiener RS. Physician approaches to conflict with families surrounding end-of-life decision-making in the intensive care unit. A qualitative study. *Ann Am Thorac Soc*. 2018;15(2):241–249.
58. Lobo SM, De Simoni FHB, Jakob SM, et al. Decision-making on withholding or withdrawing life support in the ICU: a worldwide perspective. *Chest*. 2017;152(2):321–329. https://doi.org/10.1016/j.chest.2017.04.176kon. [published correction appears in Chest. 2021 Oct;160(4):1576-1577].
59. Cox CE, Ashana DC, Haines KL, et al. Assessment of clinical palliative care trigger status vs actual needs among critically ill patients and their family members. *JAMA Netw Open*. 2022;5(1):e2144093. https://doi.org/10.1001/jamanetworkopen.2021.44093.
60. VandeKieft GK. End-of-life care: medical aid in dying. *FP Essent*. 2020;498:32–36.
61. Grassi L, Folesani F, Marella M, et al. Debating euthanasia and physician-assisted death in people with psychiatric disorders. *Curr Psychiatry Rep*. 2022;24(6):325–335. https://doi.org/10.1007/s11920-022-01339-y.
62. Surges SM, Garralda E, Jaspers B, et al. Review of European guidelines on palliative sedation: a foundation for the updating of the European Association for Palliative Care Framework. *J Palliat Med*. 2022;25(11):1721–1731. https://doi.org/10.1089/jpm.2021.0646.
63. National POLST Coalition. About POLST. Accessed Februar 24, 2023. https://polst.org/about/.
64. Robert R, Le Gouge A, Kentish-Barnes N, et al. Terminal weaning or immediate extubation for withdrawing mechanical ventilation in critically ill patients (the ARREVE observational study). *Intensive Care Med*. 2017;43(12):1793–1807. https://doi.org/10.1007/s00134-017-4891-0. [published correction appears in Intensive Care Med. 2017 Nov 24].
65. Sullivan MF, Kirkpatrick JN. Palliative cardiovascular care: the right patient at the right time. *Clin Cardiol*. 2020;43(2):205–212. https://doi.org/10.1002/clc.23307.
66. Cherny NI, Radbruch L. Board of the European association for palliative care. European association for palliative care (EAPC) recommended framework for the use of sedation in palliative care. *Palliat Med*. 2009;23(7):581–593. https://doi.org/10.1177/0269216309107024.
67. Arantzamendi M, Belar A, Payne S, et al. Clinical aspects of palliative sedation in prospective studies. A systematic review. *J Pain Symptom Manage*. 2021;61(4). https://doi.org/10.1016/j.jpainsymman.2020.09.022. 831-844.e10.
68. AMA code of medical ethics' opinions on sedation at the end of life. *Virtual Mentor*. 2013;15(5):428–429.
69. Song MK, Metzger M, Ward SE. Process and impact of an advance care planning intervention evaluated by bereaved surrogate decision-makers of dialysis patients. *Palliat Med*. 2017;31(3):267–274. https://doi.org/10.1177/0269216316652012.

70. Levoy K, Tarbi EC, De Santis JP. End-of-life decision making in the context of chronic life-limiting disease: a concept analysis and conceptual model. *Nurs Outlook*. 2020;68(6):784–807. https://doi.org/10.1016/j.outlook.2020.07.008.
71. Wittenberg E, Reb A, Kanter E. Communicating with patients and families around difficult topics in cancer care using the COMFORT communication curriculum. *Semin Oncol Nurs*. 2018;34(3):264–273. https://doi.org/10.1016/j.soncn.2018.06.007.
72. Wu Y, Yao J, Zhao J, Wang L. Effect of high quality nursing on alleviating negative emotions in patients with advanced lung cancer. *Am J Transl Res*. 2021;13(10):11958–11965. Published 2021 Oct 15.
73. White DB, Angus DC, Shields AM, et al. A randomized trial of a family-support intervention in intensive care units. *N Engl J Med*. 2018;378(25):2365–2375. https://doi.org/10.1056/NEJMoa1802637.
74. Bone N, Swinton M, Hoad N, Toledo F, Cook D. Critical care nurses' experiences with spiritual care: the SPIRIT study. *Am J Crit Care*. 2018;27(3):212–219. https://doi.org/10.4037/ajcc2018300.
75. Collins A. "It's very humbling": the effect experienced by those who facilitate a legacy project session within palliative care. *Am J Hosp Palliat Care*. 2019;36(1):65–71. https://doi.org/10.1177/1049909118787772.
76. Hesse M, Forstmeier S, Ates G, Radbruch L. Patients' priorities in a reminiscence and legacy intervention in palliative care. *Palliat Care Soc Pract*. 2019;13:2632352419892629. https://doi.org/10.1177/2632352419892629.
77. Zhang YY, Zhang C, Han XR, Li W, Wang YL. Determinants of compassion satisfaction, compassion fatigue and burn out in nursing: a correlative meta-analysis. *Medicine*. 2018;97(26):e11086. https://doi.org/10.1097/MD.0000000000011086.
78. Peters E. Compassion fatigue in nursing: a concept analysis. *Nurs Forum*. 2018;53(4):466–480. https://doi.org/10.1111/nuf.12274.
79. Cross LA. Compassion fatigue in palliative care nursing: a concept analysis. *J Hosp Palliat Nurs*. 2019;21(1):21–28. https://doi.org/10.1097/NJH.0000000000000477.
80. Running A, Tolle LW, Girard D. Ritual: the final expression of care. *Int J Nurs Pract*. 2008;14(4):303–307. https://doi.org/10.1111/j.1440-172X.2008.00703.x.
81. Nalayeh H. Addressing the cultural, spiritual and religious perspectives of palliative care. *Ann Palliat Med*. 2018;7(Suppl 1):AB016. https://doi.org/10.21037/apm.2018.s016.
82. Ohr S, Jeong S, Saul P. Cultural and religious beliefs and values, and their impact on preferences for end-of-life care among four ethnic groups of community-dwelling older persons. *J Clin Nurs*. 2017;26(11–12):1681–1689. https://doi.org/10.1111/jocn.13572.
83. García-Navarro EB, Medina-Ortega A, García Navarro S. Spirituality in patients at the end of life-is it necessary? A qualitative approach to the protagonists. *Int J Environ Res Public Health*. 2021;19(1):227. https://doi.org/10.3390/ijerph19010227.
84. Krikorian A, Maldonado C, Pastrana T. Patient's perspectives on the notion of a good death: a systematic review of the literature. *J Pain Symptom Manage*. 2020;59(1):152–164. https://doi.org/10.1016/j.jpainsymman.2019.07.033.
85. Balboni TA, Prigerson HG, Balboni MJ, Enzinger AC, VanderWeele TJ, Maciejewski PK. A scale to assess religious beliefs in end-of-life medical care. *Cancer*. 2019;125(9):1527–1535. https://doi.org/10.1002/cncr.31946.
86. Chakraborty R, El-Jawahri AR, Litzow MR, Syrjala KL, Parnes AD, Hashmi SK. A systematic review of religious beliefs about major end-of-life issues in the five major world religions. *Palliat Support Care*. 2017;15(5):609–622. https://doi.org/10.1017/S1478951516001061.
87. Mahmoud S, Moughrabi SM, Khasawneh WF. Dying in isolation: an islamic perspective on end-of-life care during COVID-19. *J Hosp Palliat Nurs*. 2022;24(6):321–327. https://doi.org/10.1097/NJH.0000000000000905. [published online ahead of print, 2022 Sep 9].
88. Cloyes KG, Hull W, Davis A. Palliative and end-of-life care for lesbian, gay, bisexual, and transgender (LGBT) cancer patients and their caregivers. *Semin Oncol Nurs*. 2018;34(1):60–71. https://doi.org/10.1016/j.soncn.2017.12.003.
89. Maingi S, Bagabag AE, O'Mahony S. Current best practices for sexual and gender minorities in hospice and palliative care settings. *J Pain Symptom Manage*. 2018;55(5):1420–1427. https://doi.org/10.1016/j.jpainsymman.2017.12.479.

5

Organ Donation

Chelsea Sooy, BSN, RN, CCTC
Melissa A. Kelley, RN, CPTC

INTRODUCTION

For more than 50 years, solid organ transplantation has been the only definitive treatment option for patients living with end-stage organ failure. However, there are many challenges associated with organ transplantation. In particular, the number of people who need an organ transplant far exceeds the number of organs available for donation. More than 100,000 people in the United States are active on the national transplant waiting list, and every 10 minutes another person is added.[1] While data are constantly changing, as of 2022, the Organ Procurement and Transplantation Network (OPTN) reported there were 42,889 organ transplants performed (Figs. 5.1 and 5.2). Of these transplants, 36,421 were from deceased donors and 6468 were from living donors.[2] The number of patients active on the transplant waiting list fluctuates due to inactivity as a result of infection, severity of illness, or death. As of 2022, more than 1 million organ transplants had been performed in the United States, with more than half occurring within the previous 15 years.[2] Medical innovation, advances in technology, and growing public support for organ donation have led to an increasing number of transplants each year.

Critical care nurses work collaboratively with organ procurement organizations (OPOs) and transplant teams throughout the continuum of care to identify a potential organ donor, facilitate brain-death testing (when indicated), provide emotional support for donor families, and manage the donor in preparation for organ procurement or recovery.[3] This chapter provides an overview of the organ donation process throughout all phases of care: evaluation, referral, brain-death testing, donor management, and transplant criteria for select organs. Care of the organ recipient is not discussed in this chapter, as care for these patients is highly specialized.

TYPES OF DONATIONS

Organ Donation

In 1968, the Uniform Anatomical Gift Act (UAGA) was passed in the United States and has been adopted by all states and the District of Columbia. This law established a legal framework for individuals to authorize an anatomical gift of their organs, tissues, and eyes after death. The anatomical gift, according to the legislation, cannot be rescinded by another individual without the consent of the donor.[4]

The National Organ Transplant Act of 1984 called for the OPTN to be created and run by a private, non-profit organization under federal contract. This Act established the OPTN to provide oversight for transplantation and organ donation and to develop and maintain a national registry for organ sharing and matching. The United Network for Organ Sharing (UNOS) was first awarded the national OPTN contract in 1986 and continues as the only organization to operate the OPTN. Multiple resources are available from UNOS for healthcare providers, transplant professionals, and members of the public seeking information on organ donation and transplantation. These resources are available at https://unos.org/.

There are 56 non-profit, certified OPOs that serve the United States. Each OPO provides organ donation services to designated geographical areas and provides public education, professional development, and bereavement care to donor families. The Centers for Medicare & Medicaid Services (CMS) certifies all OPOs and monitors their performance.[5] OPOs must abide by the regulations set by CMS and the unique requirements of the state in which it resides.

Despite these national efforts, donor organs remain scarce, therefore limiting transplantation. In 1998, CMS imposed requirements for hospital reporting to increase organ donation. Any hospital that receives reimbursement from CMS must notify the local OPO in all cases of impending death.[6] Many hospitals have developed clinical criteria, or triggers, to ensure identification and appropriate referral of potential organ donors to the OPO. Clinical triggers will vary by OPO but may include the loss of neurological reflexes, a low Glasgow Coma Scale score, discussion of withdrawing or ceasing life-support, consulting palliative care, referral to hospice, or family members initiating a discussion about donation.

Tissue Donation

Though not the focus of the chapter, critical care nurses may play a role in tissue and eye donor referral. Tissue and eye donation, although not life-saving, greatly improve a person's quality of life. A single tissue donor may enhance the lives of more than 75 people, and one eye donor can restore sight for two people.[6] Tissue recovery occurs after organ recovery is complete, but it is also an option for patients who have a cardiac time of death and do not meet criteria for organ donation. Tissue donation includes bone, skin, blood vessels, heart valves, cartilage, and tendons. There are a multitude of uses for these tissues, and advancements are ongoing. Cornea donation restores vision, and whole eye donation can be used to repair injuries to the eye. Hospitals are required by CMS to have a formal arrangement with a tissue and eye bank for the referral of potential donors.[6-8] The referral process for tissue and eye donors involves contacting the local tissue and eye bank once the patient has a cardiac time of death. The tissue coordinator asks the nurse questions related to medical suitability and then calls the family for authorization, when applicable.

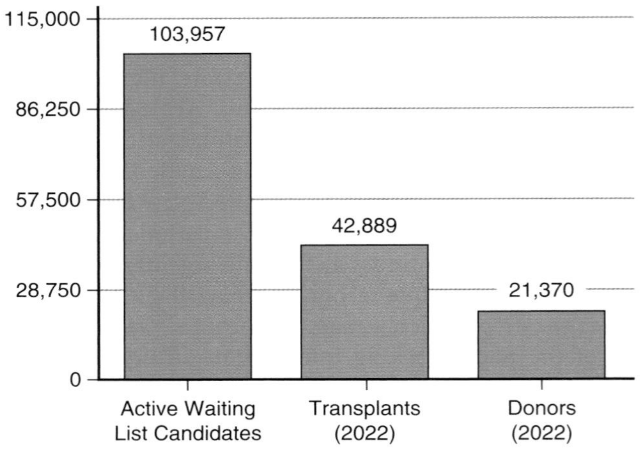

Fig. 5.1 The great imbalance between organ supply and demand. (Based on Organ Procurement and Transplantation Network [OPTN] data. https://optn.transplant.hrsa.gov/data/view-data-reports/national-data/. Accessed November 17, 2023.)

CLINICAL JUDGMENT ACTIVTY

After stabilization in the emergency department, an intubated and mechanically ventilated patient's emergent head computed tomography (CT) scan shows massive intracranial hemorrhage, significant midline shift, edema, and blood within the ventricles. The patient's neurologic examination is declining, despite aggressive efforts to maximize recovery. Determine the appropriate time frame to initiate a referral to the local organ procurement organization.

TYPES OF ORGAN DONORS

Organ donation may occur in one of three donor types: living donor, brain dead, or donation after circulatory death (DCD). Table 5.1 describes the types of organ donors and the most common organs donated.[8-10]

Living Donor

Living donation is done only after clinical evaluation identifies an appropriate match between the donor and recipient. A living donor does not have to be biologically related to or know the recipient (i.e., altruistic/nondirected living donor; see Table 5.1). To qualify, the donor must meet several criteria:

- Be at least 18 years old and willing to donate.
- Have good physical and mental health (medical conditions such as uncontrolled high blood pressure, diabetes, cancer, or certain infections could prevent donation).
- Be well informed regarding risks, benefits, and potential outcomes, including complications for the donor and recipient.

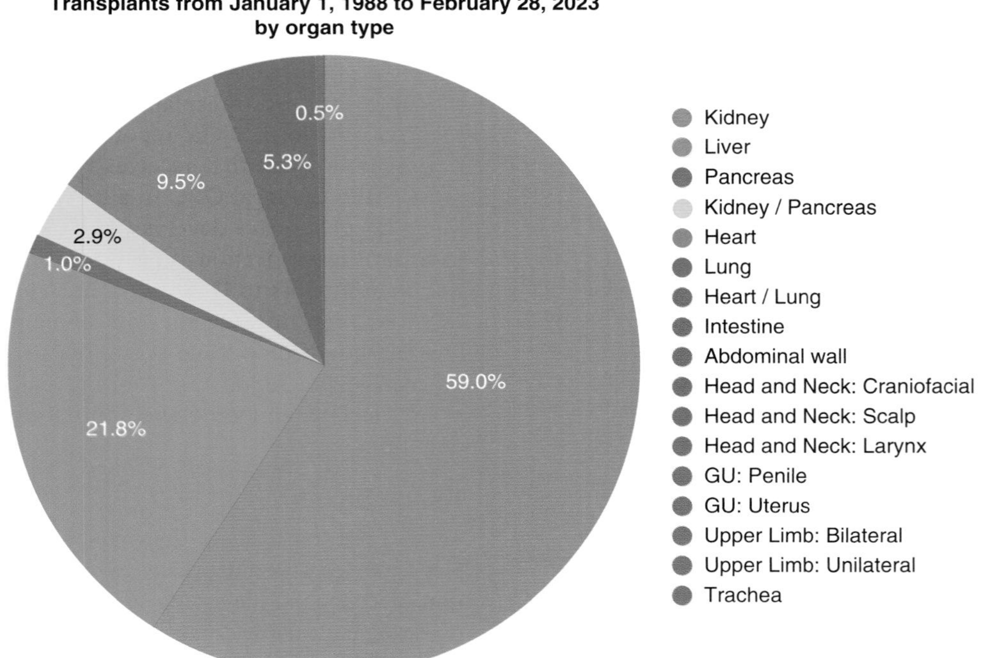

Fig. 5.2 Transplants from 1988 to 2023 by organ type. (From United Network for Organ Sharing. Data and Trends. https://optn.transplant.hrsa.gov/data/view-data-reports/build-advanced/. Accessed March 15, 2023.)

TABLE 5.1 Types of Organ Donors in the United States

Donor Type	Description	Organs Donated
Brain dead	Declared dead by neurological criteria due to head trauma, cardiopulmonary arrest, ischemic stroke, or intracranial hemorrhage.	Heart, lung, liver, kidney, pancreas, intestine, VCA
Donation after circulatory death (also called donation after cardiac death, asystolic, and non–heart-beating donors)	Donation after withdrawal of life-sustaining therapy. Donor must become asystolic within a prescribed period following withdrawal of mechanical ventilation and vasoactive medications.	Heart, lung, liver, kidney, pancreas
Living donor	An organ or part of an organ offered by a healthy individual to a patient with end-organ disease. Living donors may be related or unrelated.	Kidney, one or two lobes of the liver, a lung or part of a lung, part of a pancreas, part of the intestine
	Nondirect/altruistic: donation of an organ or part of an organ by a healthy individual to a stranger. Directed: donation of an organ or part of an organ by a healthy individual to a specified individual.	Kidney, liver lobe

VCA, vascularized composite allograft (refers to multiple tissues such as the abdominal wall, face, penis, uterus, upper limb).
Data from Organ Procurement and Transplantation Network. *Policy*. https://optn.transplant.hrsa.gov/. Accessed February 21, 2024.

- Have a good support system.
- Be able to take time off from work or school for the diagnostic workup, as well as up to 3 weeks after the surgery.

The OPTN has policies that mandate advocacy, screening, and care for the living donor. Every living donor is assigned an independent living donor advocate (ILDA) who functions independently of the transplant team to avoid any conflict of interest. Evaluation of a living donor typically begins after the intended recipient is active on the transplant waiting list and includes a full medical and psychosocial evaluation, including the motivation for donation. The decision to donate must be completely voluntary, without any coercion or financial incentive. Individual transplant centers may allow flexibility in the screening criteria based on need and the health of the donor. Gender and race are not factors in determining a successful match, but donors must have a blood type compatible with the intended recipient. After evaluation, the living donor donation is coordinated by the transplant team.

Brain Dead Donor

Historically, death was defined as the cessation of blood flow when the heart permanently stopped beating in response to a catastrophic illness or injury. During the 1950s, critical care units were created with the introduction of ventilators, sustaining the circulatory function of patients with fatal brain injuries. This led to exploration of the concept of brain death. This concept dates back to 1959 with the introduction of "coma dépassé," a state beyond coma indicating loss of brain reflexes and respiratory drive. In 1968, the Ad Hoc Committee of the Harvard Medical School described "irreversible coma" (what is now considered brain death), establishing criteria that remains the foundation for current brain death testing and diagnosis.[9]

BOX 5.1 Mechanisms of Death in Potential Organ Donors in the United States

- Asphyxiation
- Blunt injury
- Cardiovascular event
- Drowning
- Drug intoxication
- Electrocution
- Head trauma
- Penetrating trauma (i.e., gunshot wound, stab wound)
- Intracranial hemorrhage or stroke
- Status epilepticus
- Sudden unexpected infant death

Brain death/death by neurologic criteria (BD/DNC) include permanent coma, absence of reflexes, and apnea. A permanent coma may be structural (i.e., traumatic brain injury, intracranial hemorrhage) and/or anoxic (i.e., drug overdoses, cardiopulmonary arrest).[9] Box 5.1 identifies several common mechanisms of death in this population.

BD/DNC testing and clinical diagnosis occur while cardiopulmonary function and end-organ perfusion are artificially maintained (i.e., mechanical ventilation, infusion of vasoactive medications, maintenance of intravascular volume, treatment of electrolyte derangements). Updated guidelines for BD/DNC, published in 2023, lay out the determination of brain death in four steps: (1) BD/DNC prerequisites (Table 5.2), (2) neurologic examination (Table 5.3), (3) ancillary tests (Table 5.4), and (4) documentation. The guidelines state a minimum of one neurologic examination is required; however, the risk of a false-positive determination can be reduced with a second independent examination. The examination may be completed by appropriately credentialed attending physicians with adequate training and competency. Depending on local laws and institutional standards,

TABLE 5.2 Brain Death/Death by Neurologic Criteria Prerequisites

Steps	Clinical Evaluation
1. Establish that the patient has sustained a catastrophic, permanent brain injury with an etiology known to cause BD/DNC	Per patient history, physical examination, neuroimaging, and laboratory tests, the clinician: • Excludes the effect of CNS depressant medication. • Recognizes that prior use of targeted temperature management (TTM) may delay drug metabolism. • Verifies no recent administration of neuromuscular blockade medications. • Verifies no severe electrolyte, acid-base, or endocrine disturbances. • Verifies no confounding factors present that may "mimic" brain death, such as locked-in syndrome, fulminant Guillain-Barré syndrome, severe hypothermia, post–cardiac arrest syndrome, massive baclofen/anticholinergic overdose, severe overdose of CNS depressants, massive overdose of valproic acid or tricyclic antidepressants, or severe snake envenomation.
2. Allow an appropriate observation period prior to BD/DNC evaluation	• Hypoxic ischemic brain injury—observe for at least 24 hours prior to BD/DNC evaluation • Based on brain injury pathophysiology observe for a sufficient amount of time prior to BD/DNC evaluation • After medical or surgical intervention to treat elevated ICP, wait a sufficient amount of time (based on pathophysiology of the brain injury and neuroimaging) prior to BD/DNC evaluation
3. Achieve normal core temperature	A warming blanket is often needed to maintain normothermia. Vasodilation following catecholamine depletion leads to additional heat loss as blood flow increases to the periphery and causes additional heat loss after final brainstem herniation. Evaluation should be delayed for at least 24 hours if the core temperature was ≤35.5°C.
4. Achieve normal blood pressure	Hypovolemia and loss of peripheral vascular tone are often present, which may be corrected with IV fluids, vasopressors, or inotropic medications. Neurologic examination is most reliable with a systolic blood pressure ≥100 mm Hg and a mean arterial blood pressure ≥75 mm Hg.
5. Perform neurologic examination	One neurologic exam, although controversial, is now considered sufficient for diagnosing brain death in most states. Brain death must be pronounced and documented by a physician.

BD/DNC, Brain death/death by neurologic criteria; *CNS*, central nervous system; *ICP*, intracranial pressure.
Data from Greer DM, Kirschen MP, Lewis A, et al. Pediatric and adult brain death/death by neurologic criteria consensus guideline: report of the AAN Guidelines Subcommittee, AAP, CNS, and SCCM. *Neurology*. 2023. https://doi.org/10.1212/WNL.0000000000207740. [published online ahead of print, 2023 Oct 11].

TABLE 5.3 Examination for Brain Death/Death by Neurologic Criteria

Neurologic Assessment	Clinical Evaluation
Coma	• Patient lacks all evidence of responsiveness. • Noxious stimuli should not produce a motor response.
Absence of brainstem reflexes	• Absence of pupillary response to bright light. Usually, the pupils are fixed and dilated (4-9 mm). Constricted pupils suggest the possibility of drug intoxication. • Absence of ocular movements using oculocephalic testing and oculovestibular reflex testing. • Oculocephalic testing: Once the integrity of the cervical spine is ensured, the head is briskly rotated horizontally and vertically. There should be no movement of the eyes relative to head movement. • Oculovestibular reflex testing (caloric testing): After the patency of both external auditory canals is confirmed, the patient's head is elevated to 30 degrees. The external auditory canal of each ear is irrigated (one ear at a time) with approximately 50 mL of ice water. Movement of the eyes should be absent during 1 minute of observation. • Absence of corneal reflex: Demonstrated by touching the cornea with a piece of tissue paper, a cotton swab, or squirts of water. No eyelid movement should be seen. • Absence of facial muscle movement to a noxious stimulus: Deep pressure on the condyles at the level of the temporomandibular joints and deep pressure at the supraorbital ridge should produce no grimacing or facial muscle movement. • Absence of the pharyngeal and tracheal reflexes: The pharyngeal or gag reflex is tested after stimulation of the posterior pharynx with a tongue blade or suction device. The tracheal reflex is tested by examining the cough response to tracheal suctioning. The catheter should be inserted into the trachea and advanced to the level of the carina, followed by one or two suctioning passes.

TABLE 5.3 **Examination for Brain Death/Death by Neurologic Criteria—cont'd**

Neurologic Assessment	Clinical Evaluation
Apnea	• Absence of a breathing drive is tested with a CO_2 challenge, with documentation of an increase in $PaCO_2$ above normal levels. • Prerequisites: (1) normotensive, (2) euvolemic, (3) absence of hypoxia, (4) normal arterial pH (7.35–7.45), and (5) eucapnia ($PaCO_2$ 35–45 mm Hg). An exception to eucapnia is the patient who is known to be hypercarbic, in which case their baseline $PaCO_2$ is the target. **Procedure:** 1. Adjust vasopressors to a systolic blood pressure ≥100 mm Hg. 2. Preoxygenate for at least 10 minutes with 100% oxygen to a PaO_2 >200 mm Hg. 3. Reduce ventilation frequency to 10 breaths/min to eucapnia. 4. Reduce positive end-expiratory pressure (PEEP) to 5 cm H_2O (oxygen desaturation with decreasing PEEP may suggest difficulty with apnea testing). 5. If pulse oximetry oxygen saturation remains >95%, obtain a baseline blood gas (PaO_2, $PaCO_2$, pH, bicarbonate, base excess). 6. Disconnect the patient from the ventilator. 7. Preserve oxygenation (e.g., place an insufflation catheter through the endotracheal tube, close to the level of the carina, and deliver 100% O_2 at 6 L/min). 8. Look closely for respiratory movements for 8-10 minutes. Respiration is defined as abdominal or chest excursions and may include a brief gasp. 9. Abort if systolic blood pressure decreases to <100 mm Hg or mean arterial pressure <75 mm Hg despite titration of vasopressors, inotropes, and/or intravenous fluids. 10. Abort if hemodynamic instability with cardiac arrhythmia. 11. Abort if oxygen saturation measured by pulse oximetry is <85% for >30 seconds. 12. If no respiratory drive is observed, repeat arterial blood gas (PaO_2, $PaCO_2$, pH, bicarbonate, base excess) after approximately 8 minutes. 13. If respiratory movements are absent, arterial $PaCO_2$ is ≥60 mm Hg (or 20 mm Hg increase in arterial $PaCO_2$ over a baseline normal arterial $PaCO_2$) and the arterial pH < 7.30, the apnea test result is positive (i.e., supports the clinical diagnosis of brain death). 14. If the test is inconclusive but the patient is hemodynamically stable during the procedure, it may be repeated for a longer period (10-15 minutes) after the patient is again adequately preoxygenated.

CO_2, carbon dioxide; *$PaCO_2$*, partial pressure of carbon dioxide; *PaO_2*, partial pressure of oxygen.
Data from Greer DM, Kirschen MP, Lewis A, et al. Pediatric and adult brain death/death by neurologic criteria consensus guideline: report of the AAN Guidelines Subcommittee, AAP, CNS, and SCCM. *Neurology*. 2023. https://doi.org/10.1212/WNL.0000000000207740. [published online ahead of print, 2023 Oct 11].

advanced practice providers may be allowed to perform BD/DNC evaluations. Ancillary testing is recommended when the neurologic examination or an apnea test cannot be performed or the interpretation of the findings is uncertain. Though there are other ancillary neurodiagnostic tests, the ones most commonly found in clinical practice due to their availability are cerebral angiography, radionuclide cerebral perfusion scan, and transcranial Doppler ultrasonography.[9] The legal time of death is documented when brain death is determined based on the aforementioned criteria.[9-10]

Although the above criteria must be met to declare a patient brain dead, state laws and hospital policies may require additional criteria. Some states require that two physicians complete the neurologic examination and write separate notes of brain death. In this case, the time of the second brain death note is the time of death. There are also differing requirements regarding timing of the neurologic examination(s).

Federal and state laws require the hospital staff to contact the OPO after determination of brain death.[6] However, the OPO is usually contacted before brain death declaration in response to clinical triggers, allowing evaluation of the potential donor before brain death declaration.

Brain death is still not completely understood by some healthcare professionals and the general public. For example, a patient who is dead by neurological criteria may appear to be "alive" only because the ventilator is moving air in and out of the lungs, causing the chest to rise and fall. The patient has a pulse and warm skin because artificial support is being provided, such as mechanical ventilation, vasoactive and inotropic medications, and intravenous (IV) fluids. Once any of these therapies are removed, the patient does not have the ability to maintain respirations or circulation on their own due to the absence of brainstem function. Caring for the brain dead donor is complex and can be emotionally demanding for the critical care nurse. Therefore implementing strategies to mitigate the challenges of

TABLE 5.4 Ancillary Neurodiagnostic Testing in Brain Death Determination

Test	Description	Advantages	Disadvantages	Normal Findings	Findings in Brain Death
Four-vessel cerebral angiography	Injection of radiopaque contrast into blood supply to the brain	Short time to obtain results; easy to read; definitive when consistent with brain death clinical criteria	Requires transport of an unstable patient. Invasive; radiopaque contrast may compromise kidney function. Blood flow may persist after clinical evidence of brain death if terminal injury not associated with ICP elevation (hypoxic injury, craniectomy).	Blood flow into all areas of brain, contrast documented in large blood vessels of brain	No blood flow into the brain
Radionuclide cerebral perfusion scanning	IV injection of radioisotope tracer	Less invasive; rapid interpretation; no radiopaque contrast load on kidneys	Requires transport of unstable patient. May yield radiographic evidence of flow in clinical examination consistent with brain death (craniotomy defect, absence of significant ICP elevation).	Images show uptake of radioisotope tracer in viable brain tissue	Absence of radioisotope tracer uptake in brain tissue (Fig. 5.3)
Transcranial Doppler ultrasonography	Ultrasound used to assess cerebral blood flow	Easy to perform at bedside; noninvasive; widely available	Skull thickness may interfere with testing; operator dependent	Sharp systolic upstroke and stepwise deceleration with positive end-diastolic flow	Oscillating flow or systolic spikes in the proximal large intracranial arteries (i.e., internal carotid, middle and anterior cerebral, posterior cerebral, basilar, and vertebral arteries)

CNS, central nervous system; *ICP,* intracranial pressure.

Adapted from Lau VI, Arntfield RT. Point-of-care transcranial Doppler by intensivists. *Crit Ultrasound J.* 2017;9(1):21. doi:10.1186/s13089-017-0077-9;37(3):408-414. doi:10.3174/ajnr.A4548; Greer DM, Kirschen MP, Lewis A, et al. Pediatric and adult brain death/death by neurologic criteria consensus guideline: report of the AAN Guidelines Subcommittee, AAP, CNS, and SCCM [published online ahead of print, 2023 Oct 11]. *Neurology.* 2023;10.1212/WNL.0000000000207740. doi:10.1212/WNL.0000000000207740

caring for the brain dead donor are vital to the health and well-being of the critical care nurse (see Nursing Self-Care Box).

Confounding factors must be evaluated prior to brain death testing because equivocal results can confuse clinicians and family members regarding brain death (Table 5.5). Hypothermia, high-dose central nervous system depressants, and massive drug or toxin ingestion may severely depress consciousness and interfere with valid brain death testing. Thus these conditions must be reversed prior to brain death testing.

Any discussion of death touches on cultural, personal, and religious perspectives and must be addressed carefully. The concept of brain death also requires careful, sensitive communication with families and consistent messages from multiprofessional team members. The primary care team is responsible

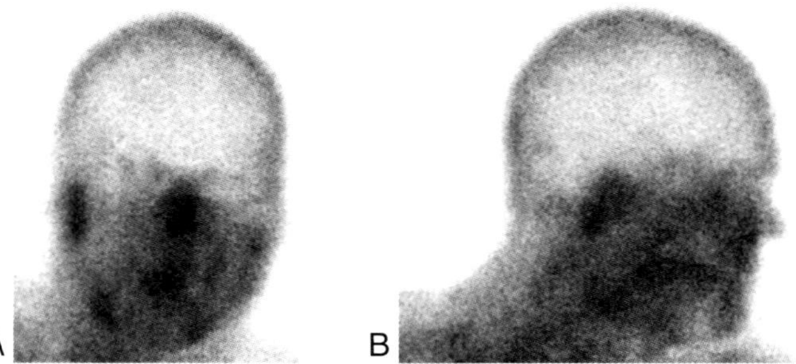

Fig. 5.3 Radionuclide Brain Perfusion Study Consistent with Brain Death. **A**, Anterior posterior view. **B**, Lateral view. Lighter color indicates absence of isotope uptake and absence of perfusion. Darker color indicates isotope uptake and presence of perfusion to the neck and face (nose).

for ensuring the family has a clear understanding that death of the patient has in fact occurred by neurological criteria (see the section Care of the Donor Family). Once the family understands death has occurred and the patient is considered medically suitable for organ donation, a designated requestor from the OPO approaches the family. The OPO-designated requestor is responsible for discussing end-of-life decisions and organ donation with the patient's family after brain death declaration and for obtaining authorization for organ donation. This discussion occurs separately from family discussions with the primary care team. Separating these discussions is called decoupling and has been found to significantly increase organ donation authorization rates.[11-12]

NURSING SELF-CARE

Overcoming the Challenges of Caring for the Brain Dead Donor

Challenges:

- Lack of understanding about the diagnosis or concept of brain death.
- Insufficient knowledge about the management of a brain dead donor and the stress of maintaining circulation until time of donation.
- Effectively interacting and communicating with the donor's family.
- Psychological, mental, and emotional challenges of caring for the brain dead donor.
- Personal religious or culture beliefs may not support organ donation.

Strategies to Overcome the Challenges:

- Provide respectful and dignified care to the brain dead donor's body, as this promotes positive feelings in the nurse.
- Promote a healthy work environment where nurses are encouraged to ask questions and seek clarity regarding the care of the brain dead donor and understanding brain death.
- Seek education on the concept of brain death, brain death testing, the donor process, effective management of the brain dead donor, conflict resolution, and communication strategies.
- Develop relationships across disciplines and units to facilitate effective communication, role clarification, and stress reduction during the organ donation process.
- Use social and spiritual support to help cope with the strain of these situations and separate work from personal life.

From Yazdimoghaddam H, Manzari ZS, Mohammadi E. Nurses' challenges in caring for an organ donor brain dead patient and their solution strategies: a systematic review. *Iran J Nurs Midwifery Res.* 2020;25(4):265-272. https://doi.org/10.4103/ijnmr.IJNMR_226_18; Yazdimoghaddam H, Manzari ZS, Heydari A, Mohammadi E. Improving psychological security and empowerment: new model for nurses toward the care of potential organ donors. *J Educ Health Promot.* 2021;10:101. https://doi.org/10.4103/jehp.jehp_657_20.

CHECK YOUR UNDERSTANDING

1. A patient is admitted with a catastrophic intracranial hemorrhage. After pursuing aggressive treatment for 3 days, the patient has been weaned off of all sedatives and analgesics. Assessment findings include fixed and dilated pupils, no response to painful stimuli, absence of a gag reflex during suctioning, and no respirations over the ventilator's set rate. Which one or more of the following interventions should the nurse recommend the multiprofessional care team implement?
   A. Goals of care discussions with the family
   B. Brain death testing
   C. Surgical consult for tracheostomy
   D. Discussion of organ donation with the family

Authorization for organ donation may be obtained through donor designation (i.e., first-person authorization for donation) or from the legal authorized representative, which is typically a family member. First-person authorization for the anatomical gift occurs when the person signs up for organ donation via the registry. If donor designation exists, the OPO designated requestor discloses the registry information to the family.[6] Authorization from the legal next of kin is not required in this instance for organ donation, but it is important that the family is supported emotionally and involved with the donation process. If donor designation is not present and the patient's organ and tissue donation wishes are not documented, the legal authorized representative needs to be made aware of the end-of-life options. In these cases, the OPO-designated requestor provides compassionate grief support and explains the options, which include organ and tissue donation.[11-12]

Donation After Circulatory Death

Prior to the widespread use of ventilators, organ donation was completed by DCD with only the liver and kidneys recovered; however, with improvements in technology, artificial perfusion systems have paved the way for hearts and lungs to be recovered from DCD donors (see Table 5.1).[3,13-14] DCD is an option for patients who do not meet criteria for brain death and the family has made the decision to compassionately extubate when the prognosis is grave. It is normally a family-driven process because it is triggered by their decision to withdraw life-sustaining measures.

Suitability for DCD donation is determined by several factors. The patient must have a diagnosis in which no meaningful recovery is expected. Brain death criteria is usually not met; however, the patient must be dependent on life-sustaining medical interventions, such as mechanical ventilation or vasoactive medications.

TABLE 5.5 Potential Confounding Factors Affecting Brain Death/Death by Neurologic Criteria Testing

Confounding Factors	Clinical Implications
High cervical spinal cord injury	Can yield absent responses to brainstem testing with preserved brain or brainstem function. Cough and gag reflexes, motor responses to noxious stimulation, intrinsic respiratory drive and valid apnea testing require intact spinal cord function.
Complex spinal reflex movements	Arm adduction or elbow flexion may resemble purposeful movement. Muscle stretch reflexes, abdominal muscle movements, facial twitching, persistent Babinski reflexes, and toe flexion from plantar stimulation may be elicited by mechanical stimulation of the spinal cord or sensory nerve roots. "Lazarus sign" (shoulder adduction, elbow flexion, arm lifting, possible crossing of hands) may also occur.
Muscle fasciculations	Fasciculations of extremities, chest, and abdomen may occur, beginning shortly after terminal brainstem herniation with duration up to 2-3 days. May falsely imply brain or brainstem function.
Ventilator auto-triggering: Overbreathing of ventilator set rate in absence of intrinsic respiratory drive	May falsely imply residual brainstem function and preservation of intrinsic respiratory drive. May delay or abort formal brain death protocols.
Interventions for suspected cardiogenic ventilator auto-triggering	Identify or rule out indications of intrinsic respiratory drive on clinical evaluation and ventilator waveform analysis. Analyze ventilator flow and pressure waveforms concurrently with clinical evaluation. Adjust ventilator trigger settings to eliminate auto-triggering. Match precordial motion with cardiac cycle, pulse palpation, auditory tone (beep), and QRS on bedside monitor, as well as corresponding oscillations on ventilator flow and pressure waveforms (done collaboratively at the bedside by critical care nurse, respiratory therapist, and physician).
Targeted temperature management (TTM)	TTM can blunt brainstem reflexes temporarily and is more pronounced in patients who received sedation before or during TTM. If core temperature was ≤35.5°C, wait at least 24 hours after rewarming to 36°C prior to BD/DNC evaluation.

BD/DNC, Brain death/death by neurologic criteria; *CNS,* central nervous system; *EEG,* electroencephalogram; *NMB,* neuromuscular blockade.

Adapted from Greer DM, Shemie SD, Lewis A, et al. Determination of brain death/death by neurologic criteria: the World Brain Death Project. *JAMA.* 2020;324(11):1078-1097. https://doi.org/10.1001/jama.2020.11586; Wijdicks EF, Varelas PN, Gronseth GS, Greer DM; American Academy of Neurology. Evidence-based guideline update: determining brain death in adults: report of the Quality Standards Subcommittee of the American Academy of Neurology. *Neurology.* 2010;74(23):1911-1918. https://doi.org/10.1212/WNL.0b013e3181e242a8.

Once the family begins end-of-life discussions with the multiprofessional team, if the OPO is not already following the patient, they are notified. For a patient to be considered a candidate for DCD, the OPO staff must determine if the patient will have a cardiac time of death within a designated time frame. That time frame may vary slightly depending on the evaluating agency. Determining if the patient meets criteria for DCD requires collaboration between the OPO and the primary care team. The multiprofessional team, including the OPO team, assesses medical suitability for organ donation and the patient's cardiopulmonary status. Some factors that may affect a patient's suitability for DCD include organ function, hemodynamics, age, and neurological function. In most instances, a respiratory assessment is done collaboratively with the physician, nurse, respiratory therapist, and the OPO team that is caring for the donor. The assessment includes the degree of ventilator assistance required to maintain oxygenation, oxygen requirements, and intrinsic respiratory drive. This data helps determine how likely the patient is to experience circulatory death within an appropriate time frame after the withdrawal of life-sustaining measures. Each OPO and transplant center may have slightly different criteria for determining if a patient meets criteria for DCD. If the patient is deemed suitable for DCD, a designated requestor presents the option of DCD to the patient or family. The decision to withdraw life support is made first and is independent of the decision to donate. The patient or the legal next of kin must authorize organ donation.[6]

CARE OF THE DONOR FAMILY

The relationship between the critical care team and the family is an important factor in a family's decision to donate organs of a loved one.[11-12] Developing trust between the multiprofessional team and the patient's family is important throughout the critical care hospitalization. Families often have many questions, concerns, or fears about organ donation that may affect willingness to donate.[11-12] Collaboration between the OPO and the primary care team provides accurate and timely answers to the family's questions. Emotional support and grief counseling is paramount throughout the process.

Donor families have special needs that result from both the death of a loved one and their decision to donate. The multiprofessional and OPO teams establish a unique relationship with the grieving family as they assist in navigating end-of-life processes. The teams work collaboratively to meet the needs of the family as well as guide them through the decision-making process that includes: organ and tissue donation, medical examiner and coroner involvement, funeral planning, and grief counseling resources.[11-12] Advocacy, honesty, and empathy help to develop trust between the patient's family and the OPO designated requestor. Building trust starts with assessing and acknowledging the family's cultural, ethnic, and religious beliefs regarding death. Understanding the perspectives of the family of a potential donor better prepares critical care nurses for discussions about brain death and organ donation (see Evidence-Based Practice box).[11-12]

EVIDENCE-BASED PRACTICE

Interventions to Increase Organ Donation

Problem

Many initiatives have been implemented worldwide in an effort to increase organ donation; unfortunately, it is unclear which of these initiatives are effective. The aim of this study was to identify which of these initiatives increase the number of organ donors.

Clinical Question

Which initiatives aimed at healthcare professionals are most effective in increasing the number of organ donors?

Evidence

In this systematic review, the authors analyzed 22 studies published before April 24, 2019. Statistically significant effects on the rate of identification, family consent, and/or donation were found in 14 of the studies. One or more of these outcomes were positively impacted by the following interventions: training emergency personnel in organ donation, an electronic support system to identify and/or refer potential donors, a collaborative care pathway, donation request by a trained professional, and additional family support in the critical care unit by a trained nurse.

Implications for Nursing

Although data may be limited, collaboration between the critical care unit and other departments (e.g., neurology, emergency medicine, neurosurgery) to identify potential organ donors through the use of clinical triggers increases donation. Training healthcare professionals and providing additional support to potential donor families may also increase the number of organ donors. Nursing knowledge of the organ donation process, including support for families of potential donors, is an important component of increasing consent for organ donation.

Level of Evidence

C—Systematic review

Reference

Witjes M, Jansen NE, van der Hoeven JG, Abdo WF. Interventions aimed at healthcare professionals to increase the number of organ donors: a systematic review. *Crit Care.* 2019;23(1):227.

EVALUATION OF THE POTENTIAL ORGAN DONOR

The evaluation of the organ donor is a data collection process that allows transplant centers to choose the best recipient for each organ, improving patient safety and graft survival. An OPO coordinator is assigned to the patient and has the primary responsibilities of managing the donor, evaluating the organs for transplant, and assisting in the placement of transplantable organs. The OPO coordinator evaluates the potential donor through extensive history gathering and physical assessments.

Medical and Social Histories

The process begins when the OPO coordinator obtains extensive medical and social histories from the patient's medical records and family. A medical history screening includes the presence or absence of any health condition(s) that may affect the function of a transplantable organ like diabetes mellitus, hypertension, or chronic obstructive pulmonary disease (COPD). Although active cancer does not automatically disqualify a potential donor, consideration may be given to when and how long the potential donor has been in remission, the tumor type, treatment, and follow-up.[15]

A social history is also obtained and identifies any history of cigarette use, heavy alcohol use, drug use, as well as sexual history. The goal is to identify any risk factors for potential transmission of bloodborne illnesses including HIV, hepatitis C virus (HCV), and hepatitis B virus (HBV). HIV, HCV, and severe acute respiratory syndrome coronavirus-2 (SAR-CoV-2, the virus that causes coronavirus disease 19) were contraindications to donation at one time, but now those organs are being safely transplanted.[16] There are very few contraindications to donation; however, the OPO coordinator relays this information to the recipient transplant center to assist in their selection of the best recipient for the transplantable organ.

Physical Assessment and Diagnostics

A physical assessment is another part of the donor evaluation process. Coordinators are looking for signs of infection, previous surgeries, injuries, tattoos, scars, or needle marks that follow the path of the veins to supplement the obtained medical and social histories. Another important part of the physical assessment is an accurate height and weight. Measurement of the organs from a computerized tomography (CT) scan or chest x-ray may also be used as a tool to match organs to waiting recipients.

The donor's blood type (ABO) is a critical factor in matching to waiting recipients. Other laboratory tests are indicators of current organ function and include basic metabolic, hepatic, and coagulopathy panels; complete blood count; urinalysis; and an arterial blood gas test. Cultures of blood, sputum, and urine may be ordered. Transplant labs identify the donor's human leukocyte antigen (HLA) histocompatibility, which is useful in predicting organ rejection in the recipient. HLA can be obtained from blood or a lymph node recovered from the donor. Serological testing screens the potential donor for transmissible diseases, including COVID-19, HIV, hepatitis A virus, HBV, HCV, Epstein-Barr virus (EBV), cytomegalovirus (CMV), toxoplasmosis, and sexually transmitted infections.[3] Other evaluative tools that may be used to determine the function of an organ are bronchoscopies, echocardiograms, cardiac catheterizations, liver biopsies, and ultrasound. These evaluation tools may be used for both brain dead and DCD donors.

! CLINICAL ALERT

All major religions, including Islam, Christianity, Judaism, and Hinduism, support organ donation as a charitable helping act.

CHECK YOUR UNDERSTANDING

2. Determine which of the following patients would be considered medically suitable for organ donation if their prognosis was grave and/or they met brain death criteria:
   A. 55-year-old assault victim with a subdural hematoma and history of hepatitis C
   B. 40-year-old patient positive for COVID-19
   C. 75-year-old patient with a status of post-cardiac arrest and a history of breast cancer 25 years ago
   D. All of the above

Matching Organs to Waiting Recipients

When a potential donor organ becomes available, the OPO coordinator enters demographic and medical data into DonorNet, an electronic medical record system for organ allocation, created and managed by UNOS. This includes the donor's height, weight, blood type, serology, HLA histocompatibility, and the evaluations of each organ system. Lists are generated electronically based on this information, which the OPO coordinator then uses to communicate the donor's information with the transplant center. The transplant team reviews the donor's information and determines if the organ is an appropriate match for their recipient, then enters an accept or decline code into DonorNet. The process continues until all transplantable organs are allocated.

DONOR MANAGEMENT

Donation Following Brain Death

To avoid any conflict of interest, the OPO has no direct involvement in the management of the potential donor until brain death is formally declared. Once this occurs, the OPO has a trained staff member approach the family to discuss organ and/or tissue donation. If agreeable, authorization for donation is obtained. Once this authorization is obtained, the OPO directs management of the brain dead donor (Box 5.2).[17]

Preserving Organ Function. Care of the brain dead donor is focused on preserving organ function and viability by maintaining hemodynamic and pulmonary stability, normothermia, and normal laboratory parameters. Consequences of brain death include autoregulatory loss resulting in intense vasoconstriction from catecholamine release, followed by vasodilation from catecholamine depletion. This results in relative hypovolemia, hypotension, and potential for cardiac dysrhythmias (e.g., bradycardia). Loss of hypothalamus function causes inability to regulate temperature. Loss of pituitary function results in decreased antidiuretic hormone secretion, causing diabetes insipidus with massive volume loss and electrolyte imbalances, as well as depletion of cortisol, thyroid-stimulating hormone, and thyroid hormones. Decreased insulin levels and increased insulin resistance occur, further contributing to acid-base imbalance and fluid and electrolyte depletion. Optimal donor management effectively replaces neurohormonal regulation, modulates the proinflammatory state, replaces intravascular volume, and supports vasomotor tone as well as cardiac contractility.[18-19] Table 5.6 outlines medications used in donor management.

BOX 5.2 Focus of Donor Management

Rule of 100, states that a patient's heart rate, temperature, systolic blood pressure and hourly urine output stay around 100 for adult donor management.

- Maintain normothermia
- Maintain blood pressure
- Maintain euvolemia (i.e., treat polyuria, optimize fluid and electrolyte levels)
- Provide appropriate mechanical ventilation
- Treat anemia
- Treat coagulopathy and thrombocytopenia
- Maintain normal serum glucose level
- Maintain normal acid-base balance

CLINICAL JUDGMENT ACTIVITY

A patient becomes increasingly hypoxemic and hemodynamically unstable after being admitted with an intracranial hemorrhage. Brain death testing has not yet been completed, nor has the family been approached about organ donation. Ventilator management is provided to maintain adequate oxygenation. Despite three vasoactive medications, hemodynamic stability continues to decline with a mean arterial pressure of 50 mm Hg. Determine the appropriate treatment to recommend to the provider to support blood pressure and tissue perfusion.

Standardized order sets can be used, focusing on optimizing fluid, electrolyte, and acid-base balances, in addition to oxygenation to preserve organs for donation. A pulmonary artery catheter or central venous catheter may be used to provide hemodynamic parameters, including central venous pressure, pulmonary artery occlusion pressure, cardiac output, and cardiac index. Alternatively, devices that use pulse contour methods for hemodynamic assessment (see Chapter 9) provide stroke volume variation (SVV), pulse pressure variation (PPV), continuous cardiac output, and other hemodynamic parameters. These parameters help guide volume replacement and the use of vasoactive and inotropic medications.

CLINICAL ALERT

Many hospitals have created "interim order sets" that treat the physiological consequences of brain death while the patient is undergoing brain death testing. These order sets help to maintain hemodynamic stability and preserve organ function.

Organ Recovery. Once all organs have been accepted for placement, the OPO coordinator works with the donor hospital to set an operating room (OR) time for organ recovery. The organ recipients are called into their respective hospitals to begin the preoperative process. The recipient hospitals send a surgical team to the donor hospital to recover the accepted organ(s). They may request that a local transplant surgeon recover the organ if one is available. Timing and communication are critical to the recovery process. Organs have a limited time they can be out of the body, so the recipient team(s) must be ready to implant immediately upon arrival of the recovered organ.

TABLE 5.6 PHARMACOLOGY

Medications Commonly Used in Donor Management

Medication	Action/Use	Dose/Route	Side Effects	Nursing Implications
		ANTIHYPERTENSIVES		
Esmolol (Brevibloc)	Cardiac selective beta-1 blocker used to control tachycardia and decrease myocardial oxygen consumption.	*Continuous infusion:* Loading dose, 500 mcg/kg IV over 1 min (optional) Maintenance, 25-50 mcg/kg/min IV, titrate, max 200 mcg/kg/min IV	Bradycardia Heart block Hypotension Infusion site reactions	Rapid onset Short acting (except with increased doses and prolonged duration) Monitor continuous blood pressure
Nicardipine (Cardene)	Calcium channel blocker causing arterial vasodilation used to control severe blood pressure elevations.	*Continuous infusion:* Maintenance, 2.5-5 mg/h IV, titrate, max 15 mg/h IV	Hypotension	Administer through large peripheral vein or central line (venous irritant). Monitor continuous blood pressure.
Nitroprusside (Nipride)	Direct vasodilator used to control severe blood pressure elevations.	*Continuous infusion:* Maintenance, 0.25-0.5 mcg/kg/min IV, titrate, max 10 mcg/kg/min (limit doses >3 mcg/kg/min to avoid cyanide toxicity)	Precipitous hypotension Sinus tachycardia/ bradycardia	Rapid onset Monitor continuous blood pressure. Protect from light and monitor for color change. Monitor for cyanide (dose related) and thiocyanate (in renal failure) toxicity.
		INOTROPES AND VASOPRESSORS		
Dobutamine	Stimulates $beta_1$ receptors to increase contractility and heart rate to increase cardiac output.	*Continuous infusion:* Maintenance, 2.5-5 mcg/kg/min IV, titrate, max 20 mcg/kg/min IV	Hypotension Tachyarrhythmias	Monitor heart rate, blood pressure, cardiac output/index, and clinical signs of tissue perfusion. Do not titrate to blood pressure.
Dopamine	Stimulates alpha and beta receptors *Moderate doses (2-10 mcg/kg/min): more beta-1 activity to increase cardiac contractility and heart rate* *High doses (10-20 mcg/kg/min): more alpha activity to increase blood pressure through vasoconstriction*	*Continuous infusion:* Maintenance, 5 mcg/kg/min IV, titrate, max 20 mcg/kg/min IV	Tachyarrhythmias (most proarrhythmic vasopressor)	Administer through central line if possible; for peripheral administration must be large vein (vesicant). Monitor continuous blood pressure.
Norepinephrine (Levophed)	Stimulates alpha receptors to cause vasoconstriction to increase blood pressure. Stimulates beta-1 receptors to increase contractility, heart rate, and coronary blood flow.	*Continuous infusion:* Maintenance, 2-20 mcg/min IV, titrate, no true max dose	Dysrhythmias Peripheral ischemia	Administer through central line if possible; for peripheral administration must be large vein (vesicant). Monitor continuous blood pressure.
Phenylephrine	Stimulates alpha receptors to cause vasoconstriction to increase blood pressure.	*Continuous infusion:* Maintenance, 20-300 mcg/min IV	Ischemia (e.g., peripheral, mesentery) Reflex bradycardia	Weak alpha agonist Monitor heart rate and blood pressure. Administer through central line if possible; for peripheral administration must be large vein (vesicant).
Vasopressin (Vasostrict)	Stimulates smooth muscle contraction to cause vasoconstriction: 1. Augments effects of other vasopressor medications. 2. Replacement therapy for ADH depletion in treatment of DI to control urine output and preserve circulating blood volume.	*Continuous infusion:* Maintenance, 0.01-0.04 units/min IV	Generally well tolerated	Monitor urine output, serum electrolytes, serum/urine osmolality, and volume status.

Continued

TABLE 5.6 PHARMACOLOGY—cont'd

Medications Commonly Used in Donor Management

Medication	Action/Use	Dose/Route	Side Effects	Nursing Implications
		HORMONE REPLACEMENT		
Desmopressin (DDAVP)	Replacement therapy for ADH depletion in treatment of DI to control urine output and preserve circulating blood volume.	*Intravenous:* Bolus, 1-4 mcg IV over 1 min, 1–2 mcg IV q6h (higher doses may be used); may be scheduled or PRN for urine output	Hypertension from hypervolemia Hyponatremia	Monitor urine output, serum sodium, serum/urine osmolality, volume status. Repeat bolus dosing based on urine output.
Levothyroxine (T_4) (Synthroid)	Replacement therapy for thyroid hormone depletion following loss of pituitary function Augments metabolism at cellular and tissue level, improving cardiovascular and acid-base balance.	*Continuous infusion:* Bolus, 20 mcg IV Maintenance, 10-20 mcg/h IV, titrate	Dysrhythmias Hypertension	Data supporting clinical benefits is conflicting. Administration considered in hemodynamically unstable patients with peripheral hypoperfusion and decreased cardiac output. Monitor blood pressure and tissue perfusion. May facilitate decreasing doses of vasopressors and inotropes.
Methylprednisolone (Solu-Medrol)	Decreases inflammatory state after brainstem herniation. Replacement therapy for cortisol depletion.	*Intravenous/Continuous infusion:* Bolus, 1000 mg, 15 mg/kg, or 250 mg IV x1 Maintenance, may follow bolus with 50–100 mg/h IV	Hyperglycemia	Titrate vasoactive medications in response to therapy.
		OTHER MEDICATIONS		
Insulin Regular	Treats hyperglycemia from stress response and high-dose steroid administration.	*Continuous infusion:* Protocol-directed, titrated to point-of-care serum blood glucose goal	Hypoglycemia Hypokalemia	Monitor blood glucose levels and titrate infusion dose per protocol.
Isotonic crystalloid (e.g., 0.9% NS or Lactated Ringer's)	Provides replacement for intravascular volume depletion (continuous infusion or rapid bolus)	*Continuous infusion:* Initial volume and titration based on volume replacement needs	Hemodilution Pulmonary edema	Monitor urine output and overall volume status.

ADH, antidiuretic hormone; *DI,* diabetes insipidus; *NS,* normal saline; *T_4,* thyroxine.
Data from Dhar R, Stahlschmidt E, Marklin G. A randomized trial of intravenous thyroxine for brain-dead organ donors with impaired cardiac function. *Prog Transplant.* 2020;30(1):48-55; Korte C, Garber JL, Descourouez JL, et al. Pharmacist's guide to management of organ donors after brain death. *Am J Health Syst Pharm.* 2016;72(22):1829-1839; Kotloff RM, Blosser S, Fulda G, et al. Management of the potential organ donor in the ICU: Society of Critical Care Medicine/American College of Chest Physicians/Association of Organ Procurement Organizations consensus statement. *Crit Care Med.* 2015;43(6):1291-1325.

Total recovery of donor organs can take an average of 3 to 6 hours. The recovery time per donor organ varies based on the specific organ and needs of the recovery team(s) and recipient(s). In general, for a brain dead donor, all recovery teams arrive at the donor hospital and begin the recovery process. Patient identification is confirmed, authorization and brain death declaration are verified, and the patient is prepped and draped for the procedure. A time out is done and a message from the family may be read, or a moment of silence is taken to respect the donor and their gift of life. An incision is made from the sternum to the pubis. The abdominal and thoracic recovery teams inspect the organs to confirm they are transplantable based on anatomy and function. Recipient hospitals are notified if the organs are transplantable, and the recipients are prepped for surgery. Once the preliminary dissection of each organ is complete, the surgeons place cannulas and flush each organ with a cold perfusion solution that maintains organ viability. The heart is recovered first, followed by lungs, liver, pancreas, intestines, and kidneys. Each organ is packaged and labeled according to UNOS standards and transported to the recipient hospital by the recovery team. An exception is the kidneys, which may be shipped via a medical courier to the recipient hospital. Tissue and eye procurement are completed after organ recovery. Postoperatively, the donor body is closed, and postmortem care is completed. Once all organs are recovered, the OPO coordinator updates the family and provides supportive care. The coordinator updates anyone involved in the care of the body postoperatively, including hospital staff, medical examiners, coroners, funeral homes, and tissue and eye banks.

Donation After Circulatory Death

DCD donors are managed by the primary team per their unique clinical needs until cardiac time of death occurs after the compassionate withdrawal of life support. Withdrawal typically occurs in the OR, but there may be another designated location near the OR such as the Postanesthesia Care Unit (PACU). Some hospitals allow the family to be present in the OR when the withdrawal of life support occurs. They are escorted into the OR by an OPO family care coordinator while the critical care nurse provides comfort measures and end-of-life care to the patient. Life-sustaining measures are withdrawn (e.g., extubation, discontinuing vasoactive medications) and comfort medications are given per the orders of the primary medical team. Once the declaration of death is made per hospital policy, either the family is escorted from the OR or the donor is transferred to the OR. Typically, for DCD organs to be viable for transplantation, time of death must occur between 30 and 60 minutes from withdrawal of life support. The time frame varies based on the organ being recovered and the policy of the recipient hospital. Though it varies based on OPO policy, once the patient is asystolic, the surgical team waits an allotted time prior to starting the organ recovery process. Warm ischemic time (WIT) is the amount of time the organ is not adequately oxygenated and not preserved in a cold solution. Cold ischemic time (CIT) is how long the organ is in a cold storage solution for transport to the recipient. The longer the WIT, the less likely the organ will function when transplanted. In general, the liver needs to have less than 45 minutes of WIT and kidneys less than 60 minutes.[20] Cardiothoracic surgeons may be willing to have longer WITs for hearts and lungs, but this varies considerably based on multiple factors (i.e., recipient need, donor health, surgeon preference). If the patient does not have a cardiac time of death within the required time frame to permit the recovery of organs, the patient is transferred to a predetermined critical care unit or designated palliative care bed, where the planned organ donation process stops and end-of-life care continues, including family support.[17]

 **CLINICAL JUDGMENT ACTIVITY**

A patient with a catastrophic brain injury continues to experience a decline in their neurologic assessment. The patient's pupils become fixed and dilated, and all brainstem reflexes are lost. Discuss strategies on how to communicate this change to the patient's family.

TRANSPLANT CANDIDATE EVALUATION

A comprehensive evaluation of each potential transplant candidate is performed to assess medical and surgical alternatives and determine the best criteria for a matching donor offer. Donor size, medical history, and previous infections are important considerations in assessing donor suitability. Acuity of illness of the potential recipient typically determines placement on the waiting list. For example, liver transplant candidates who have severe, acute liver failure with multisystem complications are highest on the waiting list.

Donor-derived infections are another challenge for transplant recipients. Although potential donors who are febrile are carefully screened for potential infections that could be transmitted, infections can be missed if the donor's history is incomplete. Depending on medical and social histories, a donor may be identified as having risk criteria for HIV, HCV, and HBV (Box 5.3); however, because of medical advances, these infections are not contraindications to donation.[21] Donor-derived infections that have been transmitted to recipients include CMV, EBV, HIV, lymphocytic choriomeningitis virus, West Nile virus, HBV, HCV, herpes simplex, and Chagas disease.[22] All recipients are tested for HIV, HCV, and HBV within 1 to 2 months after transplant. Liver transplant recipients are additionally tested for HBV 11 to 13 months after transplant to ensure disease transmission does not occur from the donor. It is mandatory to report any donor-derived infections to the OPO and UNOS so they can be reviewed by the Centers for Disease Control and Prevention.[22] At the time of the organ offer, the potential recipient is informed of donor information that could impact the recipient posttransplant.

CLINICAL EXEMPLAR

Quality and Safety

A 21-year-old patient was admitted to the critical care unit the previous evening at 2100 with a traumatic brain injury after falling from a cliff. The patient was declared brain dead the next morning at 0900, and mechanical ventilation was removed. The family arrives from out of town and inquires about organ donation. The nurse contacts the organ procurement organization (OPO). After sharing the sequence of events, the nurse learns that organ donation is not an option because the patient is off mechanical ventilation. The nurse requests a meeting to identify strategies to avoid this from occurring in the future. The OPO staff member conducts a retrospective review of the medical record and OPO database and discovers the hospital never called in a referral. A meeting was arranged with the OPO staff member and the critical care unit team to review this case, the Centers for Medicaid and Medicare Services (CMS) regulations, and best practices for timely referrals of potential organ donors. Protocols and policies on brain death and OPO notification are reviewed and revised, and unit-based education is completed.

Lung Transplantation

Lung transplantation is the treatment of choice for patients with end-stage lung disease when no other treatment options are available. The most common indications are COPD, interstitial lung disease, cystic fibrosis, pulmonary arterial hypertension, lymphangioleiomyomatosis, thoracic malignancy, acute respiratory distress syndrome, and urgent retransplantation for graft failure.[23] A total of 3,131 new candidates were added to the lung waiting list and there were 2,692 lung transplants performed in 2022.[2] Posttransplant 1-year survival was 89.4% in transplant recipients in 2019, and 5-year survival was 61.2% in transplant recipients in 2015.[22] Efforts to increase the number of lung

BOX 5.3 Donor Risk Factors

Donors are at risk of acute transmission of HIV, HBV, or HCV. Includes but not limited to the following, if the behavior occurred within the past 30 days:

- Sex with a person known or suspected to have HIV, HBV, or HCV infection.
- Males who have sex with males.
- Sex with a person in exchange for money or drugs.
- Sex with a person who had sex in exchange for money or drugs.
- Sex with a person who has injected drugs by IV, intramuscular, or subcutaneous route for nonmedical reasons.
- Been in jail, prison, or a juvenile correctional facility for more than 72 consecutive hours.
- Child breastfed by a mother with known HIV infection.
- Child born to a mother infected with HIV, HBV, or HCV infection.
- Risk factors that cannot be determined or an unknown medical or social history.

HBV, hepatitis B virus; *HCV*, hepatitis C virus.

transplant recipients have resulted in a variety of lung transplantation options, including heart-lung, single lung, double lung en bloc, and living donor lobar. Considerations in selecting the type of lung transplantation include the specific disease process, the need for cardiac transplantation, and donor availability.[24]

Lung transplantation typically uses deceased donors. However, it is possible for two living donors to each donate one lobe. This is high-risk; hence, a living donor lung transplant has not been completed since 2013.[2] The ideal deceased donor meets the following criteria[23,25]:

- Aged less than 55 years
- Smoking history less than 20 pack-years
- Clear chest radiograph
- PaO_2 greater than 300 mm Hg on 100% fraction of inspired oxygen and 5 cm H_2O positive end-expiratory pressure (PEEP)
- No history of significant chronic lung disease, current sepsis, or aspiration; absence of chest trauma; and no prior cardiopulmonary surgery
- No organisms on sputum Gram stain
- Absence of purulent secretions on bronchoscopy

Few donors fit the ideal criteria, and strict criteria can extend time on the waiting list and lead to increased waiting list mortality. Advances in posttransplant care have allowed transplant centers to expand criteria in an effort to expand the donor pool.[7] It is important to identify risk factors for lung dysfunction, including donor smoking history, elevated oxygen requirements, history of cardiopulmonary bypass, large-volume blood transfusion, and obesity in the recipient.[26] Thorough donor evaluation plus proper management and recovery can decrease posttransplant lung dysfunction and allow greater utilization of expanded criteria.[26]

Kidney Transplantation

Any patient with end-stage renal disease (ESRD) should be considered for kidney transplantation. Successful kidney transplantation can greatly improve the patient's quality of life because they are free from the restrictions of dialysis. Almost 90,000 patients are on the national waiting list for kidney transplantation.[2] As of 2020, more than 250,000 kidney transplant recipients were alive with sustained kidney function, including pediatric recipients.[27]

Kidneys are one of the few organs that can be donated whole from a living donor. Living donors may be related or unrelated, with the most desirable source being a related donor who matches the recipient closely. If a potential living donor does not match the recipient, the two may enter into a paired exchange program. A paired exchange program allows a living donor to be matched to another potential recipient whose living donor is not a good match because of blood type or preformed antibodies against a donor. Prospective living donors undergo physical and psychosocial evaluations and are screened for blood type, tissue-specific antigens, HLA histocompatibility, and preexisting kidney disease or other medical problems that would be contraindications to donation. The transplant center must determine the donor is healthy enough to tolerate surgery and maintain kidney function after donation. Living donors are also screened to ensure the absence of coercion or financial incentives driving the donation decision. The number of living donors is slowly increasing due to public outreach education, national commitment to donation, and the continued development and growth of living donor programs within active transplant centers. Of the 25,500 kidney transplants performed in 2022, nearly a quarter came from living donors.[2]

Heart Transplantation

Heart transplantation is the primary treatment for patients with advanced heart failure who continue to have limitations on exertion despite guideline-directed medical therapy. Indications for heart transplant evaluation include severe cardiovascular disease causing progressive ventricular dysfunction, severe hypertensive or viral cardiomyopathy, and congenital heart disease that cannot be surgically repaired. The upper age limit for heart transplant candidacy is 70 years, but carefully selected patients greater than 70 may be considered.[28] Over 3000 candidates are on the national waiting list for heart transplantation.[2] In 2022, 4,111 heart transplants were performed. Of recipients who underwent heart transplantation in 2019, 7.4% died within 6 months; however, 1-year survival was 90.6%. Of those who underwent transplant in 2017, 3-year mortality was 14%.[29]

Because of the limited availability of donor hearts, another focus of care is optimal management of end-stage heart failure. Additional treatment options include pharmacological therapies and mechanical assist devices to maximize cardiac output and tissue perfusion. Mechanical assist devices include cardiac resynchronization therapy with biventricular pacing to increase efficiency of the cardiac cycle, intraaortic balloon pump, and implanted right-ventricular and left-ventricular assist devices. These interventions support the heart and augment regional blood flow and tissue perfusion. The limited availability of donor organs and improvements in the left ventricular assist device (LVAD) has increased this device's utilization as destination therapy rather than bridge to transplantation. The survival of patients on LVAD support is approximately 50% at 5 years.[28]

Innovations in organ procurement and preservation, acceptance of expanded criteria donors, use of donors with HCV, and hearts recovered from DCD have expanded the donor pool. Criteria used to determine suitability of a potential donor heart include age; cause of death; clinical factors such as smoking, drug use, laboratory values (troponin, creatine kinase MB), use of vasoactive medications, and echocardiography results; and timing and use of hormonal resuscitation protocols. If the potential organ donor suffered a cardiac arrest, evaluation of heart function, donor management, and downtime are all considered. The potential donor's family history of cardiac disease is reviewed when evaluating extended criteria.

Expanded donor criteria include older hearts (>55 years), hearts with an ischemic time of more than 4 hours, and use of hearts from donors who died of a drug overdose. In the past, donor hearts with medical comorbidities such as diabetes and hypertension, left ventricular hypertrophy, wall motion abnormalities requiring high doses of inotropic medications, refractory shock, or ventricular dysrhythmias were declined. However, because of the significant shortage of transplantable organs, donor hearts previously thought to be unacceptable have been used with positive recipient outcomes.

CHECK YOUR UNDERSTANDING

3. An OPO coordinator is reviewing the history of a potential donor. Determine which of the following histories would improve the likelihood that the organs will be further evaluated for donation:
   A. Recent smoking history
   B. Low levels of low-density lipoprotein (LDL)
   C. Diabetes
   D. Hypertension

Liver Transplantation

Liver transplantation is the standard treatment for patients with progressive, irreversible acute or chronic liver disease for which there are no other medical or surgical options. Alcohol-associated liver disease and liver disease due to nonalcoholic steatohepatitis are the leading indications for the transplant waiting list, whereas the proportions of acute liver failure, cholestatic liver disease, and HCV have declined.[30] Patients with hepatocellular carcinoma (HCC) have nearly doubled over the past decade, comprising 10.9% of new waiting list registrations in 2020.[15] There are over 10,000 candidates on the national waiting list for liver transplantation.[2] In 2022, 9,528 liver transplants were performed, with 603 from living donors. Short- and long-term outcomes after liver transplantation continue to improve. For transplants performed in 2019, graft failure occurred in 5.9% of deceased donor recipients at 6 months and 7.9% at 1 year.[30]

Living and expanded criteria donors are more widely accepted as potential options for patients in need of a liver transplant. Expanded criteria include patients of advanced age, livers recovered from DCD donors, and livers with steatosis or intrahepatic fat.[15] The number of living donor transplants has increased slowly over the past 2 decades.[30] The increase in living donors has been largely driven by a rise in the number of unrelated directed donors (see Table 5.1).[15] Other efforts to increase the number of recipients include reduced-size liver (living donor left lobe) and split-liver (one liver divided between an adult and a child) transplantation.

CASE STUDY

A 36-year-old patient has prolonged cardiopulmonary arrest after a fall from 8 m. Return of spontaneous circulation was achieved on scene, where IV access was established and the patient was intubated. The patient remained unconscious in transit to the emergency department (ED). Neurologic assessment revealed pupils dilated at 5 mm and sluggish in response to light; myoclonic movements; and preserved but decreased cough, gag, and corneal reflexes. Urgent head computed tomography (CT) was significant for severe, diffuse cerebral edema and compression of the ventricles.

During the late evening hours of hospital day 2, the patient became hypertensive and bradycardic, then the blood pressure dropped precipitously to a mean arterial pressure of 58 mm Hg despite maximal dosing of vasopressors. Neurologic evaluation revealed pupils fixed and dilated and absent cough, gag, and corneal reflexes. The critical nature of the patient's condition was discussed with the family, and the concept of potential brain death was introduced by the multiprofessional team. The family had many questions about treatment, injury, and prognosis, as well as the meaning of "brain death." The OPO coordinator was contacted.

Clinical brain death/death by neurologic criteria examinations were performed on hospital day 3. Clinical examination findings were consistent with brain death, and the patient was pronounced dead according to neurologic criteria at that time. The multiprofessional team communicated with the family throughout the testing process.

Once the family members understood what brain death meant, the OPO designated requestor discussed the option of organ donation with the family. The patient's family authorized organ donation, seeing it as a way to have something positive come from this painful tragedy.

Questions

1. What assessment findings are most significant and indicative of potential brain death?
2. What interventions are a priority to maintain cardiovascular stability?
3. With a deteriorating neurologic examination, determine the three indications that are appropriate to begin formal brain death/death by neurologic criteria determination.
4. If the patient was unable to tolerate apnea testing and became hemodynamically unstable during testing, what alternative testing could the nurse recommend? Describe these tests, as well as their advantages and disadvantages.
5. Review the benefits and potential outcomes of separating discussions of brain death from those of organ donation.

KEY POINTS

- The Uniform Anatomical Gift Act established a legal framework for individuals to authorize an anatomical gift of their organs, tissues, and eyes after death.
- Solid organ transplantation is the only definitive treatment for patients with end-organ disease; unfortunately, donor organs are scarce, despite national efforts to increase donation.
- The critical care nurse should be aware of the clinical triggers for organ donation as established by their OPO, which may include the loss of neurological reflexes, a low Glasgow Coma Scale score, discussion of withdrawing or ceasing life support, consulting palliative care, referral to hospice, or family members initiating a discussion about donation.
- Organ donation occurs in one of three donor types: living donor, brain dead donor, or donation after circulatory death.
- Living donors complete a full medical and psychosocial evaluation to ensure they are appropriate for donation and that they are not being coerced.
- Criteria for BD/DNC include permanent coma, absence of reflexes, and apnea. Once brain death is declared and the family is aware of the diagnosis, the OPO designated requestor approaches the family to discuss organ donation.
- DCD is an option for patients with a grave prognosis whose end-of-life care involves compassionate extubation and whose death is expected to occur within a specified time frame postextubation.
- Authorization for organ donation is obtained either through first-person authorization for donation or from the legal authorized representative.
- Donor families have unique needs that require support from the critical care team and the OPO.
- Evaluation of a potential donor is a strenuous process that requires an accurate history and thorough physical exam.
- Brain death leads to several hormonal, metabolic, and systemic changes that may require volume, electrolyte, and hormone replacement and vasopressor support to preserve the organs.
- Regardless of the donor type, organs have a limited time they can be out of the body; therefore timely and efficient recovery is paramount.
- Each organ has unique donor criteria, and transplantation of each organ has varying success and survivability.

REFERENCES

1. Health Resources and Services Administration. Organ Donation Statistics. https://www.organdonor.gov/learn/organ-donation-statistics. Updated March 2022. Accessed January 27, 2023.
2. Build advanced - OPTN. Organ Procurement and Transplantation Network. https://optn.transplant.hrsa.gov/data/view-data-reports/build-advanced/. Accessed November 17, 2023.
3. Anwar AS, Lee JM. Medical management of brain-dead organ donors. *Acute Crit Care*. 2019;34(1):14–29. https://doi.org/10.4266/acc.2019.00430.
4. Health Resources and Services Administrations' Federal Advisory Council. U.S. Department of Health and Human Services. U.S. Department of Health and Human Services Recommendations 19-28. https://www.hrsa.gov/advisory-committees/organ-transplantation/recommendations/19-28. Updated June 2021. Accessed March 9, 2023.
5. Organ procurement organizations: Increasing organ donations. UNOS. https://unos.org/transplant/opos-increasing-organ-donation/. Published January 11, 2022. Accessed September 29, 2022.
6. Policies. Organ Procurement and Transplantation Network. https://optn.transplant.hrsa.gov/media/eavh5bf3/optn_policies.pdf. Accessed September 29, 2022.
7. *Organ Procurement Organizations (OPO) Agreements with Hospitals*. Centers for Medicare and Medicaid Services; 2013. CMS Quality Safety and Oversight Memo 13-48-OPO. Accessed. https://www.cms.gov/Medicare/Provider-Enrollment-and-Certification/SurveyCertificationGenInfo/Policy-and-Memos-to-States-and-Regions-Items/Survey-and-Cert-Letter-13-48. Accessed September 29, 2022.
8. Donate Life America. Living donation. https://www.donatelife.net/types-of-donation/living-donation/. Published August 25, 2021. Accessed September 29, 2022.
9. Greer DM, Kirschen MP, Lewis A, et al. Pediatric and adult brain death/death by neurologic criteria consensus guideline: report of the AAN Guidelines Subcommittee, AAP, CNS, and SCCM. *Neurology*. 2023. https://doi.org/10.1212/WNL.0000000000207740. [published online ahead of print, 2023 Oct 11].
10. Greer DM, Shemie SD, Lewis A, et al. Determination of brain death/death by neurologic criteria: The World Brain Death Project. *JAMA*. 2020;324(11):1078–1097. https://doi.org/10.1001/jama.2020.11586.
11. Chandler JA, Connors M, Holland G, Shemie SD. "Effective" requesting: a scoping review of the literature on asking families to consent to organ and tissue donation. *Transplantation*. 2017;101(5S Suppl 1):S1–S16. https://doi.org/10.1097/TP.0000000000001695.
12. Shemie SD, Robertson A, Beitel J, et al. End-of-life conversations with families of potential donors: leading practices in offering the opportunity for organ donation. *Transplantation*. 2017;101(5S Suppl 1):S17–S26. https://doi.org/10.1097/TP.0000000000001696.
13. Potter KF, Cocchiola B, Quader MA. Donation after circulatory death: opportunities on the horizon. *Curr Opin Anaesthesiol*. 2021;34(2):168–172. https://doi.org/10.1097/ACO.0000000000000960.
14. Egan TM, Haithcock BE, Lobo J, et al. Donation after circulatory death donors in lung transplantation. *J Thorac Dis*. 2021;13(11):6536–6549. https://doi.org/10.21037/jtd-2021-13.
15. Ahmed O, Doyle MBM. Liver transplantation: expanding the donor and recipient pool. *Chin Clin Oncol*. 2021;10(1):6. https://doi.org/10.21037/cco-20-212.
16. Woolley AE, Singh SK, Goldberg HJ, et al. Heart and lung transplants from HCV-infected donors to uninfected recipients. *N Engl J Med*. 2019;380(17):1606–1617. https://doi.org/10.1056/NEJMoa1812406.
17. Kumar L. Brain death and care of the organ donor. *J Anaesthesiol Clin Pharmacol*. 2016;32(2):146–152. https://doi.org/10.4103/0970-9185.168266.

18. Yu WS, Son J. Donor Selection, Management, and Procurement for Lung Transplantation. *J Chest Surg*. 2022;55(4):277–282. https://doi.org/10.5090/jcs.22.068.
19. Lazzeri C, Bonizzoli M, Guetti C, Fulceri GE, Peris A. Hemodynamic management in brain dead donors. *World J Transplant*. 2021;11(10):410–420. https://doi.org/10.5500/wjt.v11.i10.410. PMID: 34722170; PMCID: PMC8529942.
20. Reich DJ, Mulligan DC, Abt PL, et al. ASTS recommended practice guidelines for controlled donation after cardiac death organ procurement and transplantation. *Am J Transplant*. 2009;9(9):2004–2011. https://doi.org/10.1111/j.1600-6143.2009.02739.
21. Jones JM, Kracalik I, Levi ME, et al. Assessing solid organ donors and monitoring transplant recipients for Human Immunodeficiency Virus, Hepatitis B Virus, and Hepatitis C Virus Infection - U.S. Public Health Service Guideline, 2020. *MMWR Recomm Rep*. 2020;69(4):1–16. https://doi.org/10.15585/mmwr.rr6904a1.
22. Wolfe CR, Ison MG, AST Infectious Diseases Community of Practice. Donor-derived infections: Guidelines from the American Society of Transplantation Infectious Diseases Community of Practice. *Clin Transplant*. 2019;33(9):e13547. https://doi.org/10.1111/ctr.13547.
23. Leard LE, Holm AM, Valapour M, et al. Consensus document for the selection of lung transplant candidates: an update from the International Society for Heart and Lung Transplantation. *J Heart Lung Transplant*. 2021;40(11):1349–1379. https://doi.org/10.1016/j.healun.2021.07.005.
24. Chambers DC, Zuckermann A, Cherikh WS, et al. The International Thoracic Organ Transplant Registry of the International Society for Heart and Lung Transplantation: 37th adult lung transplantation report - 2020; focus on deceased donor characteristics. *J Heart Lung Transplant*. 2020;39(10):1016–1027. https://doi.org/10.1016/j.healun.2020.07.009.
25. Valapour M, Lehr CJ, Skeans MA, et al. OPTN/SRTR 2020 annual data report: lung. *Am J Transplant*. 2022;22(Suppl 2):438–518. https://doi.org/10.1111/ajt.16991.
26. Costa J, Benvenuto LJ, Sonett JR. Long-term outcomes and management of lung transplant recipients. *Best Pract Res Clin Anaesthesiol*. 2017;31(2):285–297. https://doi.org/10.1016/j.bpa.2017.05.006.
27. Lentine KL, Smith JM, Hart A, et al. OPTN/SRTR 2020 Annual data report: kidney. *Am J Transplant*. 2022;22(Suppl 2):21–136. https://doi.org/10.1111/ajt.16982.
28. Mehra MR, Canter CE, Hannan MM, et al. The 2016 International Society for Heart Lung Transplantation listing criteria for heart transplantation: a 10-year update. *J Heart Lung Transplant*. 2016;35(1):1–23. https://doi.org/10.1016/j.healun.2015.10.023.
29. Colvin M, Smith JM, Ahn Y, et al. OPTN/SRTR 2020 Annual Data Report: heart. *Am J Transplant*. 2022;22(Suppl 2):350–437. https://doi.org/10.1111/ajt.16977.
30. Kwong AJ, Ebel NH, Kim WR, et al. OPTN/SRTR 2020 Annual Data Report: liver. *Am J Transplant*. 2022;22(Suppl 2):204–309. https://doi.org/10.1111/ajt.16978.

6

Comfort and Sedation

Mamoona Arif Rahu, PhD, MSN, RN, CCRN, TCRN

INTRODUCTION

Critically ill patients often have alterations in comfort secondary to pain, agitation, and delirium. The patient's perception, expression, and tolerance of pain, agitation, and delirium vary because of different psychological, social, and cultural influences. Often interrelated, pain, agitation, and delirium may be difficult to differentiate because the physiological and behavioral findings can be similar. The relationship between pain and agitation is cyclical, with each exacerbating the other.[1,2] Pain that is inadequately treated leads to greater agitation, and agitation is associated with higher pain intensity. Agitation contributes to the perception of pain by activating pain pathways, altering the cognitive evaluation of pain, increasing aversion to pain, and increasing the reports of pain. If pain and agitation are unresolved and escalate, the patient often experiences feelings of powerlessness, suffering, and psychological changes such as delirium.[3] In addition, pain, agitation, and delirium can lead to patient morbidity and increased length of hospital stay.[2,4,5] Therefore, it is important for healthcare providers to assess and manage signs and symptoms appropriately.

The American College of Critical Care Medicine/Society of Critical Care Medicine (SCCM) has updated comprehensive guidelines for integrated, evidence-based, and patient-centered protocols for preventing and treating pain, agitation/sedation, delirium, immobility, and sleep disruption (PADIS) in critically ill adult patients.[1] The PADIS guidelines have been successfully integrated into the elements of the care bundle to facilitate the **A**ssessment, prevention, and management of pain; **B**oth spontaneous awakening and breathing trials; **C**hoosing the appropriate analgesia and sedation; **D**elirium monitoring and management; **E**arly exercise and mobility (rehabilitation), and **F**amily engagement, commonly known as the ICU Liberation Bundle *(A-F bundle)* (Table 6.1).[1,6] The committee recommends the use of validated tools and assessments, nonpharmacological and pharmacological therapies, and coordinating care that aligns patients' goals. This chapter focuses on these evidence-based assessment, prevention, and management strategies for the critically ill patient experiencing acute pain, agitation, delirium, or a combination of the three.

DEFINITIONS

Pain

Pain is a subjective experience leading to variable tolerability; therefore, the patient is the true authority on the pain that is being experienced. A revised definition of pain from the International Association for the Study of Pain considers biological, psychological, and social well-being in an individual's pain experience (Box 6.1).[7]

Agitation

Agitation is a state marked by aggression, intense sensation of unease, disorganized thinking, and an inability to cope with overstimulation.[8,9] Patients exhibit signs of increased emotional distress, restlessness or thrashing, combative or violent behavior, and pulling or removing devices that interfere with care and place themselves and others at potential risk for harm. Agitation is not a benign state, and unrelieved agitation leads to greater morbidity and mortality, especially after critical illness.[10,11]

Delirium

Delirium (acute brain dysfunction) is characterized by an acutely changing or fluctuating mental status, inattention, disorganized thinking, and altered levels of consciousness. Categorized according to the level of alertness and level of psychomotor activity, delirium is divided into three clinical subtypes: hyperactive, hypoactive, and mixed (Table 6.2).

Patients with *hyperactive delirium* are agitated, disoriented, combative, and have increased motor movement (e.g., picking or pulling on medical equipment).[12] These patients place themselves or others at risk of injury because of their altered thought processes and resultant behaviors. Psychotic features such as hallucinations, delusions, and paranoia may be observed. Patients may believe that members of the nursing or medical staff are attempting to harm them. Though the most easily recognized, the prevalence of hyperactive delirium is less common than the following two subtypes, with a prevalence of 4% in the critically ill population.[13]

Hypoactive delirium is often referred to as quiet delirium, as patients are characterized by a lack of motor movement, the absence of behavioral problems, and a perceived cooperativeness. Without active monitoring via a validated clinical instrument, these patients are often undiagnosed and underestimated. It is also the most prevalent subtype, occurring in more than 17% of critical care patients.[12]

The *mixed subtype* describes the fluctuating nature of delirium. Some agitated patients with hyperactive delirium may receive sedatives to calm them and then may emerge from

TABLE 6.1 A-F Bundle

Assess, prevent, and manage pain	• Patient's self-report of pain is the gold standard.
	• Use validated behavioral pain scales when the patient is unable to self-report pain:
	  o Behavioral Pain Scale (BPS)
	  o Critical-Care Pain Observation Tool (CPOT)
	• Pain should be treated before a sedative agent is considered.
	• Use pharmacological and nonpharmacological measures to achieve pain management goals.

Both spontaneous awakening trial (SAT) and spontaneous breathing trial (SBT)	• The coordination of SAT and SBT requires a collaborative approach among providers, nurses, respiratory therapists, and pharmacists to assess the patient and administer the appropriate type and amount of sedation, safely allow the patient to wake up daily, and evaluate the patient's ability to breathe independently of the ventilator. • Decrease sedatives until the patient is responsive. • Complete the SAT screen. If the patient passes the screening, perform the SAT. • Complete the SBT safety screen. If the patient passes the screening, perform the SBT. • If the patient passes the SBT, consider extubation.

Choice of analgesia and sedation	• Treat pain first. Use the patient's self-report or validated behavioral pain scales to assess and manage pain.
	• Use standardized tools to assess and manage sedation:
	  o Richmond Agitation-Sedation Scale (RASS)
	  o Sedation-Agitation Scale (SAS)
	• Promote comfort by ensuring adequate pain control, anxiolysis, and prevention and treatment of delirium.
	• Use both pharmacological and nonpharmacological interventions. Identify target goals for analgesia and sedation.

Delirium assessment and management	• Monitor patient throughout the day (before and after SAT) for the presence of delirium.
	• Use validated tools to assess for delirium:
	  o Confusion Assessment Method for the ICU
	  o Intensive Care Delirium Screening Checklist
	• Identify and treat cause(s) of delirium or altered mental status:
	  o Infection or sepsis
	  o Dehydration, hypoglycemia
	  o Sleep deprivation
	  o Alcohol, benzodiazepine, or home medication withdrawal
	  o Medications: anticholinergics, benzodiazepines, opiates, steroids
	• Treat with nonpharmacological measures first:
	  o Decrease nighttime disturbances to enhance sleep.
	  o Increase mobility efforts (physical-occupational therapy).
	  o Allow patient to use eyeglasses and hearing aids.
	  o Encourage interactions with family and friends.

Early mobility and exercise	• Collaborate with respiratory, physical, and occupational therapists to develop a mobility protocol. • Evaluate and assess all patients for progressive mobility needs. • Begin with passive range of motion and progress activity as tolerated to the patient's highest level of mobility. • Use available assist devices as needed.
Family engagement and empowerment	• Engage the family early and often in the patient's plan of care.

Adapted from Barr J, Fraser GL, Puntillo K et al. American College of Critical Care Medicine. Clinical practice guidelines for the management of pain, agitation, and delirium in adult patients in the intensive care unit. *Crit Care Med.* 2013;41(1):263-306.; Devlin JW, Skrobik Y, Gelinas C et al. Clinical practice guidelines for the prevention and management of pain, agitation/sedation, delirium, immobility, and sleep disruption in adult patients in the ICU. *Crit Care Med.* 2018;46:e825-e873.

sedation in a hypoactive state. This subtype of delirium occurs in approximately 10% of critical care patients.[13]

PHYSIOLOGY

Physiology of Pain

All pain results from a signal cascade within the body's neurological network. Pain is initiated by signals that travel through the peripheral nervous system to the central nervous system (CNS) for processing.[14] Pain is classified as *acute, chronic,* or *acute on chronic; malignant* or *nonmalignant;* and *nociceptive* or *neuropathic.* In all forms of acute pain, the sympathetic nervous system (SNS) is activated quickly, and several physiological responses occur (Box 6.2). In contrast, some forms of chronic pain may result in less activation of the SNS and a different clinical presentation, such as degenerative changes (i.e., arthritis), sensory abnormalities (i.e., neuropathies), and psychosocial stressors (i.e., depression, posttraumatic stress disorder [PTSD], poor social support).[15]

The sensation of pain is carried to the CNS by activation of two separate pathways (Fig. 6.1). The fast (i.e., sharp, acute) pain signals are transmitted to the spinal cord by rapidly conducting, thinly myelinated A-delta fibers. A-delta fibers are activated by high-intensity physical (i.e., hot and cold) stimuli that are important in initiating rapid reactions and reflex withdrawal. Conversely,

BOX 6.1 Revised IASP Definition of Pain

Pain

An unpleasant sensory and emotional experience associated with, or resembling that associated with, actual or potential tissue damage.

- Pain is always a personal experience that is influenced to varying degrees by biological, psychological, and social factors.
- Pain and nociception are different phenomena. Pain cannot be inferred solely from activity in sensory neurons.
- Through their life experiences, individuals learn the concept of pain.
- A person's report of an experience as pain should be respected.
- Although pain usually serves an adaptive role, it may have adverse effects on physical function, as well as social and psychological well-being.
- Verbal description is only one of several behaviors used to express pain; inability to communicate does not negate the possibility that a person experiences pain.

Adapted from Raja SN, Carr DB, Cohen M et al. The revised International Association for the Study of Pain definition of pain: concepts, challenges, and compromises. *Pain.* 2020;161(9):1976-1982.

TABLE 6.2 Clinical Subtypes of Delirium

Subtype	Characteristics
Hyperactive	Agitation Restlessness Attempts to remove catheters or tubes Hitting Biting Emotional lability
Hypoactive	Withdrawal Flat affect Apathy Lethargy Decreased responsiveness
Mixed	Concurrent or sequential appearance of some features of both hyperactive and hypoactive delirium

BOX 6.2 Physiological Responses to Pain and Agitation

- Constipation
- Cool extremities
- Diaphoresis
- Hypertension
- Increased cardiac output
- Increased glucose production (gluconeogenesis)
- Mydriasis (pupillary dilation)
- Nausea
- Pallor and flushing
- Sleep disturbance
- Tachycardia
- Tachypnea
- Urinary retention

slow (i.e., burning, chronic) pain is transmitted by the unmyelinated, polymodal C fibers, which are activated by a variety of high-intensity mechanical, chemical, hot, and cold stimuli.[16]

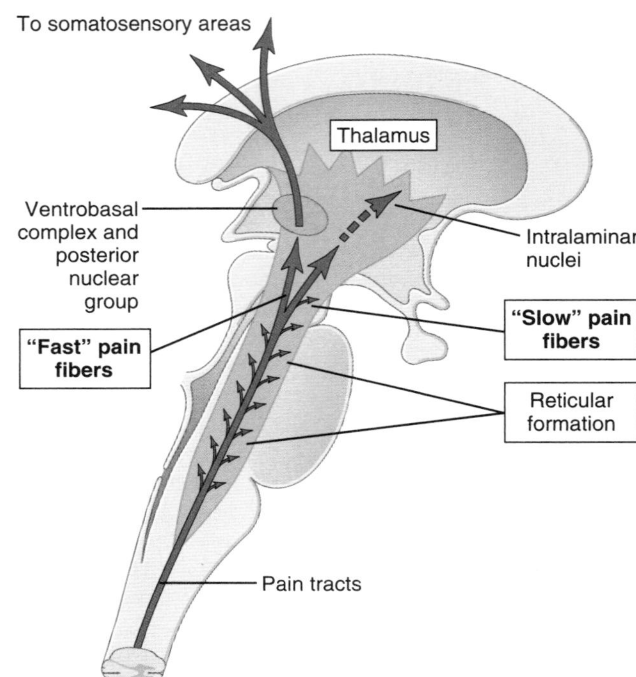

Fig. 6.1 Transmission of pain signals into the brainstem, thalamus, and cerebral cortex by way of the "fast" pain pathway and "slow" pain pathway. (From Guyton A, Hall J. *Textbook of Medical Physiology.* 14th ed. Philadelphia, PA: Saunders; 2021.)

The most abundant receptors in the nervous system for pain recognition are nociceptors, whose cell bodies are in the dorsal root ganglia. The sensation of pain received by peripheral endings of sensory neurons is called *nociception.* The nociceptive pain is divided into somatic and visceral. Nociceptive pain is detected by specialized transducers attached to A-delta and C fibers. *Somatic pain* results from irritation or damage to the nervous system that is well localized. *Visceral pain* is diffuse, poorly localized, and often referred.

Nociceptors differ from other nerve receptors in the body in that they adapt very little to the pain response. If the stimulus for pain is not removed, the body continues to experience pain until the stimulus is discontinued or other interventions (e.g., analgesic agents) are initiated. This is a protective mechanism so that the body tissues being damaged are removed from harm. Identifying the correct pain-inducing stimulus is important in the effective management of pain, and removal of the stimulus should always precede other treatment measures. If pain is not effectively managed, the brain can activate the "fight or flight" response, leading to increased agitation and restlessness.

CHECK YOUR UNDERSTANDING

1. A patient with a history of alcohol use disorder reports a sudden onset of severe epigastric pain that radiates to their back. Based on assessment findings, determine the type of pain the patient is experiencing:
   A. Visceral pain
   B. Somatic pain
   C. Neuropathic pain
   D. A-delta pain

Physiology of Agitation

The neurobiology of the agitation pathway is a more complex process, because no actual tissue injury is thought to occur. Agitation is a behavior that is regulated by multiple brain regions, including the cortex, basal ganglia, thalamus, and limbic system. These regions interact to generate and regulate arousal, attention, and emotional behavioral responses.[17,18]

In a healthy person, agitation is an adaptive mechanism used to increase mental and physical performance levels to allow a person to move away from potential harm. When the SNS is activated, the person becomes more vigilant of the environment, especially to potential dangers. Once dangers are recognized, the person makes a choice whether to flee the situation or combat the possible threat (i.e., "fight-or-flight" response).

Physiology of Delirium

The exact pathophysiological mechanisms involved in the development and progression of delirium are unknown; however, acute delirium is common in critically ill patients with an incidence of approximately 22% and a prevalence of 31%. Mechanically ventilated patients are at even greater risk for acquiring delirium.[13] Untreated delirium may result in longer duration of mechanical ventilation, longer critical care unit and hospital stay, and increased rates of self-extubation compared to those of patients without delirium.[13,19]

Risk factors specific to the development of delirium in the critical care unit include coma, preexisting dementia, history of hypertension or alcoholism, and a high severity of illness at admission (i.e., hypoxemia, metabolic disturbances, electrolyte imbalances, head trauma).[6,19–22] Evidence indicates patient risk for delirium doubles when on mechanical ventilation for more than 24 hours.[20] Older patients are especially at risk for delirium.[12,23] Medications with anticholinergic properties, benzodiazepines, opioids, and other psychotropic medications are associated with an increased risk of developing delirium, yet these medications are commonly given to critically ill patients.[23]

 **CLINICAL JUDGMENT ACTIVITY**

Determine key assessment characteristics and behaviors observed in each of the delirium subtypes.

1. Hyperactive
2. Hypoactive
3. Mixed

PATHOPHYSIOLOGY OF PAIN, AGITATION, AND DELIRIUM

Physical

Pain is a common cause of agitation in critically ill patients. Pain stimulates the release of stress hormones and can activate the SNS, leading to an increase in heart rate, blood pressure, and agitation. Catecholamine levels increase, which may place a significant burden on the cardiovascular system, especially in a critically ill patient. Activation of the SNS results in tachycardia and hypertension, which leads to increased myocardial oxygen demand. Recurrent cardiac events and increased level of agitation have a bidirectional impact, meaning uncontrolled agitation may exacerbate cardiovascular disease, or vice versa.[24]

Pain, agitation, and delirium can cause hyperventilation (tachypnea) that can be stressful to the patient, because rapid breathing requires significant effort with the use of accessory muscles. Hyperventilation may cause respiratory alkalosis, resulting in impaired tissue perfusion. If the patient is mechanically ventilated, an increased respiratory rate leads to feelings of breathlessness. As the patient "fights" the mechanical ventilator (dyssynchrony), further alveolar damage ensues, and the endotracheal or tracheostomy tube creates a "choking" sensation and increased agitation.

A frequent issue in mechanically ventilated patients is dyspnea, which is often underrecognized and undertreated by healthcare providers. Dyspnea is highly associated with agitation and pain and may be improved by managing the underlying condition, adjusting the ventilator settings, and administering bronchodilators or opioids.[10,25,26]

Psychological

Many critically ill patients report feelings of panic and fear.[27,28] Pain and agitation exacerbate reports of lack of sleep; nightmares; and feelings of bewilderment, isolation, and loneliness. Approximately half of critically ill patients recall having pain, anxiety, and fear as stressful experiences during their hospitalization in the critical care unit.[9,10,29] In addition, the presence of comorbid conditions such as delirium, substance abuse, and withdrawal can exacerbate the response to pain and increase the likelihood of agitation.

Delirium has been associated with sleep disturbances, abnormal psychomotor activity, and emotional disturbances (i.e., fear, anxiety, anger, depression, apathy, euphoria).[1,23,30] Unrecognized and untreated delirium is a predictor of negative clinical outcomes in critically ill patients, including increased mortality, critical care unit and hospital length of stay, cost of care, and long-term cognitive impairment consistent with a dementia-like state.[30,31]

ASSESSMENTS

Assessment of Pain

Quality pain management begins with a thorough assessment, ongoing reassessment, and documentation to facilitate treatment and communication among healthcare providers. Pain assessment is challenging in patients who cannot communicate. Factors that can alter the ability to communicate in critically ill patients include endotracheal intubation, altered level of consciousness, restraints, sedation, and neuromuscular blockade.

The PADIS guidelines recommend evaluation of both physiological and behavioral responses to pain in patients who are unable to communicate. Optimal pain assessment in adult critical care settings is essential, because nurses often underrate and undermedicate the patient's pain. Inaccurate pain assessments and resulting inadequate treatment of pain in critically ill adults can lead to significant physiological consequences.[1]

The "gold standard" for assessing pain is the patient's self-report of the pain experience. If a patient can respond, ask the patient to describe the pain being experienced or to provide a numeric score to indicate the level of pain. Observe signs of agitation such as restlessness or physiological cues of pain. Typical physiological responses related to pain are detailed in Box 6.2. In a healthy person, these responses are adaptive mechanisms and result from activation of the SNS.

As part of the assessment of pain, consider premedication, note what procedures cause pain, and evaluate the effectiveness of interventions to prevent or relieve pain. Implement nonpharmacological interventions such as reorientation and reassurance. When possible, ask patients about any use of herbal remedies, complementary and alternative medical therapies, prescription or over-the-counter medications, medical cannabis, or illicit drugs to treat chronic pain. These products may lead to adverse drug interactions, especially in older adults who are more likely to be taking multiple medications.

Pain Measurement Tools for Patients Who Can Communicate. To assess pain, ask the patient to identify several characteristics associated with the pain: precipitating factors, severity, location (including radiation to other sites), duration, and any alleviating or aggravating factors.

One of the most common methods used to determine pain severity is the Numeric Rating Scale, in which the patient is asked to rate their pain on a scale from 0 to 10 (administered either verbally or visually). A score of 0 indicates no pain, and a score of 10 indicates the worst pain the patient could possibly imagine. Use the pain rating method only with patients who are cognitively aware of their surroundings and can follow simple commands. It is possible for patients with mild-to-moderate dementia to self-report pain, but this ability decreases with progression of the disease. Numeric rating is not an appropriate method to assess pain in patients who are disoriented or have severe cognitive impairment.

Another widely used subjective pain measurement tool is the Visual Analog Scale (VAS). The VAS is a 10-cm line that looks similar to a timeline. The scale may be drawn horizontally or vertically, and it may or may not be numbered. If numbered, 0 indicates no pain, whereas 10 indicates the most pain (Fig. 6.2). To use the VAS, hold up the scale and ask the patient to point to or place an "X" on the line at the location that correlates to their pain level. The VAS can also be used to evaluate a patient's level of anxiety, with 0 representing no anxiety and 10 representing the most anxiety. The VAS is used only with patients who are alert and able to follow directions.

Reassess the pain score after medications or other pain-relieving measures have been provided to evaluate the effectiveness of interventions. Institutional policies provide guidelines for the method and frequency of pain assessment.

It is imperative to identify ways to communicate effectively with patients who have limited communication abilities. Several writing tablets and computer applications (apps) are available for patients to use to communicate their pain level. The Patient Communicator app by the SCCM[32] was designed to assist critical care providers to communicate with patients who are unable to speak because of mechanical ventilation, hearing loss, or speech limitations. The Patient Communicator app allows patients to identify where on the body they are feeling sensations, as well as the severity of those sensations.

Pain Measurement Tools for Patients Unable to Communicate. Assessment of pain in a noncommunicative patient requires identification of an optimal pain scale using the behavioral-physiological tools. The PADIS guidelines recommend use of behavioral assessment tools in critically ill adults unable to self-report pain and in whom behaviors are observable. Vital signs are not valid indicators for pain and should be used only as cues to initiate further assessment.

Observe behaviors using either the Behavioral Pain Scale in intubated (BPS)[33] or nonintubated (BPS-NI)[34] patients or the Critical-Care Pain Observation Tool (CPOT) for either population.[35] Both tools demonstrate the greatest validity and reliability for monitoring pain in noncommunicative patients.[1,6] As appropriate, involve the family in the pain assessment process.

Widely used and validated, the BPS was developed to assess pain in the critically ill adult who is nonverbal and unable to communicate (Table 6.3). The BPS, comprising the original BPS and the BPS-NI, includes three behavioral indicators: facial expression, movement of upper limbs, and compliance with ventilation for intubated patients or vocalization for nonintubated patients. Each indicator is rated from 1 to 4, with a total BPS score ranging from 3 to 12 and a score greater than 5 indicating significant pain.[6]

The CPOT (Table 6.4) includes four behavioral categories: facial expression, body movements, muscle tension, and compliance with the ventilator for intubated patients or vocalization for extubated patients. Items in each category are scored from 0 to 2, with a total CPOT score ranging from 0 to 8; scores greater than 2 indicate significant pain (see Clinical Exemplar box).[6]

CHECK YOUR UNDERSTANDING

2. A patient was admitted to the critical care unit after coronary artery bypass grafting. As they emerge from anesthesia, the patient is agitated, not making eye contact, and unresponsive to questions. What is the appropriate tool to assess the patient's pain?
   A. Critical-Care Pain Observation Tool
   B. FACES Scale
   C. Visual Analog Scale
   D. Numeric pain scale

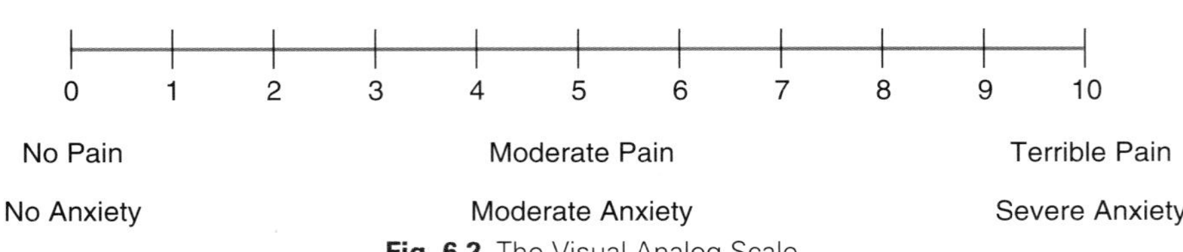

Fig. 6.2 The Visual Analog Scale.

CLINICAL EXEMPLAR

Person-Centered Care

In a 24-bed trauma critical care unit, a nurse recognized the challenges of assessing pain in the intubated patient who was unable to communicate. After discussing with other members of the team, the nurse identified that many were struggling to effectively assess pain in this population, and each person had their own approach and triggers for treating pain. In addition, the current pain management order sets used vital signs to trigger administration of as-needed pain medications in this population. The nurses were wary of this practice, as vital signs can be altered by other medications and treatments provided in the critical care unit.

A multiprofessional workgroup was assembled to investigate solutions to the problems identified. After reviewing the literature and seeking feedback from other unit team members, the Critical-Care Pain Observation Tool (CPOT) was selected for implementation. The CPOT was built into the electronic health record, and the pain management order sets were updated to reflect this new tool as a reason for administration of pain medications. If the CPOT total score was greater than 2, the nurse was able to administer the lowest effective dose of the ordered pain medication. If after 15 minutes, the CPOT score remained greater than 2, the nurse could repeat the same dose of pain medication. A premedication dose was also added to the order set, allowing the nurse to premedicate the patient prior to pain-producing activities (i.e. repositioning, suctioning, mobility). An education plan was developed to train nurses on how to use the CPOT and the new pain management order set. The education plan included videos, pocket cards, and in-person education.

At the next team meeting, the nurses and other multiprofessional team members discussed how they felt empowered to effectively manage pain in patients who are unable to communicate. The nurses felt they were using less sedation, as they were able to better recognize when their patients are in pain. The team members were excited and wanted to implement another practice change so that they could continue to improve the care of their severely injured patient population.

CLINICAL JUDGMENT ACTIVITY

Differentiate between subjective and objective tools when assessing pain and provide examples of each.

Assessment of Agitation and Sedation

Agitation typically produces hyperactive psychomotor functions, including tachycardia, hypertension, and movement. Patients are usually sedated to limit this hyperactivity, as it often interferes with the ability to effectively care for the patient. The goal is to maintain light levels of sedation, which are associated with shorter mechanical ventilation duration and critical care unit length of stay.[1] By using lower doses of medications, the patient is less likely to experience medication accumulation or adverse effects. These adverse effects include longer hospital stays, delayed ventilator weaning, immobility, increased rates of ventilator-associated pneumonia, and a higher incidence of delirium.[1,6,36,37] The level of sedation can be measured using objective tools or scales to monitor depth of sedation and brain function. An ideal sedation scale is simple to compute and record, accurately describes the degree of sedation or agitation within well-defined categories, guides the titration of therapy, and is valid and reliable in both ventilated and nonventilated critically ill patients.

TABLE 6.3 The Behavioral Pain Scale (BPS) for Intubated and Nonintubated Patients

Item	Description	Score
Facial expression	Relaxed	1
	Partially tightened (e.g., brow lowering)	2
	Fully tightened (e.g., eyelid closing)	3
	Grimacing	4
Upper limbs	No movement	1
	Partially bent	2
	Fully bent with finger flexion	3
	Permanently retracted	4
Compliance with mechanical ventilation (intubated)	Tolerating movement	1
	Coughing but tolerating ventilation most of the time	2
	Fighting ventilator	3
	Unable to control ventilation	4
	OR	
Vocalization (nonintubated)	No pain vocalization	1
	Infrequent moaning (≤3/min) and not prolonged (≤3 s)	2
	Frequent moaning (>3/min) or prolonged (>3 s)	3
	Howling or verbal complaints including Ow!, Ouch! or breath-holding	4

From Payen JF, Bru O, Bosson JL etal. Assessing pain in critically ill sedated patients by using a behavioral pain scale. *Crit Care Med.* 2001;29:2258-2263.

CHECK YOUR UNDERSTANDING

3. Activation of the SNS occurs with agitation. Determine which of the following physiological symptoms may occur with agitation:
   A. Drowsiness
   B. Increased heart rate
   C. Decreased respiratory rate
   D. Vertigo

Sedation Measurement Tools. The PADIS guidelines recommend two valid and reliable sedation scales for targeting sedation: the Richmond Agitation-Sedation Scale (RASS)[38] and the Sedation-Agitation Scale (SAS).[1,39] The goal of sedation is to either maintain light levels of sedation or use daily awakening trials to reduce sedative exposure.[1] Ultimately, the appropriate target level of sedation depends on the patient's disease process, the therapeutic interventions required, or the type of mechanical support needed.

The RASS is a 10-point scale, ranging from 4 (combative) through 0 (calm, alert) to −5 (unarousable). The patient is assessed for 30 to 60 seconds in three steps, using discrete criteria (Table 6.5). The RASS is useful in detecting changes in sedation status over consecutive days of hospitalization and correlates with the administered dose of sedative and analgesic medications.[38,40]

The SAS (Table 6.6) describes patient behaviors seen in the continuum of sedation to agitation. Scores range from 1 (unarousable) to 7 (dangerously agitated). Both scales have strong interrater reliability and internal consistency.[6]

TABLE 6.4 Critical-Care Pain Observation Tool

Indicator	Score
Facial Expression	
• Relaxed, no muscle tension	0
• Tense facial muscles (brow lowering, orbit tightening, and levator contraction)	1
• Grimacing with tense facial muscles	2
Body Movements	
• Absence of movements	0
• Protection	1
• Restlessness	2
Muscle Tension in Upper Extremities	
• Relaxed	0
• Tense, rigid	1
• Very tense or rigid	2
Compliance With the Ventilator	
• Tolerating ventilator or movement	0
• Coughing but tolerating ventilator	1
• Fighting ventilator	2
OR	
Nonventilated, Vocalization	
• No sound	0
• Sighing, moaning	1
• Crying out, sobbing	2
Total Score	

Data from Gelinas C, Fillion L, Puntillo KA et al. Validation of critical-care pain observation tool in adult patients. *Am J Crit Care.* 2006;15:420-427.

Continuous Monitoring of Sedation. No technological device provides the bedside nurse with an absolute measurement of the patient's pain or agitation. Although various devices that assess the patient's brain activity are available, guidelines recommend that objective measures of brain function (i.e., electroencephalography [EEG] and Bispectral Index Score [BIS]) be used only in specific populations.[1,6] Continuous electroencephalography (cEEG) monitoring may be used to assess levels of consciousness in patients requiring sedation and in patients with nonconvulsive seizures or elevated intracranial pressures (ICP).[1,41] The cEEG records spontaneous brain activity that originates from the cortical pyramidal cells on the surface of the brain by placing electrodes on the patient's head. The cEEG generally changes from a low-amplitude, high-frequency signal while the patient is awake to a high-amplitude, low-frequency signal when the patient is deeply anesthetized. Monitoring cEEG allows for real-time assessment of brain function; however, it requires specific expertise and is resource and labor intensive.[42]

Proprietary commercial monitors are readily available to aid in the clinical assessment of sedated patients.[41,43,44] These devices include the BIS and the Patient State Index (PSI). These monitors derive different frontal EEG and electromyogram (EMG) frequency bands. They are noninvasive devices indicated for sedation titration in patients receiving deep sedation (RASS <−3) or neuromuscular blockade, as we have limited ways to evaluate depth of sedation in these populations.[1,43,44]

TABLE 6.5 Richmond Agitation-Sedation Scale (RASS)

Term	Score
Combative—Overtly combative or violent; immediate danger to staff	+4
Very agitated—Pulls on or removes tubes or catheters or has aggressive behavior toward staff	+3
Agitated—Frequent nonpurposeful movements; fights ventilator	+2
Restless—Anxious or apprehensive but movements are not aggressive or vigorous	+1
Alert and calm	0
Drowsy—Not fully alert, but has sustained (>10 sec) awakening, with eye contact, to voice[a]	−1
Light sedation—Briefly awakens, (<10 sec) with eye contact, to voice[a]	−2
Moderate sedation—Any movement (but no eye contact) to voice[a]	−3
Deep sedation—No response to voice, but any movement to physical stimulation[a]	−4
Unarousable—No response to voice or physical stimulation	−5

[a]In a loud voice, state patient's name and direct patient to open eyes and look at speaker.

From Sessler CN, Gosnell MS, Grap MJ et al. The Richmond Agitation-Sedation Scale: validity and reliability in adult intensive care unit patients. *Am J Respir Crit Care Med.* 2002;166:1338-1344.

TABLE 6.6 Sedation-Agitation Scale

Score	Characteristic	Examples of Patient's Behavior
7	Dangerously agitated	Pulls at endotracheal tube, tries to remove catheters, climbs over bed rail, strikes at staff, thrashes from side to side
6	Very agitated	Does not calm despite frequent verbal reminding of limits, requires physical restraints, bites endotracheal tube
5	Agitated	Anxious or mildly agitated, attempts to sit up, calms down in response to verbal instructions
4	Calm and cooperative	Calm, awakens easily, follows commands
3	Sedated	Difficult to arouse, awakens to verbal stimuli or gentle shaking but drifts off again, follows simple commands
2	Very sedated	Arouses to physical stimuli but does not communicate or follow commands, may move spontaneously
1	Unarousable	Minimal or no response to noxious stimuli, does not communicate or follow commands

From Riker RR, Fraser GL, Simmons LE et al. Validating the Sedation-Agitation Scale with the Bispectral Index and Visual Analog Scale in adult ICU patients after cardiac surgery. *Intensive Care Med.* 2001;27:853-858.

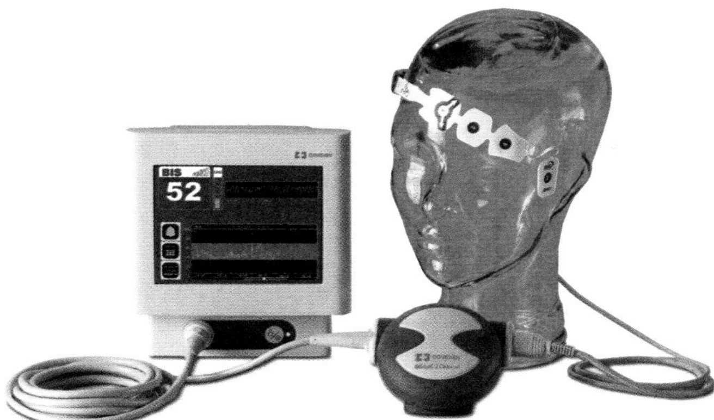

Fig. 6.3 The Bispectral Index Score (BIS) monitor and electrode. (Reproduced with permission from Nellcor Puritan Bennett LLC, Boulder, CO, doing business as Covidien.)

These devices provide a noninvasive, objective analysis of the level of wakefulness. To obtain a signal, four electrodes are placed across the patient's forehead and attached to a monitor (Fig. 6.3). These devices digitize the raw EEG signal and apply a complex algorithm that results in a numeric score ranging from 0 (isoelectric EEG) to 100 (fully awake).[1,43,44] A value greater than 90 typically indicates full consciousness, a score of 40 to 60 represents deep sedation, and a score of 0 represents complete EEG suppression. Studies have shown a moderate-to-strong correlation between BIS and sedation scales when the patient cannot be clinically assessed for depth of sedation; however, the optimal target for the critically ill patient remains unknown based on the current evidence.[43–46]

Assessment of Delirium

All patients in critical care should be assessed for delirium given the risk for its development and the subsequent increase in mortality and morbidity.[1] Two of the most frequently used and validated instruments are the Confusion Assessment Method for the ICU (CAM-ICU)[47] and the Intensive Care Delirium Screening Checklist (ICDSC).[48] The CAM-ICU (Box 6.3) is designed to be a serial assessment tool for use by bedside nurses and providers. It is easy to use, takes only 2 minutes to complete, and requires minimal training. The first step is to assess consciousness using any validated sedation scale; however, the RASS is incorporated into the CAM-ICU, as this was the tool used to validate the instrument. A patient is considered delirium positive on the CAM-ICU if the following are present: acute mental status change (feature 1) and inattention (feature 2), plus either disorganized thinking (feature 3) or an altered level of consciousness (feature 4).[47]

The ICDSC is a screening checklist of eight items based on *Diagnostic and Statistical Manual of Mental Disorders* (DSM) criteria (Table 6.7). After consciousness is assessed, the patient is screened for seven indicators of delirium. The patient is scored throughout the shift, as not all components need to be present at the same time. One point is given for each positive sign of delirium identified. The scores range from 0 to 8 points, and a patient with more than 4 points is defined as delirium positive.[48]

BOX 6.3 Confusion Assessment Method for the Critical Care Unit

Step 1. Level of Consciousness: RASS

Assess RASS. If RASS is ≥–3, proceed to CAM-ICU; otherwise, the patient is "unable to assess" and should be reevaluated later.

Step 2. Content of Consciousness: CAM-ICU

Feature 1: Acute Change or Fluctuating Course of Mental Status

Is the mental status different from baseline?

OR

Has mental status fluctuated in the past 24 hours as evidenced by scores on a sedation/level of consciousness scale (i.e., RASS/SAS), GCS, or previous delirium assessment?

AND

Feature 2: Inattention

Conduct the Letters Attention Test (or Picture Test, available in Training Manual*). Say to the patient, "I am going to read you a series of 10 letters. Whenever you hear the letter 'A,' indicate by squeezing my hand." Read letters 3 seconds apart from one of the following sequences.

S A V E A H A A R T or **C A S A B L A N C A** or **A B A D B A D A A Y**

Errors are counted when patient fails to squeeze on the letter "A" and when the patient squeezes on any letter other than "A." More than 2 errors is considered present.

AND

Feature 3: Altered Level of Consciousness

Considered present if the RASS score is anything other than alert and calm (zero).

OR

Feature 4: Disorganized Thinking

Ask a series of yes/no questions:

1. Will a stone float on water?
2. Are there fish in the sea?
3. Does one pound weigh more than two pounds?
4. Can you use a hammer to pound a nail?
   Errors are counted when the patient incorrectly answers a question.

Ask the patient to follow a two-part simple command:

1. "Hold up this many fingers" (Hold two fingers in front of the patient).
2. "Now, do the same thing with the other hand." If patient is unable to complete the entire command, it is considered an error. If the patient is unable to move both arms, for the second part of the command, ask the patient to "Add one more finger."
   An error is counted if the patient is unable to complete the entire command.

Patient considered positive for delirium when Features 1 and 2 present along with either Feature 3 or 4.

GCS, Glasgow Coma Scale; *RASS*, Richmond Agitation-Sedation Scale; *SAS*, Sedation-Agitation Scale.

*Additional resources, including the Training Manual, can be found at https://www.icudelirium.org/medical-professionals/delirium/monitoring-delirium-in-the-icu.

CLINICAL JUDGMENT ACTIVITY

What factors or characteristics increase the risk of pain, agitation, and delirium in critically ill patients?

TABLE 6.7 Intensive Care Delirium Screening Checklist[a]

Screening	Score
1. **Altered level of consciousness.** a. Deep sedation/coma entire shift (SAS 1, 2; RASS −4, −5) = unable to assess b. Agitation at any time (SAS 5, 6; RASS 1-4) = 1 point c. Normal wakefulness entire shift (SAS 4; RASS 0) = 0 points d. Light sedation (SAS 3; RASS −1, −2, −3) = 1 point (no sedatives) or 0 points (recent sedatives)	____
2. **Inattention.** Difficulty following instructions, easily distracts, does not reliably squeeze hands to spoken letter A (e.g., SAVEAHAART)	____
3. **Disorientation.** Disoriented to person, place, time, situation, caregivers	____
4. **Hallucination-delusion psychosis.** Responds positively to having hallucinations or is afraid of people or things around them	____
5. **Psychomotor agitation or retardation.** Exhibits hyperactivity requiring sedatives or restraints to prevent harm or exhibits hypoactive behaviors	____
6. **Inappropriate speech or mood.** Exhibits inappropriate emotions or interactions, incoherent speech, apathy, or overly demanding behavior	____
7. **Sleep-wake cycle disturbance.** Frequent awakening, less than 4 hours of sleep at night, or sleeping much of the day	____
8. **Symptom fluctuation.** Fluctuation of any of the above over a 24-hour period	____
Total Shift Score (0-8)	____

[a]Assess the patient over the entire shift, as not all behaviors may be present at the same time. Assess level of consciousness first. If the patient is deeply sedated or comatose, the patient is unable to be screened for delirium. Items 1 to 4 require a focused assessment, whereas items 5 to 8 are based on observations throughout the shift. A score of 4 to 8 is positive for delirium.

RASS, Richmond Agitation-Sedation Scale; *SAS*, Sedation-Agitation Scale.

Adapted from Bergeron N, Dubois MJ, Dumont M et al. Intensive Care Delirium Screening Checklist: evaluation of a new screening tool. *Intensive Care Med.* 2001;27:859-864; and screening tools at https://www.icudelirium.org/medical-professionals/delirium/monitoring-delirium-in-the-icu.

MANAGEMENT OF PAIN, AGITATION, AND DELIRIUM

Pain, agitation, and delirium are closely related and can be difficult to differentiate given their similar presentation and assessment findings. The complex interplay of pain, agitation, and delirium requires a multicomponent, multiprofessional approach, and the management strategies for each often overlap.

Nonpharmacologic Management

Nonpharmacological approaches to manage pain, agitation, and delirium should be used early in an effort to avoid or reduce analgesic and sedative requirements and the risk of developing delirium (refer to the Collaborative Care Plan found in Chapter 1, Overview of Critical Care Nursing). Pain, agitation, and delirium are exacerbated by the continuous noise of alarms, equipment, and personnel; bright ambient lighting; and excessive stimulation from inadequate analgesia, frequent assessments, repositioning, lack of mobility, and physical restraints.[1,2,10,34,49]

Nonpharmacological interventions such as environmental manipulation and complementary and alternative therapies can reduce pain, agitation, and the risk of delirium.

Currently, delirium does not have a pharmacological treatment; therefore, the use of multicomponent, nonpharmacological interventions that focus on reducing modifiable risk factors for delirium; improving cognition; and optimizing sleep, mobility, hearing, and vision are vital.[1]

Environmental Manipulation. At times, the critical care environment can feel sterile or hostile to the patient and their family. Interventions to improve the environment consist of frequent patient orientation, family participation, increasing physical activity, avoiding restraints, listening to music, reducing vision and hearing impairments (i.e., eyeglasses, hearing aids), noise reduction, facilitating sleep (i.e., offer eye covers/earplugs), and effective lighting (i.e., natural light during the day, reduced lighting in the evening). Placing calendars and clocks within sight of the patient can assist in reorientating the patient and decrease agitation and confusion.

Altering the patient's room to create a more comforting environment may be beneficial. Ask family members to bring in pictures of family members and other small keepsakes to provide diversions from the stressful critical care environment. Technology, such as tablet computers, can provide another mechanism for sharing photos, music, and virtual chats with loved ones. Depending on a unit's design, position the bed so that it faces a window so the patient can see outside and orient to the time of day. Some critical care units are designed to conceal monitoring equipment behind cabinetry to provide a homelike atmosphere. Patients may benefit from being moved to a different room. Physically moving the patient to a different location prevents the patient from becoming tired of the surroundings, and it may provide some sense of clinical improvement for the patient and family.[50,51]

Use the least restrictive measures when patients are confused or agitated, because unnecessary use of restraints or medication may exacerbate pain, agitation, and delirium. Apply splints, mittens, or binders to restrict movement if the patient is pulling at catheters, drains, or dressings. Remove any type of tubing as soon as possible, particularly nasogastric tubes, which are irritating to agitated patients. If these measures are not successful, medication may be necessary to reduce agitation, but this does not actually treat the delirium.[20]

Family engagement is one of the most important strategies to decrease the patient's pain, agitation, or delirium.[52] The patient's family is often able to interpret patient behaviors for the nursing staff, especially those associated with pain or agitation. Encourage family members to participate in the care whenever the patient's condition allows it (Chapter 2, Patient and Family Response to the Critical Care Experience). Examples of family participation include coaching during breathing exercises, assisting with passive and active range of motion, reorienting the patient, and providing hygiene measures.

Complementary and Alternative Therapy. Four complementary therapies that critical care nurses can independently initiate are guided imagery, music, animal-assisted therapy, and essential oils and aromatherapy.

Guided Imagery. Guided imagery is a mind-body intervention intended to relieve stress and to promote a sense of peace and tranquillity. It involves a form of directed daydreaming that provides relaxation and distraction and purposefully focuses thoughts. Guided imagery is a strategy that all nurses can easily incorporate into their daily practice during most procedures and interventions, such as dressing changes and ventilator weaning. Box 6.4 provides directions on using guided imagery. Combine guided imagery with other complementary therapies to decrease pain and tension.[53] Benefits of a guided imagery program include reduced stress and anxiety, decreased pain and narcotic consumption, decreased length of stay, enhanced sleep, and increased patient satisfaction.[53,54]

Music Therapy. Music therapy offers patients a diversionary technique for pain and agitation. Some institutions have staff members dedicated solely to music therapy. When appropriate, a music therapist comes to the patient's bedside in the critical care unit and offers one-on-one therapy.

Music therapy may be effective in reducing pain and anxiety if patients are able to participate.[53,55] Music therapy is an ideal intervention for patients with low-energy states who fatigue easily, such as those who require ventilatory support, because it does not require the focused concentration necessary for guided imagery. When patients can select their own music, there is a significant reduction in anxiety and sedative exposure during ventilator support.[56,57]

Musical selections without lyrics that contain slow, flowing rhythms that duplicate pulses of 60 to 80 beats/min decrease anxiety in the listener. Music can also provide an alternative focus on a pleasant, comforting stimulus, rather than on stressful environmental stimuli or thoughts. Careful scrutiny of musical selections and of personal preferences for what is considered relaxing is important for success.[58]

Animal-Assisted Therapy. Animal-assisted therapy (AAT) involves interactions between patients and trained animals accompanied by human owners or handlers. This interaction has been shown to alleviate distress through neurohormonal feedback mechanisms.[59] By allowing 15 to 30 minutes of AAT, patients can improve their orientation, increase their attention span, and decrease their risk of delirium.[60] AAT improves the patient's physiological and emotional well-being, builds motivation, reduces anxiety levels, eases suffering, and may reduce cortisol, norepinephrine, and epinephrine levels.[59,60]

Essential Oils and Aromatherapy. Essential oils and aromatherapy are effective when used as an adjunctive therapy for pain management.[61] When the aroma of essential oils stimulates cilia of the nasal passages, an electrical signal is sent to the olfactory bulb causing serotonin, endorphin, and noradrenaline release.[53] In a study of critically ill patients, use of essential oils with lavender and Citrus aurantium resulted in a significant decrease in pain.[61] Essential oils that assist with pain management include lavender, Citrus aurantium, German chamomile, sweet marjoram, dwarf pine, rosemary, and ginger.[61,62] Essential oils and aromatherapy are noninvasive and individualized to the patient's preference. However, ensure that patients do not have allergies or other adverse reactions to scents before using aromatherapy. Review institutional policy for use of aromatherapy prior to initiating this intervention.

BOX 6.4 Practicing Guided Imagery

Have the patient imagine a scenario in which they are on a warm beach, in their favorite place, or with someone they love. Prompt the patient through the following steps:

1. **Get comfortable**—Get into a relaxed position.
2. **Breathe from your belly**—Use diaphragmic deep breathing and close your eyes, focusing on "breathing in peace and breathing out stress." This means letting your belly expand and contract with your breath.
3. **Choose a scene**—Imagine yourself there.
4. **Immerse yourself in sensory details**—Involve all of your senses. What does it look like? How does it feel? What special scents are involved?
5. **Relax**—Enjoy your "surroundings" and let yourself be far from what stresses you.
6. **Returning**—When you're ready to come back to reality, count back from 10 or 20 and tell yourself that when you get to 1, you'll feel serene and alert and enjoy the rest of your day. When you return, you'll feel calmer and refreshed, like returning from a mini-vacation, but you won't have left the room!

Pharmacologic Management

Many critically ill patients require medications to relieve pain, agitation, or both. The appropriate management of pain and agitation may result in improved pulmonary function, earlier ambulation and mobilization, decreased stress response with lower catecholamine concentrations, and lower oxygen consumption, leading to improved outcomes. According to the PADIS guidelines, an assessment-driven protocol should make treating pain a priority over providing sedatives and include clear guidance on medication choice and dosing.[1] Table 6.8 summarizes pharmacological therapies commonly used in the treatment of pain and agitation. At this time, there are no pharmacological interventions to treat delirium; however, medications may be used to help manage the signs and symptoms associated with delirium. Table 6.9 illustrates an order set for pain, agitation, and delirium.

Opioids. Opioids bind to opioid receptors within the body, inactivating the receptors and therefore inhibiting ascending or mitigating descending pain signals as they travel along the nervous system pathways from the periphery, dorsal root ganglion, spinal cord, or brain.[63]

Prior to opioid administration, determine the patient's history of ever receiving an opioid. Opioid-naive patients are at higher risk for oversedation, respiratory depression, and aspiration, especially if they receive opioids in inappropriate dosages

TABLE 6.8 PHARMACOLOGY

Medications Frequently Used in the Treatment of Pain, Agitation, Delirium, and Neuromuscular Blockade[a]

Medication	Action/Use	Dose/Route	Side Effects	Nursing Implications
Opioids				
Fentanyl (Sublimaze [IV], Duragesic [patch])	Opioid; inhibits ascending pain pathway in CNS; ↑ pain threshold; alters pain perception	*Intravenous*: Bolus, 25-100 mcg q1-2h IV *Continuous infusion:* Initial, 25-50 mcg/h IV Maintenance, titrate to clinical end point *Patch:* 12.5-25 mcg/h TD; higher dose may be required every 72 h.	Constipation Decreased gastric motility Muscle rigidity Respiratory depression	Monitor BP, heart rate, and respiratory status. *Patch:* Apply to upper torso. Avoid direct heat (e.g., heating blanket), which accelerates fentanyl release. Apply to a new site q72h. *Antidote*: Naloxone.
Hydromorphone (Dilaudid)	Opioid; inhibits ascending pain pathway in CNS; increases pain threshold; alters pain perception	May be given scheduled or PRN *Oral*: Tablet, 2-4 mg q4-6h Solution, 2.5-10 mg q3-6h *Intravenous*: Bolus, 0.2-1 mg q2-3h IV *Intramuscular/subcutaneous:* 1-2 mg q4-6h	Constipation Decreased gastric motility Hypotension Itching Nausea Respiratory depression Seizures	Monitor BP, heart rate, and respiratory status. Monitor liver function. Administer lower doses in older patients. Hydromorphone high potency injection should never be administered to opioid-naive patients. *Antidote*: Naloxone.
Morphine (Duramorph, MS Contin, Roxanol)	Opioid; depresses pain impulse transmission at spinal-cord level by interacting with opioid receptors	May be given scheduled or PRN *Subcutaneous/Intramuscular:* 2.5-15 mg q2-6h *Oral:* Immediate-release tablets or oral solution, 10-30 mg q3-4h Extended-release tablets, 15-30 mg q8-12h *Rectal:* 10-20 mg q4h *Intravenous:* Bolus, 2.5-15 mg q3-4h over 4-5 min *Continuous infusion:* 0.8-10 mg/h *Epidural:* Initial, injection of 5 mg in lumbar region; may give 1-2 mg more after 1h to a maximum of 10 mg Maintenance, 2-4 mg/24h *Intrathecal:* 0.2-1 mg one time; repeat doses not recommended	Constipation Decreased gastric motility Hypotension Itching or rash Nausea and vomiting Respiratory depression Urinary retention	Titrate infusion slowly. Monitor BP, heart rate, and respiratory status. Administer lower doses in older adults. Gradually taper to avoid withdrawals. Avoid in patients with renal failure due to accumulation and toxicity. *Antidote*: Naloxone.
Oxycodone hydrochloride (Roxicodone, Oxycontin)	Opioid agonist selectively blocking mu receptor; alters pain perception	May be given scheduled or PRN *Oral:* 5-15 mg q 4-6 h, no true maximum dose Extended release capsules are not equivalent to non-extended release tablets	Constipation Drowsiness Gastric upset Respiratory depression	Evaluate renal function as accumulation of effects is possible. Use lower dosages in patients with hepatic impairment. Initiate lower dose with geriatric patients. Take with food *Antidote:* Naloxone

TABLE 6.8 PHARMACOLOGY—cont'd

Medications Frequently Used in the Treatment of Pain, Agitation, Delirium, and Neuromuscular Blockade[a]

Medication	Action/Use	Dose/Route	Side Effects	Nursing Implications
Nonopioids Adjuvant				
Acetaminophen (Tylenol, Ofirmev [IV])	Nonnarcotic analgesic; blocks pain impulses peripherally that occur in response to inhibition of prostaglandin synthesis; no antiinflammatory properties Used for mild-to-moderate pain Antipyretic	May be given scheduled or PRN *Oral/Rectal:* 325-650 mg q4-6h, not to exceed 4 g/day *Intravenous:* Bolus, (Patient ≥50 kg), 650 mg IV q4h *or* 1000 mg IV q6h, not to exceed 4 g/day Bolus, (Patient <50 kg), 12.5 mg/kg IV q4h *or* 15 mg/kg IV q6h, not to exceed 75 mg/kg in 24h or 3.75 g/day Infuse IV over at least 15 min	Blood dyscrasias Hepatic toxicity occurs with high doses (>4 g/day) Renal failure with prolonged high dosage	Monitor renal and liver function. Assess other medications for acetaminophen content (e.g., Percocet). Treat overdose with acetylcysteine, gastric lavage.
N-methyl-D-aspartate (NMDA) Receptor Antagonist				
Ketamine (Ketalar)	Nonbarbiturate general anesthetic; interrupts association pathways of the brain selectively; produces a somatesthetic sensory blockade Used for the management of acute pain, continuous and procedural sedation, and rapid sequence intubation	Given the wide variety of critical care uses, collaborate with your critical care pharmacy specialist and provider to determine the appropriate indication and dosage.	Anaphylaxis Apnea Emergence reactions Excess oral secretions Hypertension Nausea and vomiting	Monitor BP, heart rate, and respiratory status. Protect the patient's airway, as vomiting is a common side effect. Psychological manifestations vary and may involve unpleasant hallucinations, confusion, and excitement.
Nonsteroidal Antiinflammatory Drugs (NSAIDs)				
Ibuprofen (Advil, Motrin) (IV: Caldolor)	Inhibits COX-1, COX-2 by blocking arachidonate Used for mild-to-moderate pain Reduces inflammation Antipyretic	May be given scheduled or PRN *Oral:* 200-800 mg q4-6h; maximum 2.4-3.2 g/day *Intravenous:* 400-800 mg IV over ≥30 min q6h; maximum 3.2 g/day	Bleeding GI ulcers Thrombocytopenia Tinnitus	Monitor complete blood count. Monitor renal and liver function. Patients should be well hydrated before IV ibuprofen administration. Black Box Warning: GI Bleeding – Assess for bleeding, bruising, ulceration, perforation of stomach.
Ketorolac (Toradol)	Inhibits prostaglandin synthesis Used to treat pain Reduces inflammation	*Intravenous/Intramuscular:* Maximum duration 5 days 15-30 mg q6h; maximum 120 mg/day Patients ≥65 years of age, renal impairment, or patient <50 kg, 15 mg q6h; maximum 60 mg/day	Acute kidney injury Dyspepsia GI bleed, ulceration, perforation Headache Nausea	Monitor complete blood count. Monitor renal and liver function. Do not use to treat perioperative pain associated with cardiac surgery. Do not administer epidural or intrathecal route because solution contains alcohol.
Neuropathic Drugs				
Gabapentin (Neurontin)	Mechanism unknown Used to treat neuropathic pain May be used for alcohol use disorder	*Oral:* 100-900 mg/day in 2-3 divided doses; may titrate to 900-3600 mg/day to clinical end point	Changes in vision CNS depression Confusion Peripheral edema	Slow onset Monitor for signs and symptoms of depression, mood changes, or suicidal thoughts. Wean slowly.
Pregabalin (Lyrica)	GABA analog; strongly binds to the alpha 2-delta site in CNS tissues; effects noradrenergic and serotonergic pathways in the brainstem, modulating pain transmission in the spinal cord used to treat neuropathic pain	*Oral:* Initial, 75-150 mg/day Maintenance, may increase q3 days based on response and tolerability, maximum 300-600 mg/day	Angioedema CNS depression Dizziness Peripheral edema Visual disturbances	Monitor for signs and symptoms of depression, mood changes, or suicidal thoughts. Assess for allergic reactions. Wean slowly.

Continued

TABLE 6.8 PHARMACOLOGY—cont'd

Medications Frequently Used in the Treatment of Pain, Agitation, Delirium, and Neuromuscular Blockade[a]

Medication	Action/Use	Dose/Route	Side Effects	Nursing Implications
Epidural Analgesics				
Bupivacaine (Marcaine)	Local anesthetic/analgesic; blocks generation and conduction of nerve impulses May be used for postoperative pain	Concentration of 0.25%-0.75% (25-150 mg) provides partial to complete motor block	Constipation Hypotension Itching Nausea and vomiting Respiratory paralysis Tinnitus Urinary retention	Assess dermatomes for sensation and movement. Monitor renal and liver function. Ensure medication is preservative free.
Ropivacaine (Naropin)	Local anesthetic/analgesic; blocks generation and conduction of nerve impulses; used for postoperative pain management	Dosing varies based on area to be anesthetized. Lumbar/thoracic epidural infusion, 6-14 mL/h of 0.2% solution	Bradycardia Hypotension Nausea Paresthesia Pruritus Rigors Vomiting	Assess dermatomes for sensation and movement. Monitor renal and liver function.
Treatment of Agitation				
Midazolam (Versed)	Benzodiazepine; depresses subcortical levels in the CNS Used for acute agitation, procedural sedation, and rapid sequence intubation	*Continuous infusion:* Initial, 1-5 mg IV over 2-3 min, q10-15 min PRN Maintenance, 1-8 mg/h IV	CNS depression Hypotension Paradoxical agitation Respiratory depression	Use a valid sedation scale to monitor effect. Only use continuous infusion with mechanically ventilated patients. Titrate infusion up or down by 25%-50% of the initial infusion rate to ensure adequate titration of sedation level and to prevent tolerance development. Use the lowest dose to achieve desired effect. Monitor BP and respiratory status. Slowly wean medication after prolonged therapy (decrease by 10%-25% every few hours). Avoid in older adults with delirium or at high risk for delirium; assess frequently for confusion, delirium. Lower doses may be needed for patients >65 years.
Lorazepam (Ativan)	Benzodiazepine; potentiates the actions of GABA Used to reduce anxiety and provide sedation Sedation in mechanically ventilated patients (unlabeled)	May be given scheduled or PRN *Oral:* Initial, 2-3 mg/day given q4-12h; maximum dose 10 mg/day *Intramuscular:* 0.05 mg/kg IM; 4 mg IM maximum *Intravenous:* Bolus, 0.02-0.04 mg/kg IV or 1-4 mg q2-6h; maximum dose 4 mg IV; inject no faster than 2 mg/min *Continuous infusion:* 0.5-8 mg/h IV, titrate to clinical end point	Hyperosmolar metabolic acidosis (IV prolonged infusion) Hypotension (less than midazolam) Paradoxical agitation Respiratory depression	Administer lower doses in older adults. Monitor BP and respiratory status. Assess acid-base status with prolonged infusion. Avoid smaller veins to prevent thrombophlebitis. Only use continuous infusion if patient is mechanically ventilated. Higher than recommended dose infusions have been associated with tubular necrosis, lactic acidosis, and hyperosmolar states because of the polyethylene glycol and propylene glycol solvents.

TABLE 6.8 PHARMACOLOGY—cont'd

Medications Frequently Used in the Treatment of Pain, Agitation, Delirium, and Neuromuscular Blockade[a]

Medication	Action/Use	Dose/Route	Side Effects	Nursing Implications
Propofol (Diprivan)	Nonbenzodiazepine; depresses the CNS by activation of GABA receptor Used for sedation in mechanically ventilated patients and procedural sedation	*Continuous infusion:* Initial, 5 mcg/kg/min; increase dose in 5-10 mcg/kg/min increments q5-10 min to clinical end point Maintenance, infusion rate of 5-50 mcg/kg/min (or higher) Administration should not exceed 4 mg/kg/h unless the benefits outweigh the risks	Bradyarrhythmias CNS depression Fever Hypertriglyceridemia Hypotension Respiratory depression Sepsis	Patient should be intubated and mechanically ventilated. Avoid rapid bolus administration to reduce respiratory depression. Monitor BP and hemodynamic status. Change infusion set q12h. Emulsion is preservative free and may support growth of microorganisms. Monitor plasma lipid and triglyceride levels.
Dexmedetomidine (Precedex)	Selective alpha$_2$-adrenoreceptor agonist Used to reduce anxiety and provide sedation	*Continuous infusion:* 0.2-0.7 mcg/kg/h IV, titrate maximum 1.5 mcg/kg/h to clinical end point	Bradycardia Hypotension Nausea	Give only by continuous infusion. Monitor heart rate and blood pressure. May use in patients not mechanically ventilated. Does not suppress respiratory drive. Prolonged use may lead to withdrawal syndrome upon discontinuation.
Agitation in Delirium				
Haloperidol (Haldol)	Neuroleptic; depresses cerebral cortex, hypothalamus, and limbic system Typical antipsychotic May be used to treat symptoms of alcohol withdrawal	*Oral:* 0.5-10 mg q6h; maximum 30 mg/day *Intramuscular:* 2-10 mg q15min to q6h IM *Intravenous:* Bolus, 2-10 mg q15 min to 6h IV	Drowsiness Euphoria/agitation, paradoxical agitation Extrapyramidal symptoms Neuroleptic malignant syndrome Prolonged QT interval Tachycardia	Measure QTc interval at start of therapy and periodically. Use with caution when patient is receiving other QT prolonging agents. Administer anticholinergic for extrapyramidal symptoms. Consider a lower dose in older adults.
Quetiapine (Seroquel)	Antagonist to multiple neurotransmitter receptors in the brain Used to treat agitation and acute psychosis (unlabeled use), schizophrenia, bipolar affective disorder	*Oral/Enteral Tube:* 25-50 mg q8-12h, maximum 400-800 mg/day	Agitation Dizziness Drowsiness Extrapyradmidal symptoms Increased risk of suicidal thoughts Orthostatic hypotension Prolonged QT interval	Check potassium and magnesium levels. Monitor QTc intervals. Monitor orthostatic blood pressure.
Risperidone (Risperdal)	Atypical antipsychotic; exact mechanism unknown Used to treat anxiety, schizophrenia, bipolar disorders; unlabeled use for acute psychosis and agitation	*Oral/Enteral Tube:* 2 mg/day as single dose or in divided doses. Increase dose to maximum 4-8 mg/day (varies based on indication)	Blurred vision Drowsiness Extrapyramidal symptoms Insomnia Nausea Orthostatic hypotension Prolonged QT interval	Often given at bedtime. Monitor QTc intervals. Monitor orthostatic blood pressure.

Continued

TABLE 6.8 PHARMACOLOGY—cont'd

Medications Frequently Used in the Treatment of Pain, Agitation, Delirium, and Neuromuscular Blockade[a]

Medication	Action/Use	Dose/Route	Side Effects	Nursing Implications
Neuromuscular Blockade Agents				
Atracurium (Tracrium)	Nondepolarizing neuromuscular blocker	*Intravenous:* Bolus, 0.4-0.5 mg/kg IV Maintenance, 5-10 mcg/kg/min IV; maximum 17.5 mcg/kg/min IV titrated to clinical end point	Hypotension Rash Tachycardia	Ensure adequate airway. Can no longer use pain or sedation scales for titration. Ensure adequate pain management and deep sedation prior to administration. Safer than other paralytic agents in patients with hepatic or renal failure. Obtain train-of-four prior to initiating NMB, then as ordered to monitor level of paralysis.
Cisatracurium (Nimbex)	Nondepolarizing neuromuscular blocker	*Intravenous*: Bolus, 0.15-0.2 mg/kg IV Maintenance, 0.15-0.20 mg/kg IV; maximum 0.02 mcg/kg/min IV titrated to clinical end point	Bradycardia Flushing Hypotension Tachycardia	Ensure adequate airway. Can no longer use pain or sedation scales for titration. Ensure adequate pain management and deep sedation prior to administration. Obtain train-of-four prior to initiating NMB, then as ordered to monitor level of paralysis.
Rocuronium	Nondepolarizing neuromuscular blocker	*Intravenous:* Bolus, 0.5-1 mg/kg prn *Continuous infusion:* 10-12 mcg/kg/min, titrate to clinical end point	Hypotension Myasthenia gravis risk with prolonged use Tachycardia	Ensure adequate airway Can no longer use pain and sedation scales for titration Ensure adequate pain management and deep sedation prior to administration Obtain train of four prior to initiating NMB then as ordered to monitor level of paralysis.
Succinylcholine	Depolarizing neuromuscular blocker; short-term use; commonly used for rapid sequence inductions	*Intravenous:* Bolus, 0.3-1.1 mg/kg IV; maximum dose 150 mg IV	Hyperkalemia Muscle fasciculations	Secure airway. Can no longer use pain or sedation scales for titration. Ensure adequate pain management and deep sedation prior to administration. Avoid in patients with elevated serum potassium and glaucoma. Obtain train-of-four prior to initiating NMB, then as ordered to monitor level of paralysis.
Reversal Agents				
Naloxone (Narcan)	Opioid antagonist Used to treat opioid-induced respiratory depression and opioid overdose	*Intravenous/Subcutaneous/Intramuscular:* 0.4-2.0 mg; repeat q2-3 min to maximum of 10 mg *Continuous Infusion:* Initial, 0.005 mg/kg IV Maintenance, 0.0025 mg/kg/hr IV *Nasal:* One spray (4 or 8 mg) q2-3 min	Diaphoresis Dyspnea Dysrhythmias Nausea/vomiting Opioid withdrawal Seizures	Assess respiratory status. Anticipate withdrawal symptoms within 2h for those with dependence or addiction. Severity of withdrawal symptoms may vary depending on length of time opioids were taken.

TABLE 6.8 PHARMACOLOGY—cont'd

Medications Frequently Used in the Treatment of Pain, Agitation, Delirium, and Neuromuscular Blockade[a]

Medication	Action/Use	Dose/Route	Side Effects	Nursing Implications
Flumazenil	Benzodiazepine receptor antagonist Used to reverse the sedative effects of benzodiazepines	*Intravenous:* 0.2 mg over 30 sec; wait 30 sec, then give 0.3 mg over 30 sec if consciousness does not occur; further doses of 0.5 mg can be given over 30 sec at intervals of 1 min up to cumulative dose of 3 mg	Ataxia Blurred vision Dizziness Dyspnea Nausea Palpitations Seizures Tinnitus Vomiting	Monitor respiratory depression, benzodiazepine withdrawal, and other residual effects of benzodiazepines for at least 2 h. Do not use in patients with a history of seizures, head injury, or those who have ingested a tricyclic antidepressant.

[a]All dosages are for adult patients; this table does not account for typical dose adjustments used with older adults or those undergoing alcohol withdrawal.

*Not all medications may be given via an enteral access; check with pharmacist.

bid, two times per day; *BP,* blood pressure; *CNS,* central nervous system; *GABA,* gamma-aminobutyric acid; *GI,* gastrointestinal; *IM,* intramuscular; *NMB,* neuromuscular blockade; *NG,* nasogastric; *PO,* by mouth; *PR,* per rectum; *PRN,* as needed; *q,* every; *RASS,* Richmond Agitation-Sedation Scale; *TD,* transdermal.

From Collins, Shelly R. *Elsevier's 2023 Intravenous Medications.* 39th ed. St. Louis, MO: Elsevier; 2023; Skidmore-Roth L. *Mosby's 2023 Nursing Drug Reference.* 36th ed. St. Louis, MO: Elsevier; 2023.

(Box 6.5). The selection of an opioid is based on its pharmacological effects and potential for adverse outcomes. The benefits of opioids include rapid onset, ease of titration, lack of accumulation, and low cost. Intravenous (IV) opioids are considered as the first-line medication class of choice to treat nonneuropathic pain in critically ill patients.[6] However, using a multimodal analgesic approach that includes administering analgesic medications from one or more pharmacological classes in an effort to target different receptors is recommended by the guidelines.[1,6] As an example, nonopioid analgesics may be used to decrease the number of opioids and their side effects.[1] The most commonly used opioids in critically ill patients are fentanyl, morphine, and hydromorphone. Fentanyl is a highly lipophilic synthetic opioid analgesia that has the fastest onset and the shortest duration, but repeated dosing may cause accumulation and prolonged effects in some patients.[64] Morphine has a longer duration of action. Side effects may include hypotension as a result of vasodilation and prolonged sedation in patients with renal insufficiency due to active metabolites. Hydromorphone is similar to morphine in its duration of action, but it does not have active metabolites.

Fentanyl may also be administered by a transdermal patch in hemodynamically stable patients with chronic pain. The patch provides consistent medication delivery, but the extent of absorption varies depending on permeability, temperature, perfusion, and thickness of the skin. Fentanyl patches are not recommended for acute analgesia because it takes 12 to 24 hours to achieve peak effect and, once the patch is removed, another 12 to 24 hours until the medication is no longer present in the body.

Adverse effects of opioids are common. Respiratory depression is a concern in nonintubated patients or those on minimal ventilator settings. Hypotension may occur in hemodynamically unstable patients or in hypovolemic patients. A depressed level of consciousness and hallucinations leading to increased agitation are observed in some patients. Constipation, gastric retention, and ileus may occur, but empiric bowel regimens may prevent these side effects (see Chapter 7, Nutritional Therapy).

Renal or hepatic insufficiency may alter opioid and metabolite elimination. Titration to the desired response and assessment of prolonged effects are necessary. Older adult patients may have reduced opioid requirements, as many are opioid naive. Administration of a reversal agent such as naloxone is not recommended after prolonged analgesia. It can induce withdrawal and may cause nausea, cardiac stress, and dysrhythmias.

Preventing pain is more effective than treating established pain. When patients are administered opioids on an "as-needed" basis, they may receive less than the prescribed dose, and delays in treatment may occur. Administer analgesics on a continuous or scheduled intermittent basis, with supplemental bolus doses as required. Establish a pain management plan for each patient to include appropriate pain assessment, realistic goals of treatment, and efficacy of the medications administered. As the patient's clinical condition changes, this pain management plan requires reevaluation.

Adjuvants to Opioid Therapy. A multimodal analgesic approach is essential in the management of pain in the critical care unit. Nonopioid analgesics such as acetaminophen, nefopam, ketamine, neuropathic agents, and nonsteroidal antiinflammatory drugs (NSAIDs) decrease pain intensity and opioid consumption for pain management in critically ill adults.[1,6]

Acetaminophen. The most commonly used pain reliever is *acetaminophen,* which belongs to a class of medications called *analgesics* (pain relievers) and *antipyretics* (fever reducers). The exact mechanism of action of acetaminophen is not known. It may reduce the production of prostaglandins in the brain. Acetaminophen is used to treat mild-to-moderate pain, such as pain associated with prolonged bed rest. In combination with an opioid, acetaminophen has a greater analgesic effect than higher doses of an opioid alone. The IV form of acetaminophen (Ofirmev) is used for the treatment of acute pain and fever in adults and children. Administer acetaminophen cautiously in patients with hepatic dysfunction. Acetaminophen is an active

TABLE 6.9 Pain, Agitation, and Delirium Order Set

Sedation Orders: Ventilated Patient in Critical Care Unit
- Assess level of sedation q4h
- Target RASS Score _____
- SAT protocol twice daily, or as directed by provider
- SBT safety screen twice daily, or as directed by provider

Pain Management
- Pain assessment
- Rule out and correct reversible causes
- Opioids are the agents of choice for treatment of nonneuropathic pain
- Medications
  - Fentanyl
  - Morphine
  - Hydromorphone

Agitation Management
- Agitation assessment by RASS
- Minimize benzodiazepine usage
- Nonbenzodiazepine agents (propofol, dexmedetomidine) are preferred
- Medications
  - Midazolam
  - Lorazepam
  - Propofol
  - Dexmedetomidine

Delirium Management
- Nonpharmacological therapy
  - Mobility protocol
  - Maximize sleep-wake conditions (sleep protocol)
  - Minimize benzodiazepine use
  - Eyeglasses and hearing aids
  - Encourage family participation in patient reorientation
- PT evaluation and treatment
- OT evaluation and treatment
- Medications to treat agitation related to delirium
  - Haloperidol
  - Quetiapine
  - Risperidone

Diagnostic Tests
- In patients prescribed antipsychotics for the management of delirium symptoms, 12-lead ECG at baseline to assess QTc-interval.

ECG, electrocardiogram; *OT*, occupational therapy; *PT*, physical therapy; *QTc*, QT corrected for heart rate; *RASS*, Richmond Agitation-Sedation Scale; *SAT*, spontaneous awakening trial; *SBT*, spontaneous breathing trial.

ingredient in many other preparations (i.e., hydrocodone/acetaminophen [Vicodin, Lortab]); therefore, it is important to ensure that the maximum daily dosage is not exceeded.

Ketamine. Ketamine is classified as an anesthetic agent that can be used for amnesia and sedation in critical care, but it is often used at subanesthetic doses for pain management. Low-dose ketamine as an adjunct to opioid therapy controls moderate-to-severe pain and reduces the risk of sedation or respiratory depression compared to opioids and other CNS depressants. It has a wide safety margin with minimal cardiopulmonary depression, potentially improves blood pressure, and can concomitantly be administered with opioids and other pain medications. Patients might appear awake with preserved airway reflexes and respiratory drive but are unable to respond to sensory input.[65,66]

BOX 6.5 Definitions of Opioid-Naive and Opioid-Tolerant

Opioid-naive—patients who have received opiates for less than 1 week, are not chronically receiving opioid analgesics on a daily basis, and have not received opioid doses for 1 week or longer at the dosages listed below.

Opioid-tolerant—patients who have received at least one of the following for 1 week or longer:
- 60 mg oral morphine/day
- 25 mcg transdermal fentanyl/hour
- 30 mg oral oxycodone/day
- 8 mg oral hydromorphone/day
- 25 mg oral oxymorphone/day
- An equianalgesic dose of another opioid

Neuropathic Medications. The PADIS guidelines also recommend using neuropathic pain medication (e.g., gabapentin, carbamazepine, pregabalin) with opioids for neuropathic pain management in critically ill adults, Guillain-Barré syndrome, or recent cardiac surgery patients. These medications reduce opioid consumption within 24 hours of their initiation but require patients to have a functioning gastrointestinal tract with enteral access or the ability to swallow.[1]

Nonsteroidal Antiinflammatory Drugs. NSAIDs provide analgesia by inhibiting cyclooxygenase, a critical enzyme in the inflammatory cascade. NSAIDs have the potential to cause significant adverse effects, including gastrointestinal bleeding, bleeding secondary to platelet inhibition, and renal insufficiency. The risk of developing NSAID-induced renal insufficiency is higher in patients with hypovolemia or renal hypoperfusion, in older adults, and in patients with preexisting renal impairment. Do not administer NSAIDs to patients with asthma or aspirin sensitivity.

NSAIDs are available in oral, liquid, and IV forms (i.e., aspirin, ibuprofen, and ketorolac). IV administration may reduce opioid requirements. NSAIDs are active ingredients in many other preparations (e.g., hydrocodone/ibuprofen [Vicoprofen]); therefore, it is important to ensure that the maximum daily dosage is not exceeded. When these medications are given, patients are at increased risk of acute kidney injury. Monitor blood urea nitrogen, creatinine, liver function tests, potassium, hemoglobin, hematocrit, blood glucose, white blood cell count, and platelets to assist in determining the most appropriate NSAID for the patient.[67] Collaboration with the clinical pharmacist is essential.

Patient-Controlled Analgesia. Patient-controlled analgesia (PCA) is a medication delivery system in which the patient controls when medication is given. Using a special type of infusion pump (Fig. 6.4) that has a "locked" supply of opioid medication, either a basal rate, on-demand bolus dosing, or a combination of the two may be ordered. When the patient feels pain or just before any pain-inducing therapy, the patient can depress a button on the pump that delivers a prescribed bolus of medication. A PCA requires patient participation; therefore, not all critically ill patients are

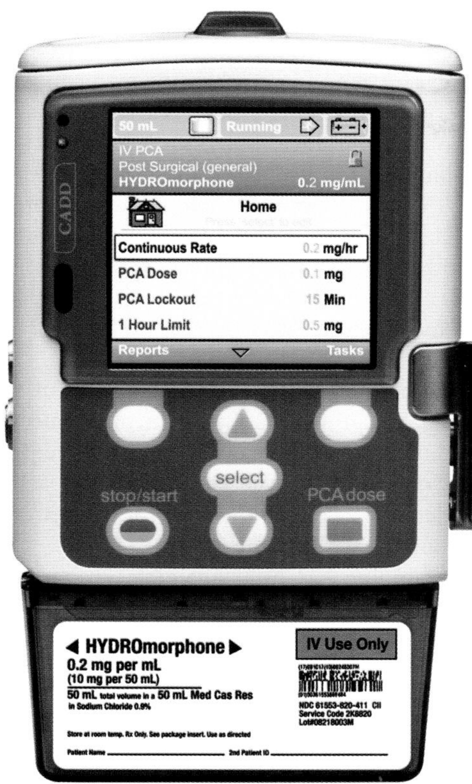

Fig. 6.4 A patient-controlled analgesia infusion pump. (Courtesy Smiths Medical ASD, Inc., St. Paul, MN.)

able to use a PCA due to the severity of illness or altered mental status. Opioids delivered by PCA pump result in stable drug concentrations, good quality of analgesia, less sedation, less opioid consumption, and potentially fewer side effects. Typical patient criteria for PCA therapy are listed in Box 6.6.[68]

Elastomeric Infusion Pump. An elastomeric infusion pump catheter is indicated for the delivery of medications, typically long-acting regional anesthetics (i.e., ropivacaine, bupivacaine), to or around surgical wound sites for preoperative, perioperative, and postoperative pain management. The ON-Q pain pump (I-Flow Corporation, Lake Forest, CA) is an elastomeric infusion pump that delivers medication at a flow rate determined by the pressure in the elastomeric reservoir, the flow restriction in the infusion circuit, and the viscosity of the fluid (Fig. 6.5). These elastomeric devices are currently used in the extrathoracic, paraspinous space to create a continuous intercostal nerve block. ON-Q has been used on adult patients with blunt trauma and three or more unilateral rib fractures and was associated with significantly improved pulmonary function, pain control, and shortened length of stay in patients with rib fractures.[69]

Epidural Analgesia. Opioids, dilute local anesthetic agents, or both can also be delivered through a catheter placed in the epidural or intrathecal caudal space or via nerve blockade to interrupt the transmission of pain. The discovery of opioid

BOX 6.6 Criteria for Patient-Controlled Analgesia Therapy

- Patient with acute, chronic, postoperative, or labor pain.
- Patients who are unable to tolerate oral medications.
- Patients with normal motor skills able to depress the medication delivery button.
- Patient with the mental capacity to participate and understand the concepts of dosing, time frames for administration, lockout periods, and expected pain relief.

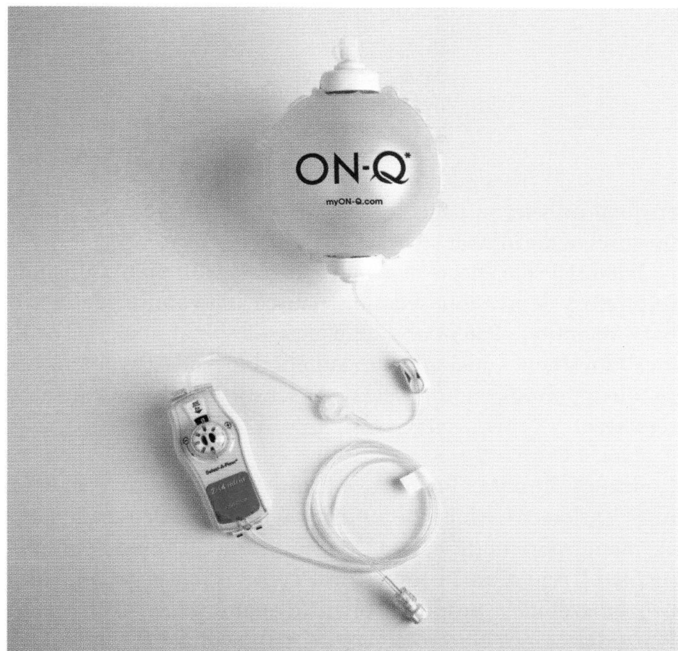

Fig. 6.5 ON-Q pain pump. (Courtesy Avanos, Irvine, CA.)

receptors in the spinal cord was considered a major breakthrough in the management of pain associated with traumatic injury of the chest and abdomen. Patients with such injuries do not want to cough, breathe deeply, ambulate, or participate in pulmonary exercises because these activities are too painful. Eventually, atelectasis, hypoxemia, respiratory failure, and pneumonia result. Epidural analgesia provides great relief for patients with multiple rib fractures and improves pulmonary function.[70] Other patients, such as those of specific postsurgical populations, may benefit from epidurals.[71]

The administration of epidural agents has many benefits in addition to pain relief (Table 6.10).[6] Some of the most commonly used epidural local anesthetics are bupivacaine, levobupivacaine, and ropivacaine.

Patients receiving epidural analgesia are carefully assessed to determine the appropriateness of spinal analgesia. Contraindications include coagulopathies, cardiovascular instability, sepsis, spine injury, infection or injury to the skin at the proposed insertion site, patient refusal, and the inability to lie still during catheter insertion.[72] In addition, it is difficult to place an

TABLE 6.10 Potential Benefits of Epidural Analgesia

System	Response
Pulmonary	↑ Vital capacity ↑ Functional residual capacity Improved airway resistance
Cardiac	Coronary artery vasodilation ↓ Blood pressure, heart rate
Gastrointestinal	Less nausea and vomiting Faster return of gastrointestinal function
Neurological	↓ Total opioid requirement ↓ Sedation
Activity	Earlier extubation Earlier mobilization ↓ Length of stay

epidural catheter in patients who are obese or have compression fractures of the lumbar spine.

Potential side effects of spinal analgesia with opioids include respiratory depression, sedation, nausea and vomiting, and urinary retention. Potential side effects of spinal analgesia with local anesthetics include sympathetic blockade (hypotension, venous pooling), motor weakness, sensory block, and urinary retention.

Sedative Agents. Prior to administering sedative agents, interventions to reduce the patient's agitation such as pain management, reorientation, and sleep promotion should be implemented.[1] Agitation in the critical care setting is treated with benzodiazepines, propofol, or dexmedetomidine (Table 6.8). Benzodiazepines bind to receptors that facilitate the inhibitory effects of gamma-aminobutyric acid (GABA) leading to sedative, hypnotic, and amnestic effects. Although they are not considered analgesics, they do moderate the anticipatory pain response. Benzodiazepines vary in their potency, onset, and duration of action, distribution, and metabolism. The patient's age, prior alcohol use, concurrent medication therapy, and current medical condition affect the intensity and duration of medication activity. Older adult patients and patients with renal or hepatic insufficiency may exhibit slower clearance of benzodiazepines, which may contribute to a significant delay in elimination.

Titrate benzodiazepines to a predefined end point, for example, a specific depth of sedation using either the RASS or SAS. Sedation may be maintained with intermittent doses of lorazepam, diazepam, or midazolam; however, patients requiring frequent doses to maintain the desired effect may benefit from a continuous infusion titrated to the lowest effective dose. Monitor patients receiving continuous infusions for oversedation, respiratory depression, and delirium.

Propofol is a sedative preferred over benzodiazepines to improve clinical outcomes in mechanically ventilated patients.[1] Propofol is an IV general anesthetic; however, propofol has no analgesic properties. It has a rapid onset and short duration of sedation once it is discontinued. Adverse effects include hypotension, bradycardia, and pain when the medication is infused through a peripheral IV site. Propofol is available as an emulsion in a phospholipid substance, which provides 1.1 kcal/mL from fat, and it should be counted as a caloric source (see Chapter 7, Nutritional Therapy). Given the lipid content of propofol, the bottle and tubing should be exchanged every 12 hours to avoid bacterial growth. Long-term or high-dose infusions may result in a rare side effect, propofol infusion syndrome, which is characterized by metabolic acidosis, dysrhythmias, renal failure, and hyperkalemia.[67]

Dexmedetomidine is a potent anesthetic agent with selective alpha-2 agonist properties. Given the mechanism of action, dexmedetomidine is not indicated for patients requiring deep sedation. As only lighter levels of sedation are achieved and respiratory depression does not occur, dexmedetomidine can be used in nonintubated patients.[73]

Dexmedetomidine has mild analgesic properties, reduces concurrent analgesic and sedative requirements, and produces anxiolytic effects comparable to those of the benzodiazepines. In addition, dexmedetomidine may actually improve sleep architecture.[1] Bradycardia and hypotension may develop, especially in the presence of hypovolemia or severe ventricular dysfunction and in older adults. This may be significant enough to suspend dexmedetomidine and initiate an alternative sedative agent. Overall, administration of dexmedetomidine or propofol, rather than a benzodiazepine regimen, in critically ill adults has shown to reduce critical care unit length of stay and the duration of mechanical ventilation.[74]

CHECK YOUR UNDERSTANDING

4. A patient is receiving deep sedation with hydromorphone and propofol. How should the nurse assess the patient's CAM-ICU status?
   A. Positive
   B. Negative
   C. Unable to Assess

Tolerance and Withdrawal. Patients who require prolonged, high-dose opioid or sedative therapy to maintain sedation may develop physiological dependence and tolerance to the medication. Collaborate with the clinical pharmacist and provider to develop a plan for tapering the medications slowly and systematically and consider other medications. Stopping these medications abruptly may lead to withdrawal symptoms. Opioid withdrawal symptoms include pupillary dilation, sweating, rhinorrhea, tachycardia, hypertension, tachypnea, vomiting, diarrhea, increased sensitivity to pain, restlessness, and anxiety. Signs of benzodiazepine withdrawal include tremor, headache, nausea, sweating, fatigue, anxiety, agitation, increased sensitivity to light and sound, muscle cramps, sleep disturbances, and seizures. To avoid these symptoms, wean medications slowly and titrate medications up if symptoms develop.[75]

Special Consideration

Invasive Procedures. Many invasive procedures, including nasogastric tube insertion; tracheal suctioning; bronchoscopy, central venous, or arterial catheter insertion; chest tube insertion; wound care; and removal of tubes, lines, and sheaths, take place in the critical care unit. All of these minimally invasive and invasive procedures have the likelihood of inducing pain or agitation. If pain or agitation occurs during a procedure, the length and difficulty of the procedure may increase, inaccurate data may be obtained, and physical harm can result.[1] To avoid negative outcomes, assess and manage the patient's comfort and agitation before, during, and after such procedures. Many times, the patient is kept in a conscious state during the procedure to avoid the risk of complications such as respiratory depression and hypotension. Therefore, sedative or analgesic agents, or both, are given in a way such that the patient appears sedate yet is able to verbalize. This type of sedation has been referred to as *procedural sedation* or *conscious sedation*.

Nursing care during these procedures involves monitoring vital signs, including pulse oximetry, ensuring a patent airway, and observing for adverse effects of medications. With the advent of the electronic health record, customized pain assessment forms can be developed to improve clinical efficiency and documentation.

Neuromuscular Blockade. Neuromuscular blockade (NMB) agents impede the transmission of nerve impulses at the myoneural junction, paralyzing skeletal muscles and sparing cardiac and smooth muscles. The use of NMB agents is indicated for general anesthesia in the operating room, endotracheal intubation, dyssynchrony during mechanical ventilation, elevated intracranial pressure, and minimally invasive and invasive procedures at the bedside (e.g., bronchoscopy, tracheostomy).

During endotracheal intubation, the use of a rapidly acting NMB agent (rapid-sequence intubation) allows the airway to be secured quickly and without trauma. Following intubation, some patients are dyssynchronous with mechanical ventilation despite adequate sedation and alternative ventilator modes (see Chapter 10, Ventilatory Assistance, and Chapter 15, Acute Respiratory Failure).[76] NMB agents may improve chest wall compliance, reduce peak airway pressures, and prevent ventilator dyssynchrony by reducing or suppressing patient effort. The result is improved gas exchange with increased oxygen delivery and decreased oxygen consumption.[76]

NMB agents do not possess any sedative or analgesic properties. Any patient who receives NMB agents is neither able to communicate nor produce any voluntary muscle movement, including breathing. Therefore, ensure that any patient receiving these agents receives appropriate pain management and deep sedation prior to NMB administration. Adequate pain and sedation necessitates the initiation of continuous infusions of analgesic and sedative medications. Objective measures of brain function (e.g., BIS) are useful in managing sedation in patients receiving NMB agents, as subjective assessments are unobtainable (see Evidence-Based Practice box).[1,6]

EVIDENCE-BASED PRACTICE

Problem

Neuromuscular blocking (NMB) agents are commonly used in the critical care setting. Nurses are unable to effectively monitor depth of sedation when patients are receiving NMB agents because sedation scales require assessment of a patient's movement in response to stimulus. Managing sedation then becomes a challenge in this population. If the patient is not adequately sedated, the patient may be aware during paralysis, which can lead to posttraumatic stress disorder. Alternatively, oversedation has been linked to an increase in mortality among this population.

Clinical Question

Does BIS monitoring correlate to clinical sedation scales in a broad population of nonparalyzed, critically ill adults?

Evidence

PubMed, Embase, Cochrane Library, Scopus, and OpenGrey were searched using keywords and subject headings for the concepts of consciousness monitors, sedation scales (i.e., RASS, Ramsay Sedation Scale [RSS], or SAS), and critical care units. There were no date or language restrictions. Twenty-four studies that enrolled 1235 patients met inclusion criteria for the systematic review and meta-analysis. The overall correlation between BIS and RASS, RSS, and SAS was 0.68 (95% confidence interval, 0.61-0.74). Subgroup analysis by sedation scale indicated that the correlations between BIS and RASS, RSS, and SAS were 0.66 (95% confidence interval 0.58-0.73), 0.76 (95% confidence interval 0.69-0.82), and 0.53 (95% confidence interval 0.42-0.63), respectively.

Overall, BIS demonstrated moderate-to-strong correlation with clinical sedation scales in critically ill adults. The findings suggest that BIS monitoring potentially provides clinically relevant information regarding depth of sedation in critically ill patients receiving NMB therapy; however, mapping specific BIS values to validated clinical sedation scales is hindered by the substantial heterogeneity across studies.

Implication for Nursing

Future studies should evaluate whether BIS monitoring is safe and effective in improving outcomes among patients receiving NMB therapy. The optimal target BIS range during NMB treatment remains unknown. This highlights the importance of ensuring adequate pain and sedation prior to initiating NMB therapy. Though the BIS appears to be a useful tool, it is only one assessment finding among many that should be evaluated as a whole and trended to determine adequate sedation. Additional findings that may indicate inadequate sedation include tearing, tachycardia, hypertension, and diaphoresis. Based on the study findings, the authors recommend developing sedation algorithms for this population that do not allow for sedation to be titrated below a certain level, regardless of the BIS value or the implementation of NMB holidays. During NMB holidays, the NMB would be suspended to clinically evaluate the level of sedation.

Level of Evidence

A—Systematic review and meta-analysis

Reference

Heavner MS, Gorman EF, Linn DD, Yeung SYA, Miano TA. Systematic review and meta-analysis of the correlation between bispectral index (BIS) and clinical sedation scales: toward defining the role of BIS in critically ill patients. *Pharmacotherapy.* 2022;42(8):667–676. https://doi.org/10.1002/phar.2712.

If the patient is receiving NMB therapy, closely monitor for skin breakdown, corneal abrasions, and the development of venous thrombi. Nursing care for patients receiving NMB therapy is presented in Box 6.7.

BOX 6.7 Nursing Care of the Patient Receiving Neuromuscular Blockade

- Perform train-of-four testing before initiation, 15 minutes after dosage change, then every 4 hours to monitor the degree of paralysis
- Ensure appropriate pain and sedation management prior to initiation of NMB
- Lubricate eyes to prevent corneal abrasions
- Ensure prophylaxis for venous thromboembolism
- Reposition the patient every 2 hours, as tolerated
- Monitor skin integrity
- Provide oral hygiene
- Maintain mechanical ventilation
- Monitor breath sounds; suction airway as needed
- Provide passive range of motion
- Monitor heart rate, respiratory rate, blood pressure, and oxygen saturation
- Place indwelling urinary catheter to monitor urine output
- Monitor bowel sounds; monitor for abdominal distention
- Advocate for early discontinuation when NMB in no longer indicated

NMB, neuromuscular Blockade

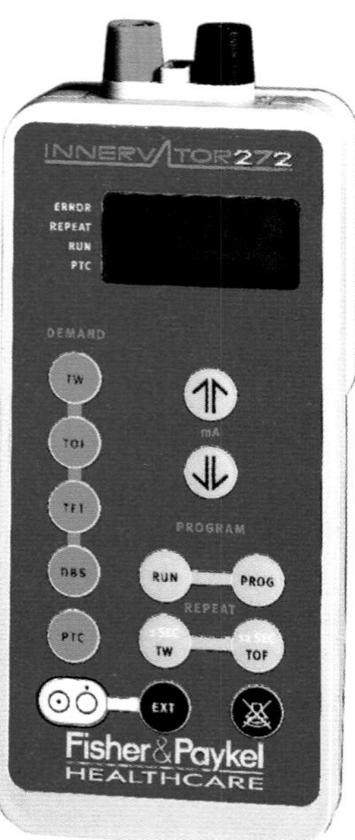

Fig. 6.6 A train-of-four peripheral nerve stimulator. (Courtesy Fisher and Paykel Healthcare, Auckland, New Zealand.)

Assess the level or degree of paralysis by using a peripheral nerve stimulator to determine a train-of-four (TOF) response. The TOF procedure evaluates the level of NMB to ensure the lowest dose of NMB medication is administered to achieve a goal of two out of four twitches. The ulnar nerve and the facial nerve are the most frequently used sites for peripheral nerve stimulation. The peripheral nerve stimulator delivers four low-energy impulses, and the number of muscular twitches is assessed. A baseline TOF is established prior to administration of any NBM agents by starting at the lowest milliamp (mA) and titrating up until four out of four twitches are observed from the chosen nerve location. This information should be recorded in the patient's electronic health record and handed off during shift change. Four twitches of the thumb or facial muscle indicate incomplete NMB in the presence of NMB therapy. The absence of twitches indicates complete NMB. An example of a peripheral nerve stimulator is shown in Fig. 6.6.

Several NMB agents are available; those most frequently used are outlined in Table 6.8. Succinylcholine (paralytic), when administered with etomidate (sedative), is frequently used for rapid-sequence intubation because of its short half-life. However, do not administer succinylcholine in the presence of hyperkalemia, because ventricular dysrhythmias and cardiac arrest may occur. These medications should not be given to patients with a family history of malignant hyperthermia.

Substance Use Disorders. The opioid endemic in the United States continues to worsen, creating a unique challenge for managing pain and sedation in the critical care environment.[77] Critically ill patients who have a history of substance or drug use disorders pose special challenges from managing symptoms of withdrawal to medication tolerance. Drug use disorder combined with alcohol use disorder has been associated with an increased need for mechanical ventilation and a longer critical care stay.[78] Patients with a history of substance use disorders may require higher and more frequent dosing for many analgesics, sedatives, and hypnotic medications. If pain is not managed effectively, an inflammatory cascade can be triggered and has been found to increase morbidity, hospital length of stay, and cost.[79]

Assess all patients with a history of alcohol use for symptoms of alcohol withdrawal syndrome (AWS), particularly in the first 24 to 48 hours. AWS usually presents within 72 to 96 hours after the patient's last alcohol intake. The initial symptoms, such as disorientation, agitation, tachycardia, and delirium tremens (shaking of the extremities or digits), may be mild. If untreated, symptoms can progress to severe confusion, hallucinations, paranoid-like behavior, seizures, convulsions, and even death. AWS assessment tools, such as the Clinical Institute Withdrawal Assessment for Alcohol, Revised (CIWA-Ar), are available.[80] The CIWA-Ar is used to determine the severity of withdrawal symptoms as they are actively experienced but does not predict which patients are at risk for withdrawal. This tool relies on patient communication for information on nausea and vomiting, anxiety, tactile and auditory disturbances, and headache. Unfortunately, CIWA-Ar is not validated in mechanically ventilated patients and should not be used in this population. Assess agitation symptoms using the RASS or SAS, and whenever feasible with CIWA-Ar, to match medication dosing and symptom severity and improve outcomes. The most important treatment of AWS is prevention, which has been shown to improve morbidity and mortality and decrease hospital and critical care unit lengths of stay. Benzodiazepines are commonly used for the prevention and treatment of AWS, though other medications and adjuncts may be of benefit.[81,82] Collaborate with the clinical pharmacist and multiprofessional team to determine the best regimen for the patient. Fluid resuscitation; correction of electrolyte deficiencies; and parenteral administration of thiamine, multivitamin, and folate are usually performed daily to treat underlying comorbidities and prevent complications associated with alcohol use.

Lifespan Considerations. Consider the impact of lifespan changes when managing pain, agitation, and delirium. Older adult patients often have a high prevalence of pain, and they might experience many painful conditions (e.g., neoplasms, injuries, and other external causes and diseases of the musculoskeletal and connective tissue systems). Some older adult patients believe pain is a normal process of aging and is something they must learn to accept as normal.[31] Patients older than 65 years of age may pose special concerns because of physiological characteristics, the presence of comorbid conditions, use of multiple medications, physical frailty, and cognitive and sensory deficits. Older adults are also more vulnerable to alcohol and substance use disorders, and they may be more vulnerable to toxicity from analgesics.[83] Renal function and creatinine clearance rate are often decreased in older adults, resulting in a longer elimination half-life of medications.

Treatment of pain and agitation in pregnant people requires consultation with the clinical pharmacist to consider both the mother and baby. Refer to the Lifespan Considerations box for additional strategies related to management of pain and agitation.

LIFESPAN CONSIDERATIONS

Older Adults

- Speak slowly and clearly when evaluating pain and agitation.
- Verify any underlying cognitive deficits (e.g., dementia, Alzheimer's disease, cerebrovascular accident).
- Ensure that scales or other assessment tools have a large font.
- Provide sensory resources to facilitate engagement in pain assessment (i.e., glasses, hearing aids).
- Stoic behavior may be the patient's normal baseline; therefore, assess for nonverbal cues to pain (facial grimace or withdrawal).
- Observe for changes in behavior, such as confusion or agitation. Older adult patients are at risk of developing delirium.
- Older adult patients may be resistant to taking additional medications; therefore, offer nonpharmacological strategies to manage agitation or pain.
- Older adult patients may not ask for as-needed medications in a timely fashion. Collaborate with the clinical pharmacist to identify the need for routine scheduling of medications.
- Assess renal and liver function and collaborate with the clinical pharmacist and provider to adjust medication dosages.
- Assess for paradoxical effects of medications in older adults (e.g., benzodiazepines often cause agitation).

Pregnant People

- Collaborate with the clinical pharmacist regarding the safety of medications for managing sedation and agitation in pregnant people and to identify benefits versus risks.
- If opioids are administered during pregnancy, the infant must be assessed and monitored for neonatal abstinence syndrome. Collaborate with the obstetrician and neonatologist.

CASE STUDY

A 52-year-old patient is in the surgical critical care unit after liver transplantation the day prior. The patient has a 15-year history of hepatic cirrhosis secondary to alcohol use disorder. The patient is intubated and is receiving multiple vasopressor medications for hypotension. During the initial assessment, the patient follows simple commands and denies pain or agitation with simple head nods. An hour later, the patient is kicking their legs and places their arms outside the side rails. Attempts by the nurse to reorient the patient result in the patient pulling at their endotracheal tube. Soft wrist restrains are applied to prevent self-extubation. At this time, the patient does not follow any simple commands. The patient continually shakes their head back and forth. Facial grimacing is noted, and the patient is biting down on the endotracheal tube, which is causing the ventilator to sound the high-pressure alarm. The monitor displays sinus tachycardia at a rate of 140 beats/min, and the patient has become dyssynchronous with the ventilator. Medication infusions include epinephrine (3 mcg/min), norepinephrine (15 mcg/min), dopamine (2 mcg/kg/min), and fentanyl (100 mcg/h). The only other medications are the patient's immunosuppressive medication regimen.

Questions

1. Based on the above assessment findings, determine the patient's pain score, agitation/sedation level, and delirium status using the following objective tools:

Tool	Score
Behavioral Pain Scale (BPS)	
Critical-Care Pain Observation Tool (CPOT)	
Richmond Agitation-Sedation Scale (RASS)	
Sedation-Agitation Scale (SAS)	
Confusion Assessment Method for the Intensive Care Unit (CAM-ICU)	

2. Based on the findings of the assessment tools, what appears to be the reason for the change in condition?
3. What factors may have predisposed the patient to this change in condition?
4. What possible nonpharmacological interventions are indicated for this patient?
5. What pharmacological interventions should the nurse recommend to address the patient's current condition?
6. What assessment findings would the nurse expect to find if interventions were effective? If ineffective, how should the nurse proceed?

KEY POINTS

- Pain, agitation, and delirium are interrelated concepts that are common in critically ill patients.
- The PADIS guidelines provide a clear, evidence-based road map to manage pain, agitation, and delirium in critically ill patients.
- If not effectively managed, pain, agitation, and delirium can increase morbidity and mortality in the critically ill population.
- The patient is the true authority on the pain they experience; therefore, the patient's self-report is the current "gold standard" for assessing pain.
- There are several tools for assessing pain, agitation, and delirium in critical care, including assessments for nonverbal patients. The Numeric Rating Scale, VAS, CPOT, BPS, RASS, SAS, CAM-ICU, and ICDSC are the tools that have been found valid and reliable for critically ill patients.
- Given the interrelationships among pain, agitation, and delirium, their management is complex, with pharmacological and nonpharmacological interventions that often overlap.
- Nonpharmacological approaches to manage pain, agitation, and delirium should be used early and include manipulation of the environment, as well as complementary and alternative therapies (i.e., guided imagery, music therapy, animal-assisted therapy, aromatherapy).
- Currently, there are no pharmacological interventions to treat delirium, but there are medications to manage the symptoms associated with delirium.
- The management of pain can be complex, and there is a variety of treatment regimens and modalities to improve patient comfort; therefore, regimens should be person-centered and tailored to the individual.
- Continue to assess the patient, develop and implement a plan of care, and monitor and evaluate the patient's response to treatment until the symptoms are adequately managed. The goal should not be to eradicate symptoms in all patients, as this may not be feasible, but to improve their comfort.

REFERENCES

1. Devlin JW, Skrobik Y, Gelinas C, et al. Clinical practice guidelines for the prevention and management of pain, agitation/sedation, delirium, immobility, and sleep disruption in adult patients in the ICU. *Crit Care Med.* 2018;46:e825–e873.
2. Teece A, Baker J, Smith H. Identifying determinants for the application of physical or chemical restraint in the management of psychomotor agitation on the critical care unit. *J Clin Nurs.* 2020;29(1–2):5–19.
3. Ormseth CH, LaHue SC, Oldham MA, Josephson SA, Whitaker E, Douglas VC. Predisposing and precipitating factors associated with delirium: a systematic review. *JAMA Netw Open.* 2023;6(1):e2249950. https://doi.org/10.1001/jamanetworkopen.2022.49950.
4. Askari Hosseini SM, Arab M, Karzari Z, Razban F. Post-traumatic stress disorder in critical illness survivors and its relation to memories of ICU. *Nurs Crit Care.* 2021;26(2):102–108.
5. Martillo MA, Dangayach NS, Tabacof L, et al. Post intensive care syndrome in survivors of critical illness related to Coronavirus disease 2019: cohort study from a New York City critical care recovery clinic. *Crit Care Med.* 2021;49(9):1427–1438.
6. Barr J, Fraser GL, Puntillo K, et al. American College of Critical Care Medicine. Clinical practice guidelines for the management of pain, agitation, and delirium in adult patients in the intensive care unit. *Crit Care Med.* 2013;41(1):263–306.
7. Raja SN, Carr DB, Cohen M, et al. The revised International Association for the Study of Pain definition of pain: concepts, challenges, and compromises. *Pain.* 2020;161(9):1976–1982.
8. Aubanel S, Bruiset F, Chapuis C, et al. Therapeutic options for agitation in the intensive care unit. *Anaesth Crit Care Pain Med.* 2020;39(5):639–646.
9. Hatch R, Young D, Barber V, Griffiths J, Harrison DA, Watkinson P. Anxiety, depression and post traumatic stress disorder after critical illness: a UK-wide prospective cohort study. *Crit Care.* 2018;22(1):310.
10. Takashima N, Yosihno Y, Sakaki K. Quantitative and qualitative investigation of the stress experiences of intensive care unit patients mechanically ventilated for more than 12 hr. *Jpn J Nurs Sci.* 2019;16(4):468–480.
11. de Jager TAJ, Dulfer K, Radhoe S, et al. Predictive value of depression and anxiety for long-term mortality: differences in outcome between acute coronary syndrome and stable angina pectoris. *Int J Cardiol.* 2018;1(250):43–48.
12. Smit L, Wiegers EJA, Trogrlic Z, et al. Prognostic significance of delirium subtypes in critically ill medical and surgical patients: a secondary analysis of a prospective multicenter study. *J Intensive Care.* 2022;10(1):54.
13. Krewulak KD, Stelfox HT, Leigh JP, Ely EW, Fiest KM. Incidence and prevalence of delirium subtypes in an adult ICU: a systematic review and meta-analysis. *Crit Care Med.* 2018;46(12):2029–2035.
14. Guyton A, Hall J. *Textbook of Medical Physiology.* 14th ed. Philadelphia, PA: Saunders; 2021.
15. Cohen SP, Vase L, Hooten WM. Chronic pain: an update on burden, best practices, and new advances. *Lancet.* 2021;397(10289):2082–2097.
16. Allen J. Pain, temperature, regulation, sleep, and sensory dysfunction. In: Rogers J, ed. *McCance and Huether's Pathophysiology: The Biologic Basis for Disease in Adults and Children.* 9th ed. St. Louis, MO: Elsevier; 2022:474–508.
17. Stollings JL, Devlin JW, Lin JC, et al. Best practices for conducting interprofessional team rounds to facilitate performance of the ICU Liberation (ABCDEF) Bundle. *Crit Care Med.* 2020;48(4):562–570.
18. Miller CWT, Hodzic V, Weintraub E. Current understanding of the neurobiology of agitation. *West J Emerg Med.* 2020;21(4):841–848.
19. Canet E, Amjad S, Robbins R, et al. Differential clinical characteristics, management and outcome of delirium among ward compared with intensive care unit patients. *Intern Med J.* 2019;49(12):1496–1504. https://doi.org/10.1111/imj.14287.
20. Zhou Q, Zhou X, Zhang Y, et al. Predictors of postoperative delirium in elderly patients following total hip and knee

arthroplasty: a systematic review and meta-analysis. *BMC Musculoskelet Disord.* 2021;22(1):945.
21. Prendergast NT, Tiberio PJ, Girard TD. Treatment of delirium during critical illness. *Annu Rev Med.* 2022;73:407–421.
22. Villani ER, Franza L, Cianci R. Delirium in head trauma: looking for a culprit. *Rev Recent Clin Trials.* 2022;17(4):245–249.
23. Vondeling AM, Knol W, Egberts TCG, Slooter AJC. Anticholinergic drug exposure at intensive care unit admission affects the occurrence of delirium. A prospective cohort study. *Eur J Intern Med.* 2020;78:121–126.
24. Angermann CE, Ertl G. Depression, anxiety, and cognitive impairment: comorbid mental health disorders in heart failure. *Curr Heart Fail Rep.* 2018;15(6):398–410.
25. Binks AP, Desjardin S, Riker R. ICU clinicians underestimate breathing discomfort in ventilated subjects. *Respir Care.* 2017;62(2):150–155.
26. Campbell M. Dyspnea. *Crit Care Nurs Clin North Am.* 2017;29(4):461–470.
27. Roberts M, Bortolotto SJ, Weyant RA, et al. The experience of acute mechanical ventilation from the patient's perspective. *Dimens Crit Care Nurs.* 2019;38(4):201–212.
28. Malinowski A, Benedict NJ, Ho MN, et al. Patient-reported outcomes associated with sedation and agitation intensity in the critically ill. *Am J Crit Care.* 2020;29(2):140–144.
29. Lewandowska K, Mędrzycka-Dąbrowska W, Pilch D, et al. Sleep deprivation from the perspective of a patient hospitalized in the intensive care unit-qualitative study. *Healthcare (Basel).* 2020;8(3):351.
30. Balas MC, Weinhouse GL, Denehy L, et al. Interpreting and implementing the 2018 pain, agitation/sedation, delirium, immobility, and sleep disruption clinical practice guidelines. *Crit Care Med.* 2018;46(9):1464–1470.
31. Ho LYW. A concept analysis of coping with chronic pain in older adults. *Pain Manag Nurs.* 2019;20(6):563–571.
32. Society of Critical Care Medicine. ICU Patient Communicator Application. https://www.sccm.org/MyICUCare/THRIVE/Patient-and-Family-Resources/Patient-and-Family. Accessed October 30, 2022.
33. Payen JF, Bru O, Bosson JL, et al. Assessing pain in critically ill sedated patients by using a behavioral pain scale. *Crit Care Med.* 2001;29:2258–2263.
34. Chanques G, Payen JF, Mercier G, et al. Assessing pain in non-intubated critically ill patients unable to self report: an adaptation of the Behavioral Pain Scale. *Intensive Care Med.* 2009;35:2060–2067.
35. Gelinas C, Fillion L, Puntillo KA, et al. Validation of the critical-care pain observation tool in adult patients. *Am J Crit Care.* 2006;15:420–427.
36. Ortiz D. Assessment and management of agitation, sleep, and mental illness in the surgical ICU. *Curr Opin Crit Care.* 2020;26(6):634–639.
37. Pham T, Heunks L, Bellani G, et al. Weaning from mechanical ventilation in intensive care units across 50 countries (WEAN SAFE): a multicentre, prospective, observational cohort study. [published online ahead of print, 2023 Jan 20] [published correction appears in Lancet Respir Med. 2023;11(3):e25] *Lancet Respir Med.* 2023;S2213-2600(22). 00449-0. https://doi.org/10.1016/S2213-2600(22):00449-0.
38. Sessler CN, Gosnell MS, Grap MJ, et al. The Richmond Agitation-Sedation Scale: validity and reliability in adult intensive care unit patients. *Am J Respir Crit Care Med.* 2002;166:1338–1344.
39. Riker RR, Fraser GL, Simmons LE, et al. Validating the sedation-agitation scale with the bispectral index and visual analog scale in adult ICU patients after cardiac surgery. *Intensive Care Med.* 2001;27:853–858.
40. Rasheed AM, Amirah MF, Abdallah M, et al. Ramsay sedation scale and Richmond agitation sedation scale: a cross-sectional study. *Dimens Crit Care Nurs.* 2019;38(2):90–95.
41. Herman ST, Abend NS, Bleck TP, et al. Critical Care Continuous EEG Task Force of the American Clinical Neurophysiology Society. Consensus statement on continuous EEG in critically ill adults and children, part I: indications. *J Clin Neurophysiol.* 2015;32(2):87–95.
42. Katyal N, Singh I, Narula N, et al. Continuous electroencephalography (CEEG) in neurological critical care units (NCCU): a review. *Clin Neurol Neurosurg.* 2020;198:106145.
43. Stewart JA, Särkelä MOK, Wennervirta J, Vakkuri AP. Novel insights on association and reactivity of Bispectral Index, frontal electromyogram, and autonomic responses in nociception-sedation monitoring of critical care patients. *BMC Anesthesiol.* 2022;22(1):353.
44. Idei M, Seino Y, Sato N, et al. Validation of the patient State Index for monitoring sedation state in critically ill patients: a prospective observational study. *J Clin Monit Comput.* 2023;37(1):147–154.
45. Heavner MS, Gorman EF, Linn DD, Yeung SYA, Miano TA. Systematic review and meta-analysis of the correlation between bispectral index (BIS) and clinical sedation scales: toward defining the role of BIS in critically ill patients. *Pharmacotherapy.* 2022;42(8):667–676.
46. Pérez GA, Pérez JAM, Álvarez ST, et al. Modelling the PSI response in general anesthesia. *J Clin Monit Comput.* 2021;35(5):1015–1025.
47. Ely EW, Margolin R, Francis J, et al. Evaluation of delirium in critically ill patients: validation of the confusion assessment method for the intensive care unit (CAM-ICU). *Crit Care Med.* 2001;29(7):1370–1379.
48. Bergeron N, Dubois MJ, Dumont M, et al. Intensive care delirium screening checklist: evaluation of a new screening tool. *Intensive Care Med.* 2001;27:859–864.
49. Park S, Na SH, Oh J, et al. Pain and anxiety and their relationship with medication doses in the intensive care unit. *J Crit Care.* 2018;47:65–69.
50. Kotfis K, van Diem-Zaal I, Williams Roberson S, et al. The future of intensive care: delirium should no longer be an issue. *Crit Care.* 2022;26(1):200.
51. Saha S, Noble H, Xyrichis A, et al. Mapping the impact of ICU design on patients, families and the ICU team: a scoping review. *J Crit Care.* 2022;67:3–13.
52. Goldfarb M, Debigaré S, Foster N, et al. Development of a family engagement measure for the intensive care unit. *CJC Open.* 2022;4(11):1006–1011.
53. Hamlin AS, Robertson TM. Pain and complementary therapies. *Crit Care Nurs Clin North Am.* 2017;29(4):449–460.
54. Hadjibalassi M, Lambrinou E, Papastavrou E, Papathanassoglou E. The effect of guided imagery on physiological and psychological outcomes of adult ICU patients: a systematic literature review and methodological implications. *Aust Crit Care.* 2018;31(2):73–86.
55. Golino AJ, Leone R, Gollenberg A, et al. Impact of an active music therapy intervention on intensive care patients. *Am J Crit Care.* 2019;28(1):48–55.

56. Bamikole PO, Theriault BM, Caldwell SL, Schlesinger JJ. Patient-directed music therapy in the ICU. *Crit Care Med.* 2018;46(11):e1085.
57. Chlan LL, Heiderscheit A, Skaar DJ, Neidecker MV. Economic evaluation of a patient-directed music intervention for ICU patients receiving mechanical ventilatory support. *Crit Care Med.* 2018;46(9):1430–1435.
58. Umbrello M, Sorrenti T, Mistraletti G, Formenti P, Chiumello D, Terzoni S. Music therapy reduces stress and anxiety in critically ill patients: a systematic review of randomized clinical trials. *Minerva Anestesiol.* 2019;85(8):886–898.
59. Marcus DA. The science behind animal-assisted therapy. *Curr Pain Headache Rep.* 2013;17(4):322.
60. Malik J. Animal-assisted interventions in intensive care delirium: a literature review. *AACN Adv Crit Care.* 2021;32(4):391–397.
61. Karimzadeh Z, Azizzadeh Forouzi M, Tajadini H, Ahmadinejad M, Roy C, Dehghan M. Effects of lavender and Citrus aurantium on pain of conscious intensive care unit patients: a parallel randomized placebo-controlled trial. *J Integr Med.* 2021;19(4):333–339.
62. Pehlivan S, Karadakovan A. Effects of aromatherapy massage on pain, functional state, and quality of life in an elderly individual with knee osteoarthritis. *Jpn J Nurs Sci.* 2019;16(4):450–458.
63. Pergolizzi Jr JV, LeQuang JA, Berger GK, Raffa RB. The basic pharmacology of opioids informs the opioid discourse about misuse and abuse: a review. *Pain Ther.* 2017;6(1):1–16.
64. Kovacevic MP, Szumita PM, Dube KM, DeGrado JR. Transition from continuous infusion fentanyl to hydromorphone in critically ill patients. *J Pharm Pract.* 2020;33(2):129–135.
65. Brown K, Tucker C. Ketamine for acute pain management and sedation. *Crit Care Nurse.* 2020;40(5):e26–e32.
66. Pruskowski KA, Harbourt K, Pajoumand M, et al. Impact of ketamine use on adjunctive analgesic and sedative medications in critically ill trauma patients. *Pharmacotherapy.* 2017;37(12):1537–1544.
67. Skidmore-Roth L. *Mosby's 2023 Nursing Drug Reference.* 36th ed. St. Louis, MO: Elsevier; 2023.
68. Pastino A, Lakra A. Patient controlled analgesia. In: *StatPearls.* Treasure Island (FL): StatPearls; 2023. Publishing; January 29.
69. Truitt MS, Mooty RC, Amos J, Lorenzo M, Mangram A, Dunn E. Out with the old, in with the new: a novel approach to treating pain associated with rib fractures. *World J Surg.* 2010;34(10):2359–2362. https://doi.org/10.1007/s00268-010-0651-9.
70. Lynch N, Salottolo K, Foster K, et al. Comparative effectiveness analysis of two regional analgesia techniques for the pain management of isolated multiple rib fractures. *J Pain Res.* 2019;24(12):1701–1708.
71. Dieu A, Huynen P, Lavand'homme P, et al. Pain management after open liver resection: procedure-specific postoperative pain management (PROSPECT) recommendations. *Reg Anesth Pain Med.* 2021;46(5):433–445. https://doi.org/10.1136/rapm-2020-101933.
72. Leslie V, Freeman BS. Combined spinal-epidural anesthesia. In: Freeman BS, Berger JS, eds. *Anesthesiology Core Review: Part One Basic Exam.* McGraw Hill; 2014. Accessed February 13, 2023.
73. Weerink MAS, Struys MMRF, Hannivoort LN, et al. Clinical pharmacokinetics and pharmacodynamics of dexmedetomidine. *Clin Pharmacokinet.* 2017;56(8):893–913.
74. Hughes CG, Mailloux PT, Devlin JW, MENDS2 Study Investigators. Dexmedetomidine or propofol for sedation in mechanically ventilated adults with sepsis. *N Engl J Med.* 2021;384(15):1424–1436.
75. Arroyo-Novoa CM, Figueroa-Ramos MI, Puntillo KA. Opioid and benzodiazepine iatrogenic withdrawal syndrome in patients in the intensive care unit. *AACN Adv Crit Care.* 2019;30(4):353–364.
76. Renew JR, Ratzlaff R, Hernandez-Torres V, Brull SJ, Prielipp RC. Neuromuscular blockade management in the critically Ill patient. *J Intensive Care.* 2020;8:37.
77. National Center for Injury Prevention and Control. *Understanding Drug Overdoses and Death*Updated February 14 Centers for Disease Control and Prevention; 2022. Accessed March 28, 2023.
78. Secombe PJ, Stewart PC. The impact of alcohol-related admissions on resource use in critically ill patients from 2009 to 2015: an observational study. *Anaesth Intensive Care.* 2018;46(1):58–66.
79. Karamchandani K, Klick JC, Linskey Dougherty M, Bonavia A, Allen SR, Carr ZJ. Pain management in trauma patients affected by the opioid epidemic: a narrative review. *J Trauma Acute Care Surg.* 2019;87(2):430–439. https://doi.org/10.1097/TA.0000000000002292.
80. Sullivan JT, Sykora K, Schneiderman J, Naranjo CA, Sellers EM. Assessment of alcohol withdrawal: the revised clinical institute withdrawal assessment for alcohol scale (CIWA-Ar). *Br J Addict.* 1989;84(11):1353–1357.
81. Seshadri A, Appelbaum R, Carmichael 2nd SP, et al. Prevention of alcohol withdrawal syndrome in the surgical ICU: an American association for the surgery of trauma critical care committee clinical consensus document. *Trauma Surg Acute Care Open.* 2022;7(1):e001010. https://doi.org/10.1136/tsaco-2022-001010. Published 2022 Nov 21.
82. Day E, Daly C. Clinical management of the alcohol withdrawal syndrome. *Addiction.* 2022;117(3):804–814. https://doi.org/10.1111/add.15647.
83. Hoel RW, Giddings Connolly RM, Takahashi PY. Polypharmacy management in older patients. *Mayo Clin Proc.* 2021;96(1):242–256.

PART II

Tools for the Critical Care Nurse

7

Nutritional Therapy

Jan Powers, PhD, RN, CCNS, CCRN, NE-BC, FCCM, FAAN

INTRODUCTION

The approach to nutrition has evolved from a secondary and supportive treatment focused on preservation of lean muscle mass to a therapeutic intervention that prevents harm, protects immune function, and facilitates healing.[1,2] The critical care nurse and multiprofessional team members are responsible for optimizing the patient's nutritional status in an effort to reduce the risks of adverse outcomes and malnutrition. The true prevalence of malnutrition in hospitalized patients is unknown; however, studies have cited rates ranging from 20% to 50% of patients on admission.[3] Nosocomial malnutrition, or a declining nutritional status during the hospital stay, occurs in 10% to 65% of inpatient adults, regardless of their prehospital nutritional status.[3] The incidence increases significantly in critically ill patients, with up to 80% developing malnutrition.[4] Malnutrition is associated with increased readmission rates, length of stay, healthcare costs, and mortality.[4,5] Critically ill patients have an increased risk of malnutrition and related complications due to alterations in protein and energy metabolism. During critical illness, the rate of muscle protein breakdown is greatly increased; this catabolic state leads to a worsened inflammatory response and muscle wasting.[6] The gastrointestinal (GI) system is not only important for nutritional needs but also plays an essential role in protecting against infection. Trauma, burns, sepsis, or other critical illnesses are often exacerbated by a frequent inability to tolerate oral nutrition.[1]

This chapter reviews the GI system's function related to nutrition and the basic assessment of a patient's nutritional status. Nutrient formulas and supplements, goals of therapy, practice guidelines for enteral nutrition (EN) and parenteral nutrition (PN), and complications related to nutritional therapy are also discussed. Though the focus of this chapter is on the importance of ensuring patient nutrition and hydration, the nurse must also ensure their own nutritional health (see Nursing Care box).

ANATOMY AND PHYSIOLOGY

Alimentary Canal

The main organs of digestion form the alimentary canal, which extends from the mouth to the anus (Fig. 7.1). The alimentary canal facilitates the acquisition of nutrients through a combination of mechanical and chemical digestive processes starting in the mouth. Mastication, the process of chewing, creates a bolus of food that is then broken down via enzymatic reactions.[7] The average person secretes approximately 1 to 1.5 L

NURSING SELF-CARE

Nurse Health and Nutrition

- According to the American Nurses Association's Healthy Nurse Campaign:
  - 16% of nurses met prescribed dietary goals.
  - 16% consumed five or more servings of fruits or vegetables per day.
  - 35% consumed three or more servings of whole grains.
- The core elements that make up a healthy dietary pattern include:
  - Consuming all of the following:
    - Vegetables and fruits of all types
    - Grains, at least half of which are whole grain
    - Dairy, including fat-free or low-fat options (lactose-free versions and fortified soy beverages and yogurt as alternatives)
    - Protein foods (i.e., lean meats, poultry, and eggs; seafood; beans, peas, and lentils; nuts, seeds, and soy products)
    - Oils, including vegetable oils and oils in food, such as seafood and nuts
  - Adequate hydration: Recommended daily intake of water is eight 8-oz glasses water (or about 2 L).
  - Limit the following:
    - Alcoholic beverages
    - Foods and beverages high in added sugars
    - Saturated fat
    - Sodium
- Strategies to improve nutrition and hydration:
  - Create a culture that promotes healthy eating (i.e., allowing time for scheduled breaks, cross coverage).
  - Packing your own meals is a great way to assure healthy foods and prevent the temptation of unhealthy snacks or fast food places.
  - Bring a water bottle to work and track water intake.
  - Avoid dehydrating drinks (those high in sugar).

Data from American Nurses Association. *Executive Summary: American Nurses Association Health Risk Appraisal.* 2017. Accessed December 26, 2023. https://www.nursingworld.org/~495c56/globalassets/practiceandpolicy/healthy-nurse-healthy-nation/ana-healthriskappraisalsummary_2013-2016.pdf; Perkins A. Nurse health: nutrition. *Nursing Made Incredibly Easy.* 2021;19(2):13-16; U.S. Department of Agriculture and U.S. Department of Health and Human Services. *Dietary Guidelines for Americans, 2020-2025.* December 2020. 9th ed. Accessed December 26, 2023. https://www.dietaryguidelines.gov/sites/default/files/2020-12/Dietary_Guidelines_for_Americans_2020-2025.pdf.

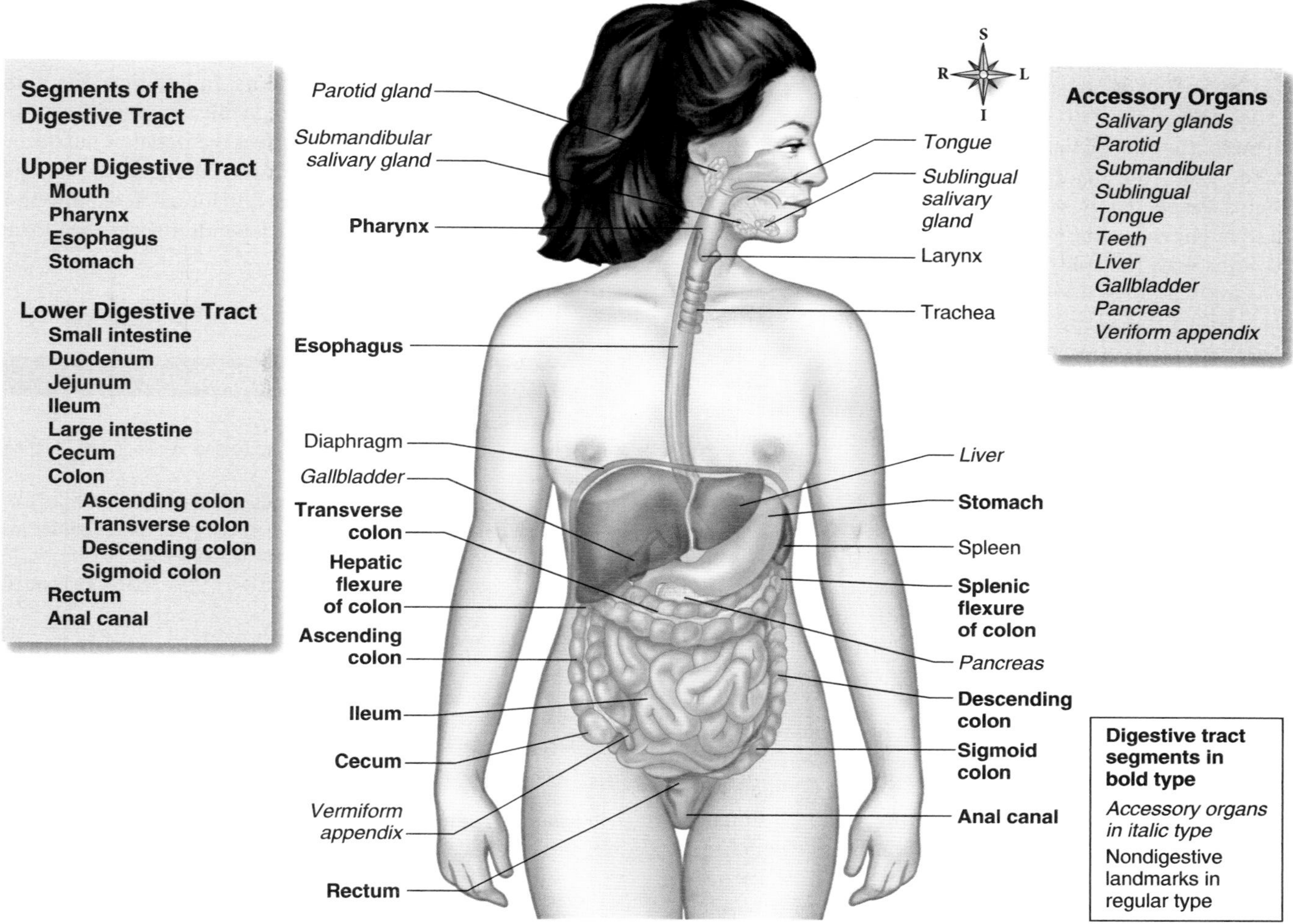

Fig. 7.1 Digestive organs. Organs of the alimentary tract are labeled in *boldface font*, while the accessory organs are labeled in *italic font*. (From Patton KT, Bell F, Thompson T, Williamson P. *Anatomy and Physiology*. 11th ed. St. Louis, MO: Elsevier; 2022.)

of saliva daily, which facilitates the digestion of starches and lubrication of masticated food.[7] Upon swallowing, or deglutition, the food bolus travels from the pharynx via voluntary and involuntary movements to the esophagus and through the esophageal sphincter to the stomach. Through peristalsis and the concurrent secretions of gastrin, hydrochloric acid, mucus, and pepsinogen, the stomach creates a semifluid mixture of food, secretions, and water, called chyme. Chyme is then slowly released into the small intestine at a rate that facilitates digestion and absorption.[7] Most absorption occurs in the small intestine through the epithelium via enzymatic breakdown: peptides are split into amino acids, disaccharides into monosaccharides, and fats into glycerol and fatty acids.[7,8] The large intestine uses large circular movements to propel the chyme forward, while absorbing most water and electrolytes in the proximal half of the colon.[7] The distal half of the colon stores feces until excretion occurs through the anus.

Accessory Organs

Multiple accessory organs also participate in absorption, digestion, and excretion. These accessory organs include the parotid, submandibular, and sublingual salivary glands; tongue; teeth; liver; gallbladder; pancreas; and vermiform appendix (Fig. 7.1). The salivary glands, tongue, and teeth assist in the production of saliva, mastication, and deglutition. These processes aid in the digestion and absorption of nutrients.

The liver regulates the appetite center in the brain, secretes bile, and aids in the metabolism of macronutrients. Hepatocytes, or liver cells, form bile, which flows through multiple ducts in the liver that eventually join with the cystic duct of the gallbladder, forming the common bile duct. Bile backs up into the gallbladder, where it is stored and concentrated. When chyme enters the small intestine, the gallbladder contracts, releasing bile into the duodenum. Bile aids in fat digestion and absorption. In addition, the liver stores iron and vitamins B_{12}, A, and D. Glycogen, a storage form of carbohydrate in the liver, is broken down, releasing glucose into the bloodstream. The pancreas also contributes to carbohydrate digestion and glycemic control.[7]

The acinar cells of the pancreas secrete the digestive enzymes amylase, lipase, and protease, which aid in the breakdown of the macronutrients: carbohydrates, fats, and proteins, respectively. After release from the acinar cells, the digestive enzymes enter the pancreatic duct. The pancreatic duct joins with the common bile duct, and pancreatic secretions empty into the duodenum. The pancreas secretes bicarbonate to neutralize the acidity of gastric juices entering the duodenum.[7]

The pancreatic islets are made up of beta cells, which secrete insulin, and alpha cells, which secrete glucagon. Insulin is the hormone that controls carbohydrate metabolism by allowing glucose to enter cells and be used as energy, lowering the serum blood glucose level. Glucagon is a hormone that increases the serum blood glucose level by stimulating gluconeogenesis, the production of glucose from fat or protein sources, as well as the breakdown of glycogen. The pancreas also secretes the hormones somatostatin, ghrelin, and pancreatic polypeptide, which contribute to digestion via their effects on endocrine secretions of the pancreas; gastrointestinal motility; and appetite, hunger, and satiety cues.[7]

The vermiform appendix has often been classified as an organ that no longer serves a functional purpose in the body; however, it is still considered an accessory organ to the digestive system due to its communication with the cecum. It functions as a storage and reproduction site for nonpathogenic bacteria, contributing to the normal flora of the large intestine. In digesting insoluble fiber, these bacteria release gases, contributing to the production of flatus.

The alimentary tract and its accessory organs are essential to the use of nutrients from foods ingested. During critical illness, function of the alimentary tract may be compromised due to insults from injury, inability to consume food orally, and concomitant medications and interventions. Because of the inherent risks of critical illness, the nutritional status of patients must be continually assessed and monitored.

ASSESSMENT

Critical illness causes a hypercatabolic stress state, increasing the inflammatory response and metabolic demands of the patient (refer to the Collaborative Care Plan found in Chapter 1, Overview of Critical Care Nursing).[2] An initial nutritional screening is recommended for hospitalized patients within 24 hours of admission; however, critically ill patients are at a higher risk for nutritional status deterioration, necessitating a full nutritional assessment.[1,9] Critical illness and an inability to mount an adequate inflammatory response can worsen as patients become immunocompromised and are more susceptible to poor outcomes.[2] Therefore, timely and adequate nutritional support is important to minimize nutrition-related complications and optimize patient response.[2] The objective of the nutritional assessment in the critically ill patient is to document baseline subjective and objective nutrition parameters, determine nutrition risk factors, identify deficits, and establish estimated needs for patients. In addition, the nutritional assessment serves to discern medical, psychosocial, and socioeconomic factors that may affect the patient's nutritional status and administration of nutritional therapy (see Lifespan Considerations box).[4,10-13] Several nutritional screening tools exist, but the adoption of each depends on the healthcare facility.

LIFESPAN CONSIDERATIONS

Older Adults

- Problems chewing or swallowing caused by poor dentition and ill-fitting dentures result in decreased intake.
- Chronic diseases that decrease the appetite or the ability to obtain and prepare appropriate and adequate meals (e.g., dementia, chronic obstructive pulmonary disease, osteoarthritis, heart failure, loss of functional mobility).
- Food insecurity, defined as limited access to a reliable source of nutritious, affordable food in sufficient quantity:
  - Fixed and/or decreased income level
  - Social isolation (e.g., living alone) and decreased physical mobility
  - Barriers to access to food (e.g., lack of transportation, minimal availability of meal delivery services)
- Medication side effects and/or interactions that may affect intake by altering appetite, flavor, taste, and/or odor perceptions.

Pregnant People

- Hyperemesis gravidarum may require:
  - Enteral nutrition (EN)
  - If EN fails, administration of total parenteral nutrition (TPN) may be considered but increases the risk of morbidity and complications.
  - IV fluid hydration
- Increasing nutritional needs based on trimester:
  - First trimester: does not require additional caloric intake
  - Second trimester: additional 340 calories per day
  - Third trimester: additional 450 calories per day
  - First 20 weeks: no additional protein required; second 20 weeks: additional 25 g per day
- Glycemic control:
  - Critical illness increases the risk for hyperglycemia, with a higher demand on insulin in pregnant people; monitor blood glucose frequently.
  - Evaluate for gestational diabetes, as indicated.
- Increased risk for foodborne illnesses secondary to a weakened immune system.
- Encourage patient to consume a balanced diet and initiate or continue prenatal vitamins to facilitate fetal health and development.

Pathophysiological Considerations

Considerations must be taken in evaluating disease states that may affect nutritional needs, onset of nutritional support, and tolerance. Some conditions may increase nutritional needs, alter the route and method of administration, and contribute to providers delaying initiation of nutritional support. For example, patients with inadequate perfusion on vasopressors or an altered level of consciousness require different nutritional therapy than awake, alert patients.

In some instances, these delays in nutritional support are based on inconclusive or insufficient evidence. Research demonstrates the benefits of EN compared with PN in patients with acute pancreatitis; however, initiation is often delayed, even though evidence supports early EN in this population (see Evidence-Based Practice box).[14]

EVIDENCE-BASED PRACTICE

Early Enteral Nutrition Compared With Late Enteral Nutrition or Parenteral Nutrition in Acute Pancreatitis

Problem

Acute pancreatitis is an inflammatory disease of the pancreas that, if left untreated, results in increased infection and multiorgan dysfunction. Historically, patients with acute pancreatitis were often kept at a nothing by mouth (NPO) status for several days before initiating nutritional support. Research has demonstrated a reduction in complications with the use of early enteral nutrition (EN) instead of delayed EN or parenteral nutrition (PN) in patients with acute pancreatitis; however, the optimal timing of initiation of EN has not been established.

Clinical Question

Should early EN be used (within 24–48 hours of admission) in patients with acute pancreatitis instead of delayed EN or PN?

Evidence

A prospective study was completed with 120 patients with acute, moderate, or severe pancreatitis (67 were assigned to early EN, and 53 were assigned to delayed EN or PN). Patients with moderate or severe acute pancreatitis who received early EN were found to have a decreased length of hospital stay, decreased infections, and decreased pain when compared to those with delayed EN or PN. There were no significant differences between groups for organ failure or mortality.

For patients with moderate or severe acute pancreatitis, it is recommended to start EN within 48 hours of admission. Early EN is beneficial and safe in patients with acute pancreatitis.

Implications for Nursing

During multiprofessional rounds, address nutritional support and recommend early initiation of EN in patients with moderate to severe acute pancreatitis. By advocating for early EN, the nurse supports optimal patient outcomes.

Level of Evidence

B – Prospective, controlled trial

Reference

Venkat S, Subramaniam R, Raveendran V. Early enteral nutrition in acute pancreatitis: how beneficial is it? *Int Surg J.* 2021;8:3279–3284.

Bowel Sounds

Auscultate the abdomen to assess contractility of the GI tract; an accurate assessment requires auscultation for 20 minutes. Clinical utility of bowel sound auscultation is questionable, and bowel sounds are only detected in 40% of patients. Bowel sounds alone provide neither information on mucosal/barrier integrity nor information on absorption; therefore, the presence or absence of bowel sounds should not be the only criteria used to determine GI functioning.[1,15] Reduced or absent bowel sounds may indicate a worse prognosis; however, this should not delay initiation of EN.[1]

Calculating Nutritional Needs

Determining nutritional needs for patients is a pivotal part of the nutritional assessment. Calculation of caloric, protein, and fluid requirements is standard when completing a nutritional assessment. Reference standards for the intake of vitamins, minerals, and trace elements have been published. Enteral formulas are designed to provide the recommended daily intake for vitamins and minerals when infusing at goal rate. Supplemental vitamins and minerals may be given to critically ill patients to facilitate healing, improve skin integrity, and address real or potential deficiencies.

Indirect calorimetry (IC) is considered the most accurate method of determining energy expenditure.[16] Calorie requirements are determined by measuring an individual's oxygen consumption and carbon dioxide production over a period of time. Oxygen consumption is then converted into resting energy expenditure using the Weir formula and a standardized constant respiratory quotient.[17] Collaborative guidelines from the American Society for Parenteral and Enteral Nutrition (ASPEN) and the Society of Critical Care Medicine (SCCM) recommend the use of IC to predict a patient's estimated energy requirements; however, the quality of evidence is low.[1] Several factors associated with critical illness such as high positive end-expiratory pressure (PEEP), dialysis, agitation, and use of sedatives may limit the accuracy of IC.[16] Furthermore, the availability of IC is often limited by high cost, limited access to the equipment, and a lack of adequate training on how to use the equipment effectively.[1]

In the absence of IC, ASPEN recommends using a published predictive equation or a simplistic weight-based equation to provide a range of calories per kilogram (kcal/kg) to meet the patient's energy requirements (Table 7.1).[1,17] More than 200 equations have been published, with the accuracy of these equations ranging from 40% to 75% when compared with IC. Resting energy expenditure (REE) represents the number of calories required by the body for a 24-hour nonactive period. Even though predictive equations remain the most common estimation method for REE, most have been developed in healthy adults, resulting in large variations and errors when used in critically ill patients.[16] Research has not yet identified a superior equation, as multiple factors affect the reliability of each equation in the critical care setting. For example, predictive equations are less accurate in patients who are overweight or obese when compared to patients with a normal body weight. Regardless of the method used to determine energy requirements, weekly monitoring and reassessment of estimated needs to optimize protein and energy requirements is recommended in the critically ill patient.[1]

TABLE 7.1 Estimated Nutritional needs

Caloric Requirements	Protein Requirements	Considerations
Low BMI (<18.5 kg/m²)		
30-45 kcal/kg/day (based on actual body weight)	1.2-2 g/kg/day	While energy requirements are higher in the intubated patient, it is not recommended to exceed 30 kcal/kg of body weight in daily nutritional support.
Normal BMI (18.5-24.9 kg/m²)		
25-30 kcal/kg/day (based on actual body weight)	1.2-2 g/kg/day	Protein requirement increased during critical illness.
Overweight (BMI 25-29.9 kg/m²)		
25-30 kcal/kg/day (based on actual body weight)	1.2-2 g/kg/day	Protein requirement increased during critical illness.
Obesity (BMI 30-40 kg/m²)		
11-14 kcal/kg/day (based on actual body weight)	2 g/kg/day	Hypocaloric, high-protein feedings to preserve lean body mass in the critically ill patient.
Morbid Obesity (BMI >40 kg/m²)		
22-25 kcal/kg/day (based on ideal body weight)	2.5 g/kg/day	Hypocaloric, high-protein feedings to preserve lean body mass in the critically ill patient.

BMI, Body mass index.

Protein needs are increased due to illness and other factors, such as wounds and interventional therapies; therefore, 1.2 g/kg or more of protein daily is recommended for critically ill patients (Table 7.1).[1,17] Evaluate the calorie and protein status of a patient by monitoring skin integrity, weight, and physical signs of muscle and fat wasting. The serum protein markers (i.e., albumin, prealbumin, total protein, and transferrin) are not validated methods for assessing nutrition adequacy and should not be used to evaluate nutritional status in the critical care unit.[1,18]

OVERVIEW OF NUTRITIONAL THERAPY

Evidence is insufficient to determine if one route of nutrition is superior to another when evaluating impact on mortality, ventilator-free days, and adverse events.[19] EN preserves immune function and health of the alimentary tract and lowers the risk of infection via the use of oral access versus central venous access. In addition, 70% to 80% of immune cells are present in the gut, and nutrition plays a key role with the gut microbiota, immune response, and infectious disease prevention.[20] Therefore, EN remains the preferred route per critical care guidelines for nutritional therapy.[1] PN may be started if adequate EN is not achieved by the first week of critical illness.[21]

CHECK YOUR UNDERSTANDING

1. A patient is intubated and on low-dose vasopressors. There are no issues with gastrointestinal tract continuity. What is the priority nutrition intervention?
   A. Obtain enteral access
   B. Auscultate for bowel sounds
   C. Recommend total parenteral nutrition
   D. Obtain ordered labs to identify potential nutritional deficits

Enteral Nutrition

Optimizing. Most critically ill patients may safely receive and should begin EN within 24 to 48 hours of admission.[1] Studies evaluating early EN (within 24 hours) versus delayed EN found benefits associated with decreased pneumonia, mortality, critical care unit length of stay, and maintaining GI tract integrity.[1,22] Exclusions to initiating early EN include diagnoses such as bowel obstruction, hemodynamic instability requiring high dose vasopressors, GI bleeding, bowel ischemia, or intraabdominal hypertension.[23,24] Many facilities have protocols to begin EN as early as medically feasible, with multiprofessional consults implemented as needed to maximize therapy. Protocols are essential to facilitate early EN and empower nurses to advocate for or initiate feedings as appropriate. Research studies show substantial benefit for earlier initiation of EN and the ability to achieve nutrition goals when protocols are used.[25,26] In addition, nursing can promote optimal nutrition intake by advocating for decreased fasting times prior to procedures.

Enhanced Recovery After Surgery. Traditionally, patients are kept at nothing by mouth (NPO) status from midnight prior to surgery until, at times, multiple days postoperatively. This is often due to waiting for the return of bowel function or resolution of postoperative ileus prior to beginning nutrition. Research suggests that reducing fasting times for procedures is associated with improvement in patient outcomes and nutritional status. Current recommendations support reduced fasting times, and enhanced recovery after surgery (ERAS) protocols have been developed; however, there is a disconnect in the implementation into current practice.[27]

Evidence has shown that a 2-hour fast from liquids and a 6-hour fast from solids is adequate for gastric emptying to avoid pulmonary aspiration during general anesthesia.[28] Research finds that resuming oral nutrition or EN within 24 hours postoperatively not only is safe and tolerated but also improves recovery. Early initiation of gastric feeding may improve ileus and expedite the return of bowel function.[27-29]

Method of Delivery. EN can be delivered by three methods: trophic, targeted hourly rate, and volume-based feeding (VBF). Trophic feeding provides patients with less than their estimated nutritional needs due to an actual or perceived risk of intolerance. In some cases, patients are started on trophic feeds and advanced to a goal volume or rate, as tolerated. Trophic feeding rates are most often between 10 and 30 mL/h. Feeding not only provides nutrients but also helps protect the gut and improve immune functioning. If unable to provide full-dose nutrients, or if using PN, trophic feedings can be beneficial.[23] Even with intolerance, starting early EN at a low rate is beneficial in protecting mucosal integrity, mobility, and immune function, whereas absence of nutrients results in mucosal atrophy and apoptosis, causing an impairment in barrier and immunological function.[20,30]

In the targeted hourly rate method, a goal *rate* for EN administration is calculated based on the daily estimated nutritional need. Initiation of EN either occurs at a trophic rate and advances to the hourly goal or is initiated at the hourly goal rate. The rate then remains at the specified hourly volume (e.g., 45 mL/h). This method does not typically account for missed EN secondary to procedures, nursing care, or diagnostic tests; therefore, the patient is at risk for suboptimal nutritional therapy. Certain tests or procedures may not require fasting; avoid withholding EN unnecessarily. Clarify with the provider who is ordering or performing the procedure how long to hold EN or whether holding EN is necessary. Upon procedure completion, resume nutritional support promptly. Compensating for missed EN via VBF can help optimize the patient's nutritional status.

Upon implementing the VBF method, the provider orders the appropriate EN as a goal *volume* to be infused over 24 hours. Increases in the hourly rate occur in response to interruptions in EN therapy, with the goal of compensating for gaps in EN therapy. For example, if the goal volume is 1200 mL and the patient's EN is held for 12 hours for a procedure, the patient has 12 hours remaining in the day to achieve the goal volume. Recalculate the rate of administration based on the remaining hours (1200 mL divided by 12 hours) and run the EN at 100 mL/h for the remainder of the day. With this method, patients receive more prescribed calories and protein than with the target hourly rate method (see Clinical Exemplar box).[31]

VBF protocols are safe in critically ill trauma patients and may be more effective at delivering energy and protein than the targeted hourly rate method.[31,32] However, caution should be exerted with higher doses of EN in the early phase of critical illness, as there may be negative effects from GI dysfunction.[30]

CLINICAL EXEMPLAR

Quality and Safety

Nutritional support is essential in acute illness to mitigate the effects of the inflammatory and catabolic state. The Society of Critical Care Medicine (SCCM) and American Society for Parenteral and Enteral Nutrition (ASPEN) guidelines recommend providing more than 80% of prescribed nutritional needs to critically ill patients. ASPEN and SCCM recommend the use of enteral nutrition (EN) delivery protocols due to the known failure of standard delivery mechanisms. Prest and colleagues retrospectively evaluated the use of a PEP uP protocol (enhanced protein-energy provision via the enteral route feeding protocol) to assess efficacy in providing improved nutritional support. The PEP uP protocol was implemented in a surgical trauma critical care unit. Prior to implementing PEP uP, standard practice varied based on the dietitian and provider recommendations, no standard formula was used, and rates were started at 10 mL/h and increased 10 mL every 4 to 6 hours. If feedings were held, they were restarted at 10 mL/h. Using the PEP uP protocol, patients were prescribed standard semi-elemental formula; EN was started on day 1 at 25 mL/h and increased on day 2 to the goal rate. Standard protocol steps included: (1) using a 24-hour volume goal (i.e., volume-based feeding [VBF]) instead of a targeted hourly goal rate; (2) using semidigested formulas; (3) using prophylactic protein supplements and motility agents; and (4) increasing the threshold for gastric residual volume (GRV) to greater than 300 mL. Patients on the PEP uP protocol achieved 80% of daily energy needs 57% of the time compared to 26.9% before the protocol was implemented. Patients also received 80% of their protein needs 57.4% of the time, up from 18.6% preprotocol. Patients on the PEP uP protocol also had less occurrences of hypoglycemia and hyperglycemia and used less PN. In the trauma intensive care unit, implementation of a volume-based feeding protocol was safe and effective and improved delivery of EN.

Reference

Prest PJ, Justice J, Bell N, McCarroll R, Watson C. A volume-based feeding protocol improves nutrient delivery and glycemic control in a surgical trauma intensive care unit. *JPEN*. 2020;44(5):880–888.

CLINICAL JUDGMENT ACTIVITY

What strategies can you use to reduce interruptions in the delivery of enteral feeding?

Route of Delivery. EN can be administered through a number of options, with the optimal access depending on the patient's acute and long-term nutritional support needs. Fig. 7.2 shows many of the common EN access devices (i.e., feeding tubes). Often, the intubated patient receives an orogastric tube (OGT) for stomach decompression after intubation. The OGT can easily be transitioned from a decompressive device to EN access. Nasogastric tubes (NGTs) are another gastric tube option; however, NGTs increase the risk of sinusitis by 200% in intubated patients.[33] The placement of all blindly inserted gastric tubes should be confirmed via radiographic study prior to use, then checked every 4 hours during continuous feeding based on external tube length (see Clinical Alert box).[34,35]

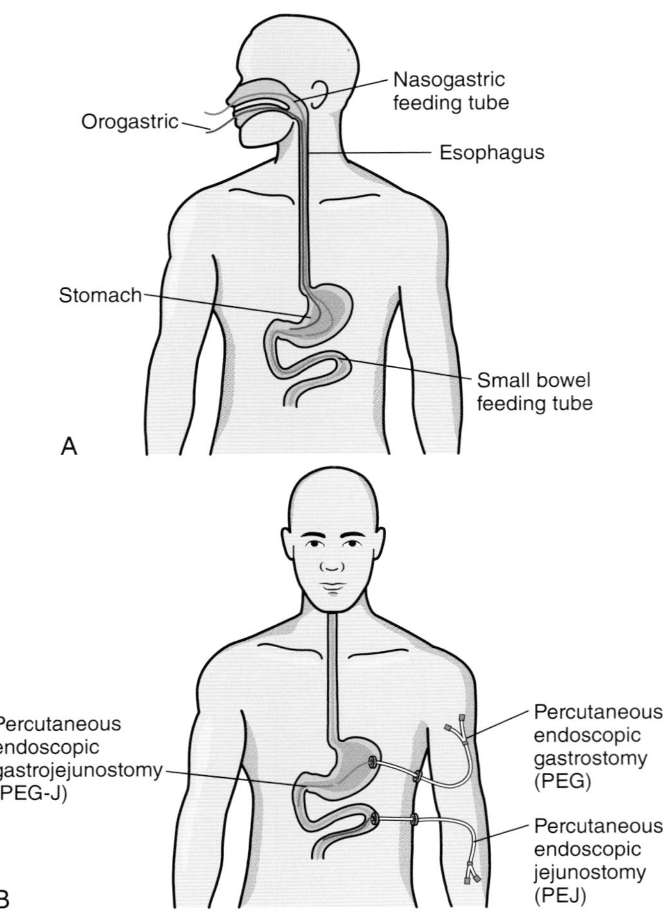

Fig. 7.2 Common enteral nutrition access used in critical care. **A**, Oral and nasal access devices. **B**, Percutaneous access devices.

! CLINICAL ALERT

Assessment of Feeding Tube Placement

Misplaced feeding tubes increase the risk of complications, including nutrition delays, aspiration pneumonia, and pneumothorax. Radiographic confirmation of correct tube placement is expected before initiation of tube feedings or administration of medications. Tube placement must also be verified if the tube becomes dislodged and requires reinsertion. Auscultatory or pH testing methods are unreliable for assessing tube placement. Patients with the highest risk of placement complications are intubated patients and those with an altered level of consciousness or an impaired gag reflex.

Patients at high risk for aspiration or EN intolerance should receive postpyloric feeding tubes in the small bowel for reduced aspiration and regurgitation.[1] Small bowel feeding tubes (SBFTs) are safe and do not increase the likelihood of complications when compared to gastric feeding tubes.[36] Use of SBFTs requires additional training to safely achieve postpyloric placement.[37] Assistive devices that offer direct or indirect visualization during tube placement are available (e.g., electromagnetic placement device [EMPD], camera assistive).[37] EMPD is the most commonly used device/method used to track the location of the SBFT through the use of an electromagnetic signal, which allows the nurse to determine the location and trajectory of the SBFT.[38]

The use of an assistive device versus blind placement is recommended to decrease risk of complications during insertion. Regardless of the method or technique used to place feeding tubes, the healthcare clinician should be trained and deemed competent before placing the feeding tube.[37]

Long-term (typically longer than 4 to 5 weeks) nutritional access is considered based on the patient's swallowing ability, aspiration risks, goals of care or wishes, and ability to meet nutritional requirements. Feeding tubes can be inserted externally through the stomach or jejunum. A percutaneous endoscopic gastrostomy (PEG) tube is inserted under local to moderate sedation, allowing enteral feedings to begin within 4 hours of placement.[5] If a patient does not tolerate gastric feedings, a percutaneous endoscopic gastrojejunostomy (PEG-J) tube can be placed, allowing jejunal feeding and bypassing the stomach. The PEG portion is often used for medication administration to facilitate adequate absorption, and the PEG-J portion is used for continuous EN. Another postpyloric long-term feeding tube option is the surgically placed percutaneous endoscopic jejunostomy (PEJ) tube; however, endoscopic placement is available to certain patients based on clinical disposition. PEJ tubes have significantly better long-term patency than PEG-J tubes, which tend to recoil back into the stomach. Additional long-term access can be achieved via surgical approaches for gastric tube or jejunostomy tube placement.

Types of Enteral Nutrition. In addition to the method and route of EN administration, the formula and supplements prescribed can affect nutritional therapy. Various formulas and supplements for EN exist and can be tailored to specific disease states. Tables 7.2 and 7.3 discuss the common formulas and supplements used in critical care.

Tolerance. Upon initiating EN, intolerance to therapy is evaluated. Intolerance is often defined as abdominal distension, constipation, emesis, or nausea/vomiting. In years past, gastric residual volume (GRV) was used to evaluate intolerance; however, current guidelines do not recommend routine monitoring of GRV. Research found that GRVs greater than 250 mL did not increase the patient's risk of aspiration or pneumonia. Monitoring GRV compromised EN delivery, increased nursing workload, and led to an increase in enteral device clogging.[1] The recommendation is to not check the GRV; however, in facilities still using GRV, EN should not be held unless GRV is greater than 500 mL.[1,39] In patients with postpyloric enteral access, GRV should not be assessed given the location, pliability, and small bore of the tube.

Critically ill patients are often on medications that decrease motility, such as analgesics and sedatives, increasing the risk of EN intolerance. To reduce the risk of intolerance in this population, a proactive bowel regimen should accompany the initiation of EN, unless contraindicated. If patients become constipated or demonstrate signs and symptoms of intolerance,

TABLE 7.2 Common Formulas

Type	Description	Calories (kcal/mL)	Disease States
Standard (Jevity, Nutren, Fibersource HN, Isosource)	Fiber containing, average osmolality	1; 1.2; 1.5; 2	Patient with minimal or no comorbid conditions
Low residue (Osmolite, Nutren, Isosource HN)	No fiber, low osmolality	1; 1.2; 1.5	Surgical patients, GI conditions
Elemental (Vital, Vivonex, Peptamen)	Fully hydrolyzed protein	1.2; 1.5	Patients with intolerance, GI surgery, or trauma
Peptide based (Pivot, Impact)	Partially hydrolyzed protein	1.5	SIRS, ARDS, improves protein absorption
Diabetes specific (Glucerna, Diabetisource)	Lower carbohydrate content, higher protein	1; 1.2; 1.5	Improves glucose control for diabetics or patients with hyperglycemia
Renal specific (Suplena, Nepro)	Lower in sodium, phosphorus, and potassium; high and low protein formulations available; carbohydrate controlled	1.8	Chronic kidney disease or end-stage renal disease; high-protein formula used for patients on dialysis and low-protein formula used for patients not requiring dialysis

ARDS, Acute respiratory distress syndrome; *GI,* gastrointestinal; *SIRS,* systemic inflammatory response syndrome.

TABLE 7.3 Common Supplements

Supplement	Details
Protein	Whole grams of protein provided as a powder, gel, or liquid to increase protein content of enteral nutrition (EN) Often provide 10-20 g protein/serving
Insoluble fiber	Add to EN to provide prebiotics or to bulk Decrease incidence of loose bowel movements or diarrhea
Arginine/glutamine	Add to promote wound and pressure injury healing

promotility medications may be considered. Common medications used for motility and bowel regimens are outlined in Table 7.4.

Patients on EN may also develop diarrhea, which can be perceived as intolerance to EN. However, the most common cause of diarrhea is liquid medications containing sorbitol. Other common causes could be contamination, disease process, antibiotic-related, or *Clostridium difficile*. Rarely is EN formula the cause; however, consultation with the dietitian may be helpful to determine opportunities to change the rate or type of formula.[40,41]

Post-pyloric access is preferred in patients with demonstrated gastric EN intolerance.[1] If gastric EN intolerance persists, the nurse should recommend diverting the enteral access to lower in the GI tract.

CLINICAL JUDGMENT ACTIVITY

Upon assessing the patient, the nurse notes the patient's abdomen is distended. When reviewing the record, the nurse determines that the patient's last bowel movement was 4 days ago. How should the nurse proceed?

Nursing Considerations. During administration of EN, elevate the patient's head of bed to 30 degrees or higher to prevent aspiration. Placing the head of bed higher than 30 degrees requires frequent integumentary assessments and patient repositioning to reduce the risk of pressure injury. Avoid unnecessary interruptions of EN for procedures or repositioning. The amount of EN delivered during repositioning will not increase risk for aspiration. This is especially true for enteral access devices in the small bowel; these feedings should not be withheld for repositioning.[42]

Whenever medications are administered via an enteral feeding tube, always use an enteral (ENFit) syringe and flush the tube with 30 mL of water before and after each medication is administered. Patients requiring fluid restriction may receive 15 mL for flushes. Additional flushes may be required for viscous medications or preparations (i.e., protein solutions). If the patient's EN is to be placed on hold, flush the feeding tube to prevent a buildup of residue in the tube and reduce the risk of clogging.[35,43]

Liquid medication formulations may be preferred for administration via the enteral feeding tube; however, they increase the risk of diarrhea, as many liquid medications use sorbitol as an excipient. If enough sorbitol is consumed, the sugar alcohol can have a laxative effect. Sustained-release medications must not be crushed and given via a feeding tube because of the potential for overdose. Bioavailability of some medications may be reduced when administered with enteral feedings.[43] EN may require temporary discontinuation before and after medication administration. For example, current recommendations for administration of phenytoin are to stop enteral feedings 1 to 2 hours before and after administration.[43] This method may not always be optimal, especially for malnourished patients. Other options include monitoring and adjusting phenytoin dosages based on serum drug levels while the patient is receiving EN or transitioning the patient to IV therapy during continuous EN administration. Once EN is discontinued, the drug dosage

TABLE 7.4 **PHARMACOLOGY**

Medications Frequently Used for Motility and Bowel Regimens

Medication	Action and Use	Dose and Route	Side Effects	Nursing Implications
Bisacodyl (Dulcolax)	Laxative; stimulant	*Oral/Enteral:* 5-15 mg daily *Rectal:* 10 mg suppository daily	Cramping Diarrhea Nausea Rectal burning Vomiting	Educate patient on avoiding long-term use (>1 wk). Ensure patient hydration.
Docusate sodium (Colace)	Laxative; stool softener	*Oral/Enteral:* 50-400 mg divided 1-2 times daily	Cramps Diarrhea Nausea	Do not break or crush tablet. Product may take up to 3 days to soften stool. Ensure patient hydration.
Erythromycin	Prokinetic	*Oral/Enteral:* 250-500 mg tid	Cardiac toxicity Tachyphylaxis	Use liquid form for tubes; do not break or crush tablet. Monitor for allergic reactions.
Metoclopramide (Reglan)	Prokinetic	*Intravenous:* 10 mg IV q6h May give 10 mg IV for small bowel feeding tube insertion CrCl <40, 5 mg IV q6h	Diarrhea EPS Fatigue Neuroleptic malignant syndrome Neutropenia Sedation Seizures Suicidal ideation	Increased risk of hypertension if combined with MAOIs. EPS risk increases with prolonged and high-dose use. Monitor for QT prolongation (especially with renal patients). Avoid in combination with haloperidol because of increased risk for tardive dyskinesia, EPS, and prolonged QT intervals. More likely with treatment >3 months and with geriatric patients.
Polyethylene glycol (Miralax)	Laxative; osmotic	*Oral/Enteral:* 17 g daily to bid	Abdominal distension Diarrhea Nausea Stomach cramping	Dissolve in 4-8 ounces of water or beverage of patient's choice.
Senna (Senokot)	Laxative; stimulant	*Oral/Enteral:* 17.2 mg daily to bid	Abdominal cramping Diarrhea Nausea	Ensure patient hydration.

bid, Two times a day; *CrCl*, creatinine clearance; *EPS*, extrapyramidal symptoms; *MAOIs*, monoamine oxidase inhibitors; *tid*, three times a day; *wk*, week.

Data from Chapman MJ, Fraser RJ, Kluger MT, et al. Erythromycin improves gastric emptying in critically ill patients intolerant of nasogastric feeding. *Crit Care Med.* 2000;28:2334-2337; Skidmore-Roth L. *Mosby's 2023 Nursing Drug Reference.* 36th ed. St. Louis, MO: Elsevier; 2023.

or route of administration is readjusted. When administering medications via a feeding tube, collaborate with the pharmacist to ensure safe and effective medication administration.

The location of enteral access in the alimentary tract may also affect bioavailability of some medications.[43] In patients receiving medications via a small bowel or jejunostomy tube, care should be given to ensure that all medications are effectively absorbed in the small bowel. For example, antacid medications such as pantoprazole or famotidine are ineffective when administered directly into the small intestine given their mechanism of action. Open communication and collaboration with the pharmacist is essential. Communication with the multiprofessional team to effectively reconcile the medication administration record during transitions between oral and feeding tube administration will facilitate safe and effective therapy.

CHECK YOUR UNDERSTANDING

2. What intervention(s) would be most appropriate for the nurse when caring for a patient with feeding intolerance? (Select all that apply)
   A. Stop feeding
   B. Request prokinetic agents
   C. Ask the dietitian to change the enteral formula
   D. Request an order to place a postpyloric feeding tube

CLINICAL JUDGMENT ACTIVITY

Determine the types of enteral nutrition–drug interactions that may cause complications.

Parenteral Nutrition

Optimizing. PN is a form of nutrition that supplies protein, fat, minerals, electrolytes, and carbohydrates via the IV route. In patients for whom EN is contraindicated because of the structure or function of the alimentary tract (e.g., discontinuity, obstruction), assess them early for the provision of PN. A multiprofessional approach to PN implementation may reduce the associated risks, including those of hyperglycemia, electrolyte imbalances, immune suppression, increased oxidative stress, and potential infectious morbidity.

PN should be withheld for the first 7 days of a critical care admission if the patient is well nourished or at low risk for malnutrition and EN is not feasible.[1,44] If the patient cannot receive EN and is found to be severely malnourished or have a high nutritional risk, initiate PN as soon as possible after admission. In patients receiving EN, consider PN if nutritional goals are not met after 7 days of EN.[44] Do not use PN unnecessarily, as its initiation and the treatment itself are not without risks. However, if PN is indicated, initiate the nutrition early to maximize benefits. If possible, consider trophic feeds to reduce the risk of sepsis and wean the patient from PN as soon as possible.[19]

Delivery Route and Types. There are two types of PN, total and peripheral, with total PN (TPN) being more common given the concentrated dosing and lower fluid volume. Peripheral PN (PPN) is not indicated for use in the adult population. PPN does not provide full nutritional support to patients and has the risk of compromising peripheral veins.

TPN involves the administration of a highly concentrated dextrose solution (≥10%) with a high osmolarity (>900 mOsm/L).[45] Because of the high concentration of dextrose, patients receiving TPN have an increased risk of hyperglycemia and require frequent glucose monitoring and management. The caustic nature of the hyperosmolar fluid requires central venous access through a peripherally inserted central catheter (PICC), port, or subclavian, jugular, or femoral central venous access. Central venous access increases the patient's risk of nosocomial infection (i.e., central line–associated bloodstream infection [CLABSI]). Decrease this risk by implementing CLABSI prevention bundles and adhering to hand hygiene practices (refer to the Collaborative Care Plan found in Chapter 1, Overview of Critical Care Nursing).

Lipids. Lipids or fatty acids are infused with TPN to prevent essential fatty acid deficiency. Provision of lipids should not exceed 30% of a patient's total caloric intake from TPN. In patients receiving lipids, monitor triglyceride levels and withhold lipids if levels are elevated. Some medications use lipids as an emulsifier (e.g., the sedative propofol [Diprivan]), and lipids are often held until discontinuation of these medications to prevent hypertriglyceridemia. Lipids can be infused concurrently with TPN or separately. Lipids have generally been thought to increase the risk of infection. More recent research refutes this notion, noting the risk may vary based on the type of lipid emulsion preparation. However, it is important to closely monitor patients receiving lipids for infection as well as hypertriglyceridemia.[46,47]

CHECK YOUR UNDERSTANDING

3. A healthy, well-nourished patient was admitted to the critical care unit 8 days ago after a motor vehicle collision. The patient has been hemodynamically unstable, on high-dose vasopressors. The patient has returned to the operating room multiple times to address a severe bowel injury. The surgeons are concerned about the patient's bowel continuity. She has remained NPO since admission. Which assessment findings would indicate initiation of total parenteral nutrition (TPN) is appropriate?
   A. Potential bowel discontinuity
   B. NPO for 8 days in a healthy, well-nourished patient
   C. High-dose vasopressor use
   D. All of the above when combined

Nursing Considerations. Use a dedicated port in the central venous access device to administer TPN and lipids. Preferably, do not administer other medications via the same port as TPN.

Monitor and evaluate electrolytes closely in patients receiving TPN, as these patients' high nutritional risk predisposes them to refeeding syndrome. Refeeding syndrome is a potentially life-threatening electrolyte fluctuation in response to aggressive administration of nutritional therapy in a previously malnourished patient.[17] The guidelines recommend a slow titration of TPN to the feeding goal over a 3- to 4-day period in at-risk patients.[1] Electrolyte monitoring and repletion is especially important, and in severe cases of refeeding, nutritional support has to be reduced to allow adequate electrolyte repletion.[48,49]

Ideally, a patient who has been receiving TPN is transitioned to EN when possible. Ensure that the patient is receiving more than 80% of estimated caloric needs from EN or an oral diet prior to discontinuing TPN.[35] When the TPN is discontinued, especially if done abruptly, monitor for signs and symptoms of hypoglycemia.

 **CLINICAL JUDGMENT ACTIVITY**

Outline factors to consider when selecting a type of nutritional support.

Monitoring and Evaluating the Nutrition Care Plan

A multiprofessional approach is essential when developing and reviewing the nutrition plan of care to ensure best practices and evidence-based therapies are implemented (see Evidence-Based Practice box; the Collaborative Care Plan found in Chapter 1, Overview of Critical Care Nursing).[1] Laboratory and diagnostic studies can be useful in the assessment and administration of nutritional therapy (see Laboratory Alert box). In addition, assessment of daily weights, fluid balance, and functional status can assist in evaluating the adequacy of energy and protein provision. If goals are not being met, reassessment of the plan is necessary to help the patient achieve optimal nutrition outcomes. Assessment of weight loss, abnormal laboratory values, and the appearance of dehydration or fluid overload are indicators that the nutrition care plan may need to be adjusted.

EVIDENCE-BASED PRACTICE

Nutritional Support in Critical Illness

Problem

Critically ill patients are at high risk for malnutrition secondary to the catabolic stress state associated with critical illness. Nutritional therapy is essential to attenuate the metabolic response to stress, prevent cellular injury, and modulate immune responses.

Clinical Question

What are recommended practices to optimize nutritional therapy in critically ill patients?

Evidence

The Society of Critical Care Medicine (SCCM) and the American Society for Parenteral and Enteral Nutrition (ASPEN) convened an expert panel to review available evidence related to nutritional therapy in critically ill patients. They evaluated primarily randomized controlled trials and meta-analyses to rate the evidence; however, they also included cohort trials, observational studies, and retrospective studies. Guidelines were reviewed and updated in 2021. If data were limited, the group achieved consensus on the best clinical practice recommendations. Evidence thus varied for each of the many recommendations. Recommendations relevant to the majority of critically ill patients are:

- Nutritional assessment
  - Determine risk using valid assessment tools (NRS-2002 or NUTRIC).
  - Adjust assessment based on comorbid conditions.
  - Determine energy requirements.
    - Indirect calorimetry (IC)
    - Predictive equations
    - Simplistic formula of 25 to 30 kcal/kg
  - Ensure adequate protein intake.
- Enteral nutrition (EN)
  - Start EN within 24 to 48 hours if patient is unable to maintain oral intake.
  - The presence of bowel sounds is not required to start EN.
  - Gastric feedings can be safely administered to most patients.
  - Consider postpyloric feedings in those at high risk for aspiration or those who have a history of intolerance to gastric feedings.
  - Those at low nutritional risk do not require specialized nutritional therapy.
  - Advance nutrition for those at high risk to the target goal, as tolerated, over 24 to 48 hours.
- Monitor tolerance to EN
  - Avoid unnecessary interruptions.
  - Gastric residual volume (GRV) should not be used to assess aspiration risk.
  - If GRV is assessed, avoid holding EN for volumes less than 500 mL.
  - Assess for aspiration risk and implement interventions to reduce aspiration.
  - Do not interrupt EN for diarrhea; assess and treat potential causes of diarrhea.
- Selection of EN formula
  - Use standard polymeric formulas.
  - Avoid routine use of specialty formulas in medical patients.
  - Avoid routine use of disease-specific formulas in the surgical patient.
  - Consider formulas containing fiber or peptides for persistent diarrhea.
- Parenteral nutrition (PN)
  - Avoid administration for the first 7 days of admission in low-risk patients.
  - Start PN as soon as possible when EN is contraindicated in patients at high nutritional risk.
  - Consider supplemental PN if the patient is unable to meet at least 60% of energy and protein requirements after 7 days of EN.
  - Use a nutritional therapy team to manage PN.
- Obesity
  - Start early EN within 24 to 48 hours.
  - Administer high-protein, hypocaloric feedings to preserve lean muscle mass.

Implications for Nursing

These guidelines provide a broad range of recommendations for the critically ill patient. Collaborate with members of the multiprofessional team to implement the recommendations according to patient assessment. In addition, implement the following recommended nutrition bundle in critically ill patients:

- Assess critically ill patients on admission for nutritional risk; calculate energy and protein requirements to determine goals of therapy.
- Start EN within 24 to 48 hours after admission; increase goals over the first week.
- Initiate interventions to reduce aspiration risk and improve tolerance of EN.
- Implement EN protocols.
- Do not use GRV as part of routine monitoring.
- Initiate PN early when EN is not feasible or is insufficient in meeting nutritional goals.
- Maintain head of bed elevation at 30 to 45 degrees, unless contraindicated.

Level of Evidence

D—Professional standards developed from evidence

Reference

Taylor BE, McClave SA, Martindale RG, et al. Guidelines for the provision and assessment of nutrition support therapy in the adult critically ill patient: Society of Critical Care Medicine (SCCM) and American Society for Parenteral and Enteral Nutrition (ASPEN). *Crit Care Med.* 2016;44(2):159–211.

Compher C, Bingham AL, McCall M, et al. Guidelines for the provision of nutrition support therapy in the adult critically ill patient: the American Society for Parenteral and Enteral Nutrition. *J Parenter Enteral Nutr.* 2022;46:12–41.

LABORATORY ALERT

Laboratory Test	Normal Range	Critical Value[a]	Significance
Prealbumin	15-36 mg/dL	<10.7 mg/dL	Serum levels fluctuate quickly (1.9-day half-life). More reliable indication of protein synthesis and catabolism than albumin. Affected by inflammatory process, so may make interpretation difficult; not a validated method for evaluating nutrition status. Increased with chronic kidney disease. Decreased with malnutrition, inflammation, and infection.
Albumin	3.5-5 g/dL	<3.5 g/dL	Half-life between 18 and 21 days. Not a reliable indication of protein synthesis or catabolism. Many disease states decrease serum albumin levels, including inflammatory processes, liver disease, acute reaction, and nephrotic syndrome.
Triglycerides (TGs)	Male: 40-160 mg/dL Female: 35-135 mg/dL	>400 mg/dL	**Hypotriglyceridemia:** Malnutrition **Hypertriglyceridemia:** TGs act as a storage form of energy, and when excess builds up in the bloodstream, it is deposited into tissue. May consider withholding lipids from TPN; implement alternative sedative regimens, as indicated (i.e., propofol is suspended in lipids).
Sodium	136-145 mEq/L	<120 mEq/L >160 mEq/L	Many factors and disease states affect serum sodium levels. **Hyponatremia:** May affect neurological function; indicative of the syndrome of inappropriate antidiuretic hormone secretion (SIADH); may be caused by excessive free water or inadequate dietary provision of sodium. **Hypernatremia:** May affect neurological function; sign of dehydration, inadequate free water intake, excessive sodium in IV fluids.
Potassium	3.5-5 mEq/L	<2.5 mEq/L >6.5 mEq/L	Levels are affected by acid-base balance, sodium resorption, and aldosterone. **Hypokalemia:** Caused by GI losses, medications, or inadequate dietary intake/IV supplementation when NPO, hypothermia. **Hyperkalemia:** Caused by dehydration, certain medications, renal impairment.
Magnesium	1.3-2.1 mEq/L	<0.5 mEq/L >3.0 mEq/L	Most organ functions depend on magnesium, and levels must be closely monitored in cardiac patients. **Hypomagnesemia:** Caused by malnutrition, malabsorption. **Hypermagnesemia:** Most often caused by renal disease or excessive intake of magnesium.
Phosphate	3-4.5 mg/dL	<1.0 mg/dL	**Hypophosphatemia:** Caused by phosphate shifting from extracellular to intracellular, renal phosphate wasting, GI losses, intracellular losses, or malnutrition. **Hyperphosphatemia:** Caused by renal disease or excessive dietary intake.
Glucose	74-106 mg/dL (fasting)	<50 mg/dL >450 mg/dL	**Hypoglycemia:** Often a result of insulin overdose, concomitant medications, or starvation. **Hyperglycemia:** True elevation indicates diabetes; however, there are many causes. Can be elevated due to stress, pregnancy, IV fluids containing dextrose, and/or medications (e.g., steroids).

[a]Critical values vary by facility and laboratory.
GI, Gastrointestinal; *NPO,* nothing by mouth; *TPN,* total parenteral nutrition.
Data from Pagana KD, Pagana TJ, Pagana TN. *Mosby's Diagnostic and Laboratory Test Reference.* 16th ed. St. Louis, MO: Elsevier, Inc.; 2023.

CASE STUDY

A 50-year-old female admitted after an out-of-hospital cardiac arrest with return of spontaneous circulation and intubation in the field. Targeted temperature management (TTM) was initiated, her blood pressure was being supported by high dose vasopressors, and an analgosedation regimen was initiated. On hospital day 3, TTM was discontinued, and vasopressors were weaned. She is neurologically intact. Objective data include the following: height, 164 cm; weight, 92 kg; body mass index (BMI), 34.2 kg/m^2; history of stable nutritional intake at home per the family. Laboratory data include a potassium level of 4.1 mEq/L, magnesium level of 2.5 mEq/L, and prealbumin level of 8 mg/dL. Urine output has been approximately 50 mL/h, and bowel sounds are hypoactive. During multiprofessional rounds, the nurse advocates for enteral nutrition (EN) via the orogastric tube (OGT) given the patient's inability to wean from the ventilator. The dietitian recommends a polymeric formula with hypocaloric and high-protein content, which is ordered at a targeted hourly rate by the provider. Two days later, on hospital day 5, the nursing assessment reveals bloating and distension. Based on discussions with the family and chart review, the nurse determines the patient has not had a bowel movement in 6 days.

Questions

1. What combination of assessment findings determines the patient's nutritional status and EN tolerance?
2. Given the patient's gastrointestinal (GI) signs and symptoms, what should the nurse recommend during multiprofessional rounds?
3. How should the nurse justify the preferred route of intake in this critically ill patient?
4. What assessment findings would indicate the interventions were effective and the patient is meeting her nutritional goals?

KEY POINTS

- EN is the preferred mode of nutrition for a patient unable to take nutrition by mouth.
- Radiographic confirmation of blindly placed enteral tubes is needed prior to initiating enteral feeding; reassess placement every 4 hours by examining external tube length.
- Gastric residual volume should not be routinely monitored to assess enteral feeding tolerance.
- Monitor for signs of tolerance by assessing gastric distention, constipation, nausea, and vomiting.
- Analgesic and sedative medications may slow gastric motility, increasing risk of intolerance.
- PN should only be considered in patients in whom EN is not possible.

REFERENCES

1. Taylor BE, McClave SA, Martindale RG, et al. Guidelines for the provision and assessment of nutrition support therapy in the adult critically ill patient: Society of Critical Care Medicine (SCCM) and American Society for Parenteral and Enteral Nutrition (ASPEN). *Crit Care Med*. 2016;44(2): 159–211.
2. Sharma K, Mogensen KM, Robinson MK. Pathophysiology of critical illness and role of nutrition. *Nutr Clin Pract*. 2019;34(1):12–22. https://doi.org/10.1002/ncp.10232.
3. Cass AR, Charlton KE. Prevalence of hospital-acquired malnutrition and modifiable determinants of nutritional deterioration during inpatient admissions: a systematic review of the evidence. *J Hum Nutr Diet*. 2022;35(6):1043–1058. https://doi.org/10.1111/jhn.13009.
4. Osooli F, Abbas S, Farsaei S, Adibi P. Identifying critically ill patients at risk of malnutrition and underfeeding: a prospective study at an academic hospital. *Adv Pharm Bull*. 2019;9(2):314–320. https://doi.org/10.15171/apb.2019.037.
5. Lew CCH, Yandell R, Fraser RJL, Chua AP, Chong MFF, Miller M. Association between malnutrition and clinical outcomes in the intensive care unit: a systematic review. *J Parenter Enteral Nutr*. 2017;41(5):744–758. https://doi.org/10.1177/0148607115625638.
6. van Gassel RJJ, Baggerman MR, van de Poll MCG. Metabolic aspects of muscle wasting during critical illness. *Curr Opin Clin Nutr Metab Care*. 2020;23(2):96–101. https://doi.org/10.1097/MCO.0000000000000628.
7. Turner KC. Structure and function of the digestive system. In: McCance KL, Huether SE, eds. *Pathophysiology: The Biologic Basis for Disease in Adults and Children*. 9th ed. St. Louis, MO: Elsevier; 2022:1285–1317.
8. Kiela PR, Ghishan FK. Physiology of intestinal absorption and secretion. *Best Pract Res Clin Gastroenterol*. 2016;30(2):145–159. https://doi.org/10.1016/j.bpg.2016.02.007.
9. The Joint Commission Standards Interpretation Group. Nutritional and functional screening - requirement. The Joint Commission. https://www.jointcommission.org/standards/standard-faqs/hospital-and-hospital-clinics/provision-of-care-treatment-and-services-pc/000001652/. Published November 17, 2022. Accessed January 13, 2023.
10. Norman K, Haß U, Pirlich M. Malnutrition in older adults-recent advances and remaining challenges. *Nutrients*. 2021;13(8):276. https://doi.org/10.3390/nu13082764.
11. Roberts SB, Silver RE, Das SK, et al. Healthy aging-nutrition matters: start early and screen often. *Adv Nutr*. 2021;12(4):1438–1448. https://doi.org/10.1093/advances/nmab032.
12. American College of Obstetricians and Gynecologists. *Your Pregnancy and Childbirth: Month to Month*. 7th ed. Washington, DC: American College of Obstetricians and Gynecologists; 2021.
13. Erick M, Cox JT, Mogensen KM. ACOG practice bulletin 189: nausea and vomiting of pregnancy. *Obstet Gynecol*. 2018;131(5):935. https://doi.org/10.1097/AOG.0000000000002604.
14. Venkat S, Subramaniam R, Raveendran V. Early enteral nutrition in acute pancreatitis - how beneficial is it? *Int Surg J*. 2021;8:3279–3284.
15. Deane AM, Ali Abdelhamid Y, Plummer MP, Fetterplace K, Moore C, Reintam Blaser A. Are classic bedside exam findings required to initiate enteral nutrition in critically ill patients: emphasis on bowel sounds and abdominal distension. *Nutr Clin Pract*. 2021;36(1):67–75. https://doi.org/10.1002/ncp.10610.
16. Delsoglio M, Achamrah N, Berger MM, Pichard C. Indirect calorimetry in clinical practice. *J Clin Med*. 2019;8(9):1387. https://doi.org/10.3390/jcm8091387.
17. Mahan LK, Raymond JL. *Krause's Food and the Nutrition Care Process*. 15th ed. St. Louis, MO: Elsevier, Inc.; 2020.
18. Keller U. Nutritional laboratory markers in malnutrition. *J Clin Med*. 2019;8(6):775. https://doi.org/10.3390/jcm8060775.
19. Lewis S, Schofield-Robinson O, Alderson P, Smith A. Enteral versus parenteral nutrition and enteral versus a combination of enteral and parenteral nutrition for adults in the intensive care unit. *Cochrane Database Syst Rev*. 2018;6(6):CD012276. https://doi.org/10.1002/14651858.CD012276.pub2.
20. Wiertsema SP, van Bergenhenegouwen J, Garssen J, Knippels LMJ. The interplay between the gut microbiome and the immune system in the context of infectious diseases throughout life and the role of nutrition in optimizing treatment strategies. *Nutrients*. 2021;13(3):886. https://doi.org/10.3390/nu13030886.
21. Al-Dorzi HM, Arabi YM. Nutrition support for critically ill patients. *J Parenter Enteral Nutr*. 2021;45(S2):47–59. https://doi.org/10.1002/jpen.2228.
22. Tian F, Heighes PT, Allingstrup MJ, et al. Early nutrition provided within 24 hours of ICU admission: a meta-analysis of randomized controlled trials. *Crit Care Med*. 2018;46(7):1049–1056.
23. Reintam BA, Starkopf J, Alhazzani W, et al. Early enteral nutrition in critically ill patients: ESICM clinical practice guidelines. *Intensive Care Med*. 2017;43(3):380–398.
24. Wischmeyer PE. Enteral nutrition can be given to patients on vasopressors. *Crit Care Med*. 2020;48(1):122–125. https://doi.org/10.1097/CCM.0000000000003965.
25. Ventura AM, Waitzberg DL. Enteral nutrition protocols for critically ill patients: are they necessary? *Nutr Clin Pract*. 2015;30(3):351–362. https://doi.org/10.1177/0884533614547765.
26. Orinovsky I, Raizman E. Improvement of nutritional intake in intensive care unit patients via a nurse-led enteral nutrition feeding protocol. *Crit Care Nurse*. 2018;38(3):38–44. https://doi.org/10.4037/ccn2018433.
27. Jovanović G, Jakovljević DK, Lukić-Šarkanović M. Enhanced recovery in surgical intensive care: a review. *Front Med (Lausanne)*. 2018;5:256. https://doi.org/10.3389/fmed.2018.00256.

28. Practice guidelines for preoperative fasting and the use of pharmacologic agents to reduce the risk of pulmonary aspiration: application to healthy patients undergoing elective procedures: an updated report by the American Society of anesthesiologists task force on preoperative fasting and the use of pharmacologic agents to reduce the risk of pulmonary aspiration. *Anesthesiology*. 2017;126(3):376–393. https://doi.org/10.1097/ALN.0000000000001452.
29. Weimann A, Braga M, Carli F, et al. ESPEN practical guideline: clinical nutrition in surgery. *Clin Nutr*. 2021;40(7):4745–4761. https://doi.org/10.1016/j.clnu.2021.03.031.
30. Reintam Blaser A, Deane AM, Preiser JC, Arabi YM, Jakob SM. Enteral feeding intolerance: updates in definitions and pathophysiology. *Nutr Clin Pract*. 2021;36(1):40–49. https://doi.org/10.1002/ncp.10599.
31. Prest PJ, Justice J, Bell N, McCarroll R, Watson C. A volume-based feeding protocol improves nutrient delivery and glycemic control in a surgical trauma intensive care unit. *J Parenter Enteral Nutr*. 2020;44(5):880–888.
32. Heyland DK, Lemuix M, Shu L, et al. What is "best achievable" practice in implementing the enhanced protein-energy provision via the enteral route feeding protocol in intensive care units in the United States? results of a multicenter, quality improvement collaborative. *J Parenter Enteral Nutr*. 2018;42(2):308–317. 35.
33. Metheny NA, Hinyard LJ, Mohammed KA. Incidence of sinusitis associated with endotracheal and nasogastric tubes: NIS database. *Am J Crit Care*. 2018;27(1):24–31.
34. American Association of Critical-Care Nurses. AACN practice alert: initial and ongoing verification of feeding tube placement in adults. *Crit Care Nurs*. 2016;36(2):e8–e13.
35. Boullata JI, Carrera AL, Harvey L, et al. ASPEN safe practices for enteral nutrition therapy. *J Parenter Enteral Nutr*. 2017;41(1):15–103.
36. Liu Y, Wang Y, Zhang B, Wang J, Sun L, Xiao Q. Gastric-tube versus post-pyloric feeding in critical patients: a systematic review and meta-analysis of pulmonary aspiration- and nutrition-related outcomes. *Eur J Clin Nutr*. 2021;75(9):1337–1348. https://doi.org/10.1038/s41430-021-00860-2.
37. Powers J, Brown B, Lyman B, et al. Development of a competency model for placement and verification of nasogastric and nasoenteric feeding tubes for adult hospitalized patients. *Nutr Clin Pract*. 2021;36(3):517–533. https://doi.org/10.1002/ncp.10671.
38. Powers J, Luebbenhusen M, Spitzer T, et al. Verification of an electromagnetic placement device compared with abdominal radiograph to predict accuracy of feeding tube placement. *J Parenter Enteral Nutr*. 2011;35(4):535–539.
39. Metheny NA. Monitoring adult patients for intolerance to gastric tube feedings. *Am J Nurs*. 2021;121(8):36–43. https://doi.org/10.1097/01.NAJ.0000767356.16777.f1.
40. Pitta MR, Campos FM, Monteiro AG, Cunha AGF, Porto JD, Gomes RR. Tutorial on diarrhea and enteral nutrition: a comprehensive step-by-step approach. *J Parenter Enteral Nutr*. 2019;43(8):1008–1019. https://doi.org/10.1002/jpen.1674.
41. Parrish CR, McCray S. Part II enteral feeding: eradicate barriers with root cause analysis and focused interventions. nutrition issues in gastroenterology, series #184. *Practical Gastroenterology*. 2019:14–33.
42. DiLibero J, Lavieri M, O'Donoghue S, DeSanto-Madeya S. Withholding or continuing enteral feedings during repositioning and the incidence of aspiration. *Am J Crit Care*. 2015;24(3):258–261. https://doi.org/10.4037/ajcc2015482.
43. Boullata JI. Enteral medication for the tube-fed patient: making this route safe and effective. *Nutr Clin Pract*. 2021;36(1):111–132. https://doi.org/10.1002/ncp.10615.
44. Compher C, Bingham AL, McCall M, et al. Guidelines for the provision of nutrition support therapy in the adult critically ill patient: The American Society for Parenteral and Enteral Nutrition. *J Parenter Enteral Nutr*. 2022;46:12–41.
45. Boullata JI, Gilbert K, Sacks G, et al. ASPEN clinical guidelines: parenteral nutrition ordering, order review, compounding, labeling and dispensing. *J Parenter Enteral Nutr*. 2014:1–44.
46. Mayer K, Klek S, García-de-Lorenzo A, et al. Lipid use in hospitalized adults requiring parenteral nutrition. *J Parenter Enteral Nutr*. 2020;44(Suppl 1):S28–S38. https://doi.org/10.1002/jpen.1733.
47. Tota A, Serra A, Raoul P, Gasbarrini A, Rinninella E, Mele MC. Lipid-enriched parenteral nutrition and bloodstream infections in hospitalized patients: is it a real concern? *Medicina (Kaunas)*. 2022;58(7):885. https://doi.org/10.3390/medicina58070885.
48. Friedli N, Odermatt J, Reber E, Schuetz P, Stanga Z. Refeeding syndrome: update and clinical advice for prevention, diagnosis and treatment. *Curr Opin Gastroenterol*. 2020;36(2):136–140. https://doi.org/10.1097/MOG.0000000000000605.
49. McKnight CL, Newberry C, Sarav M, Martindale R, Hurt R, Daley B. Refeeding syndrome in the critically ill: a literature review and clinician's guide. *Curr Gastroenterol Rep*. 2019;21(11):58. https://doi.org/10.1007/s11894-019-0724-3.
50. Kirkland LL, Shaughnessy E. Recognition and prevention of nosocomial malnutrition: a review and a call to action. *Am J Med*. 2017;130(12):1345–1350.

8

Dysrhythmia Interpretation and Management

Angela D. Pal, PhD, APRN, ACNP-BC, CHSE

INTRODUCTION

The interpretation of cardiac rhythm disturbances or dysrhythmias is an essential skill for nurses employed in patient care areas where electrocardiographic monitoring occurs. The ability to rapidly analyze a rhythm disturbance and initiate appropriate treatment improves patient safety and optimizes successful outcomes. The critical care nurse is often the healthcare professional responsible for the continuous monitoring of the patient's cardiac rhythm and has the opportunity to provide early intervention that can prevent an adverse clinical situation. This responsibility requires not only a mastery of interpreting dysrhythmias, but also the ability to identify the unique monitoring needs of each patient. The terms *dysrhythmia* and *cardiac arrhythmia* refer to an abnormal cardiac rhythm that deviates from normal sinus rhythm (NSR). The term *dysrhythmia* is used throughout this text. This chapter reviews basic cardiac dysrhythmias, etiological factors, clinical significance, and appropriate treatments to aid the critical care nurse in mastering dysrhythmia recognition. The goal is to provide an essential understanding of electrocardiography for analyzing and interpreting cardiac dysrhythmias.

Electrocardiography is the process of creating a visual tracing of the electrical activity of the cells in the heart. This tracing is called an *electrocardiogram* (ECG). The critical care nurse understands the need for cardiac monitoring, lead selection, and rhythm interpretation. Part of the difficulty in learning rhythm interpretation is that many of the terms used are synonymous. Throughout this chapter, these terms are clarified within the discussion of general concepts of dysrhythmia interpretation.

CARDIAC PHYSIOLOGY REVIEW

Cardiac Physiology

The ECG detects a summation of electrical signals generated by specialized cells of the heart called *pacemaker cells.* Pacemaker cells have the property of *automaticity,* meaning these cells can generate a stimulus or an action potential without outside stimulation. This electrical signal is conducted through specialized fibers of the conduction system to the mechanical or muscle cells of the heart where a cardiac contraction is generated. Thus, there must be an electrical signal for the mechanical event of contraction to occur. The coordinated electrical activity followed by a synchronous mechanical event constitutes the *cardiac cycle.*

The heart's conduction system (Fig. 8.1) is responsible for the *cardiac cycle* (Fig. 8.2), which begins with an impulse that is generated from a small, concentrated area of pacemaker cells high in the right atrium called the *sinoatrial* (SA) *node* or *sinus node.* The SA node has the fastest rate of discharge and thus is the dominant pacemaker of the heart. The SA node impulse quickly passes through the internodal conduction tracts and the Bachmann's bundle, conductive fibers in the right and left atria. The impulse rapidly reaches the atrioventricular (AV) node located in the area called the *AV junction,* between the atria and the ventricles. Here, the impulse is slowed to allow time for ventricular filling during relaxation or ventricular *diastole.* The AV node has pacemaker properties and can discharge an impulse if the SA node fails. The electrical impulse is then rapidly conducted through the bundle of His to the ventricles via the left and right bundle branches. The left bundle branch further divides into the left anterior fascicle and the left posterior fascicle. The bundle branches divide into smaller and smaller branches, finally terminating in tiny fibers called *Purkinje fibers* that reach the myocardial muscle cells, or myocytes. The bundle of His, the right and left bundle branches, and the Purkinje fibers are also known as the *His-Purkinje system.* The ventricles have pacemaker capabilities if the SA or AV nodes cease to generate impulses.

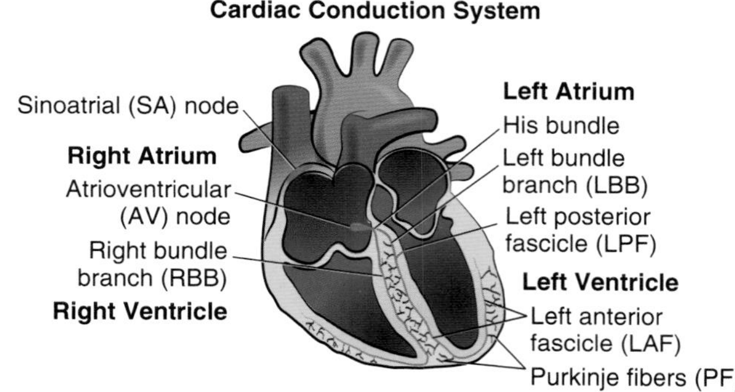

Fig. 8.1 The electrical conduction system of the heart.

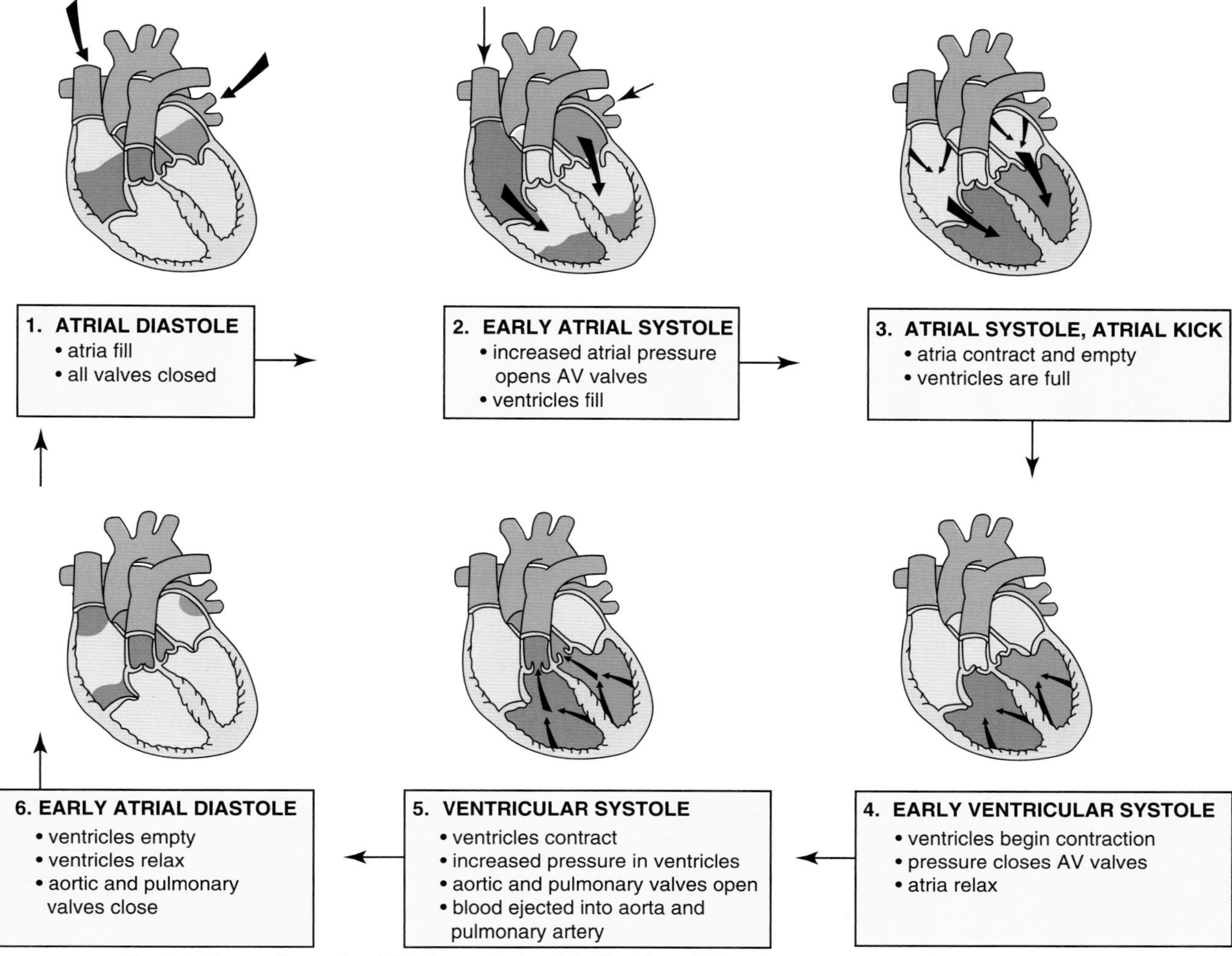

Fig. 8.2 The cardiac cycle. *AV,* Atrioventricular. (Modified from Hubert RJ, VanMeter KC. *Gould's Pathophysiology for Health Professions.* 6th ed. St. Louis, MO: Elsevier; 2018.)

The electrical signal stimulates the atrial muscle, called atrial *systole,* and causes the atria to contract simultaneously and eject their blood volume into the ventricles. Concurrently, the ventricles fill with blood during ventricular diastole. During atrial systole, a bolus of atrial blood is ejected into the ventricles. This step is called the *atrial kick,* and it contributes approximately 30% more blood to the cardiac output of the ventricles. The inflow or AV valves (tricuspid and mitral) close because of the increasing pressure of the blood volume in the ventricles. By this time, the electrical impulse reaches the Purkinje fibers, and the muscle cells have become stimulated and cause ventricular contraction. The outflow valves (aortic and pulmonic) open because of increased pressure and volume in the ventricles, allowing for ejection of the ventricular blood, called *ventricular systole.* At the same time ventricular systole is occurring, atrial diastole, or filling, is occurring. The atria are relaxed and filling with blood from the periphery (deoxygenated) and the lungs (oxygenated). Then, because of the rhythmic pacing of the heart, the muscle cells are again stimulated, the atria contract, and atrial blood is ejected once again into the ventricles. This process of electrical stimulation and mechanical response occurs rhythmically 60 to 100 times per minute in a healthy adult heart. The coordination of the electrical and mechanical events in the upper and lower chambers of the heart results in the emptying and filling of these chambers, and the valves open and close because of pressure changes. These physiological actions result in what is known as *cardiac output,* which continually adjusts to the needs of the body's tissues (see Fig. 8.2).

Cardiac Electrophysiology

Specialized cardiac pacemaker cells possess the property of *automaticity* and can generate an electrical impulse on their own. Nonpacemaker or muscle cells must receive an outside stimulus in normal circumstances to generate a response. The response generated by either the pacemaker or the muscle cells, once stimulated, is called the *action potential.* The cardiac action potential consists of phases related to depolarization, repolarization, and the resting or polarized state of the cell. Although this summary describes the action potential of a single cell, imagine that this is occurring in millions of cardiac cells almost simultaneously, resulting in the coordinated contractions of the atria and ventricles.

During the resting state of the cell, there is a difference in polarity, or charge, between the extracellular and intracellular environments that is maintained by the cell membrane. Specialized pumps prevent ions from passing through the cell membrane by diffusion. The inside of the cell is predominantly negatively charged, whereas the outside is positively charged. The resting membrane potential occurs when the cell is in the polarized or resting state. The polarized cell has a higher concentration of positive ions, including sodium outside the cell, causing the extracellular environment to be positive. The interior of the cell is more negative, and the concentration of potassium is higher. The voltage in the interior of the cardiac muscle cell during resting membrane potential is −90 mV, whereas that of the pacemaker cells in the SA and AV nodes is −65 mV.

The stimulation of a cardiac muscle cell by an electrical impulse changes the permeability of the myocardial cell membrane. Sodium ions rush into the cell via sodium channels in the cell membrane, and potassium ions flow out of the cell, resulting in a more positively charged cell interior (Fig. 8.3). The action potential describes the flow of ions inside and outside the cell, as well as the voltage changes that occur. The first phase of the action potential occurs when the cell membrane becomes permeable to sodium molecules. When the membrane potential reaches −65 mV, also known as *threshold,* more channels in the cell membrane open up and allow sodium ions to rush into the cell; the cell interior quickly reaches +30 mV, resulting in *depolarization.* After this fast phase of sodium influx, the plateau phase of the action potential occurs when calcium channels open and calcium flows into the cell. This slower phase allows for a longer period of depolarization, resulting in sustained muscle contraction.

The next event of the action potential occurs when the cell returns to the resting state. This process is called *repolarization* and results from ions returning to the outside (calcium and sodium) and the inside (potassium) of the cell. Sodium and potassium pumps within the cell membrane maintain this concentration gradient across the cell membrane when the cell is polarized. These pumps require energy in the form of adenosine

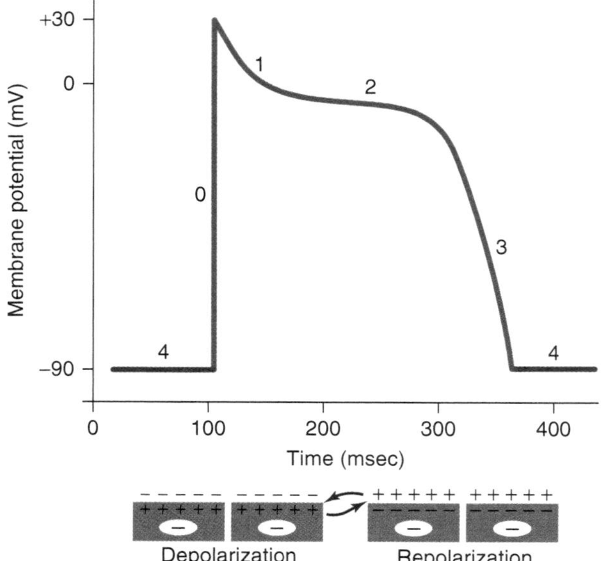

Fig. 8.3 Cardiac action potential.

triphosphate (ATP). Now the cell has returned to its resting state with a polarity of −90 mV once again. Depolarization of adjacent cells occurs simultaneously as the stimulus moves across the cardiac muscle, allowing for almost instantaneous depolarization of the entire muscle mass and resultant contraction (Fig. 8.4).

Pacemaker cells can reach threshold and depolarize without an outside stimulus. The cell membrane becomes suddenly permeable to sodium during the resting state and reaches threshold, resulting in spontaneous depolarization. Resting membrane potential for these automatic cells is −65 mV, and threshold is reached at approximately −50 mV.

The SA node reaches threshold at a rate of 60 to 100 times per minute. Because this is the fastest pacemaker in the heart, the SA node is the dominant pacemaker of the heart. The AV node and His-Purkinje pacemakers are latent pacemakers that reach threshold at a slower rate but can take over if the SA node fails or if sinus impulse conduction is blocked. The AV node has an inherent rate of 40 to 60 beats/min, and the His-Purkinje system can fire at a lower rate of 15 to 20 beats/min with an upper rate limit of 40 beats/min.

Autonomic Nervous System. The rate of spontaneous depolarization of the pacemaker cells is influenced by the autonomic nervous system. The sympathetic nervous system releases catecholamines, causing the SA node to fire more quickly in response to epinephrine and norepinephrine, which increases the heart rate. The parasympathetic nervous system releases acetylcholine, which slows the heart rate. During normal circumstances, these substances modulate each other, and the cardiac response allows for appropriate changes in cardiac output to meet the varying demands of the body (Fig. 8.5).

Causes Of Dysrhythmias

Dysrhythmias may occur when automaticity of the normal pacemaker cells of the heart is either stimulated or suppressed. For example, if the SA node fails to fire, latent pacemakers from the AV node or ventricles may fire as a backup safety mechanism. The SA node may fire more rapidly because of the influence of circulating catecholamines. Cells, either within or outside the normal conduction system, may take on characteristics of pacemaker cells and begin firing because of electrolyte imbalances, ischemia, injury, necrosis, or myocardial stretch caused by hypertrophy. *Ectopic beats* or *ectopic rhythms* arise from cells that normally do not have pacemaker capabilities. Slowed conduction can create alternative conductive pathways that produce abnormally fast heart rhythms. If conduction is sufficiently decreased, latent pacemakers may take over this function.

CHECK YOUR UNDERSTANDING

1. What are two significant considerations when a patient's heart rate increases, manifesting with symptoms?
   A. Venous return diminishes and cardiac filling increases, resulting in hypotension.
   B. Venous return increases and cardiac filling decreases, stimulating compensatory hypertension.
   C. Ventricular filling decreases and coronary perfusion is reduced, precipitating possible angina.
   D. Ventricular filling increases and coronary perfusion is increased.

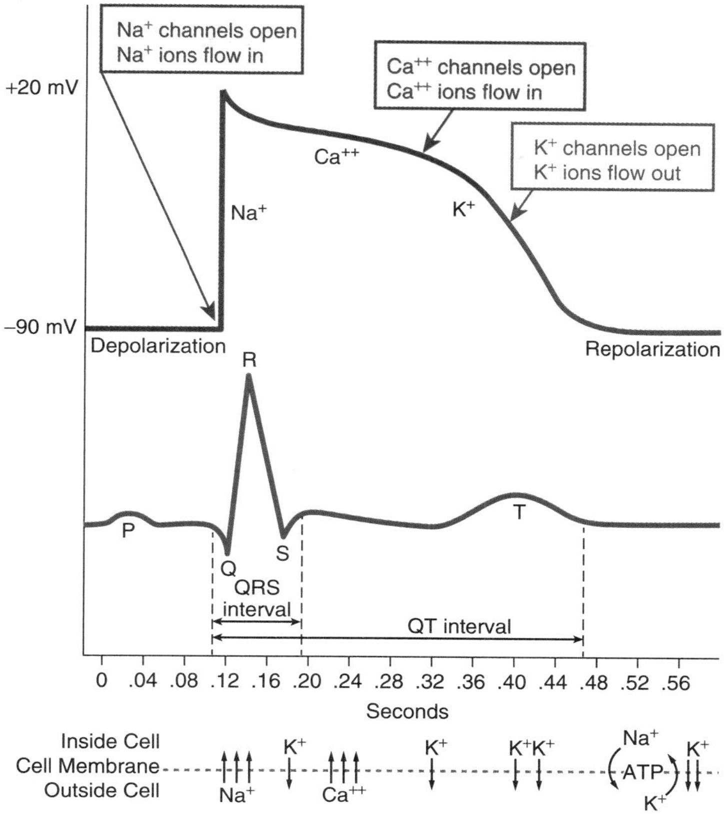

Fig. 8.4 Cardiac action potential with the electrocardiogram and movement of electrolytes. *ATP*, Adenosine triphosphate; *Ca++*, calcium; *K+*, potassium; *Na+*, sodium.

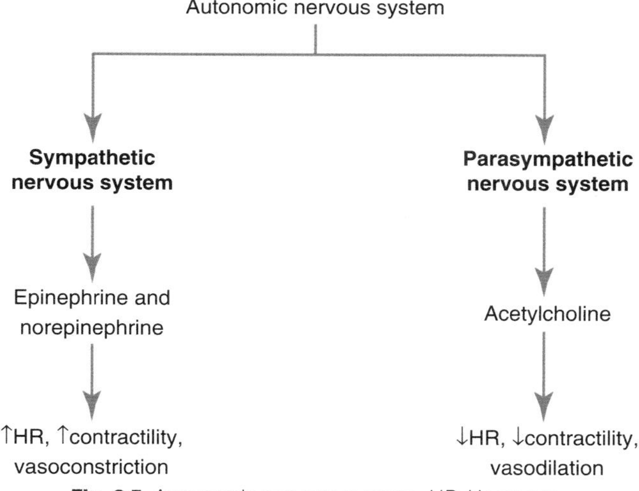

Fig. 8.5 Autonomic nervous system. *HR*, Heart rate.

CARDIAC MONITORING

Overview of Electrocardiogram Monitoring

The first ECG of the human heart was recorded in 1887 by British physiologist Augustus Waller via a capillary electrometer.[1] The PQRST complex (p-wave, QRS complex, t-wave) was later described by Willem Einthoven, who expanded on Waller's work. Einthoven proceeded to commercially produce a string galvanometer that was popularized in the early 1900s because he advocated for the use of the ECG in the clinical setting. Einthoven won the Nobel Prize in Physiology for Medicine in 1924 for inventing the electrocardiograph. Many other scientists continued to advance Waller and Einthoven's work, including the addition of the chest leads to provide additional information of the myocardium, and later the 12-lead ECG. Today, the 12-lead ECG machine is a diagnostic tool considered an essential mainstay of health care.

Continuous ECG monitoring did not become common practice until the 1960s, when the first cardiac care units were developed. Early cardiac monitoring consisted of monitoring for a heart rate that was too fast or too slow and for life-threatening dysrhythmias, including ventricular tachycardia (VT), ventricular fibrillation (VF), and asystole.[1] Today, cardiac monitoring is increasingly sophisticated. Technologies allow for continuous monitoring of 12 leads and of multiple patients at one time, and trending of many physiological variables can be performed over any time frame. Cardiac monitoring is also performed outside the critical care unit, including in the home setting. Box 8.1 lists priority patient populations for dysrhythmia monitoring.

The 12-Lead Electrocardiogram

The 12-lead ECG is an important diagnostic tool that provides information about myocardial ischemia, injury, cell necrosis, electrolyte disturbances, increased cardiac muscle mass (hypertrophy), conduction abnormalities, and abnormal heart rhythms.

BOX 8.1 Indications for Cardiac Monitoring

- Immediate recognition of sudden cardiac arrest
- Recognition of deteriorating conditions
- Syncope (of suspected cardiac origin) and palpitations (to guide appropriate management)
- Early recognition of ischemia
- Chest pain or coronary artery disease
- Major cardiac interventions (including open heart surgery, mechanical circulatory support, transcatheter structural interventions)
- Arrhythmias
  - Ventricular tachycardia
  - Atrial tachyarrhythmias
  - Chronic atrial fibrillation
  - Sinus bradycardias
  - Atrioventricular block
- Arrhythmic syndromes: Wolff-Parkinson-White syndrome
- After electrophysiology procedures or ablations
- After pacemaker or implantable cardioverter-defibrillator (ICD) implantation
- Semipermanent transvenous pacing
- Preexisting rhythm devices
- Moderate-to-severe imbalance of potassium or magnesium
- Drug overdose
- Intraaortic balloon counterpulsation
- Acute decompensated heart failure
- Infective endocarditis
- Stroke
- Conditions requiring critical care admission
- Procedures that require moderate sedation or anesthesia

Data from American Heart Association. 2017 Update to practice standards for electrocardiographic monitoring in hospital settings: a scientific statement from the American Heart Association. *Circulation.* 2017;136:e273-e344.

Electrodes applied to the skin transmit the electrical signals of the movement of the cardiac impulse through the conduction system. This signal passes through patient's skin, muscle, and bone and finally through electrodes and wires outside of the patient's body to be amplified by the ECG machine and either transcribed to ECG paper or displayed digitally. The ECG machine records the summation of the waves of depolarization and repolarization occurring during the cardiac cycle. During the polarized or resting state, a flat, or *isoelectric,* line is inscribed that means that no current or electrical activity is occurring.

The 12-lead ECG provides a view of the electrical activity of the heart from 12 different views, both frontally and horizontally. Cardiac electrical activity is not one-dimensional; thus, observation in two planes provides a more complete view in the horizontal and vertical planes. When assessing the 12-lead ECG or a rhythm strip, it is helpful to understand that the electrical activity is viewed in relation to the positive electrode of that particular lead. The positive electrode is the "viewing eye" of the camera. When an electrical signal is aimed directly at the positive electrode, an upright inflection off the isoelectric line is visualized. If the impulse is moving away from the positive electrode, a negative deflection off the isoelectric line is seen. If the signal is perpendicular to the imaginary line between the positive and negative poles of the lead, the tracing is equiphasic, with equally positive and negative deflection (Fig. 8.6). A tracing may be observed on a monitor, displayed digitally on a computer screen, or recorded on paper.

The electrical activity of normal conduction occurs downward between the right arm and the left leg, called the *mean*

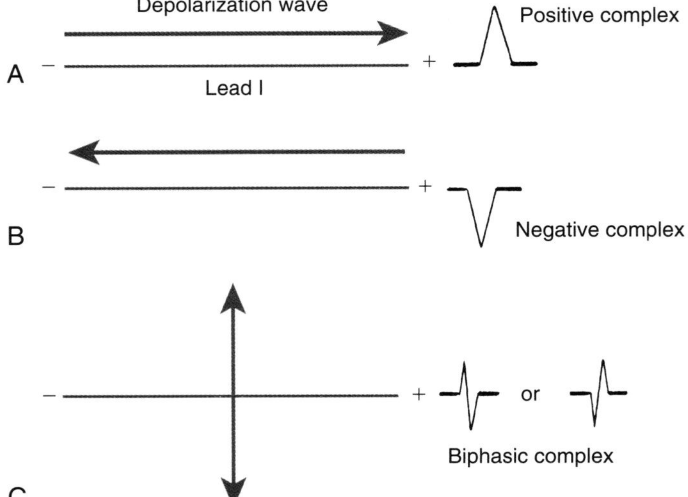

Fig. 8.6 **A,** A positive complex is seen in any lead if the wave of depolarization spreads toward the positive pole of the lead. **B,** A negative complex is seen if the depolarization wave spreads toward the negative pole (away from the positive pole) of the lead. **C,** A biphasic (partly positive, partly negative) complex is seen if the mean direction of the wave is at a right angle. These apply to the P wave, QRS complex, and T wave (From Goldberger AL, Goldberger ZD, Shvilkin A. *Goldberger's Clinical Electrocardiography: A Simplified Approach.* 10th ed. St. Louis, MO: Elsevier; 2024.)

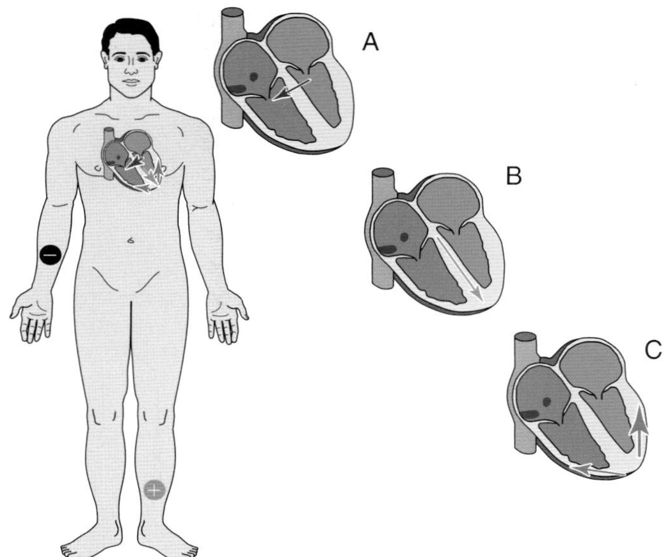

Fig. 8.7 Direction of normal current flow through the ventricles. A, Activation of the septum beginning on the left side of the septum, moving across toward the right side of the septum. B, Activation moves down and to the left within the septum between both ventricular chambers. C, Activation throughout the Purkinje system.

cardiac vector or direction of current flow. Thus, the positive electrode reflects this electrical activity by an upright inflection if the flow of current is directed at that positive electrode or a negative deflection if moving away from that positive electrode. The wave of current flow of the cardiac cycle or the vector is inscribed on the ECG paper in relation to the lead vector that is being viewed. The lead reflects the magnitude and the direction of current flow (Fig. 8.7).

The 12-lead ECG consists of three standard bipolar limb leads (I, II, and III), three augmented unipolar limb leads (aV_R, aV_L, and aV_F), and six precordial unipolar leads (V_1, V_2, V_3, V_4, V_5, and V_6). Bipolar leads consist of a positive and a negative lead, whereas the unipolar leads consist of a positive electrode and the ECG machine itself.

Standard Limb Leads. The standard three limb leads are I, II, and III. Limb leads are placed on the arms and legs. These leads are bipolar, meaning that a positive lead perspective is on one limb and a negative lead perspective is on another limb. Lead I records the magnitude and direction of current flow between the negative lead on the right arm and the positive lead on the left arm (Fig. 8.8A). Lead II records activity between the negative lead on the right arm and the positive lead on the left leg. (Fig. 8.8B) Lead III records activity from the negative lead on the left arm to the positive lead on the left leg (Fig. 8.8C). The normal ECG waveforms are upright in these leads, with lead II often producing the most upright waveforms. The bipolar limb leads form Einthoven's triangle (Fig. 8.9A). This is an equilateral upside-down triangle with the heart in the center.

Augmented Limb Leads. The augmented limb leads are unipolar, meaning they record electrical flow in only one direction (Fig. 8.9B). A reference point is established in the ECG machine, and electrical flow is recorded from that reference point toward the right arm (aV_R), left arm (aV_L), and left foot (aV_F) (Fig. 8.9C). The *a* in the names of these leads means *augmented;* because these leads produce small ECG complexes, they must be augmented, or enlarged. The *V* means *voltage,* and the subscripts *R, L,* and *F* stand for *right arm, left arm,* and *left foot,* where the positive electrode is located. The augmented limb leads are displayed by using the electrodes already in place for the limb leads.

The addition of the augmented limb leads to Einthoven's triangle forms a hexaxial reference figure when the six frontal plane leads are intersected in the center of each lead (Fig. 8.9D). The figure is used to determine the exact direction of current flow, called *axis determination,* a requisite skill of 12-lead ECG analysis. Assessment of axis deviation is an advanced skill and not addressed in this chapter. Fig. 8.9D shows that leads I and aV_L are in proximity, as are leads II, III, and aV_F. Therefore, the QRS patterns of leads that are close together usually appear similar. Because current flow is directed between the left arm and left foot, leads I, II, III, aV_L, and aV_F, the waveforms are usually positive if conduction is normal.

Precordial Leads. The six precordial leads (also called *chest leads*) are positioned on the chest wall directly over the heart. These leads provide a view of cardiac electrical activity from a horizontal plane rather than the frontal plane view of the limb leads. Precise placement of these leads is crucial for providing an accurate representation and for comparison with previous and future ECG tracings. A misplaced V *(chest)* lead can result in erroneous or missed diagnoses of acute coronary syndrome and lethal dysrhythmias, as well as incorrect interpretation of ST segment changes. The precordial leads are unipolar, with a positive electrode and the AV node as a center reference (Fig. 8.10). Landmarks for placement of these leads are the intercostal spaces, the sternum, and the clavicular and axillary lines.

Grouping of Leads. Each lead provides a view of the electrical activity of the heart from a different angle. Two or more leads that view the current flow in the heart from the same angle can be grouped together and are considered anatomically contiguous. Anatomical regions are described as *septal, anterior, lateral,* and *inferior.* Septal leads are V_1 and V_2; anterior leads are V_3 and V_4; lateral leads are I, aV_L, V_5, and V_6; and inferior leads are II, III, and aV_F.[2] Assessing leads that localize these regions of the heart assists in identifying the location of myocardial ischemia, injury, and infarct. Posterior and right ventricular electrodes are not commonly part of the standard 12-lead ECG; however, if indicated, newer ECG machines can record tracings from these areas. The 15-lead ECG is an additional assessment that is warranted if the patient is suspected of having an inferior myocardial infarction, because right ventricular and posterior involvement are common with this type of infarct (Fig. 8.11).

Continuous Cardiac Monitoring. Continuous cardiac monitoring is conducted in a variety of patient care settings, including the emergency department, ambulances, high-risk obstetric units, cardiac catheterization and electrophysiology

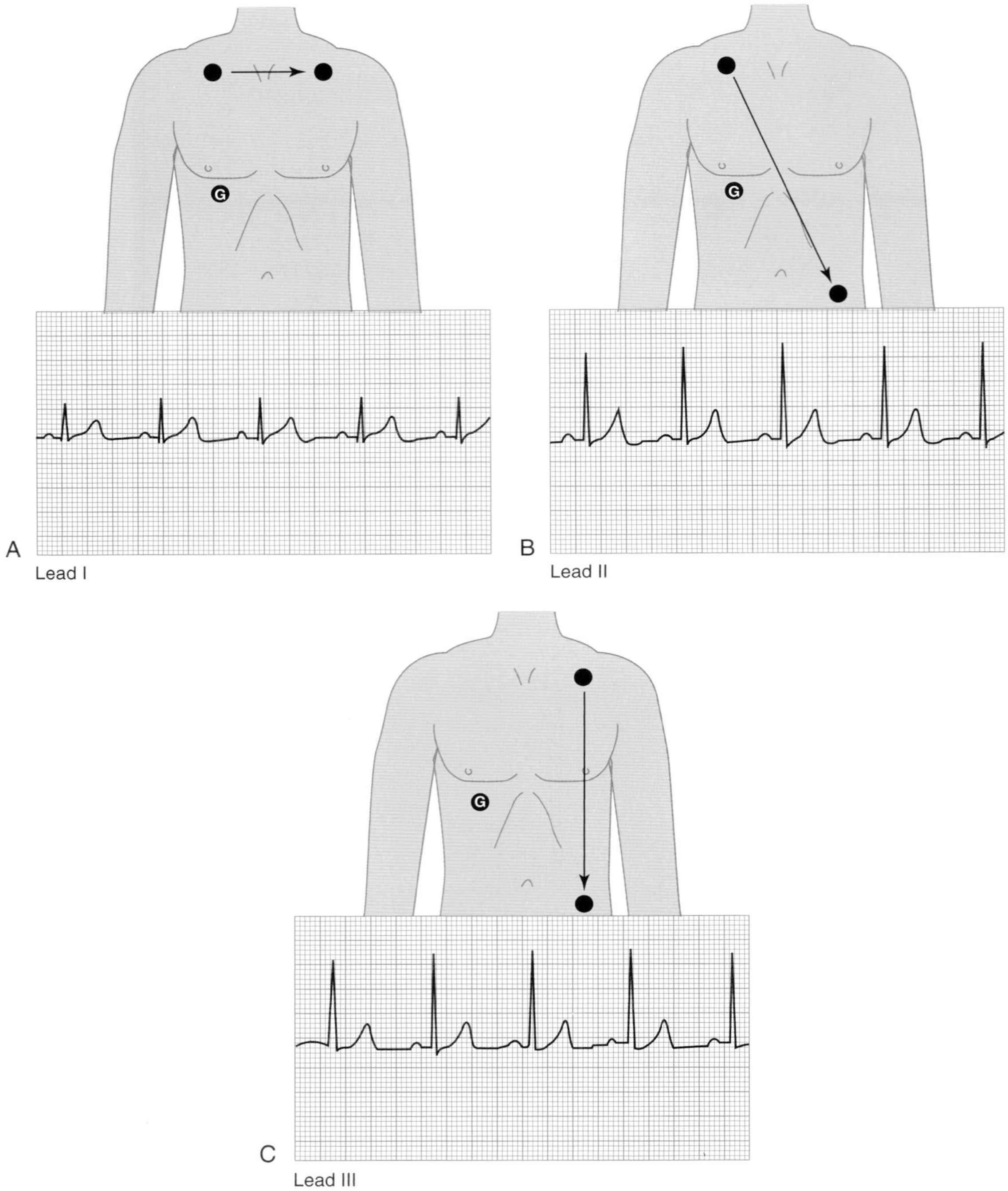

Fig. 8.8 Standard bipolar limb leads. **A**, Lead I. **B**, Lead II. **C**, Lead III.

laboratories, critical care units, operating rooms, postanesthesia care units, endoscopy suites, progressive care units, and outpatient settings. Depending on the sophistication of the monitoring system, any of the 12 leads can be monitored continuously. The most critical elements of cardiac monitoring are in skin preparation, lead placement, and appropriate lead selection.

Skin Preparation and Lead Placement. Adequate skin preparation of electrode sites requires clipping the hair, cleansing the skin, and drying the skin. Cleansing includes washing with soap and water, or alcohol, to remove skin debris and oils.

The three-lead monitoring system depicts only the standard limb leads. These leads are marked as *RA, LA,* and *LL.* The right and left arm leads (RA and LA) are placed just above the right and left clavicles, and the leg lead (LL) is placed on the left abdominal area below the level of the umbilicus (Fig. 8.12A). Five-lead monitoring systems that monitor all of the limb leads and one chest lead are commonly available. Instead of placing the limb leads on the arms and legs, these leads are placed just above the right and left clavicles and on the right and left abdomen below the level of the umbilicus. The precordial or chest lead is placed in the selected V lead position, usually V_1 (Fig. 8.12B). Some five-lead systems can derive a 12-lead tracing (Fig. 8.13).

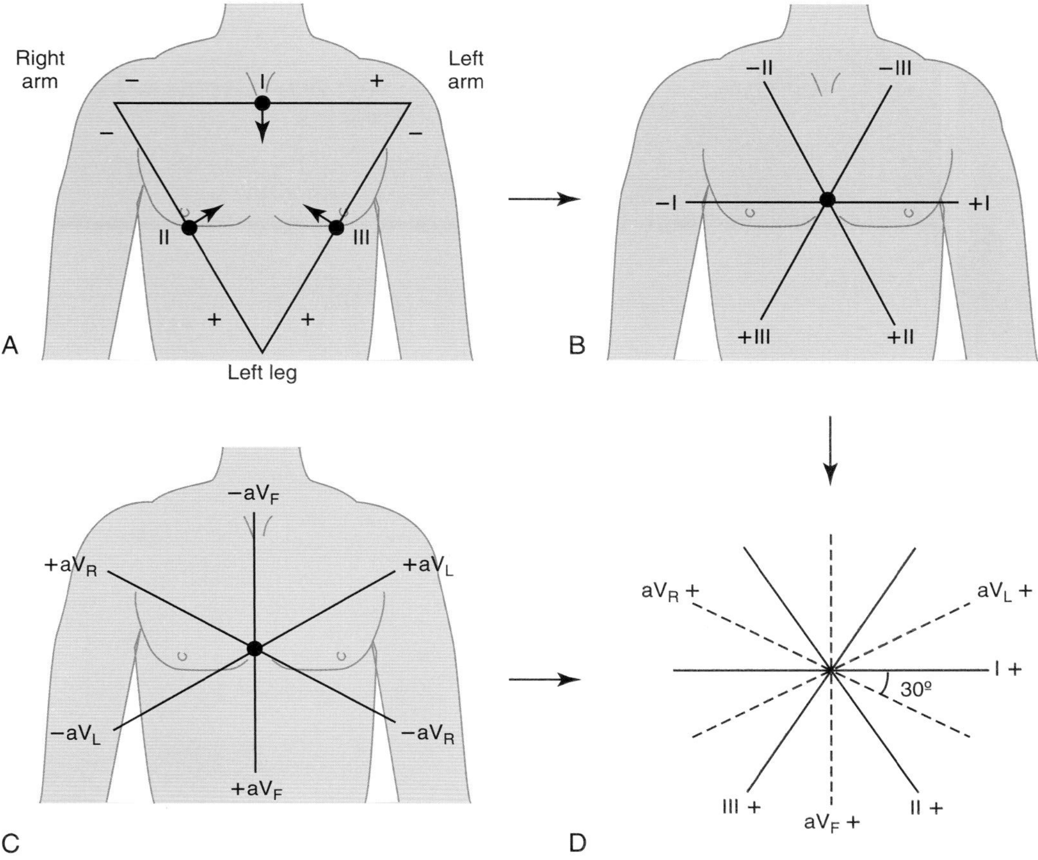

Fig. 8.9 A, Einthoven's triangle. B, The triangle is converted to a triaxial diagram by shifting leads I, II, and III so they intersect at a common point. C, Triaxial lead diagram showing the relationship of the three augmented (unipolar) leads, aV_R, aV_L, and aV_F. Notice that each lead is represented by an axis with a positive and negative pole. D, The hexaxial reference figure combining the three axis leads from part B with the three axis leads from part C, producing the hexaxial reference.

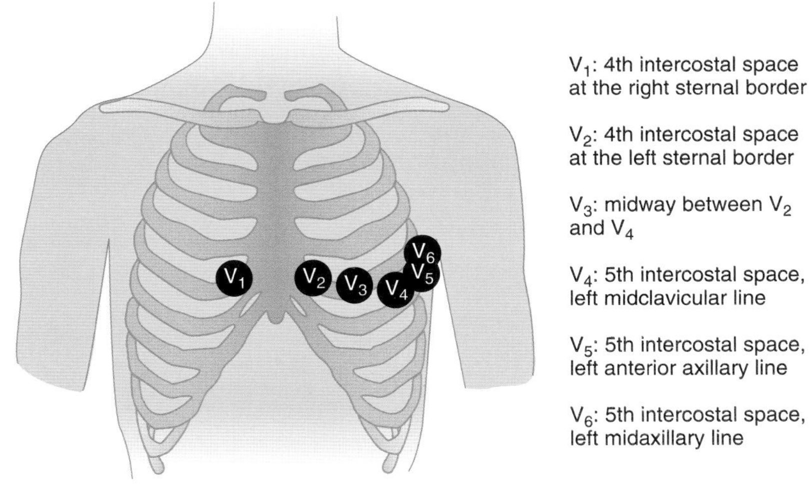

Fig. 8.10 Precordial chest leads.

Before application, check the electrodes to ensure that the gel is moist. Attach the electrode to the lead wire and place it in the designated location. Following electrode placement, assess the signal to ensure that the waveform is clear and not disrupted by artifact. At the beginning of each shift, assess that electrodes are placed in the correct anatomical positions. Change electrodes based on institutional policy.

Determine lead selection by the patient's diagnosis and the risk for an ischemic cardiac event, dysrhythmia, or other factors. Typically, the first lead selected is V_1 for dysrhythmia

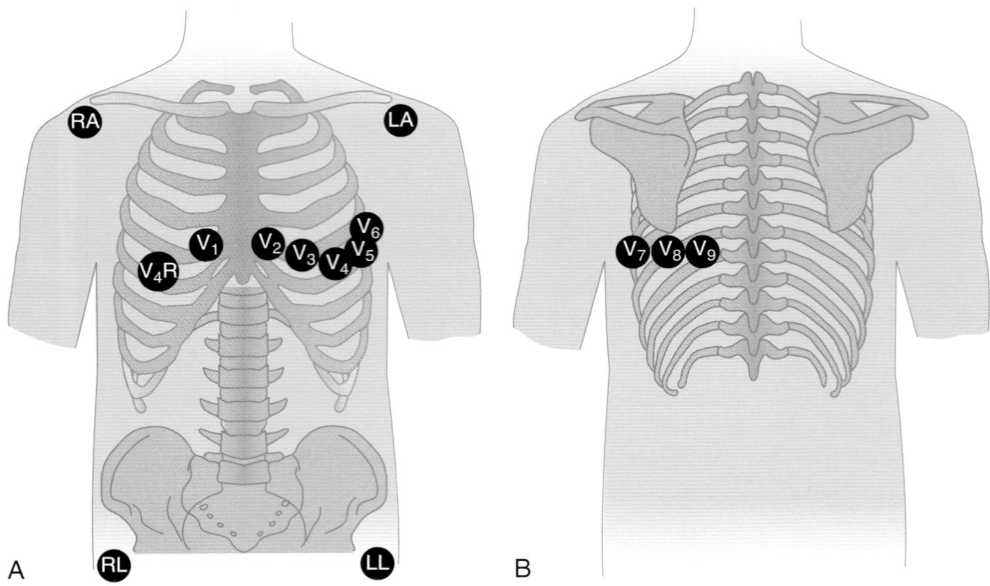

Fig. 8.11 Lead placement for a 15-lead electrocardiogram (ECG). **A**, Anterior leads. **B**, Posterior leads. *LA*, Left arm; *LL*, left leg; *RA*, right arm; *RL*, right leg; V_1-V_9, chest leads for 15-lead ECG.

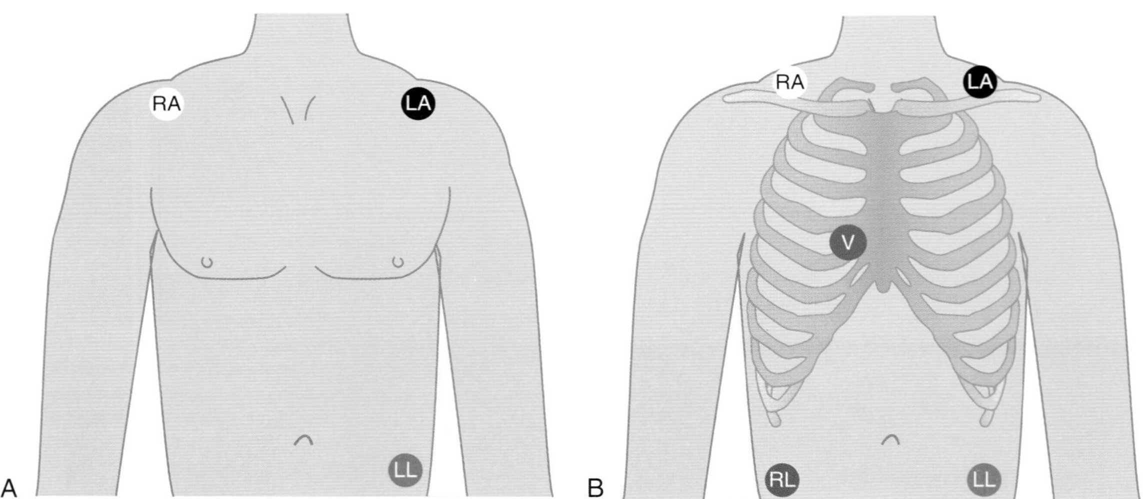

Fig. 8.12 **A**, Three-lead electrocardiographic (ECG) monitoring system. **B**, Five-lead monitoring system with V lead placed in the V_1 position. *LA*, Left arm; *LL*, left leg; *RA*, right arm; *RL*, right leg; *V*, chest lead.

monitoring. If the system is able to simultaneously monitor a second lead, selection of this lead is based on the patient's diagnosis and individual needs. A limb lead is usually selected, such as III, because of the easy visualization of P waves; however, if the patient has a history of ischemia, the second lead can be based on the patient's 12-lead ECG, identifying the lead showing the greatest ischemic change. For dysrhythmia monitoring in a system that provides continuous monitoring of two leads, V_1 and III are the standard recommendations.[3,4]

In most settings, a 6-second strip of the patient's rhythm is obtained and documented in the patient's chart at intervals from every 4 to 8 hours, based on the patient acuity level and institutional policy. In addition, it is essential to document a rhythm strip any time a change in rhythm is noted. If the patient experiences chest discomfort or other signs of myocardial ischemia or a dysrhythmia, obtain a 12-lead ECG. Many ECG machines can print a continuous 12-lead rhythm recording, allowing for assessment of a dysrhythmia from 12 different views. This is a helpful tool when assessing new onset symptoms or rhythm such as heart block, atrial dysrhythmia, or wide QRS complex tachycardia.

ST-segment monitoring allows for continuous monitoring for changes that may reflect myocardial ischemia.[4] The decision about which lead is selected is based on the "ST-segment fingerprint" noted on the 12-lead ECG. The lead that demonstrates the ST change warrants the lead that is monitored. ST-segment monitoring is warranted in patients with acute coronary syndrome, those at risk for silent ischemia, and those who have undergone cardiac interventions such as angioplasty and stent placement.[4]

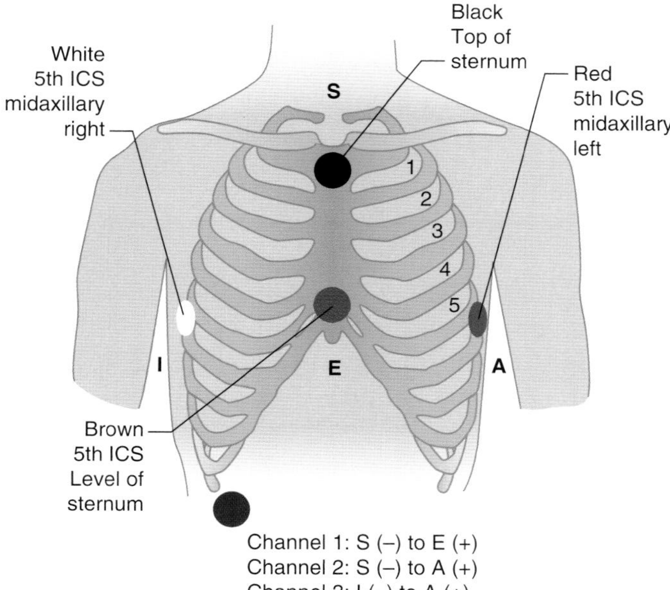

Fig. 8.13 5-Lead electrocardiographic (ECG) monitoring system with 12-lead capability. *ICS,* Intercostal space.

DYSRHYTHMIA ANALYSIS AND INTERPRETATION

Basics of Dysrhythmia Analysis

Measurements. ECG paper contains a standardized grid where the horizontal axis measures time and the vertical axis measures the voltage or amplitude (Fig. 8.14). Larger boxes are circumscribed by darker lines and smaller boxes by lighter lines. The larger boxes contain five smaller boxes on the horizontal line and five on the vertical line, for a total of 25 per large box. Horizontally, the smaller boxes denote 0.04 seconds each, or 40 milliseconds (ms); the larger box contains five smaller horizontal boxes and thus equals 0.20 seconds, or 200 ms. Along the uppermost aspect of the ECG paper are vertical hash marks that occur every 15 large boxes. The area between these marks equals 3 seconds. Some ECG paper has markings every second.

The monitoring standard is to use a 6-second rhythm strip for analysis and documentation of cardiac rhythms. A 6-second strip consists of two 3-second intervals or a span of three hash marks. The measurement of time on the ECG tracing represents the speed of depolarization and repolarization in the atria and ventricles and is printed at 25 mm/sec.

Amplitude is measured on the vertical axis of the ECG paper (Fig. 8.14). Each small box is equal to 0.1 mV in amplitude. Waveform amplitude indicates the amount of electrical voltage generated in the various areas of the heart. Low-voltage and small waveforms are expected from the small muscle mass of the atria. Large-voltage and large waveforms are expected from the larger muscle mass of the ventricles.

Waveforms and Intervals. The normal ECG tracing is composed of P, Q, R, S, and T waves (Fig. 8.15). These waveforms rise from a flat baseline called the *isoelectric line.*

P wave. The P wave represents atrial depolarization. It is usually upright in leads I and II and has a rounded, symmetrical shape. The amplitude of the P wave is measured at the center of the waveform and normally does not exceed three boxes, or 3 mm, in height. Normally, a P wave indicates that the SA node initiated the impulse that depolarized the atrium. However, a change in the shape of the intrinsic or baseline P wave may indicate the impulse arose from a site in the atria other than the SA node.

PR interval. The downslope of the P wave returns to the isoelectric line for a short time before the beginning of the QRS complex. The interval from the beginning of the P wave to the next deflection from the baseline is called the *PR interval.* The PR interval measures the time it takes for the electrical impulse to depolarize the atria, travel to the AV node, and pauses there briefly before entering the bundle of His. The normal PR interval is 0.12 to 0.20 seconds, three to five small boxes wide (Fig. 8.15). When the PR interval is longer than normal, the speed of conduction is delayed in the AV node. When the PR interval is shorter than normal, the speed of conduction is abnormally fast.

QRS complex. The QRS complex represents ventricular depolarization (Fig. 8.15). Atrial repolarization also occurs simultaneously to ventricular depolarization, but because of the larger muscle mass of the ventricles, visualization of atrial repolarization is obscured by the QRS complex. The classic QRS complex begins with a negative, or downward, deflection immediately after the PR interval. The first negative deflection after the P wave is called the *Q wave.* A Q wave may or may not be present before the R wave. If the first deflection from the isoelectric line is positive, or upright, the waveform is called an *R wave, representing early depolarization.* The size of the R wave varies across leads.

The R wave is positive and tall in those leads where the direction of current is going toward the positive electrode lead. All limb leads, except for aV_R, normally have tall R waves. In the precordial leads, the R wave begins small and progressively becomes taller and more positive, going from small in V_1 to a maximal size in V_5. This change in size is called *R-wave progression* and occurs because the direction of current flow is moving more directly toward the positive electrode of V_5 (Fig. 8.16). The R-R interval is the distance between two consecutive R waves. This interval is used in determining the heart rate in irregular rhythms and calculation of the QT interval.

The *S wave* is a negative waveform that follows the R wave. The S wave deflects below the isoelectric line. Some patients may have a second positive waveform in their QRS complex. If so, that second positive waveform is called *R prime* (R′).

The term *QRS complex* designates the waveforms representing ventricular depolarization. In reality, the complex may be an R wave, a QS wave, or other wave, depending on the lead viewed or any abnormalities that are present. Fig. 8.17 depicts the various shapes of the QRS complex and nomenclature.

If a Q wave is present on the 12-lead ECG (not the cardiac monitor), it must be determined whether it represents a pathological condition or is normal. A pathological Q wave has a width

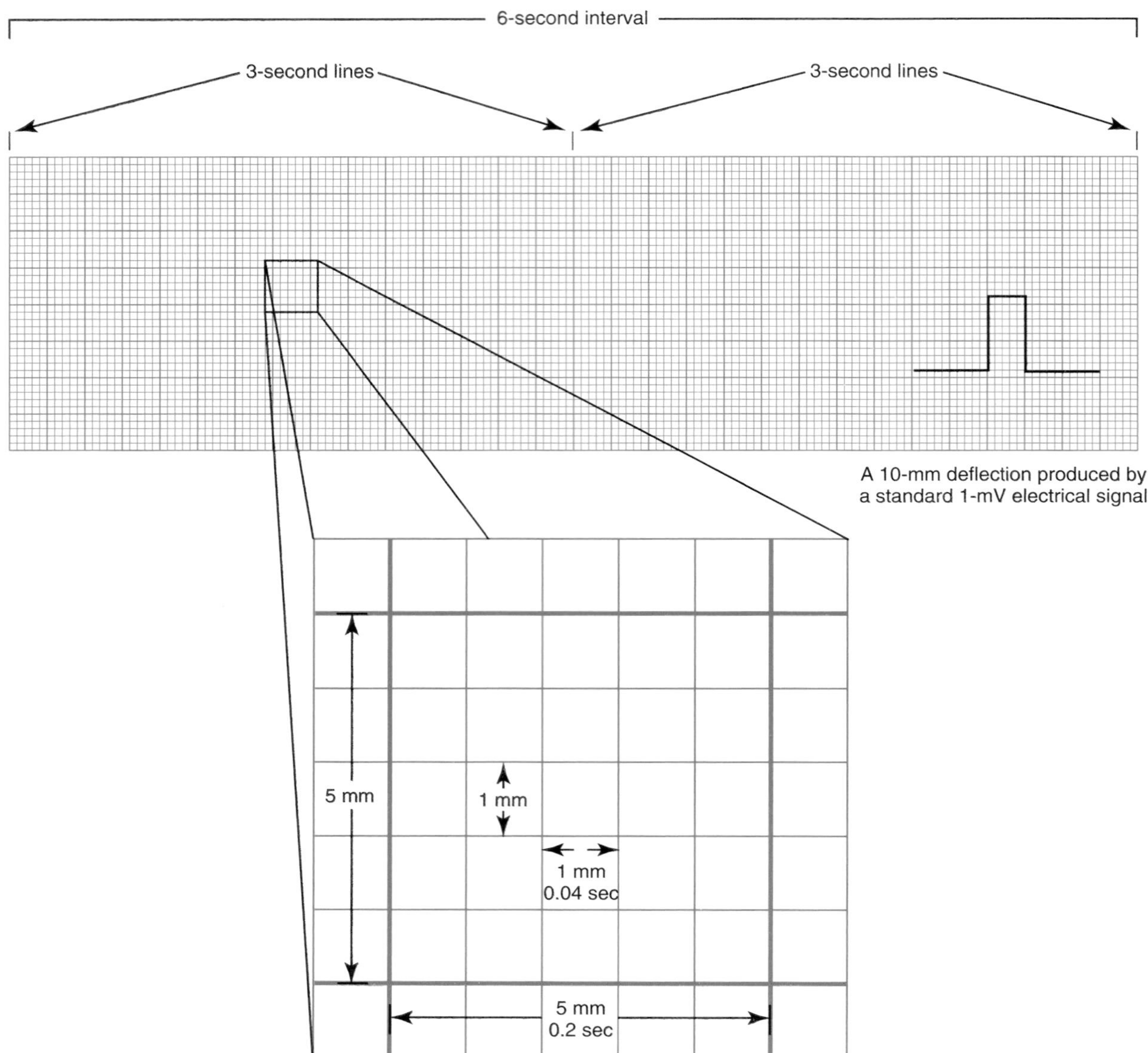

Fig. 8.14 Electrocardiogram paper records time horizontally in seconds or milliseconds. Each large box contains 25 smaller boxes, with 5 on the horizontal axis and 5 on the vertical axis. Each small horizontal box is 0.04 seconds, whereas each large box is 0.20 seconds in duration. Vertically, the graph depicts size or voltage in millivolts (mV) and in millimeters (mm). Fifteen large boxes equal 3 seconds, and 30 large boxes equal 6 seconds, used in calculating heart rate. (From Wesley K. *Huszar's ECG and 12-Lead Interpretation*. 6th ed. St. Louis, MO: Elsevier; 2022.)

of 0.04 seconds and a depth that is greater than one-fourth the height of the R wave amplitude. Pathological Q waves are found on ECGs of individuals who have had myocardial infarctions, and they represent myocardial muscle death (Fig. 8.18).

QRS interval. The QRS interval is measured from where it leaves the isoelectric line of the PR interval to the end of the QRS complex (Fig. 8.15). The waveform that initiates the QRS complex (whether it is a Q wave or an R wave) marks the beginning of the interval. The normal width of the QRS complex is 0.06 to 0.10 seconds. This width equals 1.5 to 2.5 small boxes. A QRS width greater than 0.10 seconds may signify a delay in conduction through the ventricles potentially caused by a variety of factors, including myocardial infarction, atherosclerosis of the aging conduction system, or cardiomyopathy.

T wave. The *T wave* represents ventricular repolarization (Fig. 8.15). T-wave amplitude is measured at the center of the waveform and is usually no higher than five small boxes, or 5 mm. In contrast to P waves, which are usually symmetrical, T waves are usually asymmetrical. Changes in T-wave amplitude or direction can indicate electrical disturbances resulting from an electrolyte imbalance or from myocardial ischemia or injury. For example, hyperkalemia can cause tall, peaked T waves, and ischemia may cause a flattened T wave or an inverted or upside-down T wave.

When learning dysrhythmia interpretation, it can be difficult to differentiate the P wave from the T wave. Understanding that the P wave normally precedes the QRS complex and the T wave normally follows the QRS complex aids in identification of these waveforms. In addition, the T wave usually has greater width and amplitude than the P wave, because the atria are smaller muscle masses and therefore produce smaller waveforms than do the larger ventricles.

ST segment. The ST segment connects the QRS complex to the T wave and is usually isoelectric, or flat. However, in some conditions, the segment may be depressed (fall below baseline) or elevated (rise above baseline). The point at which the QRS complex ends and the ST segment begins is called the *J* (junction) *point*. ST-segment change is measured 0.04 seconds after the J point. To identify ST-segment elevation, use the isoelectric portion of the PR segment as a reference for baseline. Next, note whether the ST segment is level with the PR segment (Fig. 8.15). If the ST segment is above or below the baseline, count the number of small boxes above or below at 0.04 seconds after the J point.[4] A displacement in the ST segment can indicate myocardial ischemia or injury. If ST displacement is noted and is a new finding, obtain a 12-lead ECG and notify the provider. Assess the patient for signs and symptoms of myocardial ischemia or infarction.

QT interval. The QT interval is measured from the beginning of the QRS complex to the end of the T wave (Fig. 8.15). This interval measures the total time taken for ventricular depolarization and repolarization. Abnormal prolongation of the QT interval increases vulnerability to lethal ventricular dysrhythmias, fibrillation, or torsades de pointes. Normally, the QT interval becomes longer with slower heart rates and shortens with faster heart rates, thus requiring a correction of the value. Generally, the QT interval is less than half the R-R interval.

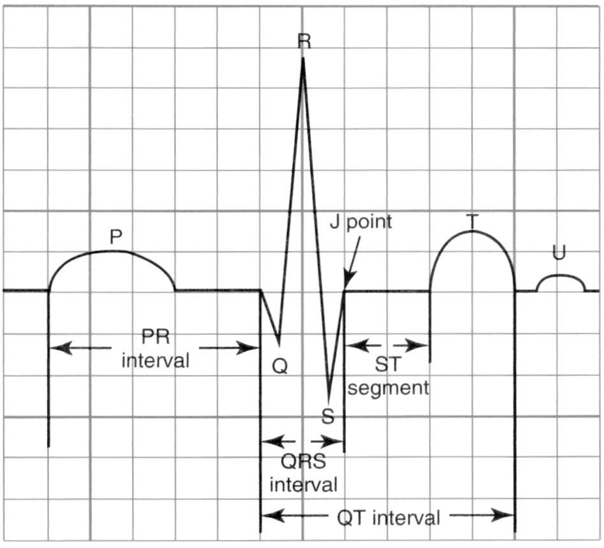

Fig. 8.15 Electrocardiogram waveforms.

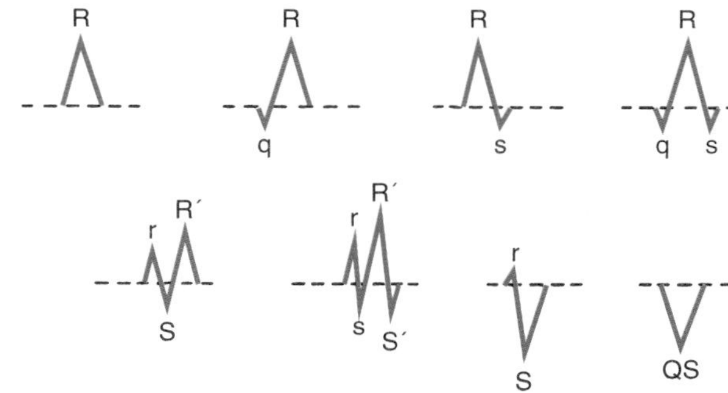

Fig. 8.17 Nomenclature for QRS complexes of various shapes: Different types of QRS complexes. An R wave is a positive waveform. A negative deflection before the R wave is a Q wave. The S wave is a negative deflection after the R wave. If the waveform is tall or deep, the letter naming the waveform is a capital letter. If the waveform is small in either direction, the waveform is labeled with a lowercase letter.

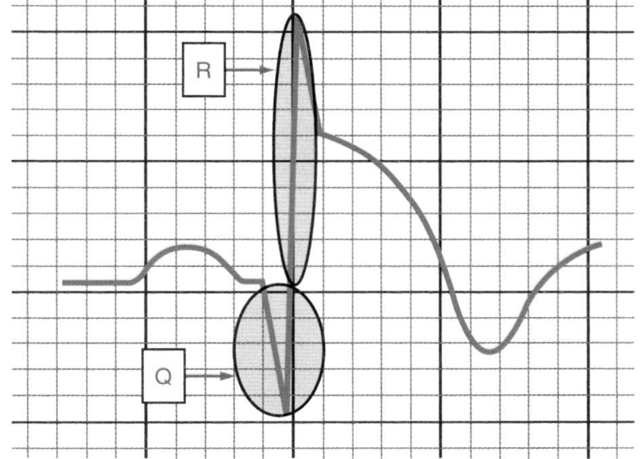

Fig. 8.18 Pathological Q wave is greater than one-fourth the height of the R wave.

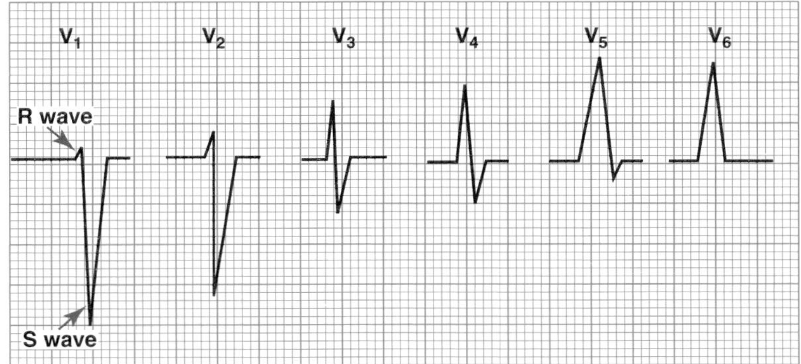

Fig. 8.16 The normal 12-lead precordial R wave progression.

A preferred calculation that corrects for varying heart rates is a calculated QT interval, or *QTc*, which is based on the QT interval divided by the square root of the R-R interval. QT and QTc are routinely measured when analyzing a rhythm strip. A healthy QTc is less than 0.45 seconds in men and 0.46 seconds in women.[4] Many monitoring systems can calculate the QTc if the R-R interval is measured. QTc accuracy is based on a regular rhythm. In irregular rhythms such as atrial fibrillation, an average QTc may be necessary, because the QT interval varies from beat to beat.

Risk of a lethal heart rhythm called *torsades de pointes* occurs if QTc is prolonged more than 0.50 seconds.[4,5] Observe for prolonged QT intervals when medications that prolong the QT interval are started, doses are increased, or in cases of overdose.

U wave. A final waveform that is occasionally noted on the ECG is the *U wave*. If present, this waveform follows the T wave, and it represents repolarization of a small segment of the ventricles or delayed repolarization. The U wave is usually small, rounded, and less than 2 mm in height (Fig. 8.15). Larger U waves may be present in patients with hypokalemia, hypertrophic cardiomyopathy, left ventricular hypertrophy, and digoxin toxicity.

EVIDENCE-BASED PRACTICE

Implementation of Practice Standards for Electrocardiographic Monitoring

Problem

Electrocardiographic (ECG) monitoring of patients in hospitals is not often validated beyond initial competency assessment. Implementation of the American Heart Association (AHA) practice standards is influenced by the nurses' knowledge and affects quality of care and patient outcomes.

Clinical Question

What are the recommendations regarding ECG monitoring and nurses' sustained knowledge that influence quality of care and patient outcomes?

Evidence

The Practical Use of the Latest Standards of Electrocardiography (PULSE) randomized clinical trial was conducted over 6 years in 65 cardiac units at 17 hospitals. Baseline data were assessed, and outcomes were measured at time 2 after group 1 hospitals received the intervention and at time 3 after group 2 hospitals received the intervention. Measurement periods were 15 months apart. The two-part intervention consisted of an online ECG monitoring education program and strategies to sustain practice change. Nursing knowledge was measured by a validated online test in 3,013 nurses. Quality of care related to ECG monitoring was assessed by 4,587 patients through on-site observation, and patient outcomes were determined by mortality, in-hospital myocardial infarction, and not surviving a cardiac arrest in 95,884 hospital admissions. Nurses' knowledge in both groups improved significantly immediately after intervention but did not demonstrate a sustained effect at 15 months. Quality measures improved and were sustained, including accurate electrode placement, appropriate ECG and ST segment monitoring, and accurate rhythm interpretation significantly improved and were sustained after 15 months. In addition, in-hospital myocardial infarction declined significantly and was sustained after intervention.

Implications for Nursing

Education courses to enhance nursing knowledge and strategies to improve the quality of care and patient outcomes using standards of ECG monitoring can aid in making practice changes. Further research is needed to identify the best strategies to influence sustained change beyond 15 months.

Level of Evidence

B—Randomized controlled trial

Reference

Funk M, Fennie KP, Stephens KE, et al. Association of implementation of practice standards for electrocardiographic monitoring with nurses' knowledge, quality of care, and patient outcomes: findings from the Practice Use of the Latest Standards of Electrocardiography (PULSE) trial. *Circ Cardiovasc Qual Outcomes*. 2017;10:e003132.

Dysrhythmia Interpretation

Analysis of a cardiac rhythm must be conducted systematically to correctly interpret the rhythm. Proper dysrhythmia analysis includes assessment of the following:

- Atrial and ventricular rates
- Regularity of rhythm
- Measurement of PR, QRS, and QT/QTc intervals
- Shape or morphological characteristics of waveforms and their consistency
- Identification of the underlying rhythm and any dysrhythmia in addition to the underlying rhythm
- Patient tolerance of the rhythm
- Clinical implications of the rhythm

Rate. The rate represents how fast the heart is depolarizing. Under normal conditions, the atria and the ventricles depolarize in a regular sequence. However, each can depolarize at a different rate. P waves are used to calculate the atrial rate, and QRS waves or R waves are used to calculate the ventricular rate. Rate can be assessed in various ways:

Six-second method. A quick and easy estimate of heart rate can be accomplished by counting the number of P waves or QRS waves within a 6-second strip to obtain atrial and ventricular heart rates per minute. This is the optimal method for irregular rhythms. Identify the lines above the ECG paper that represent 6 seconds and count the number of P waves within the lines; then add a zero to identify the atrial heart rate estimate for 1 minute. Next, identify the number of QRS waves in the 6-second strip and again add a zero to identify the ventricular rate (Fig. 8.19).

Large box method. In this method, two consecutive P and R waves are located. Count the number of large boxes between the highest points of two consecutive P waves; divide that number of large boxes into 300 to determine the atrial rate. Count the number of large boxes between the highest points of two consecutive R waves; divide that number of large boxes into 300 to determine the ventricular rate (Fig. 8.20). This method is accurate only if the rhythm is regular. If one large box is between the two R waves, the rate is 300 beats/min (300 ÷ 1 = 300); two large boxes equal 150 (300 ÷ 2 = 150) and so on. A mnemonic can be used to simplify this method. Memorize *300-150-100-75-60-50-42-38*.

Small box method. The small box method is used to calculate a more exact rate of a regular rhythm. In this method, locate two consecutive P and QRS waves. Count the number of small

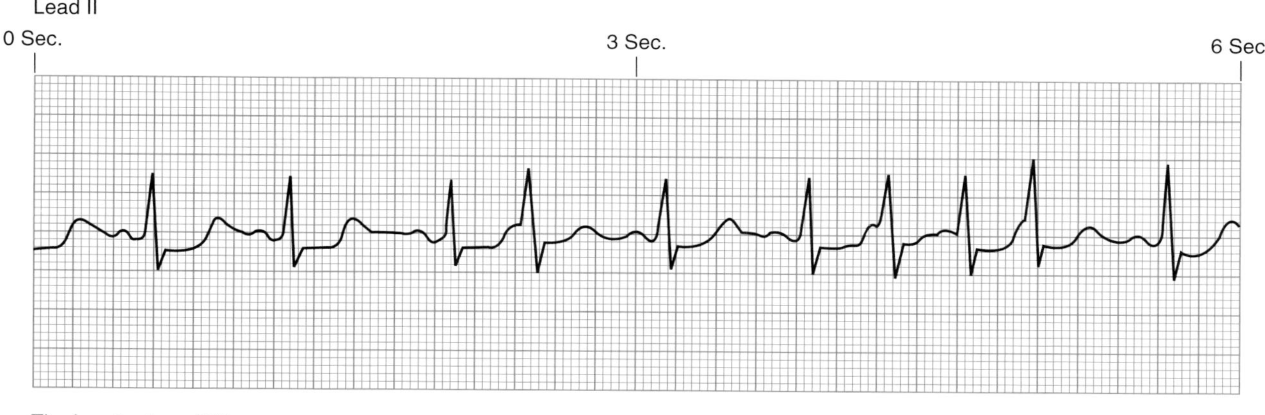

Fig. 8.19 Six-second method of rate calculation.

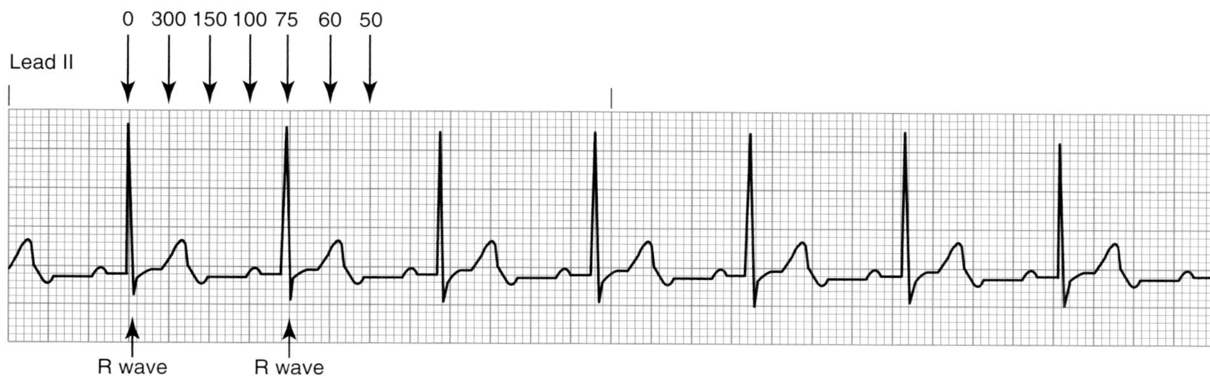

Big Box Method of Heart-Rate Calculation

- Identify an R wave on a solid vertical line.
- Count the number of big boxes between the first and the following R waves.
- Divide 300 by the number of big boxes between R waves or count the cadence (300...150...100...75...60) representing the big boxes between R waves.

NOTE: Since the position of the second R wave occurs with the arrow reading 75, the heart rate in this example is approximately 75 beats/min.

Fig. 8.20 Large box method of heart-rate calculation.

boxes between the highest points of these consecutive P waves; divide that number into 1500 to determine the atrial rate. Count the number of small boxes between the highest points of two consecutive QRS waves; divide that number into 1500 to determine the ventricular rate (Fig. 8.21). This method is accurate only if the rhythm is regular. Charts are available to calculate heart rate based on the rule of 1500.

Cardiac monitors continuously display heart rates. However, always verify the accuracy of the displayed rate using one of the rate calculation methods described.

Regularity. Regularity is assessed by using electronic or physical calipers or a piece of paper and pencil. To determine atrial regularity, identify the P wave and place one caliper point on the peak of the P wave. Locate the next P wave and place the second caliper point on its peak. The second point is left stationary, and the calipers are flipped over. If the first caliper point lands exactly on the next P wave, the atrial rhythm is regular. If the point lands one small box or less away from the next P wave, the rhythm is essentially regular. If the point lands more than one small box away, the rhythm is considered irregular. Electronic calipers on some monitoring systems are used in the same way. For example, Fig. 8.22 depicts use of electronic calipers in measuring the PR interval.

The same process can be performed with a simple piece of paper. Place the paper parallel and below the rhythm line, make a hash mark below the first and second P waves, then move the paper over to determine if the distance between the second and third P waves is equal to that between the first and second P waves. When an atrial rhythm is regular, each P wave is an equal distance from the next P wave.

This process is also used to assess ventricular regularity, except that a line marking the peak of two consecutive R waves is used. One pencil line is placed under one R wave, and the other pencil line is placed under the next R wave. Then, the paper is moved to the second and third R waves to determine if the R wave comes as expected. Then, the paper is moved down the rhythm strip to determine if the subsequent R waves land

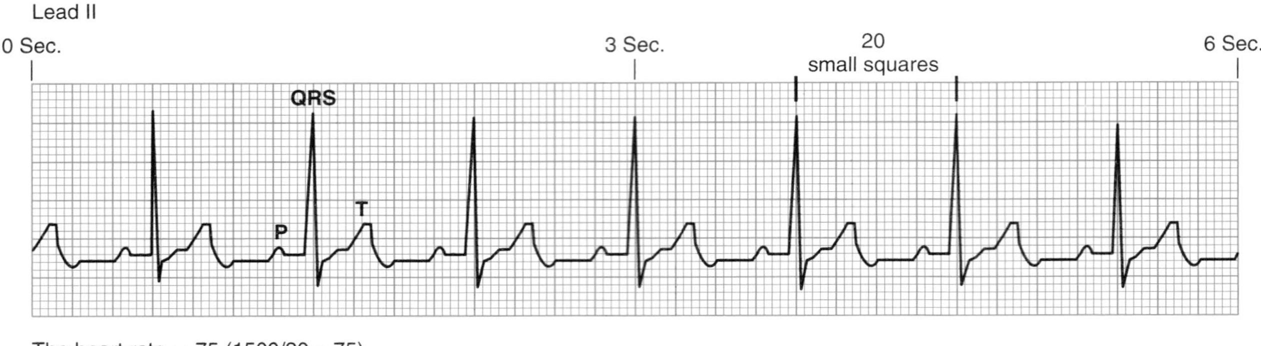

Fig. 8.21 Small box method of heart-rate calculation.

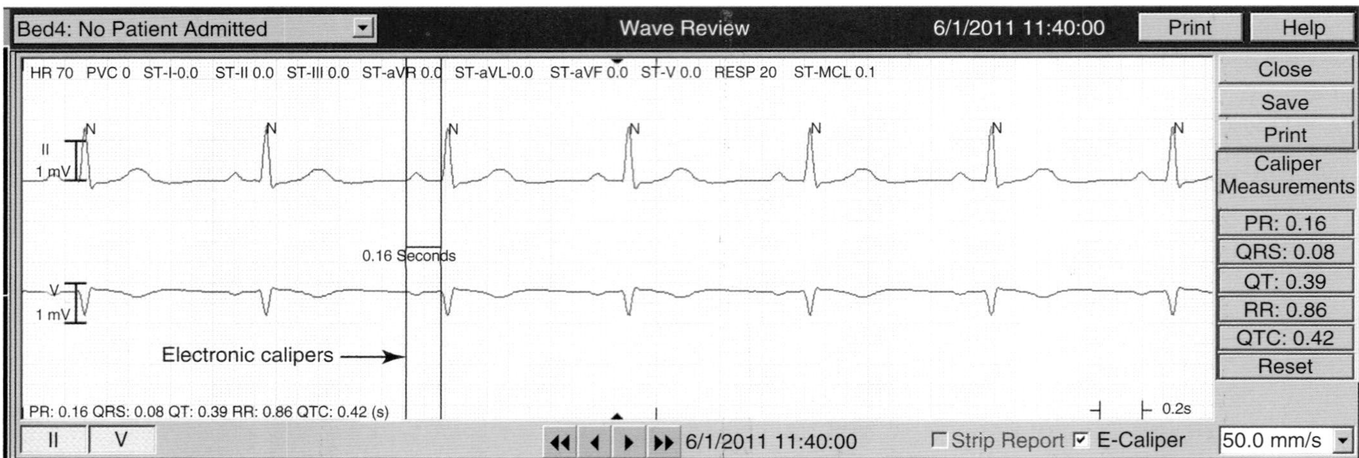

Fig. 8.22 Electronic calipers. *HR,* Heart rate; *PVC,* premature ventricular contraction; *RR,* respiratory rate; *mV,* millivolts; *mm/s,* millimeters per second. https://www.ncbi.nlm.nih.gov/books/NBK507823/ (Courtesy Philips Healthcare, Andover, MA.)

on the hash mark. If the hash mark is more than one small box away from the next R wave, the rhythm is irregular (Fig. 8.23).

Irregular rhythms can be regularly irregular or irregularly irregular. Regularly irregular rhythms have a pattern. Irregularly irregular rhythms have no pattern and no predictability. Atrial fibrillation is an example of an irregularly irregular rhythm.

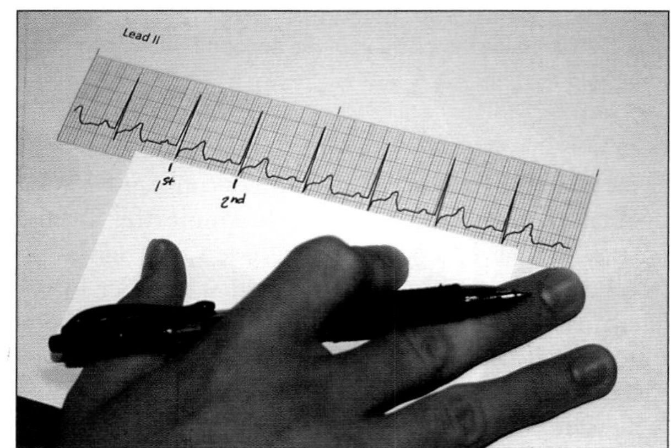

Fig. 8.23 Use of paper and pencil to assess regularity.

Measurement of PR, QRS, and QT/QTc Intervals. PR, QRS, and QT/QTc intervals are measured and documented as part of rhythm analysis. In some dysrhythmias, intervals such as the PR interval may change; thus, all PR intervals are measured to ensure they are consistent. QRS intervals can lengthen in response to new bundle branch blocks or with ventricular dysrhythmias. QT/QTc intervals can lengthen in response to certain medications as well as electrolyte imbalances. Intervals are measured with calipers or paper and pencil as previously described by identifying the number of small boxes and multiplying by 0.04 seconds. If the end of the interval being measured falls between boxes, add 0.02 to the measurement, as this is the time allowed for half of a box of measurement.

Morphological Characteristics of Waveforms. Assess the P, QRS, and T waves of the rhythm strip for shape and consistency. All waveforms should look alike in a normal ECG. Abnormal shapes may indicate that the stimulus that caused the waveform came from an ectopic focus or that there is a delay or block in conduction creating a bundle branch block. It is important to also confirm that a P wave precedes the QRS complex and that the T wave follows the QRS complex. Several dysrhythmias are characterized by abnormal location or sequencing of waveforms, such as the P waves in complete heart block.

BOX 8.2 Symptoms of Decreased Cardiac Output

- Change in level of consciousness
- Chest discomfort
- Hypotension
- Shortness of breath; respiratory distress
- Pulmonary congestion; crackles
- Rapid, slow, or weak pulse
- Dizziness
- Syncope
- Fatigue
- Restlessness

Identification of Underlying Rhythm and Any Dysrhythmia. Identify the underlying rhythm first. After this step, determine the dysrhythmia that disrupts the underlying rhythm. Next, identify patient tolerance of the rhythm and clinical implications. Once an abnormal heart rhythm is identified, the priority is to assess the patient for any symptoms that may be related to the dysrhythmia (Box 8.2). Assess for hemodynamic deterioration: obtain vital signs, assess for alterations in level of consciousness, auscultate lung sounds, and ask the patient if dyspnea or chest discomfort are present. Instability is manifested by any of the following: hypotension, acutely altered mental status, signs of shock, ischemic chest discomfort, or acute heart failure. In addition, obtain a 12-lead ECG to aid in identifying the dysrhythmia.

The next step is to determine if there are causes of the dysrhythmia that can be treated immediately. An example is a patient with a fast, wide complex tachycardia who has a pulse but low blood pressure. The immediate priority is to treat the patient's fast heart rhythm with a therapy such as emergent cardioversion, but the next critical step is to identify potential causes of the dysrhythmia, such as hypokalemia, hypomagnesemia, hypoxemia, or ischemia.

BASIC DYSRHYTHMIAS

Basic dysrhythmias are classified based on their site of origin, including:

- SA node
- Atrial
- AV node or junctional
- Ventricular
- Heart blocks of the AV node

The following discussion reviews the ECG characteristics and provides examples of each dysrhythmia. Specific criteria that can be used to recognize and identify dysrhythmias are presented systematically for each one. The discussion includes typical causes, patient responses, and appropriate treatment. Medications used to treat common dysrhythmias are described in Table 8.1.

The learner who is new to identification of dysrhythmias will benefit from extensive practice in reading rhythm strips and collaborating with experienced colleagues who are adept at rhythm interpretation. Maintaining a pocket notebook (or using handheld devices with cardiac rhythm applications) with ECG criteria for each rhythm helps the learner memorize the criteria specific for common dysrhythmias. Other suggested learning aids are to complete a classroom or online course in basic rhythm interpretation. Finally, mastering the identification of dysrhythmias requires practice, practice, and more practice. Another essential assessment skill is recognition of hemodynamic instability related to decreased cardiac output associated with some dysrhythmias (Box 8.2).

Normal Sinus Rhythm

Normal sinus rhythm (NSR) reflects normal conduction of the sinus impulse through the atria and ventricles. Any deviation from sinus rhythm is a dysrhythmia; thus, it is critical to remember and understand the criteria that determine NSR. Sinus rhythm is initiated by an impulse in the SA node. The generated impulse propagates through the conductive fibers of the atria, reaches the AV node where there is a slight pause, and then spreads throughout the ventricles, causing depolarization and resultant cardiac contraction in a timely and organized manner (Fig. 8.24).

Rhythm analysis.

- *Rate:* Atrial and ventricular rates are the same and range from 60 to 100 beats/min in the adult patient.
- *Regularity:* Rhythm is regular or essentially regular.
- *Interval measurements:* PR interval is 0.12 to 0.20 seconds. QRS interval is 0.06 to 0.10 seconds.
- *Shape and sequence:* P and QRS waves are consistent in shape. P waves are small and rounded. A P wave precedes every QRS complex, which is then followed by a T wave.
- *Hemodynamic effect:* Patient is hemodynamically stable.

Dysrhythmias of the Sinoatrial Node

Sinus Tachycardia. Tachycardia is defined as a heart rate faster than 100 beats/min. Sinus tachycardia results when the SA node fires faster than 100 beats/min (Fig. 8.25). Sinus tachycardia is a normal response to stimulation of the sympathetic nervous system. Sinus tachycardia is also a normal finding in children younger than 6 years of age.

Rhythm analysis.

- *Rate:* Both atrial and ventricular rates are faster than 100 beats/min, up to 160 beats/min, but may be as high as 180 beats/min.
- *Regularity:* Onset is gradual rather than abrupt. Sinus tachycardia is regular or essentially regular.
- *Interval measurements:* PR interval is 0.12 to 0.20 seconds (at higher rates, the P wave may not be readily visible). QRS interval is 0.06 to 0.10 seconds. QT may shorten.
- *Shape and sequence:* P and QRS waves are consistent in shape. P waves are small and rounded. A P wave precedes every QRS complex, which is then followed by a T wave.
- *Patient response:* The fast heart rhythm may cause a decrease in cardiac output because of the shorter filling time for the ventricles. Vulnerable populations are those with ischemic heart disease who are adversely affected by the shorter time for coronary filling during diastole.
- *Causes:* Hyperthyroidism, hypovolemia, heart failure, anemia, exercise, use of stimulants, fever, and sympathetic response to fear or pain and anxiety may each cause sinus tachycardia.
- *Care and treatment:* The dysrhythmia itself is not treated, but the cause is identified and treated appropriately. For example, pain medications are administered to treat pain, or antipyretics are given to treat fever.

TABLE 8.1 PHARMACOLOGY

Antiarrhythmic Medication Classifications

Class[a]	Description	Examples
IA	Inhibits the fast sodium channel Prolongs the action potential duration; increases QT interval Used to treat atrial and ventricular dysrhythmias Most proarrhythmic of Class I's, limiting their use	Quinidine, procainamide, disopyramide
IB	Inhibits the fast sodium channel Shortens the action potential duration; shortens QTc interval Used to treat ventricular dysrhythmias only	Lidocaine, mexiletine
IC	Inhibits the fast sodium channel Shortens the action potential duration of only Purkinje fibers; does not affect QT interval Used to treat supraventricular tachyarrhythmias and ventricular tachyarrhythmias Has proarrhythmic effects	Flecainide, propafenone
II	Causes beta-adrenergic blockade	Metoprolol, esmolol, propranolol, atenolol, timolol, carvedilol, sotalol
III	Inhibits the potassium channels Prolongs the action potential duration; potential to prolong QT interval Used to treat atrial and ventricular tachyarrhythmias Has proarrhythmic effects	Amiodarone, dronedarone, sotalol, bretylium, ibutilide, dofetilide
IV	Inhibits the slow inward movement of calcium to slow impulse conduction, especially in the atrioventricular node Used to treat supraventricular tachyarrhythmias and ventricular tachyarrhythmias without structural heart disease	Diltiazem, verapamil
V	Opens the potassium channel	Adenosine, digoxin, magnesium sulfate

[a]Class I, sodium channel blockers; Class II, beta-adrenergic blockers; Class III, potassium channel blockers; Class IV, calcium channel blockers; Class V, antiarrhythmics.

Adapted from Gahart B, Nazareno A, Ortega MQ. Collins, S. *Elsevier's 2022 Intravenous Medications: A Handbook for Nurses and Health Professionals*. St. Louis, MO: Elsevier; 2022.

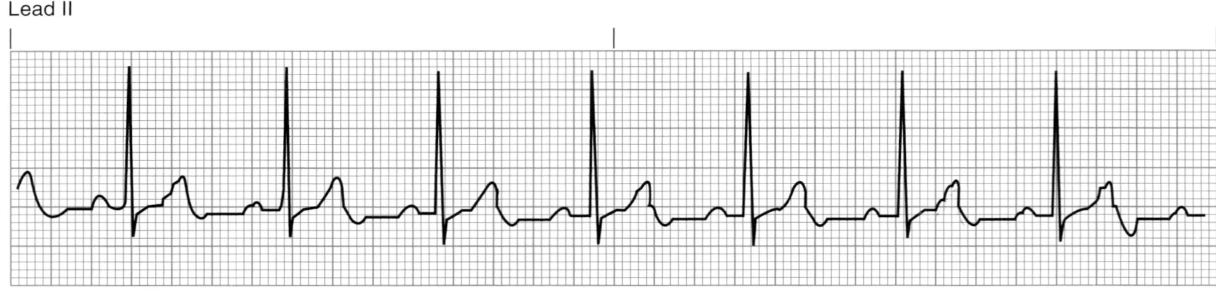

Fig. 8.24 Normal sinus rhythm.

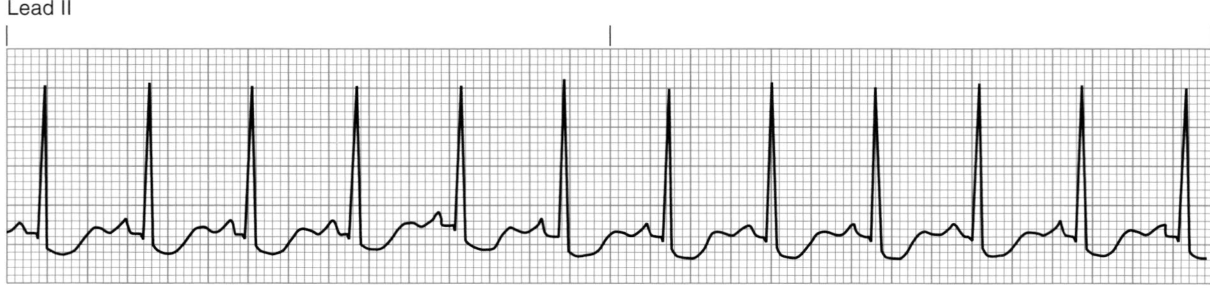

Fig. 8.25 Sinus tachycardia.

Sinus Bradycardia. Bradycardia is defined as a heart rate less than 60 beats/min. Sinus bradycardia may be a normal heart rhythm for some individuals such as athletes, or it may occur during sleep. Although sinus bradycardia may be asymptomatic, it may cause instability if it results in a decrease in cardiac output. The key is to assess the patient and determine if the bradycardia is accompanied by signs of instability (Fig. 8.26).

Rhythm analysis.

- *Rate:* Both atrial and ventricular rates are less than 60 beats/min.
- *Regularity:* Rhythm is regular or essentially regular.
- *Interval measurements:* Measurements are normal, but QT may be prolonged.
- *Shape and sequence:* P and QRS waves are consistent in shape. P waves are small and rounded. A P wave precedes every QRS complex, which is then followed by a T wave.
- *Patient response:* The slowed heart rhythm may cause a decrease in cardiac output, resulting in hypotension and decreased organ perfusion.
- *Causes:* Vasovagal response; medications such as digoxin or AV nodal blocking agents, including calcium channel blockers and beta-blockers; myocardial ischemia or infarction; normal physiological variant in the athlete; disease of the SA node; increased intracranial pressure; hypoxemia; and hypothermia may cause sinus bradycardia.
- *Care and treatment:* Assess for hemodynamic instability related to the bradycardia. If the patient is symptomatic, interventions include administration of atropine. If atropine is not effective in increasing heart rate, then transcutaneous pacing, dopamine infusion, or epinephrine infusion may be administered.[2,6] Atropine is avoided for treatment of bradycardia associated with hypothermia.

Sinus Arrhythmia. Sinus arrhythmia is a cyclical change in heart rate that is associated with respiration. The heart rate slightly increases during inspiration and slightly slows during exhalation because of changes in vagal tone. The ECG tracing demonstrates an alternating pattern of faster and slower heart rate that changes with the respiratory cycle (Fig. 8.27).

Rhythm analysis.

- *Rate:* Atrial and ventricular rates are between 60 and 100 beats/min.
- *Regularity:* This rhythm is cyclically irregular, slowing with exhalation and increasing with inspiration.

CLINICAL PEARLS

Clinical Indications Suggesting Symptomatic Findings

- Anxiety
- Chest pain or pressure
- Dizziness
- Fainting or near-fainting
- Fatigue
- Lightheadedness
- Pounding in the chest
- Shortness of breath
- Weakness

- *Interval measurements:* Measurements are normal.
- *Shape and sequence:* P and QRS waves are consistent in shape. P waves are small and rounded. A P wave precedes every QRS complex, which is then followed by a T wave.
- *Patient response:* This rhythm is tolerated well.
- *Care and treatment:* No treatment is required.

Sinus Pauses. Sinus pauses occur when the SA node either fails to generate an impulse (sinus arrest) or the impulse is blocked and does not exit from the SA node (sinus exit block). The result of the SA node not firing is a pause without any electrical activity.

Sinus arrest. Failure of the SA node to generate an impulse is called *sinus arrest*. The arrest results from a lack of stimulus from the SA node. The sinus beat following the arrest is not on time because the SA node has been reset and the next sinus impulse begins a new rhythm. The result is that no atrial or ventricular depolarization occurs for one heartbeat or more (Fig. 8.28A). If the pause is long enough, the AV node or ventricular backup pacemaker may fire, resulting in escape beats. These beats are called *junctional escape* or *ventricular escape beats*. Typically, the SA node resumes normal generation of impulses following the pause.

Sinus exit block. Sinus exit block also results in a pause, but the P wave following the pause in rhythm is on time or regular because the SA node does not reset. The sinus impulse simply fails to "exit" the SA node (Fig. 8.28B).

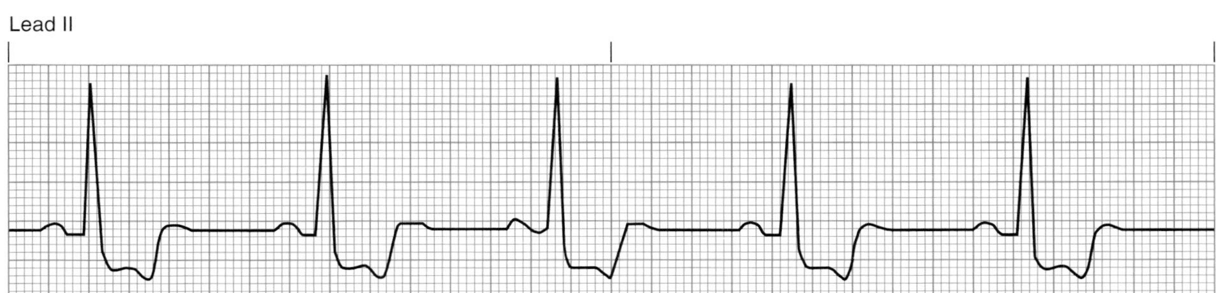

Fig. 8.26 Sinus bradycardia.

Rhythm analysis.

- *Rate:* Atrial and ventricular rates are usually between 60 and 100 beats/min, but any pause may result in a heart rate less than 60 beats/min.
- *Regularity:* The rhythm is irregular for the period of the pause but regular when sinus rhythm resumes. In SA exit block, the P wave following the pause occurs on time. In sinus arrest, the P wave following the pause is not on time.
- *Interval measurements:* Measurements of conducted beats are normal.
- *Shape and sequence:* P and QRS waves are consistent in shape. P waves are small and rounded. A P wave precedes every QRS complex, which is then followed by a T wave.
- *Patient response:* Single pauses in rhythm may not be significant, but frequent pauses may result in a severe bradycardia. The patient with multiple pauses may experience signs and symptoms of decreased cardiac output (Box 8.2).
- *Causes:* Hypoxemia; ischemia or damage of the SA node related to myocardial infarction; AV nodal blocking medications such as beta-blockers, calcium channel blockers, and digoxin; and increased vagal tone may cause sinus exit block.
- *Care and treatment:* If the patient is symptomatic, treatment may be needed, including temporary and permanent insertion of a pacemaker. Collaborate with the provider and pharmacist to explore causes and discuss the need to adjust medications.

Dysrhythmias of the Atria

Normally, the SA node is the dominant pacemaker initiating the heart rhythm; however, cells outside the SA node within the atria can create an ectopic focus that can cause a dysrhythmia. An ectopic focus is an abnormal beat or a rhythm that occurs outside the normal conduction system. In this case, atrial dysrhythmias arise in the atrial tissue.

CLINICAL JUDGMENT ACTIVITY

You are working in the critical care unit, and a patient's heart rate suddenly decreases from 88 to 50 beats/min. Identify potential reasons for the decreased heart rate. Prioritize assessment and interventions.

Premature Atrial Contractions. A premature atrial contraction (PACs) is a single ectopic beat arising from atrial tissue, not the

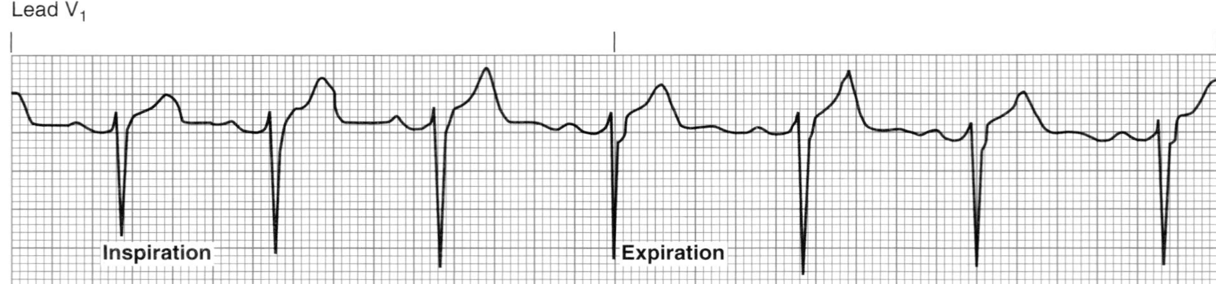

Fig. 8.27 Sinus arrhythmia. The heart rate increases slightly with inspiration and decreases slightly with expiration.

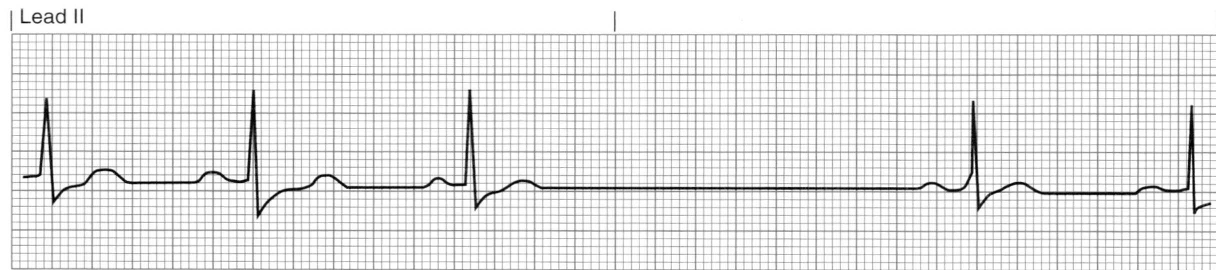

A Sinus arrest

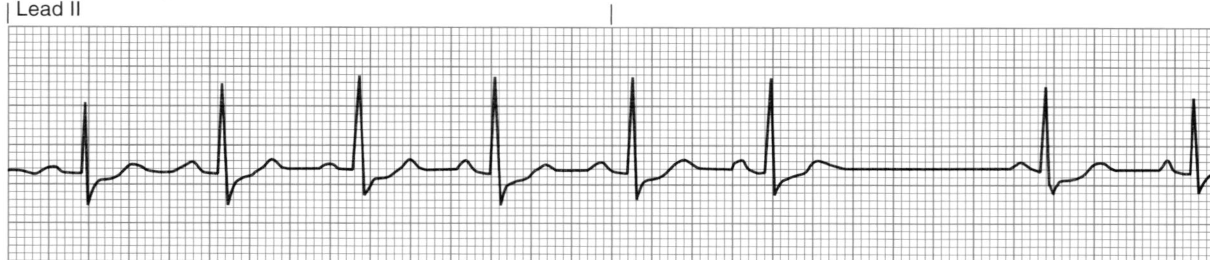

B Sinus exit block

Fig. 8.28 A, Sinus arrest. B, Sinus exit block.

SA node. The PAC occurs earlier than the next normal beat and interrupts the regularity of the underlying rhythm. The P wave of the PAC has a different shape than the sinus P wave because it arises from a different area in the atria; it may follow or be in the T wave of the preceding normal beat. If the early P wave is in the T wave, this T wave will look different from the T wave of a normal beat. Following the PAC, a pause occurs, and then the underlying rhythm typically resumes. The pause is noncompensatory, which means when measuring the P-P intervals for atrial regularity, the P wave following the pause does not occur on time. Box 8.3 discusses how to distinguish compensatory and noncompensatory pauses. PACs are common but denote an irritable area in the atria that has developed the property of automaticity (Fig. 8.29A).

Nonconducted PACs are beats that create an early P wave but are not followed by a QRS complex. The ventricles are unable to depolarize in response to this early stimulus because they are not fully repolarized from the normally conducted beat preceding the PAC (Fig. 8.29B). This creates a pause, but a P wave occurs either in or after the T wave. Therefore, comparing the shapes of the normal PQRST is a critical requirement in rhythm analysis. The frequency of occurrence of PACs varies (Box 8.4).

Rhythm analysis.

- *Rate:* The rate matches that of the underlying rhythm.
- *Regularity:* The PAC interrupts the regularity of the underlying rhythm for a single beat. The PAC is followed by a noncompensatory pause (Box 8.3).
- *Interval measurements:* The PAC may have a different PR interval than the normal sinus beat, usually shorter.
- *Shape and sequence:* The P wave of the PAC is typically a different shape than the sinus P wave. The T wave of the preceding beat may be distorted if the P wave of the PAC lies within it.
- *Patient response:* Premature atrial contractions are usually well tolerated, although the patient may complain of palpitations.
- *Causes:* Stimulants such as caffeine or tobacco, agitation, anxiety, myocardial hypertrophy or dilation, myocardial ischemia, lung disease, hypokalemia, and hypomagnesemia may cause PACs. It may also be a normal variant.
- *Care and treatment:* Increasing numbers of PACs may occur before atrial fibrillation or atrial flutter. No treatment is indicated for PACs.

CHECK YOUR UNDERSTANDING

2. You are asked to look at a patient's rhythm strip and notice that there are no P waves in the rhythm. Your understanding of the rhythm is that the patient may have:
   A. Sinus rhythm
   B. Sinus arrhythmia
   C. Junctional rhythm
   D. Premature atrial contractions

Atrial Tachycardia. Atrial tachycardia is a rapid rhythm that arises from an ectopic focus in the atria. Because of the fast rate, atrial tachycardia can be life-threatening. The ectopic atrial focus generates impulses more rapidly than the AV node can conduct while still in the refractory phase from the previous impulse, and these impulses are not transmitted to the ventricles. Therefore, more P waves may be seen than QRS complexes and T waves. This refractoriness serves as a safety mechanism to prevent the ventricles from contracting too rapidly. The AV node may block impulses in a set pattern, such as every second, third, or fourth beat. However, if the ventricles respond to every

BOX 8.3 Compensatory Versus Noncompensatory Pause

- Analyze a rhythm strip with a premature beat using calipers or paper and pencil.
- Locate two consecutive normal beats just before the premature beat and place the caliper points or pencil marks on the R wave of each normal beat.
- Flip the calipers (or paper) over, to where the next normal beat should have occurred. The premature beat occurs early.
- Avoid losing placement and flip the calipers (or paper) over one more time. If the point of the calipers or the mark on the paper lands exactly on the next normal beat's R wave, the SA node compensated for the one premature beat and kept its normal rhythm.
- If the caliper point or pencil mark does not land on the next normal beat's R wave, the SA node did not compensate and had to establish a new rhythm, resulting in a noncompensatory pause.

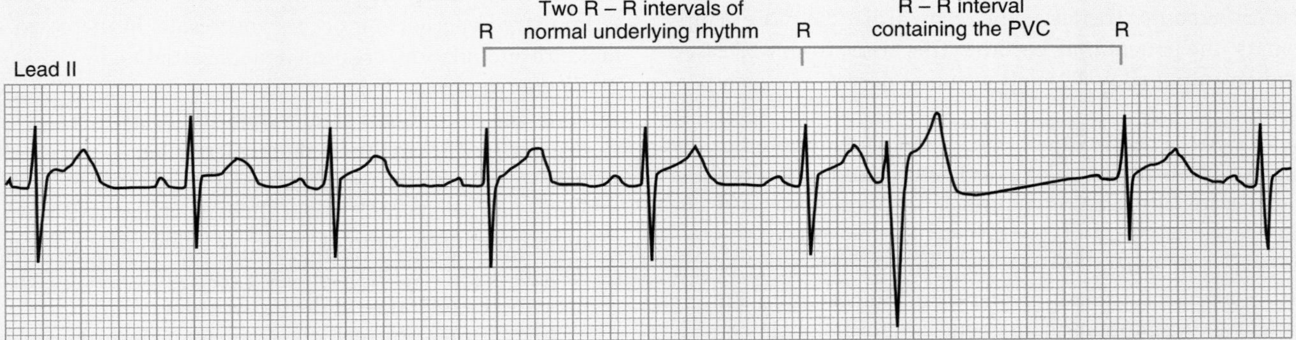

Compensatory pause; sinus rhythm with premature ventricular contraction (PVC). The pause following the PVC is compensatory. From Paul S, Hebra JD. *The Nurse's Guide to Cardiac Rhythm Interpretation: Implications for Patient Care.* Philadelphia: Saunders; 1998.

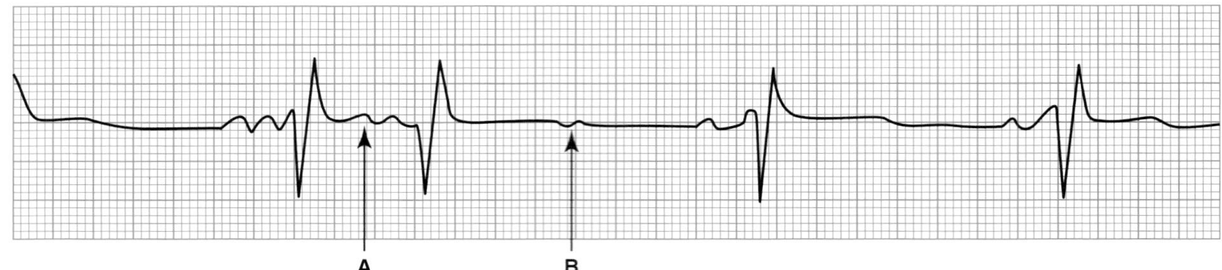

Fig. 8.29 A, Premature atrial contractions (PACs) shown in the third beat. B, A nonconducted PAC.

BOX 8.4 Names Given to Early Beats

- An early beat that occurs every other beat is called bigeminy.
- An early beat that occurs every third beat is called trigeminy.
- An early beat that occurs with frequency is given the name of the underlying rhythm, and then the naming of the frequency of early beats follows that name. An example is sinus rhythm with bigeminal premature atrial contractions.

ectopic atrial impulse, it is called 1:1 conduction, one P wave for each QRS complex. Because the P wave arises outside the SA node, the shape is different from the sinus P wave (Fig. 8.30).

If an abnormal P wave cannot be visualized on the ECG but the QRS complex is narrow, the term *supraventricular tachycardia (SVT)* is often used. This is a generic term that describes any tachycardia that is not ventricular in origin; it is also used when the source above the ventricles cannot be identified, usually because the rate is too fast.

Rhythm analysis.

- *Rate:* The rate ranges from 150 to 250 beats/min.
- *Regularity:* The rhythm is regular if all P waves are conducted.
- *Interval measurements:* The PR interval is different from the sinus PR interval. If the ectopic P wave arises near the junction, the PR interval may be shortened. If close to the SA node, it is nearer the normal PR interval in duration.
- *Shape and sequence:* The P wave shape is different from that of the sinus P wave. The QRS complex is narrow unless there is a bundle branch block. If the P wave of the ectopic rhythm occurs in the T wave, this may alter the shape.
- *Patient response:* The faster the tachycardia, the more symptomatic the patient may become. This arises from decreased cardiac output (Box 8.2) and resultant decreased organ perfusion.
- *Causes:* Atrial tachycardia can occur in patients with healthy hearts as well as those with cardiac disease. Causes include digitalis toxicity, electrolyte imbalances, lung disease, ischemic heart disease, and cardiac valvular abnormalities.
- *Care and treatment:* Assess the patient's tolerance of the tachycardia. If the rate is greater than 150 beats/min and the patient is symptomatic, emergent cardioversion is considered. *Cardioversion* is the delivery of a synchronized electrical shock to the heart by an external defibrillator (Chapter 11, Rapid Response Teams and Code Management). Medications that may be used include adenosine, beta-blockers, calcium channel blockers, and amiodarone.[2,5]

Wandering Atrial Pacemaker. Wandering atrial pacemaker is a dysrhythmia characterized by at least three different ectopic atrial foci followed by a QRS complex at a rate less than 100 beats/min. At least three different P-wave shapes are noted. P waves in wandering atrial pacemaker can be upright, inverted, flat, pointed, notched, or slanted in different directions. The PR interval varies because the impulses originate from different locations within the atria, taking various times to reach the AV node (Fig. 8.31).

Rhythm analysis.

- *Rate:* Rate is less than 100 beats/min.
- *Regularity:* The rate may be slightly irregular.
- *Interval measurements:* PR intervals vary based on the sites of the ectopic foci.
- *Shape and sequence:* At least three different P shapes are noted. The QRS complex is narrow and followed by a T wave.
- *Patient response:* Patients usually tolerate this rhythm unless the rate increases.
- *Causes:* May occur in lung disease, such as chronic obstructive pulmonary disease, or be a normal variant in the young and in older adults.
- *Care and treatment:* No treatment is usually indicated.

Multifocal Atrial Tachycardia. Multifocal atrial tachycardia is essentially the same as wandering atrial pacemaker, except the heart rate exceeds 100 beats/min (Fig. 8.32). At least three ectopic P waves are noted. This dysrhythmia is found almost exclusively in the patient with chronic obstructive pulmonary disease. Pulmonary hypertension occurs and results in increased atrial pressure and dilation, creating irritable atrial foci.

Rhythm analysis.

- *Rate:* The heart rate is greater than 100 beats/min.
- *Regularity:* The rhythm is slightly irregular.
- *Interval measurements:* PR intervals vary.
- *Shape and sequence:* P waves differ in shape. A P wave precedes every QRS complex, which is followed by a T wave.
- *Patient response:* The response varies and is determined by the patient's tolerance of the tachycardia.
- *Causes:* Chronic obstructive pulmonary disease causes dilation of the atria with resultant ectopic foci from the stretched tissue.
- *Care and treatment:* The treatment goal is to optimize the patient's pulmonary status.

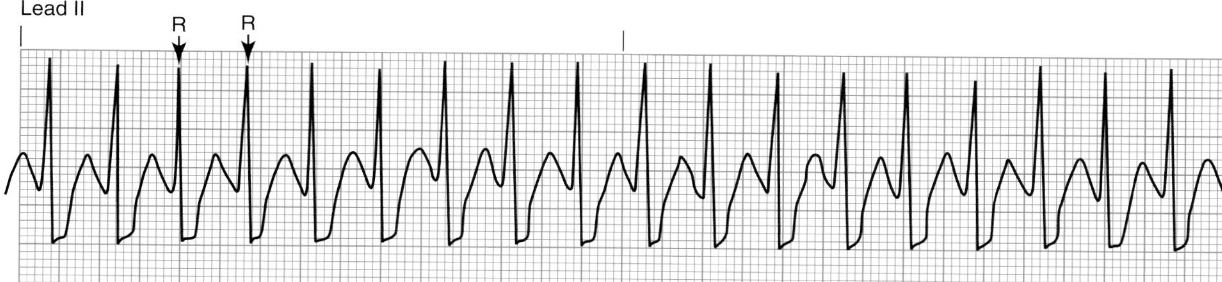

Fig. 8.30 Atrial tachycardia with 1:1 conduction. *R,* R wave of the QRS complex.

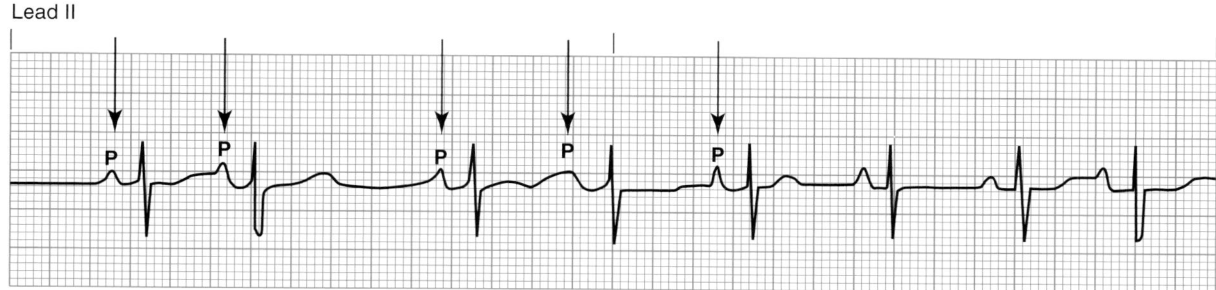

Fig. 8.31 Wandering atrial pacemaker. *Arrows* indicate different shapes of P waves.

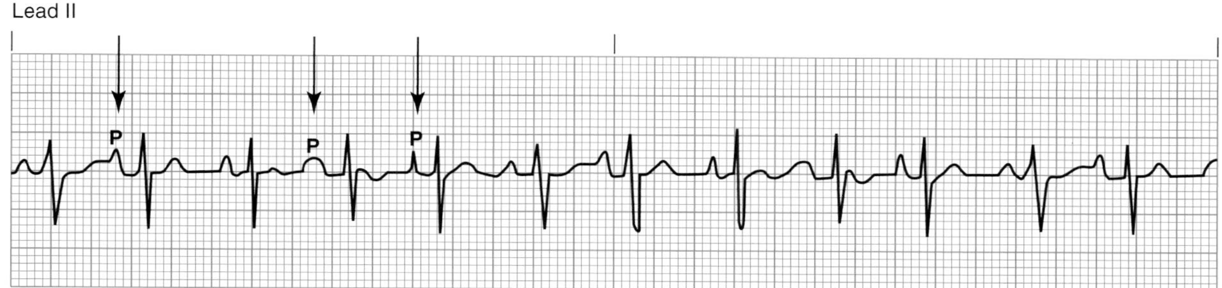

Fig. 8.32 Multifocal atrial tachycardia. *Arrows* indicate different shapes of P waves.

Atrial Flutter. Atrial flutter arises from a single irritable focus in the atria. The atrial focus fires at an extremely rapid, regular rate, between 240 and 320 beats/min, known as *type I flutter.* An ECG tracing with a rate faster than 340 beats/min is designated as *type II flutter;* the mechanism remains undefined. The P waves are called *flutter waves* and have a sawtooth appearance (Fig. 8.33A). The ventricular response may be regular or irregular based on how many flutter waves are conducted through the AV node. The number of flutter waves to each QRS complex is called the conduction ratio. The conduction ratio may remain the same or vary depending on the number of flutter waves that are conducted to the ventricles. The description of atrial flutter might be constant at 2:1, 3:1, 4:1, 5:1, and so forth, or it may be variable. Flutter waves occur through the QRS complex and the T wave and often alter their appearances (Fig. 8.33A). It is helpful to identify the best lead for visualizing the flutter waves in atrial flutter and use this as the second monitor lead.

Rhythm analysis.

- *Rate:* Atrial rate is between 240 and 320 beats/min but is typically 300 beats/min (one large box between flutter waves; see Fig. 8.33B). Ventricular rate is determined by the conduction ratio of the flutter waves.
- *Regularity:* Flutter waves are regular, but the QRS complex and T waves may not be regular depending on the conduction ratio of the atrial flutter.
- *Interval measurements:* No PR interval is present. QRS and QT intervals are normal unless distorted by a flutter wave.
- *Shape and sequence:* P or flutter waves are consistent in shape and look like teeth on a saw blade. QRST waves are altered in shape by the flutter waves.
- *Patient response:* Usually the patient is asymptomatic unless atrial flutter results in a tachycardia called rapid ventricular response (RVR). Atrial flutter with RVR occurs when atrial impulses cause a ventricular response greater than 100 beats/min.
- *Causes:* Lung disease, ischemic heart disease, hyperthyroidism, hypoxemia, heart failure, and alcoholism can cause atrial flutter.
- *Care and treatment:* Alterations in atrial blood flow leading to blood stasis can cause clot formation. Patients identified with atrial flutter of 48 hours in duration or longer

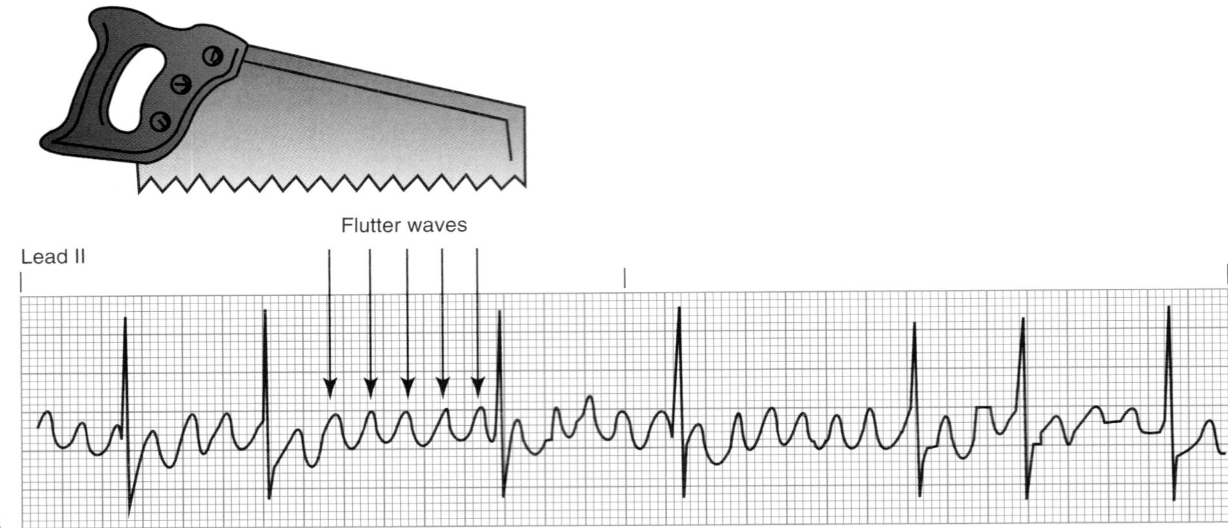

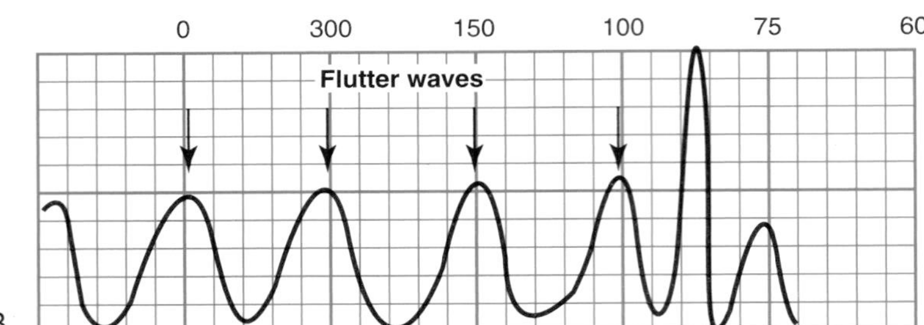

Fig. 8.33 Atrial flutter. A, Flutter waves show a sawtooth pattern at an atrial rate of 250 to 350 beats/min. B, Enlarged view shows one large box between flutter waves.

or unknown duration usually receive chronic antithrombotic therapy (with warfarin, a factor Xa inhibitor, or a direct thrombin inhibitor) unless contraindicated. Patients with atrial flutter less than 48 hours in duration should be assessed for the risk of stroke using the CHA_2DS_2-VASc score. If a patient is at risk for stroke, then heparin, a factor Xa inhibitor, or a direct thrombin inhibitor is recommended before cardioversion.[7] The CHA_2DS_2-VASc score is a calculated score that can provide the risk of stroke in patients with atrial fibrillation and atrial flutter and includes age, sex, heart failure history, hypertension history, stroke/transient ischemic attacks/thromboembolism history, vascular disease history, and diabetes. Rate control is accomplished with medications that block the AV node. Elective cardioversion may be performed once the patient has been taking anticoagulants for approximately 3 weeks before and 4 weeks after cardioversion.[7] Interventional electrophysiological treatments, including ablation of the irritable focus, may be indicated.[7]

Atrial Fibrillation. Atrial fibrillation is the most common dysrhythmia observed in clinical practice. Atrial fibrillation arises from multiple ectopic foci in the atria, causing chaotic quivering of the atria and ineffectual atrial contraction. The AV node is bombarded with hundreds of atrial impulses and conducts these impulses in an unpredictable manner to the ventricles. The atrial rate may be as high 700, and no discernible P waves can be identified, resulting in a wavy baseline and an extremely irregular ventricular response. This irregularity is called *irregularly irregular* (Fig. 8.34). The ineffectual contraction of the atria results in loss of atrial kick. If too many impulses conduct to the ventricles, atrial fibrillation with RVR may result and compromise cardiac output. When atrial fibrillation occurs sporadically, it is called *paroxysmal atrial fibrillation*.

If the atrial impulse is conducted through the ventricles in a normal fashion, the QRS complex is narrow and appears normal, although the rhythm is irregularly irregular. However, if the impulse reaches one of the bundle branches before full repolarization, the QRS complex is widened in classic bundle branch block morphological finding. The widened QRS is due to the delay caused by the bundle branch block and results in slowed conduction through either the right or the left ventricle, depending on which bundle branch has not fully repolarized. When this event occurs, the impulse is said to be aberrantly conducted (Fig. 8.35).

In atrial fibrillation, aberrantly conducted beats are referred to as *Ashman beats*. Ashman beats are more likely

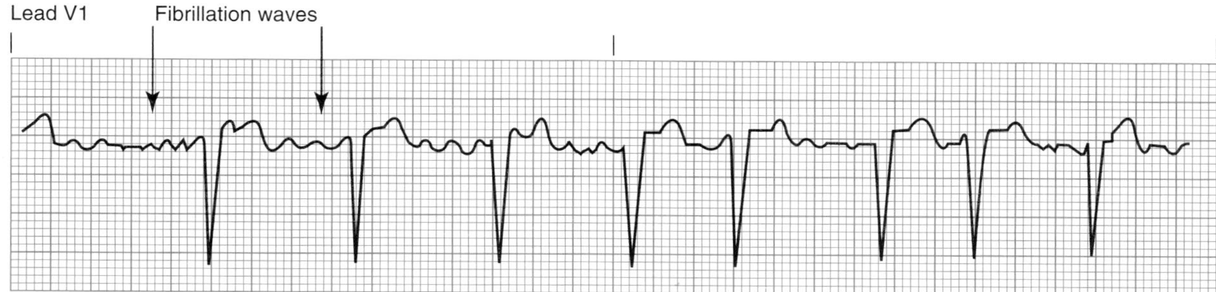

Fig. 8.34 Atrial fibrillation.

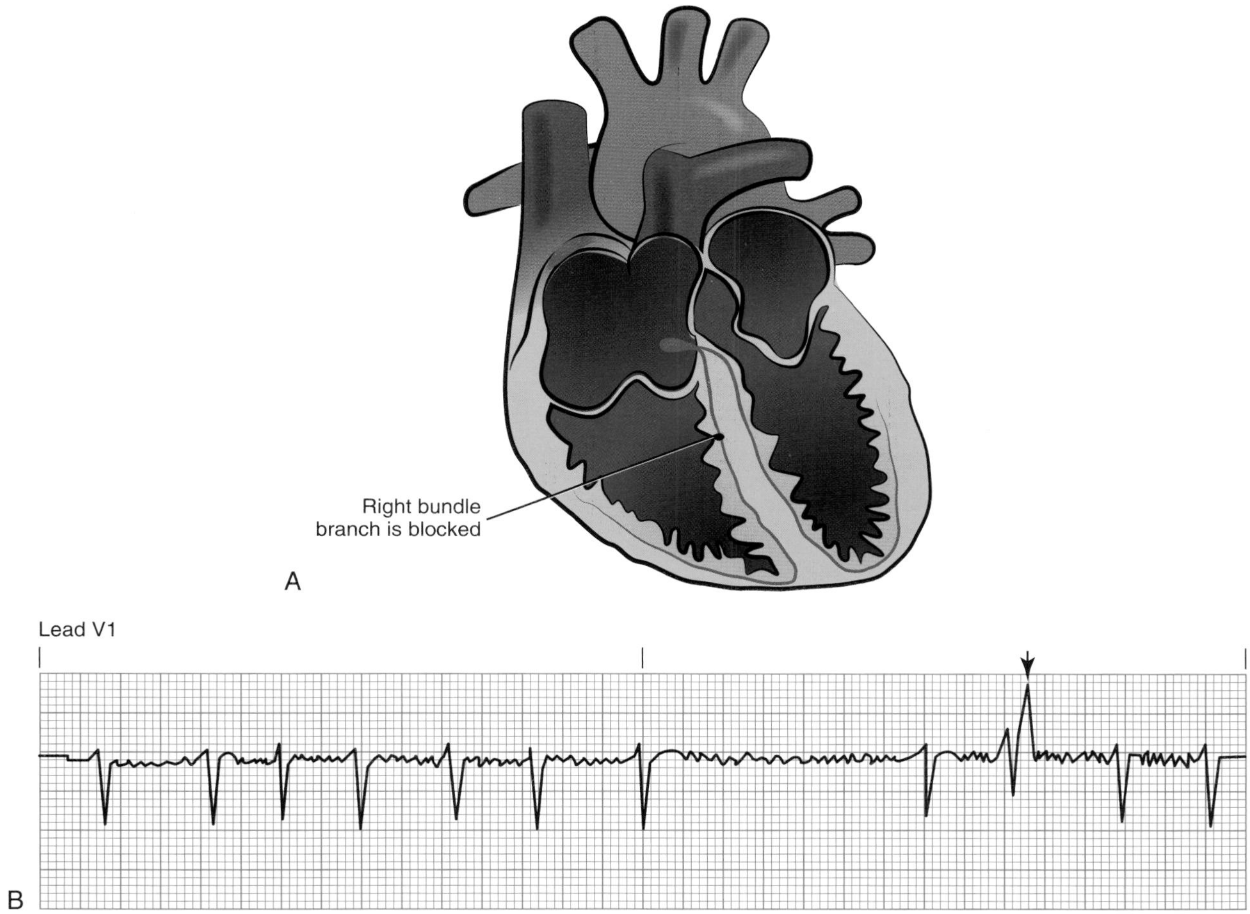

Right bundle branch is blocked

A

Lead V1

B

Fig. 8.35 Atrial fibrillation with aberrant conduction. **A**, The site in the right bundle branch that has not repolarized in time. **B**, The manifestation of the QRS complex (aberrantly conducted beat) in the ninth beat *(arrow)* caused by the nonrepolarized tissue.

to occur when an atrial impulse arrives at the AV node just after a previously conducted impulse (Fig. 8.35; note that the ninth beat has this appearance). Ashman beats are often seen when the rate changes from slower to faster, referred to as a long-short cycle. Ashman beats are not clinically significant.

One complication of atrial fibrillation is thromboembolism. The blood that collects in the atria is agitated by fibrillation, and normal clotting is accelerated. Small thrombi, called *mural thrombi,* begin to form along the walls of the atria. These clots may dislodge, resulting in pulmonary embolism or stroke.

Rhythm analysis.

- *Rate:* Atrial rate is uncountable; ventricular rate may vary widely.
- *Regularity:* Ventricular response is irregularly irregular.
- *Interval measurements:* PR interval is absent. The QRS complex and QT interval are normal in duration unless a bundle branch block exists.
- *Shape and sequence:* No recognizable or discernible P waves are present. The isoelectric line is wavy. QRS waves are

consistent in shape unless aberrantly conducted. The QRS complex is followed by a T wave.

- *Patient response:* The patient may or may not be aware of the atrial fibrillation. If the ventricular response is rapid, the patient may show signs of decreased cardiac output or worsening of heart failure symptoms.
- *Causes:* Ischemic heart disease, valvular heart disease, hyperthyroidism, lung disease, heart failure, and aging may cause atrial fibrillation.
- *Care and treatment:* As with atrial flutter, alterations in blood flow and hemostasis may predispose the patient to clot formation. If there are no contraindications, the patient is prescribed anticoagulants based on the risk according to a calculation of the CHA_2DS_2-VASc score. After at least 3 weeks of antithrombotic therapy, elective cardioversion can be considered followed by 4 more weeks of antithrombotic therapy.[7] Anticoagulation with warfarin, a factor Xa inhibitor, or a direct thrombin inhibitor are useful for cardioversion, provided that contraindications to the selected medication are absent. Always determine the ventricular rate and document it. High ventricular rates or ventricular rates not tolerated by the patient are controlled by administration of AV nodal blocking agents. As with atrial flutter, ablation may be attempted. Symptomatic tachycardia is usually treated with medications because of the risk of thromboembolism. Emergent cardioversion is considered if the tachycardia is associated with hemodynamic instability.[7]

CLINICAL JUDGMENT ACTIVITY

Discuss why patients with pulmonary disease are prone to atrial dysrhythmias.

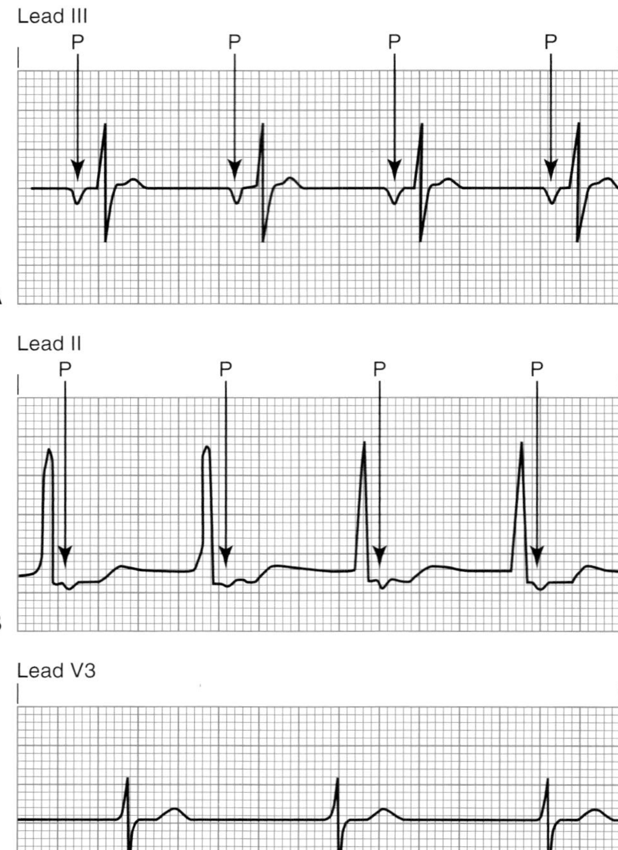

Fig. 8.36 P waves in junctional dysrhythmias. **A,** Backward conduction with inverted P wave. **B,** Forward and backward conduction with retrograde P wave. **C,** Forward conduction with absent P wave.

Dysrhythmias of the Atrioventricular Node

Dysrhythmias of the AV node are called *junctional rhythms,* which include junctional escape rhythm, premature junctional contractions (PJCs), accelerated junctional rhythm, junctional tachycardia, and paroxysmal SVT. Several ECG changes are common to all junctional dysrhythmias. These changes include P wave abnormalities and PR interval changes.

P-Wave Changes. Because of the location of the AV node—in the center of the heart—impulses generated may be conducted forward, backward, or both. With the potential of forward, backward, or bidirectional impulse conduction, three different P waveforms may be associated with junctional rhythms:

1. When the AV node impulse is conducted backward, the impulse enters the atria first. Conduction back toward the atria allows for at least partial depolarization of the atria. When depolarization occurs backward, an inverted P wave is created in leads where the P wave is usually upright. Once the atria have been depolarized, the impulse then moves down the bundle of His and depolarizes both ventricles normally (Fig. 8.36A). A short PR interval (<0.12 seconds) is noted.
2. When the impulse is conducted both forward and backward, *P waves may be present after the QRS complex.* In this type of conduction, the impulse first moves into the ventricles, depolarizing them and creating a QRS complex. Because the impulse is also conducted backward, some atrial depolarization occurs, and a late P wave is noted after the QRS complex (Fig. 8.36B).
3. When the AV node impulse moves forward, P waves may be absent because the impulse enters the ventricle first. The atria receive the wave of depolarization at the same time as the ventricles; thus, because of the larger muscle mass of the ventricles, there is no P wave (Fig. 8.36C).

Junctional Escape Rhythm. Junctional escape rhythms occur when the dominant pacemaker, the SA node, fails to fire. A junctional escape rhythm has an inverted P wave and short PR interval preceding the QRS complex, a P wave that follows the QRS complex (retrograde), or no visible P wave. The escape rhythm may consist of many successive beats (Fig. 8.37A), or it may occur as a single escape beat that follows a pause, such as a sinus pause (Fig. 8.37B).

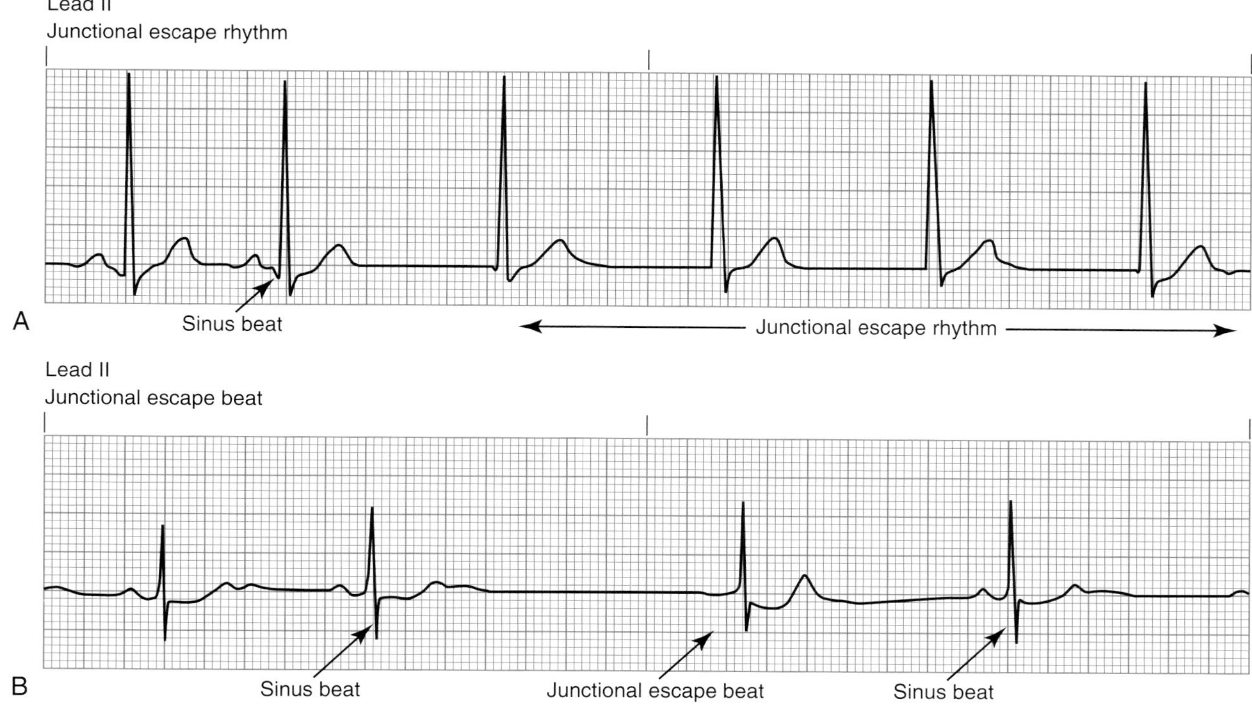

Fig. 8.37 A, Junctional escape rhythm. B, Junctional escape beat.

Rhythm analysis.

- *Rate:* Heart rate is 40 to 60 beats/min.
- *Regularity:* The rhythm is regular.
- *Interval measurements:* If a P wave is present before the QRS complex, the PR interval is shortened to less than 0.12 ms. QRS complex is normal.
- *Shape and sequence:* P waves may be inverted, follow the QRS complex, or be absent.
- *Patient response:* The patient is assessed for tolerance of the bradycardia.
- *Causes:* The escape rhythm results from loss of SA node activity.
- *Care and treatment:* Determine the patient's tolerance of the bradycardia. Alert the provider of the change in rhythm. If symptomatic, administer atropine; consider transcutaneous pacing, dopamine infusion, or epinephrine infusion.[2]

Accelerated Junctional Rhythm and Junctional Tachycardia. The normal intrinsic rate for the AV node and junctional tissue is 40 to 60 beats/min, but rates can accelerate. An accelerated junctional rhythm has a rate between 60 and 100 beats/min (Fig. 8.38A), and the rate for junctional tachycardia is greater than 100 beats/min (Fig. 8.38B).

Rhythm analysis.

- *Rate:* Accelerated junctional rhythm is 60 to 100 beats/min. Junctional tachycardia rhythm is greater than 100 beats/min.
- *Regularity:* The rhythm is regular.
- *Interval measurements:* If a P wave is present before the QRS complex, the PR interval is shortened less than 0.12 ms. The QRS complex is followed by a T wave, and both are normal in shape.
- *Shape and sequence:* The P wave may have a variety of configurations: precede the QRS complex, be inverted, not visible, or follow the QRS complex.
- *Patient response:* A patient may have a decrease in cardiac output and hemodynamic instability, depending on the rate.
- *Causes:* Sinoatrial node disease, ischemic heart disease, electrolyte imbalances, digitalis toxicity, and hypoxemia can be causes.
- *Care and treatment:* Assess and treat the tachycardia if the patient is hemodynamically unstable. Alert the provider to the change in rhythm.

Premature Junctional Contractions. Irritable areas in the AV node and junctional tissue can generate premature beats that are earlier than the next expected beat (Fig. 8.39). These premature beats are similar to PACs but with characteristics of a junctional beat. The regularity of the underlying rhythm is interrupted by the premature junctional beat. The PJC is followed by a noncompensatory pause.

Rhythm analysis.

- *Rate:* The rate is that of the underlying rhythm.
- *Regularity:* The underlying rhythm is interrupted by a premature beat that momentarily disrupts regularity.
- *Interval measurements:* The PJC is early; thus, it is next to the T wave.
- *Shape and sequence:* The P wave may have a variety of configurations: precede the QRS complex, be inverted, not visible, or follow the QRS complex. The QRS complex is followed by the T wave, and both are normal in shape.
- *Patient response:* The rhythm is well tolerated, but the patient may experience palpitations if the PJCs occur frequently.
- *Causes:* PJCs may be a normal variant; may be caused by digitalis toxicity, ischemic or valvular heart disease, or heart failure; or may be a response to endogenous or exogenous catecholamines such as epinephrine.
- *Care and treatment:* No treatment is indicated.

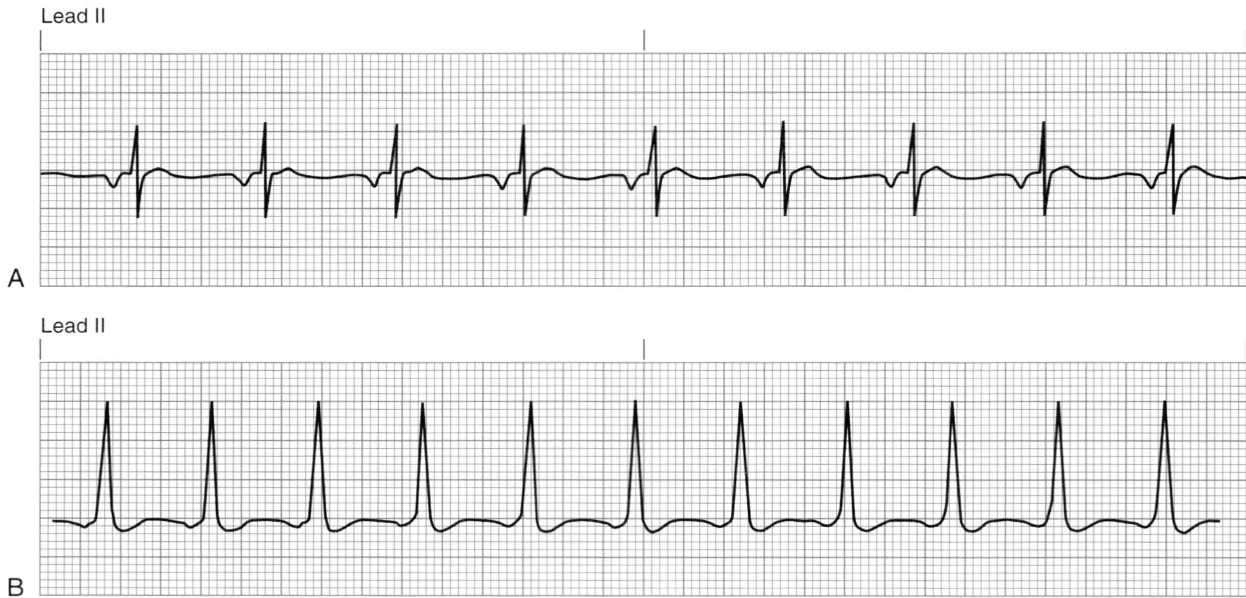

Fig. 8.38 A, Accelerated junctional rhythm. B, Junctional tachycardia.

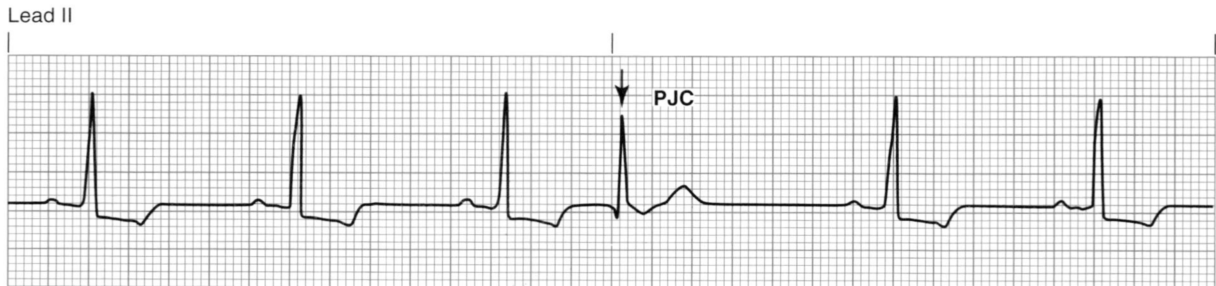

Fig. 8.39 Sinus rhythm with premature junctional contraction *(PJC)*.

Paroxysmal Supraventricular Tachycardia. Paroxysmal supraventricular tachycardia (PSVT) occurs above the ventricles, and it has an abrupt onset and cessation. It is initiated by either a PAC or a PJC. An abnormal conduction pathway through the AV node or an accessory pathway around the AV node results in extreme tachycardia. The QRS complex is typically narrow, and a P wave may or may not be present. The primary criteria are those of the abrupt onset and cessation of the dysrhythmia (Fig. 8.40).

Rhythm analysis.

- *Rate:* Heart rate is 150 to 250 beats/min.
- *Regularity:* The rhythm is regular.
- *Interval measurements:* If the P wave is present, the PR interval is shortened. Other intervals are normal.
- *Shape and sequence:* P wave (if present) and QRS complex are consistent in shape. The QRS complex is narrow and followed by a T wave.
- *Patient response:* The patient may be asymptomatic or symptomatic.
- *Causes:* PSVT often occurs in healthy, young adults without structural heart disease. It may be precipitated by increased catecholamines, stimulants, heart disease, electrolyte imbalances, and anatomical abnormality.
- *Care and treatment:* If the patient is asymptomatic, vagal maneuvers may be attempted. If the patient is symptomatic and the heart rate is greater than 150 beats/min, emergent cardioversion is considered. Adenosine or AV nodal blocking agents are usually administered. Once stabilized, the patient is referred for further evaluation by an electrophysiologist.[8]

CHECK YOUR UNDERSTANDING

3. The patient's cardiac monitor is alarming. The heart rate is 200 beats/min, and the QRS complex is very narrow. The patient states that he feels lightheaded, and BP is 80/40 mm Hg. You understand your priority is to:
   A. Continue to observe the patient.
   B. Anticipate assisting to administer adenosine.
   C. Get a complete set of vital signs.
   D. Assess if it is time to change the IV access site.

Dysrhythmias of the Ventricle

Ventricular dysrhythmias arise from ectopic foci in the ventricles. Because the stimulus depolarizes the ventricles in a slower, abnormal way, the QRS complex appears widened and has a bizarre shape. The QRS complex is wider than 0.12 seconds and often wider than 0.16 seconds. The polarity of the T wave can be opposite that of the QRS complex.

Depolarization from abnormal ventricular beats rarely activates the atria in a retrograde fashion. Consequently, most ventricular dysrhythmias have no apparent P waves. However, if a P wave is

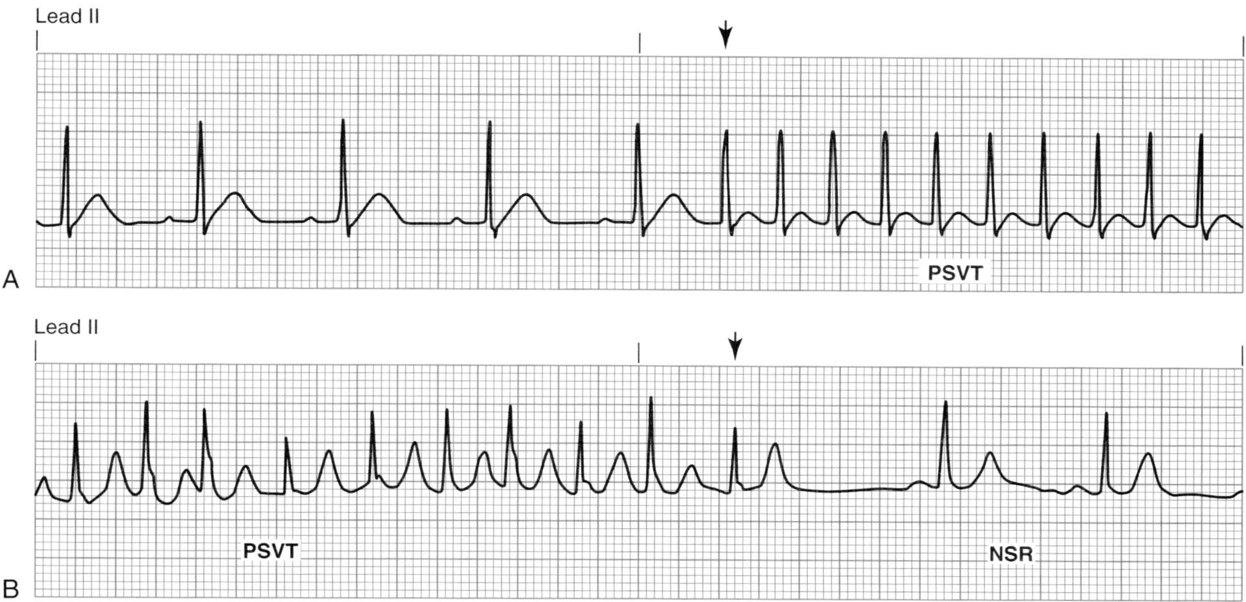

Fig. 8.40 Paroxysmal supraventricular tachycardia (PSVT). **A,** The abrupt onset initiated by a premature junctional contraction *(arrow).* **B,** The abrupt cessation of the PSVT *(arrow). NSR,* Normal sinus rhythm.

present, it is usually seen in the T wave of the following beat or it has no relationship to the QRS complex and is dissociated from the ventricular rhythm. Ventricular dysrhythmias can be life-threatening; thus, fast recognition and intervention are imperative.

Premature Ventricular Contractions. Premature ventricular contractions (PVCs) are a common ventricular dysrhythmia. PVCs are early beats that interrupt the underlying rhythm; they can arise from a single ectopic focus or from multiple foci within the ventricles. A single ectopic focus produces PVC waveforms that look alike, called unifocal PVCs (Fig. 8.41A and C). Waveforms of PVCs arising from multiple foci are not identical and are called multifocal PVCs (Fig. 8.41B). PVCs do not generally reset the SA node, so the next sinus beat following the pause occurs on time. This is called a *compensatory pause.*

PVCs may occur in a predictable pattern, such as every other beat, every third beat, or every fourth beat. Box 8.4 lists the nomenclature for early beats. Bigeminal PVCs are noted in Fig. 8.41A. PVCs can also occur sequentially. Two PVCs in a row are called a *couplet* (Fig. 8.41C), and three or more in a row are called *nonsustained VT.*[9]

The peak of the T wave through the downslope of the T wave is considered the vulnerable period, which coincides with partial repolarization of the ventricles. If a PVC occurs during the T wave, VT may occur. When the R wave of PVC falls on the T wave of a normal beat, it is referred to as the *R-on-T phenomenon* (Fig. 8.42).

PVCs may occur in healthy individuals and usually do not require treatment. The nurse must determine if PVCs are increasing in number by evaluating the trend and assess the patient for symptoms and hemodynamic status. If PVCs are increasing, the nurse should evaluate for potential causes such as electrolyte imbalances, myocardial ischemia or injury, and hypoxemia. Runs of nonsustained VT may be a precursor to development of sustained VT.

Rhythm analysis.

- *Rate:* The rate matches the underlying rhythm.
- *Regularity:* The rhythm is interrupted by the premature beat.
- *Interval measurements:* There is no PR interval, and the QRS complex is greater than 0.12 seconds.
- *Shape and sequence:* The QRS complex of the PVC is wide and bizarre looking. The T wave may be oriented opposite the direction of the QRS complex of the PVC.
- *Patient response:* Patients may experience palpitations and may become symptomatic if the PVCs occur frequently.
- *Causes:* Hypoxemia, ischemic heart disease, hypokalemia, hypomagnesemia, acid-base imbalances, and increased catecholamine levels can cause PVCs.
- *Care and treatment:* Treat the cause if PVCs are increasing in frequency.

Ventricular Tachycardia. VT is a rapid, life-threatening dysrhythmia originating from a single ectopic focus in the ventricles. It is characterized by at least three PVCs in a row. VT occurs at a rate greater than 100 beats/min, but the rate is usually approximately 150 beats/min and may be up to 250 beats/min. Depolarization of the ventricles is abnormal and produces a widened QRS complex (Fig. 8.43). The patient may or may not have a pulse.

The wave of depolarization associated with VT rarely reaches the atria. Hence, P waves are usually absent. If P waves are present, they have no association with the QRS complex. The SA node may continue to depolarize at its normal rate, independent of the ventricular ectopic focus. P waves may appear to be randomly scattered throughout the rhythm, but the P waves are actually fired at a consistent rate from the SA node. This is called AV dissociation, another clue that the rhythm is VT. Occasionally, a P wave will "capture" the ventricle because of the timing of atrial depolarization, interrupting the VT with a

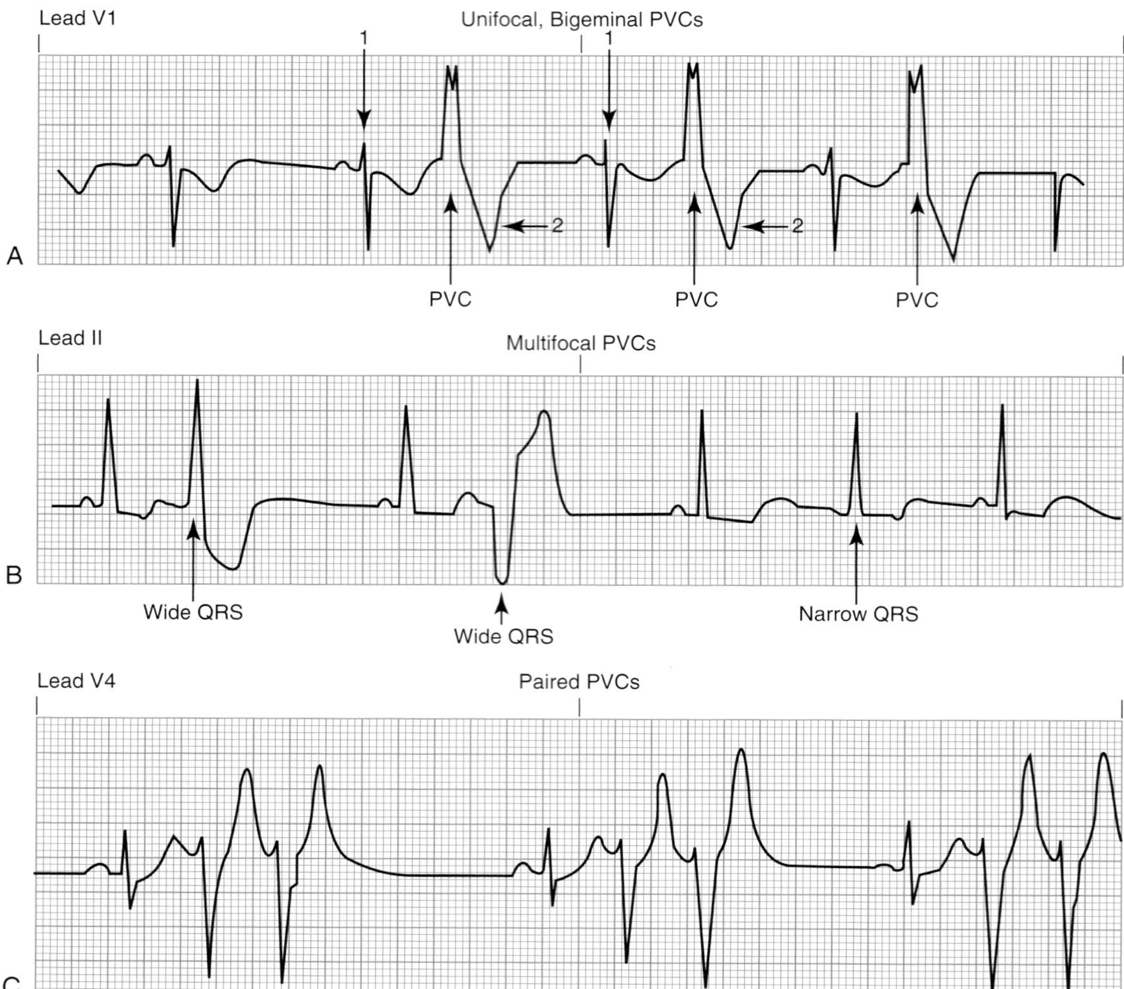

Fig. 8.41 Premature ventricular contractions (PVCs). **A**, Sinus rhythm with unifocal PVCs. The sinus beat is *1; 2* points to the presence of an inverted T wave. **B**, Sinus rhythm with multifocal PVCs; note the different configuration of the PVCs, indicating generation from more than one focus. **C**, The PVCs are in pairs and look the same, indicating that they are from the same foci.

single capture beat that appears normal and narrow. Then, the VT recurs. Capture beats are a diagnostic clue to differentiating wide complex tachycardias.

Torsades de pointes ("twisting about the point") is a type of VT caused by a prolonged QT interval, and it is often caused by magnesium deficiency.[9] Unlike VT, in which the QRS complex waveforms have similar shapes, torsades de pointes is characterized by the presence of both positive and negative complexes that move above and below the isoelectric line. This lethal dysrhythmia is treated as pulseless VT.[2,9] It can often be prevented by routine measurement of the QT/QTc intervals, especially if the patient is receiving medications that prolong the QT interval. Increases in QT/QTc intervals are reported to the provider, potential medication-related causes are explored, and magnesium levels are monitored and corrected (Fig. 8.44).

Rhythm analysis.

- *Rate:* The heart rate is 110 to 250 beats/min.
- *Regularity:* The rhythm is regular unless capture beats occur and momentarily interrupt the VT.
- *Interval measurements:* There is no PR interval. The QRS complex is greater than 0.12 seconds and often wider than 0.16 seconds.
- *Shape and sequence:* QRS waves are consistent in shape but appear wide and bizarre. The polarity of the T wave is opposite to that seen in the QRS complex.
- *Patient response:* If enough cardiac output is generated by the VT, a pulse and blood pressure are present. If cardiac output is impaired, the patient has signs and symptoms of low cardiac output and may experience a cardiac arrest.
- *Causes:* Hypoxemia, acid-base imbalance, exacerbation of heart failure, ischemic heart disease, cardiomyopathy, hypokalemia, hypomagnesemia, valvular heart disease, genetic abnormalities, and QT prolongation are all possible causes of VT.
- *Care and treatment:* Determine whether the patient has a pulse. If no pulse is present, provide emergent basic and advanced life-support interventions, including defibrillation.[2,9] If a pulse is present and the blood pressure is stable, the patient can be treated with IV amiodarone or procainamide. Cardioversion is used as an emergency measure if the patient continues to have a pulse but becomes hemodynamically unstable.[2,9]

Ventricular Fibrillation. VF is a chaotic rhythm characterized by a quivering of the ventricles, which results in total loss of

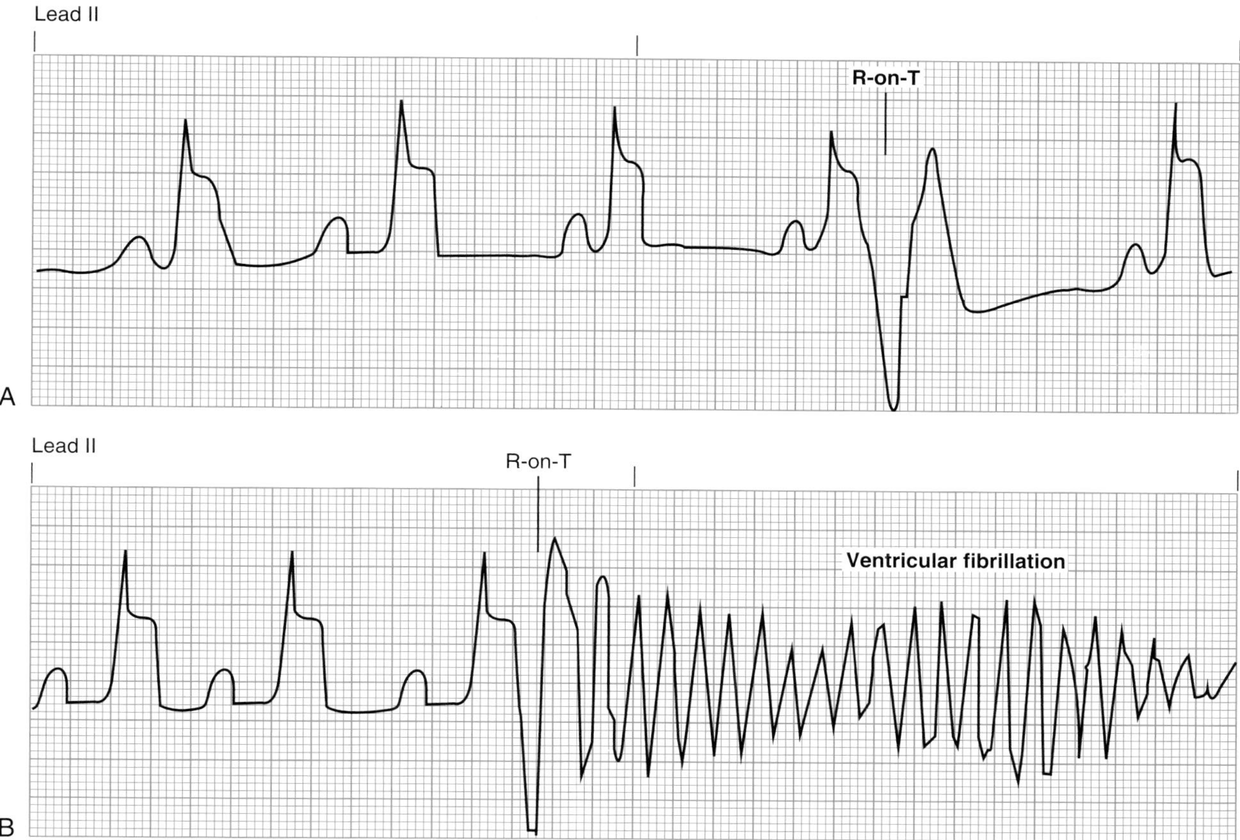

Fig. 8.42 R-on-T phenomenon. A, Single premature ventricular contraction (PVC) on T wave. B, PVC causing ventricular fibrillation.

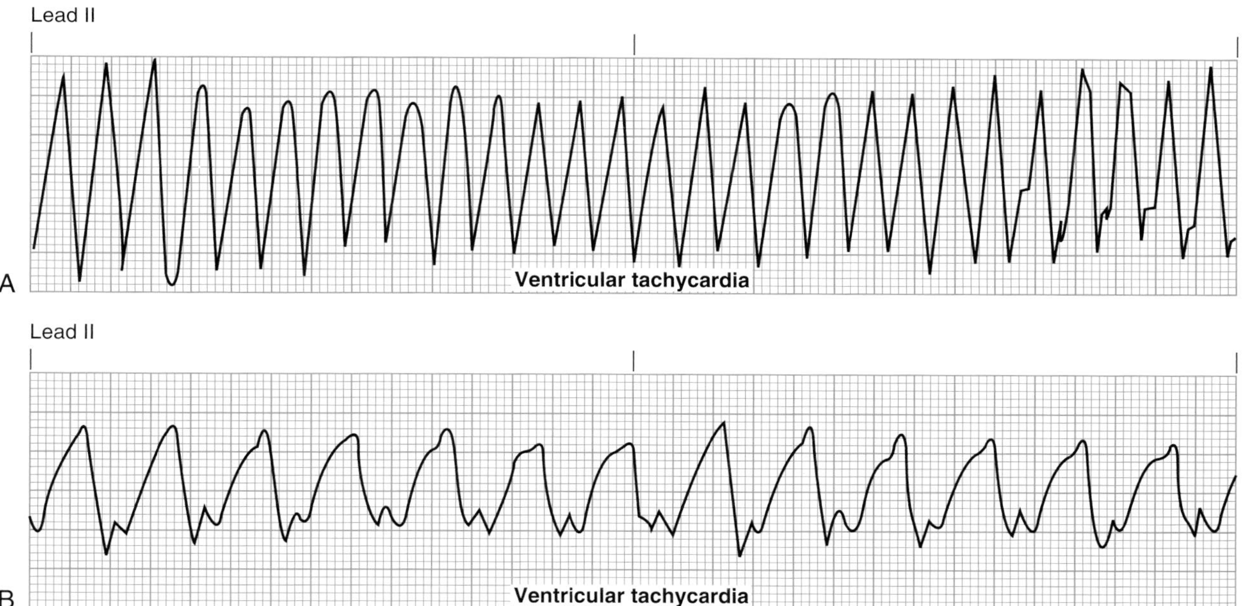

Fig. 8.43 Ventricular tachycardia (VT). A, One example of VT with a narrower QRS complex. B, Another example of VT with a wider QRS complex.

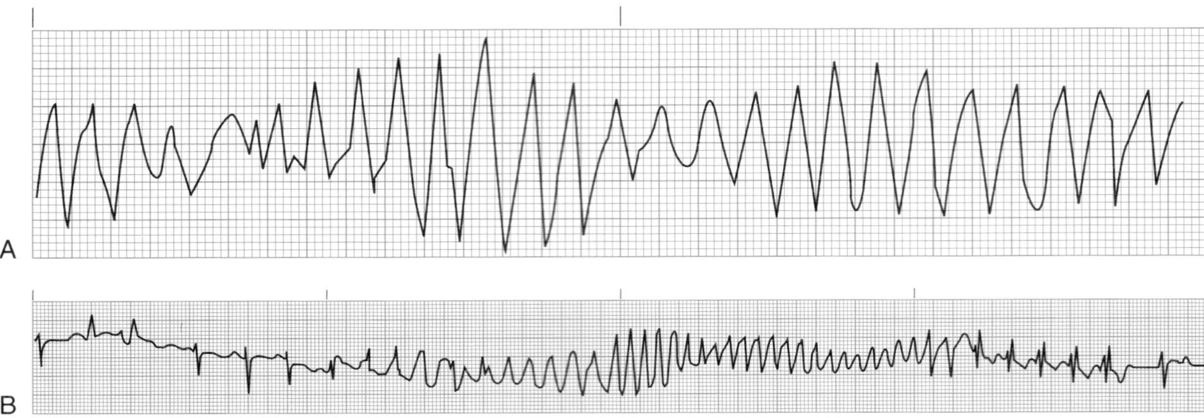

A is presented at 100% for a 6-second strip. B has been reduced to 55% of actual size to be able to see a longer waveform over 12 seconds, showing how a patient goes into and comes out of rhythm.

Fig. 8.44 Torsades de pointes.

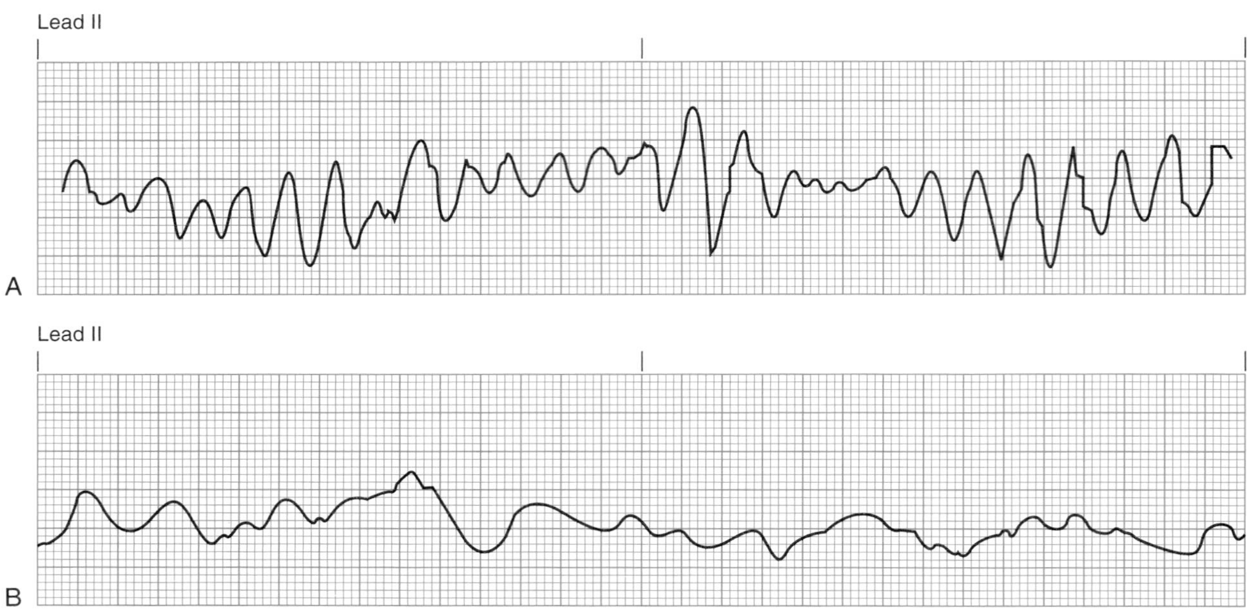

Fig. 8.45 Ventricular fibrillation. A, Coarse. B, Fine.

cardiac output and pulse. VF is a life-threatening emergency, and the more immediate the treatment, the better the chance of survival. VF produces a wavy baseline without a PQRST complex (Fig. 8.45).

Because a loose lead or electrical interference can produce a waveform similar to VF, it is always important to immediately assess the patient for pulse and consciousness.

Rhythm analysis.

- *Rate:* Heart rate is not discernible.
- *Regularity:* Heart rhythm is not discernible.
- *Interval measurements:* There are no waveforms.
- *Shape and sequence:* The baseline is wavy and chaotic, with no PQRST complexes.
- *Patient response:* The patient is in cardiac arrest.
- *Causes:* VF can be caused by ischemic and valvular heart disease, electrolyte and acid-base imbalances, and QT prolongation.
- *Care and treatment:* Begin immediate basic life support (BLS) and advanced cardiovascular life support (ACLS) interventions.[2,9]

Idioventricular Rhythm or Ventricular Escape Rhythm. Idioventricular rhythm is an escape rhythm that is generated by the Purkinje fibers. This rhythm emerges only when the SA and AV nodes fail to initiate an impulse. The Purkinje fibers are capable of an intrinsic rate of 20 to 40 beats/min. Because this last pacemaker is in the ventricles, the QRS complex appears wide and bizarre with a slow rate (Fig. 8.46). An idioventricular rhythm is considered a lethal dysrhythmia because the Purkinje fiber pacemakers may cease to fire, resulting in asystole. A single ventricular escape beat may occur following a pause if the junctional escape pacemaker does not fire (Fig. 8.46). If the rate is between 40 and 100 beats/min, this rhythm is called *accelerated idioventricular rhythm* (AIVR). This wide-complex rhythm is

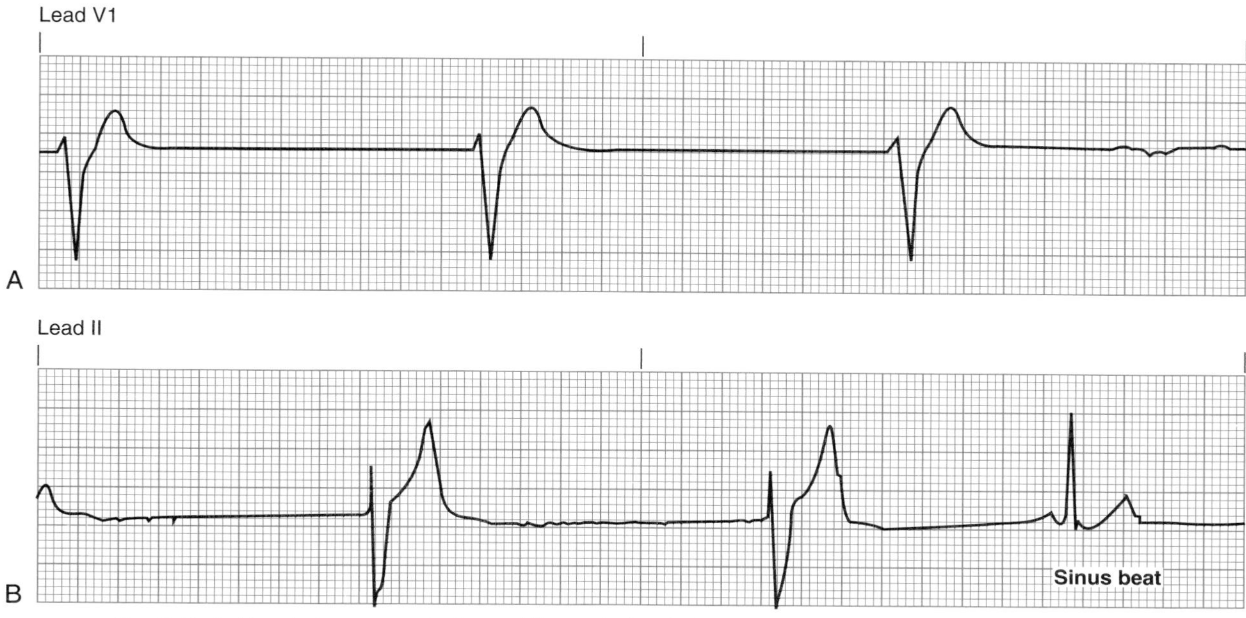

Fig. 8.46 A, Ventricular escape rhythm or idioventricular rhythm. B, Two ventricular escape beats followed by a sinus beat.

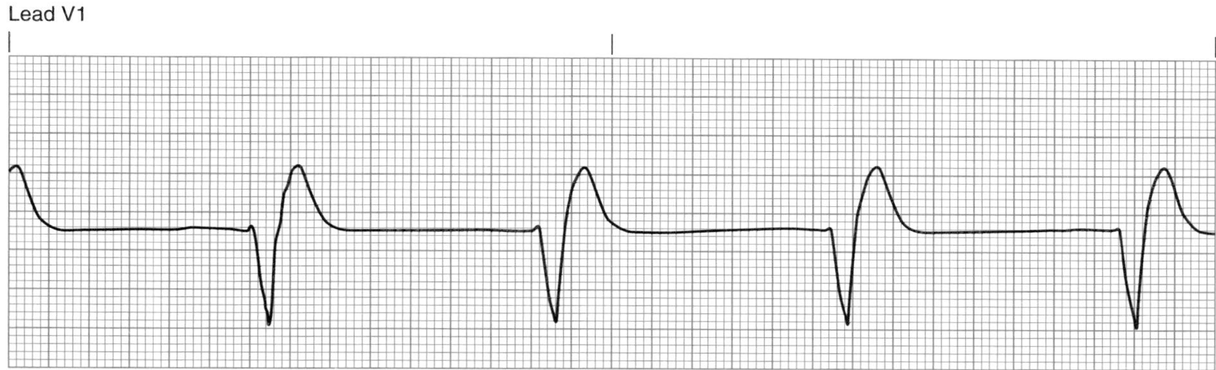

Fig. 8.47 Accelerated idioventricular rhythm (AIVR).

often seen after reperfusion of a coronary artery by thrombolytics; percutaneous coronary interventions, such as angioplasty or stent placement; and cardiac surgery (Fig. 8.47).

Rhythm analysis.

- *Rate:* The rate of idioventricular rhythm is 20 to 40 beats/min, and the rate of AIVR is 40 to 100 beats/min.
- *Regularity:* The rhythm is regular.
- *Interval measurements:* No P waves are present, and the QRS complex is greater than 0.12 seconds.
- *Shape and sequence:* QRS waves are wide and bizarre in shape. The QRS complex is followed by a T wave of opposite polarity.
- *Patient response:* The extreme bradycardia may cause the same symptoms as any severe bradycardia. This mechanism is the last backup pacemaker, and asystole may occur.
- *Causes:* Failure of the SA and AV nodal pacemakers causes idioventricular rhythm.
- *Care and treatment:* Initiate BLS and ACLS protocols. Consider emergent transcutaneous pacing.[2]

Asystole. Asystole is characterized by complete cessation of electrical activity. A flat baseline is seen, without any evidence of P, QRS, or T waveforms. A pulse is absent, and there is no cardiac output; cardiac arrest has occurred (Fig. 8.48A).

Asystole often occurs following VF or ventricular escape rhythm. Following a ventricular escape rhythm, this rhythm is referred to as ventricular standstill (Fig. 8.48B). Pulse should be assessed immediately, because a lead or electrode coming off may mimic this dysrhythmia. During cardiac arrest situations, if asystole occurs when another rhythm has been monitored, a check of two leads should occur to confirm asystole.

Rhythm analysis.

- *Rate:* Heart rate is absent.
- *Regularity:* Heart rhythm is absent.
- *Interval measurements:* PQRST waveforms are absent.
- *Shape and sequence:* Waveform presents as a flat or undulating line on the monitor.
- *Patient response:* The patient is in cardiac arrest.
- *Causes:* Asystole is usually preceded by another dysrhythmia such as VF or ventricular escape rhythm.
- *Care and treatment:* Initiate BLS and ACLS protocols.[2]

NURSING SELF-CARE

Alarms are essential for monitors to alert nurses to dysrhythmias. Poorly set alarms can result in erroneous or false alarms that desensitize clinicians and can lead to delayed response or inaction to alarms. The volume of alarms, especially alarms that do not require intervention, creates fatigue, or alarm fatigue.

Strategies to reduce cardiac monitor alarm fatigue

Interventions for bedside nurses

- Prepare skin appropriately for ECG electrodes.
- Ensure proper ECG electrode placement and change every 24 hours and PRN.
- Verify alarm settings regularly (beginning of shift, change in patient status, change in caregiver).
- Ensure alarm parameters are appropriate for individual patients and current status as per hospital and unit policies.

Nursing administration/leaders

- Develop interprofessional teams (including staff nurses) to create polices & procedures according to current evidence/data.
- Establish default alarm settings appropriate for the unit's patient population.
- Provide continuous education for nurses and staff on devices with alarms and alarm monitoring.
- Ensure appropriate patient selection for monitoring.
- Consider implementation of an alarm notification system (monitor technicians, pagers, phones, etc.).

American Association of Critical-Care Nurses. Practice alert. Managing alarms in acute care across the lifespan: electrocardiography and pulse oximetry. *Crit Care Nurse*. 2018;38(2):e16-e20; Storm, J, Chen, HC. The relationships among alarm fatigue, compassion fatigue, burnout and compassion satisfaction in critical care and step-down nurses. *J Clin Nurs*. 2021;30(3-4):443-453. https://doi.org/10.1111/jocn.15555.

Atrioventricular Blocks

Atrioventricular block, which is also known as *heart block*, refers to an inability of the AV node to conduct sinus impulses to the ventricles in a normal manner. Atrioventricular blocks can cause a delay in conduction from the SA node through the AV node or completely block conduction intermittently or continuously. Atrioventricular blocks may arise from normal aging of the conduction system or be caused by damage to the conduction system from ischemic heart disease.

Four types of AV block exist, each categorized in terms of degree. The four types of blocks are first-degree, second-degree type I, second-degree type II, and third-degree. The greater the degree of block, the more severe the consequences. First-degree block has minimal consequences, whereas third-degree block may be life-threatening.

First-Degree Atrioventricular Block. *First-degree AV block* describes consistent delayed conduction through the AV node or the atrial conductive tissue but does make it through to the ventricles. It is not actually a block, but instead a delay. It is represented on the ECG as a prolonged PR interval. It is a common dysrhythmia in older adults and in patients with cardiac disease. As the normal conduction pathway ages or becomes diseased, impulse conduction becomes slower than normal (Fig. 8.49).

Rhythm analysis.

- *Rate:* Heart rate is determined by the underlying rhythm.
- *Regularity:* The underlying rhythm determines regularity.
- *Interval measurements:* PR interval is prolonged and is greater than 0.20 seconds. QRS complex and QT/QTc measurements are normal.
- *Shape and sequence:* P and QRS waves are consistent in shape. P waves are small and rounded. A P wave precedes every QRS complex, which is followed by a T wave.
- *Patient response:* Atrioventricular block is well tolerated.
- *Causes:* Aging and ischemic and valvular heart disease can cause AV block.
- *Care and treatment:* No treatment is required.

Second-Degree Heart Block. *Second-degree heart block* refers to AV conduction that is intermittently blocked. Two types of second-degree block may occur, and each has specific diagnostic criteria for accurate diagnosis.

Second-degree atrioventricular block type I also called *Mobitz I* or *Wenckebach phenomenon,* is represented on the ECG as a progressive lengthening of the PR interval until there is a P wave without a QRS complex. The AV node progressively delays conduction to the ventricles, resulting in progressively longer PR intervals until finally a QRS complex is dropped. The PR interval following the dropped QRS complex is shorter than the PR interval preceding the dropped beat. By not conducting this one beat, the AV node recovers and is able to conduct the next atrial impulse (Fig. 8.50). If dropped beats occur frequently, it is useful to describe the conduction ratio, such as 2:1, 3:1, or 4:1.

Rhythm analysis.

- *Rate:* The rate is slower than the underlying rhythm because of the dropped beat.
- *Regularity:* P-P intervals stay the same, but R-R intervals shorten until the dropped beat.
- *Interval measurements:* The PR interval becomes progressively longer until a QRS complex is dropped. The PR interval before the dropped QRS complex is longer than the PR interval of the next conducted PQRST waveforms.
- *Shape and sequence:* P and QRS waves are consistent in shape. P waves are small and rounded. A P wave precedes every QRS complex, which is followed by a T wave, except for the dropped beats.
- *Patient response:* This rhythm is usually well tolerated unless there is an underlying bradycardia or frequent dropped beats.
- *Causes:* Aging, AV nodal blocking medications, acute inferior wall myocardial infarction or right ventricular infarction, ischemic heart disease, digitalis and other AV nodal blocking agent toxicity, and excess vagal response are all possible causes.
- *Care and treatment:* A 12-lead ECG is obtained to document rhythm, rate, and conduction. This type of block is usually well tolerated, and no treatment is indicated unless the dropped beats occur frequently. If the patient is symptomatic, medications that may contribute to the rhythm are discontinued. A temporary and/or permanent pacemaker may be indicated if the cause is not resolved.

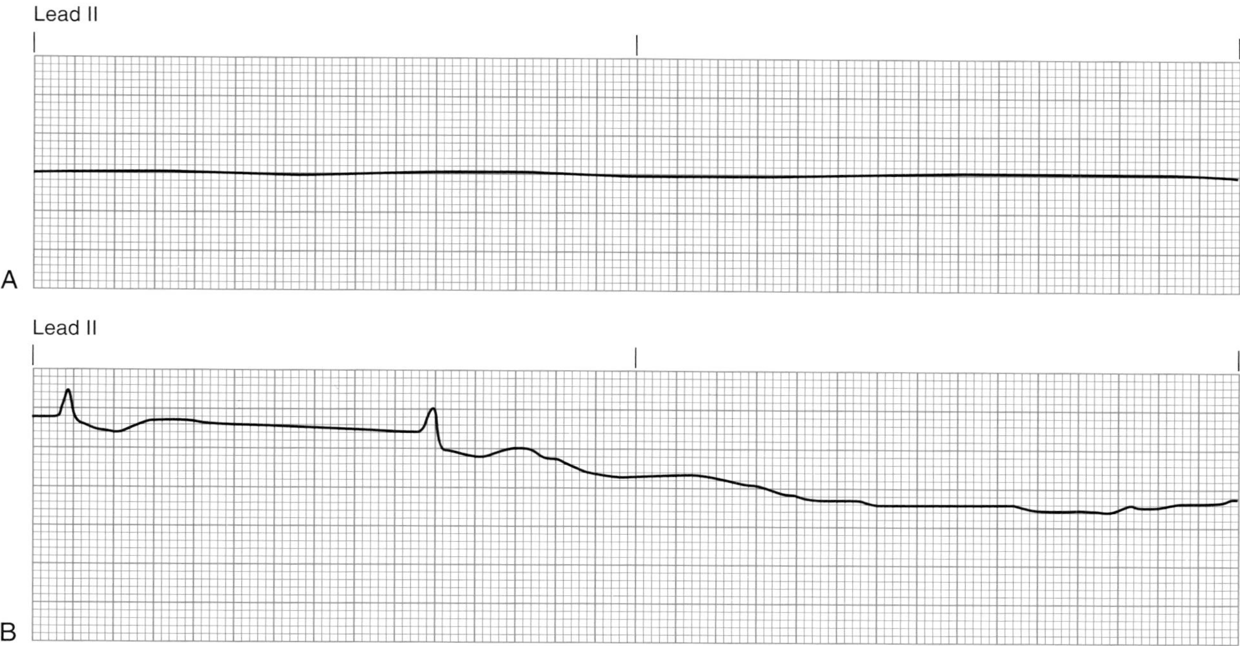

Fig. 8.48 A, Asystole. B, Ventricular standstill.

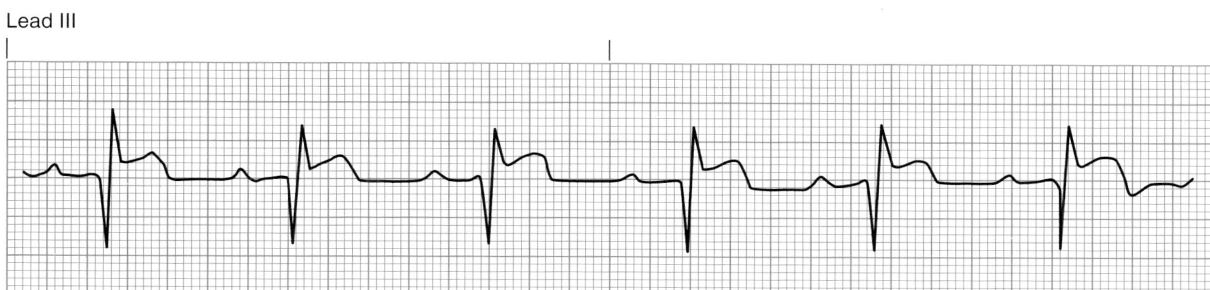

Fig. 8.49 First-degree atrioventricular block.

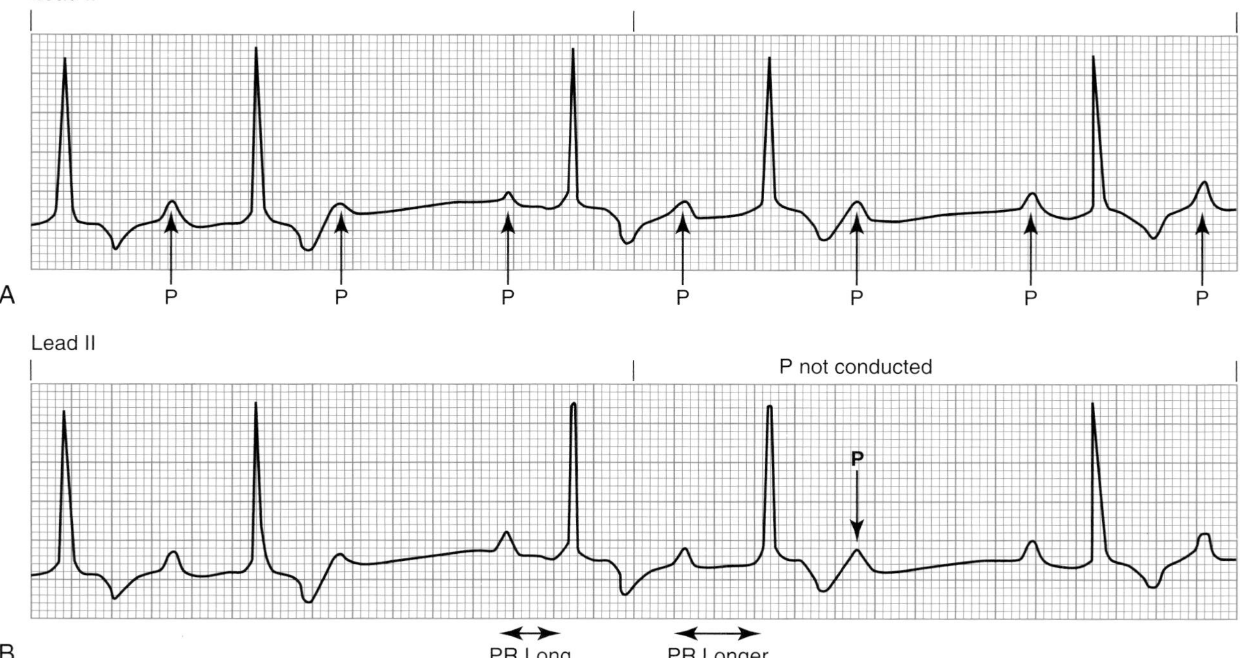

Fig. 8.50 Second-degree atrioventricular block type I (Mobitz I, Wenckebach). A, Shows every other P wave as a nonconducted beat, yet for the P waves that are conducted, the PR interval is prolonged. B, Shows how the PR interval is long on the labeled example, followed by a PR interval that is longer on the labeled example and then by a P wave that is not conducted.

Second-degree AV block type II (Mobitz II) is a more critical type of heart block that requires early recognition and intervention. The conduction abnormality occurs below the AV node, either in the bundle of His or the bundle branches. A P wave is generated but is not conducted to the ventricles for one or more beats. The PR interval remains the same throughout, except for the dropped beat(s) (Fig. 8.51). Second-degree AV block type II is often associated with a bundle-branch block and a corresponding widened QRS complex; however, narrow QRS complexes may be observed. Second-degree AV block type II can progress to the more clinically significant third-degree block and may cause the patient to be symptomatic.

Rhythm analysis.

- *Rate:* Heart rate is slower than the underlying rhythm because of the dropped beats.
- *Regularity:* P waves are regular, but QRS complexes are occasionally absent.
- *Interval measurements:* Intervals are constant for the underlying rhythm. PR intervals of the conducted beats do not change. QRS complexes may be widened because of a bundle branch block.
- *Shape and sequence:* P and QRS waves are consistent in shape. P waves are small and rounded. QRS complexes are missing.
- *Patient response:* The patient may tolerate one missed beat, but symptoms may occur if frequent beats are missed.
- *Causes:* Heart disease, increased vagal tone, conduction system disease, ablation of the AV node, and inferior and right ventricular myocardial infarctions are possible causes of second-degree AV block type II.
- *Care and treatment:* The patient may require emergent treatment with transcutaneous or transvenous pacing followed by insertion of a permanent pacemaker if the cause is not resolved.[2,6]

Third-Degree Heart Block. Third-degree block is often called complete heart block because no atrial impulses are conducted through the AV node to the ventricles. The block in conduction can occur at the level of the AV node, the bundle of His, or the bundle branches. In complete heart block, the atria and ventricles beat independently of each other because the AV node is completely blocked to the sinus impulse, and it is not conducted to the ventricles. An escape rhythm arises from the junctional tissue or the ventricles: the atria beat at one rate, and the ventricles beat at a different rate. The atrial rate is dictated by the SA node. The ventricular rate is slow, and usually only a ventricular or junctional escape rhythm is present. No communication exists between the atria and ventricles. Third-degree block is a type of AV dissociation (Fig. 8.52).

One hallmark of third-degree heart block is that the P waves have no association with the QRS complexes and appear throughout the QRS waveform. Both the P-P and R-R intervals are regular, but the rates for each are different because they have no relationship to each other. Whenever a rhythm strip appears to have no consistent, predictable relationship between P waves and QRS complexes, third-degree block is considered.

Rhythm analysis.

- *Rate:* The atrial rate is greater than the ventricular rate.
- *Regularity:* P-P intervals are regular and R-R intervals are regular, but they are not associated with each other.
- *Interval measurements:* There is no PR interval in the absence of conduction. The QRS complex is often widened greater than 0.12 seconds, with a ventricular escape rhythm.
- *Shape and sequence:* P and QRS waves are consistent in shape. P waves are small and rounded. The QRS complex is followed by a T wave. There is no relationship between the P waves and QRS complexes.
- *Patient response:* Patients may become symptomatic because of the bradycardia of the escape rhythm.
- *Causes:* Ischemic heart disease, acute myocardial infarction, and conduction system disease are possible causes of third-degree heart block.

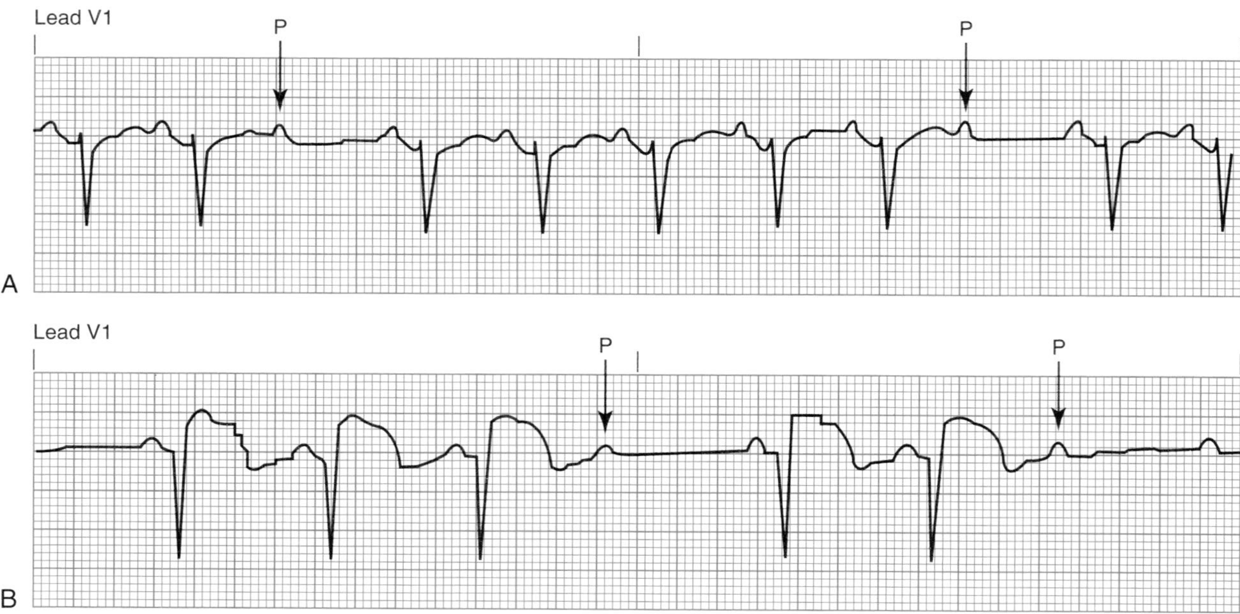

Fig. 8.51 Second-degree atrioventricular block type II (Mobitz II). A, The PR interval is constant; at the third and ninth P waves, there is no QRS complex following the P wave. B, No QRS complex follows the fourth and seventh P waves. Note for the P waves that are conducted, the PR interval is constant.

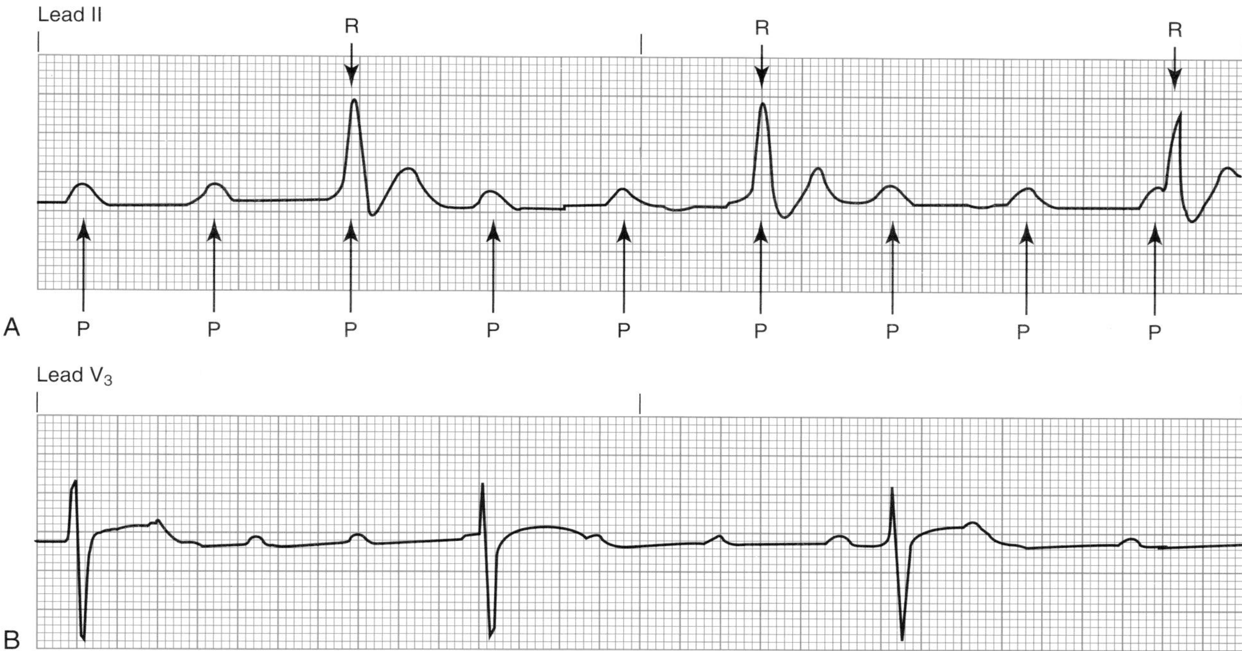

Fig. 8.52 Third-degree atrioventricular block (complete heart block). **A,** P waves regular and present throughout at an atrial rate of 94 beats/min and ventricular rhythm of 30 beats/min. The P waves are not associated with the QRS complexes. **B,** Similar tracing; atrial rate of 100 beats/min and ventricular rate of 30 beats/min.

- *Care and treatment:* If the patient has symptomatic bradycardia and is unstable, then atropine is given to increase the heart rate. Additional medications may be needed for continued instability or specific causes of third-degree block. Additionally, treatment includes transcutaneous or transvenous pacing and implanting a permanent pacemaker.[2,6]

CLINICAL JUDGMENT ACTIVITY

A 65-year-old female with type 2 diabetes presents to the emergency department; symptoms include complaints of sudden-onset shortness of breath with neck and shoulder pain. Her blood pressure is 185/95 mm Hg, and her heart rate is 155 beats/min. What will your priority assessment focus be? How will you initially manage this patient? What medical intervention would you anticipate? List serious signs and symptoms of hemodynamic instability in a patient with a tachydysrhythmia.

CARDIAC PACING DEVICES

Types of Cardiac Pacemakers

A cardiac pacemaker delivers electrical current to the myocardium to stimulate depolarization when the heart rate is too slow or the heart is unable to initiate or conduct a native beat. A pacemaker is often implanted to treat symptomatic bradycardia, which may occur from a number of different pathophysiological conditions. Most common reasons for pacemaker therapy are second-degree AV block type II, third-degree AV block, and sick sinus syndrome. The need for a pacemaker may be temporary (e.g., after an acute myocardial infarction or cardiac surgery) or permanent. Battery-operated external pulse generators are used to provide electrical energy for temporary transvenous pacemakers. Implanted permanent pacemakers are used to treat chronic conditions. These devices have a battery life of up to 10 years, which varies based on the manufacturer.

It is important that patients be assessed for the need for pacing. Unnecessary pacing may lead to worsened outcomes, including heart failure, rehospitalization, increased mortality, and new onset of atrial fibrillation.[6]

Temporary Pacemakers. Types of temporary pacemakers include the following[2,6]:

- *Transcutaneous:* Electrical stimulation is delivered through the skin via external electrode pads connected to an external pacemaker (a defibrillator with pacemaker functions; see Chapter 11, Rapid Response Teams and Code Management).
- *Transvenous:* A pacing catheter (Fig. 8.53) is inserted percutaneously into the right ventricle, where it contacts the endocardium near the ventricular septum. It is connected to a small external pulse generator (Fig. 8.54) by electrode wires. Note the electrical ports on the pacing catheter, which are covered by black caps in Fig. 8.53. These are connected to the pulse generator, whereupon pacing thresholds are set for each specific patient.
- *Epicardial:* Pacing wires are inserted into the epicardial wall of the heart during cardiac surgery (Fig. 8.55); wires are brought through the chest wall and can be connected to a pulse generator, if needed (Fig. 8.56). Note that only two pacing wires are shown in Fig. 8.55; however, in cardiac bypass surgery patients, four wires are often placed through the chest wall of the patient, two wires from the atrium and two wires from the ventricles. These four wires are connected to the temporary pacemaker, and pacing thresholds are set for each patient (see Clinical Exemplar box).

CLINICAL EXEMPLAR

Quality and Safety

Use of the external temporary pacemaker is standard for patients who have symptomatic bradycardia. Before pacing is started, educate the patient about indications and potential complications. Ensure a new battery has been placed in the pacemaker and verify settings with provider orders. Once the pacemaker is initiated, evaluate the pacing threshold and set the pacemaker rate at a level to optimize hemodynamic status. Trend patient assessments to ensure hemodynamic stability.

Reference

Dalia T, Amr BS. Pacemaker indications. StatPearls [Internet]. https://www.ncbi.nlm.nih.gov/books/NBK507823/. Updated August 14, 2023; Accessed February 22, 2024.

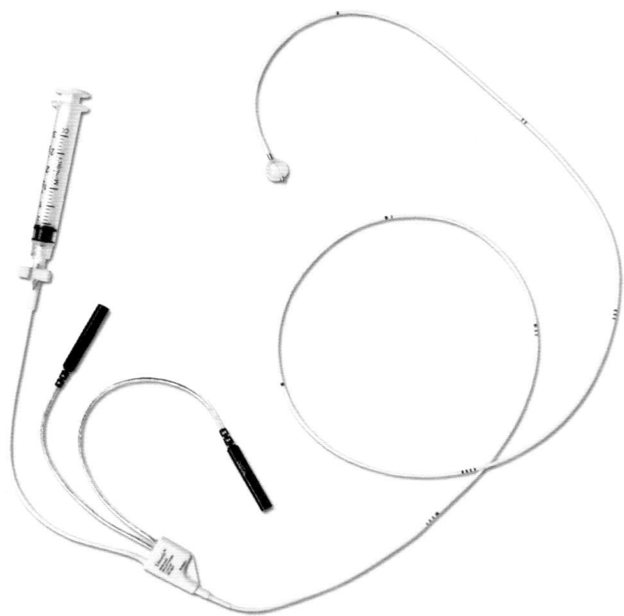

Fig. 8.53 Balloon-tipped bipolar lead wire for transvenous pacing. (From Wiegand DLM. *AACN Procedure Manual for Critical Care.* 6th ed. St. Louis, MO: Elsevier; 2011.)

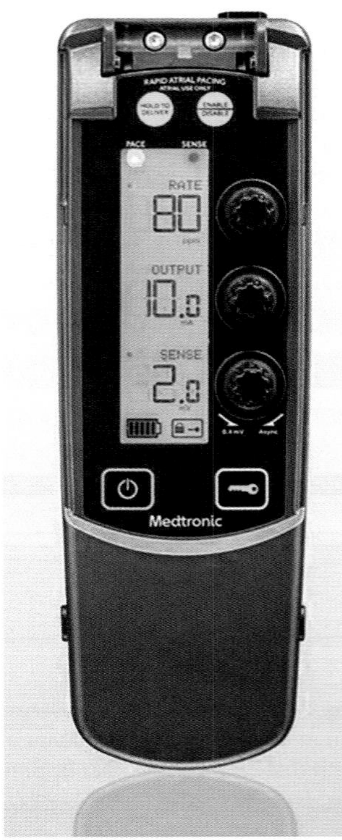

Fig. 8.54 Single-chamber temporary pulse generator. (Reproduced with permission from Medtronic Inc., Minneapolis, MN. 2022.)

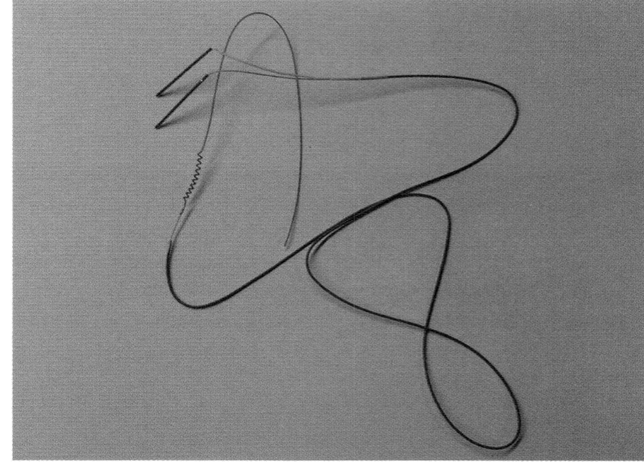

Fig. 8.55 Epicardial wires. (From Johnson, K.L. AACN Procedure Manual for Progressive and Critical Care, 8th edition. St. Louis, MO, Elsevier)

Permanent Pacemakers. Permanent pacemakers have electrode wires that are typically placed transvenously through the cephalic or subclavian vein into the heart chambers (Fig. 8.57). The leads are attached to the pulse generator, placed in a surgically created pocket just below the left clavicle.[6] Pacemakers may be used to stimulate the atrium, ventricle, or both chambers (dual-chamber pacemakers). Atrial pacing is used to mimic normal conduction and to produce atrial contraction, thus providing atrial kick. Ventricular pacing stimulates ventricular depolarization and is commonly used in emergency situations or when pacing is required infrequently. Dual-chamber pacing allows for stimulation of both atria and ventricles as needed to synchronize the chambers and mimic the normal cardiac cycle.

Permanent pacemakers may be programmed in a variety of ways, and a standardized code is used to determine the pacing mode that is programmed.[6] The North American Society of Pacing and Electrophysiology and the British Pacing and Electrophysiology Group have revised the standardized generic code for pacemakers (Table 8.2). It is important to know the programming information for the pacemaker to assess proper functioning on the rhythm strip.

Terms for Pacemaker Function

Other terms used in describing pacemaker function are rate, mode, electrical output, sensitivity, sense-pace indicator, and AV interval.

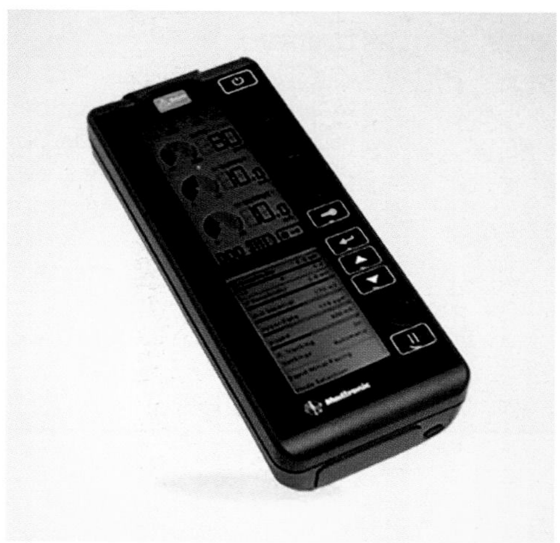

Fig. 8.56 Dual-chamber temporary pulse generator. (Reproduced with permission from Medtronic Inc., Minneapolis, MN. 2022.)

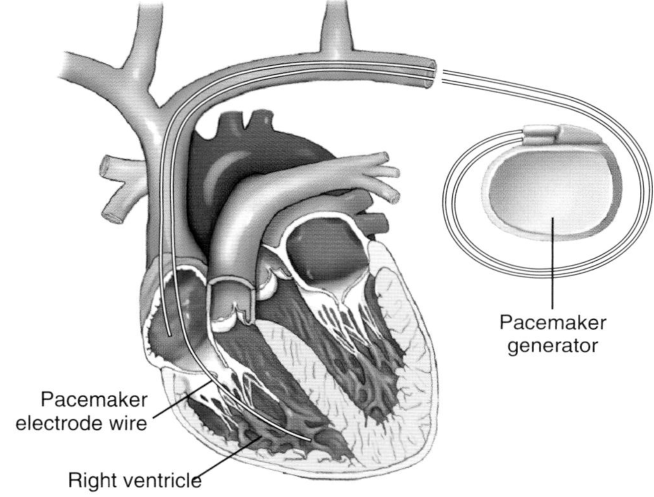

Fig. 8.57 Permanent dual-chamber (atrioventricular) pacemaker. (From Wesley K. *Huszar's ECG and 12-Lead Interpretation*. 6th ed. St. Louis, MO: Elsevier; 2022.)

Rate. The rate control determines the number of impulses delivered per minute to the atrium, the ventricle, or both. The rate is set to produce effective cardiac output and to reduce symptoms.

Mode. Pacemakers can be operated in a *demand* mode or *fixed rate (asynchronous)* mode. The demand mode paces the heart when no intrinsic or native beat is sensed. For example, if the rate control is set at 60 beats/min, the pacemaker will only pace if the patient's heart rate drops to less than 60 beats/min. The fixed rate mode paces the heart at a set rate, independent of any activity the patient's heart generates. The fixed rate mode may compete with the patient's own rhythm and deliver an impulse on the T wave (R-on-T), with the potential for producing VT or ventricular fibrillation. The demand mode is safer and is the mode of choice.

Electrical Output. The electrical output is the amount of electrical energy needed to stimulate depolarization. The output is measured in *milliamperes* (mA) and varies depending on the type of pacing. Transcutaneous pacing requires higher milliamperes than transvenous or epicardial pacing because the electrical energy must be delivered through the chest wall.

Sensitivity. The sensitivity is the ability of the pacemaker to recognize the body's intrinsic or native electrical activity. It is measured in *millivolts* (mV). Some temporary pacemakers have a sense-pace indicator. If the generator detects the patient's own beat, the "sense" indicator lights. When the generator delivers a paced beat, the "pace" light comes on. Temporary pacemakers have dials or keypads for adjusting sensitivity.

Atrioventricular Interval. The AV interval indicator is used to determine the interval between atrial and ventricular stimulation. It is used only in dual-chamber pacemakers.

Pacemaker Rhythms

Pacemaker rhythms are usually easy to identify on the cardiac monitor or rhythm strip. The electrical stimulation is noted by an electrical artifact called the *pacer spike*. If the atrium is paced, the spike appears before the P wave (Fig. 8.58). If the

TABLE 8.2 The NASPE/BPEG Generic (NBG) Pacemaker Code

Position:	I	II	III	IV	V
Category:	Chamber(s) Paced	Chamber(s) Sensed	Response to Sensing	Rate Modulation	Multisite Pacing
	O = None	**O** = None	**O** = None	**O** = None	**O** = None
	A = Atrium	**A** = Atrium	**T** = Triggered	**R** = Rate modulation	**A** = Atrium
	V = Ventricle	**V** = Ventricle	**I** = Inhibited		**V** = Ventricle
	D = Dual (A+V)	**D** = Dual (A+V)	**D** = Dual (T+I)		**D** = Dual (A+V)
Manufacturer's Designation:	**S** = Single (A or V)	**S** = Single (A or V)			

BPEG, British Pacing and Electrophysiology Group (currently known as the Heart Rhythm Society); *NASPE*, North American Society of Pacing and Electrophysiology.
From Bernstein AD, Daubert J-C, Fletcher RD, et al. The revised NASPE/BPEG generic code for antibradycardia, adaptive-rate, and multisite pacing. *J Pacing Clin Electrophysiol*. 2002;25:260-264.

ventricle is paced, the spike appears before the QRS complex (Fig. 8.59). If both the atrium and the ventricle are paced, spikes are noted before both the P wave and the QRS complex (Fig. 8.60). The heart rate is carefully assessed on the rhythm strip. The heart rate should not be lower than the rate set on the pacemaker. The pacemaker spike is usually followed by a larger-than-normal P wave in atrial pacing or a widened QRS complex in ventricular pacing. Sometimes, the P wave is not seen even though an atrial pacer spike is present. Because the heart is paced in an artificial or abnormal fashion, the path of depolarization is altered, resulting in waveforms and intervals that are also altered.

CHECK YOUR UNDERSTANDING

4. The patient calls for help stating she is not feeling well. When you inquire, the patient reports feeling weak, hot, sweaty, and like she may pass out. The patient's pulse is slow, approximately 30 beats/minute. You notice the cardiac monitor shows a rhythm in which you are unable to see a relationship between the P waves and the QRS complexes. You understand that your priority is to:
   A. Anticipate a provider order for an antiarrhythmic medication.
   B. Call a code and start cardiopulmonary resuscitation.
   C. Request a sitter for the patient as the patient may be considered a fall risk.
   D. Anticipate transcutaneous temporary pacing.

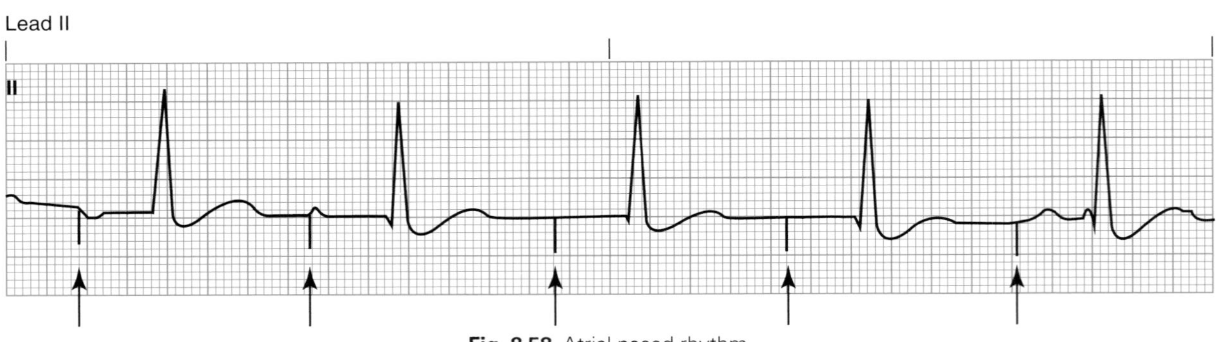

Fig. 8.58 Atrial paced rhythm.

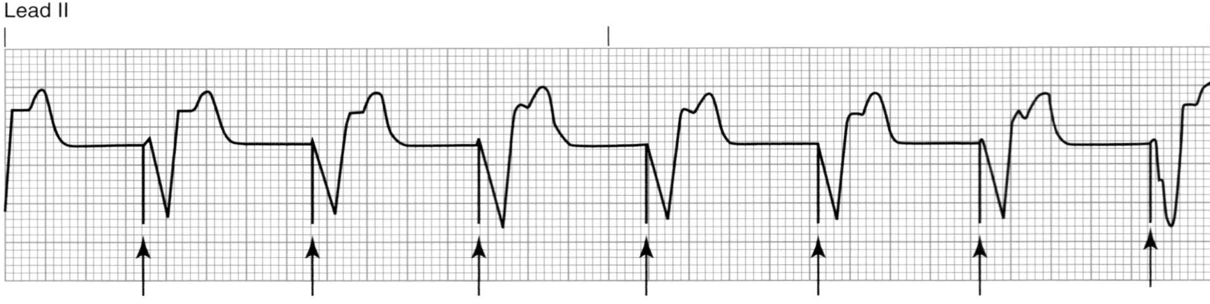

Fig. 8.59 Ventricular paced rhythm.

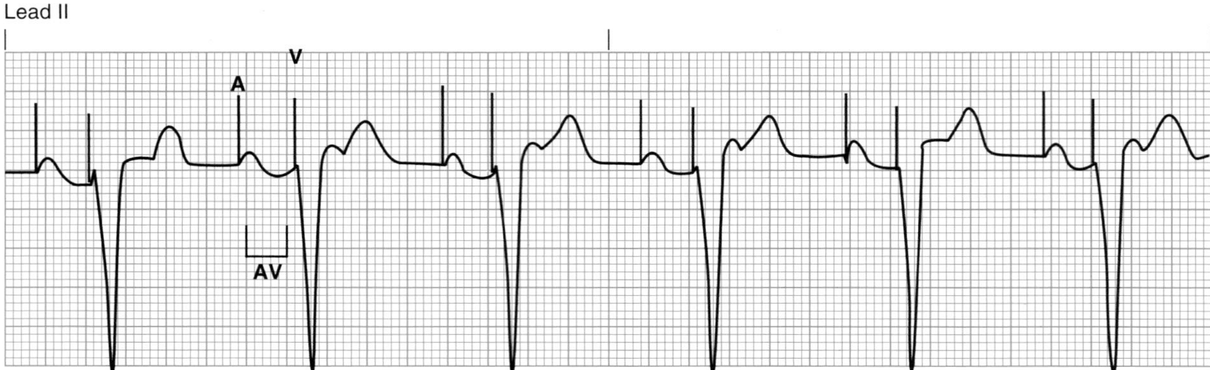

Fig. 8.60 Dual-chamber (atrioventricular) paced rhythm. *A,* Atrial pacer spike; *AV,* atrioventricular pacer interval; *V,* ventricular pacer spike.

Pacemaker Malfunction

Three primary problems can occur with a pacemaker. These problems include failure to pace (also called *failure to fire*), failure to capture, and failure to sense. If troubleshooting does not resolve pacemaker malfunction, emergency transcutaneous pacing may be needed to ensure an adequate cardiac output.

Failure to Pace. *Failure to pace* or *failure to fire* occurs when the pacemaker fails to initiate an electrical stimulus when it should fire. The problem is noted by absence of pacer spikes on the rhythm strip. Causes of failure to pace include battery or pulse generator failure, fracture or displacement of a pacemaker wire, or loose connections (Fig. 8.61).

Failure to Capture. When the pacemaker generates an electrical impulse (pacer spike) and no depolarization is noted, it is described as *failure to capture*. On the ECG, a pacer spike is noted, but it is not followed by a P wave (atrial pacemaker) or a QRS complex (ventricular pacemaker) (Fig. 8.62). Common causes of failure to capture include output (mA) set too low or displacement of the pacing lead wire from the myocardium (transvenous or epicardial leads). Other causes of failure to capture include battery failure, fracture of the pacemaker wire, or increased pacing threshold as a result of medication or electrolyte imbalance. Adjusting the output if the patient has a temporary pacemaker and placing the patient on their left side are nursing interventions to treat failure to capture. Turning the patient onto the left side facilitates contact of a transvenous pacing wire with the endocardium and septum.

Failure to Sense. When the pacemaker does not sense the patient's own cardiac rhythm and initiates an electrical impulse, it is called *failure to sense*. Failure to sense manifests as pacer spikes that fall too closely to the patient's own rhythm, earlier than the programmed rate (Fig. 8.63). The most common cause is displacement of the pacemaker electrode wire. Turning the patient to the left side and adjusting the sensitivity (temporary pacemaker) are nursing interventions to use when failure to sense occurs.

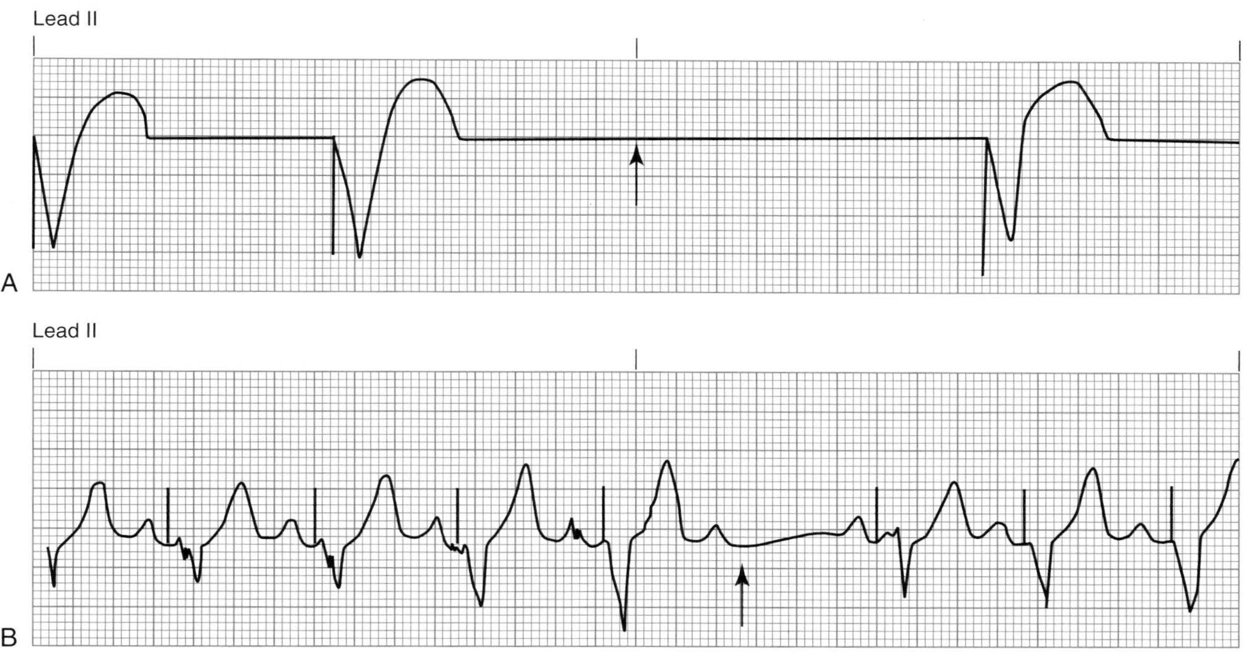

Fig. 8.61 Failure to pace or fire. A, *Arrow* indicates failure to pace from a ventricular pacemaker. B, *Arrow* indicates failure to pace from an atrial pacemaker.

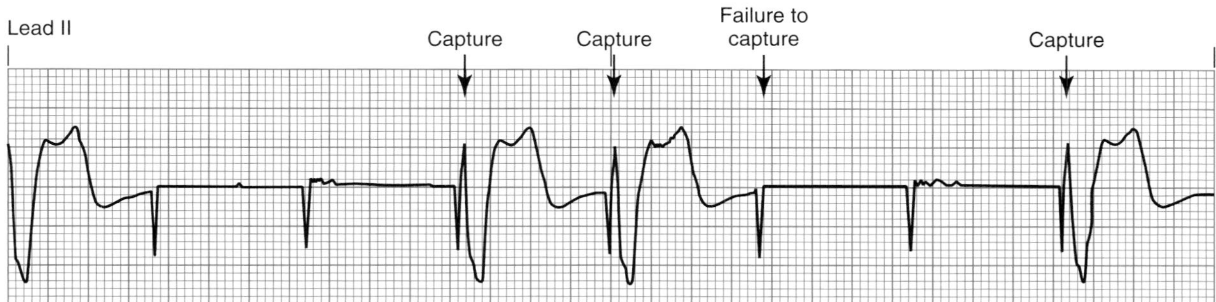

Fig. 8.62 Failure to capture: ventricular pacemaker.

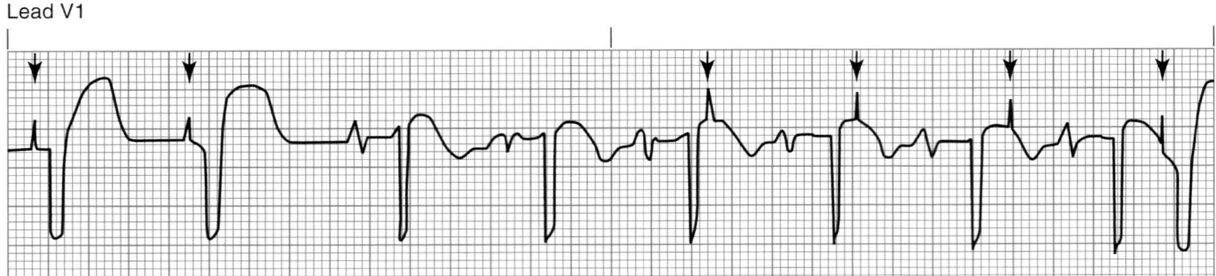

Fig. 8.63 Failure to sense. *Arrows* represent pacer spikes.

CLINICAL JUDGMENT ACTIVITY

How would you explain why tachycardia may lead to heart failure?

Other Devices With Pacemaker Capabilities

Implantable cardioverter-defibrillators (ICDs) have pacemaker capabilities.[6] The pacemaker feature of these devices is used to treat fast heart rhythms, such as VT, with antitachycardia pacing, as well as slow heart rhythms that may occur following defibrillation. Antitachycardia pacing is a short, fast burst of pacing impulses that attempt to terminate the tachycardia.

Biventricular pacemakers and ICDs have an additional electrode wire placed through the coronary sinus into the left ventricle. Additional pacing wires are in the atria and the ventricle. Pacing both ventricles simultaneously improves heart function in a certain number of patients with heart failure. Synchronous depolarization of both ventricles improves cardiac output and ejection fraction. Many patients with ICDs benefit from telemonitoring technologies.

CASE STUDY

Mr. P. is a 56-year-old male who was successfully extubated (endotracheal tube removed) 4 hours after coronary artery bypass graft surgery. However, 2 hours later, he complains of his heart racing, and it is determined that he has palpitations. The heart rate on the bedside monitor is 168 beats/min, blood pressure is 90/60 mm Hg, and respiratory rate is 26 breaths/min. The electrocardiogram (ECG) shows an irregularly irregular rhythm, a change from the sinus rhythm noted at the last assessment.

Questions

1. What are possible etiological factors of this dysrhythmia?
2. What data are you going to communicate to the provider?
3. What medications and orders do you anticipate from the provider?
4. Prioritize nursing actions and rationale for interventions.

KEY POINTS

- Critical care nurses interpret cardiac rhythms and dysrhythmias to ensure rapid analysis and appropriate treatment to improve patient safety and patient outcomes.
- The cardiac conduction cycle includes the SA node, the AV node, the bundle of His, and the Purkinje fibers. The SA node is the main pacemaker of the heart, with a rate of 60 to 100 beats/min. If the SA node fails to conduct an impulse, then the AV node will respond at a rate of 40-60 beats/min. If both the SA and AV nodes fail, then the His-Purkinje system can respond at a rate of 15 to 20 beats/min.
- The 12-lead ECG allows nurses to see 12 different views of the heart's electrical activity. ECGs provide important information of the cardiac conduction system and can show many cardiac abnormalities and dysrhythmias. Cardiac rhythm can also be viewed on a monitor at the patient's bedside.
- Interpretation of ECGs and cardiac rhythms include analysis of heart rate, heart rhythm, measurement of waveforms and intervals, assessment of morphological characteristics of waveforms, identification of the underlying rhythm and any dysrhythmias, and patient tolerance of the rhythm.
- Normal sinus rhythm is normal conduction of the impulse initiating from the SA node. These rhythms may be too fast (sinus tachycardia) or too slow (sinus bradycardia). Sinus arrhythmia is another dysrhythmia originating in the SA node that has alternating faster and slower heart rate depending on the respiratory cycle.
- Dysrhythmias may occur associated with atrial, AV, ventricular, and ectopic foci, which can result in patient symptoms requiring urgent and emergent interventions. Cardiac pacemakers are devices that deliver electrical current to the myocardium when the native heart rate is too slow or there is no conduction of an impulse. There are temporary and permanent pacemakers.

REFERENCES

1. Hannibal G. It started with Einthoven: The history of the ECG and cardiac monitoring. *AACN Adv Crit Care*. 2011;64:1–76.
2. American Heart Association (AHA). *2020 Handbook of Emergency Cardiovascular Care for Healthcare Providers*. Dallas, TX: American Heart Association; 2020.
3. American Association of Critical-Care Nurses. Practice alert: Accurate dysrhythmia monitoring in adults. *Crit Care Nurse*. 2016;36(6):e26–e34.
4. Sandau KE, Funk M, Auerbach A, et al. American Heart Association (AHA). Update to practice standards for electrocardiographic monitoring in hospital settings: a scientific statement from the American Heart Association. *Circulation*. 2017;136:e273–e344.
5. Panchal AR, Berg KM, Rios MD, et al. American Heart Association (AHA). American Heart Association focused update on advanced cardiovascular life support use of antiarrhythmic medications during and immediately after cardiac arrest. *Circulation*. 2018;138:e740–e749.
6. Kusumoto FM, Schoenfeld MH, Barrett C, Edgerton JR, Ellenbogen KA, Gold MR, et al. ACC/AHA/HRS guideline on the evaluation and management of patients with bradycardia and cardiac conduction delay: A report of the American College of Cardiology/American Heart Association Task Force on Clinical Practice Guidelines and the Heart Rhythm Society. *Heart Rhythm*. 2018:1–199.
7. January CT, Wann LS, Calkins H, et al. AHA/ACC/HRS focused update of the 2014 AHA/ACC/HRS guideline for the management of patients with atrial fibrillation: A report of the American College of Cardiology/American Heart Association Task Force on Clinical Practice Guidelines and the Heart Rhythm Society. *Circulation*. 2019;139:1–49.
8. Page R, Joglar J, Caldwell M, et al. 2015 ACC/AHA/HRS Guideline for the Management of Adult Patients With Supraventricular Tachycardia. *J Am Coll Cardiol*. 2016;67(13):e27–e115.
9. Al-Khatib S, Stevenson W, Ackerman M, et al. 2017 AHA/ACC/HRS Guideline for Management of Patients With Ventricular Arrhythmias and the Prevention of Sudden Cardiac Death. *J Am Coll Cardiol*. 2018;72(14):e91–e220.

9

Hemodynamic Monitoring

Paul Anthony Thurman, PhD, RN, ACNPC, CCNS, CCRN

INTRODUCTION

A thorough understanding of hemodynamic monitoring is essential to care for the critically ill patient. The goal of hemodynamic monitoring is to accurately assess the patient and provide therapies to optimize oxygen delivery and tissue perfusion to meet metabolic demand. This can be accomplished by monitoring the dynamic physiological relationship between many variables to determine whether oxygen delivery is adequate to meet the oxygen demands of the tissues and organs. Ensuring that the data are accurate and analyzed correctly to guide therapy and assess the outcome of interventions is a complex skill. This chapter reviews the basics of cardiovascular anatomy and physiology, the fundamentals of hemodynamic monitoring, and various modalities available to the clinician to assess and manage hemodynamic status.

REVIEW OF ANATOMY AND PHYSIOLOGY

Cardiovascular System

The cardiovascular system is a closed network of arteries, capillaries, and veins through which blood, oxygen, hormones, and nutrients are delivered to the tissues by the pumping action of the heart (Fig. 9.1). Metabolic wastes are removed from the circulating blood via the liver and kidneys. The major components of the cardiovascular system are described in the following sections.

Heart. The heart is a four-chambered organ that weighs approximately one pound and lies obliquely in the thoracic cavity. The heart is responsible for pumping oxygenated blood forward through the arterial vasculature and receiving deoxygenated blood via the venous vasculature. Four one-way valves regulate blood flow through the heart. Two atrioventricular (AV) valves (tricuspid and mitral) open during ventricular diastole, allowing blood to flow from the atria into the ventricles. At end-diastole, the atria contract and force the remaining atrial blood into the ventricles—this is commonly referred to as the "atrial kick" and contributes up to 20% of the cardiac output (CO).[1] As the ventricles begin to contract in systole, the AV valves close and the semilunar valves (pulmonic and aortic) open, allowing blood to flow into the pulmonary and systemic vasculature. At the end of ventricular systole, the semilunar valves close, and the cycle begins again (Fig. 9.2).

Arteries. Arteries are the tough, elastic vessels that carry blood away from the heart. Arteries consist of three layers: the adventitia, the media, and the intima. The adventitia is composed chiefly of longitudinally arranged collagen fibers, which make up the tough outer lining. The media consists of concentrically arranged smooth muscle. The intima consists of endothelial connective tissue that is continuous with that of the heart. The endothelial lining of the vessel is slick and smooth, allowing blood to flow freely. The elasticity of the vessels allows them to expand to accommodate volumetric changes that result with the contraction and relaxation of the heart. When the artery diameter is less than 0.5 mm, it is called an arteriole. The arterial system is a high-pressure, low-volume, high-resistance circuit responsible for delivering oxygen and nutrient-rich blood to the capillary system. Arteries have the ability to dilate or constrict in response to metabolic demand.

Capillaries. The capillaries are exchange vessels, composed of a network of low-pressure, thin-walled microscopic vessels allowing for easy passage of hormones, nutrients, and oxygen to the target tissues. They also receive metabolic wastes and carbon dioxide from the tissues and begin the process of returning deoxygenated blood to the venous portion of the cardiovascular system.

Veins. Compared with the arteries, veins are thin-walled, less elastic, fibrous, and larger in diameter; they are known as high-capacity, low-resistance vessels. The majority of the circulating blood volume is in the venous system. Veins of the extremities contain valves to assist with maintaining a one-way flow of deoxygenated blood returning to the heart. Eventually, the veins connect to larger vessels and become the superior and inferior vena cava, which empties into the right atrium. The blood flow through the cardiac veins empties directly into the right atrium through the coronary sinus. The venous system has the ability to respond to metabolic needs by vasodilation or vasoconstriction, thereby increasing or decreasing venous return. Venous return is the flow of blood back to the heart. Approximately 70% of the circulating blood volume is located in the venous system at

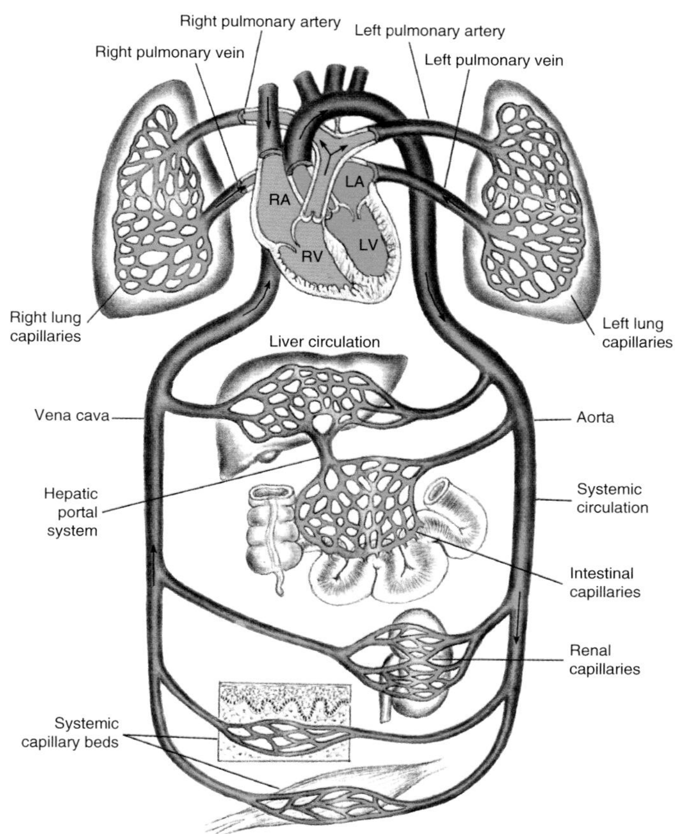

Fig. 9.1 Diagram of the cardiovascular system. *LA,* Left atrium; *LV,* left ventricle; *RA,* right atrium; *RV,* right ventricle. (From Patton K, Thibodeau S, eds. *Anthony's Textbook of Anatomy and Physiology.* 20th ed. St. Louis, MO: Elsevier; 2013.)

any given time. Venous return is affected by muscle contraction, breathing, venous compliance, and gravity.

Blood. Blood accounts for about 7% of our body weight and is estimated to total approximately 5 L. The fluid component, or plasma, makes up approximately 60% of the blood volume. The remaining 40% consists of the cellular components: erythrocytes (red blood cells), leukocytes (white blood cells), and platelets.[2,3] The red blood cell component of blood is essential for oxygen delivery to the tissues. A reduction in oxygen delivery (supply) or an increase in oxygen consumption (demand) directly affects the hemodynamic responses of the body.

Principles of Physics

According to Poiseuille's law, the rate of fluid flow through a vessel is determined by the pressure difference between the two ends of the vessel and the resistance within the lumen.[3] For any fluid to flow within a circuit, a difference in pressures within the circuit must exist. In the cardiovascular system, the driving pressure is generated by the contractile force of the heart. There is a continuous drop in pressure from the left ventricle to the tissues and a further reduction in pressure from the tissue bed to the right atrium. Without these pressure gradients, no flow occurs.

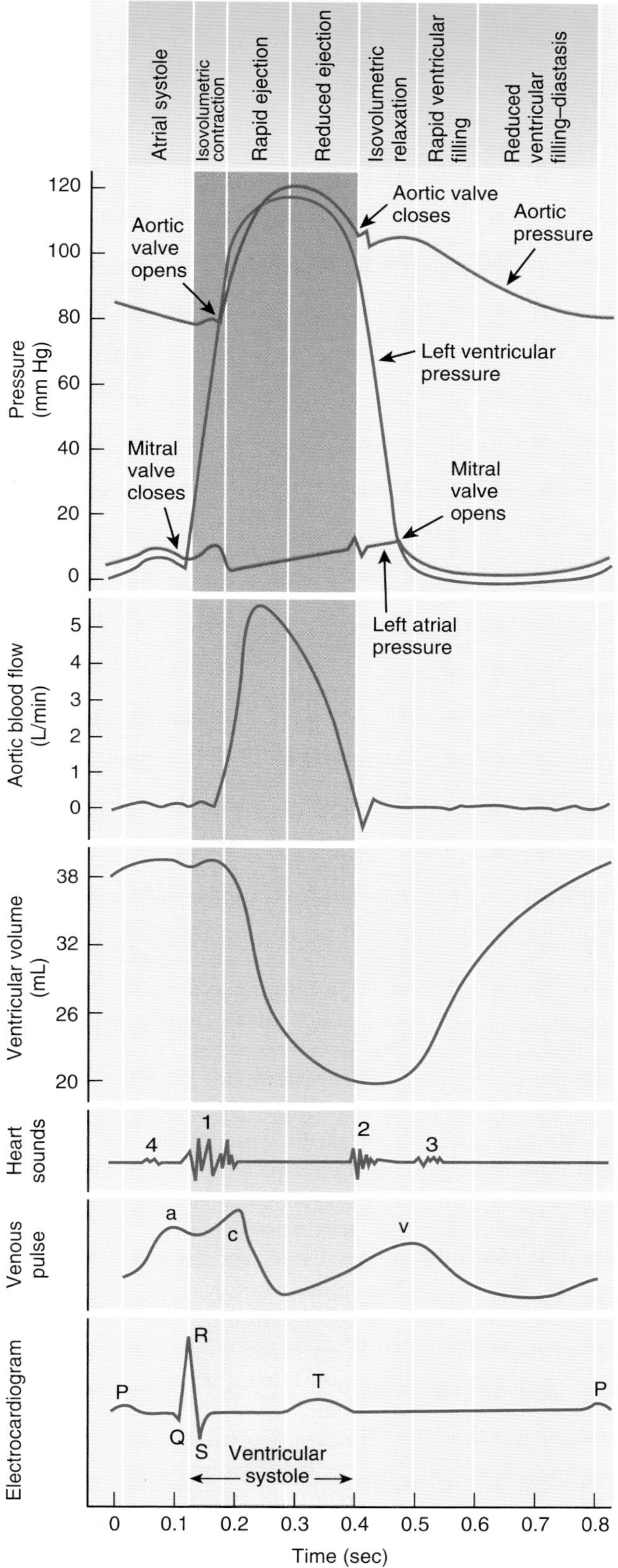

Fig. 9.2 Cardiac cycle. (From Rogers J. *McCance and Huether's Pathophysiology: The Biologic Basis for Disease in Adults and Children.* 9th ed. St. Louis, MO: Elsevier; 2023)

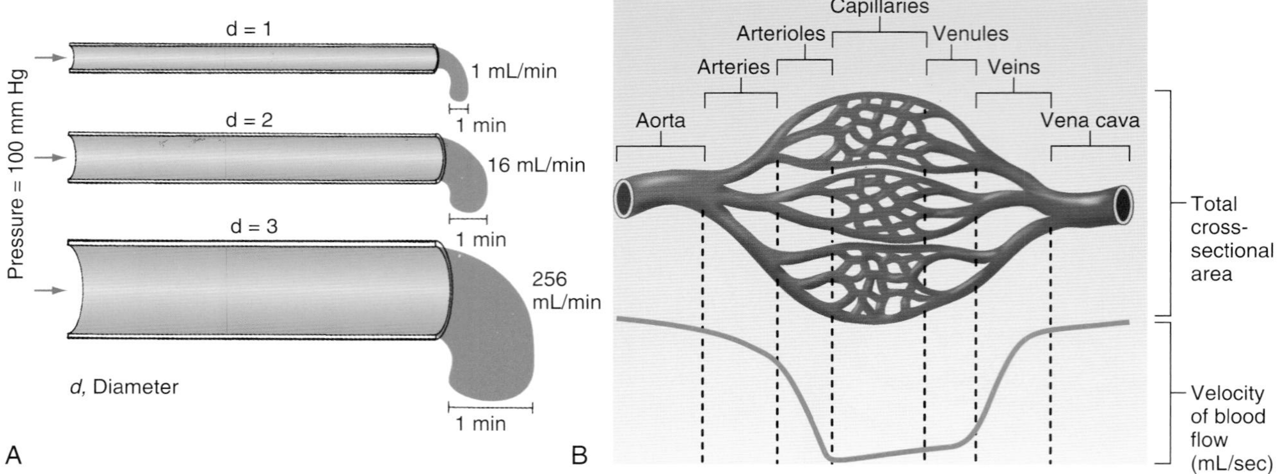

Fig. 9.3 Relationship among vessel diameter, flow, and resistance. **A**, Effect of lumen diameter on flow through vessel. **B**, Blood flows with great speed in the large arteries. However, branching of arterial vessels increases the total cross-sectional areas of the arterioles and capillaries, thus reducing the flow rate. (**A**, From McCance KL, Huether S, eds. *Pathophysiology: The Biologic Basis for Disease in Adults and Children.* 7th ed. St. Louis, MO: Elsevier; 2015; **B**, From Patton KT. *Anatomy and Physiology.* 11th ed. St. Louis, MO: Elsevier; 2022.)

Resistance is a measure of the ease with which the fluid flows through the lumen of a vessel. It is essentially a measure of friction, which depends on viscosity of the fluid and the radius and length of the vessel. A vessel with a small diameter has a greater resistance than one with a larger diameter (Fig. 9.3). Longer vessels have greater resistance to the flow of fluid within the vessel. Increased viscosity of a fluid results in increased friction within the fluid; rate of flow is inversely proportional to the fluid viscosity.[3] Consider how much easier it is to drink water through a straw than it is to drink a milkshake (viscosity). How much more difficult is it to drink a milkshake through a long, thin straw than through a wide, shorter straw (resistance)?

Highly compliant systems have low resistance; therefore, if resistance increases, compliance decreases. For example, an atherosclerotic vessel with narrowing of the intima has a reduced capacitance and compliance, leading to increased resistance and hypertension.

The body's response to metabolic demands alters the flow of blood to and from the target tissues. In response to increased metabolic demands, the circulatory system increases the volume of blood flow to the target tissues by increasing the diameter of the vessel (vasodilation), resulting in reduced resistance within the vessel.

Another determinant of flow rate is the degree of turbulence within a vessel. The rate of fluid movement in laminar flow is greater than the rate in turbulent flow.[3] A vessel lining that has excess plaque accumulation or calcification results in more turbulence, reduced flow, and reduced tissue perfusion.

Components of Cardiac Output

Cardiac output (CO) is determined by multiplying heart rate by stroke volume (SV) (Fig. 9.4). SV is the amount of blood ejected by the heart with each beat. SV is affected by preload, afterload, and contractility. Understanding hemodynamics requires a working knowledge of normal intracardiac pressures, as each chamber of the heart has a unique pressure (Fig. 9.5). In addition, a familiarity with the cardiac cycle (Fig. 9.2) assists in understanding hemodynamic concepts. Relevant concepts are defined next.

Heart rate is a major determinant of CO. Slow heart rates can result in a decreased CO, particularly if the body cannot compensate with an increase in SV. Fast heart rates can also result in decreased CO because the ventricles have less diastolic time and can result in poor ventricular filling, decreasing SV.[1] In addition, the coronary arteries fill during diastole. Fast heart rates can result in decreased coronary artery filling and subsequently in decreased coronary tissue perfusion.

Determinants of Stroke Volume. *Preload* is the degree of ventricular stretch before the next contraction. The degree of stretch is directly affected by the amount of blood present in the ventricles at end-diastole. In hemodynamic monitoring, preload is quantified by measuring ventricular end-diastolic pressures. Based on the Frank-Starling mechanism, when ventricular fibers are at maximal stretch, maximal CO results. Another way of explaining the mechanism is that, within physiological limits, the heart pumps all of the blood that is returned by the venous system.[4] Too much end-diastolic volume in the right ventricle can result in congestion of the systemic vasculature, and too much end-diastolic volume in the left ventricle can cause fluid to back up into the pulmonary vasculature. Too little blood at end-diastolic volume results in a reduction in CO. Optimizing preload or ventricular filling is the goal of many therapeutic interventions in critical care.

Afterload is the amount of resistance the ventricles must overcome to deliver the SV into the receiving vasculature. The left ventricle during systole must create the force necessary to open the aortic valve and overcome the resistance in the systemic

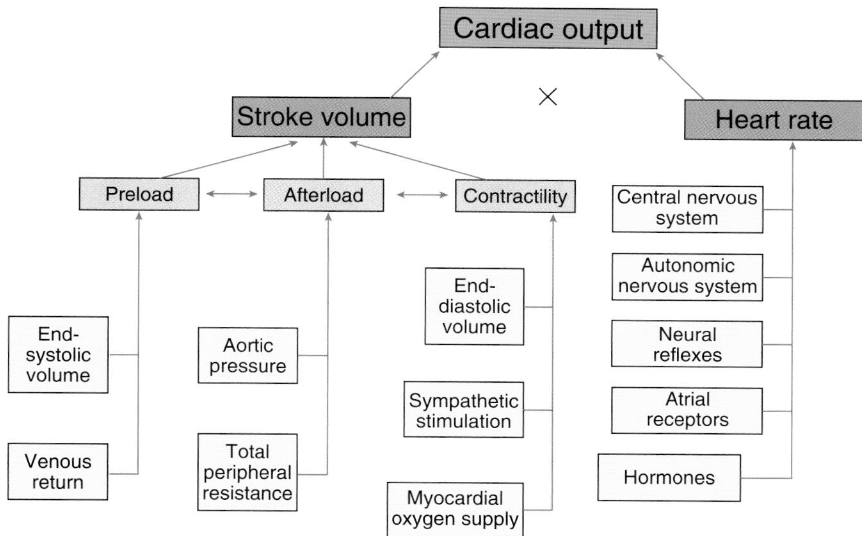

Fig. 9.4 Cardiac output components. Cardiac output is determined by heart rate and stroke volume. (From Rogers J. *McCance and Huether's Pathophysiology: The Biologic Basis for Disease in Adults and Children.* 9th ed. St. Louis, MO: Elsevier; 2023.)

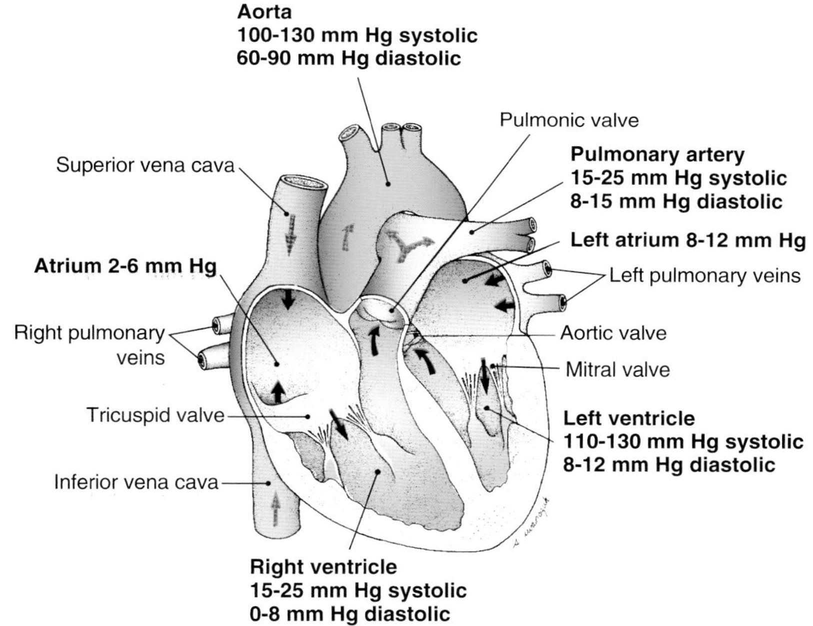

Fig. 9.5 Normal blood flow through the heart and intrachamber pressures; *arrows* indicate the normal direction of blood flow. This schematic representation of the heart shows all four chambers and valves visible in the anterior view to facilitate conceptualization of blood flow. (From Ralston SH, Penman ID, Strachan MWJ, Hobson RP. *Davidson's Principles and Practice of Medicine.* 23rd ed. Edinburgh, Scotland: Elsevier; 2018.)

circulation. The right ventricle must create enough force to open the pulmonic valve and overcome the resistance in the pulmonary circulation. Arterial systemic tone, blood viscosity, flow patterns (laminar versus turbulent), and valve competency all affect the degree of afterload the ventricle must overcome.

Contractility is the strength of myocardial muscle fiber shortening during the systolic phase of the cardiac cycle. It is the force with which the heart propels the SV forward into the vasculature. The preload influences contractility, because optimizing the preload ensures maximal stretch of the myocardial fibers according to the Frank-Starling law. Contractility is not directly measured; however, it can be expressed by the calculated values of right or left ventricular stroke work index.

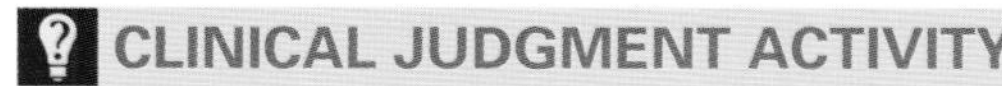

CLINICAL JUDGMENT ACTIVITY

How is stroke volume related to cardiac output?

Regulation of Cardiovascular Function

Cardiovascular anatomy and physiology are described in greater depth in Chapter 13, Cardiovascular Alterations. Function changes with aging (see Lifespan Considerations box).[5-6] The cardiovascular system is controlled through neurohormonal interactions involving the autonomic nervous system, hypothalamus, pituitary gland, adrenal glands, and kidneys. The autonomic nervous system has two branches: the sympathetic and the parasympathetic. Sympathetic nervous system (SNS) activity enhances myocardial performance by shortening the conduction time through the AV node, enhancing rhythmicity of the AV pacemaker cells, and increasing myocardial contractility. Parasympathetic nervous system (PNS) activity via the vagus nerves results in blocking of cardiac action potentials initiated by the sinus node in the atria, thus decreasing heart rate. The kidneys and adrenal glands regulate both vasomotor tone and sodium through the renin angiotensin aldosterone system (RAAS).

The cardiovascular system is also regulated by hormonal influences to maintain adequate oxygen delivery to meet the demands of the tissues. Norepinephrine acts on beta-1 receptors to increase heart rate and myocardial contractility as well as alpha-1 receptors, resulting in vasoconstriction. Epinephrine is a beta-1 and 2 adrenergic stimulator causing increased heart rate and smooth muscle (e.g., bronchioles, uterus, vasculature) relaxation, resulting in vasodilation of arterioles, particularly in skeletal muscle. Higher amounts of epinephrine produced stimulate the alpha-adrenergic receptors located in the walls of the arteriole, resulting in vasoconstriction and shunting blood to vital organs.

The right atrium secretes atrial natriuretic peptides (ANPs), and the ventricular myocardium secretes brain natriuretic peptides (BNPs) in response to stretch from the heart chambers. ANPs and BNPs cause vasodilation and diuresis and inhibit the sympathetic response and the RAAS in an attempt to decrease circulating blood volume and stress on the myocardium.

LIFESPAN CONSIDERATIONS

Older Adults

- Elasticity and compliance of the vessel walls decrease, causing the pressure within the arterial system to increase, resulting in systemic hypertension.
- The increase in impedance to the left ventricular ejection often leads to left ventricular hypertrophy. The left ventricle stiffens, impairing diastolic filling, leading to diastolic heart failure.
- The number and sensitivity of beta-adrenergic receptors in the sinoatrial node decrease with age, resulting in a decreased intrinsic and maximal heart rate.
- Fibrosis of the cardiac structures and conduction system can lead to heart block and valvular dysfunction.

Pregnant People

- Blood volume, heart rate, and stroke volume increase gradually throughout pregnancy.
- Cardiac output increases by 30%-50% by the middle of the third trimester.
- While normally systolic and diastolic blood pressures drop during pregnancy, hypertension can occur due to multiple causes and is closely monitored. Acute-onset, severe hypertension (systolic blood pressure >160 mm Hg or diastolic blood pressure >110 mm Hg) requires emergent treatment. It is most commonly caused by exacerbation of primary hypertension but can also be caused by drug or stimulant use, alcohol withdrawal, or adrenal tumors.

The RAAS is activated in the kidney in response to low blood pressure, low intravascular volume, or low sodium levels. Renin is released by the kidney and converts to angiotensin I. Angiotensin I converts to angiotensin II in the lungs. Angiotensin II is a potent vasoconstrictor, resulting in systemic arterial vasoconstriction in an attempt to increase blood pressure. Angiotensin II also activates aldosterone from the adrenal glands, resulting in retention of sodium and water at the distal convoluted tubule of the kidney in an attempt to increase blood pressure.

In addition to the systemic responses of the RAAS and the autonomic nervous system, the endothelium releases vasoactive substances that may result in vasoconstriction (i.e., endothelin-1, serotonin, and thromboxane A2) or vasodilation (i.e., nitric oxide, prostacyclin, bradykinin, and kallidin).[7]

Blood flow through the cardiovascular system to meet tissue demands is regulated globally, affecting the whole body and locally affecting specific tissue capillary systems. Global control of blood flow is regulated through changes in blood volume, changes in heart rate and contractility, and vascular resistance. Local control of blood flow occurs in the capillary bed and is regulated through the endothelium.

OVERVIEW OF HEMODYNAMIC MONITORING MODALITIES

Invasive and noninvasive hemodynamic monitoring is a major part of a comprehensive assessment of the critically ill patient. The goal in evaluating hemodynamic data is to determine if oxygen supply is meeting oxygen demands. The hemodynamic assessment aids in surveillance and early detection of oxygen imbalance, quantifying the severity of disease, and serves as a guide for assessing and adjusting therapies. Traditional hemodynamic monitoring uses specific end points to guide therapies (e.g., mean arterial pressure [MAP], CO, central venous pressure [CVP], pulmonary artery occlusion pressure [PAOP], urine output, pH, and lactate). Newer modalities, such as bedside echocardiography, mixed venous oxygen saturation (SvO_2) monitoring, central venous oxygen saturation ($ScvO_2$), and changes in the arterial pressure waveform, continually measure ever-changing bodily responses. Normal hemodynamic values are described in Table 9.1; however, these values only provide a guideline to assist in interpretation of assessment findings. The primary goal of hemodynamic monitoring is to assess and trend adequacy of tissue oxygenation and perfusion rather than to compare a patient's values to so-called "normal" parameters.

Noninvasive Monitoring

Some critically ill patients can be adequately assessed and managed with noninvasive hemodynamic monitoring. Historically, noninvasive technologies were limited to noninvasive blood pressure (NIBP) measurement, assessment of jugular venous pressure, and frequent assessments of laboratory tests, such as lactate. More recently, newer technologies such as bioimpedance analysis (BIA), applanation tonometry (AT), and the volume clamp method (VCM) are available to provide continuous noninvasive hemodynamic measures; however, accurate

TABLE 9.1 Normal Hemodynamic Values[a]

Hemodynamic Parameter	Significance	Normal Range
Cardiac output (CO)	Amount of blood pumped out by a ventricle every minute	4-8 L/min
Cardiac index (CI)	CO individualized to patient body surface area (BSA; size)	2.5-4.2 L/min/m^2
Central venous pressure (CVP)	Pressure created by volume of blood in right heart at end-diastole; used to guide assessment of fluid balance and responsiveness to fluid administration	2-6 mm Hg
Right atrial pressure (RAP)	Used interchangeably with CVP; pressure created by volume of blood in right heart at end-diastole; measured with a pulmonary artery catheter	2-6 mm Hg
Left atrial pressure (LAP)	Pressure created by volume of blood in left heart at end-diastole	8-12 mm Hg
Pulmonary artery occlusion pressure (PAOP)	Pressure created by volume of blood in left heart at end-diastole	8-12 mm Hg
Pulmonary artery pressure (PAP) (pulmonary artery systole [PAS] and pulmonary artery diastole [PAD])	Pulsatile pressure in the pulmonary artery	PAS 15-25 mm Hg PAD 8-15 mm Hg
Stroke volume (SV)	Amount of blood ejected from the ventricle with each contraction	60-130 mL/beat
Stroke index (SI)	SV individualized to BSA	30-65 mL/beat/m^2
Systemic vascular resistance (SVR)	Resistance that the left ventricle must overcome to open the aortic valve and eject a volume of blood into the systemic circulation; generally, as SVR increases, CO falls $\frac{MAP - CVP}{CO} \times 80$	770-1500 dynes/sec/cm^{-5}
Systemic vascular resistance index (SVRI)	SVR individualized to BSA	1680-2580 dynes/sec/cm^{-5}/m^2
Pulmonary vascular resistance (PVR)	Resistance that the right ventricle must overcome to open the pulmonic valve and eject a volume of blood in the pulmonary vasculature $\frac{MPAP - PAOP}{CO} \times 80$	<250 dynes/sec/cm^{-5}
Pulmonary vascular resistance index (PVRI)	PVR individualized to BSA	255-285 dynes/sec/cm^{-5}/m^2
Right cardiac work index (RCWI)	Amount of work the right ventricle performs each minute when ejecting blood; increases or decreases depending on changes in volume or pressure; used as a measure of contractility	0.54-0.66 kg-m/m^2
Right ventricular stroke work index (RVSWI)	Amount of work the right ventricle performs with each heartbeat; increases or decreases depending on changes in SV and PAP mean; used as a measure of contractility	7.9-9.7 g-m/beat/m^2
Left cardiac work index (LCWI)	Amount of work the left ventricle performs each minute when ejecting blood; increases or decreases depending on changes in CO and mean arterial pressure (MAP); used as a measure of contractility	3.4-4.2 kg-m/m^2
Left ventricular stroke work index (LVSWI)	Amount of work the left ventricle performs with each heartbeat; increases or decreases depending on changes in SV and MAP; used as a measure of contractility	50-62 g-m/beat/m^2
Right ventricular end-diastolic volume (RVEDV) and right ventricular end-diastolic pressure (RVEDP)	Measures right ventricular preload	0-8 mm Hg (RVEDP)
Left ventricular end-diastolic volume (LVEDV) and left ventricular end-diastolic pressure (LVEDP)	Measures left ventricular preload	4-12 mm Hg (LVEDP)
Mixed venous oxygen saturation (SvO_2)	Provides an assessment of balance between oxygen supply and demand. Measured in the pulmonary artery. Higher values indicate increased O_2 supply, decreased O_2 demand, or the inability to extract oxygen from blood; lower values indicate decreased O_2 supply from low hemoglobin, low CO, low SaO_2, and/or increased O_2 consumption	60%-75%
Central venous oxygen saturation ($ScvO_2$)	Similar to SvO_2 but measured in the distal portion of a central venous catheter proximal to the right atrium and before the point where the cardiac sinus returns deoxygenated blood from the myocardium, thus the reason for the discrepancy between SvO_2 and $ScvO_2$ normal ranges	65%-85%

[a]Note that normal values vary by various references.

readings are not guaranteed in low-flow states, limiting their use in shock.[8-10]

Noninvasive Blood Pressure. For decades, clinicians have used NIBP monitoring to assess patients. Typically, NIBP is used for routine examinations and monitoring. Benefits of NIBP monitoring are ease of use, quick availability, and minimal patient complications. To obtain accurate and reliable readings, an understanding of the science of pressure measurement is required. It is vitally important to select an appropriate cuff size (i.e., cuff bladder encircles 80% of the extremity). If the cuff size is too small for the patient, the pressures recorded will be falsely elevated; if the cuff size is too large, the resulting pressures will be falsely low. In addition, positioning the patient's arm at the level of the heart for measurements is also important for accurate readings.

Measurement of blood pressure may be manual or automated. Manual measurement involves a cuff and stethoscope while listening for the beginning (systolic) and ending (diastolic) of Korotkoff sounds. Measurements from automated devices use the oscillometric technique in which the amplitude of the oscillations in the lateral walls of the extremity are measured. The mean blood pressure is determined when the amplitude of the oscillations are greatest. The systolic and diastolic pressures are then calculated through proprietary algorithms from each manufacturer.[11] Evidence regarding validation of blood pressure measurements in acute care settings is limited; therefore, these measurements should be interpreted carefully, particularly in low flow states. Patients who are hemodynamically unstable, either profoundly hypotensive or profoundly hypertensive, cannot be adequately assessed using NIBP measurement. In patients who are obese with conically shaped upper arms, it is technically difficult to measure an NIBP because the cuff often does not fit appropriately or stay positioned. Blood pressure readings are also affected by the presence of cardiac dysrhythmias, respiratory variation, shivering, seizures, external cuff compression, decreased peripheral perfusion, peripheral vasoconstriction, and the patient talking or moving during the measurement. Isolated blood pressure readings are not used to guide patient management; trending of values over time and assessing the response to interventions are crucial to maximize patient outcomes.

Jugular Venous Pressure. Assessment of the jugular venous pressure is a visual assessment of the jugular veins. This assessment provides an estimate of intravascular volume, as an indirect measure of CVP, based on the amount of distention visualized. Because the internal jugular vein directly communicates with the right atrium, it can serve as a manometer to provide an estimate of the CVP. Jugular venous distension occurs when the CVP is elevated, which can occur with fluid overload, right ventricular dysfunction, superior vena cava obstruction, and right heart failure. The technique for assessing jugular venous pressure is pictured in Fig. 9.6.

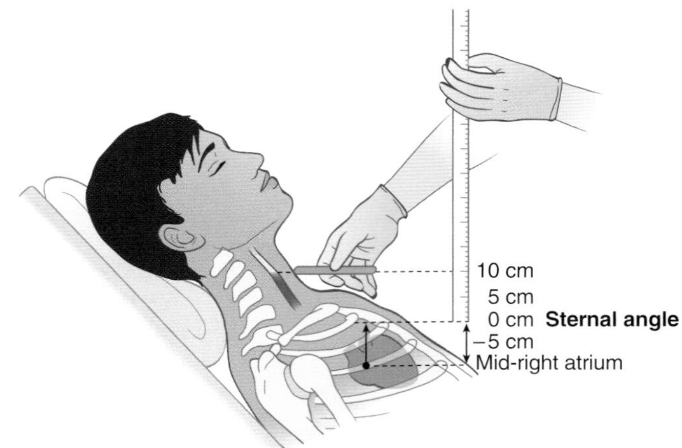

Fig. 9.6 Assessment of jugular venous pressure.

Lactate. Anything that deprives the tissues of oxygen disrupts the Krebs cycle, resulting in anaerobic metabolism and increased production of lactic acid. Measurement of lactate requires obtaining arterial or venous blood. Normal arterial lactate levels range from 0.3 to 0.8 mmol/L (3 to 7 mg/dL), and venous values range from 0.6 to 2.2 mmol/L (5 to 20 mg/dL).[12] Lactate levels may be measured to determine tissue hypoperfusion in shock, to establish adequacy of resuscitation, and to assist in the diagnosis of patients who have metabolic acidosis of unknown cause. Lactate levels may also be elevated in patients with diabetes, malignancy, alcohol intoxication, epinephrine infusions, and mitochondrial dysfunction. Clearance of lactate may be reduced in patients with liver failure.[13-15]

Bioimpedance Analysis. Information about physical and electrochemical processes in tissues are provided through measurement of exogenic bioelectric responses that change as the volume or distribution of fluids change in body regions. BIA is performed by connecting electrodes placed on the neck and thorax to the monitoring devices. A low alternating current is passed through the thorax. As the current traverses the thorax through the blood in the heart and great vessels, impedance values are calculated based on the changes in the measured electrical current. These changes allow for the calculation of SV, CO, and blood pressure.[8,16]

Applanation Tonometry and Volume Clamp Method. Continuous CO monitoring using AT occurs by strapping a transducer to an artery with a bone underneath (e.g., radial artery). Pressure is applied to compress the artery, making the transmural pressure zero, then allowing the transducer to measure the systolic and diastolic pressures that are then processed to create a pulse wave and CO. In VCM, an inflatable cuff containing infrared photodiodes and light detectors is placed around a finger. The cuff adjusts to measure the arterial blood pressure waveform and periodically clamp blood flow in the artery. The absorption of the infrared signal is utilized to measure arterial volume, generating a pulse wave. The contour of the wave is utilized to calculate SV and CO.[9,10]

BOX 9.1 Indications for Invasive Hemodynamic Monitoring

Arterial Line
- Monitoring and evaluating treatment in the hemodynamically unstable patient.
- Assess efficacy of vasoactive medications.
- Obtain frequent blood samples for arterial blood gas analysis or other laboratory tests.
- Can be used in conjunction with a stroke volume measurement device.

Central Venous Catheter
- Measure right heart filling pressures.
- Estimate fluid status.
- Guide volume resuscitation.
- Assess central venous oxygen saturation ($ScvO_2$).
- Administer large-volume fluid resuscitation or medications.
- Administration of vesicant medications.
- Access to place transvenous pacemaker.

Pulmonary Artery Catheter
- Assess left heart function with PAOP pressures.
- Identify and treat cause of hemodynamic instability.
- Assess pulmonary artery pressures.
- Assess mixed venous oxygen saturation (SvO_2).
- Directly measure cardiac output.

PAOP, Pulmonary artery occlusion pressure.

Invasive Hemodynamic Monitoring

Indications. Invasive methods of hemodynamic monitoring are used to obtain more detailed physiological information. Common indications for invasive monitoring are outlined in Box 9.1. A comprehensive hemodynamic assessment is used to guide interventions in patients with the following diagnoses: shock, cardiac tamponade, ruptured ventricular septum, heart failure, and right ventricular infarction (refer to the Collaborative Care Plan found in Chapter 1, Overview of Critical Care Nursing). In addition, hemodynamic monitoring is used with complex surgical patients to guide therapy and detect complications early.

The first step in a hemodynamic assessment is to evaluate the adequacy of tissue perfusion to determine whether the patient is in a state of shock that requires fluid resuscitation. Once preload is optimized, afterload and contractility are addressed. Hemodynamic pressure measurements may approximate volume status; however, pressure does not always equal volume in certain conditions.

Equipment Common to All Intravascular Monitoring. The basic hemodynamic monitoring system has five major components: (1) the invasive catheter, (2) high-pressure noncompliant tubing, (3) the transducer with a stopcock, (4) a pressurized flush system, and (5) the bedside monitoring system (Fig. 9.7).

The *invasive catheter* varies depending on the type of catheter, purpose, and location of insertion. The catheter can be placed into an artery, a vein, or the heart. An arterial catheter consists of a relatively small-gauge, short, pliable catheter that is placed over a guidewire or in a catheter-over-needle system. CVP or $ScvO_2$ monitoring is obtained through a central venous catheter (CVC), most commonly placed in the subclavian or internal jugular vein (Fig. 9.8). The femoral vein may be used when the thoracic veins are not available or in a trauma situation. Femoral catheters are associated with higher infection rates and should be removed as soon as possible. Pulmonary artery (PA) pressure and SvO_2 monitoring require a longer catheter that is placed into the PA (Fig. 9.9).

Noncompliant pressure tubing designed specifically for hemodynamic monitoring is used to minimize artifacts and increase the accuracy of the data transmission. Noncompliant tubing allows for the efficient transfer of intravascular pressure changes to the transducer and monitoring system. To maintain the most accurate pressure readings, the tubing should be no longer than 36 to 48 inches, with a minimum number of additional stopcocks.

The *transducer* (Fig. 9.10) translates intravascular pressure changes into waveforms and numerical data. To ensure the data are accurate, the system must be calibrated to atmospheric pressure by zeroing the transducer. A three-way stopcock attached to the transducer is generally used as the reference point for zeroing and leveling the system. This is referred to as the air-fluid interface or the zeroing stopcock.

The *flush system* maintains patency of the pressure tubing and catheter. The flush solution (usually 0.9% normal saline) is placed in a pressure bag that is inflated to 300 mm Hg to ensure a constant flow of fluid through the pressure tubing, usually 2 to 5 mL/h per lumen. The use of heparin in flush solutions has been debated for over 3 decades, with mixed results over patency.[17-24] The use of heparin carries additional risks, including the development of heparin-induced thrombocytopenia. Consider the risk-to-benefit ratio in patients requiring monitoring for more than 48 hours and patients in hypercoagulable states when determining whether to use heparin or normal saline flush solutions.

Bedside monitoring systems vary, but all have the same general function and purpose. They provide the visual display of waveforms and numerical information generated by the transducer and can store and record the data. The clinician interprets the data.

Nursing Implications. Accuracy in hemodynamic monitoring is essential for clinical decision-making (see Clinical Alert box).[25-27] Four major components for validating the accuracy of hemodynamic monitoring systems are (1) positioning the patient, (2) leveling the air-fluid interface (zeroing stopcock) to the phlebostatic axis, (3) zeroing the transducer, and (4) assessing dynamic responsiveness (performing the *square wave test*).[28] Preventing and assessing for complications (Box 9.2) are also key nursing interventions for patients with invasive hemodynamic monitoring catheters.

! CLINICAL ALERT

Hemodynamic Monitoring

Keys to success in hemodynamic monitoring are ensuring the data are accurate, conducting waveform analysis, and integrating the data with other assessment variables. Never base clinical decisions solely on one variable, and do not interpret hemodynamic values in isolation. Integration of clinical data, patient presentation, and subjective assessment are crucial to making clinical decisions to improve patient outcomes. Hemodynamic data are most beneficial when directed by established protocols with specific end points of therapy.

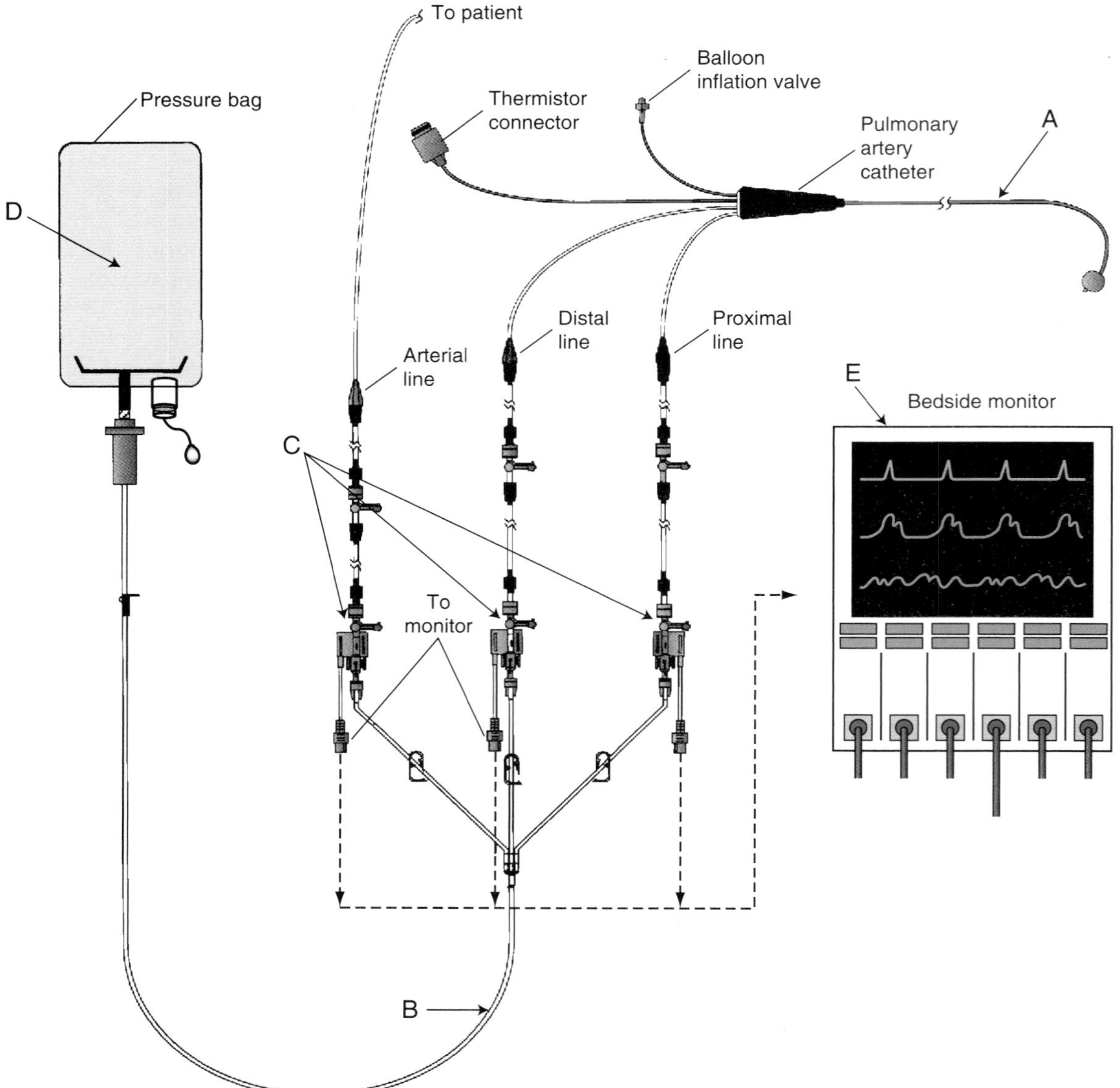

Fig. 9.7 Components of an invasive monitoring system (pulmonary artery catheter and designated arterial line) connected to one flush solution. **A**, Invasive catheter. **B**, Noncompliant pressure tubing. **C**, Transducer and zeroing stopcock. **D**, Pressurized flush system. **E**, Bedside monitoring system. (Not to scale.)

Patient Positioning. Hemodynamic data can be accurately measured with the patient in a supine or lateral position and with the head of the bed (HOB) flat or elevated as long as the air-fluid interface used to zero the transducer is level to the phlebostatic axis. HOB elevation to 30 degrees is a key factor in the prevention of complications, such as ventilator-associated pneumonia, and provides a comfortable position for most patients.[28]

Leveling the Air-Fluid Interface. Position the zeroing stopcock of the transducer system at the level of the atria for accurate readings. This external anatomical location is called the phlebostatic axis, and it is located by identifying the fourth intercostal space at the midway point of the anterior-posterior diameter of the chest wall (Fig. 9.11). A permanent marker can be used to mark the location of the phlebostatic axis on the patient to ensure that future measurements are done using the same reference point. Once the level of the phlebostatic axis is identified, secure the transducer and zeroing stopcock to the chest wall or to an IV pole positioned near the patient. The relationship of the air-fluid interface to the phlebostatic axis must be maintained so that the numerical readings transmitted to the monitor are accurate. When the transducer is affixed to the patient's chest wall, regularly assess skin integrity to prevent skin breakdown.

Because of the effects of hydrostatic pressure on the fluid-filled monitoring system, variations in the height of the transducer system by as little as 1 cm below the phlebostatic axis can result in a false result by as much as 0.73 mm Hg. Pressure measurements taken with transducers located below the point of interest (e.g., phlebostatic axis) falsely elevate the pressure

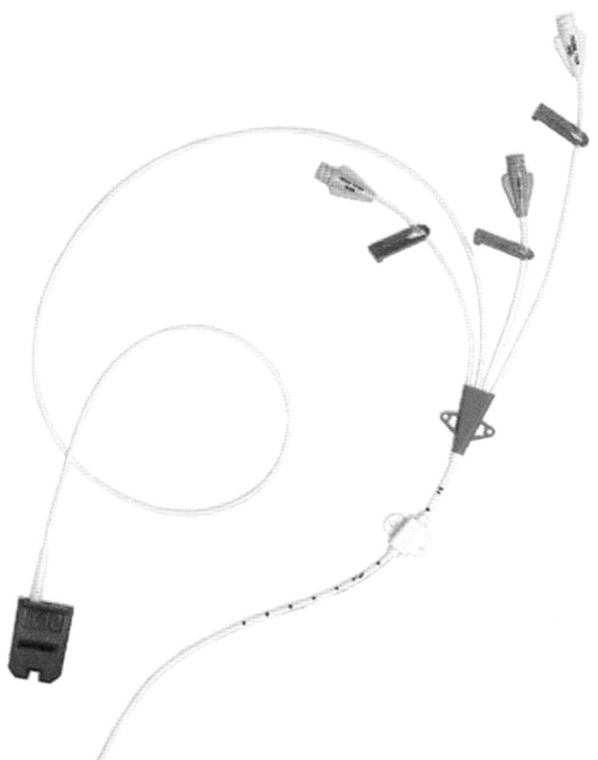

Fig. 9.8 Example of a triple-lumen central venous catheter to measure central venous pressure and oxygen saturation. (Courtesy Edwards Lifesciences, Irvine, CA.)

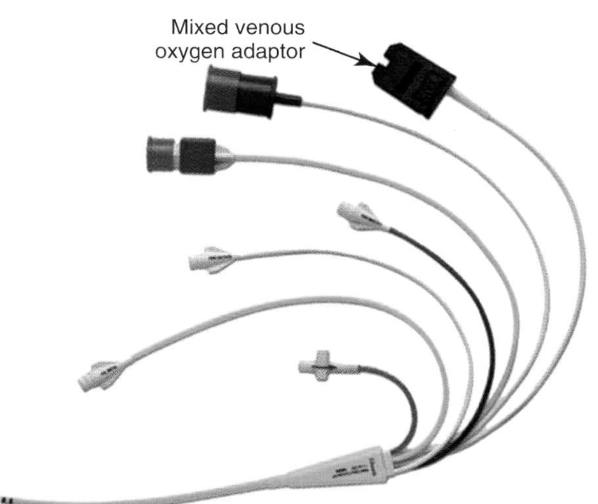

Fig. 9.9 Example of a pulmonary artery catheter with capability of monitoring mixed venous oxygenation. (Courtesy Edwards Lifesciences, Irvine, CA.)

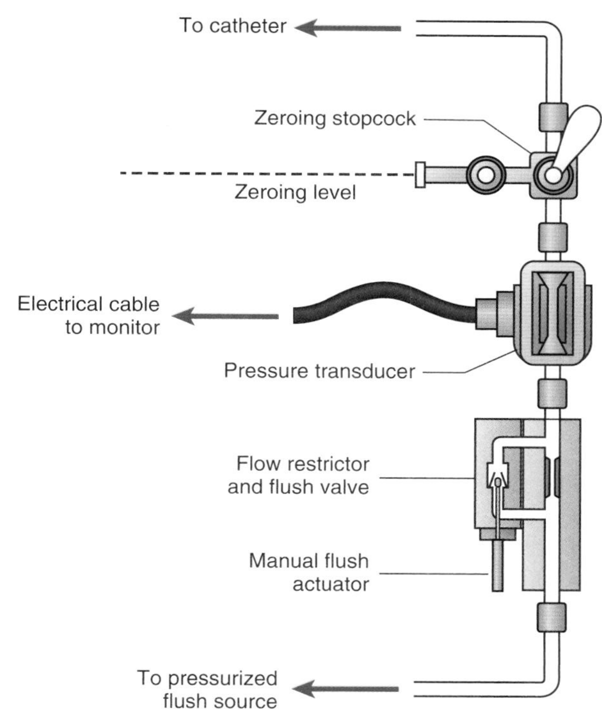

Fig. 9.10 Schematic of a typical pressure transducer. (From Kruse JA. Fast flush test. In: Kruse JA, Fink MP, Carlson RW, eds. *Saunders Manual of Critical Care*. Philadelphia, PA: Saunders; 2003.)

BOX 9.2 Potential Complications of Invasive Hemodynamic Monitoring Devices

- Vascular complications
- Thrombosis
- Hematoma
- Infection
- Bleeding
- Pneumothorax or hemothorax
- Cardiac dysrhythmias
- Pericardial tamponade

readings. If the transducer is placed above the correct landmark, the pressure readings are falsely low. Therefore, the location of the zeroing stopcock must be regularly monitored and releveled with each change in the patient's position.

Zero Referencing. The effects of atmospheric pressure on the fluid-filled hemodynamic monitoring system must be negated for accurate measurements. At sea level, the atmospheric pressure exerts a force of 760 mm Hg on any object on the Earth's surface. To eliminate the effect of the atmospheric pressure on the physiological variables, the transducer system is "zeroed" at the level of the phlebostatic axis. To accomplish this task, open the zeroing stopcock of the transducer to air (closed to the patient) and calibrate (zero) the monitoring system to read a pressure of 0 mm Hg. Each computer system has a zeroing function that is easy to perform. Zero referencing is done when the catheter is inserted, at the beginning of each shift, when repositioning the patient, and when there are significant changes in hemodynamic status.

Dynamic Response Testing. Fluid-filled monitoring systems rely on the ability of the transducer to translate the vascular pressure into waveforms and numerical data. To verify that

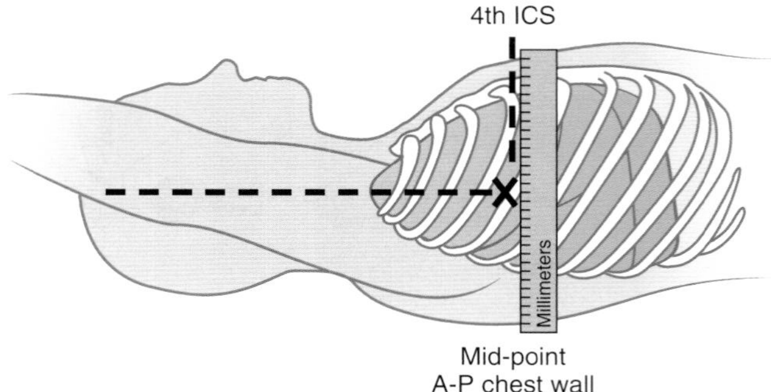

Fig. 9.11 Locating the phlebostatic axis in the supine position. *A-P*, Anterior-posterior; *ICS*, intercostal space.

the transducer system accurately represents cardiovascular pressures, perform the dynamic response, or square wave, test. This test is done by recording the pressure waveform while activating the fast-flush valve or actuator on the pressure tubing system for at least 1 second. The resulting graph should depict a rapid upstroke from the baseline with a plateau before returning to the baseline (i.e., a square wave).[28] When the pressure tracing returns to the baseline, a small undershoot should occur below the baseline, along with one or two oscillations within 0.12 seconds, before resuming the pressure waveform. If the dynamic response test meets these criteria, the system is optimally damped (Fig. 9.12**A**), and the resulting waveforms and numerical data can be interpreted as accurate. Perform the dynamic response test after catheter insertion, at least once per shift, after drawing blood from the line, and any time the system is opened. It is a simple but crucial test that must be incorporated into routine hemodynamic assessment to ensure accuracy.

The system is overdamped if the dynamic response test results in no oscillations, the upstroke is slurred, or a small undershoot is not produced (Fig. 9.12B). An overdamped system can result in a systolic pressure measurement that is falsely low and a diastolic pressure measurement that is falsely elevated.

Conversely, the system is underdamped if the dynamic response test results in excessive oscillations (Fig. 9.12C). The displayed pressure waveform and numerical data will show erroneously high systolic pressures and low diastolic pressures. Box 9.3 describes the causes of abnormal dynamic response test results and interventions for troubleshooting systems that are overdamped or underdamped.

Preventing Infection. Central line–associated bloodstream infections (CLABSIs) result in thousands of deaths each year and billions of dollars in added costs. Invasive catheters are direct portals to the circulating blood; therefore, strict infection control measures must be implemented to prevent CLABSI (refer to the Collaborative Care Plan found in Chapter 1, Overview of Critical Care Nursing). To reduce the risk for CLABSI, a central line bundle was developed that emphasizes strict hand washing, strict sterile technique with maximal barrier precautions during placement, chlorhexidine skin antisepsis, optimal catheter site selection, and daily review of line necessity.[29] Maintaining the site properly with a chlorhexidine dressing, minimizing the number of times the system is opened, using sutureless securement devices, cleansing patients with chlorhexidine baths, changing the tubing system at intervals up to 7 days, aseptic treatment of tubing infusion ports, and aseptic treatment of medications and fluids given to the patient are recommended.[29] See the Evidence-Based Practice box for more discussion related to bathing. A decreased rate of CLABSI is associated with use of the subclavian vein site, although it has the highest rate of complications resulting from pneumothorax and phrenic nerve damage. In comparison, use of the internal jugular site has a lower complication rate than the subclavian site but is associated with higher infection rates. The femoral site is the least preferred for cannulation among adult patients as a result of higher infection rates. Box 9.4 describes general strategies for managing hemodynamic monitoring systems.

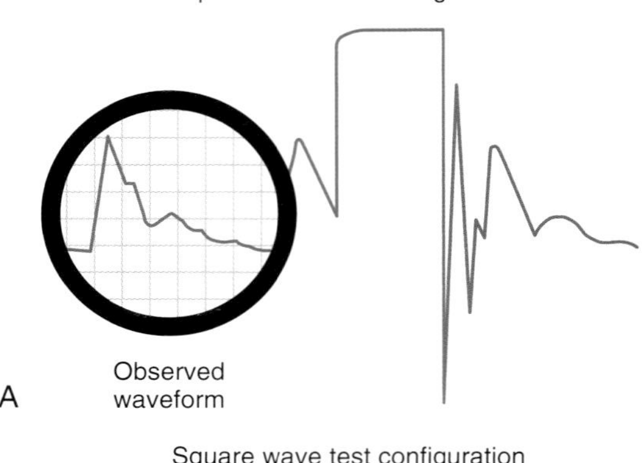

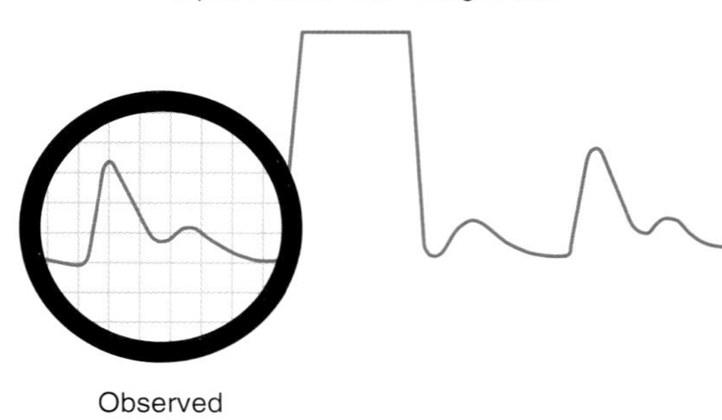

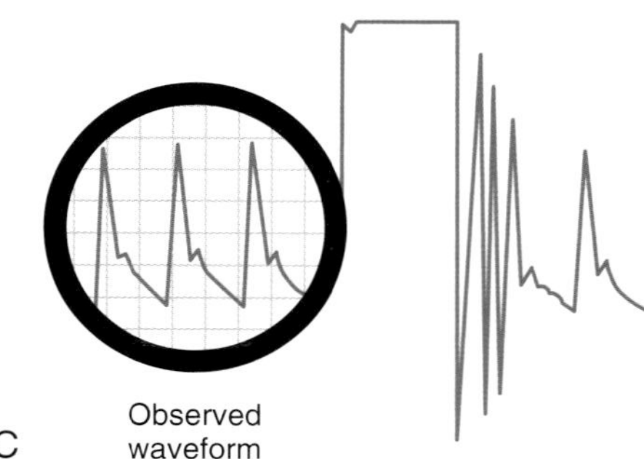

Fig. 9.12 **A**, Optimal dynamic response test. **B**, Overdamped dynamic response test. **C**, Underdamped dynamic response test.

EVIDENCE-BASED PRACTICE

Problem

Central line–associated bloodstream infections (CLABSIs) are a major complication of invasive lines. Chlorhexidine dressings have been recommended in intervention bundles to reduce CLABSI. Bathing with chlorhexidine-impregnated washcloths is another strategy that has been tested.

Clinical Question

What is the effectiveness of chlorhexidine bathing on the risk of hospital-acquired bloodstream infections (HABSI), both CLABSI and non-CLABSI, in adult critical care patients?

Evidence

The authors conducted a meta-analysis that included 26 studies with 861,546 patient-days and 5,259 hospital-acquired bloodstream infections (HABSI) to evaluate outcomes of chlorhexidine bathing. It was estimated that the bathing reduced the risk of HABSI by 40%. Bathing also reduced colonization with methicillin-resistant *Staphylococcus aureus*, gram-negative bacteria, and *Candida*. The authors note that the effectiveness of chlorhexidine bathing may be of greatest benefit in critical care unit populations with the highest risk for infection.

Implications for Nursing

Chlorhexidine bathing as part of a comprehensive HABSI reduction strategy is effective and relatively low-cost. Nurses are responsible for patient hygiene and should therefore advocate for the implementation of chlorhexidine bathing as the standard of care in the critical care setting. Monitor for any skin irritation that may be associated with chlorhexidine bathing. Allergic reactions are rare, but skin rashes, skin dryness, and pruritus are more commonly reported in the literature.

Level of Evidence

A—Systematic review and meta-analysis

Reference

Musuuza JS, Guru PK, O'Horo JC, et al. The impact of chlorhexidine bathing on hospital-acquired bloodstream infections: a systematic review and meta-analysis. *BMC Infectious Diseases*. 2019;19(1):N.PAG. https://doi.org/10.1186/s12879-019-4002-7.

REVIEW OF COMMON INVASIVE PRESSURE MONITORING

Arterial Pressure Monitoring

Arterial pressure monitoring is indicated for patients who are at risk for compromised tissue perfusion. Other indications include the need for frequent laboratory testing, hypotension or hypertension, and monitoring response to vasoactive medications. This common procedure involves cannulating an artery and recording pressures via the fluid-filled monitoring system. Although the diagnostic accuracy has been questioned, the radial artery is the site of choice because of its accessibility and collateral perfusion to the hand via the ulnar artery. Alternative sites include the femoral and brachial arteries. The radial artery should be assessed for collateral circulation by performing an Allen test or a modified Allen test (Box 9.5).[28] Cannulation can be facilitated by Doppler ultrasonography.

Invasive arterial pressure monitoring is the most accurate method of measuring the systemic blood pressure because it allows for continuous, beat-to-beat analysis of the arterial pressure. Arterial pressure monitoring is thus the method of choice in assessing blood pressure in the hemodynamically unstable patient.[28]

The normal arterial waveform (Fig. 9.13) consists of a sharp upstroke, the peak of which represents the systolic pressure. This pressure is a direct reflection of left ventricular function. Normal values for systolic pressures are less than 120 mm Hg. The lowest point on the arterial waveform represents the end-diastolic pressure and reflects systemic resistance. Normal values for diastolic pressure are less than 80 mm Hg.

BOX 9.3 Abnormal Dynamic Response Test: Causes and Interventions

Overdamped System

- Blood clots, blood left in the catheter after obtaining a blood sample, air bubbles at any point between the catheter tip and transducer
  - Flush the system or aspirate, disconnecting from the patient, if needed, to adequately flush the system to remove clots or air bubbles.
- Compliant tubing
  - Change to noncompliant tubing or commercially available tubing system.
- Loose connections
  - Ensure that all connections are secure.
- Kinks in the tubing system
  - Straighten tubing.
- Flush system integrity
  - Ensure that there is an adequate amount of flush solution.
  - Ensure that the pressure bag is at 300 mm Hg.

Underdamped System

- Excessive tubing length (normal is <36 to 48 inches)
  - Remove extraneous tubing, stopcocks, or extensions.
- Small-bore tubing
  - Replace small-bore tubing with a larger bore set.
- Cause unknown
  - Add a damping device into the system to reduce artifact.
  - Can be the result of patient anatomy and some diagnoses.
  - Change transducer.

BOX 9.4 General Nursing Strategies for Managing Hemodynamic Monitoring Systems

- Document insertion date.
- Change occlusive dressings according to institutional policy.
- Assess for signs of infection.
- Date dressing changes.
- Maintain patency of the flush system.
  - Flush the system after each use of a port.
  - Clear any blood from the tubing, ports, and stopcocks.
  - Maintain a pressure of 300 mm Hg on the flush solution using a pressure bag.
  - Ensure adequate amount of flush solution.
- Use luer locks, ensure tightened connections in the tubing and flush system.
- Keep tubing free of kinks.
- Minimize excess tubing and the number of stopcocks.
- Limit disconnecting or opening the system.
- Ensure that alarm limits are set on the monitor and alarms are turned on.
- Monitor waveforms.
- Disinfect injection ports.

BOX 9.5 Allen and Modified Allen Test Procedure

Allen Test
- Ask the patient to form a tight fist with the wrist in a neutral position.
- Occlude the radial artery by applying pressure with the thumb for approximately 10 seconds.
- Ask the patient to open the fist while the clinician maintains thumb pressure on the radial artery.
- Ulnar circulation is adequate if blanching resolves within 5 seconds and inadequate if the hand remains pale for more than 10 seconds.

Modified Allen Test
- Ask the patient to form a tight fist with the wrist in a neutral position.
- Occlude radial and ulnar arteries for approximately 10 seconds.
- Ask the patient to open the fist, revealing a blanched hand.
- Release pressure on the ulnar artery, maintaining pressure on the radial artery.
- Ulnar circulation is adequate if blanching resolves within 5 seconds and inadequate if the hand remains pale for more than 10 seconds.

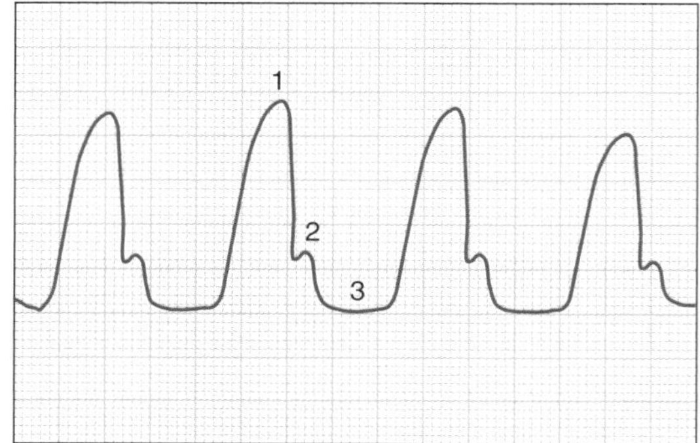

Fig. 9.13 Arterial pressure waveform obtained from an arterial line. *1,* Peak systolic pressure; *2,* dicrotic notch; *3,* diastolic pressure.

The downstroke of the arterial waveform consists of a small notch called the dicrotic notch, which represents aortic valve closure and the beginning of diastole. This is commonly considered the reference point between the systolic and diastolic phases of the cardiac system. The remainder of the downstroke is arterial distribution of blood flow through the arterial system.

Complications. The major complications of arterial pressure monitoring include thrombosis, embolism, blood loss, and infection. Embolism may occur as a result of small clot formation around the tip of the catheter or from air entering the system. Thrombosis (clot) may occur if a continuous flush solution is not properly maintained. Thrombosis and embolism may result in limb ischemia. Monitor for signs of ischemia distal to the catheter site and report any changes. Rapid blood loss can result from sudden dislodgment of the catheter from the artery or from a disconnection in the tubing connections. Maintain monitoring alarms that are individualized to the patient's parameters at all times to decrease the risk of undetected bleeding or line disconnection. Although infection is a risk of intraarterial catheters, routine replacement of the catheter is not recommended unless an infection is suspected.

BOX 9.6 Causes of Inaccurate Arterial Line Readings

- Air bubbles in the catheter system
- Failure to zero the transducer air-fluid interface
- Failure to level the transducer at the phlebostatic axis
- Blood in the catheter system
- Blood clot at the catheter tip
- Kinking of the tubing system
- Catheter tip lodging against the arterial wall
- Soft, compliant tubing
- Long tubing (>48 inches)
- Too many stopcocks (>3)

Clinical Considerations. The invasive method of obtaining blood pressure is considered to be more accurate than noninvasive methods. Although the invasive and noninvasive measurements are correlated, the invasive method measures pressure directly and the noninvasive measures the flow. In patients who are hypotensive, a serious discrepancy may exist between the blood pressures obtained by invasive and noninvasive means.[30] The pressure differences can vary widely. A study concluded that these differences may result in treatment decisions in up to 20% of critically ill patients.[30] When the noninvasive value is higher than the invasive value, suspect equipment malfunction or technical error. Check the intraarterial system. Level and zero reference the system, then perform a square wave test to evaluate accuracy. Box 9.6 lists the possible causes of inaccurate invasive blood pressure readings.

Nursing Implications. Refer to Box 9.4 for standard management of all invasive hemodynamic systems. Additional interventions specific to management of the intraarterial catheter include the following:

- Document assessment of the extremity regularly for perfusion: color, temperature, sensation, pulse, and capillary refill (normal time to refill is <3 seconds).
- Keep the patient's wrist in a neutral position and, if needed, place it on an arm board (radial artery catheters).
- When the catheter is removed, ensure adequate pressure is applied to the insertion site until hemostasis is obtained (for a minimum of 5 minutes for radial artery catheters). The time required varies depending on the type, size, and location of the catheter and on the patient's coagulation status.
- Never administer medications via an arterial line because of potential harmful complications.

Right Atrial Pressure/Central Venous Pressure Monitoring

In critically ill patients, the right atrial pressure (RAP) and CVP have been used to estimate central venous blood volume and right heart function. The CVP is pressure in the vena cava and is obtained via the distal lumen of a CVC. The RAP is the pressure in the atria and is obtained from the proximal lumen of a pulmonary artery catheter (PAC). Because no valves are present between the vena cava and right atrium, both the CVP and the RAP are essentially equal pressures. These measurements assess preload of the right side of the heart. The term RAP is used most often in this textbook. Normal RAP/CVP ranges from 2 to 6 mm Hg.

The RAP is obtained from a CVC inserted into the superior or inferior vena cava. The thoracic central veins (subclavian and internal jugular veins) are the most common insertion sites. Catheters used for RAP measurement are generally stiff and radiopaque, and they vary in length and diameter depending on the vein that is used. Shorter catheters are inserted into the subclavian and internal jugular veins, and longer catheters are used for insertion into the upper extremities or femoral vein. CVCs often have multiple lumens that facilitate pressure monitoring, administration of fluids and medications, and blood sampling. If the placement of a PAC is anticipated, a catheter with an introducer may be used.

During insertion, place the patient's bed in the Trendelenburg position to promote venous filling in the upper body for easier insertion of the catheter, unless the patient has respiratory distress or increased intracranial pressure. This position also prevents air embolism during insertion. If the Trendelenburg position is contraindicated, place a blanket roll between the patient's shoulder blades to facilitate insertion. The provider cleans the skin with an antiseptic, drapes the patient, and injects a local anesthetic to reduce pain during insertion. A needled syringe is used to puncture the vessel and to confirm placement by backward flow of blood into the syringe. The syringe is removed, and a guidewire is threaded through the needle into the vessel. The needle is then removed so that the catheter may be passed over the guidewire. Once the catheter is in place, the provider will either suture or use a sutureless device to secure the catheter, then place a dressing per institutional policy. The nurse is responsible for monitoring for dysrhythmias, air embolism, and breaches in sterile technique. If any breach occurs, interrupt the procedure to correct any unsterile items (e.g., glove, towels, catheter). After the procedure, obtain a chest radiograph to verify placement and assess for complications. Fig. 9.14 shows the position of a CVC in the right atrium, along with the corresponding waveform.

The RAP should not be solely relied upon to assess fluid status, guide fluid resuscitation, or estimate right-sided cardiac function. The RAP should be considered in conjunction with other measures of fluid responsiveness. Because the normal RAP value is low and within a narrow range, it is important to obtain an accurate reading of the RAP. Level the system at the phlebostatic axis and zero the system, then verify an optimal dynamic response test.

Measure the RAP at end-expiration and at the end of ventricular diastole. Simultaneously, obtain a graph of the cardiac rhythm (electrocardiogram [ECG]), RAP, and respiratory tracing (if available) to obtain an accurate measurement of RAP. The RAP tracing is composed of three major waveforms: *a, c* and *v* waves (Fig. 9.15). The a wave is produced by atrial contraction and follows the P wave on the ECG tracing. The c wave is produced by closure of the tricuspid valve and follows the R wave. Finally, the v wave correlates with right atrial filling and right ventricular systole; it follows the T wave on the ECG.[29]

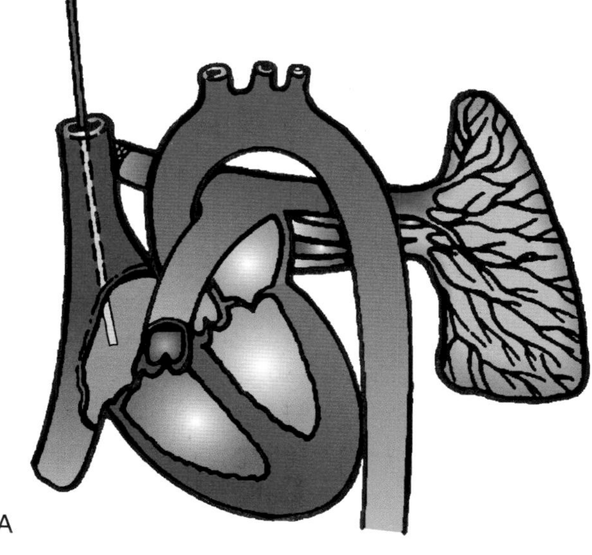

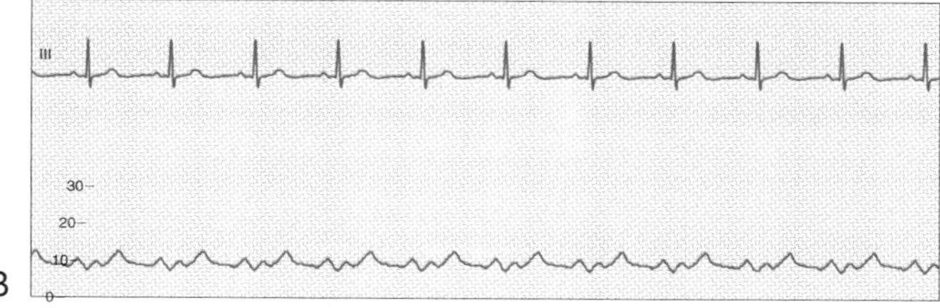

Fig. 9.14 A, Position of a central venous catheter in the right atrium. B, Cardiac rhythm and associated right atrial/central venous pressure waveform.

To measure the RAP, identify the a, c, and v waves of the RAP tracing at end-expiration (Fig. 9.15). Measure the RAP at end-expiration to ensure pleural pressure changes do not skew the numeric value. True RAP is best measured by locating the c wave and identifying the value immediately preceding the c wave (called the *pre-c measurement*). At this point, atrial contraction has occurred, and the tricuspid valve is open, providing a fluid path from the transducer to the right ventricle prior to ventricular contraction. This is known as the right ventricular end-diastolic pressure that is correlated to the right end-diastolic volume (preload). A discernable c wave may not be visible in atrial dysrhythmias. Alternatively, the average of the a wave may be computed, or the z-point method may be determined. The z-point method consists of identifying the RAP by locating the end of the QRS complex and using that as the reference point on the tracing. Box 9.7 outlines circumstances for using the different methods to determine RAP.

Complications. Maintain maximum sterile barrier precautions during insertion, because CLABSIs are common, increasing the risk of sepsis. Other complications may occur during insertion, including carotid puncture, pneumothorax, hemothorax, perforation of the right atrium or ventricle, and cardiac dysrhythmias (ventricular tachycardia/fibrillation). Obtain a chest radiograph after insertion to confirm placement and detect complications.

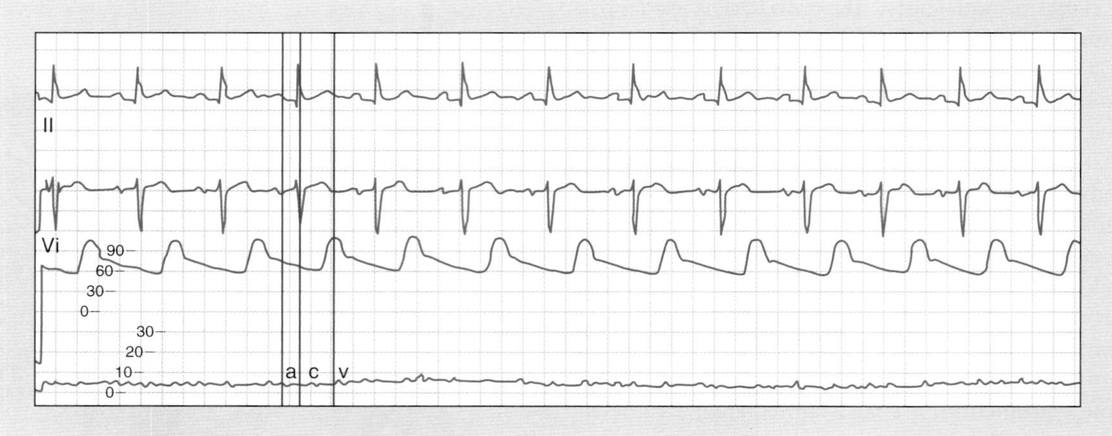

Fig. 9.15 Identifying the *a*, *c*, and *v* waveforms to determine right atrial pressure.

BOX 9.7 Methods for Determining Accurate Right Atrial Pressure

Pre-*c* Method

- Most accurate measure of right-sided preload; method of choice for numerical assessment.
- Represents the last atrial pressure before ventricular contraction.
- Difficult to use because the c wave is often unidentifiable.

Mean of the a Wave

- Clinically significant because the a wave results from atrial contraction.
- Used if the c wave cannot be identified.
- Obtain the numerical value for the top and bottom of the *a* wave; calculate the sum and divide by 2.

Z-Point Method

- Used when atrial-ventricular synchrony is not present: atrial fibrillation, third-degree heart block.
- Standardized approach results in the most reproducible value between clinicians.
- Does not account for hemodynamic effects on kidneys or liver that result from the prominent *a* or *v* waves.
- Locate the end of the QRS complex; use the numerical value associated with the exact point of intersection of the right atrial pressure waveform.

Clinical Considerations. Abnormalities in RAP are generally caused by any condition that alters venous tone, blood volume, or right ventricular contractility; however, due to the body's compensatory mechanisms, RAP may be normal when, in fact, hypovolemia may exist. Low RAP pressures also occur in relative hypovolemia because of venous vasodilation from rewarming, vasodilators, or sepsis. In all of these conditions, a decreased RAP reflects decreased blood return to the heart that is insufficient to meet the body's requirements. Confounding the interpretation of a low RAP is that the value may be negative in an individual in the upright position, even if cardiac function and volume status are normal. Consider additional techniques, such as inferior vena cava diameter and dynamic hemodynamic measures with passive leg raise, to assess volume status (discussed later in this chapter).

A high RAP measurement indicates conditions that reduce the right ventricle's ability to eject blood, thereby increasing right ventricular pressure and RAP. Such conditions include hypervolemia (seen with aggressive administration of IV fluids), severe vasoconstriction, decreased ventricular compliance, and mechanical ventilation (additional positive pressure increases RAP). Conditions causing an increased RAP also include pulmonary hypertension and heart failure.

Nursing Implications. The critical care nurse is responsible for collecting and recording patient data, ensuring the accuracy of the data, and reporting abnormal findings and trends to the provider. Analyzing the various hemodynamic parameters is a collaborative responsibility of the provider and the nurse to ensure prompt and appropriate treatment. Measurements of RAP are essential to compare with other physiological parameters and assessment findings. Other responsibilities include meticulous insertion site care, sterile dressing changes, and injection port care ("scrub the hub").

CHECK YOUR UNDERSTANDING

1. What treatment might you anticipate for an elevated right atrial pressure (RAP)?
   A. Blood transfusion
   B. Diuretics
   C. Vasopressors
   D. Coughing and deep breathing

Pulmonary Artery Pressure Monitoring

PACs are used to diagnose and manage a variety of conditions in critically ill patients. The ability to measure pressures in the PA and the left side of the heart became reality after a flow-directed PAC was invented by doctors Jeremy Swan and William Ganz in 1970.[31] Thermodilution PACs with the ability to obtain PA pressures and CO measurement became the gold standard to which all new hemodynamic monitoring methods are compared. In the last 30 years, the PAC has been redesigned to obtain a variety of hemodynamic parameters, including measurements of continuous CO (CCO), right ventricular end-diastolic volume, right ventricular ejection fraction, and SvO_2.

To determine pulmonary artery pressure (PAP), a specialized catheter is placed directly into the PA (Fig. 9.16). The PAC is a long, flexible, multilumen, balloon-tipped catheter that enables measurement of several hemodynamic parameters. The proximal port lies in the right atrium and measures RAP; it is also used to administer fluids and medications and to obtain intermittent thermodilution CO measurements. The distal port measures PAP and PAOP; SvO_2 blood samples are also drawn from this port. The thermistor port incorporates a temperature-sensitive wire that allows computer calculation of CO with the thermodilution method. Many catheters have an additional proximal infusion port for fluid and medication administration. The balloon inflation lumen provides the ability to inflate and deflate the small-volume (approximately 1.5-mL) balloon at the distal tip of the catheter. The balloon is inflated to facilitate insertion of the catheter and to measure PAOP, which provides information about the function of the left side of the heart. The concept of PAOP is discussed later in the chapter.

Several specialized PACs are available. One PAC enables transvenous pacing. This technique involves the insertion of a pacemaker wire through additional lumina in the PAC, which exits the catheter into the right ventricle to provide ventricular pacing. The CCO PAC provides continuous monitoring of CO. A PAC with a fiberoptic lumen at the tip of the catheter was developed for continuous measurement of SvO_2. The concepts of CCO and SvO_2 are discussed later in the chapter.

Nurses assist providers during PAC insertion. After the provider obtains informed consent, the nurse provides additional education on patient positioning and what the patient may feel or experience during the procedure. In addition, the nurse implements interventions to alleviate the patient's anxiety before and during the procedure.

The method of PAC insertion is similar to that for the CVC. Prior to insertion, ensure that the sterile plastic sheath is placed over the PAC. This sheath maintains catheter sterility following insertion and will be locked in place when the catheter is in its final position. Once the access port is in place, the PAC is passed freely into the vessel through the introducer. The provider inserting the catheter instructs the nurse (or other professional assisting with insertion) to inflate and deflate the balloon during the procedure to facilitate flow from the right atrium to the PA. Closed-loop communication between the inserter and the assistant is critical, as the inserter must know when the balloon is inflated and deflated. The catheter should never be withdrawn while the balloon is inflated. Complications from withdrawing an inflated balloon include pulmonary artery rupture and/or damage to the pulmonary and tricuspid valves (i.e., leaflets or chordae tendineae). The insertion technique may vary according to provider preference, brand of equipment used, and the patient's anatomy.

During PAC insertion, monitor and record respiratory rate and effort and heart rate and rhythm and assess for dysrhythmias. Monitor blood pressure and visualize and record waveforms

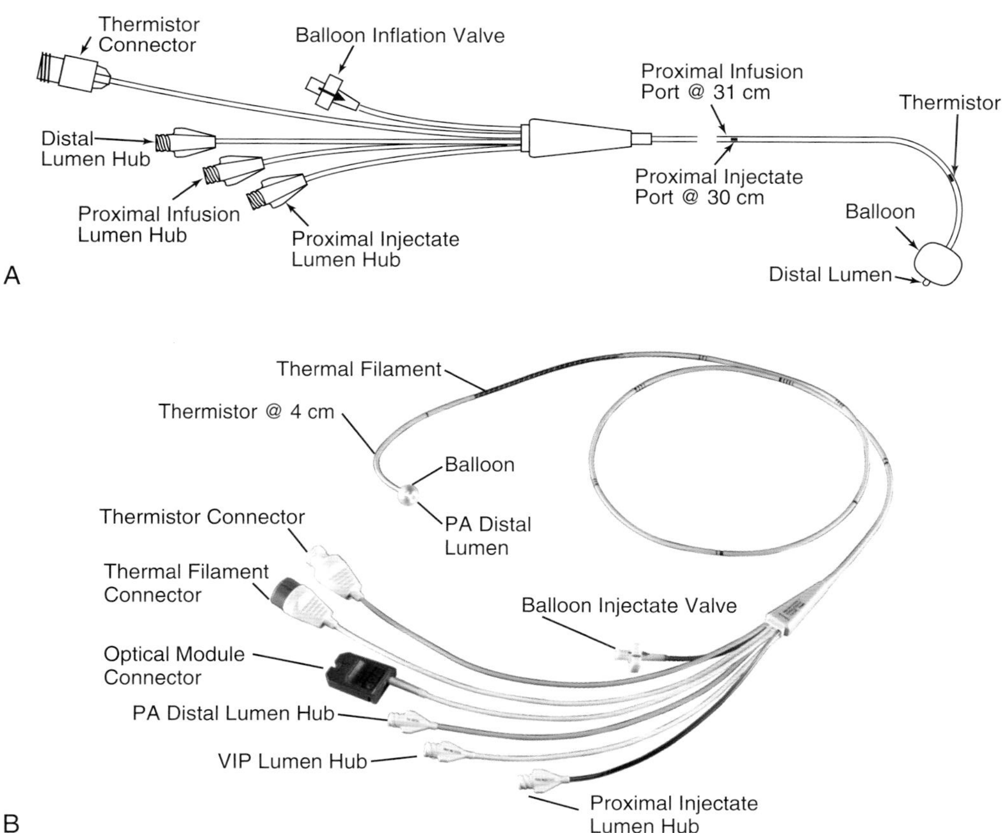

Fig. 9.16 A, A five-lumen pulmonary artery catheter containing the four-lumen components in addition to a second proximal lumen for infusion of fluid or medications. B, Combo Continuous Cardiac Output 777 catheter. (Courtesy Edwards Lifesciences, Irvine, CA.)

while the catheter is advanced. Ventricular dysrhythmias may occur as the catheter passes into and then through the right ventricle into the PA. Assist with balloon inflation during the procedure. As the catheter passes through each chamber, observe the waveform characteristics and record pressure values: RAP, right ventricular pressure, PAP, and PAOP (Fig. 9.17). The PAOP waveform signals the end of insertion, at which time the balloon is deflated. Once the balloon is deflated, the tip of the catheter settles back into the PA position. After the catheter is inserted and placement is verified, the balloon is inflated only to obtain periodic PAOP measurements; otherwise, it remains deflated to prevent complications such as pulmonary infarction and PA rupture. Nursing priorities are to accurately interpret PAC waveforms, recognize the effect of respiratory variations, prevent complications, and document hemodynamic values. Graphing the pressure waveforms and ECG tracing is also recommended.[30]

As a patient advocate, it is essential to promote patient safety throughout the procedure. Ensure that sterility is maintained, monitor the patient, and assist with balloon inflation and deflation. Because PAC insertion involves certain risks, ensure emergency medications and equipment are readily available. Complications of insertion include hemothorax; pneumothorax; perforation of the vena cava, cardiac chamber, or pulmonary artery; and cardiac dysrhythmias, especially as the PAC passes through the right ventricle. After the procedure, obtain a chest radiograph to verify placement and assess for complications. Once the position is verified, document the depth of catheter insertion at the insertion site; depth markings are noted on the PAC. Advocate for catheter removal when no longer necessary to reduce the risk of infection.

CHECK YOUR UNDERSTANDING

2. Determine which of the following cardiac functions are primarily assessed through the use of pulmonary artery catheters:
   A. Left ventricular function
   B. Pulmonary function
   C. Right atrial function
   D. Right ventricular function

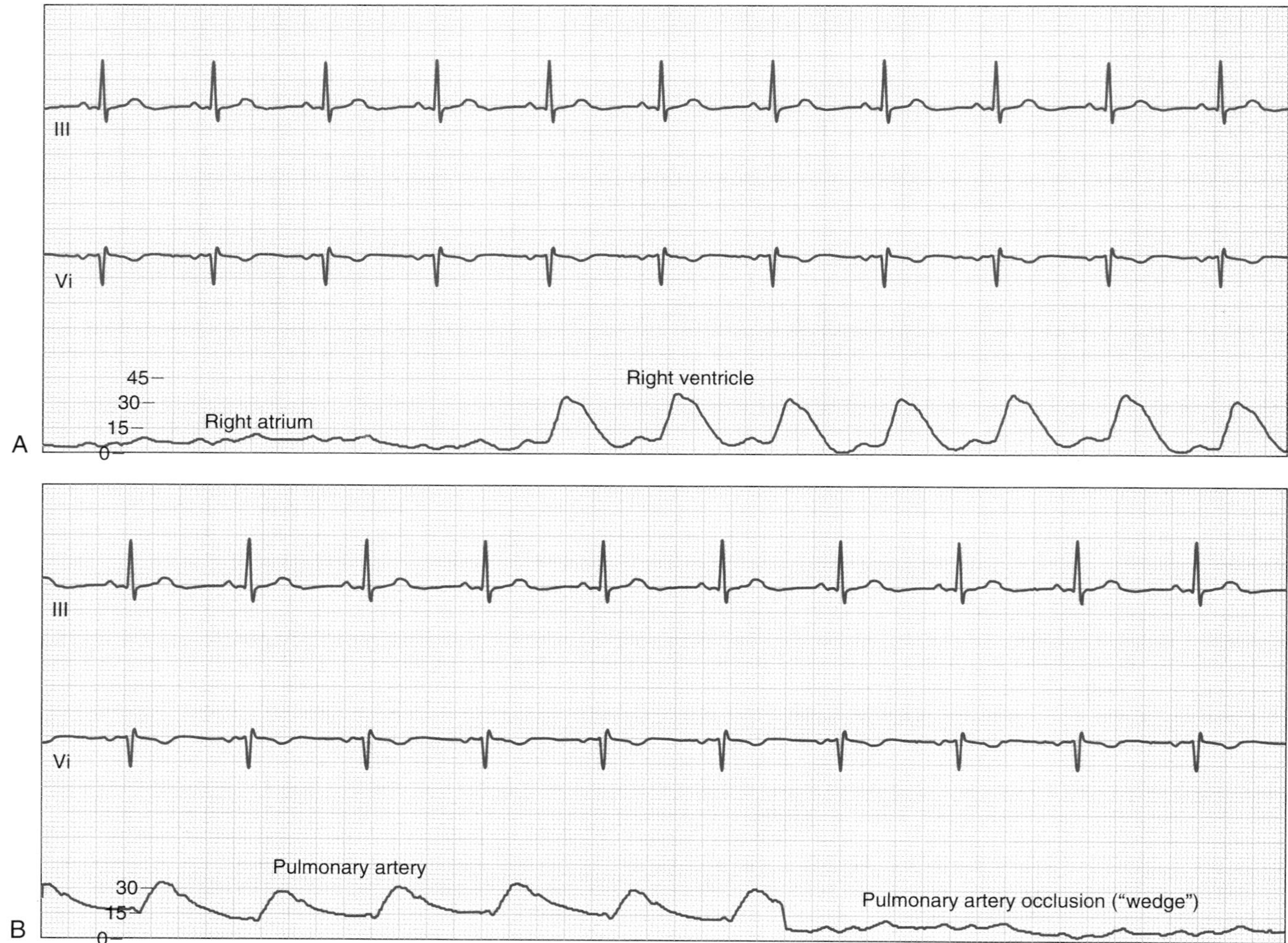

Fig. 9.17 Position of pulmonary artery catheter (PAC) and associated waveforms. A, Dual-channel tracing of cardiac rhythm with pressure waveforms obtained as the PAC is inserted into the right atrium and right ventricle. B, Dual-channel tracing of cardiac rhythm with the pulmonary artery and pulmonary artery occlusion pressure waveforms as the catheter is floated into proper position.

Hemodynamic Parameters Monitored via the Pulmonary Artery Catheter. The PAC is designed to estimate left ventricular filling pressure. Several pressures and parameters are measured or calculated by using the PAC: RAP, pulmonary artery systole (PAS), pulmonary artery diastole (PAD), mean pulmonary artery pressure (PAPm), PAOP, pulmonary and systemic vascular resistance; and CO. SvO_2 is measured if a fiberoptic catheter is inserted.

The PAS is the peak pressure created when the right ventricle ejects its SV and reflects the amount of pressure needed to open the pulmonic valve to pump blood into the pulmonary vasculature. The PAD represents the resistance of the pulmonary vascular bed as measured when the pulmonic valve is closed and the tricuspid valve is opened. The PAPm is the average pressure exerted on the pulmonary vasculature.

The PAOP is obtained when the balloon of the PAC is inflated to wedge the catheter from the PA into a small capillary. The resulting pressure reflects the left atrial pressure and left ventricular end-diastolic pressure (LVEDP) or ventricular filling pressures when the mitral valve is open. When properly assessed, the PAOP is a reliable indicator of left ventricular function. Normal PAOP is 8 to 12 mm Hg. The PAOP is measured at regular intervals as ordered by the provider or in accordance with unit protocols. To obtain the PAOP, inflate the balloon with no more than 1.5 mL of air using a PA-designated syringe, for no longer than 8 to 10 seconds, while noting the change in waveform from the PAP to the PAOP. To obtain an accurate measurement of the PAOP, print the PAOP waveform simultaneously with the ECG waveform and respiratory patterns. Compare digital measurements on the monitor to the printed measurements. Similar to RAP, obtain PAP and PAOP measurements at end-expiration. In the patient who is spontaneously breathing, pressures are highest at end-expiration and decline with inhalation (Fig. 9.18A). Obtain measurements from the waveform just before pressures decline. In the mechanically ventilated patient, pressures increase with inhalation and decrease with exhalation (Fig. 9.18B). In these patients, obtain the measurement just before the increase in pressures during inhalation. Many newer technology bedside monitors have built-in screen profiles to aid in the process of appropriately obtaining measurements in correlation to waveforms.

Clinical Considerations. Trending of PAOP provides an indirect measure of LVEDP. The PAOP is used to estimate the preload of the left heart, just as RAP/CVP is used to measure the preload of the right heart. In the absence of valvular disease and pulmonary vascular congestion, the PAD also closely approximates left ventricle function because the mitral valve is open during end-diastole. The PAD is often used as an indirect measurement of PAOP.

An increase in LVEDP (and therefore PAOP) indicates an increase in left ventricular blood volume to be ejected with the next systole. Increased PAOP may occur in patients who have fluid volume excess resulting from overzealous administration of IV fluid, as well as in patients with renal dysfunction. An increase in PAOP also provides information about impending left ventricular failure, as may be seen with myocardial infarction.

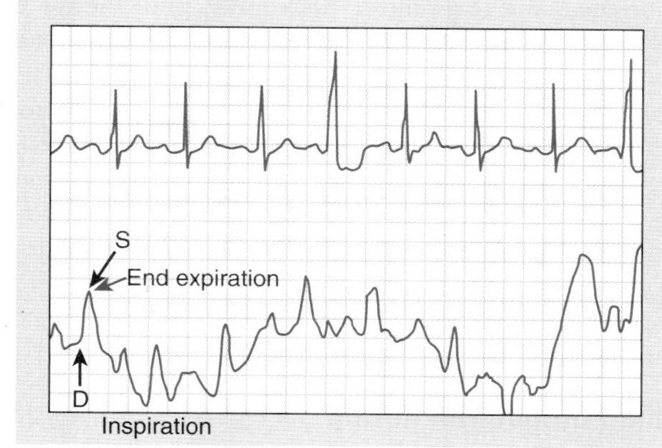

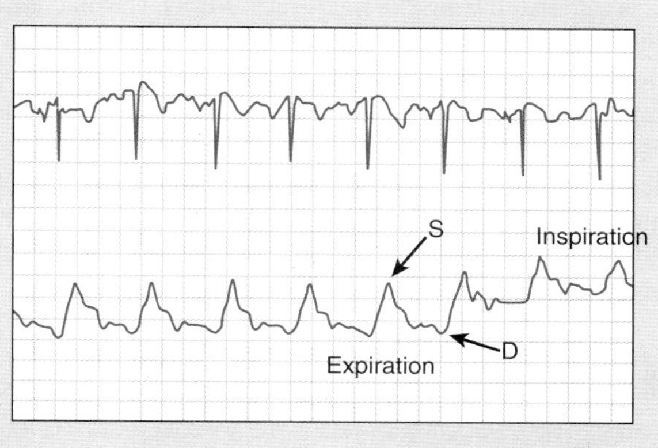

Fig. 9.18 Effect of respiration on pulmonary artery waveforms. **A**, Spontaneous breathing—Inspiration pulls down the waveform secondary to negative intrathoracic pressure. **B**, Mechanical ventilation—Inspiration pushes up the waveform secondary to positive pressure ventilation, which causes an increase in intrathoracic pressure. *D*, Diastolic pressure; *S*, systolic pressure.

A decrease in LVEDP (and a subsequently low PAOP) signals a reduction in left ventricular blood volume available for the next contraction. Conditions causing a low PAOP include those that cause fluid volume deficit, such as dehydration, excessive diuretic therapy, and hemorrhage.

Nursing Implications. Routinely monitor RAP, PAP, and PAOP to identify trends and the clinical significance of the values. The catheter position must be maintained in the PA. Assess placement, review chest radiograph results, and ensure that the balloon is deflated except during PAOP measurements. The PA pressure must be monitored continuously to ensure that the catheter has not migrated and inadvertently occluded the pulmonary artery.

Determine how much air is needed to obtain the PAOP (≤1.5 mL) and record this value. If the PAOP is obtained with a much smaller amount of air, the catheter may have migrated further into the PA. Do not inflate the balloon if this occurs. If the PAOP waveform is not seen with inflation of 1.5 mL of air, the catheter may be out of position or the balloon may have ruptured. In both of these situations, verify PAC position with a chest radiograph and observe the PAP waveform. For example, if the PAC has migrated into a small vessel, a PAOP waveform may be seen, and it should be withdrawn until the PA waveform returns. If the PAC has migrated into the right ventricle, the waveform will show higher pressure, and ventricular dysrhythmias may be noted (Fig. 9.17). If the PAD is used to estimate the PAOP, periodically compare the PAD and PAOP values to assess the accuracy of the PAD measurement, especially in patients experiencing acute hemodynamic changes. When it is determined that the PAC is no longer needed, nurses who have demonstrated competence in removing the catheter often perform the procedure as outlined in the policy and procedure manual for the unit.

Cardiac Output Monitoring

The CO is the amount of blood ejected by the heart each minute and is calculated from the heart rate and SV. Cardiac index (CI) is the CO adjusted for an individual's size or body surface area. Monitoring of CO and CI is done to assess the heart's ability to pump oxygenated blood to the tissues. CO is a measure of blood flow and is considered a reliable parameter to determine whether interventions have been successful. Causes of low and high CO are outlined in Box 9.8. Two methods are commonly used to evaluate CO via the PAC: thermodilution CO (TdCO) and CCO.

 **CLINICAL JUDGMENT ACTIVITY**

A patient's blood pressure continues to rise significantly, indicating an increase in resistance and an altered ability of the heart to eject blood. Describe the other parameters that would also be affected as a result?

Thermodilution Cardiac Output. To measure the CO via the TdCO method, the thermistor connector on the PAC is attached to a CO module on the cardiac monitor. A set volume (5 to 10 mL) of room-temperature solution of 5% dextrose in water is injected quickly and smoothly via the proximal port into the right atrium. Normal saline (0.9%) may be used in patients for whom 5% dextrose is contraindicated. The injected fluids may differ in temperature and densities that may alter measurements. Many institutions use a closed injectate delivery system to facilitate the procedure (Fig. 9.19). As the fluid bolus passes from the right atrium to the right ventricle, and subsequently the PA distal end, the difference in temperature is sensed by the thermistor located at the distal portion of the catheter (Fig. 9.20). The TdCO is calculated as the difference in temperature over time washout curve. Normal CO is represented by a smooth curve with a rapid upstroke and slow return to the baseline. The CO module calculates the area under this curve. The CO is inversely proportional to the area under the curve—patients with a high CO have a low calculated area under the curve. Therefore, the TdCO measurement is least accurate in patients with a low CO state and most accurate in those with a high CO state. Several steps must be taken to obtain accurate TdCO measurements. Box 9.9 describes these important points.

Continuous Cardiac Output. Measurement of CCO is based on the same principles as TdCO. The CCO system uses a modified PA catheter and a CO computer specific to the device. The specialized catheter has a copper filament near the proximal port that delivers pulses of energy at prescribed time intervals and

BOX 9.8 Interpretation of Abnormal Cardiac Output/Index Values

Low Cardiac Output/Index

- Heart rate that is too fast or too slow, leading to inadequate ventricular filling.
- Stroke volume reduction as a result of:
  - Decreased preload
    - Hypovolemia (e.g., hemorrhage, diuresis, dehydration)
    - Vasodilation
    - Fluid shifts (i.e., third-spacing) outside the intravascular space
  - Increased afterload
    - Vasoconstriction
    - Increased blood viscosity
  - Decreased contractility
    - Myocardial infarction or ischemia
    - Heart failure
    - Cardiomyopathy
    - Cardiogenic shock
    - Cardiac tamponade

High Cardiac Output/Index

- Heart rate elevation secondary to:
  - Increased activity
  - Anemia
  - Metabolic demands
  - Adrenal disorders
  - Fever
  - Anxiety
- Stroke volume increase as a result of:
  - Increased preload
    - Fluid resuscitation
    - Alteration in ventricular compliance
  - Decreased afterload
    - Vasodilation in sepsis
    - Decreased blood viscosity (anemia)
    - Increased contractility
    - Hypermetabolic states
    - Medication therapy

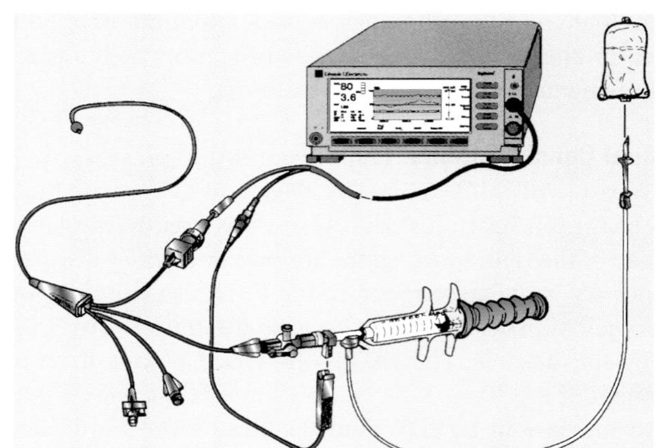

Fig. 9.19 Illustration of the closed injectate delivery system (room-temperature fluids) for thermodilution cardiac output measurement.

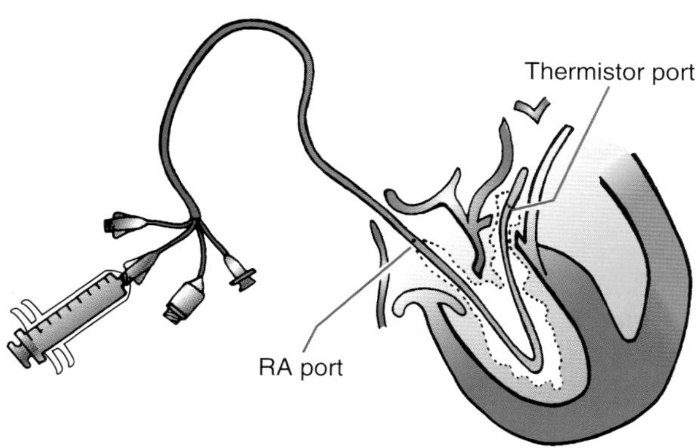

Fig. 9.20 Illustration of injection of fluid into the right atrium (RA) for cardiac output measurement.

BOX 9.9 Steps to Ensure Accurate Thermodilution Cardiac Output Measurements

- Before the procedure, assess the correct position of the PAC by verifying the waveform or measuring the PAOP.
- Enter the appropriate computation or calibration constant (per manufacturer's instruction) into the CO computer/bedside monitor. The type and size of the PAC and the volume and temperature of the injectate solution are factors that determine this value. Every manufacturer has a list of computation constants for their catheters which is printed on the device insert. It corrects for the catheter length, injectate volume and temperature.
- Assess the proximal port for patency.
- Do not infuse vasoactive drugs through the port used to obtain TdCO measurements. Rapid infusion of the injectate solution for the TdCO will result in delivery of these medications beyond the recommended dosage and cause potentially harmful side effects.
- Position the patient in the supine position with the head of bed at 0 to 30 degrees.
- Room-temperature injectate is acceptable as long as there is at least a 5.5°C difference between the temperature of the injectate and the patient's temperature. Patients with very low cardiac outputs may need iced injectate to improve the signal-to-noise ratio.
- Inject the solution smoothly and rapidly (within 4 seconds) at the end of expiration to reduce the effect of chest wall motion and intrathoracic pressure changes.
- Obtain three CO measurements and calculate the average CO (a feature on the CO computer averages the measurements). Values should be within 10% of each other. Measurements outside of 10% agreement should be discarded and repeated before averaging the results. The first CO is usually the most variable.

CO, Cardiac output; *PAC*, pulmonary artery catheter; *PAOP*, pulmonary artery occlusion pressure; *TdCO*, thermodilution cardiac output.

warms the blood as it enters the right ventricle. This temperature change is detected by the thermistor at the tip of the catheter approximately every 3 to 6 seconds. The computer interprets the temperature change and averages the CO measurements over the last 60 seconds. Fig. 9.21 shows an example of a computer interface for CCO and other hemodynamic parameters. CCO removes the potential for operator error associated with intermittent TdCO measurement. Other advantages of CCO are that no extra fluid is administered to the patient, data are

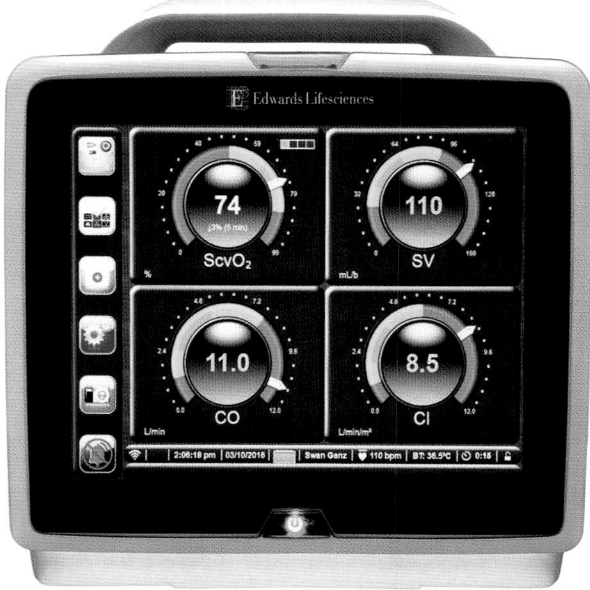

Fig. 9.21 A sample monitor interface displaying hemodynamic parameters and trends, including continuous cardiac output and central venous oxygen saturation. (Courtesy Edwards Lifesciences, Irvine, CA.)

available for trending throughout the shift, and there is no need to change the computation constant in the CO module. Patients with a CCO device can be positioned supine with the HOB elevated up to 45 degrees. Drawbacks to CCO include that the device may not accurately sense the CCO in the patient whose body temperature is greater than 40°C to 43°C, because the thermal filament heats to a maximum of 44°C. Continuous cardiac output does not reflect acute changes in CO. Because the measurements provide an average of CO over time, a delay may be common in detecting acute changes in CO of 1 L/min.[39]

Controversy Surrounding the Pulmonary Artery Catheter

Use of the PAC has decreased since evidence suggested its use was associated with increased mortality,[32] and less invasive monitoring has been developed. The PAC has limited ability to assess RAP and PAOP for preload status. PAC pressures are influenced by conditions that can increase the PAOP but do not reflect a change in preload. These include positive end-expiratory pressure and decreased ventricular compliance or a stiff ventricle. Studies have consistently shown that CVP, RAP, and PAOP are poor predictors of CO and fluid responsiveness. CVP alone is not to be used as a basis for clinical decision-making regarding fluid management.[26-27,31] PAC may be beneficial in certain populations such as those in cardiogenic shock or on mechanical circulatory support.[33-35] Other indications include diagnosing pulmonary hypertension and differentiating shock types or managing patients with mixed shock. Studies are needed to test protocols that guide therapy to determine whether the PAC can be used effectively.

Monitoring strategies are shifting to hemodynamic goal-directed therapy to guide interventions, such as administration of fluids. Many of the newer hemodynamic devices are designed to assess SV and changes in SV and other hemodynamic parameters.[36]

Balancing Oxygen Delivery and Oxygen Demand

The primary goal in caring for the critically ill is to determine whether oxygen delivery is meeting the oxygen and metabolic demands of the patient. Oxygen delivery is determined by CO and the arterial oxygen content of the blood. To determine if oxygen delivery is adequate, assess the CO, hemoglobin level, and arterial oxygen saturation (SaO_2). Oxygenated arterial blood passes through the capillary network to deliver oxygen and nutrients to the tissues. However, not all of the oxygen is used by the tissues, and residual oxygen bound to hemoglobin in the venous circulation is returned to the right heart to be oxygenated again. Venous oxygen saturation is the percent of hemoglobin saturated in the central venous circulation and provides an assessment of the amount of oxygen extracted by the tissues. The oxygen saturation of this mixed venous blood from various organs and tissues that have different metabolic needs provides a global picture of both oxygen delivery and oxygen consumption, or oxygen demand. Factors that affect venous oxygen saturation include CO, hemoglobin, SaO_2, and tissue oxygen consumption.

Oxygen delivery and consumption can be calculated using a variety of formulas (Table 9.2). Two invasive techniques are also available for clinical determination of venous oxygen saturation: SvO_2 and $ScvO_2$. SvO_2 is measured in the PA, and $ScvO_2$ is measured in the central venous system, usually the superior vena cava. Both SvO_2 and $ScvO_2$ methods use fiberoptic catheters that are connected to monitors and computers with an optical module (Figs. 9.8 and 9.9). Calibration of the system is done at insertion and if the system becomes disconnected from the optical module. To calibrate the equipment, a blood sample is obtained from either the PA (SvO_2) or the central venous catheter ($ScvO_2$), and a blood gas analysis is completed. Oxygen saturation results are used for calibration. Fig. 9.21 shows an example of the clinical information provided by one monitoring device.

Monitoring SvO_2 and $ScvO_2$ is indicated for any critically ill or injured patient who has the potential to develop an imbalance between oxygen delivery and oxygen consumption or demand. An SvO_2 between 60% and 75% indicates an adequate balance between supply and demand. The normal range for $ScvO_2$ (65% to 80%) is slightly higher, because the measurement is from the blood in the central venous circulation versus the PA. Any patient with hypoperfusion may benefit from SvO_2 or $ScvO_2$ monitoring to guide therapeutic interventions.

Many nursing interventions and clinical conditions affect the SvO_2 and $ScvO_2$. Table 9.3 highlights causes for alterations in SvO_2 values. Any changes in SaO_2, tissue metabolism, hemoglobin, or CO affect the values. For example, endotracheal suctioning may cause a transient decrease in the SvO_2 and $ScvO_2$ values if SaO_2 decreases during the procedure. Factors that increase the metabolic rate, such as shivering, fever, or an increase in physical activity, can also lead to a dramatic decrease in SvO_2 and $ScvO_2$. Values may be elevated in sepsis because the cells are unable to use the available oxygen; however, the values may also be normal or low.

When interpreting values for SvO_2 and $ScvO_2$, integrate clinical data and patient assessment to ensure good clinical

TABLE 9.3 Alterations in Mixed Venous Oxygen Saturation

Alteration	Cause	Possible Etiology
Low SvO_2 (<60%)	Decreased O_2 delivery	Hypoxia or hemorrhage, anemic states, hypovolemia, cardiogenic shock, dysrhythmias, myocardial infarction, congestive heart failure, cardiac tamponade, massive transfusions of stored blood, restrictive lung disease, ventilation/perfusion abnormalities
	Increased O_2 consumption	Strenuous activity, fever, pain, anxiety or stress, hormonal imbalances, increased work of breathing, bathing, septic shock (late), seizures, shivering
High SvO_2 (>75%)	Increased O_2 delivery	Increase in FiO_2, hyperoxygenation, shunt
	Decreased O_2 consumption	Hypothermia, anesthesia, hypothyroidism, neuromuscular blockade, early stages of sepsis
High SvO_2 (>80%)	Technical error	PAC in wedged position, fibrin clot at end of catheter, computer needs to be recalibrated

FiO_2, Fraction of inspired oxygen; *O_2,* oxygen; *PAC,* pulmonary artery catheter; *SvO_2,* mixed venous oxygen saturation.

TABLE 9.2 Hemodynamic Calculations

Parameter	Calculation	Normal Values
Mean arterial pressure	[Systolic BP + (2 × Diastolic BP)] ÷ 3	70-105 mm Hg
Arterial oxygen content (CaO_2)	[1.34 × Hgb (g/dL) × SaO_2] + [0.003 × PaO_2]	19-20 mL/dL
Venous oxygen content (CvO_2)	[1.34 × Hgb (g/dL) × SvO_2] + [0.003 × PvO_2]	12-15 mL/dL
Oxygen delivery (DO_2)	CO × CaO_2 × 10	900-1100 mL/min
Oxygen consumption (VO_2)	$C(a-v)O_2$ × CO × 10	200-250 mL/min
Oxygen extraction ratio (O_2ER)	[(CaO_2 – CvO_2)/CaO_2] × 100	22%-30%

BP, Blood pressure; *CO,* cardiac output; *Hgb,* hemoglobin; *PaO_2,* partial pressure of arterial oxygen; *PvO_2,* partial pressure of venous oxygen; *SaO_2,* arterial oxygen saturation; *SvO_2,* mixed venous oxygen saturation.

decision-making. Decreased SvO_2 and $ScvO_2$ values result from a failure to deliver adequate oxygen to the tissues or increased oxygen consumption. Physiologic reasons for elevated SvO_2 and $ScvO_2$ include:

1. Shunting, either intravascular or intracardiac, does not allow the tissues to be exposed to the oxygen being delivered to the tissue bed.
2. A shift of the oxyhemoglobin dissociation curve to the left results in an increased affinity of hemoglobin for oxygen.
3. An increased diffusion distance between the capillaries and cells is present because of interstitial edema.
4. Cells are unable to use the oxygen being delivered, a frequent phenomenon in sepsis.

CLINICAL JUDGMENT ACTIVITY

Describe how cardiac output affects the delivery of oxygen to tissues. What parameters would be the best to monitor in a patient to assess this influence?

STROKE VOLUME OPTIMIZATION

Clinicians have struggled to find a reliable and accurate method to evaluate clinical volume status. Newer technologies have been developed to measure blood flow. SV assessment may be more reliable than static measures of pressure such as RAP, PAOP, and MAP to determine cardiac performance and the need for fluids and vasoactive medications. The first step in a hemodynamic assessment is to determine whether the patient requires fluid to optimize preload and allow the heart to pump more efficiently, an inotropic medication to improve contractility, or a reduction in afterload to improve ventricular ejection. To determine fluid responsiveness (also called preload responsiveness), a volume of fluid (may also be achieved through passive leg raise) is administered to determine if SV increases. The fundamental reason to give IV fluids is to improve preload and increase SV. Fluid replacement, either colloid or crystalloid solutions, is essential to achieve and maintain adequate tissue perfusion. If fluid volume is inadequate, hypovolemia, hypotension, and inadequate perfusion of end organs will occur. Conversely, excess administration of fluids may precipitate heart failure, especially in patients with underlying cardiac disease.

Technologies allow for ongoing assessment of SV at the bedside. These include noninvasive Doppler imaging (Uscom, Sydney, Australia), esophageal Doppler imaging (Deltex Medical, Greenville, SC), endotracheally applied bioimpedance (ConMed Corporation, Lithia Springs, GA), bioreactance (Cheetah Medical, Newton Center, MA), and pulse contour methods (Edwards Lifesciences, Irvine, CA; LiDCO Ltd, Lake Villa, IL; and Pulsion Medical Systems, Feldkirchen, Germany).

CLINICAL JUDGMENT ACTIVITY

A patient who has undergone surgery has received a bed bath, requiring turning, and subsequent suctioning through the endotracheal tube. During these care activities, the patient experiences coughing and pain. What consequences will these activities and the experience of pain have on the patient's mixed venous oxygen saturation status? How should the nurse intervene?

Respiratory Variation to Assess Preload Responsiveness

Arterial Pressure Variation. Changes in arterial systolic or pulse pressure with inspiration and expiration can be used to gauge fluid responsiveness or preload responsiveness.[37] Arterial pulse pressure is defined as the difference between arterial systolic and diastolic pressure measurements. The arterial pulse pressure is affected by three variables: SV, resistance, and compliance. Because arterial resistance and compliance do not change significantly with each breath, the variation in pulse pressure is likely caused by variations in SV. A pulse pressure variation (PPV) of more than 10% to 12% is predictive of a patient's ability to respond to fluid resuscitation. Tidal volume must be adequate and constant, requiring the patient to be mechanically ventilated and sedated to suppress spontaneous ventilation. Studies evaluating PPV have been conducted using larger tidal volumes of 10 mL/kg, which is no longer the standard of care. Studies using lower tidal volumes are needed.

Stroke Volume Variation. A variation of arterial pressure variation to evaluate volume status is analysis of the degree of variation in SV. The dividing line between responders and nonresponders with regard to fluid resuscitation is an SV variability (SVV) of 10% to 15%.[37,38] Assessment of SVV requires an arterial line, a specialized transducer, and the use of a pulse contour device such as the FloTrac (discussed later in the chapter). This assessment is only predictive in the patient who is mechanically ventilated in a controlled mode with tidal volumes of more than 8 mL/kg with constant respiratory rates. Also, dysrhythmias, such as atrial fibrillation, dramatically affect SVV because the irregular rhythm results in SV changes that are independent of respiratory variability.

Bioimpedance (SonoSite, Highland Heights, OH), endotracheally applied bioimpedance (SonoSite, Highland Heights, OH), and bioreactance (Cheetah Medical, Newton Center, MA) technologies are also less invasive ways to measure hemodynamic parameters. These methods are completely noninvasive and use transcutaneous electrodes to measure parameters such as CO, blood pressure, SV, and SVV. Noninvasive devices are being used clinically to determine preload responsiveness and guide fluid resuscitation in postoperative and septic patients.[10,16]

CHECK YOUR UNDERSTANDING

3. Your patient is hypotensive with an SVV of 15%; which intervention would you expect?
   A. Initiation of dobutamine at 2 mcg/kg/min IV infusion.
   B. Administration of 500 mL of 0.9% normal saline IV.
   C. Initiation of norepinephrine at 0.05 mcg/kg/min IV infusion.
   D. Epinephrine 0.5 mg IV push.

Doppler Technology Methods of Hemodynamic Assessment

Echocardiography that uses Doppler technology has been the most commonly used method to measure SV; however, it is expensive, requires technical expertise, and is usually a one-time measurement. Technology for bedside assessment of SV and fluid responsiveness in critically ill patients is rapidly evolving. Esophageal Doppler monitoring (EDM) uses a thin silicone probe placed in the distal esophagus, allowing the clinician to evaluate descending aortic blood flow, which provides real-time assessment of left ventricular performance (Fig. 9.22). The probe is easily placed in a manner similar to an orogastric or nasogastric tube. Some patients may require sedation to tolerate the procedure. The probe is lubricated and inserted either orally or nasally with the bevel facing upward until the depth of the catheter is approximately 35 to 40 cm. Focusing the probe entails rotating, advancing, or withdrawing the probe until the loudest sound is heard from the monitor. Box 9.10 outlines indications and contraindications for EDM.

The EDM monitor interface (Fig. 9.23) provides a variety of clinical parameters, including CO and SV, derived from a proprietary algorithm. The corrected flow time (FTc), peak velocity (PV), and minute distance are obtained from the Doppler velocity measurements. The base of the waveform depicts the FTc and is indicative of left ventricular preload. The height of the waveform represents PV and reflects contractility. Normal FTc varies by age; however, an FTc of less than 330 milliseconds almost always represents an underfilled left ventricle. When both SV and PV are normal, this is indicative of hypovolemia. When FTc increases in response to a fluid challenge, hypovolemia is confirmed. If both SV and PV are low, the problem is most likely contractility or left ventricular dysfunction. In this situation, the patient does not need fluids and may respond to medications to decrease preload, decrease afterload, or increase contractility. Table 9.4 provides interpretation guidelines for waveform and numerical variations. Because EDM is minimally invasive, risk to the patient is significantly lower than with invasive monitoring.

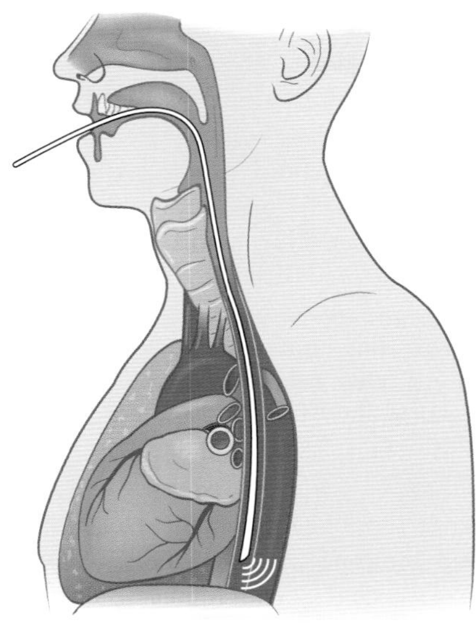

Fig. 9.22 Esophageal Doppler probe placement. (Courtesy Deltex Medical, Inc., Greenville, SC.)

BOX 9.10 Esophageal Doppler Monitoring Contraindications

Local Disease

- Esophageal stent
- Carcinoma of the esophagus or pharynx
- Previous esophageal surgery
- Esophageal stricture
- Esophageal varices
- Pharyngeal pouch

Aortic Abnormalities

- Intraaortic balloon pump
- Coarctation of the aorta

Systemic

- Severe coagulopathy

From Lough ME, Phillips R. Doppler Hemodynamic Monitoring. In: *Hemodynamic Monitoring: Evolving Technologies and Clinical Practice.* Elsevier Mosby; 2016:282-306.

Pulse Contour Methods of Hemodynamic Assessment

Several devices are available that use pulse contour analysis to determine various hemodynamic parameters, including SV and CO.[9,39] The CO derived from arterial pulse contour analysis is comparable to that obtained via PAC. Devices that use pulse

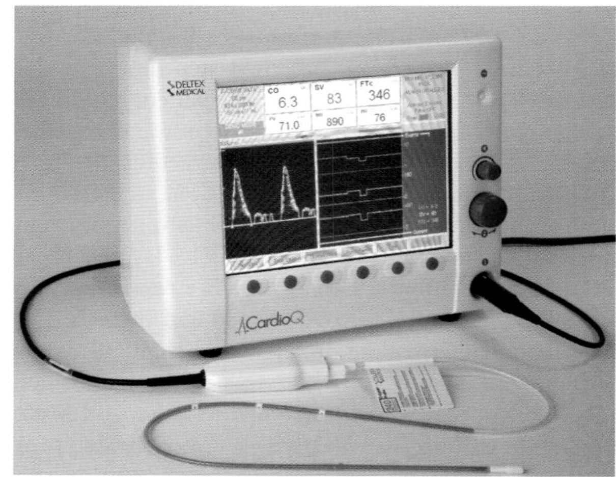

A

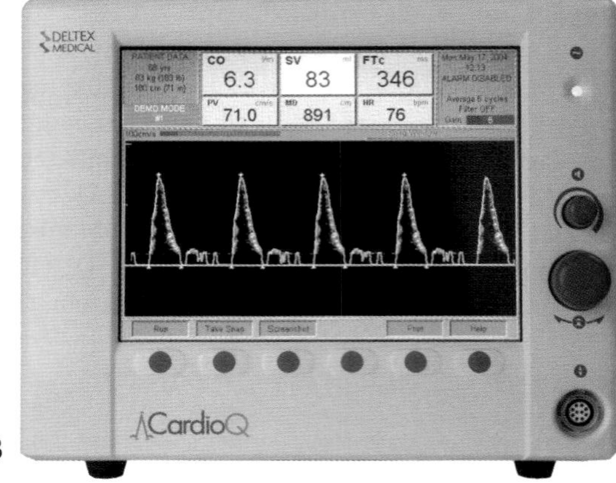

B

Fig. 9.23 A, CardioQ monitoring system for assessing cardiac output and function via the esophageal Doppler probe. B, Numerical and graphical data provided by the CardioQ device. (Courtesy Deltex Medical, Inc., Greenville, SC.)

TABLE 9.4 Interpretation Guidelines for Esophageal Doppler Monitoring

Waveform Alteration	Numerical Correlation	Interpretation
↓ Base width	↓ FTc	Hypovolemia
↑ Base width	↑ FTc	Euvolemia
↓ Waveform height	↓ PV or SV	Left ventricular failure
↑ Waveform height	↑ PV or SV	Hyperdynamic state (i.e., sepsis)
↓ Waveform height + ↓ base width	↓ FTc ↓ PV or SV	Elevated systemic vascular resistance

FTc, Corrected flow time; *PV*, peak velocity; *SV*, stroke volume.

contour analysis for assessing CO include the PiCCO (Getinge AB, Göteborg, Sweden), FloTrac and Accumen IQ (Edwards Lifesciences, Irvine, CA), and LiDCO systems (Masimo Corporation, Irvine, CA). These devices provide data for hemodynamic assessment and involve less risk than the PAC. The systems, with the exception of the PiCCO system, are generally fast to set up. They provide SVV and PPV data and are better predictors of fluid responsiveness in mechanically ventilated patients than a static measurement of RAP or PAOP. The pulse contour analysis provides an alternative to the PAC for measuring CO, even in patients who are hemodynamically unstable. For illustration purposes (Fig. 9.24), the HemoSphere advanced monitoring platform with Acumen IQ sensor (Edwards Lifesciences, Irvine, CA) provides CCO, SV, SVV, and systemic vascular resistance (SVR) data through an existing arterial line. The technology requires no manual calibration because the algorithm automatically compensates for the continuously changing effects of vascular tone on hemodynamic parameters.

The continuous measurement of SVV and PPV is only possible under full mechanical ventilation. Application of the pulse contour analysis and the derived cardiac preload parameters are limited when cardiac dysrhythmias are present. Pulse contour analysis is inaccurate in patients with significant aortic insufficiency and those with peripheral vascular disease. The use of an intraaortic balloon counterpulsation also excludes the use of this technique.

SV optimization can be used clinically to determine preload responsiveness and treat patients with low SV or low FTc. After giving a fluid challenge of either crystalloids or colloids, assess SV response. If SV improves by at least 10%, continue giving fluid boluses until the SV response is less than 10%. If no response is noted after fluid administration, collaborate with the provider to determine if other therapies are needed to correct a high afterload state (vasodilators), low contractility state (inotropic agents), or low afterload state (vasopressors).

Passive Leg Raising to Assess Preload Responsiveness

Assessing a patient's response to passive leg raising (PLR) can be used to determine whether the patient is preload responsive, indicated by an increase in SV. This allows the clinician to test for preload responsiveness before giving IV fluids. The PLR test consists of measuring the hemodynamic effects of leg elevation up to 45 degrees. The test is best performed starting from a semirecumbent position, as it allows for a larger increase in cardiac preload because it induces the shift of venous blood not only from the legs but also from the abdominal compartment. The effects of PLR occur within the first minute of leg elevation, so it is important to assess the effects in real time. Pulse contour and Doppler technologies can all be used to determine preload responsiveness with a PLR test. The maneuver is effective in spontaneously breathing patients, as well as in those on mechanical ventilation. If the patient responds with an increase in SV of more than 10%, the patient is preload responsive and a fluid bolus is indicated. Additional research is needed in the use of PLR to guide resuscitation in septic shock, as a recent meta-analysis failed to find a mortality benefit (see Clinical Exemplar).[40]

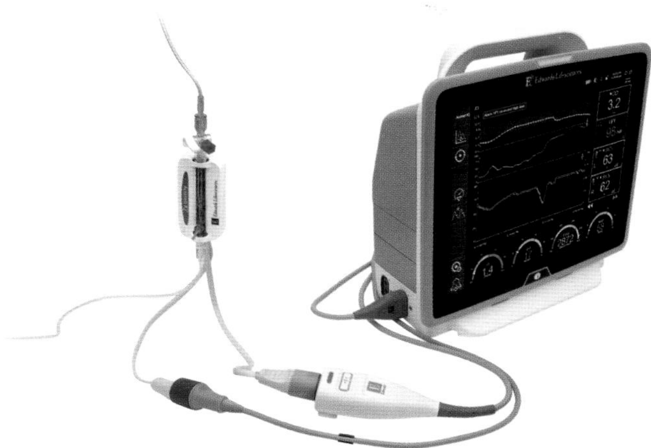

Fig. 9.24 The HemoSphere monitor and Acumen IQ sensor allow for continuous monitoring of essential hemodynamic information, including stroke volume, providing rapid insight on a minimally invasive, easy-to-use platform. (Courtesy Edwards Lifesciences, Irvine, CA.)

CLINICAL EXEMPLAR

Interprofessional Partnership

A multiprofessional team reviewing patient outcomes from the past year noticed an increase in pulmonary complications among patients who received fluid resuscitation. Based on data shared by the pharmacist on the team, there was a concern that fluid administration was not as judicious as previously thought. A nurse, who had recently returned from a conference, discussed the use of the passive leg raise as a potential solution to the problem. The multiprofessional team reviewed the literature, and based on the evidence, unanimously decided to implement the passive leg raise to guide fluid resuscitation. After educating the team at large on passive leg raise and the reason for implementing, the critical care team adopted the practice change. After 3 months, the multiprofessional team began to notice a downward trend in pulmonary complications.

CASE STUDY

A 67-year-old patient with medical history of type 2 diabetes presented to the emergency department with a chief complaint of nausea, shortness of breath, and malaise. Heart rate was 100 with blood pressure of 90/72 mm Hg. ECG demonstrated ST segment depression in leads V_{3-6}, and chest auscultation revealed crackles bilaterally. The patient was experiencing oxygen desaturation on a nonrebreather mask with subsequent intubation and mechanical ventilation with the following settings: assist/control mode, 16 breaths/min; tidal volume, 450 mL; fraction of inspired oxygen, 1.0 (100%); and positive end-expiratory pressure, 5 cm H_2O. Coronary catheterization revealed stenosis in the proximal left anterior descending (LAD) artery. Angioplasty was performed with stent placement. The left ventricle was globally hypokinetic. Right heart catheterization was performed for pulmonary artery catheter placement, then the patient was transferred to the coronary care unit. Initial vital signs and hemodynamic values are as follows:

Heart rate	105 beats/min
Blood pressure	91/74 mm Hg
Mean arterial pressure	85 mm Hg
Respiratory rate	16 breaths/min
Pulmonary artery occlusive pressure	16 mm Hg
Temperature	36.8°C (98.2°F)
Stroke volume	36 mL

The provider orders administration of 40 mg furosemide and nitroglycerin 10 mcg/min:

Heart rate	110 beats/min
Blood pressure	88/66 mm Hg
Mean arterial pressure	81 mm Hg
Pulmonary artery occlusive pressure	14 mm Hg
Stroke volume	40 mL

The nurse reports the change in stroke volume and other parameters to the provider. The provider orders to increase the nitroglycerin to 20 mcg/min and initiate dobutamine at 5 mcg/kg/min. The patient's vitals are now:

Heart rate	110 beats/min
Blood pressure	94/62 mm Hg
Mean arterial pressure	65 mm Hg
Pulmonary artery occlusive pressure	12 mm Hg
Stroke volume	50 mL

Questions

1. After reviewing the heart catheterization report and the initial hemodynamic patterns, what assumption can be made about the patient's cardiac output? What additional assessment data would assist in determining the patient's perfusion status?
2. Discuss which hemodynamic parameters you would monitor to assess efficacy of the dobutamine and why.
3. What interventions do you anticipate related to the heart rate of 110 beats/min?
4. What are your priorities in arranging nursing care based on the following options: assess arterial puncture site, pedal pulses, obtain glucose measurement, visitation by husband, completion of nursing history, daily chlorhexidine bath, endotracheal suctioning, obtaining additional routine laboratory tests?

KEY POINTS

- Driven by cardiac output, blood, oxygen, hormones, and nutrients are delivered to the tissues through an intricate network of arteries, capillaries, and veins.
- The perfusion of blood flow through the system is impacted by the length, diameter, and compliance of the vessel; turbulence within the vessel; and the viscosity of the blood.
- Cardiac output is determined by the patient's heart rate and SV. Preload, afterload, and contractility are the determinants of SV.
- Regulation of cardiac output is a complex process with neurohormonal interactions involving the autonomic nervous system, hypothalamus, pituitary gland, adrenal glands, and kidneys.
- Hemodynamic measurement may be noninvasive (e.g., blood pressure via cuff) or invasive (e.g., blood pressure via arterial catheter and transducer).
- Cardiac output is measured indirectly through an indicator over time (e.g., electrical signal, area under the arterial systolic curve, or differences of a dye concentration or temperature change).
- The accuracy of invasive hemodynamic measurements relies on the nurse to validate the patient's position, level the air-fluid interface to the phlebostatic axis, zero the transducer, and assess dynamic responsiveness.
- Oxygen consumption can be globally measured by mixed venous blood or by measurement of acid production from anaerobic metabolism (e.g., lactate). Consumption can also be locally measured in some tissues (e.g., tissue oxygen saturation). No direct measures of cellular metabolism are available.
- When compared to static measures of pressure such as RAP, PAOP, and MAP, SV assessment may be more reliable in determining cardiac performance and the need for fluids and vasoactive medications. These measures include noninvasive Doppler imaging, esophageal Doppler imaging, endotracheally applied bioimpedance, bioreactance, and pulse contour methods.
- Dynamic hemodynamic measures and hemodynamic trends may be more helpful than any single measurement.

REFERENCES

1. Hall JE, Hall ME. Cardiac muscle; the heart as a pump and function of the heart valves. In: Hall JE, Hall ME, eds. *Guyton and Hall Textbook of Medical Physiology*. 14th ed. Elsevier; 2021:113–126.
2. Hall JE, Hall ME. Regulation of body fluid compartments: extracellular and intracellular fluids; edema. In: Hall JE, Hall ME, eds. *Guyton and Hall Textbook of Medical Physiology*. 14th ed. Elsevier; 2021:305–320.
3. Hall JE, Hall ME. Overview of the circulation: pressure, flow, and resistance. In: Hall JE, Hall ME, eds. *Guyton and Hall Textbook of Medical Physiology*. 14th ed. Elsevier; 2021:171–181.
4. Hall JE, Hall ME. Cardiac output, venous return, and their regulation. In: Hall JE, Hall ME, eds. *Guyton and Hall Textbook of Medical Physiology*. 14th ed. Elsevier; 2021:245–258.

5. Singam NSV, Fine C, Fleg JL. Cardiac changes associated with vascular aging. *Clin Cardy*. 2020;43(2):92–98. https://doi.org/10.1002/clc.23313.
6. Mockridge A, Maclennan K. Physiology of pregnancy. *Anaesth Intensive Care Med*. 2022;23(6):347–351. https://doi.org/10.1016/j.mpaic.2022.02.027.
7. Maarten MB, Caroline C, Daphne M, Dirk JD, Oana S. Mechanobiology of microvascular function and structure in health and disease: focus on the coronary circulation. article. *Frontiers in Phys*. 2021;12. https://doi.org/10.3389/fphys.2021.771960.
8. Anand G, Yu Y, Lowe A, Kalra A. Bioimpedance analysis as a tool for hemodynamic monitoring: overview, methods and challenges. *Phys Measurement*. 2021;42(3). https://doi.org/10.1088/1361-6579/abe80e.
9. Pour-Ghaz I, Manolukas T, Foray N, et al. Accuracy of non-invasive and minimally invasive hemodynamic monitoring: where do we stand? *Ann Transl Med*. 2019;7(17):421. https://doi.org/10.21037/atm.2019.07.06.
10. Bein B, Renner J. Best practice & research clinical anaesthesiology: advances in haemodynamic monitoring for the perioperative patient: perioperative cardiac output monitoring. *Best Pract Res Clin Anaesth*. 2019;33(2):139–153. https://doi.org/10.1016/j.bpa.2019.05.008.
11. Muntner P, Shimbo D, Carey RM, et al. Measurement of blood pressure in humans: a scientific statement from the american heart association. *Hypertension (0194911X)*. 2019;73(5):e35–e66. https://doi.org/10.1161/HYP.0000000000000087.
12. Pagana KD, Pagana TJ, Pagana TN, Pagana KD. *Mosby's Manual of Diagnostic and Laboratory Tests*. Elsevier; 2022.
13. Marbach JA, Santo PD, Kapur N K, et al. Lactate clearance as a surrogate for mortality in cardiogenic shock: insights from the DOREMI trial. article. *J Am Heart Assoc*. 2022;11(6):e023322. https://doi.org/10.1161/JAHA.121.023322.
14. Kattan E, Hernández G. The role of peripheral perfusion markers and lactate in septic shock resuscitation. *J Intensive Med*. 2022;2(1):17–21. https://doi.org/10.1016/j.jointm.2021.11.002.
15. Richards JE, Mazzeffi MA, Massey MS, Rock P, Galvagno SM, Scalea TM. The bitter and the sweet: relationship of lactate, glucose, and mortality after severe blunt trauma. *Anesth Analg*. 2021;133(2):455–461. https://doi.org/10.1213/ANE.0000000000005335.
16. Ghosh S, Chattopadhyay BP, Roy RM, Mukherjee J, Mahadevappa M. Non-invasive cuffless blood pressure and heart rate monitoring using impedance cardiography. *Intelligent Medicine*. 2021. https://doi.org/10.1016/j.imed.2021.11.001.
17. Bolgiano CS, Subramaniam PT, Montanari JM, Minick L. The effect of two concentrations of heparin on arterial catheter patency. *Crit Care Nurse*. 1990;10(5):47–57.
18. Del Cotillo M, Grané N, Llavoré M, et al. Heparinized solution vs. saline solution in the maintenance of arterial catheters: a double blind randomized clinical trial. *Intensive Care Mede*. 2008;34(2):339–343. https://doi.org/10.1007/s00134-007-0886-6.
19. Gómez Palomar C, Gómez Palomar MJ. Comparison of the yield of arterial cannulas maintained with heparinized and nonheparinized fluids: a prospective study. *Enfermería Clínica*. 2005;15(5):262–266.
20. Jianqiu X, Tuo P, Hua J, Xiaoli X, Yan W, Dongjin W. A comparison of heparinised and non-heparinised normal saline solutions for maintaining the patency of arterial pressure measurement cannulae after heart surgery. *J Cardiothorac Surg*. 2019;14(1):1–9. https://doi.org/10.1186/s13019-019-0860-8.
21. Leeper B. Ask the Experts. *Crit Care Nurse*. 2006;26(2):137–138. https://doi.org/10.4037/ccn2006.26.2.137.
22. Maurer LR, Luckhurst CM, Hamidi A, et al. A low dose heparinized saline protocol is associated with improved duration of arterial line patency in critically ill COVID-19 patients. *J Crit Care*. 2020;60:253–259. https://doi.org/10.1016/j.jcrc.2020.08.025.
23. Robertson-Malt S, Malt GN, Farquhar V, Greer W. Heparin versus normal saline for patency of arterial lines. *Cochrane Database Syst Rev*. 2014;(5):CD007364. https://doi.org/10.1002/14651858.CD007364.pub2.
24. Ziyaeifard M, Alizadehasl A, Aghdaii N, et al. Heparinized and saline solutions in the maintenance of arterial and central venous catheters after cardiac surgery. *Anesth and Pain Med*. 2015;5(4):e28056. https://doi.org/10.5812/aapm28056.
25. Bin W, Lijuan C, Bin L, Qiongxiao H, Xuejun D. Effect of pulse indicator continuous cardiac output monitoring on septic shock patients: a meta-analysis. *Comput Math Methods Med*. 2022;2022. https://doi.org/10.1155/2022/8604322.
26. Kouz K, Michard F, Bergholz A, et al. Agreement between continuous and intermittent pulmonary artery thermodilution for cardiac output measurement in perioperative and intensive care medicine: a systematic review and meta-analysis. *Crit Care*. 2021;25(1):125. https://doi.org/10.1186/s13054-021-03523-7.
27. Scully TG, Huang Y, Huang S, McLean AS, Orde SR. The effects of static and dynamic measurements using transpulmonary thermodilution devices on fluid therapy in septic shock: a systematic review. *Anaesth & Intensive Care*. 2020;48(1):11–24. https://doi.org/10.1177/0310057X19893703.
28. Saugel B, Kouz K, Meidert AS, Schulte-Uentrop L, Romagnoli S. How to measure blood pressure using an arterial catheter: a systematic 5-step approach. *Crit Care*. 2020;24(1):172. https://doi.org/10.1186/s13054-020-02859-w.
29. Buetti N, Marschall J, Drees M, et al. Strategies to prevent central line-associated bloodstream infections in acute-care hospitals: 2022 Update. *Infect Control Hosp Epidemiol*. 2022:1–17. https://doi.org/10.1017/ice.2022.87.
30. Kaufmann T, Cox EGM, Wiersema R, et al. Non-invasive oscillometric versus invasive arterial blood pressure measurements in critically ill patients: a post hoc analysis of a prospective observational study. *J Critl Care*. 2020;57:118–123. https://doi.org/10.1016/j.jcrc.2020.02.013.
31. Headley JM, Ahrens T. Narrative history of the Swan-Ganz catheter: development, education, controversies, and clinician acumen. *AACN Adv Crit Care*. 2020;31(1):25–33. https://doi.org/10.4037/aacnacc2020992.
32. Connors Jr AF, Speroff T, Dawson NV, et al. The effectiveness of right heart catheterization in the initial care of critically ill patients. SUPPORT Investigators. *JAMA*. 1996;276(11):889–897. https://doi.org/10.1001/jama.276.11.889.
33. Bertaina M, Galluzzo A, Rossello X, et al. Prognostic implications of pulmonary artery catheter monitoring in patients with cardiogenic shock: a systematic review and meta-analysis of observational studies. *J Crit Care*. 2022;69. https://doi.org/10.1016/j.jcrc.2022.154024.
34. Radaideh Q, Abusnina W, Ponamgi S, et al. Meta-analysis of use of pulmonary artery catheter and mortality in patients with cardiogenic shock on mechanical circulatory support. *Am J Card*. 2022;180:165–166. https://doi.org/10.1016/j.amjcard.2022.06.027.
35. Radaideh Q, Abusnina W, Ismayl M, et al. Pulmonary artery catheter use and mortality in atients with cardiogenic ahock: a meta-analysis. *J Am Coll Card*. 2022;79(9):908–908. https://doi.org/10.1016/S0735-1097(22)01899-X.

36. Pinsky MR, Cecconi M, Chew MS, et al. Effective hemodynamic monitoring. *Crit Care*. 2022;26(1):294. https://doi.org/10.1186/s13054-022-04173-z.
37. Alvarado Sánchez JI, Caicedo Ruiz JD, Diaztagle Fernández JJ, Ospina-Tascón GA, Cruz Martínez LE. Use of pulse pressure variation as predictor of fluid responsiveness in patients ventilated with low tidal volume: a systematic review and meta-analysis. *Clin Med Insights: Circ, Resp & Pulm Med*. 2020;14:1–10. https://doi.org/10.1177/1179548420901518.
38. Guarracino F, Bertini P, Pinsky M,R. Cardiovascular determinants of resuscitation from sepsis and septic shock. *Crit Care*. 2019;23(1):1–13. https://doi.org/10.1186/s13054-019-2414-9.
39. Betteridge N, Armstrong F. Cardiac output monitoring. *Anaesth & Intensive Care Med*. 2022;23(2):101–110. https://doi.org/10.1016/j.mpaic.2021.10.018.
40. Azadian M, Suyee W, Abdipour A, Kim CK, Nguyen HB. Mortality benefit from the passive leg raise maneuver in guiding resuscitation of septic shock patients: a systematic review and meta-analysis of randomized trials. *J Intensive Care Med*. 2022;37(5):611–617. https://doi.org/10.1177/08850666211019713.

10

Ventilatory Assistance

Lynelle N. Baba, MS, RN, CCRN, CCNS, FAAN

INTRODUCTION

The essential nursing interventions for all patients of maintaining an adequate airway and ensuring adequate breathing (ventilation) and oxygenation provide the framework for this chapter. Respiratory anatomy and physiology are reviewed to provide a basis for discussing ventilatory assistance. Assessment of the respiratory system includes physical examination, arterial blood gas (ABG) interpretation, and noninvasive methods for assessing gas exchange. Airway management, oxygen therapy, and mechanical ventilation, as well as other important therapies in the critical care unit, are discussed.

REVIEW OF RESPIRATORY ANATOMY AND PHYSIOLOGY

The primary function of the respiratory system is gas exchange. Oxygen (O_2) and carbon dioxide (CO_2) are exchanged via the respiratory system to provide adequate O_2 to the cells and to remove CO_2, the byproduct of metabolism, from the cells. The respiratory system is divided into (1) the upper airway, (2) the lower airway, and (3) the lungs. The upper airway conducts gas to and from the lower airway, and the lower airway provides gas exchange at the alveolar-capillary membrane. The anatomical structure of the respiratory system is shown in Fig. 10.1.

Respiratory System Anatomy

Upper Airway. The upper airway consists of the nasal cavity and the pharynx. The nasal cavity conducts air, filters large foreign particles, warms and humidifies air. When an artificial airway is placed, these natural functions of the airway are bypassed. The nasal cavity is also responsible for voice resonance, smell, and the sneeze reflex. The throat, or pharynx, transports both air and food.

Lower Airway. The lower airway consists of the larynx, trachea, right and left mainstem bronchi, bronchioles, and alveoli. The larynx is the narrowest part of the conducting airways in adults and contains the vocal cords. The larynx is partly covered by the epiglottis, which prevents aspiration of food, liquid, or saliva into the lungs during swallowing. The passage through the vocal cords is the glottis (Fig. 10.2).

The trachea warms, humidifies, and filters air. Cilia in the trachea propel mucus and foreign material upward through the airway. At approximately the level of the fifth thoracic vertebra (sternal angle, or angle of Louis), the trachea branches into the right and left mainstem bronchi, which conduct air to the respective lungs. This bifurcation is referred to as the *carina*. The right mainstem bronchus is shorter, wider, and straighter than the left. The bronchi further branch into the bronchioles and finally the terminal bronchioles, which supply air to the alveoli. Mucosal cells in the bronchi secrete mucus that lubricates the airway and traps foreign materials, which are moved by the cilia upward to be expectorated or swallowed.

The alveoli are the distal airway structures and are responsible for gas exchange at the capillary level. The alveoli consist of a single layer of epithelial cells and fibers that permit expansion and contraction. The type II cells inside the alveolus secrete surfactant, which coats the inner surface and prevents it from collapsing. A network of pulmonary capillaries covers the alveoli. Gas exchange occurs between the alveoli and these capillaries.[1,2] The large combined surface area and single cell layer of the alveoli promote efficient diffusion of gases.

Lungs. The lungs consist of lobes; the left lung has two lobes, and the right lung has three lobes. Each lobe consists of lobules, or segments, that are supplied by one bronchiole. The top of each lung is the apex, and the lower part of the lung is the base.

The lungs are covered by pleurae. The visceral pleura covers the lung surfaces, whereas the parietal pleura covers the internal surface of the thoracic cage. Between these two layers the pleural space is formed, which contains pleural fluid. This thin fluid lubricates the pleural layers so that they slide across each other during breathing and holds the two pleurae together because it creates surface tension, an attractive force between liquid molecules. It is this surface tension between the two pleurae, opposing the tendency of the elastic lung to want to collapse, that leads to a pressure of −5 cm of water (H_2O) within the pleural space.[3] In disorders of the pleural space, such as pneumothorax, this negative pressure is disrupted, leading to collapse of the lung and the need for a chest tube.

Physiology of Breathing

The basic principle behind the movement of gas in and out of the lung is that gas travels from an area of higher to lower pressure. During inspiration, the diaphragm lowers and flattens, and the intercostal muscles contract, lifting the chest up and outward to

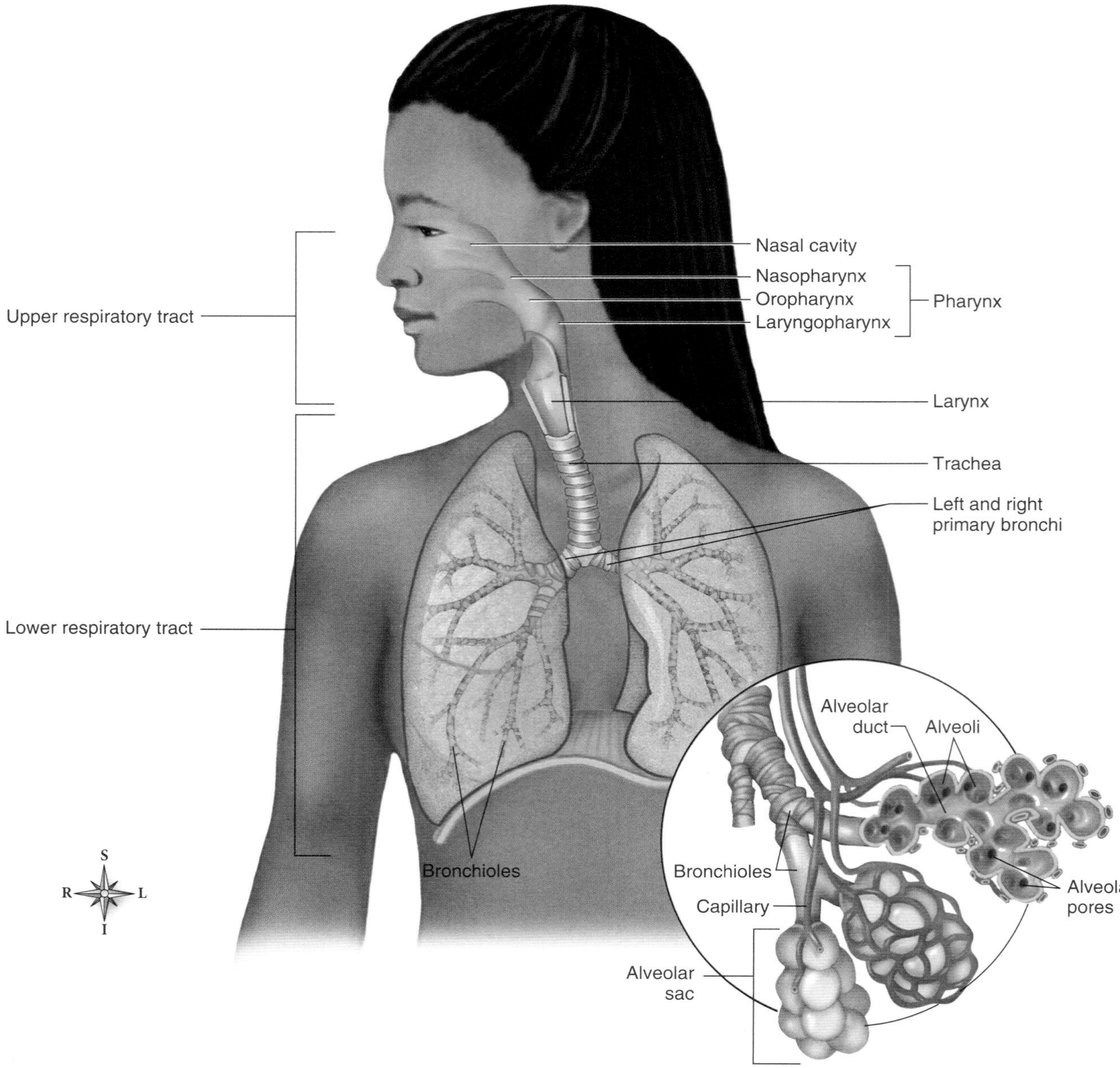

Fig. 10.1 Organization of the respiratory tract. The inset shows the alveolar sacs where the interchange of oxygen and carbon dioxide takes place through the walls of the alveoli. (From Patton KT, Thibodeau GA. *Anatomy and Physiology*. 11th ed. St. Louis, MO: Elsevier; 2022.)

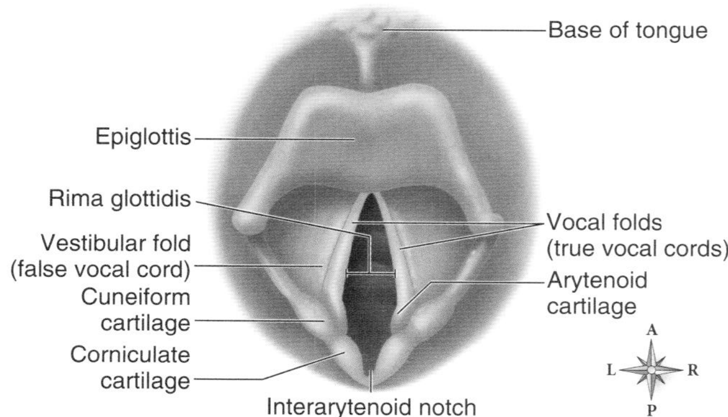

Fig. 10.2 The vocal cords and glottis. (From Patton KT, Thibodeau GA. *Anatomy and Physiology*. 9th ed. St. Louis, MO: Elsevier; 2016.)

increase the size of the chest cavity. Subsequently, intrapleural pressure becomes even more negative, and intraalveolar pressure (the pressure in the lungs) becomes negative, causing air to flow into the lungs *(inspiration)*.[3] Expiration is a passive process in which the diaphragm and intercostal muscles relax and the lungs recoil. This recoil generates positive intraalveolar pressure relative to atmospheric pressure, and air flows out of the lungs *(expiration)*.[2]

Gas exchange. The process of gas exchange (Fig. 10.3) consists of four steps: (1) ventilation, (2) diffusion at pulmonary capillaries, (3) perfusion (transport), and (4) diffusion to the cells.[2–4]

1. Ventilation is the movement of gases (O_2 and CO_2) in and out of the alveoli.

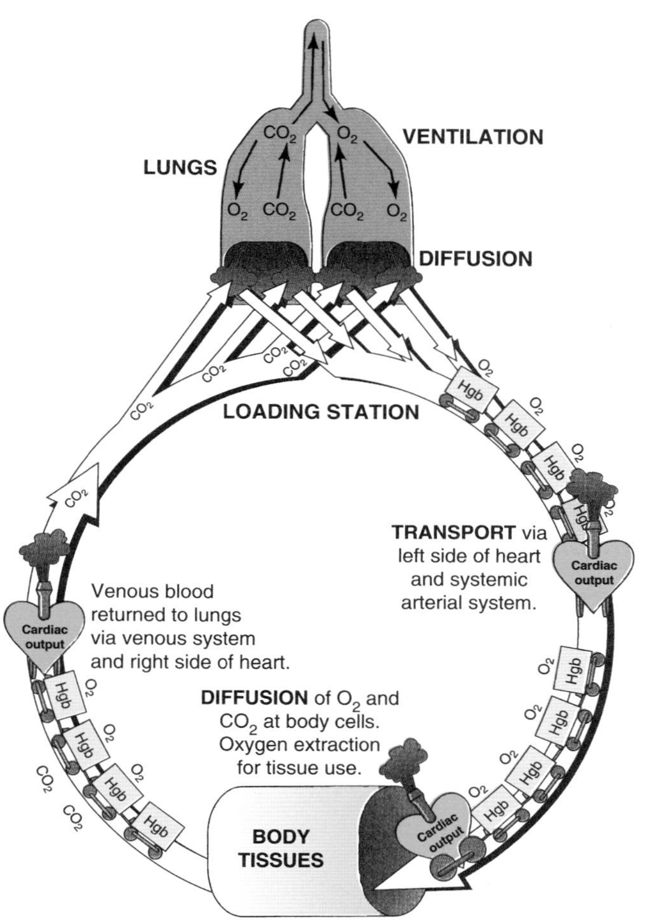

Fig. 10.3 Schematic view of the process of gas exchange. *HgB,* Hemoglobin. (Modified from Alspach J. *AACN Instructor's Resource Manual for AACN Core Curriculum for Critical Care Nursing.* 4th ed. Philadelphia, PA: Saunders; 1992.)

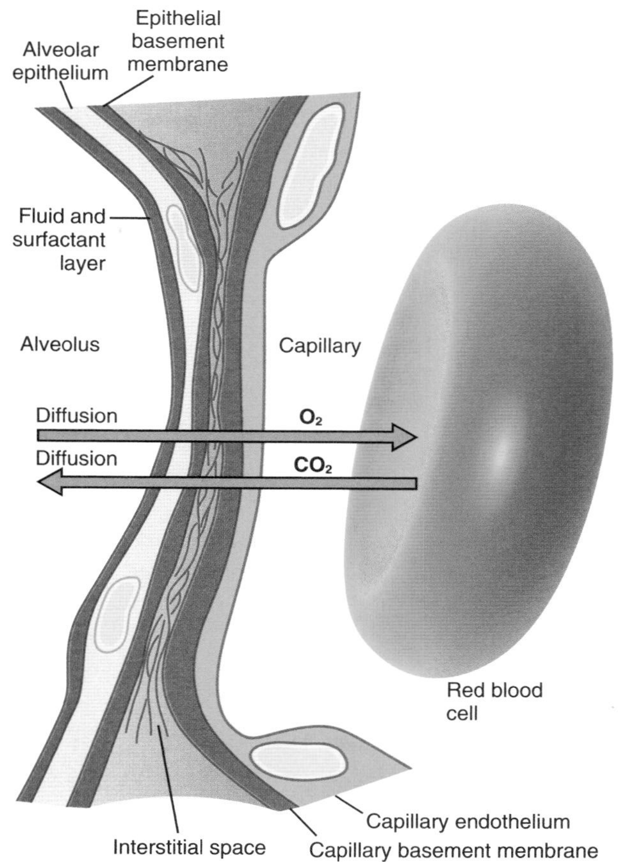

Fig. 10.4 Diffusion of oxygen and carbon dioxide at the alveolar-capillary membrane. (From Hall JE. *Guyton and Hall Textbook of Medical Physiology.* 14th ed. Philadelphia, PA: Saunders; 2021.)

2. Diffusion of O_2 and CO_2 occurs at the alveolar-capillary membrane (Fig. 10.4). The driving force to move gas from the alveoli to the capillary, and vice versa, is the difference in gas pressure across the alveolar-capillary membrane. Gas molecules move from an area of higher to lower pressure via the process of diffusion. Oxygen pressure is higher in the alveoli than in the capillaries, thus promoting O_2 diffusion from the alveoli into the blood. Carbon dioxide pressure is higher in the capillaries, thus promoting diffusion of CO_2 into the alveoli for elimination during exhalation.
3. The oxygenated blood in the pulmonary capillary is transported via the pulmonary vein to the left side of the heart, where it is then perfused, or transported to the tissues.
4. Diffusion of O_2 and CO_2 because of pressure gradients occurs at the cellular level, too. Oxygen diffuses from blood into the cells, and CO_2 leaves the cells and diffuses into the blood in a process called *internal respiration.* Carbon dioxide is transported via the vena cava to the right side of the heart and into the pulmonary capillaries, where it diffuses into the alveoli and is eliminated through exhalation.

CLINICAL JUDGMENT ACTIVITY

Based on your knowledge of clinical disorders, determine clinical conditions that could cause problems with the following steps in gas exchange:

1. Ventilation
2. Diffusion
3. Perfusion (transportation)

Regulation of Breathing. The rate, depth, and rhythm of ventilation are controlled by respiratory centers in the medulla and pons. When the CO_2 level is high or the O_2 level is low, chemoreceptors in the respiratory center, carotid arteries, and aorta send messages to the medulla to regulate respiration. In persons with normal lung function, high levels of CO_2 stimulate respiration. However, patients with chronic obstructive pulmonary disease (COPD) maintain higher levels of CO_2 as a baseline, and their ventilatory drive in response to increased CO_2 levels is blunted. In these patients, the stimulus to breathe is hypoxemia, a low level of O_2 in the blood.

Respiratory Mechanics

Work of breathing. The work of breathing (WOB) is the amount of effort required for the maintenance of a given level of ventilation. When the lungs are not diseased, the respiratory muscles can manage the WOB, and the respirations are unlabored. When lung disease is present, the respiratory pattern changes to manage the increased WOB, and the patient may use accessory muscles. As the WOB increases, more energy is expended to achieve adequate ventilation, which requires more oxygen and glucose to be consumed. If the WOB becomes too high, the muscles fatigue, respiratory failure ensues, and mechanical ventilatory support is warranted.[3–5]

Compliance. Compliance is a measure of the distensibility, or stretchability, of the lung and chest wall. The lungs are primarily made up of elastin and collagen fibers that, in disease states, become less elastic, leading to so-called stiff lungs. *Distensibility* refers to how easily the lung is stretched when the respiratory muscles work and expand the thoracic cavity. *Compliance,* a clinical measurement of the lung's distensibility, is defined as the change in lung volume per unit of pressure change.[2,5]

Various pathological conditions such as pulmonary fibrosis, acute respiratory distress syndrome (ARDS), and pulmonary edema lead to low pulmonary compliance. In these situations the patient must generate more work to breathe to create negative pressure to inflate the stiff lungs. Compliance is also decreased in obesity secondary to the increased mass of the chest wall.

In emphysema, destruction of lung tissue and enlarged air spaces cause the lungs to lose their elasticity, which increases compliance. The lungs are more distensible in this situation and require lower pressures for ventilation but may collapse during expiration, causing air to become trapped in the distal airways.

Monitoring changes in compliance provides an objective clinical indicator of changes in the patient's lung condition and ability to ventilate, especially the mechanically ventilated patient with decreased lung compliance. Compliance of the lung tissue is best measured under static conditions (no airflow) and is achieved by instituting a 2-second inspiratory hold maneuver with the mechanical ventilator.[5,6] Static compliance in patients with normal lungs usually ranges from 50 to 170 mL/cm H_2O.[2] This means that for every 1-cm H_2O change of pressure in the lungs, the volume of gas increases by 50 to 170 mL. A single measurement of compliance is not useful in monitoring patient progress; it is important to trend compliance over time.

Dynamic compliance is measured while gases are flowing during breathing; it measures not only lung compliance but also airway resistance to gas flow. The normal value for dynamic compliance is 50 to 80 mL/cm H_2O.[2] Dynamic compliance is easier to measure because it does not require breath holding or an inspiratory hold; however, it is not a pure measurement of lung compliance. A decrease in dynamic compliance may signify a decrease in compliance or an increase in resistance to gas flow.

The respiratory therapist (RT) or nurse measures compliance in the mechanically ventilated patient to identify trends in the patient's condition. Compliance can easily be obtained on most modern ventilators when the operator requests it using the menu options. Poor compliance requires higher ventilatory pressures to achieve adequate lung volume. Higher ventilatory pressures place the patient at increased risk for complications, such as volutrauma.

Resistance. *Resistance* refers to the opposition to the flow of gases in the airways. Factors that affect airway resistance are airway length, airway diameter, and the flow rate of gases. Airway resistance is increased when the airway is lengthened or narrowed, as with an artificial airway, or when the natural airway is narrowed by spasms (bronchoconstriction), the presence of mucus, or edema. Finally, resistance increases when gas flow is increased, as with increased breathing effort or when a patient requires mechanical ventilation. When resistance increases, more effort is required by the patient to maintain gas flow. If the patient is unable to generate the increased WOB, the amount of gas flow the patient produces decreases. Increasing airway resistance may result in reduced lung volume and inadequate ventilation.[2,3,6]

Lung Volumes and Capacities. Air volume within the lung is measured with an instrument called a *spirometer*. Lung volumes and capacities (two or more lung volumes added together) are important for determining adequate pulmonary function and are shown graphically in Fig. 10.5.[3] Descriptions of the lung volumes and capacities are provided in Table 10.1. Measurements of lung volumes and capacities allow the practitioner to assess baseline pulmonary function and monitor the improvement or progression of pulmonary diseases and patient response to therapy. For example, when the patient performs incentive spirometry, the nurse and RT assess the patient's inspiratory capacity and trend its improvement or decline over time and with interventions. Lung capacities decline gradually with aging.

RESPIRATORY ASSESSMENT

The ability to perform a physical assessment of the respiratory system is an essential skill for the critical care nurse. Assessment findings assist in identifying potential patient problems and in evaluating patient response to interventions. See the Lifespan Considerations box for information related to assessment of older patients and pregnant people.[7]

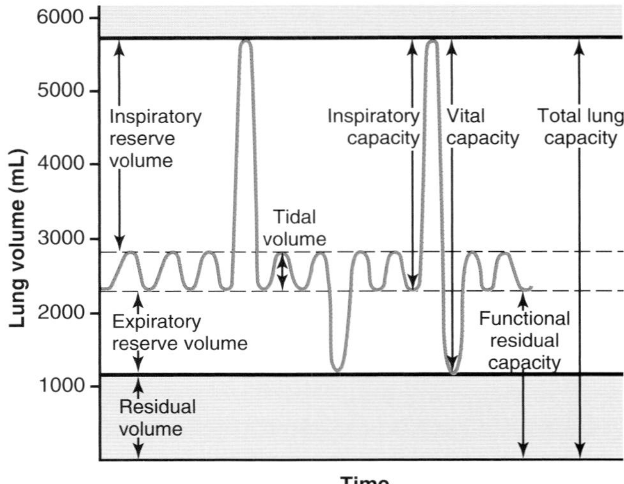

Fig. 10.5 Lung volumes and capacities. (From Hall JE. *Guyton and Hall Textbook of Medical Physiology.* 14th ed. Philadelphia, PA: Saunders; 2021.)

LIFESPAN CONSIDERATIONS[2,8]

Older Adults

- ↓ Chest wall distensibility and expansion (costal cartilage calcifies)
- ↓ Alveolar surface area (enlarged alveoli)
- ↓ Alveolar elasticity
- ↓ Vital capacity and ventilatory reserves
- ↓ Diffusing capacity
- Lower partial pressure of oxygen (PaO_2) levels on arterial blood gas
- ↓ Physiological compensatory mechanisms in response to hypercapnia or hypoxia
- ↓ Respiratory muscle strength and endurance
- ↓ Cough, gag, and exercise tolerance
- ↑ Risk for secretion retention and pneumonia, poor gas exchange, aspiration, respiratory depression caused by medications, and respiratory distress and failure

Pregnant People

- Edema and hyperemia of the upper airways
- ↓ FRC, decreased chest wall compliance
- Reduced tone of the esophagus
- ↑ Respiratory drive and larger V_T and minute ventilation due to increased progesterone
- Respiratory alkalosis with a decreased bicarbonate
- Elevated diaphragm due to the enlarging uterus (up to 5 cm)
- ↑ O_2 consumption and CO_2 production
- Common causes of respiratory failure include pneumonia, pulmonary edema, asthma exacerbation, pulmonary embolism, amniotic fluid syndrome, and pneumothorax.
- Apply mechanical ventilation as in nonpregnant people.

FRC, Functional residual capacity; *PaO_2,* partial pressure of arterial oxygen; *V_T,* tidal volume.

Health History

Ask several questions pertinent to the respiratory system when the health history is obtained:

1. Tobacco use: delivery method, amount, and number of pack-years (number of packs of cigarettes per day × number of years smoking).
2. Occupational history, such as coal mining, asbestos work, and farming, and exposure to dust, fumes, smoke, toxic chemicals, paints, and insulation.
3. History of symptoms such as shortness of breath, dyspnea, cough, anorexia, weight loss, chest pain, or sputum production; further assessment of sputum, including amount, color, consistency, time of day, and whether its appearance is chronic or acute.
4. Use of oral and inhalant respiratory medications, such as bronchodilators and steroids.
5. Use of over-the-counter or street inhalant drugs.
6. Allergies: medication, food, or environmental.
7. Dates of last chest radiograph and tuberculosis screening.

Physical Examination

Inspection. Inspection provides an initial clue for potential acute and chronic respiratory problems. Inspect the head, neck, fingers, and chest for abnormalities.

Observe the chest for shape, breathing pattern, and symmetrical chest excursion. Asymmetrical excursion is usually associated with unilateral ventilation problems. The trachea is normally in a midline position; a tracheal shift may occur with a tension pneumothorax. Signs of acute respiratory distress include labored respirations, irregular breathing pattern, use of accessory muscles, asymmetrical chest movements, chest-abdominal asynchrony, open-mouthed breathing, and gasping breaths. Cyanosis is a late sign of hypoxemia and should not be relied on as an early warning of distress. Other indications of respiratory abnormalities include pallor or rubor, pursed-lip breathing, jugular venous distension, prolonged expiratory phase of breaths, poor capillary refill, clubbing of fingers, and a barrel-shaped chest.[2]

Count the respiratory rate (RR) for a full minute in critically ill patients. The normal RR is 12 to 20 breaths/min, and expiration is usually twice as long as inspiration (inspiration-to-expiration ratio is 1:2). The normal breathing pattern is regular and even, with an occasional sigh, and is called *eupnea. Tachypnea,* a RR

TABLE 10.1 Lung Volumes and Capacities

Name	Definition	Average	Formula
VOLUMES[a]			
Tidal volume (V_T)	Volume of a normal breath	500 mL	
Inspiratory reserve volume (IRV)	Maximum amount of gas that can be inspired at the end of a normal breath (over and above the V_T)	3000 mL	
Expiratory reserve volume (ERV)	Maximum amount of gas that can be forcefully expired at the end of a normal breath	1200 mL	
Residual volume (RV)	Amount of air remaining in the lungs after maximum expiration	1300 mL	
CAPACITIES			
Inspiratory capacity (IC)	Maximum volume of gas that can be inspired at normal resting expiration; the IC distends the lungs to their maximum amount	3500 mL	$IC = V_T + IRV$
Functional residual capacity (FRC)	Volume of gas remaining in the lungs at normal resting expiration	2500 mL	$FRC = ERV + RV$
Vital capacity (VC)	Maximum volume of gas that can be forcefully expired after maximum inspiration	4700 mL	$VC = V_T + IRV + ERV$
Total lung capacity (TLC)	Volume of gas in the lungs at end of maximum inspiration	6000 mL	$TLC = V_T + IRV + ERV + RV$

[a]Volumes are average in a 70-kg young adult. There is a range of normal values that varies by age, height, body size, and sex. Volumes are less in female than male when height and age are equal.

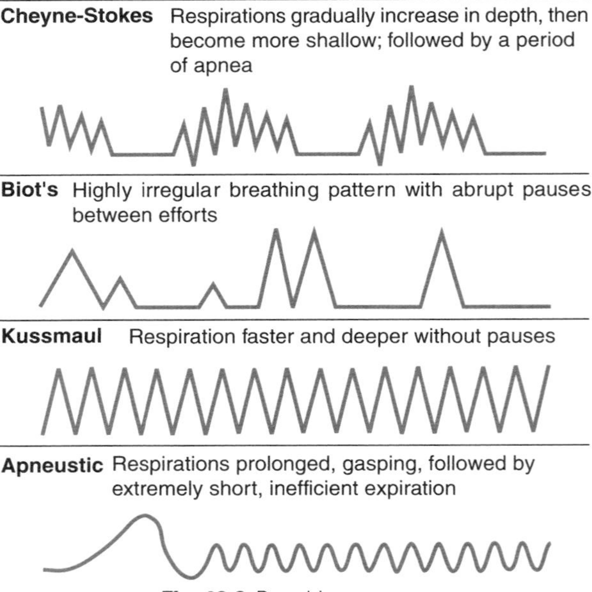

Fig. 10.6 Breathing patterns.

of greater than 20 breaths/min, may occur with anxiety, fever, pain, anemia, low partial pressure of oxygen (PaO_2), and elevated partial pressure of carbon dioxide ($PaCO_2$). *Bradypnea,* a RR of fewer than 10 breaths/min, may occur in central nervous system disorders, including administration or ingestion of central nervous system depressant medications or alcohol, severe metabolic alkalosis, and fatigue. The depth of respirations is as important as the rate and provides information about the adequacy of ventilation. Document and report alterations from normal rate and depth of respirations.

Several abnormal breathing patterns (Fig. 10.6) are possible and should be reported.[2] *Cheyne-Stokes respirations* are a cyclical respiratory pattern that occurs in central nervous system disorders and congestive heart failure. Deep, increasingly shallow respirations are followed by a period of apnea that lasts approximately 20 seconds, but the period may vary and progressively lengthen. Therefore, the duration of the apneic period is timed for trending. The cycle repeats after each apneic period. *Biot's respirations,* or cluster breathing, are cycles of breaths that vary in depth and have varying periods of apnea. Biot's respirations are seen with brainstem injury. *Kussmaul respirations* are deep, regular, and rapid (usually more than 20 breaths/min) and are commonly observed in diabetic ketoacidosis and other disorders that cause metabolic acidosis. *Apneustic respirations,* which are often associated with lesions to the pons, are gasping inspirations followed by short, ineffective expirations.

Palpation. Palpation is frequently performed simultaneously with inspection. Palpation is used to evaluate chest wall excursion, tracheal deviation, chest wall tenderness, subcutaneous crepitus, and tactile fremitus. The chest wall should not be tender to palpation; tenderness is usually associated with inflammation or trauma, including rib fractures. *Subcutaneous crepitus* or *subcutaneous emphysema* is the presence of air beneath the skin surface that has escaped from the airways or lungs. It is palpated with the fingertips and may feel like crunching rice cereal under the skin. Resist the temptation to palpate further because palpation promotes air dissection in the skin layers. Subcutaneous air indicates that air has escaped from the lungs or airways are no longer intact and may result from chest trauma, such as rib fractures, and from barotrauma.

Percussion. Percuss the chest to identify respiratory disorders such as hemothorax, pneumothorax, and consolidation. In percussion, the middle finger of one hand is tapped twice by the middle finger of the opposite hand placed against the patient's chest. The vibrations produced by tapping create different sounds, depending on the density of the underlying tissue being percussed. Five sounds may be audible on percussion: *resonance* (normal), *dullness* (tissue more dense than normal as in consolidation), *flatness* (absence of air as with an effusion), *hyperresonance* (increased amount of air as in emphysema), and *tympany* (large amount of air as in pneumothorax).[2,4]

Auscultation. Assess lung sounds at least every 4 hours in critically ill patients using the diaphragm of the stethoscope pressed firmly against the chest wall. Place the stethoscope directly on the patient's chest; sounds are difficult to distinguish if they are auscultated through the patient's gown or clothing. The friction of chest hair on the stethoscope may mimic the sound of crackles; wetting the chest hair may reduce this sound. In addition, avoid resting the stethoscope tubing against skin or objects such as sheets, bed rails, or ventilator circuitry during auscultation.[4,5]

Use a systematic sequence during auscultation, comparing sounds from one side of the chest wall with those from the other (Fig. 10.7). If possible, perform auscultation with the patient sitting in an upright position and breathing deeply in and out through the mouth. If upright positioning is not feasible, auscultate the anterior and lateral chest wall. However, take every opportunity to turn the patient and auscultate the chest posteriorly. When the patient has an artificial airway, auscultate the trachea for the presence of an air leak around the cuff of the artificial airway.[9]

Breath Sounds. Listen carefully for both normal and abnormal, or *adventitious,* breath sounds. Types of normal breath sounds include tracheal (larynx, trachea), bronchovesicular (large central airways), and vesicular (smaller airways). Be familiar with and report adventitious sounds, including crackles, rhonchi, wheezes, pleural friction rub, and stridor (Table 10.2).[5,9,10] Breath sounds may be decreased because of the presence of fluid, air, or increased tissue density. Shallow respirations can also mimic decreased breath sounds; therefore encourage the patient to take deep breaths during auscultation. Document breath sounds and report abnormalities.

Arterial Blood Gas Interpretation

The ability to interpret ABG results rapidly is an essential critical care skill. ABG results reflect oxygenation, adequacy of gas exchange (ventilation), and acid-base status. Blood for ABG analysis is obtained from either a direct arterial puncture (radial, brachial, or femoral artery) or an arterial line. Arterial blood gases aid in patient assessment and are interpreted in conjunction with the patient's physical assessment findings, clinical history, and previous ABG values. Normal and critical laboratory

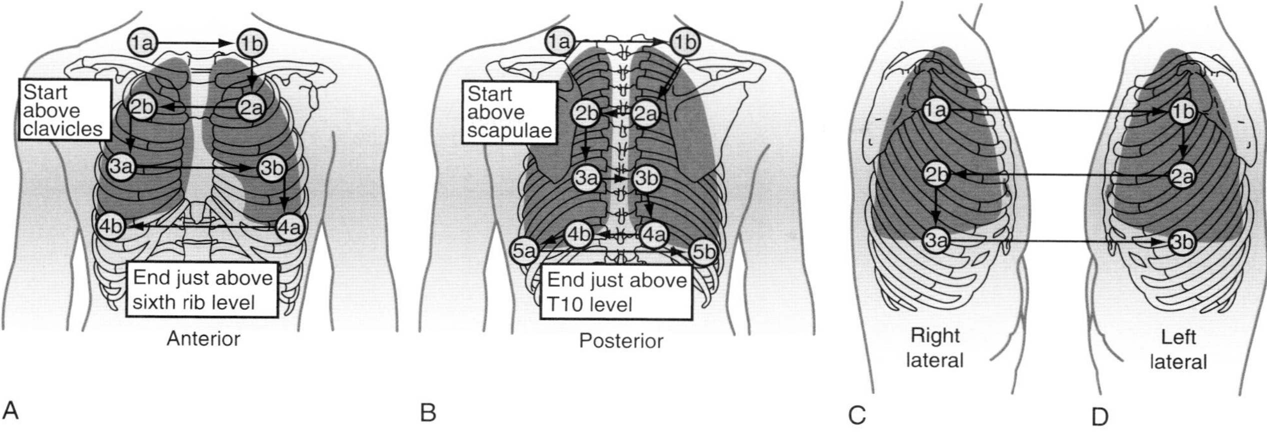

Fig. 10.7 Systematic method for palpation, percussion, and auscultation of the lungs in anterior (**A**), posterior (**B**), and lateral regions (**C** and **D**). Perform the techniques systematically to compare right and left lung fields.

TABLE 10.2 Adventitious Breath Sounds

Sound/Description	Cause	Clinical Significance	Additional Descriptors/Comments
Crackles—discontinuous, explosive, bubbling sounds of short duration	Air bubbling through fluid or mucus or alveoli popping open on inspiration	Atelectasis, fluid retention in small airways (pulmonary edema), retention of mucus (bronchitis, pneumonia), interstitial fibrosis	Fine: soft, short duration Coarse: loud, longer duration Wet or dry May disappear after coughing, suctioning, or deep inspiration if alveoli remain inflated
Rhonchi—coarse, continuous, low-pitched, sonorous, or rattling sound	Air movement through excess mucus, fluid, or inflamed airways	Diseases resulting in airway inflammation and excess mucus (e.g., pneumonia, bronchitis, or excess fluid, as in pulmonary edema)	Inspiratory and/or expiratory; may clear or diminish with coughing if caused by airway secretions
Wheezes—high- or low-pitched whistling, musical sound heard during inspiration and/or expiration	Air movement through narrowed airway, which causes airway wall to oscillate or flutter	Bronchospasm, as in asthma, partial airway obstruction by tumor, foreign body or secretions, inflammation, or stenosis	High- or low-pitched; inspiratory and/or expiratory
Stridor—high-pitched, continuous sound heard over upper airway; a crowing sound	Air flowing through constricted larynx or trachea	Partial obstruction of upper airway, as in laryngeal edema, obstruction by foreign body, epiglottitis	Potentially life-threatening
Pleural friction rub—coarse, grating, squeaking, or scratching sound, as when two pieces of leather rub together	Inflamed pleura rubbing against each other	Pleural inflammation, as in pleuritis, pneumonia, tuberculosis, chest tube insertion, pulmonary infarction	Occurs during breathing cycle and is eliminated by breath holding Need to discern from pericardial friction rub, which continues despite breath holding

values are outlined in the Laboratory Alert box. Noninvasive measures of gas exchange have reduced the frequency of ABG measurements.

! LABORATORY ALERT

Arterial Blood Gas Values[12,a,b]

Laboratory Test	Normal Range	Critical Value
pH	7.35–7.45	<7.25, >7.55
PaO_2	80–100 mm Hg	<40 mm Hg
CO_2	35–45 mm Hg	<20, >60 mm Hg
HCO_3	22–26 mEq/L	<15, >40 mEq/L
Base Excess	−2 to +2 mEq/L	−3 or +3

[a] Critical values vary by facility and laboratory.
[b] These are critical values only if they differ from baseline values (i.e., an acute change). Some patients with pulmonary disease tolerate highly "abnormal" arterial blood gas values.
CO_2, Carbon dioxide; *HCO_3*, bicarbonate; *PaO_2*, partial pressure of arterial oxygen.

Oxygenation. The ABG values that reflect oxygenation include the partial pressure of arterial oxygen (PaO_2) and the arterial oxygen saturation of hemoglobin (SaO_2). Approximately 3% of the available oxygen is dissolved in plasma. The remaining 97% of the oxygen attaches to hemoglobin in red blood cells, forming oxyhemoglobin.[2,3]

Partial pressure of arterial oxygen. The normal PaO_2 is 80 to 100 mm Hg at sea level. The PaO_2 decreases in older adults; the value for persons 60 to 80 years of age usually ranges from 60 to 80 mm Hg.

Arterial oxygen saturation of hemoglobin. The SaO_2 is the percentage of hemoglobin saturated with oxygen and is normally 92% to 99%. The SaO_2 is very important because it represents the primary way oxygen is transported to the tissues. The SaO_2 is measured directly from an arterial blood sample or continuously monitored indirectly with the use of a pulse oximeter (SpO_2).

Both the PaO_2 and the SaO_2 are used to assess oxygenation. Decreased oxygenation of arterial blood (PaO_2 <60 mm Hg) is

BOX 10.1 Signs and Symptoms of Hypoxemia

Integumentary System
- Pallor
- Cool, dry
- Cyanosis (late)
- Diaphoresis (late)

Respiratory System
- Dyspnea
- Tachypnea
- Use of accessory muscles

Cardiovascular System
- Tachycardia
- Dysrhythmias
- Chest pain
- Hypertension early, followed by hypotension
- Increased heart rate early, followed by decreased heart rate

Central Nervous System
- Anxiety
- Restlessness
- Confusion
- Fatigue
- Combativeness/agitation
- Coma

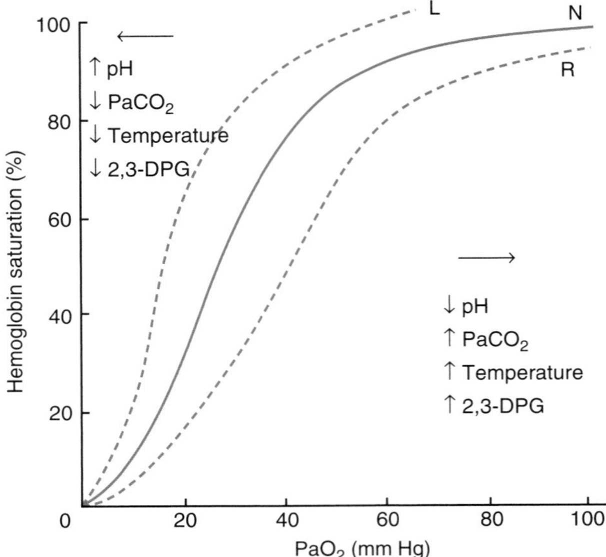

Fig. 10.8 Oxyhemoglobin dissociation curve. A partial pressure of oxygen *(PaO_2)* of 60 mm Hg correlates with an oxygen saturation of 90%. When the PaO_2 falls below 60 mm Hg, small changes in PaO_2 are reflected in large changes in oxygen saturation. Shifts in the oxyhemoglobin curve are shown. *L,* Left shift; *N,* normal; *R,* right shift. (From Weinberger SE, Cockrill BA, Mandel J. *Principles of Pulmonary Medicine.* 7th ed. Philadelphia, PA: Elsevier; 2019.)

referred to as *hypoxemia,* which may present with numerous symptoms, which are described in Box 10.1. A patient with a PaO_2 of less than 60 mm Hg requires immediate intervention with supplemental oxygen to treat the hypoxemia while further assessment is done to identify the cause. A PaO_2 of less than 40 mm Hg is life-threatening because oxygen is not available for metabolism. Without treatment, cellular death will occur.[1–3,6]

The relationship between the PaO_2 and the SaO_2 is shown in the S-shaped *oxyhemoglobin dissociation curve* (Fig. 10.8). The upper portion of the curve (PaO_2 >60 mm Hg) is flat. In this area of the curve, large changes in the PaO_2 result in only small changes in SaO_2. For example, the normal PaO_2 of 80 to 100 mm Hg is associated with an SaO_2 of 92% to 100%. If the PaO_2 decreases from 80 to 60 mm Hg, the SaO_2 decreases from 92% to 90%. Although this example reflects a drop in PaO_2, the patient is not immediately compromised because the hemoglobin responsible for carrying oxygen to all the tissues is still well saturated with oxygen.

The critical zone of the oxyhemoglobin dissociation curve occurs when the PaO_2 decreases to less than 60 mm Hg. At this point, the curve slopes sharply, and small changes in PaO_2 are reflected in large changes in the oxygen saturation (SpO_2). These changes in SaO_2 may cause a significant decrease in oxygen delivered to the tissues.[3,6,11]

As shown in Fig. 10.8, the oxyhemoglobin dissociation curve may shift under certain conditions. When the curve shifts to the right, a decreased hemoglobin affinity for oxygen exists; therefore oxygen is more readily released to the tissues. Conditions that cause a right shift include acidemia, increased temperature, and increased levels of the glucose metabolite 2,3-diphosphoglycerate (2,3-DPG), which occurs in anemia, chronic hypoxemia, and low cardiac output states. When conditions exist where the curve has shifted to the right, at any given saturation, the PaO_2 is higher than expected at the normal curve.[2]

When the curve shifts to the left, hemoglobin affinity for oxygen increases, and hemoglobin clings to oxygen. Conditions that cause a left shift include alkalemia, decreased temperature, high altitude, carbon monoxide poisoning, and a decreased 2,3-DPG level. Common causes of decreased 2,3-DPG include administration of stored bank blood, sepsis, and hypophosphatemia.[2,6] With a left shift, at any given saturation, the PaO_2 is lower than expected at the normal curve. If the patient's SpO_2 is 92%, obtain an ABG to assess for hypoxemia.

Ventilation and Acid-Base Status. Blood gas values that reflect ventilation and acid-base or metabolic status include the $PaCO_2$, pH, and bicarbonate (HCO_3^-).[2,3,11]

pH. The concentration of hydrogen ions (H^+) in the blood is referred to as the *pH.* The normal pH range is 7.35 to 7.45 (exact value, 7.40). If the H^+ level increases, the pH decreases (becomes <7.35), and the patient is said to have *acidemia.* Conversely, a decrease in H^+ level results in an increase in the pH (>7.45), and the patient is said to have *alkalemia.*

Partial pressure of arterial carbon dioxide. The $PaCO_2$ is CO_2 dissolved in arterial plasma. The $PaCO_2$ is regulated by the lungs and has a normal range of 35 to 45 mm Hg. A $PaCO_2$ of less than 35 mm Hg indicates respiratory alkalosis; a $PaCO_2$ of greater than 45 mm Hg indicates respiratory acidosis.

BOX 10.2 Causes of Common Acid-Base Abnormalities

Respiratory Acidosis: Retention of CO_2
- Hypoventilation
- CNS depression (anesthesia, narcotics, sedatives, drug overdose)
- Respiratory neuromuscular disorders
- Trauma: spine, brain, chest wall
- Restrictive lung diseases
- Chronic obstructive pulmonary disease
- Acute airway obstruction (late phases)

Respiratory Alkalosis: Hyperventilation
- Hypoxemia
- Anxiety, fear
- Pain
- Fever
- Stimulants
- CNS irritation (e.g., central hyperventilation)
- Excessive ventilatory support (bag-valve-mask, mechanical ventilation)

Metabolic Acidosis

Increased Acids
- Diabetic ketoacidosis
- Renal failure
- Lactic acidosis
- Drug overdose (salicylates, methanol, ethylene glycol)

Loss of Base
- Diarrhea
- Pancreatic or small bowel fluid loss

Metabolic Alkalosis

Gain of Base
- Excess ingestion of antacids
- Excess administration of sodium bicarbonate
- Citrate in blood transfusions

Loss of Metabolic Acids
- Vomiting
- Nasogastric suctioning
- Low potassium and/or chloride
- Diuretics (loss of chloride and/or potassium)

CNS, Central nervous system; *CO_2*, carbon dioxide.

The respiratory system controls the $PaCO_2$ by regulating ventilation (the patient's rate and depth of breathing). If the patient hypoventilates, CO_2 is retained, leading to respiratory acidosis ($PaCO_2$ >45 mm Hg). Conversely, if a patient hyperventilates, excess CO_2 is excreted by the lungs, resulting in respiratory alkalosis ($PaCO_2$ <35 mm Hg).[2] Conditions that cause respiratory acidosis and alkalosis are noted in Box 10.2.

Sodium bicarbonate. Whereas H^+ ions are an acid in the body, HCO_3^- is a base, a substance that neutralizes or buffers acids. Bicarbonate is regulated by the kidneys. The normal range is 22 to 26 mEq/L. An HCO_3^- level greater than 26 mEq/L indicates metabolic alkalosis, whereas an HCO_3^- level less than 22 mEq/L indicates metabolic acidosis. Conditions that cause metabolic acidosis and alkalosis are noted in Box 10.2.

Buffer systems. The body regulates acid-base balance through buffer systems, which are substances that minimize the changes in pH when either acids or bases are added. For example, acids are neutralized through combination with a base, and vice versa. The most important buffering system, the HCO_3^- buffer system, accounts for more than half of the total buffering and is activated as the H^+ concentration increases. Bicarbonate combines with H^+ to form carbonic acid (H_2CO_3), which breaks down into CO_2 (which is excreted through the lungs) and H_2O. The equation for this mechanism is as follows:

$$H^+ + HCO_3^- \rightarrow H_2CO_3 \rightarrow H_2O + CO_2$$

The HCO_3^- buffering system operates by using the lungs to regulate CO_2 and the kidneys to regulate HCO_3^-.[2,4]

Base excess or base deficit. The base excess or base deficit is reported on most ABG results. This laboratory value reflects the sum of all the buffer bases in the body, the total buffer base. The normal range for base deficit/base excess is −2 to +2 mEq/L. In metabolic acidosis, the body's buffers are used up in an attempt

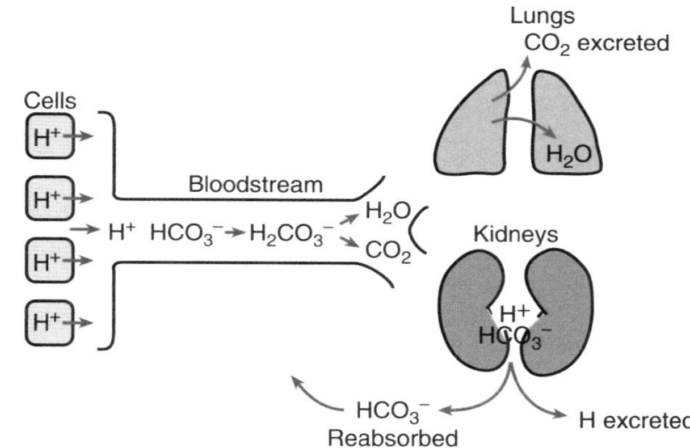

Fig. 10.9 The kidneys and lungs work together to compensate for acid-base imbalances in the respiratory or metabolic systems. *HCO_3^-*, Bicarbonate; *H_2CO_3*, carbonic acid. (Modified from Harvey MA. *Study Guide to the Core Curriculum for Critical Care Nursing.* 3rd ed. Philadelphia, PA: Saunders; 2000.)

to neutralize the acids, and a base deficit occurs. In metabolic alkalosis, the total buffer base increases, and the patient will have a base excess. All metabolic acid-base disturbances are accompanied by a change in the base excess/base deficit, making it a reliable indicator of metabolic acid-base disorders.[1,3] In pure respiratory acid-base disturbances, the base excess/base deficit is normal; however, once compensation occurs, the base excess/base deficit changes.

Compensation. Compensation involves mechanisms that normalize the pH when an acid-base imbalance occurs. The kidneys attempt to compensate for respiratory abnormalities, whereas the lungs attempt to compensate for metabolic problems. The lungs quickly respond to compensate for a primary metabolic acid-base abnormality. For example, in metabolic acidosis, the depth and rate

TABLE 10.3 **Blood Gas Interpretation**

Status	pH	$PaCO_2$	HCO_3^-	Base Excess
		RESPIRATORY ACIDOSIS		
Uncompensated	↓7.35	↑45	Normal	Normal
Partially compensated	↓7.35	↑45	↑26	↑+2
Compensated	7.35-7.45	↑45	↑26	↑+2
		RESPIRATORY ALKALOSIS		
Uncompensated	↑7.45	↓35	Normal	Normal
Partially compensated	↑7.45	↓35	↓22	↓ −2
Compensated	7.40-7.45	↓35	↓22	↓ −2
		METABOLIC ACIDOSIS		
Uncompensated	↓7.35	Normal	↓22	↓ −2
Partially compensated	↓7.35	↓35	↓22	↓ −2
Compensated	7.35-7.45	↓35	↓22	↓ −2
		METABOLIC ALKALOSIS		
Uncompensated	↑7.45	Normal	↑26	↑+2
Partially compensated[a]	↑7.45	↑45	↑26	↑+2
Compensated[a]	7.40-7.45	↑45	↑26	↑+2
		MIXED ACID-BASE DISORDERS		
Combined respiratory and metabolic acidosis	↓7.35	↑45	↓22	↓ −2
Combined respiratory and metabolic alkalosis	↑7.45	↓35	↑26	↑+2

[a]Partially compensated or compensated metabolic alkalosis generally is rarely seen clinically because of the body's mechanism to prevent hypoventilation.
HCO_3^-, Bicarbonate; *$PaCO_2$*, partial pressure of carbon dioxide.

of ventilation are increased in an effort to blow off more CO_2 (acid). Conversely, in metabolic alkalosis, the rate and depth of ventilation may be decreased in an effort to retain CO_2 (acid).[1,3]

The kidneys compensate for primary respiratory acid-base abnormalities by excreting excess H^+ and retaining HCO_3^-. The renal system activates more slowly, taking up to 2 days to regulate acid-base balance. The kidneys excrete HCO_3^- when respiratory alkalosis is present and retain HCO_3^- when respiratory acidosis is present.[3,10] The renal and respiratory systems exist in harmony to maintain acid-base balance (Fig. 10.9).

Steps in Arterial Blood Gas Interpretation. Systematic analysis of ABG values involves five steps.[4,5] Table 10.3 lists laboratory values associated with acid-base abnormalities.

Step 1: Look at each number individually and label it. Decide whether the value is high, low, or normal, and label the finding. For example, a pH of 7.50 is high and labeled as *alkalemia.*

Step 2: Evaluate oxygenation. Oxygenation is analyzed by evaluating the PaO_2 and the SaO_2. Hypoxemia is present and considered a significant problem when the PaO_2 falls to less than 60 mm Hg or the SaO_2 falls to less than 90%. A complete assessment must consider the level of supplemental oxygen a patient is receiving when the ABG is drawn.

Step 3: Determine acid-base status. Assess the pH to determine the acid-base status. A pH of 7.4 is the absolute normal. If the pH is less than 7.4, the primary disorder is acidosis. If the pH is greater than 7.4, the primary disorder is alkalosis. Therefore even if the pH is within the normal range, noting whether it is on the acid or alkaline side of 7.40 is important.

Step 4: Determine whether primary acid-base disorder is respiratory or metabolic. Assess the $PaCO_2$, which reflects the respiratory system, and the HCO_3– level, which reflects the metabolic system, to determine which one is altered in the same manner as the pH. The ABG results may reflect only one disorder (respiratory or metabolic). However, two primary acid-base disorders may occur simultaneously (mixed acid-base imbalance). For example, during cardiac arrest, both respiratory acidosis and metabolic acidosis commonly occur because of hypoventilation and lactic acidosis. Use the base excess to confirm your interpretation of the primary acid-base disturbance, especially if the disorder is mixed.

Step 5: Determine whether any form of compensatory response has taken place. *Compensation* refers to a return to a normal blood pH by means of respiratory or renal mechanisms. The system opposite the primary disorder attempts the compensation. For example, if a patient has respiratory acidosis, such as occurs in COPD (low pH, high $PaCO_2$), the kidneys respond by retaining more HCO_3^- and excreting H^+. Conversely, if a patient has metabolic acidosis, such as occurs in diabetic ketoacidosis (low pH, low HCO_3^-), the lungs respond by hyperventilation and excretion of CO_2 (respiratory alkalosis). If the $PaCO_2$ and the HCO_3^- are abnormal in the same direction, compensation is occurring.

Compensation may be absent, partial, or complete. Compensation is *absent* if the system opposite the primary disorder is within normal range. If compensation has occurred but the pH is still abnormal, compensation is referred to as *partial*. Compensation is *complete* if compensatory mechanisms are present and the pH is within normal range. The body does not overcompensate.[2] Examples of ABG compensation are shown in Box 10.3.

CLINICAL JUDGMENT ACTIVITY

Your patient has the following arterial blood gas results: pH, 7.28; PaO_2, 52 mm Hg; SaO_2, 84%; $PaCO_2$, 55 mm Hg; HCO_3^-, 24 mEq/L.

1. What is your analysis of this arterial blood gas?
2. What clinical condition or conditions do you hypothesize could cause the patient to have these arterial blood gas results?

Noninvasive Assessment of Gas Exchange

Intermittent ABG results have been the gold standard for the monitoring of gas exchange and acid-base status. Improvements in technology for noninvasive assessment of gas exchange by pulse oximetry and capnography have reduced the number of ABG samples obtained in critically ill patients.

BOX 10.3 Examples of Arterial Blood Gases and Compensation

Example 1

PaO_2	80 mm Hg (normal)
pH	7.30 (low; acidosis)
$PaCO_2$	50 mm Hg (high; respiratory acidosis)
HCO_3^-	22 mEq/L (normal)
SaO_2	95% (normal)

Interpretation: Normal oxygenation, respiratory acidosis; no compensation.

Example 2

PaO_2	80 mm Hg (normal)
pH	7.32 (low; acidosis)
$PaCO_2$	50 mm Hg (high; respiratory acidosis)
HCO_3^-	28 mEq/L (high; metabolic alkalosis)
SaO_2	95% (normal)

Interpretation: Normal oxygenation, partly compensated respiratory acidosis. The arterial blood gases are only partly compensated because the pH is not yet within normal limits.

Example 3

PaO_2	80 mm Hg (normal)
pH	7.36 (acid side of normal)
$PaCO_2$	50 mm Hg (high; respiratory acidosis)
HCO_3^-	29 mEq/L (high; metabolic alkalosis)
SaO_2	95% (normal)

Interpretation: Normal oxygenation, completely (fully) compensated respiratory acidosis. The pH is now within normal limits; therefore complete compensation has occurred.

HCO_3^-, Bicarbonate; *$PaCO_2$*, partial pressure of carbon dioxide; *PaO_2*, partial pressure of arterial oxygen; *SaO_2*, saturation of hemoglobin with oxygen in arterial blood.

Assessment of Oxygenation

Pulse oximetry. Pulse oximetry measures the saturation of oxygen in pulsatile blood (SpO_2), which reflects the SaO_2. The oxyhemoglobin dissociation curve (see Fig. 10.8) shows the relationship between SaO_2 and PaO_2 and provides the basis for pulse oximetry. The sensor that measures SpO_2 is placed on the patient's finger, toe, ear, or forehead, where blood flow is not diminished. Light emitted from the sensor is absorbed by hemoglobin with oxygen or hemoglobin without oxygen, providing the necessary information for the device to calculate the percent hemoglobin saturated with oxygen in the pulsatile (arterial) blood. Pulse oximetry is measured continuously in critically ill patients, whereas SpO_2 values are sometimes "spot checked" in patients who are less acutely ill. Pulse oximetry measurements are trended to assess the effect of pathological conditions on the adequacy of oxygenation and to monitor a patient's response to treatment (e.g., ventilator changes, suctioning, inhalation therapy, body position changes). SpO_2 only measures oxygenation and cannot be used to assess adequacy of ventilation or CO_2 levels.[13]

To obtain accurate SpO_2 readings, correctly place the appropriate type of sensor (e.g., digit, forehead, ear) on a warm, well-perfused area and ensure that an adequate pulsatile signal is detected. Several factors affect the accuracy of SpO_2 values. Artifact from patient motion or edema at the sensor site may prevent an accurate measurement. The SpO_2 measurements may be lower than the actual SaO_2 if the perfusion to the sensor site is reduced (e.g., limb ischemia due to vasopressors, cold or shock, or an inflated blood pressure cuff) or in the presence of sunlight, fluorescent light, nail polish or artificial nails, and IV dyes. The SpO_2 measurements may be higher than the actual SaO_2 reported by ABG analysis if the patient has dysfunctional hemoglobin, such as methemoglobin or carboxyhemoglobin.[3,11] Recent evidence indicates that the accuracy of pulse oximetry values is affected by the degree of skin pigmentation.[14] There is a greater risk of occult hypoxemia, or undetected hypoxemia, in individuals with darker skin tones. Future advancements in pulse oximetry technology will need to address this measurement error. In the interim, apply pulse oximetry, ensuring the accuracy principles of the technology, and request an ABG if the patient's clinical presentation does not match the reported SpO_2 Each time an ABG is obtained, simultaneously note the SpO_2 and correlation to SaO_2 values.

Assessment of Ventilation

End-tidal carbon dioxide monitoring. End-tidal carbon dioxide ($ETCO_2$) monitoring is the noninvasive measurement of alveolar CO_2 at the end of exhalation when CO_2 concentration is at its peak.[4] It reflects the alveolar CO_2 level, which in turn reflects the arterial CO_2 ($PaCO_2$), and is used to monitor and assess trends in ventilatory status. Expired gases are sampled from the patient's airway and are analyzed by a CO_2 sensor that uses infrared light to measure exhaled CO_2 at the end of inspiration. Both a numerical value and a waveform are provided for assessment of ventilation (Fig. 10.10).[15,16] The $ETCO_2$ sampling port and sensor are placed in the ventilator circuitry close to the patient's

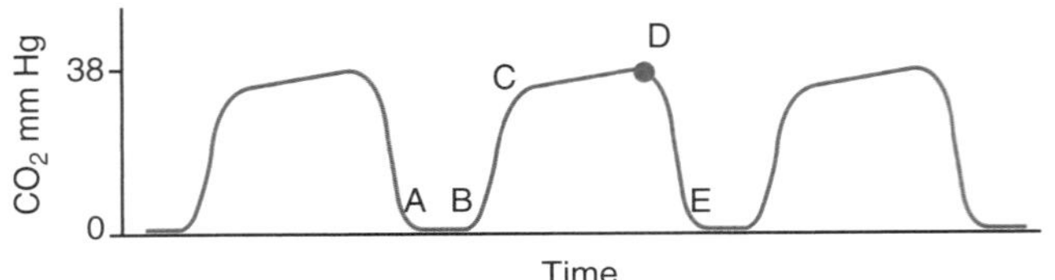

Fig. 10.10 Capnogram or graphic display of exhaled carbon dioxide (CO_2). Rise in the waveform from A to D represents CO_2 leaving the lung. Point D is where end-tidal CO_2 is measured and represents the highest concentration of exhaled alveolar CO_2.

endotracheal tube (ETT) or the tracheostomy tube. A nasal cannula with a scoop is used in patients without an artificial airway.[15]

Normally, $ETCO_2$ values average 2 to 5 mm Hg less than the $PaCO_2$ in individuals with normal lung and cardiac function.[4,15] Each time an ABG is obtained, simultaneously note the $ETCO_2$ value. $ETCO_2$ is subtracted from the $PaCO_2$, providing an index known as the *$PaCO_2$-$ETCO_2$ gradient.* The gradient is used to estimate the severity of pulmonary disease and determine the baseline correlation between $ETCO_2$ and $PaCO_2$. For example, if a blood gas shows that the $PaCO_2$ is 40 mm Hg and simultaneously the $ETCO_2$ is noted to be 36 mm Hg, the $PaCO_2$-$ETCO_2$ gradient is +4, which is within the normal range. Conversely, if the $PaCO_2$ is 56 and the $ETCO_2$ is 32, the gradient is 24, indicating significant areas of the lung that are ventilated but not perfused (dead space), affecting the exchange of CO_2 at the alveolar level. An example of a disease process that results in significant dead space is pulmonary embolism. Therapies targeted to improving the matching of ventilation to perfusion in the lung can be implemented and their effects evaluated by determining if they reduce the $ETCO_2$ gradient. Knowing the gradient also allows for noninvasive assessment of the patient's ventilation by trend monitoring the $ETCO_2$ and inferring the $PaCO_2$ by use of the gradient.[4,15] Estimate the patient's $PaCO_2$ by adding the last calculated gradient to the $ETCO_2$.

Clinical applications of $ETCO_2$ monitoring include assessment of trends in alveolar ventilation; assessment of the patient's response to ventilator changes, respiratory treatments, and procedural sedation; confirmation and continuous monitoring of proper position of the endotracheal tube, including during transport; monitoring the integrity of the ventilator circuit, including detection of disconnection; trending CO_2 in patients with increased intracranial pressure to avoid inadvertent hyperventilation; and detection of blood flow during cardiac arrest (see Chapter 11, Rapid Response Teams and Code Management).[15,17] The most common pitfall of $ETCO_2$ monitoring is believing that the value reflects only the patient's ventilatory status. Changes in exhaled CO_2 may occur because of changes not only in ventilation but also in CO_2 production (metabolism), transport of CO_2 to the lung (perfusion), and accuracy of the equipment. For example, a decreased $ETCO_2$ value could indicate decreased alveolar ventilation, a reduction in lung perfusion as in hypotension or pulmonary embolus, a reduction in metabolic production of CO_2 as in hypothermia or a return to normothermia after fever, or obstruction of the CO_2 sampling tube.[4,9,17]

Colorimetric carbon dioxide detector. Disposable colorimetric $ETCO_2$ detectors are routinely used after intubation to differentiate tracheal from esophageal intubation (Fig. 10.11). When CO_2 is detected, the color of the indicator changes, verifying correct tube placement.[10,16]

OXYGEN ADMINISTRATION

Oxygen is administered to treat or prevent hypoxemia. Oxygen may be supplied by various sources, such as piped from wall devices, oxygen tanks, or oxygen concentrators. The amount of oxygen administered to the patient is described as the fraction of inspired oxygen (FiO_2) and is reported as a decimal (e.g., FiO_2 0.5). Oxygen concentrations are reported in percentages, such as 50% oxygen. Devices can deliver low (<35%), moderate (35% to 60%), or high (>60%) oxygen concentrations.[9,18]

Oxygen delivery devices are classified into two general categories: low-flow systems (nasal cannula, simple face mask, partial-rebreather mask, and non-rebreather mask) and high-flow systems (air-entrainment or Venturi mask and high-flow nasal cannula).[10,16,18] Low-flow systems deliver oxygen at flow rates that are less than the patient's inspiratory demand for gas; total patient demand is not met. Low-flow system devices require the patient to entrain, or draw in, room air along with the delivered oxygen-enriched gas. The FiO_2 cannot be precisely controlled or predicted because it is determined not only by the amount of oxygen delivered but also by the patient's ventilatory pattern and thus the amount of air the patient entrains. For example, if the patient's ventilation increases, the delivered FiO_2 decreases because the patient entrains a larger percentage of room air. Conversely, if the patient's ventilation decreases, the oxygen delivered is less diluted, and the FiO_2 rises. In high-flow systems, the flow of oxygen-enriched gas is sufficient for the patient's total inspiratory demand. The FiO_2 remains fairly constant. In general, for delivery of a consistent FiO_2 to a patient with a variable (deep, irregular, shallow) ventilatory pattern, use a high-flow system.

The successful administration of oxygen therapy is important in treating hypoxemia. When administering oxygen, consider not only the adequacy of the flow delivered by a device but also fit and function. To ensure proper fit and function, inspect the patient's face to assess how well the oxygen delivery device is positioned and whether the airway is patent. The oxygen-connecting tubing is traced back to the gas source origin to ensure that it is connected. Finally, it is important to ensure that the gas source is oxygen, not air, and that it is turned on and set properly.

Humidification

Humidification of oxygen is recommended when oxygen flow is greater than 4 L/min to prevent the mucous membranes from drying. At lower flow rates, the patient's natural humidification system provides adequate humidity.[2,11,19] Monitor the quantity and consistency of the patient's secretions to determine the adequacy of humidification. If the secretions are thick despite adequate humidification of the delivered gases, the patient needs systemic hydration.

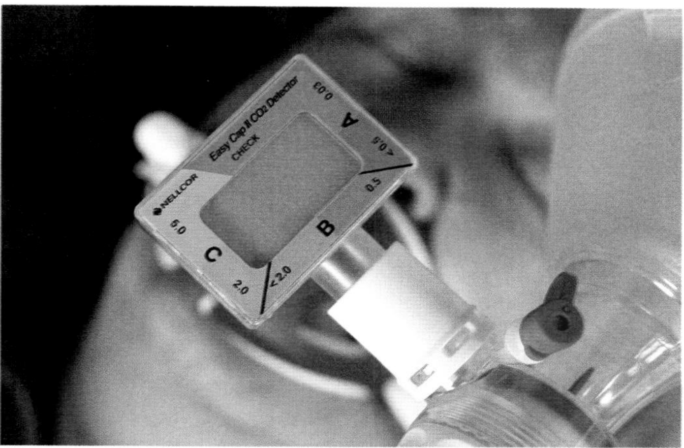

Fig. 10.11 Disposable colorimetric carbon dioxide (CO_2) detector for confirming endotracheal tube placement. Detection of CO_2 confirms tube placement in the lungs because the only source of CO_2 is the alveoli. ()

Humidification is also an important element of ventilator management. Maintain the inspired gas reaching the patient's airway at as close to 37°C (98.6°F) and 100% relative humidity as possible.[18] Two approaches are used to provide humidification. One method functions by passing the dry gas through a water-based humidification system before it reaches the patient's airway. The second method is to attach a heat-moisture exchanger (HME) to the ventilator circuit. The HME functions as an artificial "nose" to warm and humidify the patient's inspired breath with his or her own expired moisture and body heat.

During mechanical ventilation, frequently inspect the humidification unit. If a water-based humidification is used, routine checks include maintaining the water reservoir level and removing condensate from loops in the ventilator circuit. During manipulation of the circuit tubing, it is important to prevent emptying the condensate into the patient's airway. This can lead to contamination of the patient's airway as well as breathing difficulty. If an HME is used, inspect it regularly for accumulation of patient secretions in the device, which could result in partial or complete obstruction, increased airway resistance, and increased WOB.[16,20]

Oxygen Delivery Devices

Nasal Cannula. The nasal cannula is relatively comfortable to wear and easy to secure on the patient. In adult patients, nasal cannulas provide oxygen concentrations between 24% and 44% oxygen at flow rates up to 6 L/min.[10,18] An increase in oxygen flow rate by 1 L/min generally increases oxygen delivery by 4% (e.g., 2 L/min nasal cannula delivers 28% of oxygen, whereas 3 L/min provides 32%). Flow rates higher than 6 L/min are not effective in increasing oxygenation because the capacity of the patient's anatomical reservoir in the nasopharynx is surpassed. An important nursing intervention for patients receiving oxygen via nasal cannula is to assess the nares and the skin above the ears for skin breakdown. It may be necessary to pad the tubing over the ear with gauze.

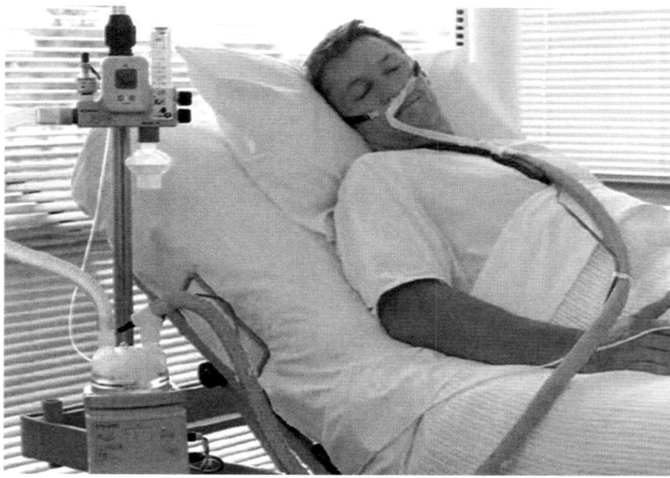

Fig. 10.12 High-flow nasal cannula setup consisting of (1) the nasal prongs patient interface, (2) a gas delivery device that regulates fraction of inspired oxygen (FiO_2), and (3) a humidifier. (Courtesy Fisher & Paykel Healthcare, Inc., Irvine, California.)

High-Flow Nasal Cannula. Oxygen delivered at rates ranging from 15 to 60 L/min is known as *high-flow therapy* and historically has been delivered with face masks. However, the delivery of high-flow therapy, which provides high concentrations of oxygen ranging from 60% to 90% and greater, is possible through a specifically designed high-flow nasal cannula (HFNC) and high-flow system that heats and humidifies the delivered gases (Fig. 10.12). Compliance with therapy is usually better with the nasal cannula because it mostly alleviates the problems associated with standard oxygen therapy, such as dry nose, dry throat, and nasal pain, and the patient can eat, drink, and talk. The high-flow system fills the patient's pharynx so that it becomes a reservoir of oxygen and generates low levels of positive end-expiratory pressure (PEEP) of approximately 1 cm H_2O for every 10 L/min of flow, preventing the cyclical opening and collapsing of the alveoli, thereby improving oxygenation.[18] The high flow rate also flushes expired CO_2 from the upper airway, which may explain why the patient's WOB may be decreased.[21,22] The humidification and heating of air preserve the consistency and volume of respiratory secretions as well as the mucosal function in gas exchange and host defense, all resulting in the potential to maximize mucociliary clearance. The breadth of applications of HFNC has led to an increasing number of clinical trials and formulation of clinical practice guidelines. HFNC is strongly recommended in hypoxemic respiratory failure with early initiation, which can result in a reduced requirement for escalation to noninvasive or invasive mechanical ventilation.[22,23] During the coronavirus disease (COVID-19) pandemic, the severe acute respiratory syndrome coronavirus-2 (SARS-CoV-2) virus spread rapidly throughout the globe, resulting in an overwhelming number of patients in hypoxemic respiratory failure and millions of deaths. The use of HFNC increased dramatically during the COVID-19 pandemic, potentially reducing the requirement for intubation and the need for critical care beds.[24] Collaborate with the RT to ensure that the water in the system remains sufficient to humidify the high flow of gas. Additionally assess the skin under the nasal cannula at the nares, the upper lip, and around the ears for signs of pressure. Apply pressure-relieving dressings as indicated at the earliest sign of pressure.

Simple Face Mask. Placing a mask over the patient's face creates an additional oxygen reservoir beyond the patient's natural anatomical reservoir. Ensure that the mask has a tight fit and the flow rate is set to at least 5 L/min to prevent rebreathing of CO_2. Oxygen is delivered at flow rates of 5 to 12 L/min, which provides concentrations of 30% to 60%. Instruct the patient about the importance of wearing the mask as applied. Clean the inside of the mask as needed and assess the skin for areas of pressure.[18,23]

Face Masks With Reservoirs. Both the partial-rebreather and the non-rebreather masks are similar to the design of a simple face mask but with the addition of an oxygen reservoir bag. The reservoir increases the amount of oxygen available to the patient during inspiration and allows for the delivery of concentrations of 35% to 60% (partial-rebreather) or 60% to 80% (non-rebreather), depending on the flowmeter setting, the fit of the mask, and the patient's respiratory pattern. The main difference between these two devices is that the non-rebreather mask has one-way valves between the mask and reservoir bag and over one of the exhalation ports. These valves ensure that the patient breathes a high concentration of oxygen-enriched gas from the reservoir with each breath (Fig. 10.13). Set the flow rate on the meter to prevent the reservoir bag from deflating no more than one-half during inspiration for the partial-rebreather and to prevent the bag from deflating for the non-rebreather.[10,18] Either mask may be used in the critically ill patient with severe hypoxemia in an effort to prevent the need for endotracheal intubation and mechanical ventilation.

Venturi or Air-Entrainment Mask. The Venturi or air-entrainment mask appears much like a simple face mask; however, it has a jet adapter placed between the mask and the tubing to the oxygen source. The jet adapters come in various sizes and are often color coded to the FiO_2 delivered. The appropriate oxygen flow rate is often inscribed on the adapter (Fig. 10.14). The Venturi mask delivers a fixed FiO_2. Because the level of oxygen can be closely

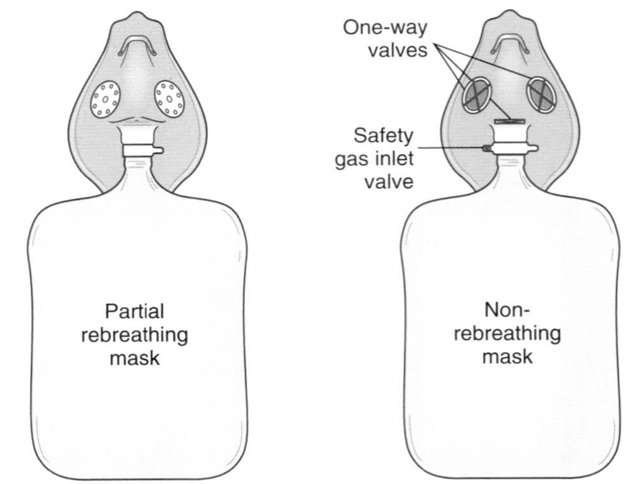

Fig. 10.13 Partial-rebreather and non-rebreather oxygen masks. (From Kacmarek RM, Dimas S, Mack CW. *The Essentials of Respiratory Care.* 4th ed. St. Louis, MO: Mosby; 2005.)

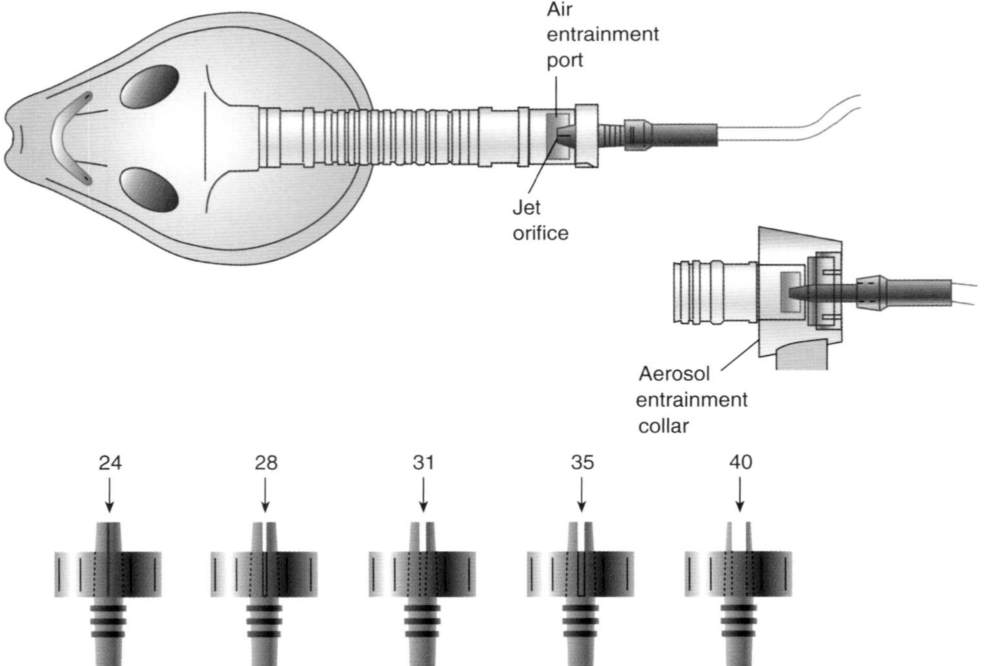

Fig. 10.14 Air-entrainment (Venturi) mask with various jet orifices. Each orifice provides a specific delivered fraction of inspired oxygen (FiO_2). (From Kacmarek RM, Stoller JK, Heur AJ. *Egan's Fundamentals of Respiratory Care.* 10th ed. St. Louis, MO: Mosby; 2013.)

regulated, the Venturi mask is commonly used in the hypoxemic patient with chronic pulmonary disease for whom the delivery of excessive oxygen could depress the respiratory drive.[9,16,18]

Aerosol and Humidity Delivery Systems. The goal of adding humidity to the inspired gases is to prevent dehydration of the airways and secretions secondary to breathing dry medical gases. The high-humidity face mask or face tent is an option for patients who do not have artificial airways (Fig. 10.15). High-flow devices used for administering humidified oxygen to patients with an artificial airway are the T-piece and the tracheostomy mask/collar. Humidity is added through a nebulizer that delivers a fixed FiO_2. Set the initial flow rate at 10 L/min and adjust it so that a constant mist is seen coming from the exhalation port.[5,9,19]

Manual Resuscitation Bag (Variable Performance). A manual resuscitation bag, or bag-valve device, is used to ventilate and oxygenate a patient manually (see Chapter 11, Rapid Response Teams and Code Management). The device is attached to a face mask or connected directly to an ETT or tracheostomy tube to ventilate the patient. When used on an emergency basis, ensure that the bag-valve device has a reservoir attached to increase the FiO_2. Set the oxygen flowmeter attached to the bag at 15 L/min.

AIRWAY MANAGEMENT

Positioning

A patent airway is essential for adequate ventilation and is a priority of nursing care. When the airway is partially or totally obstructed, the first method for reinstating a patent airway is proper head position with the head-tilt/chin-lift or jaw thrust. An airway adjunct, such as the oral or nasopharyngeal airway, may be needed to help maintain the airway.

Oropharyngeal Airways

The oropharyngeal airway, also known as an oral airway, prevents the tongue from falling back and obstructing the pharynx (Fig. 10.16A). It is indicated when the patient has a depressed level of consciousness. It may also be used to make ventilation with a manual resuscitation bag more effective or to prevent an unconscious patient from biting and occluding an ETT. It is contraindicated in a patient who is awake because it stimulates the gag reflex, resulting in discomfort, agitation, and possibly emesis. Choose the proper-size oral airway: too short an airway forces the patient's tongue back into the pharynx, and too long an airway stimulates the gag reflex.[16] The technique for inserting an oral airway is described in Box 10.4. When used, assess the lips and tongue for signs of pressure ulceration and suction the oropharynx of accumulated secretions as needed.

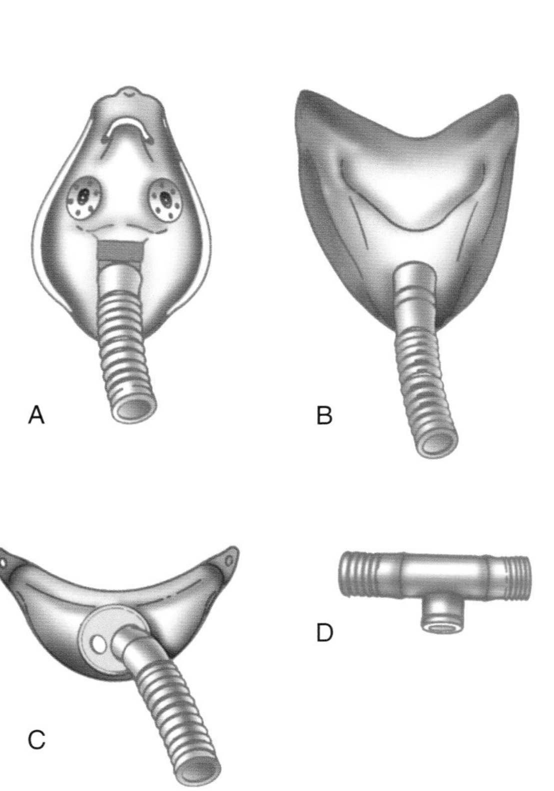

Fig. 10.15 Devices used to apply high-flow, high-humidity oxygen therapy. A, Aerosol mask. B, Face tent. C, Tracheostomy collar. D, Briggs T-piece. (From Kacmarek RM, Stoller JK, Heuer AJ. *Egan's Fundamentals of Respiratory Care.* 12th ed. St. Louis, MO: Elsevier; 2021.)

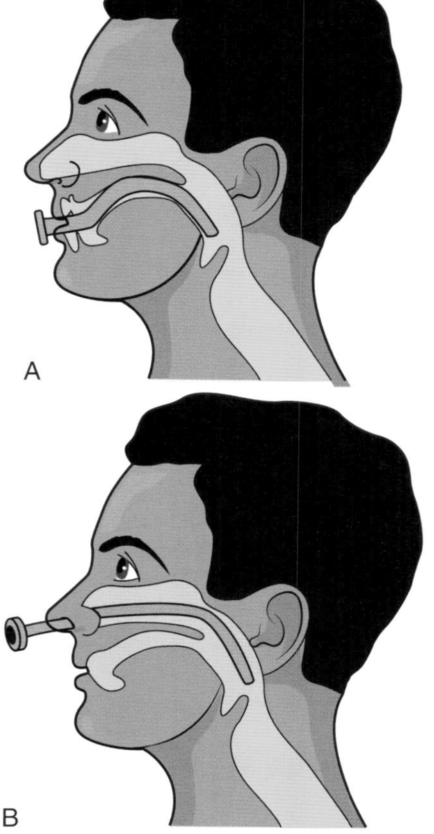

Fig. 10.16 A, Maintaining a patent airway with an oral airway. B, The nasopharyngeal airway is used to relieve upper airway obstruction and facilitate passage of a suction catheter.

Nasopharyngeal Airways

The nasopharyngeal airway, also known as a *nasal airway* or *nasal trumpet,* is a soft rubber or latex tube placed in the nose that extends to the posterior portion of the pharynx (see Fig. 10.16B). It is indicated when an oropharyngeal airway is contraindicated or too difficult to place, such as when the patient's jaw is tight during a seizure, or if oral trauma is present. Nasopharyngeal airways are better tolerated than oral airways in the conscious patient, are more comfortable, and facilitate the passage of a suction catheter during nasotracheal suctioning.

The procedure for inserting a nasal airway is described in Box 10.5. Complications of nasopharyngeal airways include insertion into the esophagus if the airway is too long, nosebleeds, and ulceration of the nares. Extended use of nasopharyngeal airways is not recommended because of an increased risk for sinusitis or otitis.[16]

BOX 10.4 Insertion of Oral Airway

1. Choose the proper size by measuring the airway on the patient. Airway should extend from the edge of the patient's mouth to the earlobe.
2. Suction mucus from the mouth using a catheter with a tonsil (e.g., Yankauer) tip.
3. Turn the airway upside down with its tip against the hard palate and slide airway into mouth until the soft palate is reached, then rotate the airway to match the curvature of the tongue into the proper position.
4. An alternative method to step 3 is to use a tongue blade to depress the patient's tongue while inserting the airway, matching its curvature to that of the tongue.
5. Advance tip to back of mouth. Ensure end of airway rests between the teeth but does not compress the lips against the teeth, which would cause injury.
6. Assess airway patency, breath sounds, and chest movement. Noises indicating upper airway obstruction should be absent.
7. Maintain proper head alignment after airway insertion.

Endotracheal Intubation

Intubation refers to the insertion of an ETT into the trachea through either the mouth or the nose. The ETT (Fig. 10.17A) is made of a polyvinyl chloride or silicone material with a distal cuff (balloon) that is inflated via a one-way valve pilot balloon. The purpose of the cuff is to facilitate ventilation of the patient by sealing the trachea and allowing air to pass through, not around, the ETT. Standard ETT cuffs are the high-volume, low-pressure type, and most cuffs are inflated with air (some tubes have a foam-filled cuff). The pilot balloon and valve are used to monitor and adjust cuff pressure.[25]

BOX 10.5 Insertion of Nasal Airway

1. Choose the proper size by positioning the airway along the side of the face. The proper-length airway extends from the nostril to the earlobe or just past the angle of the jaw.
2. Generously lubricate the tip and sides of the nasal airway with a water-soluble lubricant.
3. If time allows, lubricate the nasal passage with a topical anesthetic.
4. Insert the airway medially and downward, not upward, because the nasopharynx lies directly behind the nares. It may be necessary to rotate the airway slightly.
5. After insertion, assess airway patency, breath sounds, and chest movement.

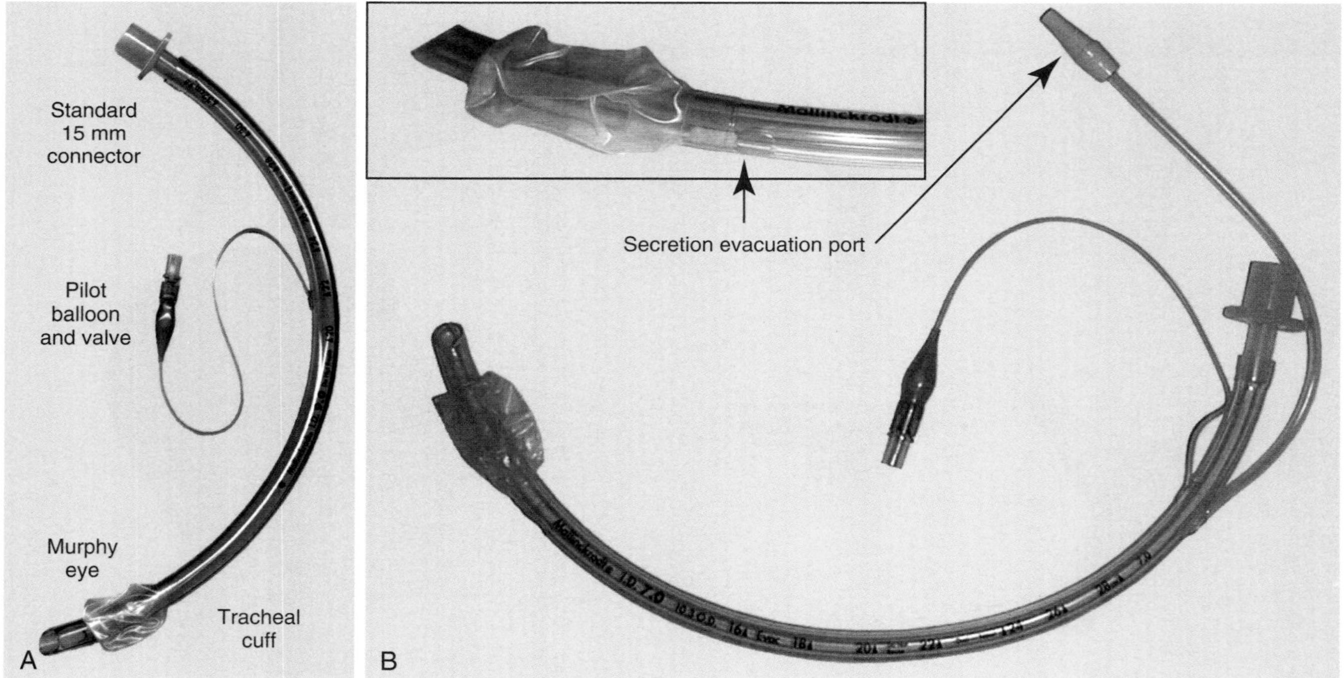

Fig. 10.17 A, Endotracheal tube. B, Hi-Lo Evac endotracheal tube. Note suction port above the cuff for removal of pooled secretions. (From Shilling A, Durbin CG. Airway management. In: Cairo JM, ed. *Mosby's Respiratory Care Equipment.* 10th ed. St. Louis, MO: Elsevier Health Sciences; 2018.)

ETTs capable of continuous suctioning of subglottic secretions have an extra suction port just above the cuff for removal of secretions that accumulate above the cuff (see Fig. 10.17B). Evidence shows a decrease in ventilator-associated events (VAE), but current data are insufficient to determine their impact on duration of mechanical ventilation, length of stay, and mortality.[26] Recent guidelines suggest considering the use of endotracheal tubes with subglottic secretion drainage ports in patients likely to require 48 to 72 hours of intubation.[27,28] Patients requiring in hospital emergency intubation and preoperative patients at risk for prolonged mechanical ventilation are reasonable candidates. It is challenging to ensure that patients who may benefit from the tube get intubated with the specialized devices, and it is not recommended to extubate followed by immediate reintubation to exchange a conventional endotracheal tube for a subglottic secretion drainage endotracheal tube. Assist in developing protocols for implementing the subglottic secretion drainage-ETT in clinical practice, such as availability of the tube on crash carts and in the emergency department. Additional interventions are required when these tubes are in place. Continuous low-pressure suction not exceeding −20 mm Hg is applied to the suction lumen. Maintain patency of the suction lumen by administering a bolus of air through the suction port as needed to relieve obstruction and maintain continuous suction.

Intubation is performed to establish an airway, assist in secretion removal, protect the airway from aspiration in patients with a depressed cough and gag, and provide mechanical ventilation. Personnel who are trained and skilled in intubation perform the procedure; these include anesthesiologists, nurse anesthetists, acute care nurse practitioners, emergency department providers, intensivists, RTs, and some paramedics. Intubation may be performed emergently on a patient in cardiac or respiratory arrest or electively in a patient with impending respiratory failure.[25]

It is important to be familiar with and be able to gather intubation equipment quickly. Know how to connect the laryngoscope blade to the handle, check to see that it illuminates properly, and change the bulb if indicated. Intubation equipment is frequently kept together in an emergency cart or special procedures box to facilitate emergency intubation (Fig. 10.18). If a patient requires intubation, notify the RT to obtain a ventilator, explain the procedure to the patient, remove dentures if present, gather all equipment, and ensure that suction equipment is in working order. During intubation, assist in positioning the patient, verify that the patient has a patent IV line for the administration of fluids and medications, and provide the necessary equipment while anticipating the needs of the individual performing the intubation.

Procedure for Oral Endotracheal Intubation. The proper-size ETT is chosen, and the cuff is inflated to check for symmetry and any leaks. The average-size ETT ranges from 7.5 to 8.0 mm for women and from 8.0 to 9.0 mm for men. It is important that the ETT not be too small because a smaller-diameter ETT substantially increases airway resistance and the patient's WOB.

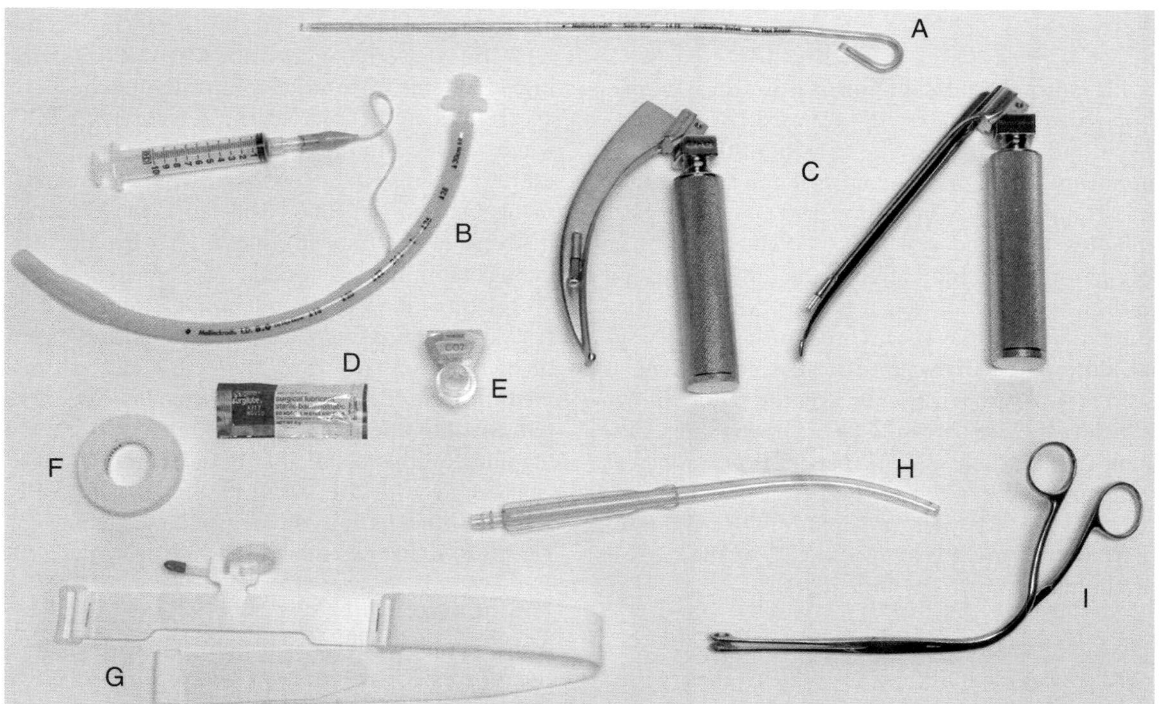

Fig. 10.18 Equipment used for endotracheal intubation: A, Stylet (disposable); B, Endotracheal tube with 10-mL syringe for cuff inflation; C, Laryngoscope handle with attached curved blade *(left)* and straight blade *(right);* D, Water-soluble lubricant; E, Colorimetric carbon dioxide detector to check tube placement; F, Tape or G, Commercial device to secure tube; H, Tonsil tip disposable pharyngeal suction device; I, Magill forceps (optional). Additional equipment, *not shown,* includes suction source and stethoscope.

A plastic-coated malleable stylet may be used to stiffen the ETT to facilitate insertion, but it should be placed carefully inside the ETT so that it does not protrude beyond the end of the ETT. The outside of the ETT is lubricated with a water-soluble lubricant to facilitate passage through the structures of the oropharynx.

The laryngoscope is attached to the appropriate size and type of blade (straight or curved) based on the patient's anatomy and the preference of the clinician performing the intubation. Blade sizes range from 0 to 4. The average-size adult is intubated with a size 3 blade. Optional equipment includes a fiberoptic laryngoscope or equipment for video-assisted intubation.

Place the patient in a "sniffing" position to facilitate visualization of the glottis, or vocal cords. Place a folded towel or bath blanket under the head to achieve this position (Fig. 10.19). Premedicate the patient as directed with a sedative and possibly a neuromuscular blocking agent (i.e., paralytic agent) to allow for easier manipulation of the mandible and visualization of the glottis. Hyperoxygenate the patient with 100% oxygen by using a bag-valve device connected to a face mask. The intubation procedure should be performed within 30 seconds. If the intubation is difficult and additional attempts are required to secure the airway, manually ventilate between each intubation attempt.

The person doing the intubation, while taking care not to damage the patient's teeth or other structures, inserts the laryngoscope blade into the patient's mouth to visualize the vocal cords. If secretions and vomitus are present, the oral cavity is suctioned. A rigid tonsil tip suction (e.g., Yankauer) is efficient in removing thick secretions and is often used. When the tube is properly inserted about 5 to 6 cm beyond the vocal cords into the trachea, the laryngoscope and stylet are removed, and the ETT cuff is inflated.[25,29,30]

Procedure for Nasotracheal Intubation. Nasotracheal intubation is rarely performed secondary to increased risk of sinusitis, otitis media, and pneumonia. The only indication is if the patient cannot be intubated orally because of oral trauma, surgery, or atypical upper airway anatomy. The two approaches to nasal intubation are blind and direct visualization.[29] The equipment for nasotracheal intubation is the same as for oral intubation with the addition of Magill forceps, which are used to guide the tube through the vocal cords in the direct visualization procedure. The naris selected for the ETT passage is prepared with a topical vasoconstricting agent to reduce bleeding from the highly vascular nares and an anesthetic agent such as water-soluble 2% lidocaine gel. The patient is positioned as indicated by the preference of the person performing the intubation: semi-Fowler, high Fowler, or supine. With nasal intubation, the correct placement level of the ETT at the naris is usually 28 cm for males and 26 cm for females.[16]

Verification of Endotracheal Tube Placement. Objective verification of correct placement of the ETT in the trachea (versus incorrect placement in the esophagus) is imperative and is performed through clinical assessment and confirmation devices. Clinical assessment includes auscultating the epigastrium and lung fields and observing for bilateral chest expansion. Failure to hear breath sounds while hearing air over the epigastrium

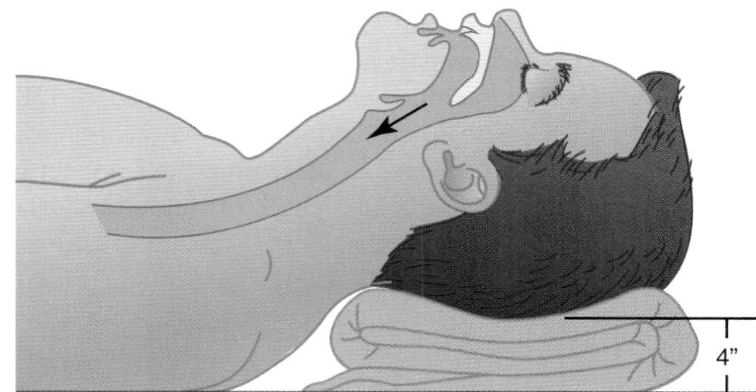

Fig. 10.19 Elevating the head with a blanket or folded towels places the patient in the "sniffing position" to facilitate endotracheal intubation.

represents esophageal rather than tracheal intubation. Breath sounds are equal bilaterally when the tube is placed correctly. Intubation of the right mainstem bronchus is common because the right mainstem is straighter than the left, and the ETT is occasionally placed deeper in the trachea than necessary. Right mainstem bronchus intubation is suspected when unilateral expansion of the right chest is observed during ventilation and the breath sounds are louder on the right than the left. Ensure that a portable chest radiograph is ordered to confirm tube placement.[10,25]

Intubation is best assessed using exhaled CO_2 analysis (capnometry) and should be performed after every intubation. If the airway is correctly placed, expired CO_2 levels will abruptly increase and may be visualized on a capnographic waveform or colorimetric display. Devices to confirm ETT placement include either a handheld or disposable $ETCO_2$ detector. The disposable $ETCO_2$ detector is attached to the end of the ETT. This device changes color when CO_2 is detected and is a highly reliable method of confirming tracheal (versus esophageal) intubation; however, the detection of $ETCO_2$ is affected when cardiac output is profoundly depressed, as in cardiac arr est.[9,10,16,25] Pulse oximetry also assists in assessing tube placement. Oxygen saturation will fall if the esophagus has been inadvertently intubated, and it may be decreased in right mainstem intubation.

The tip of the ETT should be approximately 3 to 4 cm above the carina. Once the placement is confirmed, record the centimeter depth marking at the teeth and gums or naris in the medical record. During each assessment, ensure that the tube remains in proper position as compared with the depth marking noted in the record after initial confirmation of placement. Collaborate with the RT to ensure that the ETT is properly secured with tape or a commercial device to prevent dislodging. Fig. 10.20 shows two methods for securing the ETT.

Tracheostomy

A tracheostomy tube provides an airway directly into the anterior portion of the neck. Tracheostomy tubes are indicated for long-term mechanical ventilation, long-term secretion management, protecting the airway from aspiration when the cough and gag reflexes are impaired, bypassing an upper airway obstruction that prevents placement of an ETT, and reducing the WOB associated with an ETT. The tracheostomy tube

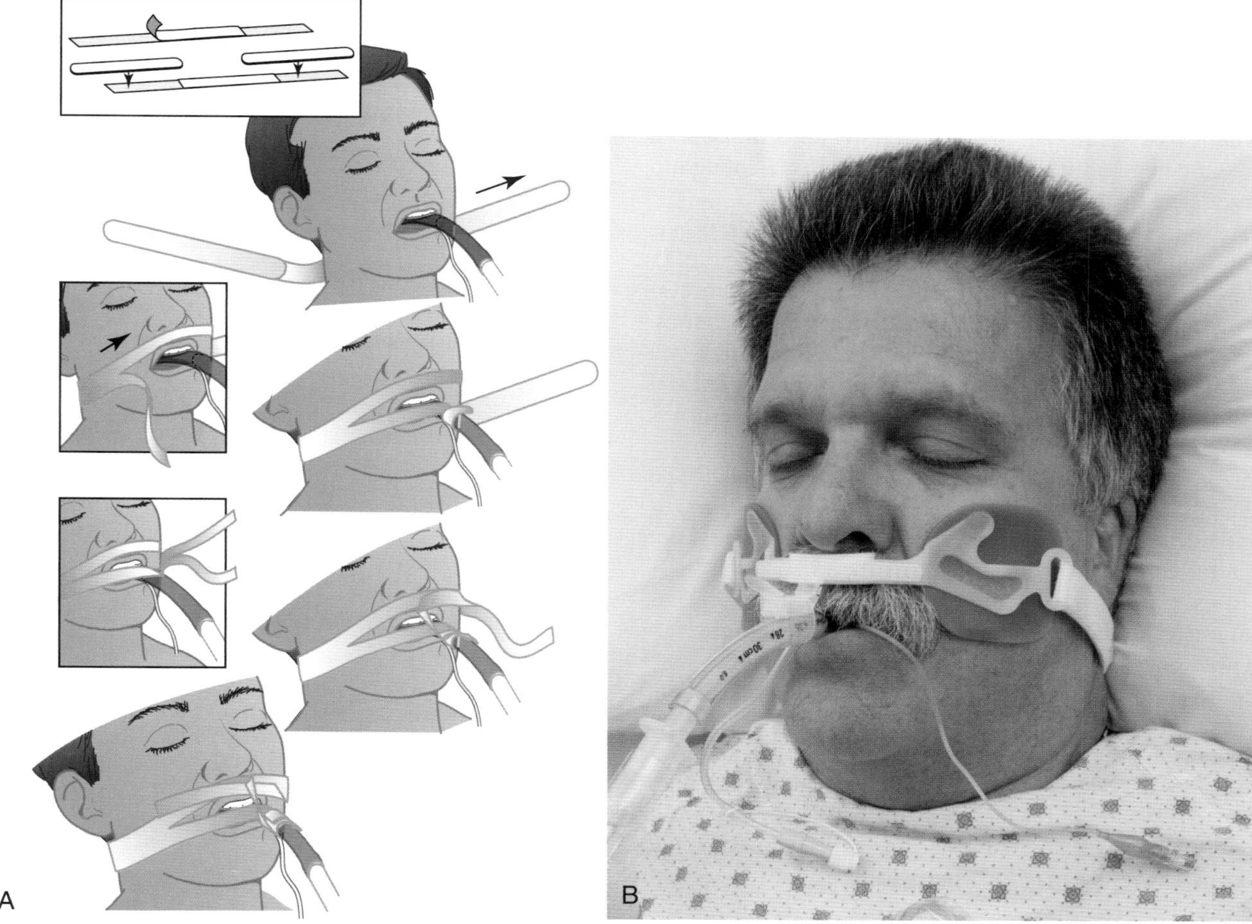

Fig. 10.20 Two methods for securing the endotracheal tube: tape (**A**) and harness device (**B**). Harness device shown is the SecureEasy Endotracheal Tube Holder. Nonelastic headgear reduces the risk of self-extubation. A soft bite block prevents tube occlusion. (**B,** Reprinted with permission, Cleveland Clinic Center for Medical Art & Photography © 2011–2019. All Rights Reserved.)

reduces the WOB because it is shorter than an ETT, and airflow resistance is less.[10,31]

A tracheostomy is the preferred airway for the patient requiring a long-term airway. It is associated with greater comfort, decreased sedative administration, less restraint use, and lower unplanned extubation (removal of the ETT). A patient may be permitted oral intake if swallowing studies demonstrate absence of aspiration. Oral hygiene is more easily performed, and some tube designs allow for talking and therefore facilitate patient communication. A speaking valve may be attached to most designs, which provides a mechanism for the patient to talk.

Optimal timing, early versus late, for when a tracheostomy should be performed is a historical controversy. A recent review indicates early tracheostomy is associated with a reduced duration of mechanical ventilation, lower incidence of VAE, and greater patient comfort.[32] These benefits are more pronounced in neurological/neurosurgical patients and are even more remarkable in patients with COVID-19, who have shown clinically significant differences in ventilator-free days, length of critical care unit stay, and hospital length of stay with early tracheostomy.[32] If mechanical ventilation and an artificial airway are projected to be needed on a long-term basis, generally defined as more than 10 days, then a decision may be made to perform a tracheostomy. The challenges are predicting which patients will require long-term mechanical ventilation and avoiding a surgical procedure in a patient for whom it may not be indicated. Furthermore, studies that evaluate the effects of early versus late timing of tracheostomy placement vary considerably in study design and definition of *early* versus *late*. A collaborative, patient-centered approach should be used in decision-making, taking into consideration the patient's and family's preferences.[32–34]

The tracheostomy traditionally was a surgical technique performed in the operating room (OR). However, a percutaneous dilational tracheostomy (PDT) procedure may be performed safely at the bedside by a trained provider. Advantages of PDT are that the patient does not have to be transported to the OR, scheduling difficulties with the OR are avoided, time required for the procedure is shorter, cost is less than an open tracheostomy, and perioperative infection rates are less. Contraindications include the inability to hyperextend the neck and patient inability to tolerate transient hypoxemia and hypercarbia. Other considerations include difficult anatomy, such as morbid obesity and coagulopathy. The PDT is performed by making a small incision into the anterior neck down to the trachea. Once this location has been reached, the provider inserts a needle and sheath into the trachea. The needle is removed, and a guidewire is passed through the sheath. A dilator is introduced over the guidewire until the patient's stoma is large enough to accommodate a tracheostomy tube.[35,36]

PDT requires teamwork, and closed-loop communication is essential. Collaboratively, the nurse and RT assist in the PDT procedure. Before the procedure, ensure that IV lines are accessible for administration of sedatives and analgesic medications. Position the patient for the procedure, including placing a roll beneath the patient's shoulders to improve neck extension, and adjust the height of the bed relative to the individual performing the procedure. Gather all supplies and ensure that sterility is maintained throughout the procedure. Monitor physiological parameters continuously, report abnormal findings immediately, and document values at least every 15 minutes throughout the PDT and for at least 1 hour after the procedure.[5,35]

The most significant postprocedure complication of PDT is accidental decannulation. When a patient undergoes a surgical tracheostomy, the trachea is surgically attached to the skin. This promotes prompt identification of the tract and reinsertion of the tracheal tube should it become dislodged. With a PDT, the trachea is not secured in this way, and a mature tract takes approximately 2 weeks to form. Accidental decannulation and attempted reinsertion of the airway during this time may result in difficulty securing the airway, bleeding, tracheal injury, and death. Oral intubation may be required if the airway becomes dislodged or needs to be replaced.

Tracheostomy Tube Designs. Tracheostomy tubes come in a variety of sizes and styles and are primarily made of plastic. Design features are shown in Fig. 10.21. The flange lies against the patient's neck and has an opening on both ends for the placement of tracheostomy ties for securing the airway. Like the ETT, some tracheostomy tubes have a distal cuff and pilot balloon. An important part of the tracheostomy system is the obturator, which is inserted into the trachea tube during insertion. The rounded end of the obturator extends just beyond the end of the tracheostomy tube and creates a smooth tip, allowing for easy entry into the stoma. The obturator is removed after tube insertion to allow for air passage through the trachea. It must be kept in a visible location in the patient's room should emergency reinsertion of a misplaced tube be necessary. In this situation the obturator is inserted into the tracheostomy to create a rounded, smooth end, promoting reentry into the stoma without tissue injury.[16]

Cuffed versus uncuffed tracheostomy tubes. Critically ill patients who need mechanical ventilation require cuffed tubes to ensure delivery of ventilation and prevent aspiration. The cuff may be a conventional low-pressure, high-volume type; a taper-shaped cuff; or it may be constructed of foam. The foam-cuff tube may prevent trauma to the airway because of the low pressure exerted on the airway, and it is sometimes used for patients who have difficulty maintaining a good seal with conventional cuffed tracheostomy tubes. Many other types of tracheostomy tubes are

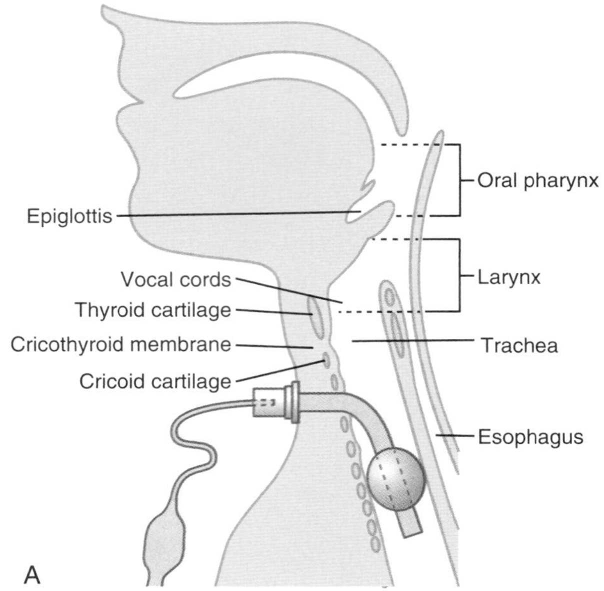

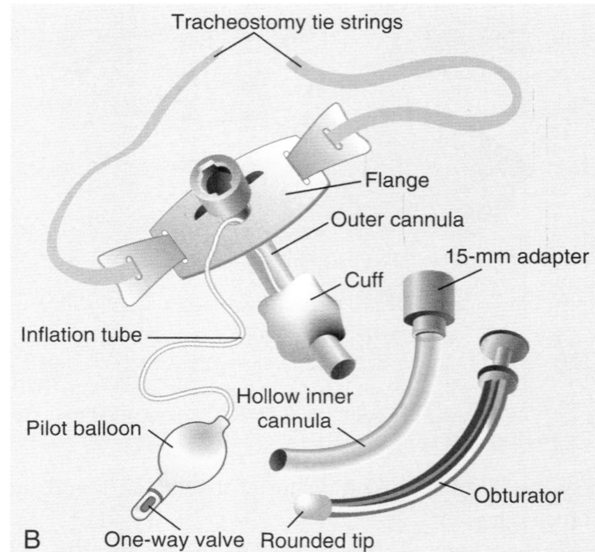

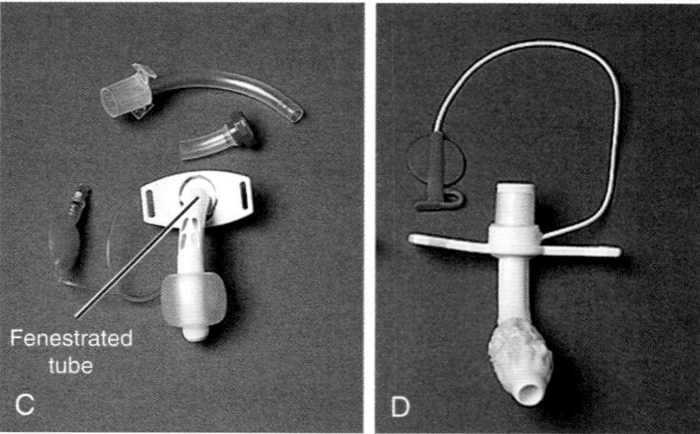

Fig. 10.21 A, General design features of the tracheostomy tube. B, Tracheostomy tube in place. C, Fenestrated tracheostomy tube (see text for description). D, Foam-cuff tracheostomy tube. (A, B, From Harding MM, Kwong J, Hager D. *Lewis's Medical-Surgical Nursing.* 12th ed. St. Louis, MO: Elsevier; 2023. C, D, From Lewis SL, Dirkson SR, Heitkemper MM et al. *Medical-Surgical Nursing.* 9th ed. St. Louis, MO: Elsevier; 2014.)

available.[29,30] An uncuffed tracheostomy tube is used for long-term airway management in a patient who does not require mechanical ventilation and is at low risk of aspiration. For example, a patient with a neurological injury may require a tracheostomy for airway management and secretion removal.[29,30,33] Metal tracheostomy tubes are uncuffed; however, they are rarely used.

Single- versus double-cannula tracheostomy tubes. Tracheostomy tubes may have one or two cannulas. A single-cannula tube does not have an inner cannula, whereas a double-cannula tube has both an inner and outer cannula. The inner cannula is removable to facilitate cleaning of the inner lumen and prevent tube occlusion from accumulated secretions. Inner cannulas can be reusable or disposable. Cuffed tracheostomy tubes with disposable inner cannulas are commonplace in the critical care unit.

Fenestrated tracheostomy tube. The fenestrated tracheostomy tube has a hole in the outer cannula that allows air to flow above the larynx. The tube functions as a standard tracheostomy tube when the inner cannula is in place. When the inner cannula is removed, the fenestrated tracheostomy tube assists in weaning a patient from the tracheostomy by gradually allowing the patient to breathe through the natural upper airway. The fenestrated tube also allows the patient to emit vocal sounds, thereby facilitating communication. To use a cuffed fenestrated tracheostomy tube for speaking or to promote breathing through the natural airway, the inner cannula is carefully removed, and the cuff is deflated. The inner cannula must be reinserted and the cuff reinflated for eating, suctioning, mechanical ventilation, or use of a bag-valve device.[9,29] It is difficult to get a proper fit for a fenestrated tracheostomy tube, which may result in increased airway resistance if the fenestrations are not properly positioned. Tubes with several fenestrations rather than a single fenestration are a lower risk. Furthermore, fenestrations may cause the formation of granulation tissue, resulting in airway compromise. Regularly assess the amount of respiratory effort the patient exerts when breathing through the fenestration.

Speaking tracheostomy valves. One-way speaking valves are available to allow patients with a tracheostomy an opportunity to verbally communicate. Although these valves can be used in both ventilated and nonventilated patients, they can be used only in patients capable of initiating and maintaining spontaneous ventilation. Examples of these adjunctive devices include the Passy-Muir Valve (Passy-Muir, Inc., Irvine, CA) and the Shiley Phonate Speaking Valve (Covidien, Boulder, CO). For the speaking valve to work correctly, deflate the cuff on the tracheostomy tube, connect the valve to the tracheostomy tube, and allow the patient to breathe and exhale through the natural airway. The valve itself is a one-way device, allowing gas to enter through it into the tracheostomy tube and to the patient. Because this is a one-way valve, exhaled gas exits the trachea via the natural airway, past the deflated cuff of the tracheostomy tube, and through the vocal cords.[29,30]

If a speaking valve is used in conjunction with mechanical ventilation, it must be used with a tracheostomy tube, not an ETT. While the valve is in place, assess the patient's respiratory stability and tolerance. Monitor the patient's SpO_2, heart rate, RR, and blood pressure; observe the patient's anxiety level and perception of the experience; and assess the WOB. The patient's ability to verbally communicate provides an opportunity for the patient to describe feelings and participate in setting goals.[37]

Endotracheal Suctioning

Patients with an artificial airway need to be suctioned to ensure airway patency because the normal protective ability to cough and expel secretions is impaired. Suctioning is performed according to a standard procedure to prevent complications such as hypoxemia, airway trauma, infection, and increased intracranial pressure in patients with head injury. Suctioning also stimulates the cough reflex and promotes the mobilization and removal of secretions.

Because suctioning is associated with complications, it is performed only as indicated by physical assessment and not according to a predetermined schedule. Indications for endotracheal suctioning include visible secretions in the tube, frequent coughing, sawtooth pattern on the flow-time waveform on the ventilator, presence of coarse crackles over the trachea, oxygen desaturation, a change in vital signs (e.g., increased or decreased heart rate or RR), dyspnea, restlessness, increased peak inspiratory pressure (PIP), high-pressure ventilator alarms in a volume mode of ventilation or decreased V_T in a pressure mode of ventilation, when the patency of the airway is questioned, when aspiration is suspected, or when a sputum specimen is indicated.[38–40]

It is common nursing practice to assess breath sounds after suctioning to determine effectiveness of the procedure. Suctioning removes secretions from the upper airways and trachea. Secretions in the lower airway that lead to adventitious sounds are rarely retrieved and therefore would not result in improved breath sounds over the lung fields. Auscultation over the trachea and reassessment of the ventilator flow-time waveform for resolution of a sawtooth pattern are recommended assessments.[38] The number of suction passes is usually one to three; however, suctioning should be continued until secretions are removed. Suction duration is limited to 10 to 15 seconds, and rest periods are provided between suction passes.[39,40]

Key points related to endotracheal suctioning are discussed in Box 10.6. Hyperoxygenate with 100% oxygen for 30 seconds before suctioning, during the procedure, and immediately after suctioning.[39,40] Most ventilators have a built-in suction mode that delivers 100% oxygen for a short period (e.g., 2 minutes).[6] If the patient is not mechanically ventilated, hyperoxygenation can also be administered with a bag-valve device. This must be done cautiously to avoid elevated peak airway pressure associated with too large a volume being delivered with manual ventilation with a resuscitation bag.[40]

The closed tracheal, or in-line, suction catheter is an alternative to the single-use suction catheter. Either the closed suction system or the open suction system can be used safely and effectively to remove secretions from the adult patient with an artificial airway.[40] The closed tracheal suction system consists of a suction catheter enclosed in a plastic sheath that is attached to the patient's ventilator circuit and airway (Fig. 10.22). Because the ventilator circuit remains closed during the suction procedure,

BOX 10.6 Key Points for Endotracheal Suctioning

- Suction only as needed as indicated by patient assessment (breath sounds, coughing), visual secretions in the artificial airway, ventilator flow-time waveform, and airway pressure assessment.[40]
- Choose the proper-size device. The diameter of the suction catheter should occlude <70% of the diameter of the artificial airway.[40]
- Assemble equipment: open suction kit with two gloves or closed suction system (CSS), sterile saline for rinsing the catheter.
- Set the suction regulator below 200 mm Hg. Efforts should be made to use the lowest suction pressure possible to effectively remove secretions.
- Use sterile technique for suctioning.
- Preoxygenate the patient via the ventilator circuit before, between, and after suctioning.
- Gently insert suction catheter. If resistance is met, pull back 1 cm before applying suction.
- Shallow suctioning prevents trauma to the mucosa. Deep suctioning is reserved only when shallow suctioning is ineffective and with consideration that it results in more adverse events.[40]
- Suction the patient no longer than 10 to 15 seconds while applying intermittent or constant suction.[40]
- Allow patient to recover between passes of the suction catheter.
- Repeat endotracheal suctioning until the airway is clear.
- Rinse the catheter with sterile saline after endotracheal suctioning is performed.
- Suction the mouth and oropharynx with a single-use suction catheter, suction swabs, or a tonsil suction device.
- Auscultate the lungs to assess effectiveness of suctioning, and document findings.
- Document the amount, color, and consistency of secretions.
- Steps specific to closed suctioning (in addition to those just noted):
  - Using the dominant hand, insert the suction catheter into the airway until resistance is met. Simultaneously, use the nondominant hand to stabilize the artificial airway.
  - Withdraw the suction catheter while depressing the suction valve; be careful not to angle the wrist of the hand while withdrawing the catheter because kinking of the catheter and loss of suction may occur.
  - Ensure that the CSS catheter is completely withdrawn from the airway. A marking is visible on the suction catheter when it is properly withdrawn.
  - Rinse the catheter after the procedure. Connect a small vial or syringe of 0.9% normal saline for tracheal instillation (without preservatives) to the irrigation port, and simultaneously instill the saline into the port while depressing the suction control.
  - Keep the CSS suction catheter out of the patient's reach to avoid accidental self-extubation.

the device assists in maintaining oxygenation, reduces symptoms associated with hypoxemia, maintains PEEP, and protects staff from the patient's secretions. Depending on the institution, closed suctioning may be used on all ventilated patients, or it may be used for specific indications, such as for clinically unstable patients receiving high levels of FiO_2 or PEEP, patients at risk for alveolar derecruitment, patients with contagious infections such as tuberculosis, or patients for whom frequent suctioning is required (e.g., six or more times per day).[10,39]

Do not routinely instill saline into the trachea during suctioning.[40,41] Saline instillation is associated with problems such as oxygen desaturation, washing organisms in the ETT into the lower airway, tachycardia, increased intracranial pressure,

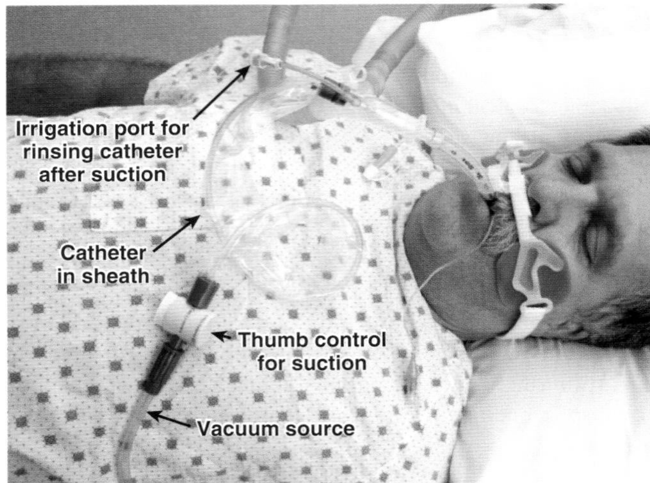

Fig. 10.22 Closed tracheal suction device. (Reprinted with permission, Cleveland Clinic Center for Medical Art & Photography © 2011–2019. All Rights Reserved.)

dyspnea, patient discomfort from excessive coughing, and bronchospasm. Purported benefits of liquefying secretions and increasing the volume of secretions removed are not proven.[41,42] Adequate patient hydration and airway humidification, rather than saline instillation, facilitate secretion removal.

BASICS OF MECHANICAL VENTILATION

The purpose of mechanical ventilation is to support the respiratory system until the underlying cause of respiratory failure can be corrected. Most ventilatory support requires an artificial airway; however, it may be applied without an artificial airway and is called *noninvasive ventilation.*

Indications

Mechanical ventilation is warranted for patients with acute respiratory failure who are unable to maintain adequate gas exchange as reflected in the ABGs. A clinical definition of respiratory failure is as follows:

- PaO_2 of 60 mm Hg or lower on an FiO_2 greater than 0.5 (oxygenation)
- $PaCO_2$ of 50 mm Hg or higher with a pH of 7.25 or less (ventilation)[3,10]

The patient may also demonstrate progressive physiological deterioration, such as rapid, shallow breathing and an increase in the WOB, as evidenced by increased use of the accessory muscles of ventilation, abnormal breathing patterns, and complaints of dyspnea. As life-saving therapy, mechanical ventilation supports the respiratory system while a treatment plan is instituted to correct the underlying abnormality.[6,10]

CHECK YOUR UNDERSTANDING

1. The patient has just undergone intubation with an ETT. Which assessment finding provides the most immediate confirmation that the tube is in the lungs?
   A. Color change from purple to yellow on the $ETCO_2$ detector
   B. Auscultating breath sounds over the lower, posterior lung fields
   C. Measurement of the centimeter marking at the lips
   D. Chest x-ray

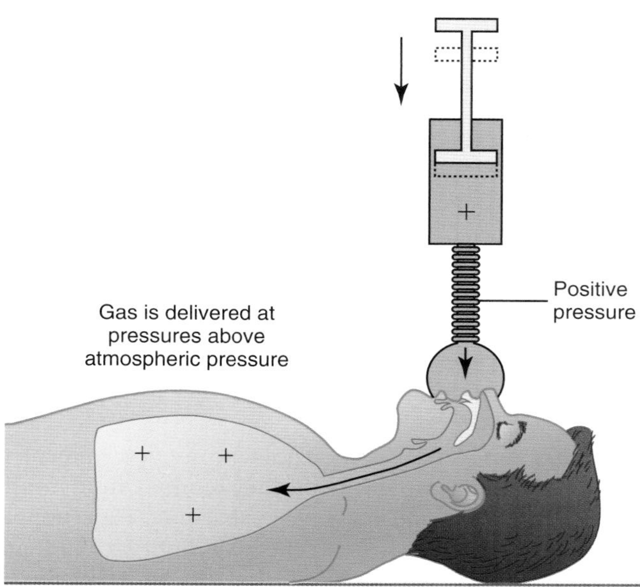

Fig. 10.23 Concept of positive-pressure ventilation.

Positive-Pressure Ventilation

In the critical care setting, most patients are treated with positive-pressure ventilation. This method uses positive pressure to force air into the lungs via an artificial airway, as illustrated in Fig. 10.23. Movement of gases into the lungs using *positive pressure* is the opposite of the pressures created in the chest during spontaneous breathing. Spontaneous ventilation begins when energy is expended to contract the muscles of respiration. This enlarges the thoracic cavity; increases *negative pressure* within the chest and lungs; and results in the flow of air, at atmospheric pressure, into the lungs. If mechanical ventilators could mimic the intrathoracic pressures that occur during spontaneous ventilation, it would be ideal. Negative-pressure ventilators, which originated with the iron lung, perform in this manner; however, these ventilators are for management of chronic conditions. Many of the complications of mechanical ventilation are related to air being forced into the lungs under positive pressure.

Ventilator Settings

Despite whether an RT is available to set up and manage the ventilator, the nurse must be familiar with how to locate values on the graphic interface unit to assess ventilator settings, patient response to ventilation, and alarms. Although the control panel of a microprocessor type of ventilator can appear overwhelming, it is important to learn to identify the common screen views that provide the settings and patient data that are integral to patient assessment. Know the basic ventilator settings: mode of ventilation, FiO_2, V_T in a volume mode of ventilation, inspiratory pressure setting in a pressure mode of ventilation, set RR rate, and PEEP. Additional settings of inspiratory-to-expiratory (I:E) ratio, sensitivity, and sigh are also discussed to provide a basis to knowledgeably communicate with the RT and provider.[5,6]

Fraction of Inspired Oxygen. The FiO_2 is set from 0.21 (21% or room air) to 1.00 (100% oxygen). The initial FiO_2 setting is based on the patient's immediate physiological needs and is set to whatever value is necessary to maintain a PaO_2 between 60 and 100 mm Hg or an SpO_2 of *at least* 90%. After the patient is stabilized, the setting is adjusted based on ABG or pulse oximetry values.

Tidal Volume. The amount of air delivered with each preset breath in a volume-controlled mode is the V_T. The V_T is dictated by body weight and by the patient's lung characteristics (compliance and resistance), and it is set to ensure that excessive stretch and pressure on the lung tissue are avoided. A starting point for the V_T setting is 4 to 8 mL/kg of ideal body weight, with the lowest value recommended in patients with obstructive airway disease or ARDS.[6,43] The parameters monitored to avoid excessive pressure are the PIP and plateau airway pressure (Pplat). These pressures should remain below 40 cm H_2O and 30 cm H_2O, respectively, to prevent ventilator-induced lung injury (VILI).[43] The V_T setting can be reduced if the resulting airway pressures are nearing the maximum. Conversely, if the airway pressures are acceptable and a larger V_T is needed to remove CO_2, it can be increased. When choosing and adjusting the V_T setting, the goal is to achieve the lowest Pplat while maintaining gas exchange and patient comfort.

Inspiratory Pressure. The inspiratory pressure setting used with pressure modes of ventilation augments the flow of gas into the lungs. When the breath begins, the preselected amount of pressure is delivered and held constant throughout inspiration, thereby promoting the flow of gas into the lungs. No tidal V_T is set. The V_T that the patient receives is determined by the compliance and resistance of the respiratory system (patient and ventilator). Lower inspiratory pressure settings are used when the patient's lungs are healthier, and high inspiratory pressures will be required when the lungs are more diseased.[5,6,10]

Respiratory Rate. The RR is the frequency of breaths (f) set to be delivered by the ventilator. The RR is set as near to physiological rates (14 to 20 breaths/min) as possible. Frequent changes in the RR are often required based on observation of the patient's WOB and comfort and assessment of the $PaCO_2$ and pH. During initiation of mechanical ventilation, many patients require full ventilatory support. The RR is selected, based on the V_T, to achieve a minute ventilation (VE) that maintains an acceptable acid-base status ($VE = RR \times V_T$). As the patient becomes capable of participating in the ventilatory work, the ventilator RR is decreased, or the mode of ventilation is changed, to encourage more spontaneous breathing.

Inspiratory-to-Expiratory Ratio. The I:E ratio is the duration of inspiration in comparison with expiration. In spontaneous ventilation, inspiration is shorter than expiration. When a patient undergoes mechanical ventilation, the I:E ratio is usually set at 1:2 to mimic the pattern of spontaneous ventilation; that is, 33% of the respiratory cycle is spent in inspiration and 66% in the expiratory phase. Longer expiratory times, an I:E ratio of 1:3 or 1:4, may be needed in patients with COPD to promote more complete exhalation and reduce air trapping.[33,44]

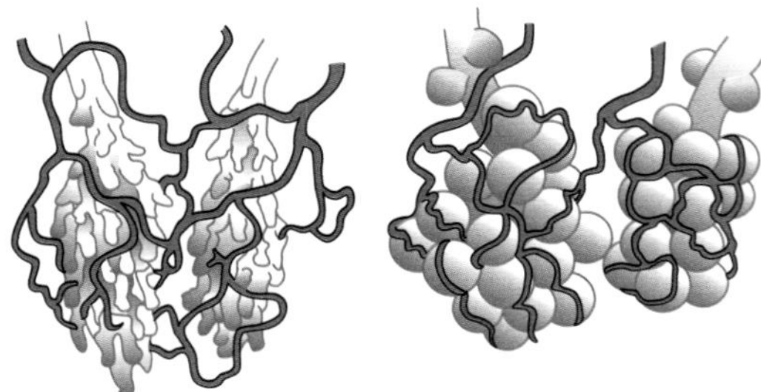

Fig. 10.24 Effect of application of positive end-expiratory pressure (PEEP) on the alveoli. (Modified from Pierce LNB. *Management of the Mechanically Ventilated Patient.* Philadelphia, PA: Saunders; 2007.)

Inverse Inspiratory-to-Expiratory Ratio. Inspiratory-to-expiratory ratios such as 1:1, 2:1, and 3:1 are called *inverse I:E ratios.* An inverse I:E ratio is used to improve oxygenation in patients with noncompliant lungs, such as in ARDS. During the traditional I:E ratio of 1:2, alveoli in noncompliant lungs may not have sufficient time to reopen during the shorter inspiratory phase and may collapse during the longer expiratory phase. An inverse I:E ratio allows unstable alveoli time to fill and prevents them from collapsing because the next inspiration begins before the alveoli reach a volume where they can collapse.[6,20]

Positive End-Expiratory Pressure. PEEP is the addition of positive pressure into the airways during expiration. PEEP is measured in cm H_2O. Initial settings for PEEP are 5 to 8 cm H_2O, although higher levels (10 to 15 cm H_2O) are usually necessary to treat refractory hypoxemia, particularly in ARDS. Because positive pressure is applied at end-expiration, the airways and alveoli are held open, and oxygenation improves. PEEP increases oxygenation by preventing collapse of small airways and maximizing the number of alveoli available for gas exchange (Fig. 10.24). By recruiting more alveoli for gas exchange and holding them open during expiration, the functional residual capacity improves, resulting in better oxygenation.[5,6,20]

Many mechanically ventilated patients routinely receive 3 to 5 cm H_2O of PEEP, referred to as *physiological PEEP.* This small amount of PEEP is thought to mimic the normal "back pressure" created in the lungs by the epiglottis in the spontaneously breathing patient that is released by the displacement of the epiglottis by the artificial airway.

PEEP is often added to decrease a high FiO_2 that may be required to achieve adequate oxygenation. For example, a patient may require an FiO_2 of 0.80 to maintain a PaO_2 of 85 mm Hg. By adding PEEP, it may be possible to decrease the FiO_2 to a level where oxygen toxicity in the lung is not a concern (<0.6) while maintaining an adequate PaO_2.[5,6,20] Monitor the PEEP level by observing the pressure level displayed on the ventilator's analog and graphic displays. When no PEEP is set, the pressure reading on the graphic display should be zero at end-expiration. When PEEP is applied, the pressure reading does not return to zero at the end of the breath, and the display shows the amount of PEEP.

Although PEEP is often essential for treatment, it is associated with adverse effects associated with an increase in intrathoracic pressure. These problems include a decrease in cardiac output secondary to decreased venous return, volutrauma or barotrauma, and increased intracranial pressure resulting from impedance of venous return from the head. Whenever the level of PEEP is increased, evaluate the patient's hemodynamic response through physical assessment and by available hemodynamic parameters. Management of decreased cardiac output secondary to PEEP includes ensuring that the patient has adequate intravascular volume (preload) and administering intravenous fluids as needed. If the cardiac output remains inadequate, an inotropic agent such as dobutamine should be considered. Optimal PEEP is defined as the amount of PEEP that affords the best oxygenation without resulting in adverse hemodynamic effects or pulmonary injury.[5,6,20]

Auto-PEEP. Auto-PEEP is the spontaneous development of PEEP caused by gas trapping in the lung resulting from insufficient expiratory time and incomplete exhalation. These trapped gases create positive pressure in the lung. Both set PEEP and auto-PEEP have the same physiological effects; therefore it is important to know when auto-PEEP is present so that it can be managed properly. Causes of auto-PEEP formation include rapid RR, high VE demand, airflow obstruction, and inverse I:E ratio ventilation. Auto-PEEP increases the WOB associated with triggering the breath. It cannot be detected by the ventilator pressure manometer until a special maneuver is performed. This maneuver involves instituting a 2-second end-expiratory pause, which allows the ventilator to read the pressure deep in the lung. The airway pressure manometer reading therefore reflects total PEEP, which is the set PEEP and auto-PEEP added together. To determine auto-PEEP, the following calculation is performed: Auto-PEEP = Total PEEP − Set PEEP.

Sensitivity. Sensitivity determines the amount of patient effort needed to initiate gas flow through the circuitry on a patient-initiated breath. The sensitivity is set so that the ventilator is "sensitive" to the patient's effort to inspire. If the sensitivity is set too low, the patient must generate more work to trigger gas flow. If it is set too high, auto-cycling of the ventilator may occur, resulting in patient-ventilator dyssynchrony, because the ventilator cycles into the inspiratory phase when the patient is not ready for a breath.[6]

Patient Data

The nurse and RT ensure that the ventilator settings are consistent with the provider's orders. The ventilator screen or graphic interface unit also provides valuable information regarding the patient's response to mechanical ventilation. These patient data include exhaled tidal volume (EV_T), PIP, and total RR.

Exhaled Tidal Volume. The EV_T is the amount of gas that comes out of the patient's lungs on exhalation. The EV_T is not a ventilator setting. It is data that indicate the patient's response to mechanical ventilation. This is the most accurate measure of the volume received by the patient and therefore is monitored at least every 4 hours and more often as indicated. Although the prescribed V_T is set on the ventilator control panel, it is not guaranteed to be delivered to the patient. Volume may be lost because of leaks in the ventilator circuit, around the cuff of the airway, or via a chest tube if there is a pleural air leak. The volume actually received by the patient, regardless of mode of ventilation, must be confirmed by monitoring the EV_T on the display panel of the ventilator. If the EV_T deviates from the set V_T by 50 mL or more, the nurse and RT must troubleshoot the system to identify the source of gas loss.

Peak Inspiratory Pressure. The PIP is the maximum pressure that occurs during inspiration. It is set in pressure modes of ventilation and is variable in volume modes of ventilation. The amount of pressure necessary to ventilate the patient increases with increased airway resistance (e.g., secretions in the airway, bronchospasm, biting the ETT) and decreased lung compliance (e.g., pulmonary edema, worsening infiltrate or ARDS, pleural space disease). The PIP should never be allowed to rise above 40 cm H_2O because higher pressures can result in VILI.[6,20,43] Monitor and record the PIP at least every 4 hours and with any change in patient condition that could increase airway resistance or decrease compliance. Increasing PIP or values greater than 40 cm H_2O should be reported immediately so that interventions can be ordered to improve lung function, ventilator settings can be adjusted to reduce the inspiratory pressure, or both.

Total Respiratory Rate. The total RR equals the number of breaths delivered by the ventilator (set rate) plus the number of breaths initiated by the patient. Assessing the total RR provides data on the patient's contribution to the WOB or whether the ventilator is performing all the work. The total RR is a very sensitive indicator of overall respiratory stability. For example, if the patient is on assist/control ventilation at a set RR of 10 breaths/min and the total RR for 1 minute is 16, the patient is initiating 6 breaths above the set rate of 10. If the patient is on volume intermittent mandatory ventilation (VIMV) at a set RR of 8 breaths/min and the total RR is 12 breaths/min with good spontaneous V_T for body weight, the patient is tolerating the mode of ventilation. If the patient's total RR increases to 26 breaths/min, this finding indicates that something has changed, and the patient needs to be reassessed for causes of the increased rate, such as fatigue, pain, or anxiety. Treatment is based on the identified cause.

MODES, ADVANCED THERAPIES, AND MONITORING OF VENTILATORY SUPPORT

Modes of Mechanical Ventilation

Modes of mechanical ventilation describe how breaths are delivered to the patient. A mode is the method by which the patient and the ventilator interact to perform the respiratory cycle. They vary in degree of patient versus ventilator effort and may provide full to partial ventilatory support. A breath is *assisted* if the ventilator performs all or some of the work. A ventilator assists breathing using either pressure or volume as the control variable, the function that is controlled during inspiration. In volume-controlled modes of ventilation, a set V_T is delivered during inspiration. In pressure-controlled modes of ventilation, pressure is set and does not vary throughout inspiration.

In addition to understanding volume and pressure control as a classification scheme for modes of ventilation, other concepts helpful in understanding varying modes of ventilation include triggering, breath classification, and breath sequence.

- Triggering indicates what initiates inspiration. Breaths may be patient triggered or ventilator triggered.
- Breaths are classified as *spontaneous* or *mandatory.* A spontaneous breath is one where the patient controls both the start and the end of inspiration, whereas a mandatory breath is a breath delivered by the ventilator, independent of the patient.

A breath sequence is a particular pattern of spontaneous and/or mandatory breaths. The three possible breath sequences are continuous mandatory ventilation (CMV), intermittent mandatory ventilation (IMV), and continuous spontaneous ventilation (CSV). CMV is commonly referred to as *assist/control.* In CMV, every breath, whether triggered by the patient or the ventilator, is assisted by the ventilator, and there are no purely spontaneous breaths. IMV is a breath sequence in which spontaneous breaths are possible between mandatory breaths. In CSV, every breath is initiated and ended by the patient. Knowledge of these terms will facilitate understanding the differences between the various modes of mechanical ventilation and how they work with the patient to perform the breath.[6,45]

Volume-Controlled Ventilation. In volume-controlled ventilation, V_T is constant for every breath delivered by the ventilator. The ventilator is set to allow airflow into the lungs until a preset volume has been reached. A major advantage of these modes is that the set V_T is delivered, regardless of changes in lung compliance or resistance. However, the PIP is variable and dependent on compliance and resistance; therefore closely monitor for elevated PIP. Volume assist/control (V-A/C; Fig. 10.25A) and VIMV (see Fig. 10.25B) are volume-controlled modes of ventilation.

Volume assist/control. The V-A/C mode of ventilation delivers a preset number of breaths of a preset V_T. The patient may trigger additional breaths between the ventilator-initiated breaths by generating a negative inspiratory effort, and the ventilator will respond by delivering an assisted breath of the preset V_T. The V_T of the assisted breaths is constant for both ventilator-initiated and patient-triggered breaths. The V-A/C mode ensures that the patient receives adequate ventilation, regardless of patient effort. It is a full ventilatory support mode; therefore it is indicated when it is desirable for the ventilator to perform the bulk of the WOB. The only work the patient must perform is the negative inspiratory effort required to trigger the ventilator on the patient-initiated breaths. This mode is useful in patients who have a normal respiratory drive but whose respiratory muscles are too weak or unable to perform the WOB (e.g., patient emerging from general anesthesia or with pulmonary disease such as pneumonia). A disadvantage of V-A/C ventilation is that respiratory alkalosis may develop if the patient hyperventilates because of anxiety, pain, a neurological issue, or other factors. Respiratory alkalosis is treated or prevented by appropriately treating the underlying cause of tachypnea or changing to a mode that allows spontaneous breaths, such as VIMV. Another disadvantage is that the

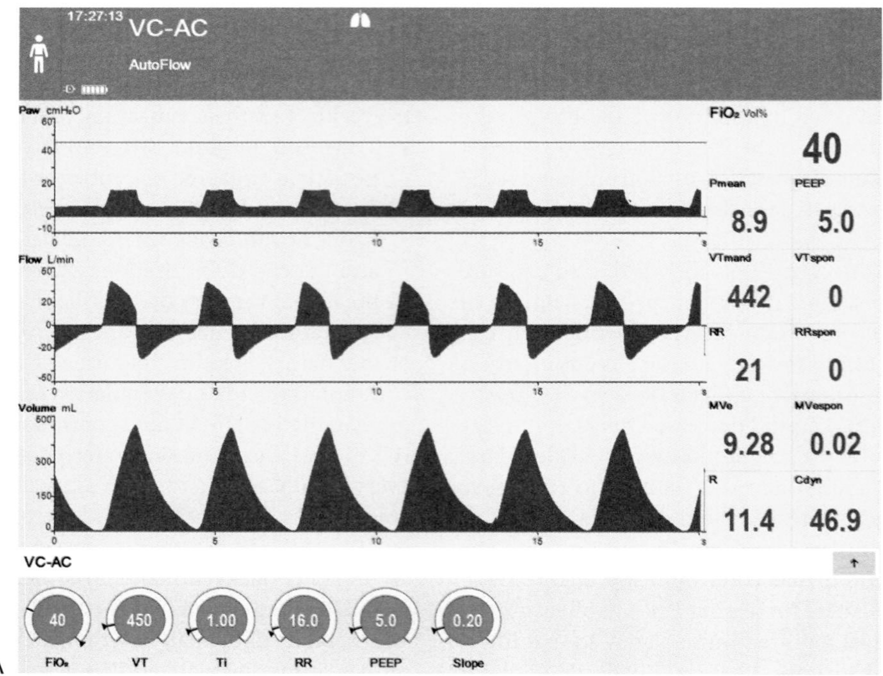

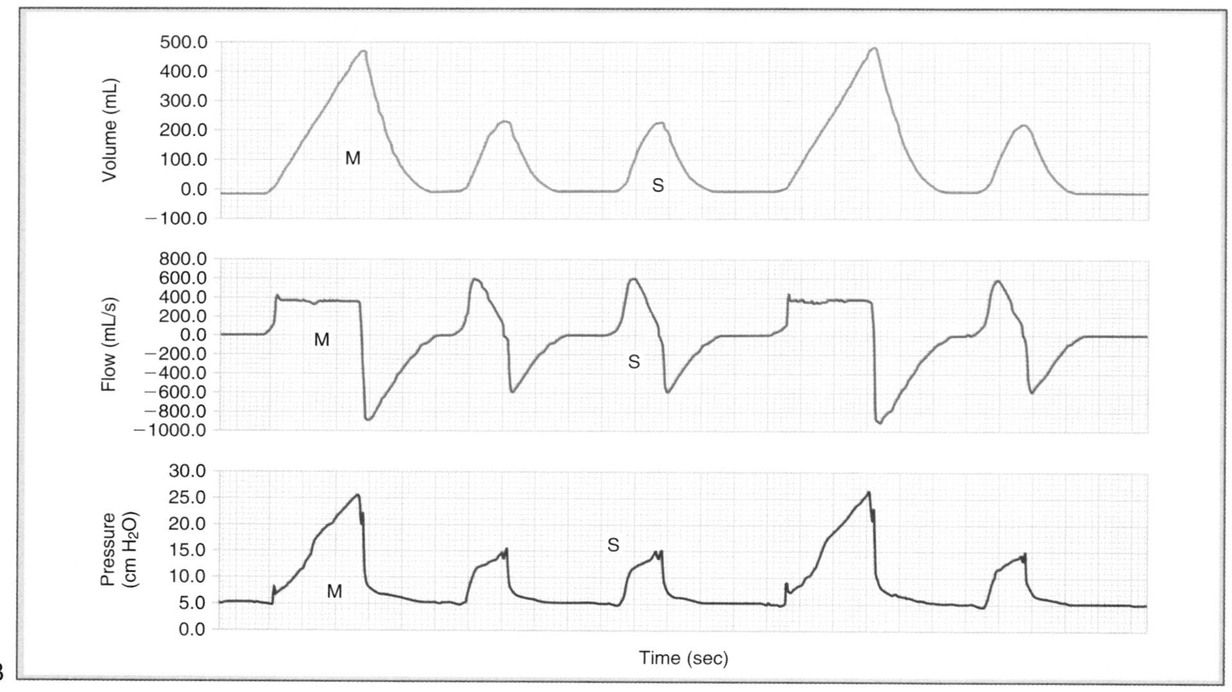

Fig. 10.25 Waveforms of volume-controlled ventilator modes. **A,** Volume assist/control *(V-A/C)* ventilation. The patient may trigger additional breaths above the set rate. The ventilator delivers the same volume for ventilator-triggered and patient-triggered (assisted) breaths. **B,** Volume intermittent mandatory ventilation (VIMV). Both spontaneous and mandatory breaths are graphed. Mandatory breaths receive the set tidal volume (V_T). V_T of spontaneous breaths depends on work the patient is capable of generating, lung compliance, and airway resistance. (**B,** From Cairo JM. *Mosby's Respiratory Care Equipment.* St. Louis, MO: Elsevier; 2018.)

patient may rely on the ventilator and not attempt to initiate spontaneous breathing if all ventilatory demands are met.

During V-A/C ventilation, check the ventilator to ensure that the parameters are set as prescribed and assess the total RR to determine whether the patient is initiating breaths, check the EV_T to ensure that the set V_T is delivered, and check the PIP to determine whether it is increasing (indicating a change in compliance or resistance, which needs to be further evaluated).

Also monitor the patient's sense of comfort and synchronization with the ventilator, oxygenation, ventilation, and the acid-base status.[6,20]

Volume intermittent mandatory ventilation. The VIMV mode of ventilation delivers a set number of breaths of a set V_T. Between mandatory breaths, the patient may initiate spontaneous breaths. The volume of the spontaneous breaths is whatever the patient can generate. If the patient initiates a breath near the time a mandatory breath is due, the ventilator will deliver a mandatory breath synchronized with the patient's spontaneous effort to prevent patient-ventilator dyssynchrony. The difference between the VIMV and V-A/C is the volume of the patient-initiated breaths. Patient-initiated breaths in V-A/C result in the patient receiving the set V_T. In VIMV, the V_T of spontaneous breaths is variable because it depends on patient effort and lung characteristics.

The VIMV mode was developed to create a mode of ventilation where the patient can participate in the WOB and begin to recondition weak respiratory muscles. The VIMV mode is indicated when it is desirable to allow patients to contribute to the WOB and assist in maintaining a normal $PaCO_2$ or when hyperventilation has occurred in the V-A/C mode. The VIMV mode may be used for weaning patients from mechanical ventilation. As the VIMV rate is lowered, the patient initiates more spontaneous breaths, assuming a greater portion of the ventilatory work. As the patient demonstrates the ability to take on even more WOB, the mandatory breath rate is decreased accordingly. However, compared with other weaning modalities, VIMV is associated with the longest weaning and lowest success rate.[46,47]

During VIMV, monitor the total RR to determine whether the patient is initiating spontaneous breaths and the patient's ability to manage the WOB. If the total RR increases, assess the V_T of the spontaneous breaths for adequacy. An adequate spontaneous V_T is 5 mL/kg of ideal body weight. A rising total RR may indicate that the patient is beginning to fatigue, resulting in a more shallow and rapid respiratory pattern. This pattern may lead to atelectasis, a further increase in the WOB, and the need for greater ventilatory support. Monitor the EV_T of both the mandatory and the spontaneous breaths to ensure that the set V_T is being delivered with the mandatory breaths and that the spontaneous V_T is adequate. As in V-A/C ventilation, assess the PIP, the patient's sense of comfort and synchronization with the ventilator, oxygenation, ventilation, and acid-base status.

Pressure Ventilation. In pressure ventilation, the ventilator is set to allow air to flow into the lungs until a preset inspiratory pressure has been reached. The V_T the patient receives is variable and depends on lung compliance and airway and circuit resistance. Patients with normal lung compliance and low resistance will have better delivery of V_T for the amount of inspiratory pressure set. An advantage of pressure-controlled modes is that the PIP can be reliably controlled for each breath the ventilator delivers. A disadvantage is that hypoventilation and respiratory acidosis may occur because delivered V_T varies; therefore the nurse must closely monitor EV_T.[9,34,44,48] Pressure modes include continuous positive airway pressure (CPAP), pressure support (PS), pressure control, pressure-controlled inverse-ratio ventilation, and airway pressure–release ventilation (APRV).

Continuous positive airway pressure. CPAP is positive pressure applied throughout the respiratory cycle to the spontaneously breathing patient (Fig. 10.26). The patient must have a reliable respiratory drive and adequate V_T because no mandatory breaths or other ventilatory assistance is given; therefore CPAP is classified as *CSV*. The patient performs all the WOB. CPAP

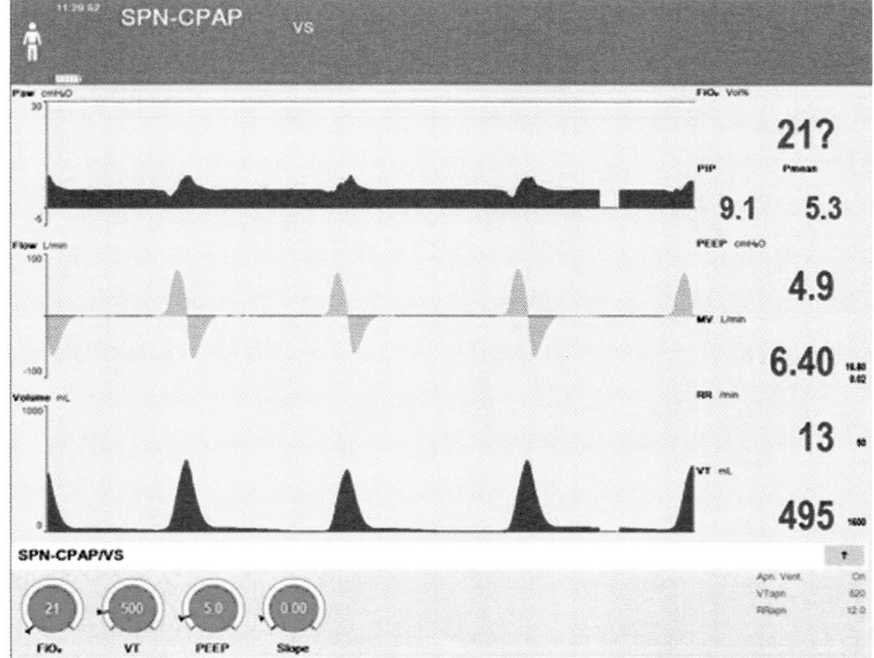

Fig. 10.26 Continuous positive airway pressure (CPAP) is a spontaneous breathing mode. Positive pressure at end-expiration splints alveoli and supports oxygenation. Note that the pressure does not fall to zero, indicating the level of CPAP.

provides pressure at end-expiration, which prevents alveolar collapse and improves the functional residual capacity and oxygenation. CPAP is identical to PEEP in its physiological effects. *CPAP* is the correct term when the end-expiratory pressure is applied in the spontaneously breathing patient. *PEEP* is the term used for the same setting when the patient is receiving any form of inspiratory assistance (e.g., V-A/C, VIMV, PS). CPAP is indicated as a mode of weaning when the patient has adequate ventilation but requires end-expiratory pressure to stabilize the alveoli and maintain oxygenation.[46] Because the ventilator is used to deliver CPAP during weaning, monitor the adequacy of the patient's EV_T, set alarms to detect low EV_T and apnea, and give backup mechanical breaths in the event of apnea.

CPAP can also be administered via a nasal or face mask. Typically, a nasal CPAP system is used to keep the airway open in patients with obstructive sleep apnea in the home setting.

Pressure support. PS is a mode of ventilation in which the patient's spontaneous respiratory activity is augmented by the delivery of a preset amount of inspiratory positive pressure. The patient must initiate every breath and determine when to end the inspiratory phase; therefore PS is classified as *CSV*. PS may be used as a stand-alone mode (Fig. 10.27) or in combination with other modes, such as IMV, to augment the V_T of the spontaneous breaths (Fig. 10.28). The positive pressure is applied throughout inspiration, thereby promoting the flow of gas into the lungs, augmenting the patient's spontaneous V_T, and decreasing the WOB associated with breathing through an artificial airway and the ventilatory circuit.[5,6,20,45] Typical levels of PS ordered for the patient are 6 to 12 cm H_2O. The V_T is variable, determined by patient effort, the amount of PS applied, and the compliance and resistance of the patient and ventilator system. Closely monitor exhaled V_T during PS; if it is inadequate, increase the level of PS. PS may increase patient comfort because the patient has greater control over the initiation and duration of each breath. PS promotes conditioning of the respiratory muscles because the patient works throughout the breath; this may facilitate weaning from the ventilator.

Pressure assist/control. Pressure assist/control (P-A/C) is a mode of ventilation in which there is a set RR, and every breath is augmented by a set amount of inspiratory pressure. If the patient triggers additional breaths beyond the set rate, those breaths are augmented by the set amount of inspiratory pressure (Fig. 10.29); therefore P-A/C is classified as *CMV*. Just as with PS, there is no set V_T. The V_T the patient receives is variable and determined by the set inspiratory pressure, the patient's lung compliance, and circuit and airway resistance. The typical pressure in P-A/C ranges from 15 to 25 cm H_2O, which is higher than a PS level because P-A/C is indicated for patients with a high PIP during traditional volume ventilation, including ARDS. Because the lungs are noncompliant in these conditions, higher inspiratory pressure levels are needed to achieve an adequate V_T. P-A/C reduces the risk of barotrauma while maintaining adequate oxygenation and ventilation. During P-A/C, be familiar with all ventilator settings: the level of pressure, the set RR, the FiO_2, and the level of PEEP. Monitor the total RR to evaluate whether the patient is initiating breaths and EV_T for adequacy of volume.

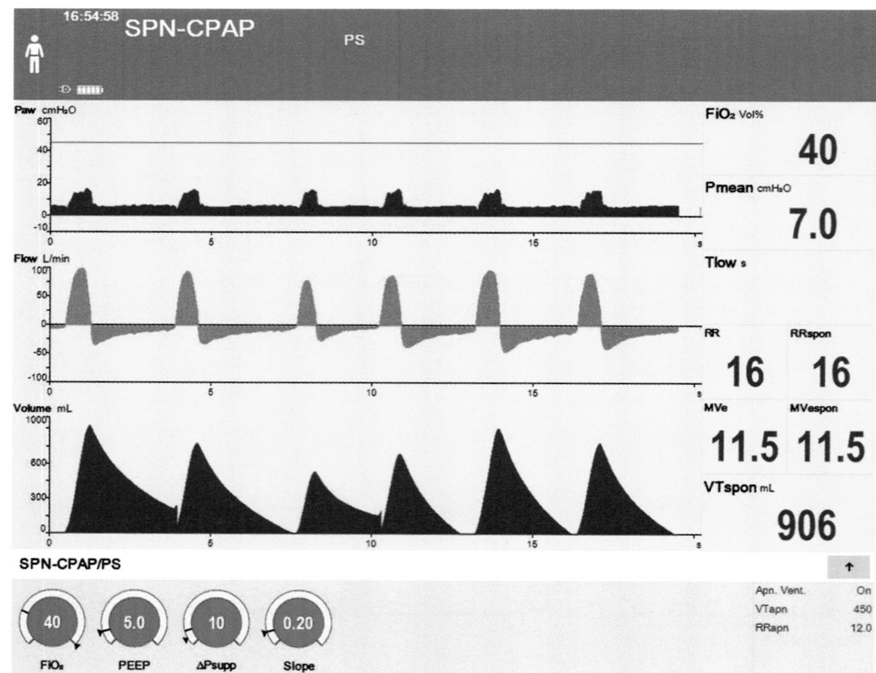

Fig. 10.27 Pressure support ventilation requires the patient to trigger each breath, which is then supported by pressure on inspiration. Inspiratory time, respiratory rate, and tidal volume (V_T) are patient dependent.

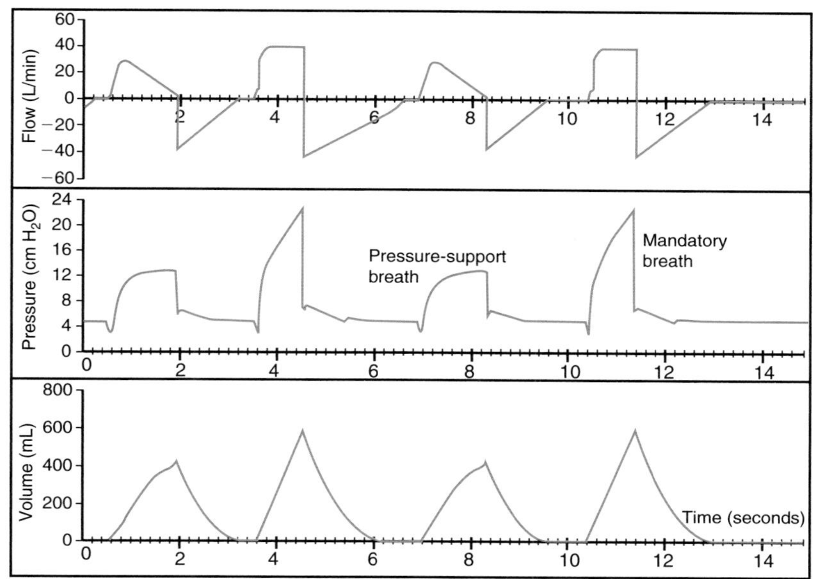

Fig. 10.28 Volume intermittent mandatory ventilation (VIMV) with pressure support (PS). VIMV breaths receive set tidal volume (V_T). Pressure support is applied to the spontaneous, patient-triggered breaths. (From Pierce LNB. *Management of the Mechanically Ventilated Patient.* Philadelphia, PA: Saunders; 2007.)

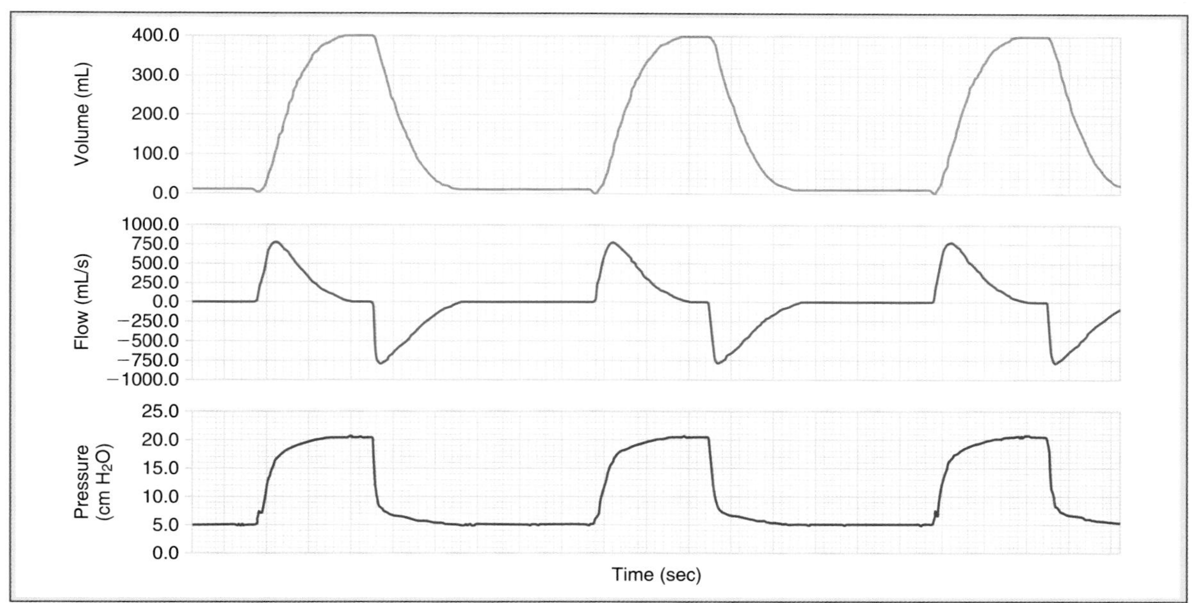

Fig. 10.29 Pressure assist/control ventilation. Patient can trigger additional breaths above the set rate. Patient- and ventilator-triggered breaths receive the same inspiratory pressure. (From Cairo JM. *Mosby's Respiratory Care Equipment.* 11th ed. St. Louis, MO: Elsevier; 2022.)

CHECK YOUR UNDERSTANDING

2. Identify and match the ventilatory mode with the type of support.

Mode	Type of Support
Volume Assist/Control	Volume-Controlled Ventilation
Pressure Support	Pressure Ventilation
Volume Intermittent Mandatory Ventilation	
Pressure Assist/Control	
Airway Pressure–Release Ventilation	

Pressure-controlled inverse-ratio ventilation. With pressure-controlled inverse-ratio ventilation (PC-IRV), the patient receives P-A/C ventilation, and the ventilator is set to provide longer inspiratory times. The I:E ratio is inversed to increase the mean airway pressure, open and stabilize the alveoli, and improve oxygenation. PC-IRV is indicated for patients with noncompliant lungs, such as in ARDS, when adequate oxygenation is not achieved despite high FiO_2, PEEP, or positioning. Although inverse-ratio ventilation can improve oxygenation, there are no clear advantages when compared with the use of higher levels of

PEEP because the reverse I:E ratio ventilation is uncomfortable, and the patient must be sedated and possibly paralyzed to prevent ventilator dyssynchrony and oxygen desaturation.

Airway pressure–release ventilation. Airway pressure–release ventilation (APRV) is a mode of ventilation that provides two levels of CPAP, one during inspiration and the other during expiration, while allowing unrestricted spontaneous breathing at any point during the respiratory cycle (Fig. 10.30). APRV starts at an elevated pressure, the CPAP level or pressure high (P_{HIGH}), followed by a release pressure, pressure low (P_{LOW}). After the airway pressure release, the P_{HIGH} level is restored. The time spent at P_{HIGH} is known as *time high* and is generally prolonged, 4 to 6 seconds. The shorter release period (P_{LOW}) is known as *time low* and is generally 0.5 to 1.1 seconds. When observing the pressure waveform, APRV is similar to PC-IRV; however, unlike PC-IRV, the patient has unrestricted spontaneous breathing. The patient is more comfortable on APRV, and deep sedation or paralysis may not be needed. APRV assists in providing adequate oxygenation while lowering PIP. It is indicated as an alternative to V-A/C or P-A/C for patients with significantly decreased lung compliance, such as those with ARDS.[6,44]

Dual-controlled modes. Dual-controlled modes, also known as *volume-assured modes,* incorporate qualities of both volume- and pressure-controlled modes. Both the desired V_T and the pressure limit are set. The ventilator delivers gas to achieve the desired V_T while ensuring that the pressure remains below the set pressure limit. The ventilator monitors the EV_T and adjusts the inspiratory pressure on a breath-by-breath basis to ensure that the V_T is delivered using the lowest possible pressure. Pressure modes with a set volume are available on many ventilators; two of the more common ones are described here.[5,6,20,44]

Pressure-regulated volume control. Pressure-regulated volume control (PRVC) is a control mode of ventilation in which the patient receives a preset number of breaths of a preset V_T that is given in the form of a pressure breath. The ventilator strives to achieve the target V_T using the lowest possible pressure. The ventilator determines the pressure needed to achieve the target breath by performing a calculation involving the pressure used for the previous breath, the target V_T, and the actual V_T of the previous breath. Inspiratory pressure is increased or decreased in a stepwise fashion to ensure the volume guarantee. If the measured V_T is too large, the pressure decreases. If it is too small, the pressure increases up to the upper pressure limit.

Volume support. Volume support (VS) is a mode of ventilation that pressure supports every breath to a level that guarantees a preset V_T. The patient triggers every breath. The ventilator determines the pressure needed to achieve the target breath as described earlier for PRVC. The difference between these two modes is that VS is a spontaneous breathing mode and no RR is set, whereas PRVC is a controlled mode with a set number of breaths delivered each minute.

Mandatory minute ventilation. Mandatory minute ventilation (MMV) is an example of a closed-loop ventilation in which the level of support changes based on the patient's level of participation. With MMV, the patient breathes spontaneously, yet a constant VE is guaranteed. The minimum ventilation is determined by the V_T and RR settings, which allows MMV to ensure that the patient always receives at least the set minimum VE (VE = VT × RR). Mandatory breaths are provided only if spontaneous breathing is not sufficient and is below the prescribed minimum ventilation. When spontaneous breathing increases, fewer mandatory breaths are provided. Thus, the patient can

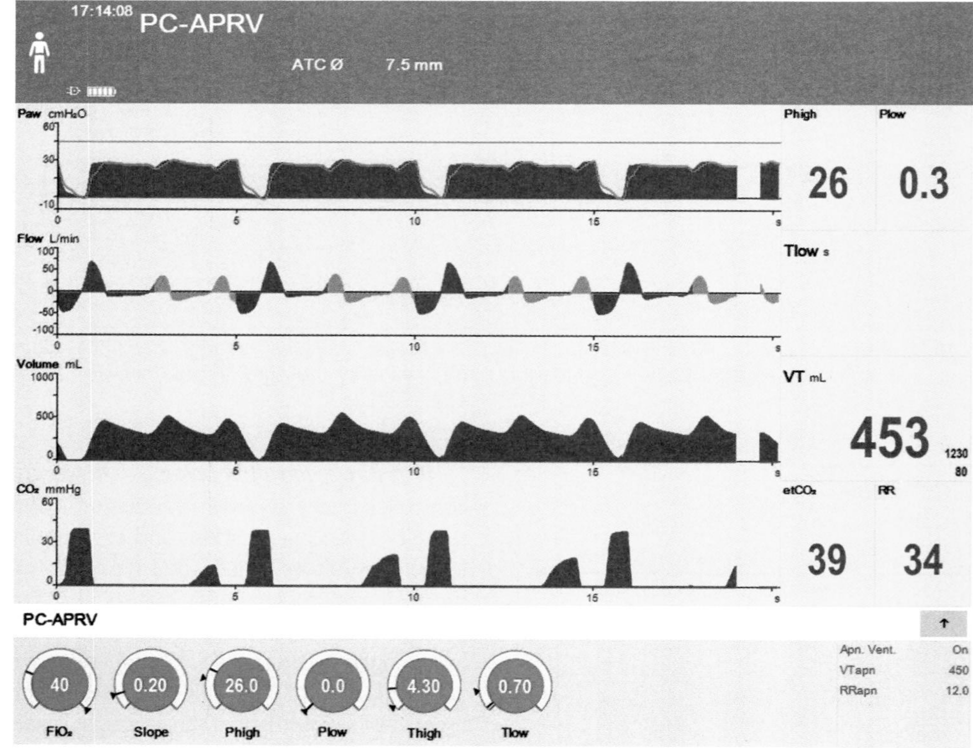

Fig. 10.30 Airway pressure–release ventilation.

gradually take over more of the WOB. If the patient's spontaneous breathing is sufficient to achieve the set VE, no further mandatory breaths are applied. Spontaneous breaths can be supported with PS. At least 5 cm H_2O of PS is typically set to assist in overcoming the resistance of the artificial airway and ventilator circuit. Additional PS is set as needed to assist the patient in achieving an adequate V_T.

Noninvasive Positive-Pressure Ventilation

Noninvasive positive-pressure ventilation (NPPV) is the delivery of mechanical ventilation without an ETT or tracheostomy tube. NPPV provides ventilation via (1) a face mask that covers the nose, mouth, or both; (2) a nasal mask or pillow; or (3) a full face mask (Fig. 10.31). Complications associated with an artificial airway, such as vocal cord injury and VAE, are reduced, and sedation needs are lessened. During NPPV, the patient can eat and speak and is free from the discomfort of an artificial airway. Treatment with NPPV may prevent the need for intubation in many patients.

NPPV is indicated for the treatment of acute exacerbations of COPD, cardiogenic pulmonary edema (along with other treatments), early hypoxemic respiratory failure in immunocompromised patients, and obstructive sleep apnea. NPPV has been used successfully in patients with asthma, pneumonia, postoperative respiratory failure, obesity hypoventilation syndrome, and other causes of acute respiratory failure. It may also be used to prevent reintubation in a patient who is experiencing respiratory distress following extubation and to provide ventilatory support while an acute problem is treated in patients for whom intubation is undesirable, such as those with "do not intubate" orders.[5,6,10,20,44] Its use is expanding beyond the critical care unit and even in settings outside of the hospital. Contraindications to NPPV include apnea and cardiovascular instability (hypotension, uncontrolled dysrhythmias, and myocardial ischemia). Relative contraindications, or factors that could contribute to noninvasive ventilation failure, include claustrophobia, impaired consciousness, high aspiration risk, viscous or copious secretions, inability to clear secretions, gastroesophageal surgery, recent craniofacial surgery, trauma, and burns.[49]

NPPV can be delivered with critical care ventilators or a ventilator specifically designed to provide NPPV (Fig. 10.32). Modes delivered can be pressure or volume; however, pressure modes are better tolerated. The most common modes of ventilation delivered via NPPV are PS or pressure control with PEEP and CPAP.

During NPPV, collaborate with the RT to ensure that the right size and type of mask is chosen and that it fits snugly enough to prevent air leaks. Monitor the mask and the skin under the mask edges for signs of pressure injury. If signs of excess pressure are noted, reposition the mask, place a layer of wound care dressing on the skin as a protective shield, or select another mask type. If mouth breathing is a problem with the nasal mask, apply a chin strap or change the mask to an oronasal or full face mask.[49] Leakage of gases around the mask edges may lead to drying of the eyes and the need for eye drops. Monitor the mouth and airway passages for excessive drying, and add a humidification system as indicated. If the patient complains of nausea or vomits, gastric insufflation may be occurring, and gastric decompression may be indicated. Also monitor the total RR, the EV_T to ensure that it is adequate, and the PIP.

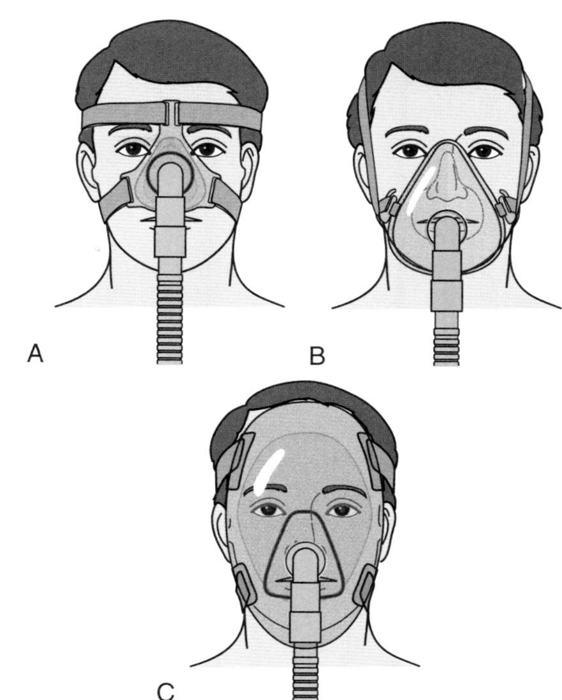

Fig. 10.31 Masks used for noninvasive positive-pressure ventilation. A, Nasal. B, Oronasal. C, Full face mask. (Redrawn from Mims BC, Toto KH, Luecke LE et al. *Critical Care Skills*. 2nd ed. Philadelphia, PA: Saunders; 2003.)

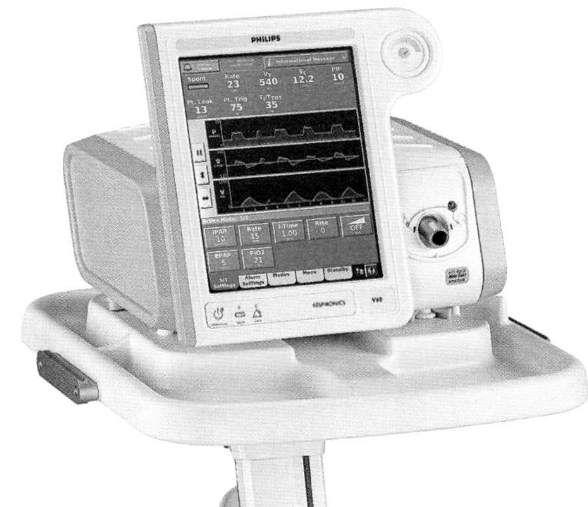

Fig. 10.32 The ventilator offers a range of conventional pressure modes, continuous positive airway pressure (CPAP), pressure-controlled ventilation (PCV), and spontaneous/timed (S/T). The volume-targeted average volume-assured pressure support (AVAPS) mode combines the attributes of pressure-controlled and volume-targeted ventilation. The optional pulse pressure variation (PPV) mode provides pressure ventilation in proportion to the patient's efforts. (Used with permission of Philips Respironics, Carlsbad, CA.)

CLINICAL JUDGMENT ACTIVITY

Your patient is being ventilated with noninvasive positive-pressure ventilation (NPPV) with a nasal mask. The patient is mouth breathing, and the ventilator is alarming low exhaled tidal volume. What actions should you take to ensure that the patient receives adequate ventilation?

Advanced Therapies for Ventilatory Support

Microprocessor ventilators offer a wide range of options for mechanical ventilation. However, other forms of ventilatory support are available. These advanced techniques are usually ordered to treat patients with respiratory failure that is refractory to conventional treatment. These techniques include but are not limited to extracorporeal membrane oxygenation (ECMO), high-frequency jet ventilation, high-frequency percussive ventilation, and inhaled nitric oxide. Specialized equipment and training are essential for these advanced treatments. ECMO is increasingly being used to treat adults with refractory hypoxemia. Some hospitals have designated ECMO units to manage these complex, critically ill patients.

High-Frequency Oscillatory Ventilation. High-frequency oscillatory ventilation (HFOV) delivers subphysiological tidal volumes at extremely fast rates (300 to 420 breaths/min). It is indicated in patients with noncompliant lungs and hypoxemia where conventional ventilation results in high airway pressures. This strategy stabilizes the alveoli and improves gas mixing, thereby improving oxygenation. The small tidal volumes limit peak pressure, preventing overdistension and protecting the lung from further injury. At the same time, collapse of the alveoli at end-expiration is limited through the creation of higher end-expiratory pressure. HFOV is delivered with a specialized ventilator that uses a diaphragm, much like a stereo speaker, driven by a piston, creating a constant flow of gases into and out of the lung (Fig. 10.33).[16] Ventilator settings control the amount, timing, and speed of piston movement. The nurse must learn new monitoring parameters when caring for a patient on HFOV.

Respiratory Monitoring During Mechanical Ventilation

Nurses and RTs collaborate to routinely monitor many parameters while a patient receives mechanical ventilation. Monitoring to assess the patient's response to treatment and to anticipate and plan for the ventilator weaning process includes physical assessment of the patient and assessment of the ventilator system: airway, circuitry, accuracy of ventilator settings, and patient data. Physical assessment includes vital signs and hemodynamic parameters, patient comfort and WOB, synchrony of patient's respiratory efforts with the ventilator, breath sounds, amount and quality of respiratory secretions, and assessment of the chest drain system if present. Evaluate ABG results, pulse oximetry, and $ETCO_2$ values to assess oxygenation and ventilation.[9,40,50] Patient data evaluated from the ventilator include EV_T (mandatory and spontaneous breaths), total RR, and PIP.

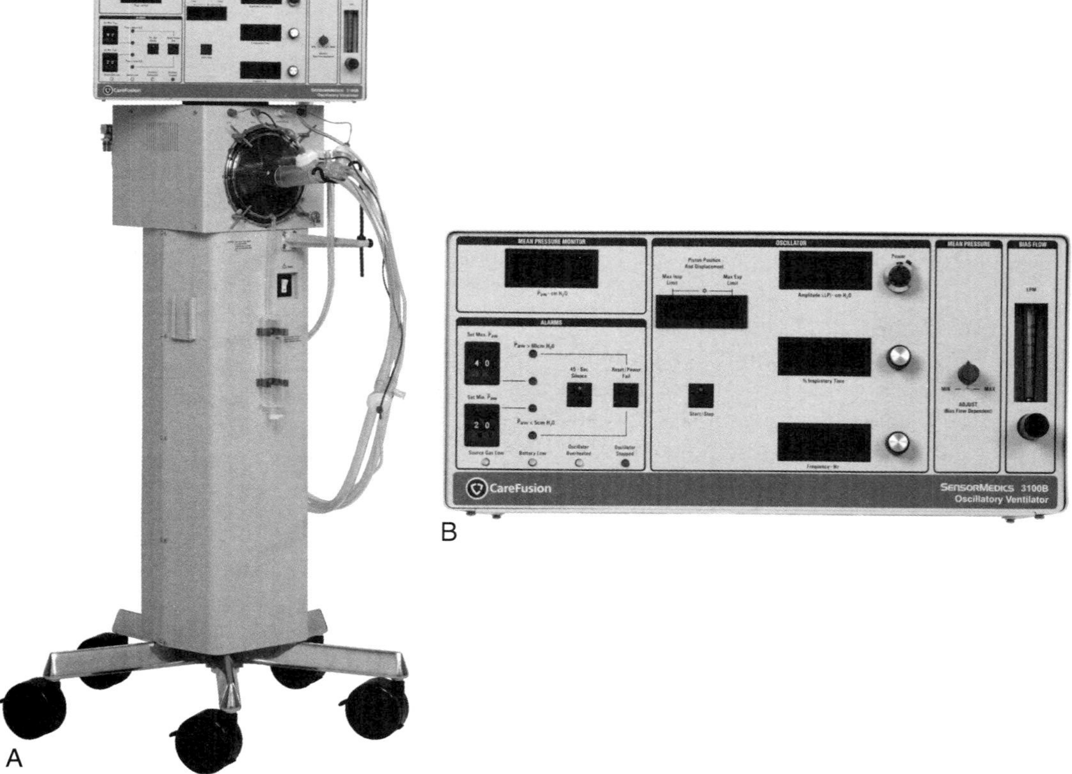

Fig. 10.33 A, Model 3100B High-Frequency Oscillatory Ventilator. B, Control panel of the 3100B. (© 2020 Vyaire Medical, Inc., Mettawa, IL; used with permission.)

Further assessment of the PIP may require direct measurements of airway resistance and static lung compliance. Check the ventilator system at least every 4 hours. The RT performs a more detailed assessment of the ventilator's functioning, including alarms and the appropriateness of alarm settings.[5,20]

Alarm Systems. Alarms are an integral part of a ventilator and warn of technical or patient events that require attention or action. Knowledge about troubleshooting alarms is essential. Follow two important rules to ensure patient safety:

1. *Never shut off alarms.* It is acceptable to silence alarms for a preset delay while working with a patient, such as during suctioning. However, alarms are never shut off.
2. *Manually ventilate the patient.* Use a bag-valve device if unable to troubleshoot alarms quickly or if equipment failure is suspected to manually ventilate the patient. Ensure that a bag-valve device is readily available at the bedside of every patient who is mechanically ventilated.

When an alarm sounds, the first thing to do is to look at the patient. If the patient is disconnected from the ventilator circuit, quickly reconnect the patient to the machine. If the circuit is connected to the airway, quickly assess whether the patient is in distress and is adequately ventilated and oxygenated. Quickly assess the patient's level of consciousness, color, airway, RR, SpO_2 level, $ETCO_2$ value, heart rate, WOB, chest wall movement, and lung sounds. Observe the ventilator display to identify the status message related to the alarm and silence the alarm while determining the cause. Immediate action is required if the patient is in acute distress with labored respirations, an abnormal breathing pattern, pallor and diaphoresis, deterioration in breath sounds, or decreasing SpO_2. Quickly disconnect the patient from the ventilator and manually ventilate the patient with a bag-valve device while a second caregiver, often the RT, further assesses the problem. If the patient is not in respiratory distress, use the assessment data gathered to proceed with problem solving. Table 10.4 provides an overview of management of common ventilator alarms.

CLINICAL JUDGMENT ACTIVITY

Your patient requires mechanical ventilation for treatment. The high peak pressure alarm has alarmed three times for a few seconds each time, even though you have just suctioned the patient. What assessment cues should be analyzed to help formulate priority hypotheses and generate solutions and potential actions?

Complications of Mechanical Ventilation. Numerous complications are associated with intubation and mechanical ventilation. Many complications can be prevented or treated rapidly through vigilant nursing care. Best practice includes implementation of the "ventilator bundle" for all mechanically ventilated patients to prevent complications and improve outcomes (see Clinical Alert box).

The absolute and relative value of each bundle component's impact on patient-centered outcomes is unclear. Recent evidence indicates that stress ulcer prophylaxis (SUP) may be harmful in some patients.[52] In the absence of updated practice guidelines, institutions should review the evidence in light of the patient populations cared for and determine their approach to application of the bundle components.

CLINICAL ALERT

Implementation of the Ventilator Bundle

The ventilator bundle of care should be implemented in all patients who receive mechanical ventilation.[28] This bundle is a group of evidence-based recommendations and has been demonstrated to improve outcomes. It is expected that all interventions in the bundle be implemented unless contraindicated. The interventions are as follows:

- Maintain head of bed elevation at 30 to 45 degrees.
- Minimize sedation, including interrupting sedation to assess readiness to wean from ventilator and extubate.
- Maintain and improve physical conditioning.
- Provide prophylaxis for venous thromboembolism.
- Use high-flow nasal oxygen or noninvasive positive-pressure ventilation (NIPPV) as appropriate whenever safe and feasible to avoid intubation and reintubation.
- Provide prophylaxis for peptic ulcer disease.
- Provide oral care at least daily with toothbrushing, or gauze if no teeth, but without chlorhexidine, which has been associated with increased mortality rates.[28,51,48]
- Provide early enteral versus parenteral nutrition.
- Change the ventilator circuit only if visibly soiled or malfunctioning (or per manufacturer instructions).

Airway problems

Endotracheal tube out of position. If not properly secured, the ETT can become dislodged during procedures such as oral care, when changing the ETT securement device, during transport, or if the patient is anxious or agitated and attempts to pull out the tube. The ETT may be displaced upward, resulting in the cuff being positioned between or above the vocal cords. Conversely, the tube may advance too far into the airway and press on the carina or move into the right mainstem bronchus. Symptoms include absent or diminished breath sounds in the left lung and unequal chest excursion. Notify the provider of these findings so that the cuff can be let down, the tube gently retracted as needed, and the cuff properly reinflated.

Whenever the ETT is manipulated, assess for bilateral chest excursion, auscultate the chest for bilateral breath sounds after the procedure, and reassess tube position at the lip. A quick check of the centimeter markings can determine whether the tube has advanced or pulled out of position. When a serious airway problem cannot be resolved quickly, attempt to manually ventilate the patient. If the patient cannot be ventilated and the tube is not obviously displaced or the patient is not biting the airway, attempt to pass a suction catheter through the airway to determine whether it is obstructed. If the catheter cannot be passed and the patient has spontaneous respirations, deflate the cuff to allow air to pass around the tube. If the patient still cannot be adequately ventilated, remove the ETT and ventilate the patient with a bag-valve device with a mask while preparing for emergent reintubation.[6,50,53]

Unplanned extubation. The patient may intentionally or inadvertently remove the airway. The two most frequent

TABLE 10.4 **Management of Common Ventilator Alarms**

Alarm	Description	Intervention
High peak pressure	Set 10 cm H_2O above average PIP Triggered when pressure increases anywhere in circuit Ventilator responds by terminating inspiratory phase to avoid pressure injury (barotrauma)	Assess for kinks in endotracheal tube or ventilator circuit and correct. Assess for anxiety and level of sedation or patient biting or gagging on tube; administer medications if warranted; use airway securing device with bite block. Observe for coughing; auscultate lung sounds for need for suctioning or bronchodilator. Use communication assistive devices for patient who is attempting to talk. Empty water from water traps if indicated. Assess for worsening pulmonary pathological conditions resulting in reduction in lung compliance (e.g., pulmonary edema) or increase in resistance (e.g., bronchospasm). Notify RT or provider if alarm persists.
Low pressure Low PEEP/CPAP	Set 10 cm H_2O below average PIP Set 3-5 cm H_2O below set PEEP/CPAP Triggered when pressure decreases in circuit	Assess for leaks in ventilator circuit or disconnection of ventilator circuit from airway; reconnect. If malfunction is noted, manually ventilate patient with bag-mask device. Notify RT to troubleshoot alarm.
Low exhaled V_T Low VE	Set 10% below the set V_T and the patient's average VE Ensures adequate alveolar ventilation	Assess for disconnection of ventilator circuit from airway; reconnect. Assess for disconnection in any part of the ventilator circuit; reconnect. Assess for leak in cuff of artificial airway by listening for audible sounds or bubbling of secretions around the airway and using device to measure cuff pressure; inflate as needed. Assess for new or increasing air leak in a chest drain system; connect if system related, notify provider if patient related. Assess for changes in lung compliance, increase in airway resistance, or patient fatigue on a pressure mode of ventilation.
High exhaled V_T High VE	Set 10% above the set V_T and the patient's average VE	Assess cause for increased RR or V_T, such as anxiety, pain, hypoxemia, metabolic acidosis; treat. Assess for excess water in tubing; drain appropriately.
Apnea alarm	Set for < 20 seconds Warns when no exhalation detected Ventilator will default to a backup, controlled mode if alarm triggers	Assess for cause of lack of spontaneous respiratory effort (sedation, fatigue, respiratory arrest, neurological condition); physically stimulate patient; encourage patient to take a deep breath; reverse sedatives or narcotics. Manually ventilate patient and notify RT or provider to modify ventilator settings to provide more support such as a mode with mandatory breaths.

CPAP, Continuous positive airway pressure; *H_2O,* water; *PEEP,* positive end-expiratory pressure; *PIP,* peak inspiratory pressure; *RR,* respiratory rate; *RT,* respiratory therapist; *VE,* minute ventilation; *V_T,* tidal volume.

methods by which self-extubation occurs are (1) by using the tongue and (2) by leaning forward or scooting downward so that the patient uses his or her hands to remove the tube.[50,53] Unplanned extubation can also occur as a result of patient care. For example, the tube can be dislodged if the ventilator circuit or closed suction catheter pulls on the ETT during procedures such as turning. Major risk factors for unplanned extubation include agitation, especially when combined with inadequate sedation, inadequate surveillance, higher levels of consciousness, and presence of physical restraints.[50,53,54] Strategies for preventing unplanned extubation are described in Box 10.7.

Laryngeal and tracheal injury. Damage to the larynx and trachea can occur because of tube movement and excess pressure exerted by the distal cuff. Prevent the patient from excessive head movement, especially flexion and extension, which result in the tube moving up and down in the airway, causing abrasive injury. An intervention for preventing tracheal damage from the cuff is routine cuff pressure monitoring (Fig. 10.34). Pressures should not exceed 25 to 30 cm H_2O (18 to 22 mm Hg).[9,10,29] Various commercial devices are available to measure cuff pressures quickly and easily.

Damage to the oral/nasal mucosa and skin. Tape or commercial devices that secure the ETT and the tube itself can cause breakdown of the lip and oral mucosa (see Fig. 10.20). Nasal intubation may result in skin breakdown on the nares and a higher risk of sinusitis. Ongoing assessment and skin care assist in preventing damage to the mouth and nose. Reposition the ETT frequently to prevent pressure necrosis. Perioral pressure injuries were the most prevalent oral complication associated with mechanical ventilation in patients with COVID-19 and most often were attributed to the duration of intubation and the devices used to secure the ETT.[55] Skin and soft tissue injuries caused by pressure from a tracheostomy have been estimated to occur in 5.5% of total cases. Device-related pressure injury from a tracheostomy tube can be attributed to inadequate moisture management and pressure from the tracheostomy plate and ties. A recent report of a quality improvement initiative described care elements that were shown to reduce these injuries to include protective foam dressing and skin barrier, careful suture placement to prevent excessive tension, suture removal at day 5 to 7, standardized stoma care and skin assessment, offloading pressure prophylactically at scheduled intervals, and clear documentation of all assessments and interventions.[56]

BOX 10.7 Strategies for Unplanned or Self-Extubation

- Provide patient education regarding the purpose of the artificial airway and reassurance that it will be removed as soon as the patient can breathe independently.
- Evaluate readiness for ventilator liberation early and often.
- Provide adequate analgesia and sedation.
- Educate staff to assess for risk factors for self-extubation.
- Monitor all intubated patients vigilantly but especially those at high risk. Request that another staff member monitor the patient if the nurse needs to leave the area. Educate the family to assist in monitoring the patient.
- Apply protective devices only as needed after less restrictive methods have been exhausted (e.g., soft wrist restraints, arm immobilizers, mittens) according to hospital standards of practice.
- Adequately secure the endotracheal tube.
- Cut the end of the endotracheal tube to 2 inches beyond the fixation point.
- Provide support for the ventilator tubing and closed suction systems; keep these items out of the patient's reach.
- Use two staff members when applying or changing an endotracheal tube securement device.
- Identify one staff member to monitor the airway during patient movement and transport.
- Use professional communication techniques that ensure extubation in a timely manner when the patient meets established criteria.

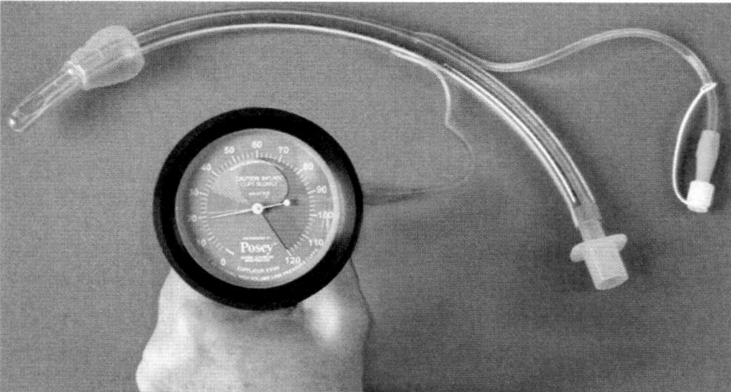

Fig. 10.34 Monitoring endotracheal tube cuff pressure. (Reprinted with permission, Cleveland Clinic Center for Medical Art & Photography © 2011–2019. All Rights Reserved.)

CHECK YOUR UNDERSTANDING

3. In which of the following situations would noninvasive ventilation be an appropriate solution?
   A. A patient with COPD and right lower-lobe pneumonia with respiratory acidosis and increased WOB.
   B. A patient with a blood pressure of 65/35, heart rate of 150 beats/min, and respiratory rate of 39 breaths/min.
   C. A patient with pneumonia who has copious amounts of purulent, thick secretions.
   D. A 65-year-old man diagnosed with ST elevation myocardial infarction (STEMI) who has cardiogenic pulmonary edema.

Pulmonary system

Trauma. *Barotrauma,* which means "pressure trauma," is injury to the lungs associated with mechanical ventilation. In barotrauma, alveolar injury or rupture occurs because of excessive pressure, excessive peak inflating volume (volutrauma), or both.[43,45,57] Barotrauma may occur when the alveoli are overdistended, such as with positive-pressure ventilation, PEEP, and high V_T. Precipitating factors include diseases in which the lung has reduced compliance, such as ARDS and pneumonia associated with high PIP and mean airway pressures. The alveoli rupture or tear so that air escapes into various parts of the thoracic cavity, causing subcutaneous emphysema (air in the tissue space), pneumothorax or tension pneumothorax, pneumomediastinum, pneumopericardium, or pneumoperitoneum. Signs and symptoms of barotrauma include decreasing SpO_2, decreased breath sounds, tracheal shift, subcutaneous crepitus, new air leak or increase in air leak in a chest drainage system, and symptoms associated with hypoxemia.

A life-threatening complication is a *tension pneumothorax.* When tension pneumothorax occurs, pressurized air enters the pleural space. Air is unable to exit the pleural space and continues to accumulate. Air in the pleural space causes an increase in intrathoracic pressure, increasing amounts of lung collapse, shifting of the heart and great vessels to the opposite thorax *(mediastinal shift),* tachycardia, and hypotension. Treatment consists of immediate insertion of a chest tube or a needle thoracostomy. Whenever a pneumothorax is suspected in a patient receiving mechanical ventilation, remove the patient from the ventilator and ventilate with a bag-valve device until a needle thoracostomy or a chest tube insertion is performed.

Lung tissue injury induced by local or regional overdistending volume is called *volutrauma.* The damage that occurs to the lung is similar to the pathological findings of early ARDS and is the result of local stress and strain on the alveolar-capillary membrane. Volutrauma results in increased permeability of the alveolar-capillary membrane, pulmonary edema, accumulation of white blood cells and protein in the alveolar spaces, and reduced surfactant production. Because it is difficult to determine the exact distribution of volume in a patient's lung, pressure is used as a surrogate for volume. The PIP is kept below 40 cm H_2O and/or the Pplat is kept at less than 30 cm H_2O as lung protective strategies to prevent both volutrauma and barotrauma.[6,20,43] Ventilator settings are adjusted to achieve these goals and may include reducing the V_T in a volume mode of ventilation or the inspiratory pressure in a pressure mode of ventilation.

Oxygen toxicity. The exposure of the pulmonary tissues to high levels of oxygen can lead to pathological changes. The degree of injury is related to the duration of exposure and to the FiO_2, not to the PaO_2. The first sign of oxygen toxicity, tracheobronchitis, is caused by irritant effects of oxygen. Prolonged exposure to high FiO_2 may lead to changes in the lung that mimic ARDS. Absorption atelectasis is another problem associated with high FiO_2. Nitrogen is needed to prevent collapse of the alveoli. When the FiO_2 is 1.0, alveolar collapse and atelectasis result from a lack of nitrogen in the distal air spaces. The goal is conservative oxygen therapy, targeting a PaO_2 of 70 to 100 mm Hg, or an SpO_2 of 90% to 92%, with an FiO_2 of 0.60 or less.[18,23] PEEP can also be adjusted to improve oxygenation in patients with collapsed alveoli.

Respiratory acidosis or alkalosis. Acid-base disturbances may occur secondary to V_T and RR settings on the ventilator. For example, if a patient is receiving V-A/C ventilation set at 10 breaths/min but the patient's RR is 28 breaths/min because of pain or anxiety, respiratory alkalosis may occur. If the ventilator is set at a low RR (e.g., 2 to 6 breaths/min) and the patient does not have an adequate drive to initiate additional breaths, respiratory acidosis may occur. Ideally the V_T and RR are set to achieve a VE that ensures a normal $PaCO_2$ level.

Infection. Patients with artificial airways who are receiving mechanical ventilation are at an increased risk of VAE because normal upper airway defense mechanisms are bypassed. The principal mechanism for the development of VAE is aspiration of colonized gastric and oropharyngeal secretions. Factors that contribute to VAE include poor oral hygiene, aspiration, contaminated respiratory therapy equipment, poor hand washing by caregivers, breach of aseptic technique when suctioning, inadequate humidification, poor systemic hydration, and decreased ability to produce an effective cough because of the artificial airway. Specific strategies to reduce VAE include the following.[31,39]

- Avoid intubation and use noninvasive mechanical ventilation when possible.
- Implement the VAE bundle (see Clinical Alert: Implementation of the Ventilator Bundle).
- Maintain and improve the patient's physical conditioning through early exercise and mobilization.
- Ensure that secretions are aspirated from above the cuff before cuff deflation or tube removal.
- Maintain the ventilator circuit and change only if visibly soiled or malfunctioning.
- Prevent drainage of ventilator circuit condensate into the patient's airway. Always discard condensate and never drain it back into the humidifier.
- Practice proper hand hygiene and wear gloves when handling respiratory secretions.

Determination of VAE has low sensitivity and specificity. The Centers for Disease Control and Prevention, along with a team of experts, has recommended surveillance for ventilator-associated conditions, including infectious and noninfectious causes. See Chapter 15, Acute Respiratory Failure.

! CLINICAL ALERT

Ventilator-Associated Events

- Following a stable period or improvement for 2 or more days on mechanical ventilation, a ventilator-associated condition (VAC) is determined by worsening oxygenation: (1) need to increase the fraction of inspired oxygen (FiO_2) or (2) need to increase positive end-expiratory pressure (PEEP).
- VAC criteria alert the caregivers that a clinically important pulmonary condition is developing, such as atelectasis, pulmonary edema, pneumothorax, pneumonia, or acute respiratory distress syndrome.
- VAC, which may be preventable, predicts poor patient outcomes, including prolonged mechanical ventilation, increased length of stay in the critical care unit, and increased hospital mortality.
- The nurse plays an important role in monitoring for trends in worsening oxygenation and gathering assessment data to help determine the underlying cause.

From Centers for Disease Control and Prevention. Device Associated Module: Ventilator-Associated Event (VAE). http://www.cdc.gov/nhsn/PDFs/pscManual/10-VAE_FINAL.pdf. Published 2023. Accessed December 8, 2023.

Dysphagia and aspiration. Artificial airways increase the risk of upper airway injury, which in turn affects upper airway mechanics and protective reflexes, resulting in a swallowing disorder.[2,42] When the patient cannot effectively transfer food, liquids, and pills from the mouth to the stomach, quality of life and functional status are affected. Patients intubated for as short as 24 hours are at risk for disordered swallowing, which can lead to aspiration, oxygen desaturation, pneumonia, and potentially reintubation. Reports of dysphagia following intubation vary widely, ranging from 3% to 62%, mostly because of varied assessment methods and instruments (see Evidence-Based Practice box). Although oral feedings may be indicated after extubation or tracheostomy, dysphagia screening and/or a dysphagia (swallowing) evaluation is recommended prior to initiating oral intake.[58] Dysphagia screening is a pass/fail series of assessments to identify individuals who may either proceed to dietary intake or require a comprehensive referral to a speech-language pathologist prior to initiating oral intake. In some institutions, a 3-ounce water swallow test followed by observation by a nurse, speech-language pathologist, or provider for clinical signs of aspiration has shown promise in identifying this potentially serious complication. This type of bedside screening for dysphagia is more common with stroke patients and is increasingly becoming the standard of care following extubation.[58] Diagnosis of a swallowing disorder is made by the speech-language pathologist using tests such as a bedside swallow evaluation or a fiberoptic endoscopic evaluation of swallow study. Review results of the swallowing evaluation and implement the treatment recommendations, such as specific food consistencies or body position when eating or drinking.

Cardiovascular system. Hypotension and decreased cardiac output may occur with mechanical ventilation and PEEP, secondary to increased intrathoracic pressure, which can result in decreased venous return. The hemodynamic effects of mechanical ventilation are more pronounced in patients with hypovolemia or poor cardiac reserve. Patients with a high PIP who receive PEEP of greater than 8 cm H_2O may need hemodynamic monitoring to assess volume status and cardiac output.[6,10,45] Management of hypotension and decreased cardiac output involves the administration of volume to ensure an adequate preload, followed by administration of inotropic agents as necessary.

Gastrointestinal system. Stress ulcers and gastrointestinal bleeding (GIB) may occur in patients who undergo mechanical ventilation, but the association with mechanical ventilation itself is unclear.[59] In the absence of any new guidelines, SUP is generally administered to patients for whom mechanical ventilation is anticipated to be 48 hours or greater. While SUP has shown a modest reduction in clinically relevant GIB, it has also been associated with a higher rate of pneumonia.[52] It is controversial whether SUP is needed after the patient is started on enteral nutrition. Initiate enteral feeding as soon as possible and monitor the patient for gross blood in the gastric aspirate and stools. Other interventions include identification and reduction of stressors, communication and reassurance, and administration of anxiolytic or sedative agents, as necessary,

EVIDENCE-BASED PRACTICE

Problem

The rates of difficulty swallowing (dysphagia) after liberation from an endotracheal tube (ETT) or postextubation dysphagia (PED) are reported to range from 3% to 62%. Patients with PED are at increased risk of aspiration due to altered glottic and subglottic sensation. As a result, PED is associated with prolonged hospital and critical care unit length of stay, increased rates of nosocomial pneumonia, and increased all-cause mortality. Given this wide reported range, it is challenging to determine the disease burden of PED and the need for qualified professionals to ensure early identification and management.

Clinical Question

First, what is the incidence of dysphagia after ETT intubation in adult critically ill patients? Second, is the wide range in reported incidence explained by differences in dysphagia assessment method, study recruitment strategies, primary reason for admission, duration of intubation, or timing of dysphagia assessment?

Evidence

A systematic review of 38 articles was conducted. From these 38 studies, 5798 patient episodes were included in the review. PED incidence ranged from 6% to 83%, with half of the studies reporting a 40% or higher incidence. Dysphagia assessment methods varied between studies and included fiberoptic endoscopic evaluation of swallowing (FEES), clinical swallowing examination by a speech pathologist, bedside dysphagia screen, patient report of symptoms, videofluoroscopy, and combinations of these. Meta-analysis identified an overall weighted incidence of PED of 41%, which equates to approximately 8.2 million people annually worldwide, demonstrating that PED is common postextubation. The findings also demonstrated that 36% of patients with PED aspirate silently and that there was no difference in the incidence of PED in patients' short-term (<48 hours) or long-term (>48 hours) intubation. Univariate and multivariate meta-regression analysis failed to identify specific factors that explain the wide variation in reported incidence of PED among the 38 studies.

Implications for Nursing

Consider all recently extubated critical care unit patients as at risk for PED and be aware of the institution's guidelines regarding the offering of food and drink postextubation. It is important for nurses to use clinical reasoning as well as any decision-making tools to perform a clinical bedside evaluation to detect dysphagia. Assessment findings that may indicate the need for further evaluation by a speech pathologist include inability to sustain alertness, produce a strong and productive cough, or manage saliva or when the vocal quality is wet/gurgly, soft, or weak. Given the scope of this clinical problem and profound negative impact on patients, there is a need for nursing to be engaged in the development and validation of bedside dysphagia screening tools.

Level of Evidence

Level C—Systematic review

Reference

McIntyre M, Doeltgen S, Dalton N, Koppa M, Chimunda T. Post-extubation dysphagia incidence in critically ill patients: a systematic review and meta-analysis. *Aust Crit Care.* 2021;34(1):67–75.

based on standardized assessment tools (see Chapter 6, Comfort and Sedation).

Nutritional support is required for all patients who require mechanical ventilation (see Chapter 7, Nutritional Therapy). Early nutritional support may reduce the severity of disease and decrease complications and length of stay.[60] The type of formula may need to be modified for ventilated patients. Excess CO_2 production may occur with high-carbohydrate feedings and place a burden on the respiratory system to excrete the CO_2, increasing the WOB. Formulas developed for the patient with pulmonary disorders may be indicated.[60] Keep the head of the bed elevated 30 to 45 degrees during enteral feeding to reduce the risk of aspiration. Another paramount problem for mechanically ventilated patients is thirst. A recent study showed that despite practical attempts to relieve thirst, no clear evidence-based strategy is available for addressing this patient problem. Nurses are in an excellent position to evaluate and report on strategies that alleviate the patient's thirst.[61]

Psychosocial complications. Several psychosocial hazards may occur because of mechanical ventilation. Patients may

NURSING SELF-CARE BOX

Calming Stress Using Controlled Lower Abdominal Breathing

Stress in the Critical Care Unit

- Caring for critically ill patients with respiratory system instability, mechanical ventilation, and communication barriers is stressful.
- The fast-paced environment of the critical care unit and constant needs of the patient and family serve as additional sources of stress for the critical care nurse.
- Stress and anxiety can contribute to shallow, upper chest breathing, which further stimulates the stress response and leads to upper back, neck, and jaw discomfort.
- The ventilator and ventilated patient can serve as external reminders to appreciate the ability to breathe spontaneously and to take controlled lower abdominal breaths. This type of breath stimulates the vagus nerve of the parasympathetic nervous system (PSNS), resulting in calm and restoring harmony and clarity of thought.

Controlled Lower Abdominal Breathing

- This technique may be done in the clinical setting, even at the patient's bedside or, if time allows, in a break or meditation room.
- Standing, place feet shoulder-width apart and parallel, knees relaxed, and allow the whole pelvic region to relax and drop down. Stand straight to allow the thoracic cavity to expand and gently lengthen the neck toward the sky.
- Fold one hand over the other on your navel to help focus your awareness to breathe into the abdomen.
- Inhale slowly to the count of 6 through the nose, dropping the diaphragm and the pelvic floor, allowing the breath to first fill your belly, then your lower chest and finally the upper chest. Exhale to the count of 6, aiming for the goal of 5 to 7 breaths/min. Aim for the breath to feel like a gentle wave rising: cresting and falling.
- Feel the calmness as the PSNS tone increases. Along with calming may come a host of responses, such as increased feelings of trust, safety, compassion, and ease.

From Deadman P. The transformative power of deep, slow breathing. *J Chinese Med.* 2018(116):56-62; Gillihan S. Yes, deep breathing will work—eventually: These five principles can help to calm your nervous system. *Psychol Today.* 2021;54(3):42-42.

experience stress and anxiety because they require a machine for breathing. If the ventilator is not set properly or if the patient resists breaths, patient-ventilator dyssynchrony may occur. The noise of the ventilator and the need for frequent procedures, such as suctioning, may alter sleep-wake patterns. In addition, the patient can become psychologically dependent on the ventilator.[62]

NURSING CARE

Nursing care of the patient who requires mechanical ventilation is complex. Use a holistic approach in patient care management. A detailed plan of care is described in the box titled Plan of Care for the Mechanically Ventilated Patient.

Communication

Communication difficulties are common because of the artificial airway. Patients identify lack of effective communication as a major stressor that elicits feelings of fear, frustration, isolation, anger, helplessness, anxiety, and sleeplessness.[62] Patients express a need to make themselves understood. They need constant reorientation, reassuring words emphasizing a caregiver's presence, and point-of-care information that painful procedures done to them are indeed necessary and helpful. Increased frequency and repetition of explanations may help the patient cope with the experience of mechanical ventilation. In addition, touch, eye contact, and positive facial expressions are beneficial in relieving anxiety. Caregivers who attempt to individualize communication with intubated patients by using a variety of methods provide patients with a greater sense of control, encourage participation in their own care, and minimize cognitive disturbances.

Head nods, mouthing words, gestures, and writing are identified as the most frequently used methods of nonverbal communication among intubated patients, but they are often inhibited by wrist restraints. Communication with gestures and lip reading can convey some basic needs; however, augmentative devices may facilitate even better communication. The term *augmentative and alternative communication strategies* describes a set of tools, technologies, and/or approaches used to solve communicative challenges in voiceless patients.[62] Although writing is sometimes used, critically ill patients are often too weak or poorly positioned to write, or they lack the concentration to spell. Greater use of communication aids such as charts, communication boards, tablet computers with a communication app, and computer-generated voice devices

PLAN OF CARE

For the Mechanically Ventilated Patient

Patient Problem

Decreased Gas Exchange. Risk factors include respiratory muscle fatigue, retained secretions, inadequate lung expansion, immobility, and metabolic factors.

Desired Outcomes

- Spontaneous ventilation with normal or baseline ABGs.
- Free of dyspnea or restlessness.
- No complications associated with mechanical ventilation.
- Patient able to manage secretions.
- Clear lung sounds.

Nursing Assessments/Interventions	Rationales
• Have bag-valve device and suctioning equipment readily available.	• Be prepared in the event of airway incompetency; maintain airway patency.
• Maintain artificial airway. • Secure ETT or tracheostomy with tape or commercial devices. • Prevent unplanned extubation (see Box 10.7).	• Ensure maintenance of an adequate airway to facilitate mechanical ventilation. • Prevent unintended removal of artificial airway.
• Assess position of artificial airway: o Auscultate for bilateral breath sounds. o Evaluate placement on chest radiograph. o Once proper position is confirmed, note position of the tube at the lip line in the medical record. o Assess depth of tube (cm markings) during routine monitoring.	• Maintain an adequate airway by ensuring that artificial airway is in the proper position.
• Monitor oxygenation and ventilation and respond to changes in: o Vital signs o Total respiratory rate o Exhaled tidal volume of ventilator-assisted and patient-initiated breaths o Oxygen saturation o End-tidal CO_2 o Mental status and level of consciousness o Signs and symptoms of hypoxemia (see Box 10.1) o ABGs	• Ensure adequate oxygenation, ventilation, and acid-base balance. • Identify when ventilator setting changes are indicated.

PLAN OF CARE—cont'd

For the Mechanically Ventilated Patient

Nursing Assessments/Interventions	Rationales
• Assess respiratory status at least every 4 hours, including initiation of assisted or spontaneous breaths in the mechanically ventilated patient.	• Ensure that patient is breathing comfortably and is not expending excessive energy on the work of breathing.
• Change position of the ETT minimally every 12 hours. o Assess and document skin condition. o Note placement of tube at lip line. o Use two staff members for procedure. o Suction secretions above the ETT cuff before repositioning tube. o After the procedure, assess position of tube at lip and auscultate for bilateral breath sounds.	• Prevent skin breakdown from the tube, tape, or airway securing device. • Prevent aspiration of oral secretions and ventilator-associated pneumonia. • Ensure that the tube remains in the proper position after manipulation.
• Monitor cuff pressure of ETT or tracheostomy and maintain within therapeutic range.	• Prevent complications associated with overinflation or underinflation of ETT cuff.
• Maintain integrity of mechanical ventilator circuit.	• Ensure safe administration of mechanical ventilation.
• Monitor ventilator settings and respond to ventilator alarms.	• Ensure adequate oxygenation and ventilation.
• Keep tubing free of moisture by draining away from the patient or using water traps to collect condensate.	• Prevent aspiration of contaminated condensate.
• Assess prescribed ventilator settings every 4 hours (mode, set rate, V_T, FiO_2, PEEP).	• Ensure that patient is receiving therapy as ordered; promote patient safety.
• Ensure that alarms are on and respond to all ventilator alarms.	• Provide immediate intervention in response to specific alarm; promote patient safety.
• Assess PIP at least every 4 hours. Collaborate with RT to adjust ventilator settings to ensure that PIP does not exceed 40 cm H_2O.	• Identify elevations in PIP, which may indicate worsening lung function.
• Implement indicated therapies to improve pulmonary compliance (secretion removal, diuresis, mobilization) and reduce resistance (bronchodilators, keep tubing drained of condensate).	• Promote adequate oxygenation and ventilation.
• Assess tolerance to ventilatory assistance and monitor for patient-ventilator asynchrony. Notify RT and provider of potential need to adjust ventilator settings: o Patient's respiratory cycle out of phase with ventilator o High-pressure and/or low-EV_T alarms o Subjective report of breathlessness o Labored respirations, especially increased effort on inspiration o Tachypnea o Anxiety, agitation	• Provide cues of condition improving or worsening; may indicate need for suctioning or need to adjust ventilator settings that are insufficient to meet patient's ventilatory needs.
• Monitor serial chest radiographs.	• Assess for correct position of ETT and improvement or worsening of pulmonary conditions.
• Implement a multiprofessional plan of care to address underlying pulmonary condition: o Evaluate response to lung expansion, bronchial hygiene, and pulmonary medication therapies. o Mobilize patient as much as possible (i.e., turning, progressive upright mobility, lateral rotation therapy). o Consider pronation therapy to treat refractive hypoxemia in ARDS. o Ensure adequate hydration, nutrition, and electrolyte balance.	• Mechanical ventilation only supports the respiratory system until the underlying condition is treated or resolved; well-coordinated team effort is essential to avoid fragmentation of care.

Patient Problem

Potential for Dyspnea. Risk factors include debilitated condition, sleep-pattern disturbances, inadequate nutrition, pain, anemia, abdominal distension, and psychological factors.

Desired Outcomes

- Liberation from mechanical ventilation.
- Adequate ABG values.
- Respiratory pattern and rate WNL.
- Effective secretion clearance.

Continued

PLAN OF CARE—cont'd

For the Mechanically Ventilated Patient

Nursing Assessments/Interventions	Rationales
• Assess patient's readiness for spontaneous breathing trial (SBT) (see Box 10.9).	• Identify readiness to begin the ventilator liberation process using validated parameters.
• Provide ventilator liberation method based on protocols and research evidence (see Box 10.8).	• Protocol-driven weaning is an effective strategy for systematic ventilator liberation that reduces ventilator days and critical care unit and hospital lengths of stay.
• Collaborate with the healthcare team to provide mechanical ventilation modes, patient coaching, and progressive mobility that supports respiratory muscle training.	• Promote respiratory conditioning that facilitates patient's ability to resume the work of breathing.
• Promote rest and comfort throughout the weaning process, especially between weaning trials; identify strategies that result in relaxation and comfort; ensure that environment is safe and comfortable.	• Facilitate mechanical ventilation liberation.
• Support patient in setting goals for weaning.	• Promote rehabilitation and give patients some control in the process.
• Collaborate with the healthcare team to determine the most effective strategies for weaning those with severe dysfunctional breathing patterns.	• Various strategies may be needed to liberate the patient; ongoing assessment is essential to determine the most effective strategy.
• Implement strategies that maximize tolerance of SBT: ○ Titrate sedation and analgesia to lowest dose possible to achieve a level at which patient is calm and cooperative with absence of respiratory depression. ○ Interrupt sedation at least twice daily to determine if it is still indicated and reduce the overall amount of sedation accumulating. Restart at half the dose and titrate as needed. ○ Schedule SBT when patient is rested. ○ Avoid other procedures during SBT. ○ Position patient upright to allow for full expansion with abdominal compression on diaphragm. ○ Monitor phosphate levels because low phosphate affects respiratory muscle function. ○ Promote normal sleep-wake cycle. ○ Limit visitors to supportive persons. ○ Coach through periods of anxiety.	• Maximize efforts to facilitate successful weaning.
○ Terminate SBT if patient is unable to tolerate the process (see Box 10.10).	○ Maintain adequate ventilation and gas exchange; prevent fatigue of respiratory muscles.
○ Consider referring patients with prolonged ventilator dependence to an alternative setting, such as a long-term acute care hospital.	○ Alternative settings specialize in weaning patients who are "difficult to wean."

ABG, Arterial blood gas; *ARDS*, acute respiratory distress syndrome; *cm H_2O*, centimeters of water; *CO_2*, carbon dioxide; *ETT*, endotracheal tube; *EV_T*, exhaled tidal volume; *FiO_2*, fraction of inspired oxygen; *PEEP*, positive end-expiratory pressure; *PIP*, peak inspiratory pressure; *RT*, respiratory therapist; *V_T*, tidal volume; *WNL*, within normal limits.

Adapted from Snyder J, Sump C. *Swearingen's All-in-One Nursing Care Planning Resource.* 6th ed. St. Louis, MO: Elsevier, 2024.

could improve communication. A picture board with icons representing basic needs and the alphabet that can be easily cleaned between patients should be available in every unit. Family members can serve as a communication link between the patient and care providers. Reassure the patient that the loss of voice is temporary and that speech will be possible after the tube is removed.

Maintaining Comfort and Reducing Distress

Intubation, mechanical ventilation, advanced methods for ventilation (e.g., inverse-ratio ventilation), and suctioning contribute to patient discomfort and distress. Patients often need both pharmacological and nonpharmacological methods to manage discomfort and treat anxiety.[63] Strategies to promote patient comfort are discussed in depth in Chapter 6, Comfort and Sedation.

Medications. Commonly used medications include analgesics, sedatives, and neuromuscular blocking agents; many patients need a combination of these drugs. Medications are chosen based on the patient's hemodynamic stability, diagnosis, and the desired treatment goals. It is essential that the nurse, RT, and physician all use the same objective sedation and analgesia scoring systems to promote unambiguous assessment and communication. Nurse-driven decision trees or algorithms to guide initiation and titration of medications to targeted sedation and analgesia goals result in fewer days on sedation and mechanical ventilation. Sedation should be interrupted at least twice daily to allow the patient to awaken and be reoriented and to determine if sedation is needed. A spontaneous breathing trial (SBT; weaning attempt) should be timed with sedation interruption.[63]

Analgesics, such as morphine and fentanyl, are administered to provide pain relief. Sedatives, such as dexmedetomidine, benzodiazepines, and propofol, are given to sedate the patient, reduce anxiety, and promote synchronous breathing with the ventilator. Benzodiazepines promote amnesia but are also associated with an increase in delirium and should be avoided if possible.[63] Patients who have acute lung injury or increased intracranial pressure or who require nontraditional modes of mechanical ventilation may require deep sedation or therapeutic paralysis with neuromuscular blocking agents (see Chapter 6, Comfort and Sedation).

When sedation is indicated, it must be titrated to a specific goal agreed upon by the multiprofessional team. Insufficient sedation may precipitate ventilator dyssynchrony and physiological alterations in thoracic pressures and gas exchange. Inadequate sedation is also associated with unplanned extubation. Oversedation and prolonged sedation are associated with a longer duration of mechanical ventilation and lengths of stay in the critical care unit and hospital.[15] Prolonged duration of mechanical ventilation predisposes the patient to an increased risk of VAE, lung injury, and other complications. Depth of sedation also contributes to delayed weaning from mechanical ventilation. Because sedation, duration of mechanical ventilation, and ventilator weaning are interrelated, ensure that the patient is maintained on the lowest dose and lightest level of sedation possible. "Daily interruption," "sedation vacation," or a "spontaneous awakening trial" to evaluate the patient's cognitive status; to reduce the overall dose of sedation; and to determine what dose, if any, is needed to achieve a calm, cooperative patient is an important nursing intervention.[63] Optimal sedation of the mechanically ventilated patient is present when patient-ventilator harmony exists and the patient remains capable of taking spontaneous breaths in readiness for weaning. Many patients achieve this state without sedative agents.

Nonpharmacological Interventions. Nonpharmacological, complementary, and alternative medicine strategies may reduce distress, promote patient-ventilator synchrony, and maintain a normal cognitive state.[64] Create a healing environment by involving the patient and family in the plan of care, reducing excess noise and light stimulation, providing a reassuring presence, and minimizing unnecessary patient stimulation to promote a normal sleep-wake cycle. Provide adequate rest and frequent reorientation to prevent delirium. Implement a progressive mobility plan to reduce deconditioning and promote endurance of the respiratory muscles to facilitate ventilator liberation. Daytime exercise may also promote a more restful nighttime sleep.

Meditation, guided imagery and relaxation, prayer, music therapy, massage, acupressure, therapeutic touch, herbal products and dietary supplements, and family presence are nonpharmacological strategies to improve patient well-being. Ask the family and patient if they are already using complementary strategies, and if so, incorporate them as possible. The goal of incorporating these therapies into practice is to reduce patient distress, promote sleep, and create a healing environment conducive to reducing ventilator days.

CLINICAL JUDGMENT ACTIVITY

You are caring for a patient who has been mechanically ventilated for 2 weeks. Physically, the patient meets all criteria to begin mechanical ventilation liberation with a spontaneous breathing trial. What parameters should you monitor to assess tolerance of weaning and the patient's ability to sustain spontaneous breathing after extubation?

Liberating Patients From Mechanical Ventilation

Mechanical ventilation is a therapy designed to support the respiratory system until the underlying disease or indication for mechanical ventilation is resolved. Weaning, or liberating, is the process of decreasing ventilator support and allowing the patient to assume a greater percentage of the work of ventilation. It may involve either an immediate shift from full ventilatory support to a period of breathing with minimal assistance (i.e., an SBT) or a gradual reduction in the amount of ventilator support. In general, patients who require short-term ventilatory support are liberated quickly.[46,64,65] Conversely, liberating patients who require long-term ventilatory support is often a slower process characterized by periods of success as well as setbacks. Once the patient demonstrates the ability to breathe without the ventilator and both airway patency and airway protection are ensured, removal of the artificial airway is considered.[66]

Evidence-Based Approaches to Liberation from Mechanical Ventilation. Based on a comprehensive review of the research, evidence-based guidelines for ventilator liberation have been developed.[46,64] Box 10.8 summarizes these guidelines. Liberation protocols define a systematic, often algorithmic process and achieve the best outcomes when implemented by the nurse and the RT. Provider-led liberation management is associated with a wide variation in timing and responsiveness to successful liberation trials.[67] Protocols should clearly define the method or screening tool to determine the patient's readiness to wean, the method and duration of the SBT, action to facilitate adequate rest if the patient does not pass the SBT, and criteria for extubation. See the Exemplar box for an example of teamwork and collaboration during the weaning process.

Assessment for Readiness to Wean (Wean Screen). Before initiating the SBT, screen the patient for readiness using parameters that have been associated with ventilator discontinuation success (Box 10.9). Screening assists in identifying patients who are ready to attempt an SBT as well as those who are not ready, thereby protecting them against the associated risks.

BOX 10.8 Evidence-Based Guidelines for Mechanical Ventilation Liberation

1. If the patient requires ventilation for longer than 24 hours, assess at least daily to identify causes for ventilator dependence.
2. Conduct a formal assessment to determine a high potential for successful liberation (see Box 10.10).
3. Conduct an SBT with inspiratory pressure augmentation (5-8 cm H_2O) rather than without (T-piece or CPAP). During the SBT, evaluate respiratory pattern, adequacy of gas exchange, hemodynamic stability, and comfort. A patient who tolerates an SBT for 30 to 120 minutes should be considered for permanent ventilator discontinuation.
4. If a patient fails an SBT, determine the cause of the failed trial. Some factors to consider include respiratory depression from sedation or analgesia, infection, fever, anxiety, sleep deprivation, anemia, pain, abdominal distension, and bowel abnormalities (diarrhea or constipation). Return the patient to a method of ventilatory support that is nonfatiguing and comfortable to provide rest. Correct reversible causes and attempt an SBT every 24 hours if the patient meets weaning criteria.
5. For patients who have been receiving mechanical ventilation for more than 24 hours, have passed an SBT, and are at high risk for extubation failure (i.e., hypercapnia, COPD, CHF, or other serious comorbidities), extubate to preventative NIV.[49]
6. For acutely hospitalized adults who have been mechanically ventilated for more than 24 hours, a physical conditioning plan using protocolized rehabilitation directed toward early mobilization should be used.[65,68]
7. Assess airway patency and the ability of the patient to protect the airway to determine whether to remove the artificial airway from a patient who has been successfully weaned. Perform a cuff leak test (CLT) in patients at high risk for postextubation stridor (i.e., traumatic intubation, intubation longer than 6 days, large ETT, female, or reintubation after unplanned extubation). For patients who fail a CLT, administer systemic steroids at least 4 hours before extubation.
8. Use protocols aimed at minimizing sedation.
9. Use either (RT and RN) personnel or computer-driven ventilator liberation protocol.[65]
10. Consider a tracheostomy when it becomes apparent that the patient will require prolonged ventilator assistance.
11. Conduct slow-paced weaning in a patient who requires prolonged mechanical ventilation. Wean a patient to 50% of maximum ventilator support before daily SBT. Then initiate SBTs with gradual increase in duration of the SBT.
12. Unless evidence of irreversible disease exists (e.g., high cervical spine injury), do not consider a patient to be ventilator dependent until 3 months of weaning attempts have failed.
13. Transfer a patient who has failed weaning attempts but is medically stable to a facility that specializes in management of ventilator-dependent patients.

CHF, Congestive heart failure; *cm H_2O*, centimeters of water; *COPD*, chronic obstructive pulmonary disease; *CPAP*, continuous positive airway pressure; *ETT*, endotracheal tube; *NIV*, noninvasive ventilation; *RN*, registered nurse; *RT*, respiratory therapist; *SBT*, spontaneous breathing trial.

BOX 10.9 Assessment Parameters Indicating Readiness to Wean

Evidence of Improvement of Underlying Cause of Respiratory Failure

- Improved chest radiograph findings
- Minimal secretions or moderate and an effective cough
- Improving breath sounds

Adequate Oxygenation Without a High FiO_2 and/or a High PEEP

- $SpO_2 \geq 92\%$ with $FiO_2 \leq 0.5$
- PEEP <9 cm H_2O

Hemodynamic Stability

- Absence of hypotension

Minimal Vasopressor Therapy or No Escalation Required, Adequate Respiratory Muscle Strength (Weaning Indices)

- Respiratory rate <25 to 30 breaths/min
- Spontaneous tidal volume 4 to 6 mL/kg IBW
- Rapid shallow breathing index <105
- Negative inspiratory force (maximum inspiratory pressure) −20 to −30 cm H_2O
- Vital capacity 10 to 15 mL/kg IBW
- Minute ventilation 5 to 10 L/min

Neurological

- Stable ICP and/or CPP, if applicable (ICP <20 mm Hg and/or CPP >60 mm Hg)

cm H_2O, Centimeters of water; *CPP*, cerebral perfusion pressure; *FiO_2*, fraction of inspired oxygen; *IBW*, ideal body weight; *ICP*, intracranial pressure; *PaO_2*, partial pressure of arterial oxygen; *PEEP*, positive end-expiratory pressure.

BOX 10.10 Criteria for Discontinuing the SBT

Respiratory

- Respiratory rate >35 breaths/min or <8 breaths/min
- Rapid shallow breathing
- Labored respirations
- Use of accessory muscles
- Abnormal breathing pattern: chest/abdominal asynchrony
- Oxygen saturation <90%

Cardiovascular

- Heart rate changes >20% from baseline
- Dysrhythmias (e.g., premature ventricular contractions, bradycardia)
- Ischemia: ST-segment elevation
- Blood pressure changes >20% from baseline
- Diaphoresis

Neurological

- Agitation, anxiety
- Decreased level of consciousness

SBT, Spontaneous breathing trial.

CLINICAL EXEMPLAR

Interprofessional Partnership

Successful patient liberation from mechanical ventilation requires a team approach. Led by a clinical nurse specialist (CNS), a hospital-established multiprofessional effort to reduce mechanical ventilator days through implementation of a spontaneous awakening trial (SAT) algorithm with spontaneous breathing trials (SBTs). The SAT and SBT protocols were revised based on current best evidence. Education was provided to all nurses, respiratory therapists (RTs), and providers. The electronic medical record was revised to mirror the protocols and facilitate provider orders, nurse and RT documentation, and patient tolerance of SAT and SBT interventions. Laminated SAT and SBT protocols were attached to ventilators and placed near charting stations. Patient sedation level and readiness to wean were discussed during multiprofessional daily rounds and the plan of care adjusted as needed, with the goal of reducing sedation to allow for extubation.

The success of the practice changes demonstrated an overall reduction in sedation (patient was less sedated using a standardized sedation assessment tool), decreased mechanical ventilation hours, and improved successful SBT with extubation. The interprofessional partnership between providers, RTs, and nurses in revising and implementing the SAT and SBT protocols led to improved practice and shorter mechanical ventilation days, thus reducing patient risks for harm.

Reference

Seyller N, Makic MBF. Clinical nurse specialist practice: impact on improving sedation practice in critical care. *Clin Nurse Spec.* 2022;36(5):264–271. https://doi.org/10.1097/NUR.0000000000000693.

Patients are usually able to attempt an SBT when the underlying disease process is resolving and they are oxygenating with minimal support, are hemodynamically stable, and are able to initiate an inspiratory effort. Assessment of the neurological, cardiovascular, and respiratory systems provides a sufficient screen in most patients requiring a ventilator for only a short period. In many settings, physiological respiratory parameters, referred to as *weaning predictors,* are also measured (see Box 10.9). The rapid shallow breathing index (RSBI) is easy to use and is the only measurement that has been shown to be a true predictor of successful liberation.

Weaning Process (Weaning Trial). Table 10.5 describes weaning methods. Evidence-based practice guidelines recommend the use of an SBT for weaning. PS, T-piece, and CPAP qualify as spontaneous breathing modes. The SBT with pressure augmentation (i.e., PS) has demonstrated a higher rate of extubation success and a trend toward lower critical care unit mortality than SBTs without pressure augmentation. An SBT for 30 to 120 minutes provides a direct assessment of spontaneous breathing capabilities and has been shown to be the most effective way to shorten the ventilator discontinuation process.[46]

Assess and monitor the patient throughout the SBT. Organize patient care to ensure vigilant assessment throughout the trial. Explain the weaning procedure to the patient and family in a manner that promotes reassurance and minimizes anxiety. Ensure that the patient is adequately rested and positioned optimally for diaphragm function and lung expansion, such as sitting. Obtain baseline parameters: vital signs, heart rhythm, SpO_2, $ETCO_2$ values, and neurological status. Monitor the patient during the SBT for tolerance of or intolerance to the procedure. Although the patient is required to increase participation in the WOB, ensure that the patient does not become fatigued and become compromised. Indicators of tolerance include an unlabored respiratory pattern, adequate oxygenation and ventilation indices, hemodynamic stability, neurological stability, and patient comfort. Box 10.10 defines the physiological parameters that constitute the integrated assessment to determine patient intolerance of the weaning process. If these signs of intolerance develop, stop the SBT and resume mechanical ventilation at ventilator settings that provide full ventilatory support.[6,20,64] However, thorough patient evaluation is necessary because reliance on a single parameter can delay ventilator liberation.

Many respiratory and nonrespiratory factors can influence weaning success. Increased oxygen demands occur with infection, fever, anemia, and pain, and asking the patient to perform another activity, such as physical therapy, during the trial can impair weaning. Other factors to assess for are decreased respiratory performance from malnutrition, overuse of sedatives or hypnotics, sleep deprivation, and abdominal distension. Factors involving equipment or technique, time of day, and method for weaning should also be examined. Psychological factors to evaluate include apprehension and fear, helplessness, and depression.[64,65] Systematically evaluate all potential factors to optimize successful weaning.

Extubation. If the patient demonstrates tolerance to the weaning procedure and can sustain spontaneous breathing for 30 to 120 minutes, the next step toward ventilator liberation is making the decision to remove the ETT. Prior to extubation, evaluate the need for airway secretion clearance; the patient must have a good cough and require suctioning no more than every 2 hours. If the patient has a tracheostomy, the patient may be liberated from the ventilator, but the tracheostomy is maintained to facilitate airway clearance. Also assess airway patency and the ability of the patient to protect the airway. Perform a cuff leak test (CLT) in patients at high risk for postextubation stridor. High risk includes traumatic intubation, intubation longer than 6 days, intubation with a large ETT, female, or reintubation after unplanned extubation. For patients who fail a CLT, administer systemic steroids at least 4 hours before extubation.[65] When the decision is made to extubate, suction the ETT thoroughly before removal. Also, suction the posterior oropharynx to remove secretions that may have pooled above the cuff, deflate the ETT cuff, and remove the ETT during inspiration. Once extubated, ask the patient to cough and speak and assess for stridor, hoarseness, changes in vital signs, or low SpO_2, which may indicate complications. Noninvasive ventilation may be used to avert reintubation in some patients.[6,10,20]

TABLE 10.5 Weaning Methods

	Description	Strategies
Spontaneous Breathing Trial (SBT) Trial of spontaneous breathing effort	Every breath is spontaneous, and patient performs all the WOB. Attempt daily if patient passes wean screen. Successful when patient remains stable for 30-120 min.	Daily trial or more often.
Reconditioning Trials Gradual exercising or reconditioning of the respiratory muscles as patient can tolerate without inducing fatigue	Alternating periods of resting on full ventilator support with advancing periods of gradually reduced support. Gradual reconditioning indicated for deconditioned patients who are unsuccessful with SBT.	Ratio of rest periods to time on trial based on patient's response. Amount of time to liberate patient varies; may be days to weeks.
Mode	**SBT Strategy**	**Difficult or Prolonged Weaning**
Pressure Support (PS) Provides inspiratory support to overcome resistance to gas flow through ventilator circuit and artificial airway	SBT = PS of 5 cm H_2O + 5 cm H_2O PEEP	Begin at level of PS that ensures nonlabored RR and V_T. Gradual reduction in PS in 2- to 5-cm H_2O increments. Gradually lengthen time interval on reduced levels of support. Discontinue when patient stable for 2 h or longer at 5 cm H_2O PS.
T-Piece Patient performs all the WOB No ventilator alarms for apnea, decreased V_T, etc. Requires high level of staff attention	Remove patient from ventilator and provide humidified oxygen via a T-piece adaptor attached to the ETT or tracheostomy tube.	May start with trial as short as 5 min. Increase time on T-piece as tolerated with adequate rest periods (6-8 h) on full ventilatory support. Discontinue when patient stable on T-piece for at least 2 h, often longer.
CPAP Useful when patient requires PEEP to maintain oxygenation Patient performs all the WOB Ventilator will provide alarms for apnea, high RR, or low EV_T	CPAP of 5 cm H_2O	CPAP of 5 cm H_2O. May start with trial as short as 5 min. Increase time on CPAP as tolerated with adequate rest periods (6-8 h) on full ventilatory support. Discontinue when patient on CPAP for at least 2 h, often longer.

cm H_2O, Centimeters of water; *CPAP,* continuous positive airway pressure; *ETT,* endotracheal tube; *EV_T,* exhaled tidal volume; *PEEP,* positive end-expiratory pressure; *RR,* respiratory rate; *V_T,* tidal volume; *WOB,* work of breathing.

CASE STUDY

Mr. P., age 65 years, was transferred to the critical care unit from the emergency department after successful resuscitation from a cardiac arrest sustained out of the hospital. Initial diagnosis based on laboratory results and electrocardiography is acute anterior myocardial infarction. It is suspected that Mr. P. aspirated gastric contents during the cardiac arrest. He opens his eyes to painful stimuli. He is orally intubated with a size 7.5-mm endotracheal tube located at the 25-cm marking at the teeth. Placement was confirmed by auscultation, end-tidal carbon dioxide, and chest radiograph. He is receiving mechanical ventilation with volume assist–control ventilation, respiratory rate set at 12 breaths/min, fraction of inspired oxygen (FiO_2) of 0.40, positive end-expiratory pressure (PEEP) of 5 cm H_2O, and tidal volume of 600 mL. An arterial blood gas drawn on arrival to the critical care unit shows the following values: pH, 7.33; partial pressure of carbon dioxide ($PaCO_2$), 40 mm Hg; bicarbonate (HCO_3^-), 20 mEq/L; partial pressure of arterial oxygen (PaO_2), 88 mm Hg; and arterial oxygen saturation (SaO_2), 99%. A decision is made to maintain the current ventilator settings. The following day, Mr. P.'s chest radiograph shows progressive infiltrates. His oxygen saturation is dropping below 90%, and he is demonstrating signs of hypoxemia: increased heart rate and premature ventricular contractions. Arterial blood gas analysis now shows pH, 7.35; $PaCO_2$, 43 mm Hg; HCO_3^-, 26 mEq/L; PaO_2, 58 mm Hg; and SaO_2, 88%. The provider orders the FiO_2 increased to 0.50 and PEEP increased to 10 cm H_2O.

Questions

1. Analyze the results of Mr. P.'s first arterial blood gas analysis. Hypothesize factors that are contributing to these results.
2. Recognize the factors that contributed to Mr. P.'s worsening condition on the day after hospital admission.
3. Analyze the arterial blood gases done on the day after the cardiac arrest.
4. Why did the provider change the ventilator settings after the second set of arterial blood gases?
5. What cues must the nurse assess for after the addition of the PEEP? Why is this especially important for Mr. P.?

KEY POINTS

- Acute respiratory failure is defined as an inability to maintain oxygenation and adequate ventilation to maintain $PaCO_2$.
- The ability to recognize a problem in the respiratory system and that a patient cannot sustain spontaneous breathing and requires an artificial airway and mechanical ventilation is an essential skill for nurses. Recognizing clinical signs of hypoxemia and hypercapnia is the first step.
- A variety of devices are used to administer supplemental oxygen and to maintain a patent natural or advanced airway.
- Invasive positive-pressure ventilation provides a range of full to partial ventilatory support. During full ventilator support, the ventilator provides all the breath, performing all the work of breathing. With partial ventilator support, the ventilatory provides a portion of the work, and the patient can assume a variable portion of the WOB.
- Noninvasive ventilation offers a viable alternative to invasive mechanical ventilation in select patients.
- The way the breath is delivered to the mechanically ventilated patient is called the *mode* of ventilation. The mode is determined by whether the breath is mandatory, IMV, or spontaneous and whether the targeted control variable is pressure or volume.
- Liberation of the patient from the mechanical ventilator is a systematic process. Best outcomes are achieved when a registered nurse and RT bedside ventilator liberation protocol is utilized.

REFERENCES

1. Patton K, Thibodeau G, Hutton A. *Anatomy and Physiology E-Book*. 1st ed. London: Elsevier Limited; 2019.
2. West JB, Luks A. *West's Respiratory Physiology: The Essentials*. 11th ed. Philadelphia, PA: Wolters Kluwer; 2021.
3. Hall JE, Hall ME. *Guyton and Hall Textbook of Medical Physiology*. 14th ed. Philadelphia, PA: Elsevier; 2021.
4. American Association of Critical Care Nurses. *AACN Core Curriculum for Progressive and Critical Care Nursing*. 8th ed. St. Louis, MO: Elsevier Health Sciences; 2022.
5. Pierce LNB. *Management of the Mechanically Ventilated Patient*. Philadelphia, PA: W.B. Saunders; 2007.
6. Cairo JM. *Pilbeam's Mechanical Ventilation: Physiological and Clinical Applications*. 7th ed. St. Louis, MO: Elsevier; 2020.
7. McCance KL, Huether SE, Brashers VL, Rote NS. *Pathophysiology: The Biologic Basis for Disease in Adults and Children*. 8th ed. St. Louis, MO: Elsevier; 2019.
8. Schwaiberger D, Karcz M, Menk M, Papadakos PJ, Dantoni SE. Respiratory failure and mechanical ventilation in the pregnant patient. *Critical Care Clinics*. 2016;32(1):85–95.
9. Oakes DF, Jones S. *Oakes' Respiratory Care Pocket Guide*. 10th ed. Zebulon, NC: Health Educator Publications, Inc.; 2021.
10. Kacmarek RM, Stoller JK, Heuer AJ. *Egan's Fundamentals of Respiratory Care E-Book*. 12th ed. St. Louis, MO: Elsevier; 2021.
11. Beachey W. *Respiratory Care Anatomy and Physiology E-Book*. 5th ed. St. Louis: Elsevier Health Sciences; 2022.
12. Pagana KD, Pagana TJ, Pagana TN. *Mosby's® Diagnostic and Laboratory Test Reference*. 15th ed. St. Louis, MO: Elsevier; 2021.
13. Lee DB. Oxygen saturation monitoring with pulse oximetry. In: Wiegand DJL-M, ed. *AACN Procedure Manual for High Acuity, Progressive, and Critical Care*. 7th ed. St. Louis, MO: Elsevier; 2017:134–141.
14. Chesley CF, Lane-Fall MB, Panchanadam V, et al. Racial disparities in occult hypoxemia and clinically based mitigation strategies to apply in advance of technological advancements. *Respiratory Care*. 2022;67(12):1499–1507.
15. Luehrs P. Continuous end-tidal carbon dioxide monitoring. In: Wiegand DJL-M, ed. *AACN Procedure Manual for High Acuity, Progressive, and Critical Care*. 7th ed. St. Louis, MO: Elsevier; 2017:103–110.
16. Cairo JM. *Mosby's Respiratory Care Equipment*. 11th ed. St. Louis, MO: Elsevier; 2022.
17. Selby ST, Abramo T, Hobart-Porter N. An update on end-tidal CO_2 monitoring. *Pediatric Emergency Care*. 2018;34(12):888–892.
18. Heuer AJ, Hilse AM. Medical gas therapy. In: Kacmarek RM, Stoller JK, Heuer AJ, eds. *Egan's Fundamentals of Respiratory Care E-Book*. 12th ed. St. Louis, MO: Elsevier; 2021:906–935.
19. Ari AFJ. Humidity and aerosol therapy. In: Cairo JM, ed. *Mosby's Respiratory Care Equipment*. 11th ed. St. Louis, MO: Elsevier; 2022.
20. Oakes DF, Jones S, Shortall SP. *Oakes' Ventilator Management Pocket Guide*. 5th ed. Zebulon, NC: Health Educator Publications, Inc.; 2022.
21. Wittenstein J, Ball L, Pelosi P, Gama de Abreu M. High-flow nasal cannula oxygen therapy in patients undergoing thoracic surgery: current evidence and practice. *Curr Opin Anaesthesiol*. 2019;32(1):44–49.
22. Rochwerg B, Einav S, Chaudhuri D, et al. The role for high flow nasal cannula as a respiratory support strategy in adults: a clinical practice guideline. *Intensive Care Med*. 2020;46(12):2226–2237.
23. Piraino T, Madden M, Roberts KJ, Lamberti J, Ginier E, Strickland SL. AARC clinical practice guideline: management of adult patients with oxygen in the acute care setting. *Respir Care*. 2022;67(1):115–128.
24. Mehmood R, Mansoor Z, Atanasov GP, et al. High-flow nasal oxygenation and its applicability in COVID patients. *SN Compr Clin Med*. 2022;4(1):49.
25. Goodrich CA. Endotracheal intubation (assist). In: Wiegand DJL-M, ed. *AACN Procedure Manual for High Acuity, Progressive, and Critical Care*. 7th ed. St. Louis, MO: Elsevier; 2017:23–31.
26. Pozuelo-Carrascosa DP, Herráiz-Adillo Á, Alvarez-Bueno C, Añón JM, Martínez-Vizcaíno V, Cavero-Redondo I. Subglottic secretion drainage for preventing ventilator-associated pneumonia: an overview of systematic reviews and an updated meta-analysis. *Eur Respir Rev*. 2020;29(155).
27. Klompas M, Li L, Kleinman K, Szumita PM, Massaro AF. Associations between ventilator bundle components and outcomes. *JAMA Intern Med*. 2016;176(9):1277–1283.
28. Klompas M, Branson R, Cawcutt K, et al. Strategies to prevent ventilator-associated pneumonia, ventilator-associated events, and nonventilator hospital-acquired pneumonia in acute-care hospitals: 2022 update. *Infect Cont Hosp Epidemiol*. 2022;43(6):687–713.
29. La Vita C. Airway management. In: Kacmarek RM, Stoller JK, Heuer AJ, eds. *Egan's Fundamentals of Respiratory Care E-Book*. 12th ed. St. Louis, MO: Elsevier; 2021:748–787.

30. Shilling AM, Thames M. Airway management devices and advanced cardiac life support. In: Cairo JM, ed. *Mosby's Respiratory Care Equipment*. 11th ed. St. Louis, MO: Elsevier; 2022:104–149.
31. Freeman BD. Tracheostomy update: when and how. *Crit Care Clin*. 2017;33(2):311–322.
32. Craven J, Slaughter A, Potter KF. Early tracheostomy: on the cutting edge, some benefit more than others. *Curr Opin Anaesthesiol*. 2022;35(2):236–241.
33. Raimondi N, Vial MR, Calleja J, et al. Evidence-based guidelines for the use of tracheostomy in critically ill patients. *J Crit Care*. 2017;38:304–318.
34. Adly A, Youssef TA, El-Begermy MM, Younis HM. Timing of tracheostomy in patients with prolonged endotracheal intubation: a systematic review. *Eur Arch Oto-Rhino-Laryngol*. 2018;275(3):679–690.
35. Ghattas C, Alsunaid S, Pickering EM, Holden VK. State of the art: percutaneous tracheostomy in the intensive care unit. *J Thorac Dis*. 2021;13(8):5261–5276.
36. Auzinger G. Early percutaneous tracheostomy during the pandemic "as good as it gets." *Crit Care Med*. 2021;49(2):361–364.
37. Santiago CRD, Porretta K, Smith O. The use of tablet and communication app for patients with endotracheal or tracheostomy tubes in the medical surgical intensive care unit: a pilot, feasibility study. *Can J Crit Care Nurs*. 2019;30(1):17–23.
38. Sole ML, Bennett M, Ashworth S. Clinical indicators for endotracheal suctioning in adult patients receiving mechanical ventilation. *Am J Crit Care*. 2015;24(4):318–325.
39. Seckel M. Suctioning: endotracheal or tracheostomy tube. In: Wiegand DJL-M, ed. *AACN Procedure Manual for High Acuity, Progressive, and Critical Care*. 7th ed. St. Louis, MO: Elsevier; 2017:69–78.
40. Blakeman TC, Scott JB, Yoder MA, Capellari E, Strickland SL. AARC clinical practice guidelines: artificial airway suctioning. *Respir Care*. 2022;67(2):258–271.
41. Ayhan H, Tastan S, Iyigun E, Akamca Y, Arikan E, Sevim Z. Normal saline instillation before endotracheal suctioning: "what does the evidence say? what do the nurses think?": multimethod study. *J Crit Care*. 2015;30(4):762–767.
42. Caparros AC. Mechanical ventilation and the role of saline instillation in suctioning adult intensive care unit patients: an evidence-based practice review. *Dimens Crit Care Nurs*. 2014;33(4):246–253.
43. Brower RG, Matthay MA, Morris A, Schoenfeld D, Thompson BT, Wheeler A. Ventilation with lower tidal volumes as compared with traditional tidal volumes for acute lung injury and the acute respiratory distress syndrome. *New Engl J Med*. 2000;342(18):1301–1308.
44. Gallagher JJ. Alternative modes of mechanical ventilation. *AACN Adv Crit Care*. 2018;29(4):396–404.
45. Pham T, Brochard LJ, Slutsky AS. Mechanical ventilation: state of the art. *Mayo Clin Proc*. 2017;92(9):1382–1400.
46. Ouellette DR, Patel S, Girard TD, et al. Liberation from mechanical ventilation in critically ill adults: an official American College of Chest Physicians/American Thoracic Society clinical practice guideline: inspiratory pressure augmentation during spontaneous breathing trials, protocols minimizing sedation, and noninvasive ventilation immediately after extubation. *Chest*. 2017;151(1):166–180.
47. Sklar MC, Burns K, Rittayamai N, et al. Effort to breathe with various spontaneous breathing trial techniques. A physiologic meta-analysis. *Am J Respir Crit Care Med*. 2017;195(11):1477–1485.
48. Vieira PC, de Oliveira RB, da Silva Mendonça TM. Should oral chlorhexidine remain in ventilator-associated pneumonia prevention bundles? *Medicina Intensiva*. 2022;46(5):259–268.
49. Frazier SK. Noninvasive positive pressure ventilation: continuous positive airway pressure (CPAP) and bilevel positive airway pressure (BiPAP). In: Wiegand DL, ed. *AACN Procedure Manual for High Acuity, Progressive, and Critical Care*. 7th ed. St. Louis, MO: Elsevier; 2017:249–260.
50. Ai ZP, Gao XL, Zhao XL. Factors associated with unplanned extubation in the intensive care unit for adult patients: a systematic review and meta-analysis. *Intensive Crit Care Nurs*. 2018;47:62–68.
51. Sozkes S, Sozkes S. Use of toothbrushing in conjunction with chlorhexidine for preventing ventilator-associated pneumonia: a random-effect meta-analysis of randomized controlled trials. *Int J Dent Hyg*. May 2023;21(2):389–397.
52. Wang Y, Ge L, Ye Z, et al. Efficacy and safety of gastrointestinal bleeding prophylaxis in critically ill patients: an updated systematic review and network meta-analysis of randomized trials. *Intensive Care Med*. 2020;46(11):1987–2000.
53. Danielis M, Chiaruttini S, Palese A. Unplanned extubations in an intensive care unit: findings from a critical incident technique. *Intensive Crit Care Nurs*. 2018;47:69–77.
54. Pengbo L, Zihong S, Jingyi X. Unplanned extubation among critically ill adults: a systematic review and meta-analysis. *Intensive Crit Care Nurs*. 2022;70:103219.
55. Khan W, Safi A, Muneeb M, Mooghal M, Aftab A, Ahmed J. Complications of invasive mechanical ventilation in critically ill Covid-19 patients—a narrative review. *Ann Med Surg*. 2022;80:104201.
56. Urquhart AE, Savage E, Danziger K, Easter T, Terala A, Nunnally M. An interprofessional approach to preventing tracheostomy-related pressure injuries. *Adv Skin Wound Care*. 2022;35(3):166–171.
57. Fan E, Del Sorbo L, Goligher EC, et al. An official American Thoracic Society/European Society of Intensive Care Medicine/Society of Critical Care Medicine clinical practice guideline: mechanical ventilation in adult patients with acute respiratory distress syndrome. *Am J Respir Crit Care Med*. 2017;195(9):1253–1263.
58. Johnson KL, Speirs L, Mitchell A, et al. Validation of a postextubation dysphagia screening tool for patients after prolonged endotracheal intubation. *Am J Crit Care*. 2018;27(2):89–96.
59. Granholm A, Zeng L, Dionne JC, et al. Predictors of gastrointestinal bleeding in adult ICU patients: a systematic review and meta-analysis. *Intensive Care Med*. 2019;45(10):1347–1359.
60. Taylor BE, McClave SA, Martindale RG, et al. Guidelines for the provision and assessment of nutrition support therapy in the adult critically ill patient: Society of Critical Care Medicine (SCCM) and American Society for Parenteral and Enteral Nutrition (A.S.P.E.N.). *Critical Care Med*. 2016;44(2):390–438.
61. Kjeldsen CL, Hansen MS, Jensen K, Holm A, Haahr A, Dreyer P. Patients' experience of thirst while being conscious and mechanically ventilated in the intensive care unit. *Nurs Crit Care*. 2018;23(2):75–81.
62. Carruthers H, Astin F, Munro W. Which alternative communication methods are effective for voiceless patients in intensive care units? A systematic review. *Intensive Critical Care Nurs*. 2017;42:88–96.
63. Devlin JW, Skrobik Y, Gelinas C, et al. Clinical practice guidelines for the prevention and management of pain, agitation/

sedation, delirium, immobility, and sleep disruption in adult patients in the ICU. *Crit Care Med*. 2018;46(9):e825–e873.
64. Frazier SK. Weaning mechanical ventilation. In: Wiegand DL, ed. *AACN Procedure Manual for High Acuity, Progressive, and Critical Care*. 7th ed. St. Louis, MO: Elsevier; 2017:277–285.
65. Girard TD, Alhazzani W, Kress JP, et al. An official American Thoracic Society/American College of Chest Physicians clinical practice guideline: liberation from mechanical ventilation in critically ill adults: rehabilitation protocols, ventilator liberation protocols, and cuff leak tests. *Am J Respir Crit Care Med*. 2017;195(1):120–133.
66. Baptistella AR, Sarmento FJ, da Silva KR, et al. Predictive factors of weaning from mechanical ventilation and extubation outcome: a systematic review. *J Crit Care*. 2018;48:56–62.
67. Hirzallah FM, Alkaissi A, do Céu Barbieri-Figueiredo M. A systematic review of nurse-led weaning protocol for mechanically ventilated adult patients. *Nurs Crit Care*. 2019;24(2):89–96.
68. Schreiber AF, Ceriana P, Ambrosino N, Malovini A, Nava S. Physiotherapy and weaning from prolonged mechanical ventilation. *Respir Care*. 2019;64(1):17–25.

11

Rapid Response Teams and Code Management

Shannan K. Hamlin, PhD, RN, AGACNP-BC, CCRN, NE-BC, FCCM,
Nicole Marie Fontenot, DNP, APRN, ACNP-BC, CCNS, CCRN,
Hsin-Mei Chen, PhD, MBA

INTRODUCTION

Code, code blue, code 99 and *Dr. Heart* are terms frequently used in hospital settings to refer to emergency situations that require life-saving resuscitation and interventions. Codes are called when patients have a cardiac or respiratory (cardiopulmonary) arrest or a life-threatening cardiac dysrhythmia that causes a loss of consciousness. The generic term *arrest* is used in this chapter to refer to these conditions. Regardless of the cause, patient survival and positive outcomes depend on prompt recognition of the situation and immediate institution of basic life support (BLS) and advanced cardiovascular life support (ACLS) measures. Code management refers to the initiation of a code and the life-saving interventions performed when a patient arrests.

Rapid response teams (RRTs) have been implemented to address changes in a patient's clinical condition before a cardiopulmonary arrest occurs. The goal of RRTs is to prevent the cardiopulmonary arrest from ever occurring. The Institute for Healthcare Improvement (IHI) and The Joint Commission (TJC) support efforts by hospitals to implement systems that enable healthcare workers to request additional assistance from specially trained individuals when the patient's condition appears to be worsening.[1]

This chapter discusses the role of RRTs in preventing cardiopulmonary arrest, the roles of the personnel involved in a code, and equipment that must be readily available to support interventions of the RRT or during a code. BLS and ACLS measures are presented, including medications commonly administered during a code. The reader should access the American Heart Association (AHA) website (https://cpr.heart.org/en/) for current recommendations for BLS and ACLS. Care of the patient after a code is also discussed in this chapter, including the use of targeted temperature management (TTM).

RAPID RESPONSE TEAMS

The RRT, available 24 hours a day, 7 days a week, consists of a group of experts typically trained in emergency response. Team members may include any combination of providers, clinical nurses, respiratory therapists, and pharmacists. The RRT is designed to bring critical care resources and interventions to clinically deteriorating patients outside of the critical care unit.[2] Locations include acute care and procedural areas (e.g., endoscopy, radiology). Activation of the RRT may be done by any member of the healthcare team, with many institutions encouraging activation by family concerned about their loved one. RRTs may also be activated for nonhospitalized patients such as visitors and hospital staff. Additionally, the use of RRTs to improve patient care by fostering end-of-life discussions between patients, their families, and healthcare providers has been introduced. Potential advantages include provision of palliative care, prevention of progression to cardiac arrest, family support, and discussions about the likelihood of success with therapies in the critical care unit.[2–6] The majority of evidence found RRTs may lead to little or no difference in unplanned critical care admissions, hospital length of stay, or mortality.[7]

Clinical Deterioration

Patient clinical deterioration is a worsening clinical state increasing the risk for morbidity, mortality, organ dysfunction, and prolonged hospital stay.[8,9] Considered a patient safety net, the RRT concept is based on three components: (1) identification of clinical deterioration that triggers early notification of a specific team of responders, (2) rapid intervention by the RRT, bringing both personnel and equipment to the patient, and (3) ongoing evaluation through data analysis to improve response and prevent worsening clinical deterioration.[2,8,10]

Failure to recognize changes in a patient's condition until major complications, including death, have occurred is referred to as *failure to rescue*.[11] Up to 50% of patients having an in-hospital cardiac arrest have signs of physiological instability as evidenced by changes in heart rate, blood pressure, and/or respiratory status 1 to 4 hours before arrest.[10,12] However, changes to vital signs are considered late-stage clinical deterioration. Before vital sign abnormalities, early signs of potential instability, including altered mental status and poor peripheral circulation, can be detected during a patient's physical assessment 24 to 48 hours before an adverse event occurs.[13]

Rapid Response Team Activation

The RRT is activated when a patient fulfills predefined criteria, including deterioration in heart rate, blood pressure, respirations, pulse oximetry saturation, mental status, urine output, and laboratory values. Some institutions use the RRT to provide proactive rounding, whereby a team member conducts rounds in the non–critical care units to identify high-risk patients and intervene preemptively. These activities have resulted in more prompt transfers to higher levels of care, fewer cardiac arrests and arrest deaths.[9,14,15]

Once the RRT is activated, personnel and equipment are brought to the patient's bedside within minutes. The RRT carries monitoring equipment, including a portable electrocardiogram (ECG) monitor, pulse oximetry monitor, oxygen delivery system, IV supplies, and medications. Point-of-care testing equipment to perform a blood glucose measurement, arterial blood gas analysis, hemoglobin and hematocrit, and a basic metabolic panel may be available. ACLS algorithms, standing medical orders, and evidence-based protocols guide RRT interventions.

CHECK YOUR UNDERSTANDING

1. It is appropriate for the nurse to call the RRT for assistance with which of the following patients?
   A. A 63-year-old patient who suddenly becomes diaphoretic, cool, clammy, and short of breath
   B. A 37-year-old patient who develops bradycardia with a sudden change in level of consciousness
   C. An 81-year-old patient with new onset chest pain
   D. All of the above

CARE TEAM AND EQUIPMENT DURING A CODE

Roles of Caregivers in Code Management

In the absence of a written order from a provider to withhold resuscitative measures, cardiopulmonary resuscitation (CPR) and a code must be initiated when a patient has a cardiopulmonary arrest (see Chapter 4, Palliative and End-of-Life Care). Ideally, the provider, family, and patient (if possible) decide whether CPR is to be performed before resuscitative measures are needed. However, it is the provider who makes the decision to terminate resuscitation efforts in progress. Decisions about resuscitation status often create ethical dilemmas for the nurse, patient, and family (see Chapter 3, Ethical and Legal Issues in Critical Care Nursing).

All personnel involved in hospital patient care should have BLS training, including how to operate an automated external defibrillator (AED). This training is also recommended for the public and can be obtained through courses offered by the AHA. Provider training for ACLS is available through the AHA and is strongly recommended for anyone working in critical care.

Prompt recognition of a patient's cardiopulmonary arrest and rapid initiation of BLS and ACLS measures are essential

TABLE 11.1 Roles and Responsibilities of Code Team Members

Team Member	Primary Role
Code leader (usually a provider)	Directs code Makes diagnoses and treatment decisions
Primary nurse	Provides information to code leader Measures vital signs Assists with procedures Administers medications
Second nurse	Coordinates use of the code cart Prepares medications Assembles equipment (intubation, suction)
Nursing supervisor	Controls the crowd Contacts the attending provider Assists with medications and procedures Ensures that a bed is available in critical care unit Assists with transfer of patient to critical care unit
Nurse or assistant	Records events on designated form
Respiratory therapist	Assists with ventilation and intubation Obtains blood sample for ABG analysis Sets up respiratory equipment/mechanical ventilator
Pharmacist or pharmacy technician	Assists with medication preparation Prepares IV infusions
Chaplain	Supports family

ABG, Arterial blood gas; *IV*, Intravenous.

for improved patient outcomes. The first person to recognize that a patient has had an arrest should call for help; instruct someone to "call a code" and obtain a defibrillator or AED; and begin CPR. One-person CPR is continued until additional help arrives.

Most hospitals have teams designated to code response. Key personnel are notified via an overhead paging system or individual pagers to assist with code management, as the code team members often work in many different departments across the hospital. The code team usually consists of a provider, critical care or emergency department nurses, a nursing supervisor, a respiratory therapist, a pharmacist or pharmacy technician, and a chaplain (Table 11.1). Some hospitals also have other crucial staff respond to codes, such as a nurse anesthetist or anesthesiologist, an ECG technician, laboratory technicians, or security guards. The code team works in conjunction with the patient's bedside nurse and primary provider, if present, to manage the patient. If a code team does not exist, any available trained personnel usually respond. Teamwork during a code is essential (see Clinical Exemplar box).

Code Leader. The person who directs, or runs, the code is responsible for making diagnoses and treatment decisions. The leader is usually a provider, preferably one who works in critical care or emergency medicine, with code experience. However, the leader may be the patient's primary or another provider who is available and qualified. If several providers are present, one assumes responsibility as the code leader and is the only person giving orders to avoid confusion and conflict. In some small hospitals, codes may be directed by a nurse trained in

ACLS. In this situation, standing orders are needed to guide and support the nurse's decision-making.

The code leader is provided information about the patient to make treatment decisions, including the reason for the patient's hospitalization, current treatments and medications, the patient's code status, and the events that occurred immediately before the code. If possible, the code leader should not perform CPR or other tasks so as to give full attention to resuscitative efforts, including assessment, diagnosis, and treatment decisions.

CLINICAL EXEMPLAR

Quality and Safety

Teamwork is essential for code teams. Advanced practice nurses on the hospital system code committee identified the need to improve multiprofessional team training for code responses. They identified that medical residents (who assume the role of code team leader) had significantly less clinical experience in codes. Additionally, the perception of teamwork among code team members could be improved. A 2-hour structured, simulated team training program was developed for nurses, respiratory therapists, and medical residents who participated in the code team on a regular basis. After each simulation, a debrief occurred to discuss successes and opportunities. The simulation was well received, and the perception of teamwork improved. The advanced practice nurses continued the simulated team training quarterly. Twelve months after adopting quarterly simulations, the advanced practice nurses observed earlier times to defibrillation, an improved rate of return of spontaneous circulation, and greater adoption of targeted temperature management.

Code Nurses

Primary nurse. The patient's primary nurse should be free to relate information to the code leader. The primary nurse may also start IV lines, measure vital signs, administer emergency medications, assist with procedures, or defibrillate the patient, as directed by the code leader (if the primary nurse is competent in ACLS).

Second nurse. The major task of the second nurse is to coordinate the use of the code cart. If a cardiac arrest is taking place outside the critical care unit, the second nurse may be a critical care nurse. This nurse must be thoroughly familiar with the layout of the code cart. This nurse locates, prepares, and labels medications and IV fluids and also assembles equipment for intubation, suctioning, and other procedures, such as central line insertion. An additional nurse or assistant records the code events on a designated form (i.e., code record) or in the electronic health record (EHR).

Nursing supervisor. The nursing supervisor responds to the code to assist in whatever manner is needed. Frequently, more people respond to a code than are needed. One job of the supervisor is to limit the number of people involved in the code to only those necessary and those there for learning purposes. This approach decreases crowding and confusion. Other responsibilities may include contacting the patient's primary provider, relaying information to the staff and family, and ensuring all necessary equipment is present and functioning. If the patient must be transferred to the critical care unit, the supervisor may also ensure that a critical care bed is available and coordinate the transfer.

Respiratory Therapist. The respiratory therapist usually assists with manual ventilation of the patient before and after intubation. The therapist may also obtain a blood sample for arterial blood gas analysis, set up oxygen and ventilation equipment, and suction the patient. In some institutions, the respiratory therapist performs intubation.

Pharmacist or Pharmacy Technician. In some hospitals, a pharmacist or pharmacy technician responds to codes to prepare medications and mix IV infusions for administration. The pharmacist may also calculate appropriate medication doses based on the patient's weight. Frequently, pharmacy staff members are also responsible for bringing additional medications if needed. At the termination of the code, pharmacy staff may replenish the code cart medications and ensure pharmacy charges to the patient's account.

Chaplain. As a code team member, the hospital chaplain can be very helpful in comforting and waiting with the patient's family. The chaplain or other support person usually takes the family to a quiet, private area for waiting and remains with them during the code. This person may also be able to check on the patient periodically to provide the family with a progress report.

Other Personnel. Depending on the resources of a hospital, additional code team members may include a laboratory technician, an ECG technician, an anesthesia provider, and security. The laboratory technician who responds to a code is responsible for operating point-of-care laboratory equipment or running specimens to the lab. An ECG technician obtains 12-lead ECGs that may be ordered to assist with diagnosis and treatment. When involved in the code team, the anesthesia provider assumes control of the patient's ventilation and oxygenation. This team member intubates the patient to ensure an adequate airway and to facilitate ventilation. If an anesthesia provider is not present, either the respiratory therapist or another provider assumes this role. Security guards may respond to help with crowd management, as well as expedite transportation if the patient must move to another level of care.

Those members of the team not directly involved in the code, such as nursing support team members and other nurses on the unit where the code is called, should focus on providing care to the remaining patients; in particular, the other patients of the primary nurse and those nurses involved directly in the code. These team members may also support the code by running errands or obtaining equipment.

CLINICAL JUDGMENT ACTIVITY

You are the second nurse to respond to a code. The first nurse is administering CPR. Outline your initial actions with supporting rationales.

Equipment Used in Codes

After the first person to recognize a code calls for help and begins life-support measures, another team member immediately brings the code cart and defibrillator to the

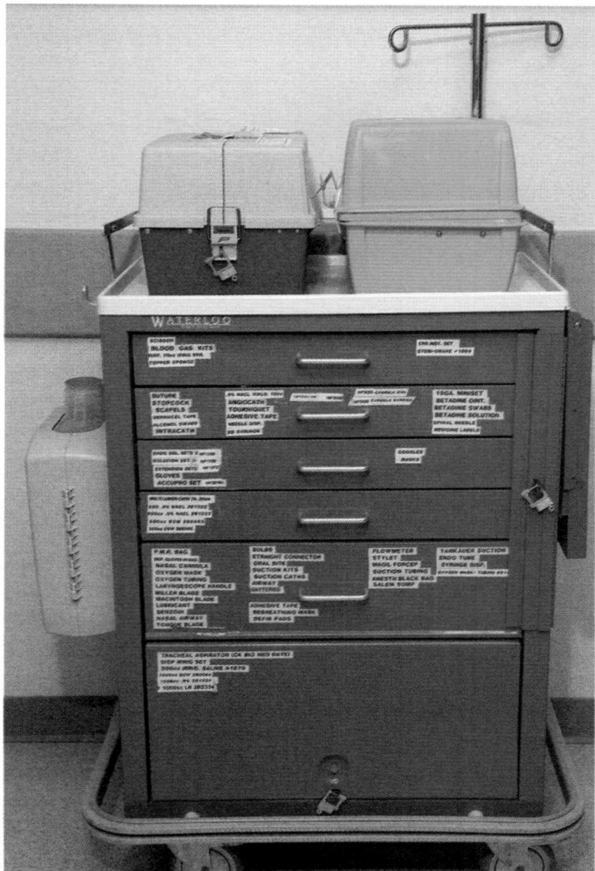

Fig. 11.1 A typical code cart.

patient's bedside (Fig. 11.1). Code carts vary in organization and layout, but they all contain the same basic emergency equipment and medications. Many hospitals have standardized code carts so that anyone responding to a code is familiar with the location of items. In other hospitals, the makeup and organization of the code cart are unique to each unit. Whether carts are standardized or unique to an individual unit, nurses responding to codes must be familiar with them.

Most carts have equipment stored on top and in several drawers. Table 11.2 lists the equipment on a typical code cart. Equipment such as cardiac boards and oxygen tanks may be attached to the cart. Larger equipment is stored on the top of the cart or in a large drawer; smaller items, such as medications and IV equipment, are in the smaller drawers.

Back or Cardiac Board. A back or cardiac board is usually located on the outside of the cart. Alternatively, some hospital bed headboards can be removed and used as a backboard. Other beds can be switched into CPR mode so that the mattress inflates to create a firm surface under the patient. High priority should be given at the beginning of the code to put a backboard under the patient, as this can improve the quality of chest compressions. Either lift or log roll the patient to one side to place the board. Care is taken to protect the patient's cervical spine if injury is suspected.

Cardiac Monitor. A monitor-defibrillator is usually located on top of the cart or on a separate cart. Monitor the patient's cardiac rhythm via the leads and electrodes or through adhesive electrode pads on this machine. A "quick look" at the patient's cardiac rhythm can also be obtained by placing the defibrillation paddles on the chest. In the hospital setting, continuous rhythm monitoring via the electrodes is preferable to intermittent use of the quick-look defibrillation paddles. The monitor must have a strip-chart recorder for documenting the patient's ECG rhythm for the code record. Monitor-defibrillator units also include capabilities for transcutaneous pacing and may include an AED. Some patient care units use an AED for initial code management.

Medications and Special Supplies. Airway management supplies are located in one of the drawers. A bag with an attached face mask (bag-valve-mask device) and oxygen tubing is usually kept on the code cart. The tubing is connected to either a wall oxygen inlet or a portable oxygen tank on the code cart. Supplemental oxygen is always used with the bag-valve-mask device. Some institutions have a separate box containing airway management supplies or the anesthesiologist or nurse anesthetist will bring an airway box or bag with them.

Another drawer contains IV supplies and solutions. Lactated Ringer's solution and 0.9% normal saline are the IV fluids most often used. Fluids used to prepare infusions include 0.9% normal saline and 5% dextrose in water (D_5W) solution in 250- and 500-mL bags.

Emergency medications fill another drawer or may be located in a separate box. These include medications given via IV push or used to compound continuous infusions. Most IV push medications are available in prefilled syringes. Several medications that are given via a continuous infusion (e.g., lidocaine, dopamine) may be available as premixed bags. Medications are discussed in depth in the section Pharmacological Intervention During a Code.

Other important items on the cart include a suction device with a canister and tubing, suction catheters, nasogastric tubes, and a blood pressure cuff. Various kits used for tracheotomy, central line insertion, and intraosseous (IO) insertion may also be stocked within the code cart.

Code Cart Maintenance. The code cart and defibrillator are usually checked by nursing staff at designated time intervals (every shift or every 24 hours) to ensure all equipment and medications are present and functional. Once the cart is fully stocked, it is locked to prevent borrowing of supplies and equipment.

Management of the code is more efficient when the nurse knows where items are on the code cart and how to use them. Many institutions require nursing staff to participate in periodic mock codes to assist in maintaining skills. Multiprofessional team simulations also provide excellent opportunities for skill development.

RESUSCITATION EFFORTS

The flow of events during a code requires a concentrated team effort. BLS is provided until the code team arrives. Once help

TABLE 11.2 Typical Contents of a Code Cart*

Item	Description
Cardiac Board/Backboard	• Often located on the back of the code cart • Place under the patient as soon as possible to improve the quality of CPR
Suction Equipment	• Portable suction machine • Extension tubing • Often located on the code cart, to be used if wall suction is not available
Sharps Container	• Container for disposing of needles, syringes, and other sharps
Monitor-Defibrillator	• Device used to monitor cardiac rhythm and deliver electrical defibrillation, cardioversion, and pacing when needed • Often sits on top of the code cart
Code Record	• Paper record, often on a clipboard, used to document the code events • May be used if the electronic health record is not available
Airway Equipment	• Oral and nasal airways • Endotracheal tube and stylet • Lubricating jelly • Laryngoscope handle with curved and straight blades • 10 mL syringe for inflating the endotracheal cuff • Tape/commercial endotracheal tube holder • Suction catheter • Oxygen flowmeter • End-tidal CO_2 detector
Oxygen Supplies and Delivery Devices	• Oxygen tank • Bag-valve-mask • Oxygen extension tubing • Face masks
IV Equipment	• IV catheters of various sizes • Tape • Syringes • Tourniquet • Gauze pads • Alcohol and/or chlorhexidine prep pads • Needles and needleless adaptors • IV fluids (NS, Lactated Ringer's solution, D_5W) • IV tubing and extension sets
Medications	• All IV push emergency medications in prefilled syringes if available • NS and sterile water for injection • IV infusion emergency medications (see Table 11.4)
Laboratory Equipment	• Arterial blood gas kit • Blood collection tubes • Needles and extension kits
Procedure Kits	• Central line insertion kits • Tracheotomy tray • Intraosseous insertion kit • Chest tube tray • Sterile gloves • Sterile scissors and hemostats • Sutures
Other Miscellaneous Equipment	• Nasogastric tubes • Chest tubes • Blood pressure cuff • Pacemaker magnet (may be in a drawer or stuck to the side of the cart) • Extra ECG recording paper • Personal protective equipment, such as nonsterile gloves, gowns, face masks, safety glasses, and shields

*Equipment and where it is stored on the code cart differ at each hospital. Learning the layout of the code carts at your hospital is important.
CO_2, Carbon dioxide; *CPR*, cardiopulmonary resuscitation; *D_5W*, 5% dextrose in water; *ECG*, electrocardiogram; *ETTs*, endotracheal tubes; *NS*, 0.9% normal saline.

arrives, CPR is continued using the two-person technique. Priorities during cardiac arrest are high-quality CPR and early defibrillation. Other tasks, such as connecting the patient to an ECG monitor, starting IV lines, attaching an oxygen source to the bag-valve-mask device, and setting up suction, are performed by available personnel as soon as possible. Depending on the patient's age and stage of life, there may be physiological changes the nurse must consider during and after resuscitative efforts (see Lifespan Considerations box).[16]

LIFESPAN CONSIDERATIONS

Older Adults

- Older adults have an increased incidence of complications from chest compressions, including rib fractures, sternal fractures, pneumothorax, and hemothorax.
- CPR is less likely to be effective in patients older than 70 years of age who have comorbidities, an unwitnessed arrest, terminal dysrhythmias (i.e., asystole or pulseless electrical activity), CPR duration greater than 15 minutes, metastatic cancer, sepsis, pneumonia, renal failure, trauma, or acute or sustained hypotension.[26]
- Hepatic or renal impairment may result in higher-than-desired serum drug concentrations and adverse drug reactions with standard therapeutic dosing regimens.
- The beta-adrenergic receptors on the myocardium are less responsive to changes in heart rate and contractility. Heart rate is less responsive to beta-blockers (i.e., propranolol, metoprolol) and parasympathetic medications (i.e., atropine). A decline in heart rate and slowing of conduction through the atrioventricular (AV) node results in a narrow therapeutic range for cardiovascular medications.

Pregnant People

- The pregnant person is placed supine on a firm backboard while using manual left uterine displacement (LUD) to relieve aortocaval compression during chest compressions.
- Chest compression rate and depth, as well as medication selection and doses, are the same as in nonpregnant patients.
- Hypoxemia is always considered as a cause of arrest. During pregnancy, oxygen reserves are lower, and metabolic demands are higher; early ventilator support may be necessary.
- After successful resuscitation, the pregnant person is placed in the full lateral decubitus position. If this is not possible due to patient monitoring, airway control, and/or IV access, continuous manual LUD is maintained.

When feasible, family members should be given the option to be bedside during resuscitation (see Chapter 2, Patient and Family Response to the Critical Care Experience).[1] Families who have been present during a code describe the benefits as knowing that everything possible was being done for their loved one, providing a sense of closure on a life shared together, and facilitating the grief process.[17,18] The activities that occur during the code are summarized in Table 11.3. Often, several activities are performed simultaneously.

The code team should be alerted to the patient's code status by the primary nurse or provider, if present. Individuals may have advance directives documenting their wishes. The advance directive provides instructions to family members, providers, and other healthcare clinicians (see Chapter 3, Ethical and Legal Issues in Critical Care Nursing, and Chapter 4, Palliative and End-of-Life Care). The patient's primary nurse should always know their patients' code status to ensure they are prepared should an emergency occur.

Many states have implemented "no CPR" options, also referred to as a Do Not Resuscitate (DNR) or Do Not Attempt Resuscitation (DNAR). The patient, who usually has a terminal illness, signs a document requesting "no CPR" if there is a loss of pulse or if breathing stops. In some states, this document directs the patient to wear a "no CPR" identification bracelet. In the event of a code, the bracelet alerts the responders that CPR efforts are prohibited and that the patient's wishes should be respected.

Basic Life Support

The goal of BLS is to support effective circulation, oxygenation, and ventilation until the return of spontaneous circulation (ROSC). Immediate CPR and rapid defibrillation with an AED for shockable rhythms are vital to improve the patient's chance of survival.[19] Therefore, all BLS providers must be trained in the use of the hospital's available AED (see Electrical Therapy section). Assessment is a part of each step, and the steps are performed in order (Box 11.1). The following summary is adapted from the 2020 AHA standards.[19,20]

Responsiveness. The first intervention is to assess responsiveness by tapping or shaking a patient and shouting, "Are you okay?" If the patient is unresponsive, call for help by shouting to fellow caregivers or by using the nurse-call system. Tell them to bring the code cart with an AED and/or defibrillator. Position the patient on his or her back, turning the head and body as a unit to prevent injury.

Circulation and Chest Compressions. The next step is to check for the presence or absence of a carotid pulse while simultaneously looking for the absence of breathing or only gasping. Take at least 5 seconds but no more than 10 seconds to check for a carotid pulse. Assess the pulse even if the patient is attached to a cardiac monitor, because artifact or a loose lead may mimic a cardiac dysrhythmia. If the pulse is absent, begin chest compressions. When able, place a firm surface (e.g., cardiac board, backboard, or headboard) under the patient.

Proper hand position is essential for performing compressions. The location for compressions is the lower half of the sternum in the center of the chest between the nipples. Place the heel of one hand on the lower half of the sternum. Place the heel of the second hand on top of the first hand so the hands are overlapped and parallel. Using both hands, begin compressions by depressing the sternum at least 2 inches (5 cm) for the average adult, letting the chest return (recoil) to its normal position between each compression. Perform compressions at a rate of at least 100 to 120 per minute ("hard and fast"). The compression-ventilation ratio is 30 compressions to two breaths.

Continue CPR until the monitor-defibrillator or AED arrives, adhesive electrode pads are placed, and the rhythm is ready to be analyzed. Provide shocks as indicated. After each shock, immediately resume CPR, beginning with

TABLE 11.3 **Flow of Events During a Code**

Priorities	Equipment from Cart	Intervention
Recognition of arrest		Assess code status Call for help, assess for absence of breathing or only gasping, initiate chest compressions
Arrival of AED		Attach AED pads, turn on, analyze rhythm, follow prompts until code team arrives
Arrival of code team, code cart, and monitor-defibrillator	Cardiac board Bag-valve-mask device with oxygen tubing Oxygen and regulator if not already at bedside	Continue chest compressions Place patient on cardiac board Ventilate with 100% oxygen and bag-valve-mask device
Identification of code leader		Assess patient; obtain history and events leading to code Assign code team roles; direct and supervise team members Identify and treat underlying cause(s)
Rhythm diagnosis	Monitor-defibrillator with ECG leads and adhesive electrode pads 12-lead ECG machine	Attach ECG leads or adhesive electrode pads (if different from AED pads); do not interrupt compressions
Follow ACLS algorithm for shockable or nonshockable rhythm	Monitor-defibrillator Code cart medications	Shockable: prompt defibrillation q2 min if indicated, epinephrine after second shock Nonshockable: epinephrine q3-5 min until ROSC
Intubation (if ventilation is inadequate and trained personnel are available)	Suction equipment Laryngoscope Endotracheal tube and intubation equipment Stethoscope $ETCO_2$ detector or waveform capnography	Connect suction equipment Intubate patient (interrupt CPR for no longer than 10 sec) Confirm tube position with waveform capnography or an $ETCO_2$ detector; by auscultating over bilateral lung fields and the epigastrium; and by observing chest movement Secure endotracheal tube Oxygenate
Venous access	Peripheral or central IV equipment IO insertion kit IV tubing, infusion fluid	Insert large-bore peripheral IV Insert IO needle if peripheral access cannot be obtained Central venous catheter may be inserted by provider
Ongoing assessment of the patient's response to resuscitative efforts		Efficacy of compressions (correct, depth, time to recoil, not slowing down) and need to swap team members Adequacy of artificial ventilation Spontaneous pulse q2 min With ROSC: spontaneous breathing and blood pressure Decision to stop if no response to therapy
Drawing arterial and venous blood specimens	Arterial puncture and venipuncture equipment	Draw specimens Treat as needed, based on results
Documentation	Code record	Accurately record events while resuscitation is in progress Record rhythm strips during the code
Controlling or limiting crowd		Dismiss those not required for bedside tasks
Family notification		Keep family informed of patient's condition Notify of outcome with sensitivity Explore options for family presence during code
Transfer of patient to critical care unit		Ensure a bed is assigned Transfer with adequate personnel and emergency equipment
Debrief		Evaluate events of code and express feelings

ACLS, Advanced cardiac life support; *AED,* automated external defibrillator; *CPR,* cardiopulmonary resuscitation; *ECG,* electrocardiogram; *$ETCO_2$,* end-tidal carbon dioxide; *IO,* intraosseous; *IV,* Intravenous; *ROSC,* return of spontaneous circulation.

compressions for 2 minutes. Minimize interruptions in chest compressions to less than 10 seconds. If available, use a device that measures the quality of CPR to ensure the appropriate rate and depth of compressions are maintained. Switch CPR providers if the quality of the compressions cannot be maintained.

Airway. There are two methods for opening the airway to provide breaths: the head-tilt/chin-lift method and the jaw-thrust maneuver (Fig. 11.2). The head-tilt/chin-lift method is performed if there is no evidence of head or neck trauma by placing one hand on the victim's forehead and tilting the head back. Place the fingers of the other hand under the bony part of the patient's lower jaw near the chin. Lift the jaw to bring the chin forward. Use the jaw-thrust if a head or neck injury is suspected. In the jaw-thrust maneuver, stand at the top of the patient's head, place palms on the patient's temples and fingers under the mandible. The mandible is lifted upward by the fingers, until the lower incisors are higher than the upper incisors, relieving airway obstruction. Usually, two people are needed to perform the jaw-thrust and provide breaths with a bag-valve-mask device.

BOX 11.1 Steps in Basic Life Support

Determine Responsiveness

- Tap and shout, "Are you all right?"
- Shout for help or activate the emergency response system; get the AED.
- Monitor chest for rise and fall; simultaneously check carotid pulse for 5 to 10 seconds.

Assess and Support Circulation

- If normal breathing with pulse, monitor until help arrives.
- If normal breathing absent with a pulse, open airway and start rescue breathing at 1 breath every 5 or 6 seconds (10 to 12 breaths/min). Check pulse every 2 minutes.
- If breathing absent with no pulse, begin cycles of CPR with chest compressions at rate of 100 to 120 compressions per minute (30 compressions to every 2 breaths).

Provide Rapid Defibrillation

- If no pulse, check for shockable rhythm with an AED.
- Provide shocks as indicated.
- Follow each shock immediately with CPR, beginning with compressions.
- Continue CPR for 2 minutes, then perform a rhythm check as prompted by the AED.
- Repeat the cycle until ACLS providers take over or patient starts to move.

ACLS, Advanced cardiac life support; *AED*, automated external defibrillator; *CPR*, cardiopulmonary resuscitation.
Data from Panchal et al. 2020 American Heart Association Guidelines for Cardiopulmonary Resuscitation and Emergency Cardiovascular Care. *Circulation*. 2020;142(suppl_2).

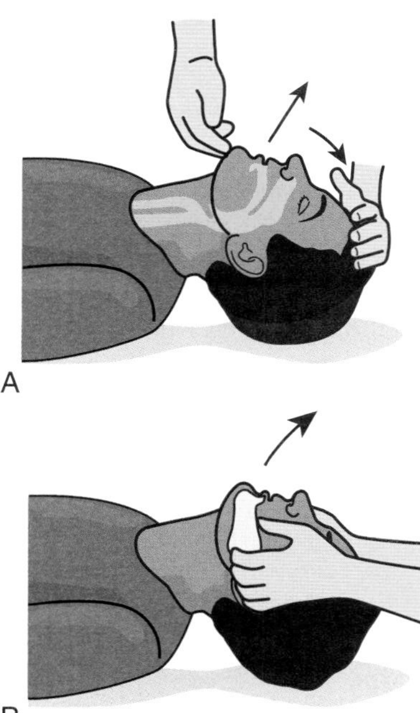

Fig. 11.2 A, Head-tilt/chin-lift technique. B, Jaw thrust maneuver.

Breathing. Devices that assist with breathing should be readily available for all hospitalized patients and require training for effective use. Bag-valve-mask devices are often available at every bedside; some hospitals may keep a barrier device, such as a pocket mask, at some bedsides.

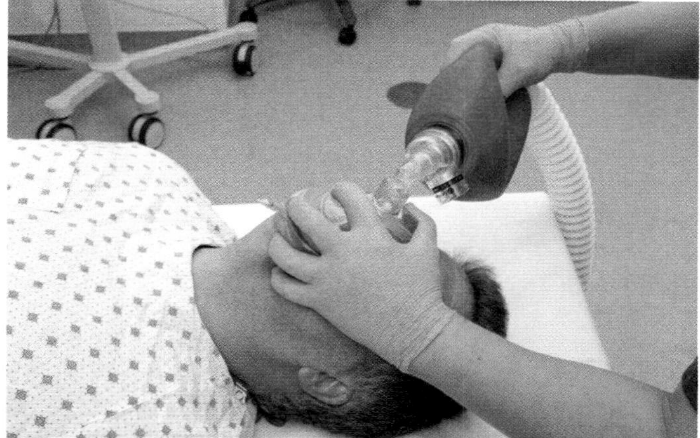

Fig. 11.3 Rescue breathing with bag-valve-mask device. (Reprinted with permission, Cleveland Clinic Center for Medical Art & Photography © 2011–2019. All rights reserved.)

Assess for the carotid pulse and respirations simultaneously. If a pulse is present without normal breathing, initiate rescue breathing. If a patient is gasping or breathing very slowly, provide ventilation support. Using the bag-valve-mask device, deliver one breath every 6 seconds, or 10 breaths/min. Continue to deliver breaths and assess the pulse every 2 minutes for 5 to 10 seconds. During CPR, deliver two breaths during a pause in compressions. In either situation, each breath is delivered over approximately 1 second, observing for visible chest rise and fall.

Ventilation of the patient with a bag-valve-mask device requires that an open airway be maintained. Frequently, an oral airway is used to keep the airway patent and to facilitate ventilation. Connect the bag-valve-mask device to an oxygen source set at 15 L/min. Position the face mask to seal over the patient's mouth and nose after the airway is opened and provide manual ventilation (Fig. 11.3).

Advanced Cardiovascular Life Support

For cardiac or respiratory emergencies, many institutions follow the AHA standards for ACLS. The tools of management are the BLS survey followed by the ACLS survey.[19,20] The ABCDs of ACLS are airway, breathing, compressions or circulation, and differential diagnosis (i.e., identifying and treating reversible causes).

Airway. Airway management involves reassessment of the original techniques established in BLS. Endotracheal intubation provides definitive airway management and is performed by properly trained personnel during the resuscitation effort.[19] The benefit of endotracheal intubation is weighed against the interruption of chest compressions. If bag-valve-mask ventilation is adequate, endotracheal intubation may be deferred until the patient fails to respond to initial CPR and defibrillation or until ROSC.

Techniques of endotracheal intubation are discussed in Chapter 10, Ventilatory Assistance. Once intubated, the patient is manually ventilated at a rate of one breath every 6 seconds or approximately 10 breaths/min with a bag-valve-mask device

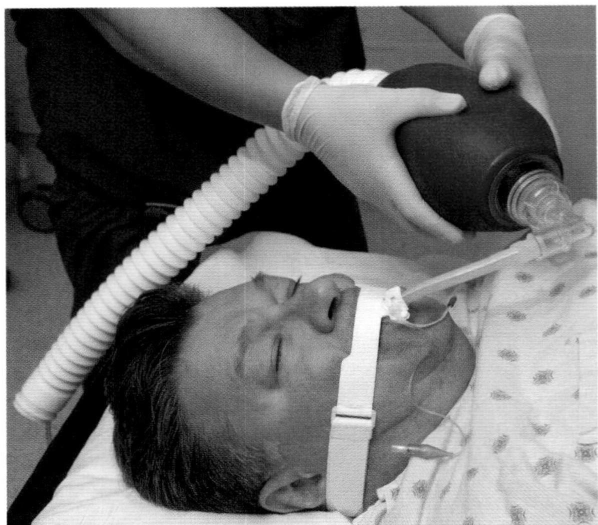

Fig. 11.4 Ventilation with a bag-valve-mask device connected to an endotracheal tube. (Reprinted with permission, Cleveland Clinic Center for Medical Art & Photography © 2011–2019. All rights reserved.)

attached to the endotracheal tube (ETT; Fig. 11.4). The bag-valve-mask device should have a reservoir and be connected to an oxygen source to deliver 100% oxygen. Chest compressions are not stopped for ventilations and are delivered continuously at a rate of 100 to 120 per minute.

Breathing. Breathing assessment determines whether the ventilatory efforts are causing the chest to rise. If the patient is intubated, confirm ETT placement by continuous waveform capnography (discussed in more detail later in this chapter) or with the use of an end-tidal carbon dioxide ($ETCO_2$) detector (Fig. 11.5).[20] Listen for bilateral breath sounds and over the epigastrium while observing chest movement with ventilation as part of the assessment. If no chest expansion is present with bag-valve-mask ventilation, the ETT is not in the trachea and must be removed immediately and reinserted. Obtain a chest radiograph after the code to confirm placement.

Circulation. Circulation initially focuses on high quality chest compressions. If ventilation is relatively constant, $ETCO_2$ reflects cardiac output and organ perfusion. Therefore, waveform capnography could be used to evaluate the effectiveness of chest compressions.[20]

If a shockable rhythm (i.e., ventricular fibrillation [VF] or pulseless ventricular tachycardia [VT]) is identified, deliver a high-energy unsynchronized shock, followed by 2 minutes of compressions with ventilation. Then, establish IV access for medication and fluid administration. IO cannulation is recommended as the primary alternative to IV access.[20] IO cannulation provides access to the bone marrow, is considered central access, and is a rapid, safe, and reliable route for administering medications, blood, and IV fluids during resuscitation. Different healthcare facilities may have a wide range of rules regarding who can insert and remove IOs; they can be managed by nurses in some facilities, and others require

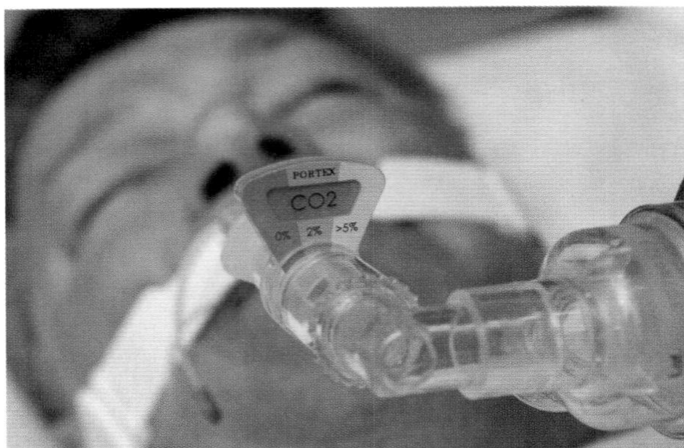

Fig. 11.5 End-tidal carbon dioxide detector connected to an endotracheal tube. Exhaled carbon dioxide reacts with the device to create a color change, indicating correct endotracheal tube placement. (Reprinted with permission, Cleveland Clinic Center for Medical Art & Photography © 2011–2019. All rights reserved.)

BOX 11.2 Reversible Causes of Cardiac Arrest

H's	T's
Hypovolemia	**T**ension pneumothorax
Hypoxia	**T**amponade, cardiac
Hydrogen ion (acidosis)	**T**oxins (drug overdose)
Hypokalemia or hyperkalemia	**T**hrombosis, pulmonary
Hypothermia	**T**hrombosis, coronary (massive myocardial infarction)

Data from Panchal et al. 2020 American Heart Association guidelines for cardiopulmonary resuscitation and emergency cardiovascular care. *Circulation*. 2020;142(suppl_2).

providers to manage them. Commercially available kits facilitate IO access in adults. Endotracheal administration of medications may be considered; however, tracheal absorption is poor, and optimal dosing is not known. Medications that can be administered through the ETT until IV access is established include epinephrine, atropine, and lidocaine.[20]

Most hospitalized patients have IV access prior to the code however assess IV access for patency before instilling medications. If the patient does not have IV access or needs additional IV access, a large-bore peripheral IV catheter is inserted. If a peripheral IV cannot be started, an IO or central line may be inserted.

Differential Diagnosis. Differential diagnosis involves identifying and treating reversible causes of the cardiopulmonary emergencies and arrest. Cardiac dysrhythmias that result in cardiac arrests have many possible causes (Box 11.2). Lethal dysrhythmias include VF or pulseless VT, asystole, and pulseless electrical activity (PEA). Other dysrhythmias that may lead to a cardiopulmonary emergency include symptomatic bradycardias and symptomatic tachycardias. Algorithms for treating these dysrhythmias have been established by the AHA.[20] Because these algorithms periodically change, they have not been reproduced here; rather, critical actions in the management of these dysrhythmias are summarized in the following sections.

Recognition and Treatment of Dysrhythmias

Ventricular Fibrillation and Pulseless Ventricular Tachycardia. In hospitalized patients who experience sudden cardiac arrest, the most common initial rhythms are VF or pulseless VT. When VF is present, the heart quivers and does not pump blood. When pulseless VT occurs, there is a rapid electrical current through the heart, but blood is not being effectively pumped to the body. The treatments for VF and for pulseless VT are the same.

Critical actions.

- Initiate the BLS survey. Begin CPR until an AED or defibrillator is available. Once an ACLS provider is present, initiate the ACLS survey. Endotracheal intubation is performed only if ventilations with a bag-valve-mask device are ineffective.
- Defibrillate as soon as possible to increase the chance of survival and a good neurological outcome. If using a biphasic defibrillator, use the defibrillator-specific dose shown to be effective for terminating VF (typically 120 to 200 J). If using a monophasic defibrillator, use 360 J for all shocks. If the type of defibrillator is unknown, use the maximum dose available. Monophasic versus biphasic defibrillation is discussed later in this chapter (see Electrical Therapy section).
- After the shock is delivered, immediately resume CPR. Continue chest compressions for 2 minutes prior to checking the rhythm.
- If VF or pulseless VT persists; resume CPR, beginning with chest compressions; recharge the defibrillator; and obtain IV or IO access. Give a second shock (with a biphasic defibrillator, use same or higher joules as for the first shock; with a monophasic defibrillator, use 360 J). Resume CPR beginning with chest compressions for 2 minutes.
- After IV or IO access is available, administer epinephrine 1 mg IV or IO every 3 to 5 minutes until ROSC is achieved. Do not stop compressions for medication administration. Check the rhythm after 2 minutes of CPR. If VF or pulseless VT persists, resume chest compressions immediately, and recharge the defibrillator.
- Give a third shock (with a biphasic defibrillator, use same or higher joules as the second shock; with a monophasic defibrillator, use 360 J). Resume CPR immediately, beginning with chest compressions, for 2 minutes.
- After the third shock, consider giving an antiarrhythmic medication (i.e., amiodarone or lidocaine); however, there is no evidence that antiarrhythmic medications given during a cardiac arrest increase survival or improve neurological outcome.[20] Dosages and administration are discussed in the section Pharmacological Intervention During a Code.
- Continue CPR for 2 minutes with pulse and rhythm checks in between. Administer epinephrine every 3 to 5 minutes throughout the code. Search for and treat the underlying cause of the arrest.

Pulseless Electrical Activity and Asystole. PEA and asystole are nonshockable rhythms. PEA is an organized electrical rhythm that does not produce mechanical contractions of the heart muscle. Asystole is the absence of electrical activity and has a poor prognosis. For either nonshockable rhythm, it is essential to identify and treat any reversible causes as soon as possible for resuscitation efforts to be successful.

Critical actions.

- Initiate the BLS survey. Begin CPR until an AED or defibrillator is available to confirm a nonshockable rhythm. Once an ACLS provider is present, initiate ACLS survey.
- Confirm asystole by ensuring the lead and cable connections are correct and the power is on. Verify asystole in another lead; an additional lead confirms or rules out the possibility of a fine VF.
- Consider possible causes and treat them (Box 11.2).
- Obtain IV or IO access. Endotracheal intubation is performed only if ventilations with a bag-valve-mask device are ineffective.
- After 2 minutes of CPR, check for a pulse and rhythm for no longer than 10 seconds. If no pulse is present, resume CPR, beginning with chest compressions, for 2 minutes.
- After IV or IO access is available, administer epinephrine 1 mg IV or IO every 3 to 5 minutes until ROSC achieved. CPR is not stopped for drug administration.
- Continue the ACLS survey while identifying underlying causes and initiating related interventions.
- Consider termination of resuscitative efforts if a reversible cause is not rapidly identified and treated and the patient fails to respond. The decision to terminate resuscitative efforts is the responsibility of the code leader and is based on consideration of many factors, including time from arrest to CPR, comorbid diseases, prearrest state, initial rhythm at time of arrest, and response to resuscitative measures. In intubated patients, failure to achieve an $ETCO_2$ of greater than 10 mm Hg by continuous waveform capnography after 20 minutes of CPR may also be considered in deciding when to end resuscitative efforts.[20]

Symptomatic Bradycardia. The category of symptomatic bradycardia encompasses two types: bradycardia with a heart rate less than 60 beats/min (e.g., third-degree heart block) and symptomatic bradycardia with any heart rate that is slow enough to cause hemodynamic compromise (Box 11.3). If bradycardia is the cause of the symptoms, the heart rate is typically less than 50 beats/min. The cause of the bradycardia must be considered. For example, hypotension associated with bradycardia may be caused by dysfunction of the myocardium or autonomic nervous system disturbance.

Critical actions.

- Perform the BLS and ACLS surveys. Maintain a patent airway and assist breathing as necessary. Provide oxygen if patient is hypoxic as determined by pulse oximetry. Monitor blood pressure, heart rate, and pulse oximetry. Obtain a 12-lead ECG and determine the cardiac rhythm. Establish IV or IO access.
- Identify and treat possible contributing factors.
- Determine whether signs and symptoms of poor perfusion are present and whether they are related to the bradycardia (Box 11.3). If adequate perfusion is present, observe and monitor.

BOX 11.3 Signs and Symptoms of Poor Perfusion Associated with Bradycardia

Signs	Symptoms
• Hypotension	• Chest pain
• Orthostatic hypotension	• Shortness of breath
• Diaphoresis	• Decreased level of consciousness
• Pulmonary congestion	• Weakness
• Pulmonary edema	• Fatigue
	• Dizziness
	• Syncope

- If poor perfusion is present, administer atropine 1 mg IV or IO every 3 to 5 minutes as needed to a total dose of 3 mg. Atropine is not indicated in second-degree atrioventricular (AV) block type II or in third-degree AV block.
- If atropine is ineffective, IV vasopressors with target beta receptor activity (e.g., epinephrine, dopamine) and/or transcutaneous (i.e., external noninvasive) pacing may be effective until transvenous temporary pacing can be initiated. For transcutaneous pacing, analgesics or sedatives may be needed because patients often find the pacing stimulus uncomfortable.

CHECK YOUR UNDERSTANDING

2. The rapid response nurse is called to the bedside of a patient who is pale, cool, and diaphoretic, complaining of chest pain and shortness of breath. The patient was admitted for syncope and increased fatigue over the last week. Upon placing the patient on the bedside monitor, what rhythm and blood pressure would the nurse most likely observe and what initial intervention should the nurse anticipate?
   A. Bradycardia, hypotension; emergent transvenous pacing
   B. Tachycardia, hypotension; passive leg raise
   C. Bradycardia, hypotension; administration of atropine 1 mg IV
   D. Tachycardia, normotensive; continue to monitor as patient is alert and oriented

Unstable Tachycardia. Tachycardia is defined as a heart rate greater than 100 beats/min. *Unstable tachycardia* occurs when the heart beats too fast for the patient's clinical condition. The treatment of this group of dysrhythmias involves the rapid recognition that the patient is symptomatic and that the signs and symptoms are caused by the tachycardia. If the heart rate is less than 150 beats/min, it is unlikely that the symptoms of instability are caused by the tachycardia. Synchronized cardioversion and antiarrhythmic therapy may be needed.[20]

Critical actions.

- Perform the BLS and ACLS surveys. Assess the patient and recognize the signs of cardiovascular instability, including increased work of breathing (e.g., tachypnea, intercostal retractions, paradoxical abdominal breathing) and hypoxia as determined by pulse oximetry. Provide supplemental oxygen, assess blood pressure, and establish IV access. Determine cardiac rhythm.
- Assess the degree of instability. If the patient has hypotension, acutely altered mental status, signs of shock, chest discomfort, or acute heart failure, prepare for synchronized cardioversion. If the ECG complex is regular and narrow, consider administration of adenosine.
- If synchronized cardioversion is indicated, premedicate with analgesics and/or a sedatives if the patient is conscious. Cardioversion is an uncomfortable procedure.
- Perform synchronized cardioversion at the appropriate energy level; often you may start with the baseline joules as set by the manufacturer of the defibrillator. Supraventricular tachycardia and atrial flutter often respond to an energy dose of 50 to 100 J. If the initial attempt fails, the energy dose is increased stepwise for subsequent attempts. In cases of unstable atrial fibrillation, start at 200 J (monophasic) or 120 to 200 J (biphasic) and increase the energy dose stepwise for subsequent cardioversion attempts. Cardioversion for monomorphic VT with a pulse should be initiated at 100 J (monophasic or biphasic) and increased stepwise for subsequent attempts.[22]
- Reassess the patient and rhythm. Further monitoring and antiarrhythmic therapy including adenosine, amiodarone, or procainamide may be considered.

Electrical Therapy

The therapeutic use of electrical current has expanded with the addition and increased use of the AED. This section addresses the use of electrical therapy in code management for the purposes of defibrillation, cardioversion, and transcutaneous pacing.

Defibrillation. The only effective treatment for VF and pulseless VT is defibrillation. VF deteriorates into asystole if not treated. VF may occur because of coronary artery disease, myocardial infarction, electrical shock, drug overdose, near drowning, or acid-base imbalance.

Definition. *Defibrillation* is the delivery of an electrical current to the heart through the use of a defibrillator (Fig. 11.6). The current can be delivered through the chest wall via external paddles or adhesive electrode pads ("hands-off" defibrillation) connected to cables. Smaller internal paddles may be used to deliver current directly to the heart during cardiac surgery when the chest is open and the heart is visualized. Defibrillation works by completely depolarizing the heart and disrupting the impulses that are causing the dysrhythmia. This allows the sinoatrial node or other pacemaker to resume control of the heart's rhythm.

Defibrillation delivers energy or current in waveforms that move between defibrillator paddles or pads. *Monophasic* waveforms deliver current in one direction; *biphasic* waveforms deliver current that flows in a positive direction for a specified duration and then reverses and flows in a negative direction. Biphasic uses fewer joules than monophasic defibrillation. Biphasic is at least as effective as monophasic defibrillation and in some reports is more effective in converting VF with fewer shocks.[20]

Procedure. Use of conductive materials during defibrillation reduces transthoracic impedance and enhances the flow of electrical current through the chest structures. Conductive materials include adhesive electrode pads and paddles with electrode paste or gel pads.

Two methods exist for paddle or adhesive electrode pad placement for external defibrillation. In the *anterior-lateral* placement, one paddle or adhesive electrode pad is placed at the second intercostal space to the right of the sternum, and the other paddle or adhesive electrode pad is placed at the fifth intercostal space, midaxillary line, to the left of the sternum (Fig. 11.7). An alternative method is *anterior-posterior placement.*[21] Adhesive electrode pads are used to facilitate correct positioning. An anterior adhesive electrode pad is placed at the left anterior precordial area, and the posterior adhesive electrode pad is placed at the left posterior-infrascapular area or at the posterior-infrascapular area (Fig. 11.8).

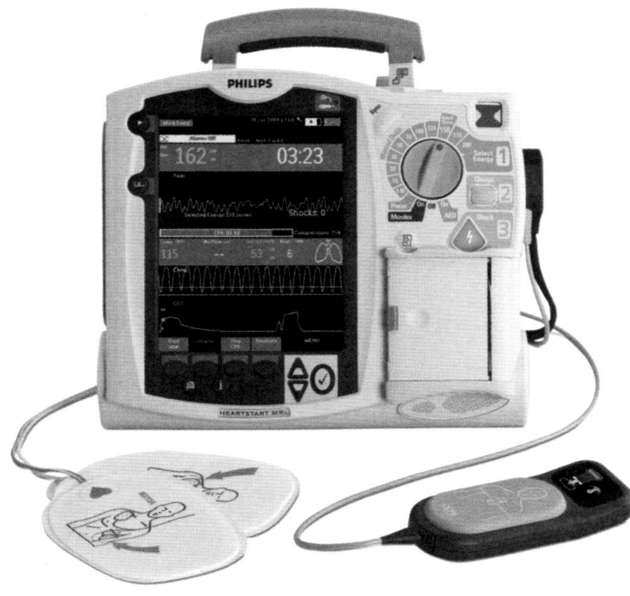

Fig. 11.6 Defibrillator. (Courtesy Philips Healthcare, Andover, MA.)

The amount of energy delivered is measured in joules, or watt-seconds. For monophasic defibrillation, 360 J is used for all shocks. For biphasic defibrillation, refer to the manufacturer's instructions for the number of joules to be delivered to the patient. If the recommended dose is unknown, use the maximum dose available.[20]

For the shock to be effective, some type of conductive medium must be placed between the pads or paddles and the skin. If paddles are used, completely cover them with gel to conduct the electricity. Commercially prepared defibrillator gel pads are available that facilitate defibrillation and prevent burns on the patient's skin that may occur when paddles are used. Adhesive electrode pads used in hands-off defibrillation also have conductive gel and are recommended instead of paddles to enhance the delivery of the electrical current.[20] Adhesive electrode pads reduce the risk of current arcing, facilitate monitoring of the patient's underlying rhythm, and allow the rapid delivery of a shock when needed.

Charge the defibrillator to the desired setting. Place the paddles firmly on the patient's chest to facilitate skin contact and reduce the impedance to the flow of current. Implement safety measures to prevent injury to the patient and personnel assisting with the procedure. Ensure that all personnel are standing clear of the bed and visually check to see that no one is in contact with the patient or bed. It is important that this step not be omitted when hands-off defibrillation is used. The announcement *"Clear. I am going to shock on three"* provides an audible check that no one is touching the patient. *"One, two, three, shocking"* is announced as the shock is delivered. Immediately after defibrillation, resume CPR, beginning with chest compressions for 2 minutes, followed by a rhythm and pulse check. Record rhythm strips during the code to document response. The procedure for defibrillation is summarized in Box 11.4.

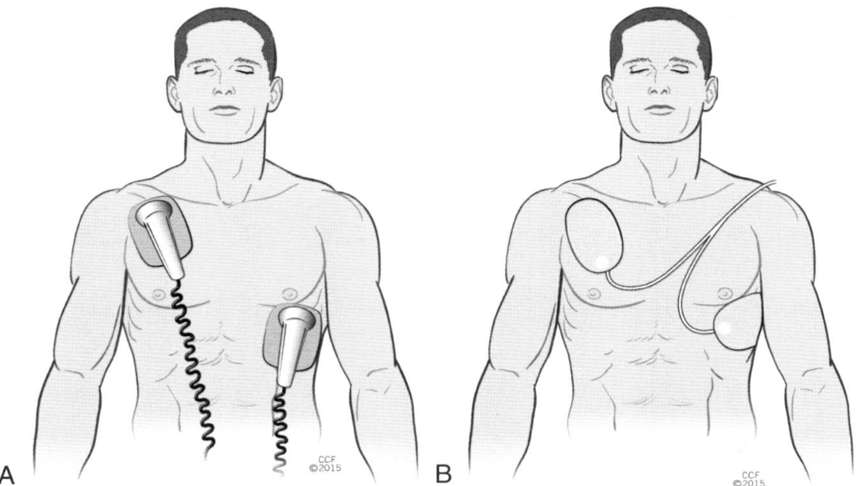

Fig. 11.7 Anterior-lateral placement of paddles or adhesive electrode pads for defibrillation. A, Paddle placement. B, Adhesive electrode pad placement.

Complications of defibrillation include burns on the skin and damage to the heart muscle. Arcing of electricity or a spark can occur if the paddles are not firmly placed on the skin, excessive conductive gel is used, or the skin is wet. Arcing has also been observed when patients have medication patches with aluminized backing (e.g., nitroglycerin, nicotine, analgesics); remove such patches and clean the area before defibrillation. Remove body jewelry, such as necklaces or nipple rings, before defibrillation to reduce the risk for arcing during the procedure.

Automated External Defibrillation. The AED extends the range of personnel trained in the use of a defibrillator and shortens the time between code onset and defibrillation. The AED is considered an integral part of emergency cardiac care.

Definition. The AED is an external defibrillator with rhythm analysis capabilities used to achieve early defibrillation (Fig. 11.9). Due to ease of use, AEDs may be placed in acute care areas, in emergency response vehicles, and public places to be used by non-ACLS certified individuals.

The AED should be used only if the patient is in cardiac arrest (unresponsive, absent or abnormal breathing, and no pulse). Confirmation that the patient is in cardiac arrest must be obtained before the AED is attached.[20]

Procedure. Apply the two adhesive electrode pads to the patient and ensure the cable is connected. Each adhesive electrode pad depicts an image of correct placement on the chest. These pads serve a dual purpose: recording the rhythm and delivering the shock. AEDs eliminate the need for training in rhythm recognition because these microprocessor-based devices analyze the surface ECG signal. The AED analyzes the patient's rhythm numerous times to confirm the presence of a rhythm for which defibrillation is indicated. The semiautomatic "shock advisory" AED charges the device and advises the operator to press a button to defibrillate. The fully automated AED requires only that the operator attach the defibrillation pads and turn on the device (Box 11.5). Both models deliver AHA-recommended energy levels for the treatment of VF or

BOX 11.4 Procedure for External Defibrillation

1. Apply adhesive electrode pads to the patient's chest and connect the cable to the defibrillator. If using paddles, either apply gel pads to the patient's chest or conductive gel to paddles.
2. Turn on the defibrillator; select the energy level.
3. If using paddles, position the paddles on the patient's chest.
4. Charge the defibrillator to the desired setting.
5. If using paddles, apply firm pressure on both paddles.
6. Shout, *"Clear. I am going to shock on three,"* and look to verify that *all* personnel are clear of the patient, bed, and any equipment connected to the patient. Disconnect the oxygen source during defibrillation.
7. Shout, *"One, two, three. Shocking."*
8. Press the "Shock" button on the defibrillator if using adhesive electrode pads. If using paddles, deliver shock by depressing buttons on each paddle simultaneously.
9. Immediately resume cardiopulmonary resuscitation, beginning with chest compression.

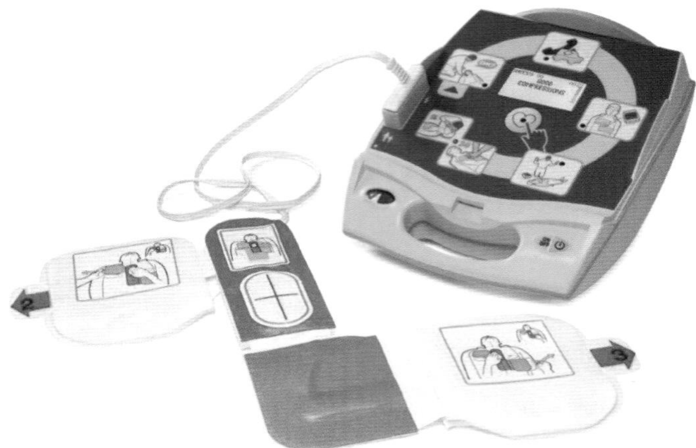

Fig. 11.9 Automated external defibrillator. (Courtesy ZOLL Medical Corporation, Chelmsford, MA.)

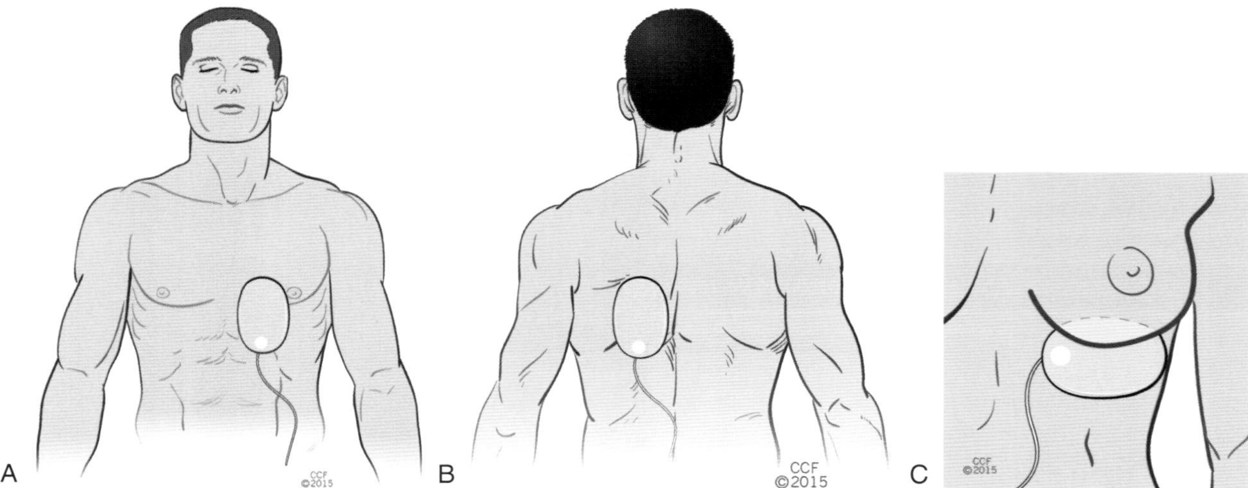

Fig. 11.8 Anterior-posterior placement of adhesive electrode pads for defibrillation or transcutaneous pacing. A, Anterior. B, Posterior. C, Anterior in females.

BOX 11.5 Procedure for Automated External Defibrillator (AED) Operation

1. Turn the power on.
2. Attach the AED connecting cable to the AED "box."
3. Attach the adhesive electrode pads to the patient. The correct position of the electrode pads is displayed on each pad (Fig. 11.7):
   - Place one pad on the upper right sternal border, directly below the clavicle.
   - Place one pad lateral to the left nipple, with the top margin of the pad a few inches below the axilla.
4. Attach the AED connecting cable to the adhesive electrode pads (if not already connected).
5. Clear personnel from the patient (no one should be touching the patient) and press the "Analyze" button to start rhythm analysis.
6. Listen or read the message "Shock indicated" or "No shock indicated."
7. If shock indicated, clear personnel from the patient and press the "Shock" button; immediately resume CPR, beginning with chest compressions.

CPR, Cardiopulmonary resuscitation

pulseless VT. They are not designed to deliver synchronous shocks and will shock VT if the rate exceeds preset values.

Cardioversion

Definition. Cardioversion is the delivery of a shock that is synchronized with the patient's cardiac rhythm. The purpose of cardioversion is to disrupt an ectopic pacemaker that is causing a dysrhythmia and to allow the sinoatrial node to take control of the rhythm. During an emergency situation, cardioversion is used to treat patients with VT, atrial flutter, atrial fibrillation, or supraventricular tachycardia who have a pulse but are developing symptoms related to poor perfusion, such as hypotension and a decreased level of consciousness. Elective cardioversion may be used to treat stable atrial flutter and atrial fibrillation.

Cardioversion is similar to defibrillation except that the delivery of energy is synchronized to occur during ventricular depolarization (peak of the QRS complex). Delivering the shock during the QRS complex prevents the shock from being delivered during repolarization (T wave), which is often called the vulnerable period. If a shock is delivered during this vulnerable period (Fig. 11.10), VF may occur. Since the purpose of cardioversion is to disrupt the rhythm rather than completely depolarize the heart, less energy is usually required. Cardioversion can be performed with energy levels as low as 50 J. The amount of energy is gradually increased until the rhythm is converted.

CLINICAL JUDGMENT ACTIVITY

A surgical patient in an acute care area has been successfully defibrillated with an AED by the nursing staff. He is being manually ventilated with a bag-valve-mask device. Determine the current nursing priorities with supporting rationales.

Procedure. The procedure for cardioversion (Box 11.6) is similar to that for defibrillation. However, the defibrillator is set in the synchronous mode for cardioversion. The R waves are sensed by the machine and are indicated by spikes or other markings on the defibrillator monitor (Fig. 11.11). Verify that all R waves are properly sensed. If using adhesive electrode pads, press the shock button and the defibrillator will not deliver a shock until synchronized with the QRS complex. If using paddles, depress the button on the defibrillator for adhesive electrode pads or both buttons on the paddles until the shock has been delivered because energy is discharged only during the QRS complex. If a patient is undergoing cardioversion in a nonemergent scenario, sedate the patient before the procedure. Record rhythm strips during cardioversion to document response.

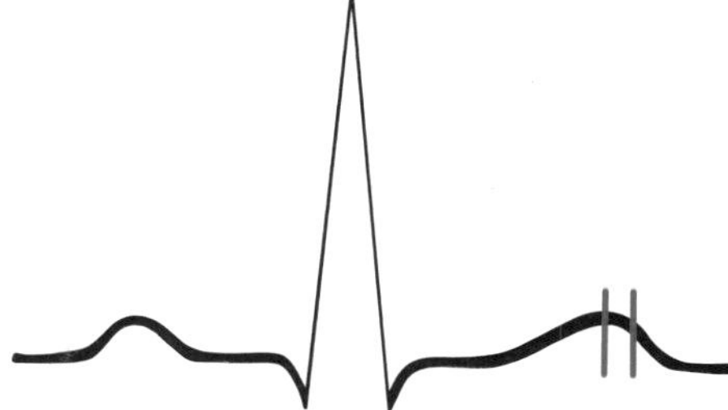

Fig. 11.10 Approximate location of the vulnerable period. (From Conover MB. *Understanding electrocardiography*. 4th ed. St. Louis, MO: Mosby; 2003.)

BOX 11.6 Procedure for Synchronized Cardioversion

1. Ensure emergency equipment is readily available.
2. Explain the procedure to the patient.
3. Attach monitor leads to the patient. Ensure the monitor displays the patient's rhythm clearly, without artifact.
4. Apply adhesive electrode pads to the patient's chest (recommended) and connect the cable to the defibrillator. If using paddles, either apply gel pads to the patient's chest or conductive gel to paddles.
5. Turn on the defibrillator to "synchronous" mode.
6. Observe the rhythm on the monitor to determine that the R wave is properly sensed and marked (usually with a spike) (see Fig. 11.11).
7. Premedicate the conscious patient with analgesics and sedatives unless unstable or rapidly deteriorating.
8. Select the appropriate energy level.
9. If using paddles, position the paddles on the patient's chest and apply firm pressure.
10. Announce, *"Charging defibrillator. Stand clear."* Press the "Charge" button on the defibrillator.
11. Shout, *"Clear. I am going to shock on three,"* and look to verify that *all* personnel are clear of the patient, bed, and any equipment connected to the patient. Disconnect the oxygen source during defibrillation.
12. Shout, *"One, two, three. Shocking."*
13. Deliver synchronized shock by pressing the "Shock" button on the defibrillator if using adhesive electrode pads. If using paddles, deliver synchronized shock by depressing buttons on each paddle simultaneously; keep the buttons depressed until the shock has been delivered.
14. After the cardioversion, observe the patient's heart rhythm and palpate pulse to determine effectiveness.

Special Situations. Patients at risk for sudden cardiac death may have an implantable cardioverter-defibrillator (ICD), with or without a permanent pacemaker, to deliver shocks directly to the heart muscle if a life-threatening dysrhythmia is detected.

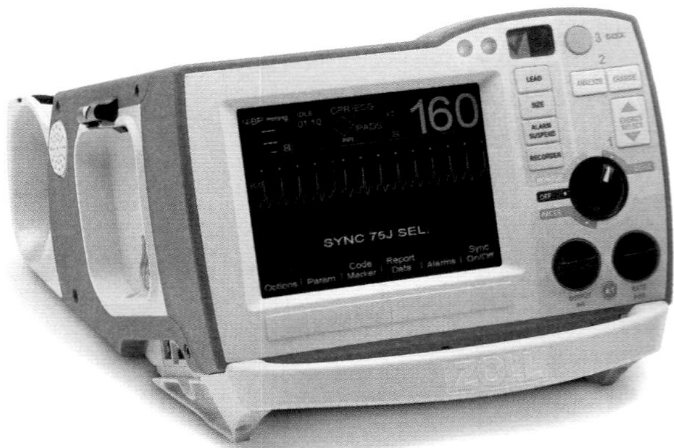

Fig. 11.11 ZOLL R Series monitor-defibrillator with marked R waves for cardioversion. (Courtesy ZOLL Medical Corporation, Chelmsford, MA.)

These devices are easily identified because they create a hard lump beneath the skin of the upper chest or abdomen. If a patient with a permanent pacemaker or ICD requires defibrillation, avoid placing the paddle or pads near the generator during the procedure. Although damage to the device rarely occurs, if paddles or pads are placed too close to the device, the device can absorb much of the current of defibrillation blocking the shock delivery, and reducing the chance of success. Place the adhesive electrode pad or paddle on either side and not directly on top of the implanted device.[20]

A patient may have an ICD with dual-chamber pacing capabilities. Be familiar, whenever possible, with the type of therapy the patient's device has been programmed to deliver. By the time VF or VT is recognized on the monitor, the ICD should recognize the rhythm. If a successful shock by the ICD has not occurred by the time the rhythm is noted on the monitor, initiate standard code protocols. If external defibrillation is unsuccessful, change the location of the adhesive electrode pads or paddles on the chest. Pads may be placed either anterior-lateral or anterior-posterior, as both are effective.

External defibrillation of a patient while the ICD is firing does not harm the patient or the ICD. ICDs and permanent pacemakers are insulated from damage caused by conventional external defibrillation. There is no danger to personnel if the ICD discharges while staff members are touching the patient. However, the shock may be felt and has been compared to the sensation of contact with an electrical outlet. Assess the pacing and sensing thresholds of the pacemaker or ICD after external defibrillation.

Transcutaneous Cardiac Pacing

Definition. Transcutaneous (i.e., external noninvasive) cardiac pacing is used during emergency situations to treat symptomatic bradycardia (i.e., hypotension, acutely altered mental status, ischemic chest pain, signs of shock, heart failure) that has not responded to atropine. Transcutaneous pacing does not correct asystole or PEA arrests. In this method of pacing, the heart is stimulated with externally applied, adhesive electrode pads that deliver the electrical impulse. Impulse conduction occurs across the chest wall to stimulate the cardiac contraction.

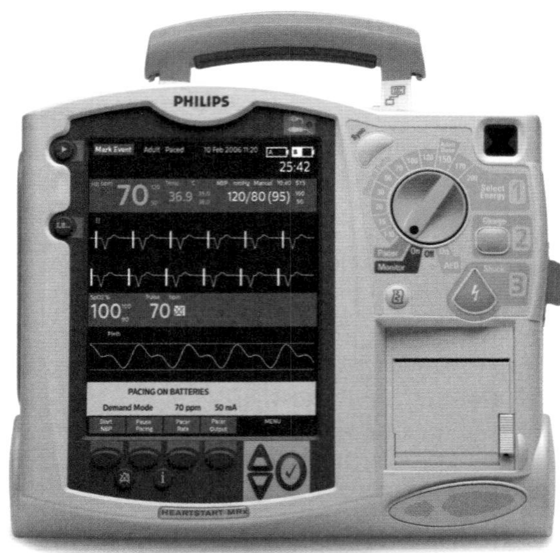

Fig. 11.12 Transcutaneous pacemaker-defibrillator. (Courtesy Philips Healthcare, Andover, MA.)

The transcutaneous pacemaker may be a freestanding unit with a monitor and a pacemaker. Most models incorporate a monitor, a defibrillator, and an external pacemaker into one system (Fig. 11.12). Transcutaneous pacemakers are easily operated in an emergent situation with minimal training without the risks associated with invasive pacemakers.

Procedure. The procedure for transcutaneous pacing (Box 11.7) involves the placement of adhesive electrode pads anteriorly and posteriorly on the patient (Fig. 11.8). Connect the electrodes to the external pacemaker, allowing for hands-off pacing. Set the pacemaker in either asynchronous or demand mode; some devices permit only demand pacing. In the asynchronous mode, the pacemaker generates a rhythm without regard to the patient's rhythm. In the demand mode, the pacemaker fires only if the patient's heart rate falls below a preset limit determined by the operator (e.g., 60 beats/min). Adjust the output, in milliamperes (mA), to stimulate a paced beat per the manufacturer's recommendations (typically 2 mA higher than the dose at which consistent capture is observed).

Assess the electrical and mechanical effectiveness of pacing. The electrical activity is verified by a pacemaker spike, followed by a broad QRS complex (Fig. 11.13). Mechanical activity is verified by palpation of a pulse during electrical activity and signs of improved cardiac output (e.g., increased blood pressure, improved skin color and temperature). If the transcutaneous pacemaker is effective, the patient may require a temporary transvenous pacemaker, depending on the cause of bradycardia.

The alert patient who requires transcutaneous pacing may experience some discomfort. Since the skeletal muscles are stimulated in addition to the heart muscle, the patient may experience a tingling, twitching, or thumping feeling that ranges from mildly uncomfortable to intolerable. Analgesics and/or sedatives may be indicated.

Cardiac Arrest After Cardiac Surgery

Cardiac arrest after cardiac surgery presents different challenges that are not addressed by ACLS algorithms. Most cardiac arrests occur within the first 24 hours after surgery from VF, cardiac tamponade, and major bleeding. If available within 1 minute from the time of arrest, defibrillation is performed for VF and pulseless VT prior to initiation of CPR. Emergency resternotomy (opening the chest) is performed to relieve tamponade and control bleeding. Epinephrine is not routinely administered unless ordered by an experienced provider. In 2017, the Society of Thoracic Surgeons published an expert consensus document for the resuscitation of patients who arrest after cardiac surgery. The protocol includes specific recommendations (Box 11.8).[22]

BOX 11.7 Procedure for Transcutaneous Pacing

1. If the patient is alert, explain the procedure.
2. Clip excess hair from the patient's chest. Do not shave hair.
3. Apply adhesive electrode pads in the anterior-posterior position (Fig. 11.8) and connect the electrode cable to the pacemaker generator.
4. Turn the unit on. Choose pacing mode (asynchronous or demand).
5. Set the pacemaker parameter for heart rate based on the provider's order or the hospital's policy.
6. Start the output (milliamperes [mA]) at 0 and increase until electrical capture (i.e., pacemaker spike followed by a QRS complex [Fig. 11.13]) is observed. Once capture is observed, set the output per the manufacture's recommendations or 2 mA above the dose at which consistent capture is observed.
7. Adjust the heart rate based on the patient's clinical response.
8. Assess the adequacy of pacing:
   - Electrical capture
   - Palpable pulse
   - Heart rate and rhythm
   - Blood pressure
   - Level of consciousness
9. Observe for patient discomfort. The patient may need analgesia and/or sedation.
10. Anticipate follow-up treatment (e.g., insertion of a temporary transvenous pacemaker).

PHARMACOLOGICAL INTERVENTION DURING A CODE OR CARDIOPULMONARY EMERGENCY

Medications that are administered during a code depend on several factors: cause of emergency or arrest, cardiac rhythm, provider's preference, and patient response. The goals of treatment are to reestablish and maintain optimal cardiac function, correct hypoxemia and acidosis, and suppress dangerous cardiac ectopic activity. In addition, medications are used to achieve a balance between myocardial oxygen supply and demand, maintain adequate blood pressure, and relieve heart failure.

Due to the rapid and profound effects these medications can have on cardiac activity and hemodynamics, continuous ECG monitoring is essential. Hemodynamic monitoring must be instituted as soon as possible after the code. Infusion pumps should be used to deliver continuous infusions because of the precise dosages and careful administration required with these medications.

BOX 11.8 Resuscitation of Patients Who Arrest After Cardiac Surgery

- Management is a multiprofessional activity with defined roles, including designated members preparing for resternotomy (i.e., instruments, sterile field).
- Perform a resternotomy within 5 minutes of arrest in the critical care setting.
- Do not delay cardiopulmonary resuscitation (CPR) for defibrillation and pacing for more than 1 minute from the onset of arrest.
- Ventricular fibrillation and pulseless ventricular tachycardia are managed with three sequential attempts at defibrillation. If unsuccessful, start CPR and administer medications as ordered by provider. Continue CPR with defibrillation until emergency resternotomy is performed.
- Asystole or extreme bradycardia is managed with pacing if pacing wires available; if unsuccessful, start CPR; transcutaneous pacing is considered, followed by emergency resternotomy.
- Pulseless electrical activity (PEA) is managed by CPR while simultaneously excluding reversible causes (e.g., tension pneumothorax, tamponade, or hemorrhage) followed by emergency resternotomy.
- Epinephrine is not routinely given due to the danger of extreme hypertension with the potential of graft failure and hemorrhage.

Data from Dunning J, Levine A, Ley J et al. The Society of Thoracic Surgeons expert consensus for the resuscitation of patients who arrest after cardiac surgery. *Ann Thorac Surg.* 2017;103(3):1005-1020.

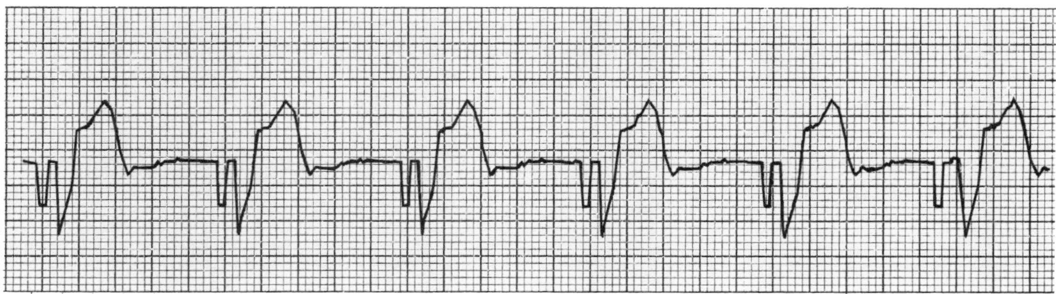

Fig. 11.13 Electrical capture of transcutaneous pacemaker. Notice the pacemaker spikes followed by a wide QRS complex and a tall T wave.

The following medications are included in ACLS guidelines and most frequently used during a code.[20] Actions, indications, and dosages for each medication, as well as side effects and nursing implications, are discussed in this section and summarized in Table 11.4.

Oxygen

Oxygen is essential to resuscitation and has several pharmacological considerations. Oxygen is used to treat hypoxemia, which exists in any cardiopulmonary emergency or arrest situation as a result of lack of adequate gas exchange, inadequate cardiac output, or both. Artificial ventilation without supplemental oxygen does not correct hypoxemia. In addition, the success of other medications and interventions, such as defibrillation, depends on adequate oxygenation and normal acid-base status.

Oxygen can be delivered by a bag-valve-mask device, a bag-valve-mask device attached to an ETT, or other airway adjuncts. During an arrest, 100% oxygen is administered.

Epinephrine (Adrenalin)

Epinephrine is a potent vasoactive agent. As a result of its alpha-adrenergic effects, epinephrine increases systemic vascular

TABLE 11.4 PHARMACOLOGY

Medications Frequently Used During a Code or Cardiopulmonary Emergency

Medication	Action/Uses	Dose/Route	Side Effects	Nursing Implications
Adenosine (Adenocard)	Slows conduction through AV node, interrupting reentry circuits *Use*: Supraventricular dysrhythmias	*Intravenous:* Push, 6 mg IV over 1-2 sec, followed by 20 mL rapid NS flush; if no response in 1-2 min, give 12 mg IV over 1-2 sec and flush; may repeat 12 mg IV over 1-2 sec dose if necessary	Bronchospasm Chest pain Dizziness Dyspnea Facial flushing Headache Light-headedness May cause asystole up to 15 sec	Half-life: 10 sec Higher dose needed with theophylline, lower dose with dipyridamole or after cardiac transplantation. Inform patient about potential effects of the medication. Defibrillator should be readily available.
Amiodarone (Cordarone)	↓ Membrane excitability, prolongs action potential to terminate VT or VF *Use*: Treatment and prophylaxis of recurrent VF and hemodynamically unstable VT; rapid atrial dysrhythmias	**Cardiac arrest** *Intravenous/Intraosseous:* Push 300 mg IV/IO, followed by 150 mg IV/IO in 3-5 min if needed **Recurrent VF/VT** *Intravenous:* Bolus, 150 mg IV over 10 min (15 mg/min); may repeat 150 mg IV q10 min as needed Maintenance, 360 mg infusion for 6 h (1 mg/min), then 540 mg for next 18 h (0.5 mg/min), for a maximum dose of 2.2 g over 24 h	Bradycardia Headache Hepatotoxicity Hypotension Pulmonary toxicity Thyroid toxicity Use with caution on preexisting conduction system abnormalities	Monitor for symptomatic sinus bradycardia; PR, QRS, and QT prolongation. Use concentration ≤2 mg/mL unless central venous catheter is used Consider in-line filter for peripheral administration
Atropine	↑ SA node automaticity and AV node conduction activity *Use*: symptomatic bradycardia	*Intravenous*: Push, 1 mg IV q3-5 min to maximum cumulative dose of 3 mg *Endotracheal*: 1-2 mg in 10 mL NS or sterile water may be given via ETT q 3-5 min	Headache Increased myocardial oxygen consumption and ischemia Tachycardia	If atropine is ineffective anticipate transcutaneous pacing, dopamine or epinephrine infusion. Ineffective in heart transplant recipients
Dopamine (Intropin)	Dose-dependent effect 2-10 mcg/kg/min stimulates beta-1 receptor (↑ contractility and HR) 10-20 mcg/kg/min: stimulates alpha receptors (vasoconstriction to increase ↑ SVR) *Use*: Symptomatic bradycardia hypotension not related to hypovolemia	*Continuous infusion:* Initial, 2-5 mcg/kg/min IV Maintenance, 5-20 mcg/kg/min Titrate by 5-10 mcg/kg/min q10 to 30 minutes to clinical end point	Anxiety Chest pain Dyspnea Headache Hypertension Palpitations Piloerection Tachyarrhythmias Vomiting	Monitor HR, BP, and ECG. If available, monitor SVR and CO/CI Treat hypovolemia. Dosing greater than 20 mcg/kg/min decreases perfusion to the kidneys. Central venous catheter preferred. Tissue necrosis if extravasation (treat with phentolamine [Regitine]).

TABLE 11.4 PHARMACOLOGY—cont'd

Medications Frequently Used During a Code

Medication	Action/Uses	Dose/Route	Side Effects	Nursing Implications
Epinephrine (Adrenalin)	Beta-1 agonist: ↑ contractility and heart rate Alpha agonist: vasoconstriction, ↑ blood pressure, improves coronary and cerebral perfusion *Use:* IV/IO push for VF, pulseless VT, PEA, asystole; continuous infusion for symptomatic bradycardia	*Intravenous/Intraosseous:* IV push, 1 mg IV/IO; may repeat q3-5 min *Endotracheal*: 2-2.5 mg in 10 mL sterile water or NS via ETT; may repeat q3-5 min *Intravenous:* Maintenance, 0.01-0.2 mck/kg/min IV or 1-15 mcg/min, titrate to clinical end point	Anxiety Chest pain Dizziness Dyspnea Headache Hypertension Ischemia (peripheral, gastrointestinal) Pallor Palpitations Pulmonary edema Sweating Tachyarrhythmias Vomiting	Monitor HR, BP, and ECG. Invasive BP monitoring recommended. Treat hypovolemia. Central venous catheter preferred for continuous infusion. Tissue necrosis if extravasation (treat with phentolamine [Regitine]).
Lidocaine (Xylocaine)	Suppresses ventricular dysrhythmias, raises fibrillation threshold *Use*: VF, pulseless VT	**VF/pulseless VT** *Intravenous/Intraosseous*: Bolus, 1-1.5 mg/kg IV/IO, followed by 0.5-0.75 mg/kg q5-10 min to max cumulative dose 3 mg/kg *Endotracheal*: 2-4 mg/kg in 10 mL sterile water or NS via ETT *Intravenous*: Maintenance, 1-4 mg/min IV, titrate to clinical end point	Bradycardia if serum lidocaine level is excessive Headache Neurological toxicity (lethargy, confusion, tinnitus, muscle twitching, paresthesia, seizures) Shivering	Lower dose for hepatic or renal impairment and in the elderly. Consider blood level monitoring for infusions >24 h (therapeutic 1.5-5 mcg/mL; toxic >9 mcg/mL)
Magnesium	Essential for enzyme reactions and sodium-potassium pump, ↓ postinfarction dysrhythmias *Use*: Torsades de pointes, hypomagnesemia	**VF/Pulseless VT** *Intravenous/Intraosseous*: Bolus, 1-2 g IV/IO over 1-2 min **VT with a pulse** *Intravenous*: Infusion, 1-2 g IV over 5-60 min, may repeat up to 4 g in 1 h Maintenance, 0.5-1 g/h, titrated to control torsades	Bradycardia Flushing Hypotension Respiratory depression	Monitor serum magnesium levels.
Norepinephrine (Levophed)	Beta-1 agonist: ↑ contractility and heart rate Alpha agonist: vasoconstrictive and ↑ blood pressure *Use*: Hypotension	*Continuous infusion:* Initial, 0.05-0.15 mcg/kg/min IV or 5-15 mcg/min IV Maintenance, titrate to clinical end point	Anxiety Chest pain Dysrhythmias Headache Hypertension Ischemia (peripheral, gastrointestinal)	Monitor BP, HR, and ECG. Central venous catheter preferred. Tissue necrosis if extravasation (treat with phentolamine [Regitine]).
Oxygen	↑ Oxygen content and tissue oxygenation *Use*: Cardiopulmonary arrest, chest pain, hypoxemia	100% in a code via bag-valve-mask device with mask or attached to ETT	None in cardiac arrest	Monitor pulse oximetry.

AV, Atrioventricular; *BP*, blood pressure; *CO/CI*, cardiac output/cardiac index; *CPR*, cardiopulmonary resuscitation; *ECG*, electrocardiogram; *ETT*, endotracheal tube; *HR*, heart rate; *IO*, intraosseous; *IV*, intravenous; *NS*, 0.9% normal saline; *PEA*, pulseless electrical activity; *q*, every; *SA*, sinoatrial; *SVR*, systemic vascular resistance; *VF*, ventricular fibrillation; *VT*, ventricular tachycardia.

Based on data from Panchal AR, Bartos JA, Cabañas JG et al. Part 3: adult basic and advanced life support: 2020 American Heart Association guidelines for cardiopulmonary resuscitation and emergency cardiovascular care. *Circulation*. 2020;142(16_suppl_2). https://doi.org/10.1161/cir.0000000000000916; Collins, Shelly R. *Elsevier's 2023 Intravenous Medications*. 39th ed. St. Louis, MO: Elsevier, Inc.; 2023.

BOX 11.9 Effects of Adrenergic Receptor Stimulation

Alpha
- Vasoconstriction

Beta-1
- Increased heart rate
- Increased contractility

Beta-2
- Vasodilation
- Relaxation of bronchial, uterine, and gastrointestinal smooth muscle

resistance through vasoconstriction, causing increased blood pressure and shunting of blood to the heart and brain. Additionally, epinephrine enhances heart rate, contractility, and automaticity of cardiac pacemaker cells through its beta-adrenergic activity (Box 11.9). Consequently, epinephrine increases myocardial oxygen demand.

 **CLINICAL JUDGMENT ACTIVITY**

A patient has an ICD or permanent pacemaker. How would care and treatment of this patient differ in a code situation?

Epinephrine is indicated immediately in PEA and asystole arrests and after the second defibrillation in VF or pulseless VT. The benefit of epinephrine in cardiac arrest is believed to be due to the increase in coronary and cerebral perfusion pressure during CPR.

During ACLS, epinephrine may be pushed IV or IO or instilled through an ETT. Once ROSC is achieved, continuous infusion epinephrine may be required to increase or maintain the heart rate or blood pressure.

CHECK YOUR UNDERSTANDING

3. On the monitor a patient has polymorphic VT. What is the priority nursing intervention?
   A. Check the patient's pulse
   B. Administer magnesium
   C. Prepare for synchronized cardioversion
   D. Recommend to the provider initiating an antiarrhythmic infusion

Atropine

Atropine is used during symptomatic bradycardia to increase heart rate by blocking parasympathetic activity on the heart. Routine use of atropine during PEA or asystole arrests is no longer recommended as it is unlikely to be of benefit.[23] For symptomatic bradycardia, atropine is administered to maintain a heart rate greater than 60 beats/min or until adequate tissue perfusion is achieved as indicated by blood pressure and level of consciousness. If atropine is ineffective in maintaining the heart rate and adequate tissue perfusion, consider transcutaneous pacing, dopamine infusion, or an epinephrine infusion. Use atropine cautiously in patients with acute coronary ischemia or myocardial infarction because the increased heart rate may worsen ischemia or increase infarction size.[19]

Amiodarone (Cordarone)

Amiodarone is a unique antiarrhythmic possessing some characteristics of all antiarrhythmic classes. It reduces membrane excitability and prolongs the action potential, slowing the refractory period, which results in the termination of VT and VF. It also has alpha- and beta-adrenergic blocking properties. Amiodarone has the added benefit of dilating coronary arteries and increasing coronary blood supply. It also decreases systemic vascular resistance, improving cardiac function in patients with impaired left ventricular function. Antiarrhythmic agents also have a propensity to exacerbate dysrhythmias, known as proarrhythmia or prodysrhythmia. Administration of amiodarone is rarely associated with prodysrhythmia.

Amiodarone IV is indicated for treatment and prevention of recurrent VF and unstable VT refractory to other treatment. Amiodarone is also given in supraventricular tachycardia for rate control or atrial fibrillation or flutter for cardioversion, especially in patients with heart failure. In cardiac arrest, amiodarone may be considered for VF and pulseless VT unresponsive to defibrillation.[24] Adverse reactions include hypotension and bradycardia, which can be prevented by slowing the administration rate or treating with fluids, vasopressors, or temporary pacing.

Lidocaine (Xylocaine)

Lidocaine is an antiarrhythmic medication that suppresses ventricular ectopic activity. It depresses the ventricular conduction system and reduces automaticity. In cardiac arrest, lidocaine may be considered for VF and pulseless VT unresponsive to defibrillation.[24] If lidocaine is successful in treating the cardiac dysrhythmia, a continuous infusion may be initiated; however, there is inadequate evidence to support that routine use will prevent recurrence.[20] Lidocaine is also used in the suppression of ventricular ectopy (premature ventricular contractions).

Decrease dosages of lidocaine in patients with impaired hepatic blood flow (as occurs in heart failure or left ventricular dysfunction) and/or renal function (glomerular filtration rate [GFR] <30 mL/min/1.73m^2) as well as in elderly patients. Monitor serum drug levels and assess the patient for central nervous system disturbances that may indicate lidocaine toxicity. Common side effects of lidocaine include lethargy, confusion, tinnitus, muscle twitching, seizures, bradycardia, and paresthesias.

Adenosine (Adenocard)

Adenosine is the initial drug of choice for the diagnosis and treatment of supraventricular dysrhythmias. Adenosine slows conduction through the AV node and interrupts AV node reentrant electrical conduction, which is the cause of most supraventricular dysrhythmias. It is effective in restoring normal sinus rhythm in patients with paroxysmal supraventricular tachycardia, including that caused by Wolff-Parkinson-White syndrome. Adenosine does not convert supraventricular rhythms that do not involve the sinoatrial or AV node, such as atrial fibrillation, atrial flutter, atrial tachycardia, and VT. However, adenosine may produce a brief AV node block, slowing the ventricular rate enough to assist in the diagnosis of these rhythms. The patient must be connected to an ECG monitor with a defibrillator readily available throughout the administration of adenosine.

Adenosine has an onset of action of 10 to 40 seconds and a duration of 1 to 2 minutes; therefore, it requires rapid administration. The initial dose is followed by a rapid 20 mL saline flush. A period of asystole lasting as long as 15 seconds may occur after administration due to suppression of AV node conduction. A second and third dose may be given 1 to 2 minutes later if the prior dose is ineffective in converting or identifying the rhythm. Common side effects include transient facial flushing (from mild dilation of blood vessels in the skin), dyspnea, coughing (from mild bronchoconstriction), and chest pain. If the patient is conscious, they should be educated on what to expect prior to administering adenosine.

Magnesium

Magnesium is essential for many enzyme reactions and for the function of the sodium-potassium pump. It also acts as a calcium channel blocker and slows neuromuscular transmission. Hypomagnesemia is associated with a high frequency of cardiac dysrhythmias, including refractory VF. Magnesium administered via the IV route may suppress or prevent recurrent torsades de pointes in patients who have a prolonged QT interval. *Torsades de pointes* is a form of VT characterized by QRS complexes that change amplitude and appearance (polymorphic) and appear to twist around the isoelectric line (Fig. 11.14). The QRS complexes may deflect downward for a few beats and then upward for a few beats. The side effects of rapid magnesium administration include hypotension, bradycardia, flushing, and respiratory depression therefore, slower rates are recommended in stable patients. Serum magnesium levels are monitored to avoid hypermagnesemia.

Sodium Bicarbonate

A patient who experiences an arrest becomes acidotic quickly. The acidosis results from two sources: no blood flow during the arrest and low blood flow during CPR. Effective ventilation with supplemental oxygen and rapid restoration of tissue perfusion by CPR and ROSC are the best mechanisms to correct these causes of acidosis.

Limited data support the administration of sodium bicarbonate during cardiac arrest.[20] Sodium bicarbonate buffers the increased numbers of hydrogen ions present in metabolic acidosis. It is beneficial in treating preexisting metabolic acidosis, hyperkalemia, and tricyclic antidepressant overdose.

When possible, bicarbonate therapy is guided by the bicarbonate concentration or calculated base deficit from arterial blood gas analysis or laboratory measurement. Do not mix or infuse sodium bicarbonate with any other medication, because it may precipitate or cause deactivation of other medications.

Dopamine (Intropin)

Dopamine may be considered in symptomatic bradycardia unresponsive to atropine. Its effects are dose related; however, the clinical effects overlap among dose ranges and may vary by patient. At doses of 2 to 10 mcg/kg/min, beta-adrenergic stimulation occurs, causing increased cardiac contractility, cardiac output, heart rate, and blood pressure. At doses greater than 10 mcg/kg/min, systemic vascular resistance markedly increases as a result of generalized vasoconstriction produced from alpha-adrenergic stimulation. At doses greater than 20 mcg/kg/min, marked vasoconstriction occurs, and myocardial workload is increased without an increase in coronary blood supply. This creates a situation that may cause myocardial ischemia. Administer the lowest dose necessary to minimize side effects and to ensure adequate perfusion of vital organs.

In addition to causing myocardial ischemia, dopamine may cause cardiac dysrhythmias such as tachycardia and premature ventricular contractions. Necrosis and sloughing of tissue may occur if the drug infiltrates; therefore, a central line is preferred. Phentolamine 5 to 10 mg in 10 to 15 mL of 0.9% normal saline can be injected around the infiltrated area to prevent necrosis.

CODE DOCUMENTATION AND POSTRESUSCITATION ACTIONS

Documentation of Code Events

Maintain a detailed chronological record of all interventions during a code. One of the first actions of the code leader is to ensure that someone is assigned to record information throughout the code. Documentation includes the time the code is called, time CPR is started, any actions taken (e.g., defibrillation, with energy used, medication administration, intubation), and patient's vitals (e.g., presence or absence of a pulse, heart rate, blood pressure, cardiac rhythm). Accurately record the time and sites of IV initiations, type and amount of fluids administered, and medications and dosages given. Record rhythm strips to document events and response to treatment. Many hospitals have standardized code records (Fig. 11.15) that list actions and medications and include spaces for entering the time of each intervention and any comments. If possible, record information directly on the code record during the code to ensure that all information is obtained. The code record identifies all those who participated in the code and becomes part of the patient's permanent record. Some institutions may document code events directly in the electronic health record instead of paper records.

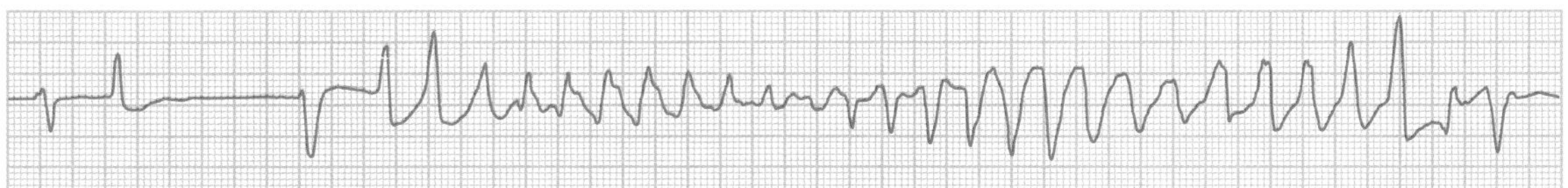

Fig. 11.14 Torsades de pointes. The QRS complex seems to spiral around the isoelectric line. (From Ralston SH, Penman ID, Strachan MWJ, Hobson RP. *Davidson's Principles and Practice of Medicine.* 24th ed. Edinburgh, Scotland: Elsevier Ltd.; 2023.)

Postresuscitation Efforts

Debriefing. The code team, including the patient's primary nurse and attending provider, may benefit from post–cardiac arrest debriefings.[27] Debriefing codes can help build a cohesive team, improve communication, and facilitate learning.[28] Additionally, debriefing codes with the code team can help team members process their experiences and reduce moral distress and burnout.

Care of the Patient After Resuscitation. Systematic post–cardiac arrest care after ROSC can improve patient survival with good quality of life.[25] Postresuscitation goals include optimizing cardiopulmonary function, transporting the patient to an appropriate critical care unit capable of providing post–cardiac arrest care, and identifying and treating the precipitating cause to prevent another arrest, including electrolyte abnormalities (see Laboratory Alert box; refer to the Collaborative Care Plan found in Chapter 1, Overview of Critical Care).[25] Key interventions to improve outcomes include advanced airway placement, maintenance of oxygenation and tissue perfusion, advanced neurological monitoring, and the use of TTM.

Advanced airway placement. An adequate airway and support of breathing must be initiated and/or maintained. The unconscious patient will require an advanced airway or endotracheal intubation. When securing the ETT, avoid ties that pass circumferentially around the patient's neck to prevent obstruction of venous return to the brain. Elevate the head of the bed to 30 degrees, if tolerated, to reduce the incidence of cerebral edema, aspiration, and pneumonia.

Waveform capnography is recommended to confirm and continuously monitor the position of the ETT, especially during patient transport.[20] Waveform capnography continuously measures the partial pressure of CO_2 at the end of expiration (i.e., $ETCO_2$), showing as a numerical value with a graphic display of the exhaled waveform over time (Fig. 11.16). A heated sensor is placed in the airway circuit between the ETT and the ventilator tubing. The exhaled gas flows directly over the sensor, providing a measurement of $ETCO_2$. The normal range of $ETCO_2$ is 35 to 40 mm Hg. When the ETT is correctly placed, a normal waveform is seen, with $ETCO_2$ rising on expiration, sustaining a plateau, and returning to baseline on inspiration (Fig. 11.16). A sudden loss of $ETCO_2$ with a waveform at baseline indicates incorrect ETT placement or cardiac arrest. The patient's airway should be assessed immediately. Waveform capnography should be used in addition to breath sound auscultation and direct visualization of the larynx to assess placement of the ETT. If it is not available, an $ETCO_2$ detector placed on the ETT (Fig. 11.5) or an esophageal detector device may be used.

Maintenance of oxygenation and tissue perfusion. Although 100% fraction of inspired oxygen (FiO_2) may have been used during the initial resuscitation, the lowest FiO_2 adequate to maintain oxygen saturation (SpO_2) at 94% or greater (as measured by pulse oximetry) and the partial pressure of oxygen (PaO_2) at approximately 100 mm Hg (as determined by arterial blood gas measurement) are used. Excessive ventilation (too fast or too much) is avoided because it may increase intrathoracic pressure and decrease cardiac output. The decrease in the partial pressure of carbon dioxide ($PaCO_2$) seen with hyperventilation can also decrease cerebral blood flow. Ventilate patients at 10 breaths/min and titrate to achieve an $ETCO_2$ of 35 to 40 mm Hg or a $PaCO_2$ of 35 to 45 mm Hg.

Continuous ECG monitoring continues after ROSC, during transport to the critical care unit, and throughout the critical care stay until no longer deemed necessary. Obtain IV access if not

! LABORATORY ALERT

Electrolyte Values

Laboratory Test	Normal Range	Critical Value[a]	Significance
Sodium (Na^+)	136-145 mEq/L	<120 or >160 mEq/L	Implications for polarization of heart muscle via K^+/Na^+ pump
Potassium (K^+)	3.5-5 mEq/L	<2.5 or >6.5 mEq/L	Affects cardiac conduction and contractility Maintains cardiac cell homeostasis ECG: **Hypokalemia:** depressed ST segment, flat or inverted T wave, presence of U wave **Hyperkalemia:** tall, peaked T wave prolonged PR interval, flattened P wave, widening of QRS (can progress to asystole)
Calcium (Ca^{++}) (total)	9-10.5 mg/dL	<6 or >13 mg/dL	Affects cardiac cell action potential and contraction ECG: **Hypocalcemia:** prolonged QT interval **Hypercalcemia:** shortened QT interval
Magnesium (Mg^{++})	1.3-2.1 mEq/L	<0.5 or >3 mEq/L	Affects contraction of cardiac muscle and promotes vasodilation that may reduce preload, alter cardiac output, and reduce systemic blood pressure ECG: **Hypomagnesemia:** ↑ cardiac irritability with cardiac dysrhythmias (torsades de pointes), tachycardia, flat or inverted T waves, ST-segment depression **Hypermagnesemia:** slowing of cardiac conduction, bradycardia, prolonged PR and QT intervals

[a]Critical values vary by facility and laboratory.
ECG, Electrocardiogram.
Data from Pagana KD, Pagana TJ, Pagana TN. *Mosby's Diagnostic and Laboratory Test Reference*. 16th ed. St. Louis, MO: Elsevier, Inc.; 2023.

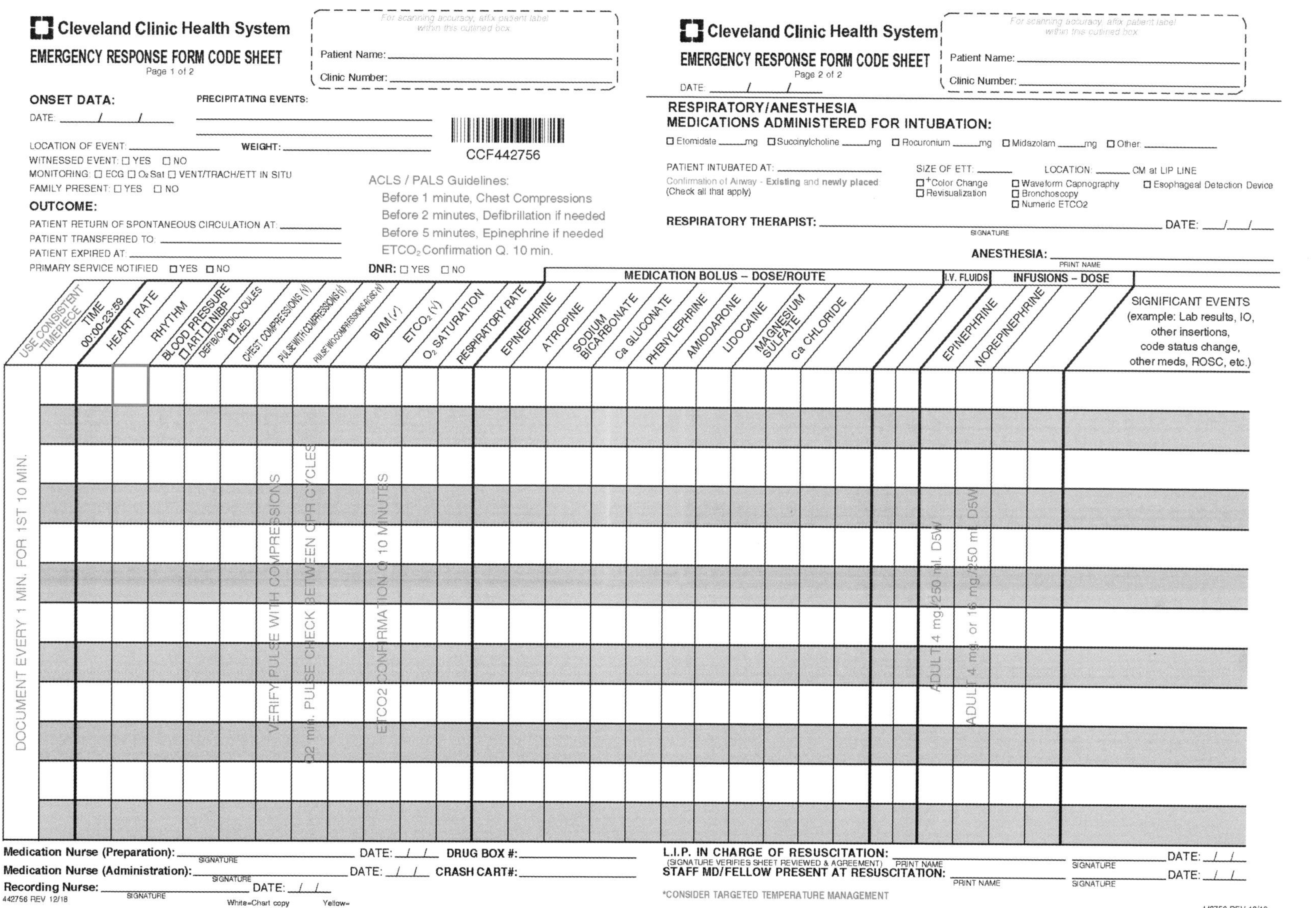
Cleveland Clinic Health System
EMERGENCY RESPONSE FORM CODE SHEET
Page 1 of 2

For scanning accuracy, affix patient label within this outlined box
Patient Name:
Clinic Number:

ONSET DATA:
DATE: / /
PRECIPITATING EVENTS:
LOCATION OF EVENT: WEIGHT:
WITNESSED EVENT: ☐ YES ☐ NO
MONITORING: ☐ ECG ☐ O_2 Sat ☐ VENT/TRACH/ETT IN SITU
FAMILY PRESENT: ☐ YES ☐ NO

CCF442756

OUTCOME:
PATIENT RETURN OF SPONTANEOUS CIRCULATION AT:
PATIENT TRANSFERRED TO:
PATIENT EXPIRED AT:
PRIMARY SERVICE NOTIFIED ☐ YES ☐ NO

ACLS / PALS Guidelines:
Before 1 minute, Chest Compressions
Before 2 minutes, Defibrillation if needed
Before 5 minutes, Epinephrine if needed
$ETCO_2$ Confirmation Q. 10 min.
DNR: ☐ YES ☐ NO

Cleveland Clinic Health System
EMERGENCY RESPONSE FORM CODE SHEET
Page 2 of 2
DATE: / /

For scanning accuracy, affix patient label within this outlined box
Patient Name:
Clinic Number:

RESPIRATORY/ANESTHESIA
MEDICATIONS ADMINISTERED FOR INTUBATION:
☐ Etomidate ___mg ☐ Succinylcholine ___mg ☐ Rocuronium ___mg ☐ Midazolam ___mg ☐ Other

PATIENT INTUBATED AT:
Confirmation of Airway - Existing and newly placed (Check all that apply)
SIZE OF ETT: LOCATION: CM at LIP LINE
☐ *Color Change ☐ Revisualization
☐ Waveform Capnography ☐ Bronchoscopy ☐ Numeric ETCO2
☐ Esophageal Detection Device

RESPIRATORY THERAPIST: SIGNATURE DATE: / /
ANESTHESIA: PRINT NAME

USE CONSISTENT TIMEPIECE | TIME 00:00-23:59 | HEART RATE | RHYTHM | BLOOD PRESSURE ☐ ART ☐ NIBP | DEFIB/CARDIO-JOULES ☐ AED | CHEST COMPRESSIONS (✓) | PULSE WITH COMPRESSIONS (✓) | PULSE W/O COMPRESSIONS-ROSC (✓) | BVM (✓) | $ETCO_2$ (✓) | O_2 SATURATION | RESPIRATORY RATE

MEDICATION BOLUS – DOSE/ROUTE: EPINEPHRINE | ATROPINE | SODIUM BICARBONATE | Ca GLUCONATE | PHENYLEPHRINE | AMIODARONE | LIDOCAINE | MAGNESIUM SULFATE | Ca CHLORIDE

I.V. FLUIDS

INFUSIONS – DOSE: EPINEPHRINE | NOREPINEPHRINE

SIGNIFICANT EVENTS (example: Lab results, IO, other insertions, code status change, other meds, ROSC, etc.)

DOCUMENT EVERY 1 MIN. FOR 1ST 10 MIN.
VERIFY PULSE WITH COMPRESSIONS
Q2 min. PULSE CHECK BETWEEN CPR CYCLES
ETCO2 CONFIRMATION Q 10 MINUTES
ADULT 4 mg/250 ml. D5W
ADULT 4 mg. or 16 mg/250 ml D5W

Medication Nurse (Preparation): SIGNATURE DATE: / / DRUG BOX #:
Medication Nurse (Administration): SIGNATURE DATE: / / CRASH CART#:
Recording Nurse: SIGNATURE DATE: / /
442756 REV 12/18 White=Chart copy Yellow=

L.I.P. IN CHARGE OF RESUSCITATION: (SIGNATURE VERIFIES SHEET REVIEWED & AGREEMENT) PRINT NAME SIGNATURE DATE: / /
STAFF MD/FELLOW PRESENT AT RESUSCITATION: PRINT NAME SIGNATURE DATE: / /
*CONSIDER TARGETED TEMPERATURE MANAGEMENT
442756 REV 12/18

Fig. 11.15 Sample of a code record used for documenting activities during a code. (Reprinted with permission, Cleveland Clinic Center for Art & Photography © 2019. All rights reserved.)

already established and verify the position and function of all IV catheters. Replace an IO catheter emergently placed during the code with IV access. If the patient is hypotensive (systolic blood pressure <90 mm Hg), administration of fluid boluses may be considered, unless volume resuscitation is already adequate. Cold fluid may be used if TTM is initiated but is no longer recommended in the prehospital setting.[26] Vasoactive medications (e.g., norepinephrine, epinephrine) may be initiated and titrated to maintain adequate perfusion (see Chapter 9, Hemodynamic Monitoring). If antiarrhythmic medications were used successfully during the code, additional doses or continuous infusions may be administered per provider discretion.

One of the most common causes of cardiac arrest is cardiovascular disease and coronary ischemia.[22] Obtain a 12-lead ECG as soon as possible to determine the presence of ST-segment elevation or a new bundle branch block. If there is a high suspicion of acute myocardial infarction, implement protocols for treatment and coronary reperfusion. Additional tubes and lines may be inserted after the code, such as an arterial line for hemodynamic monitoring, an indwelling urinary catheter to monitor hourly output, and a nasogastric tube for gastric decompression.

Advanced neurological monitoring. Neurological prognosis should not be performed during the first 72 hours after ROSC; this time frame may be extended in patients who receive TTM.[27] Serial neurological assessments, including response to verbal commands or physical stimulation, pupillary response to light, presence of corneal reflex, gag, cough, and spontaneous breaths are performed. Patients with post–cardiac arrest cognitive dysfunction may display agitation. In addition, the presence of lines and devices may result in pain, discomfort, and agitation. Intermittent or continuous sedation, analgesia, or both can be used to achieve specific goals (see Chapter 6, Comfort and Sedation). Imaging and diagnostic tests, such as head computed tomography (CT) scans or electroencephalography (EEG) monitoring, may be performed to assess neurological function.[27]

Targeted temperature management after cardiac arrest. Fever post–cardiac arrest is associated with poor neurological recovery, the degree of temperature elevation directly correlating with worsening outcomes.[28] Fever resulting from brain injury or ischemia exacerbates the degree of permanent neurological damage after cardiac arrest.[28] Patients who remain comatose (i.e., not purposefully following verbal commands) after a cardiac arrest, regardless of initial rhythm, should receive strategies for fever prevention.

TTM involves targeting a set temperature to achieve hypothermia, normothermia, or fever control. Current guidelines recommend initiating TTM by achieving and maintaining a constant temperature between 32°C and 36°C for at least 24 hours.[20] However, studies completed after guideline publication may alter future recommendations. A systematic review and meta-analysis found TTM between 32°C and 34°C did not improve patient outcomes compared to normothermia (see Evidence-Based Practice box).[29] The remainder of this section will discuss TTM as per guideline recommendations of maintaining a temperature of 32°C to 36°C and will not be applicable to institutions who utilize controlled normothermia in place of TTM.

The exact mechanism of TTM in improving neurological recovery is unknown; however, it is hypothesized to be due to reduction in the cerebral metabolic rate, thereby improving oxygen supply and reducing oxygen consumption in the ischemic brain. Currently, the optimal temperature, method, time of onset, duration, and rate of rewarming are unknown.

Multiple methods for conducting TTM are available. Commercially available automated cooling devices should be used to initiate and maintain TTM due to their ability to closely monitor patient temperature and proactively adjust device temperature to maintain the patient's target temperature. One available system uses surface cooling, where adhesive gel pads are placed around the core and thighs, with circulating water to regulate patient temperature (Fig. 11.17A). Another system uses an endovascular catheter that circulates solution through a closed system of balloons to regulate blood temperature as it circulates past the catheter (Fig. 11.17B). The use of manual cooling with ice packs, cooling blankets, and ice-cold isotonic IV fluids should be avoided due to significant fluctuations in patient temperature. These methods should only be used when automated cooling devices are unavailable and the patient is awaiting transfer to a facility with the available devices.

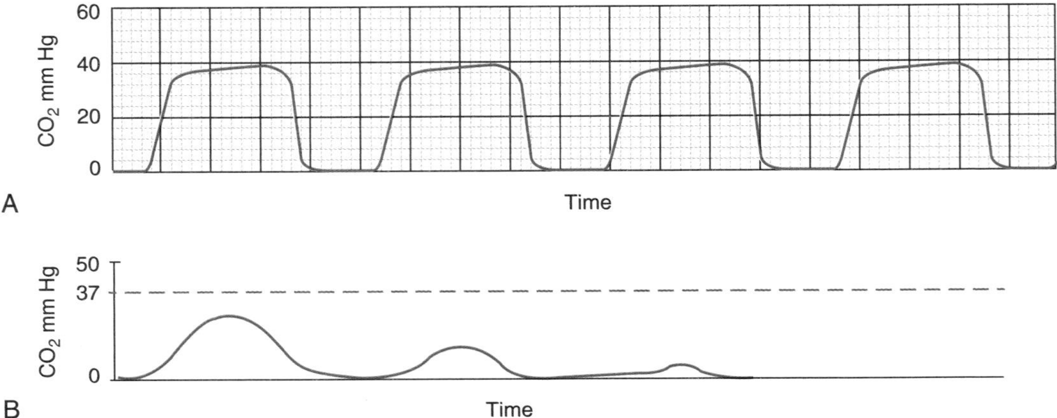

Fig. 11.16 Waveform capnography. A, Normal waveform indicating adequate ventilation pattern (end-tidal carbon dioxide [$ETCO_2$] 35 to 40 mm Hg). B, Abnormal waveform indicating airway obstruction or obstruction in breathing circuit ($ETCO_2$ decreasing).

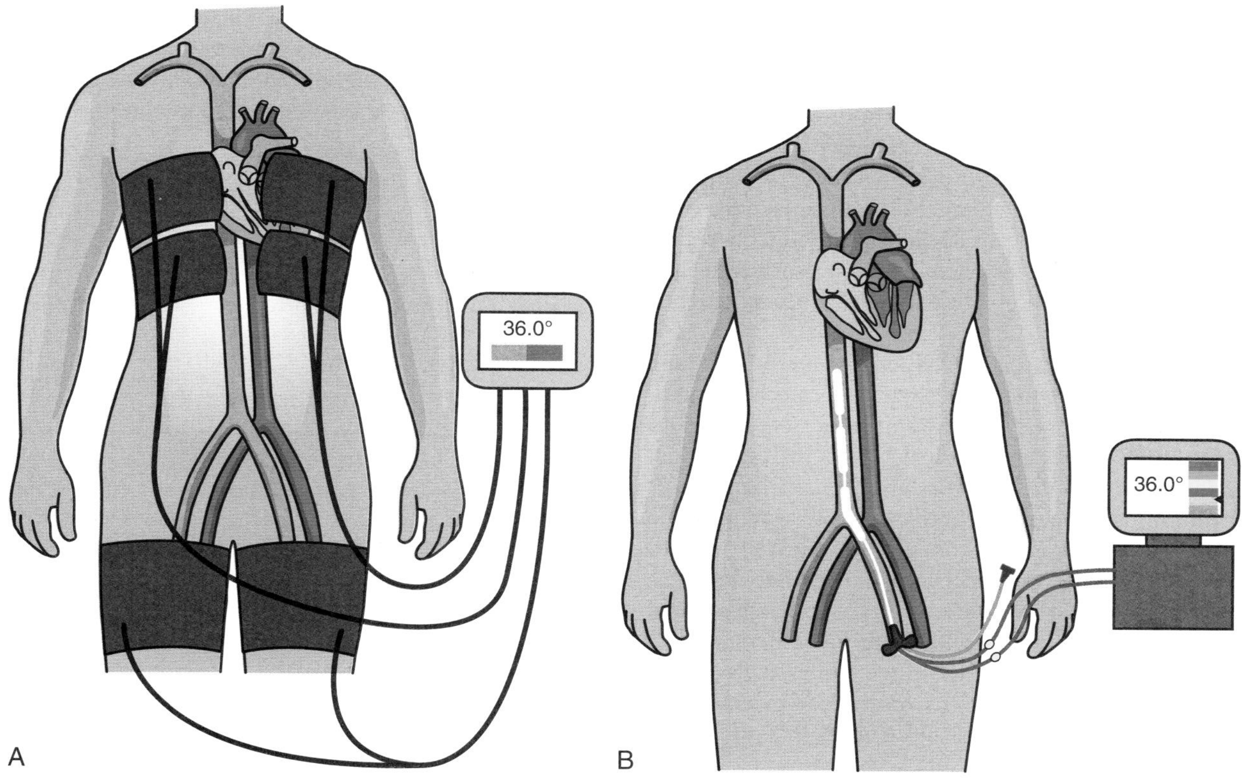

Fig. 11.17 Cooling methods. **A**, Surface-based cooling system. **B**, Endovascular catheter cooling using the femoral vein.

There are three phases of TTM: induction to the selected target core temperature, maintenance of this temperature for 24 hours, and slow rewarming to normothermia (e.g., 37°C). TTM should be initiated as soon as possible after ROSC. If the patient's post-ROSC temperature is lower than the selected target temperature, discussion should take place on how to initiate TTM to avoid rapid warming to target. The patient's core temperature is continuously monitored with the use of an esophageal thermometer, a bladder catheter with temperature probe, or a pulmonary artery catheter, if available. Axillary, oral, and tympanic temperature probes do not measure core temperature changes, and rectal temperature probes are inconsistent in their temperature measurements; therefore, none of these methods should be used during TTM.[30]

Physiological changes during TTM alter medication pharmacokinetics (PK; absorption, distribution, metabolism, and excretion) and pharmacodynamics (PD; physiological effects, mechanism of action, and relationship between medication concentration and effect). The degree of change in a medication's PK/PD is inversely correlated with the target temperature (e.g., the cooler the temperature, the more alterations in PK/PD are observed). Medication selection, dosing, and monitoring of potential medication-therapy interactions is essential to avoid potential complications.[31]

A common complication associated with TTM is shivering, predominantly during cooling and often during rewarming, as part of the normal physiological response to a change in skin temperature. Shivering increases oxygen consumption and generates heat, making it more difficult to cool the patient. Prior to treating shivering, myoclonus and seizures should be ruled out. Myoclonus, indicative of a poor neurological outcome, is defined by spontaneous and repetitive jerking movements that occur within 72 hours post–cardiac arrest.[32] Treatment of myoclonus to minimize heat generation is the same as for shivering. However, treatment for shivering or myoclonus will mask, without treating, seizures. Shivering can be prevented and/or treated with IV analgesics, sedatives, and neuromuscular blocking agents initiated in a stepwise fashion based on response and severity of shivering.[31] Counterwarming with an external warming blanket and/or socks on the patient's hands and feet are effective nonpharmacological interventions to prevent or treat shivering.[31]

Adverse effects associated with hypothermia include bradycardia, bleeding, infection, and metabolic and electrolyte disturbances.[29,31] These effects are more prominent with lower temperatures. Bradycardia occurs frequently and is only of concern if the patient is symptomatic (i.e., associated with hypotension or increasing vasopressor requirements). Since hypothermia decreases the metabolic demand, a decrease in metabolic supply with a reduced heart rate and cardiac output is often tolerated. If symptomatic bradycardia does occur, patients will not respond to typical treatment. The patient will respond to a gradual increase in the core temperature of 0.5°C to 1°C.

Hypothermia inhibits the coagulation cascade and increases the risk of bleeding. For this reason, lower target temperatures (e.g., 32°C–34°C) should be avoided in any patient with a non-compressible bleed (e.g., intracranial hemorrhage, gastrointestinal bleed). In patients receiving TTM, increased bleeding may be observed after invasive procedures (e.g., coronary angiography with antiplatelet therapy or anticoagulation) but is not associated with increased mortality.[31]

Hypothermia suppresses ischemia-induced inflammatory reactions that occur after cardiac arrest, resulting in an increased risk of infection. Bloodstream infections have occurred more frequently with the use of endovascular catheters compared with noninvasive cooling methods, but these infections have not been associated with increased mortality.[31] Infection prevention strategies must be followed, including correct central line maintenance, prevention of ventilator-associated events, and good hand hygiene.

Hyperglycemia occurs post-ROSC due to increased stress and the release of endogenous and exogenous catecholamines. Additionally, hypothermia decreases insulin secretion and insulin sensitivity. Depending on the degree of hyperglycemia, subcutaneous sliding scale corrective insulin may be used, or an IV insulin infusion may be required to achieve appropriate glycemic control. Long-acting subcutaneous insulin should be avoided, as hypothermia decreases subcutaneous perfusion, resulting in erratic medication release. During cooling, serum potassium, magnesium, phosphate, and calcium levels may decrease as a result of an intracellular shift. Replacement should be provided as needed, with avoidance of over replacement, as rewarming will cause the electrolytes to shift back to the serum.

After at least 24 hours at target temperature, rewarming proceeds slowly (0.25°C per hour) to prevent sudden vasodilation, hypotension, rebound fever, and shock.[31] After rewarming, normothermia should be maintained by leaving the devices used for TTM in place.

CLINICAL JUDGMENT ACTIVITY

Some hospitals are now considering allowing family members to be present during a code. How could the presence of family members affect the management of the code? What factors should you consider before permitting family members to be present?

CHECK YOUR UNDERSTANDING

4. Target temperature was achieved 8 hours ago in a patient post–cardiac arrest. Upon assessing the patient, the nurse notes the water temperature, which was previously stable, has been decreasing over the last 2 hours. What could this finding indicate, and what interventions would be appropriate?
   A. The system is malfunctioning and should be turned off immediately
   B. Assess the patient for shivering; initiate counterwarming and administer analgesic ordered to treat shivering
   C. Assess the patient for potential fever; administer acetaminophen as ordered, and evaluate for signs, symptoms, and sources of infection
   D. Both B and C

EVIDENCE-BASED PRACTICE

Targeted Temperature Management in Adult Cardiac Arrest

Problem

Targeted temperature management (TTM) remains a controversial topic with much debate regarding all aspects of TTM (i.e., optimal timing, target temperature, duration, method, and rewarming) for post–cardiac arrest patients. Current guidelines recommend initiating TTM by selecting and maintaining a constant temperature between 32°C and 36°C for at least 24 hours. However, ongoing trials at the time of guideline publication have since been completed, requiring an updated systematic review and meta-analysis to inform guidelines.

Question

In the post–cardiac arrest patient, what is the optimal timing, target temperature, duration, method, and rewarming for TTM?

Evidence

PubMed, Embase, and the Cochrane Central Register of Controlled Trials were searched using a combination of text and indexing search terms for cardiac arrest and TTM. Both randomized and nonrandomized controlled trials published up to June 2021 were included. A total of 39 manuscripts were included, representing 31 trials. When comparing TTM at 32°C to 36°C with normothermia (defined as core temperature of 36.5°C to 38°C), prehospital with no prehospital initiation of cooling, or different methods of achieving and maintaining TTM at 32°C to 34°C, there were no differences in favorable neurological outcomes or survival.

There is limited research evaluating the duration of TTM, and at the time of publication, there was one large trial investigating durations that was ongoing. The authors did not identify any trials assessing rewarming rates.

There were a number of limitations in the current studies. The authors noted that, in earlier studies, there was no information on avoidance of fever, whereas the more recent studies provided detailed protocols and data regarding active cooling to achieve normothermia. In addition, the four large trials were limited by prolonged times to achieve target temperature. Generalizability to inpatients may also be challenging, as the majority of the studies focused on out-of-hospital cardiac arrest. Given the limited number of studies and significant heterogeneity, the meta-analyses' results should be interpreted cautiously.

Implications for Nursing

In this meta-analysis, the authors concluded there was no improvement in clinical outcomes when target temperatures were lower; however, there were multiple limitations of the studies included. Achieving and maintaining lower TTM goals may increase the risk of adverse effects such as bradycardia, bleeding, infection, shivering, and metabolic and electrolyte disturbances, without improving outcomes for the patient. More evidence is needed to help guide the implementation of TTM to optimize patient outcomes.

The nurse managing a patient post–cardiac arrest receiving TTM should collaborate with the multiprofessional team to establish the appropriate target temperature based on the patient's clinical presentation and details of their cardiac arrest (i.e., whether it was witnessed, rhythm at time of arrest). Regardless of the target temperature, the greatest neuroprotection may be primarily related to the avoidance of hyperthermia and should continue to remain the focus of caring for this population.

Level of Evidence

A—Systematic review and meta-analysis

Reference

Granfeldt A, Holmberg MJ, Nolan JP, Soar J, Andersen LW; International Liaison Committee on Resuscitation (ILCOR) Advanced Life Support Task Force. Targeted temperature management in adult cardiac arrest: systematic review and meta-analysis. *Resuscitation*. 2021;167:160-172. https://doi.org/10.1016/j.resuscitation.2021.08.040.

Recovery and Survivorship After Cardiac Arrest

Emotional support is an important aspect of care after an arrest. Fear of death or of a recurrence of arrest is common. Survivors and family members often feel the need to discuss their experience in depth. In addition to the patient, many other people are affected when a code occurs. Family members, other patients, and staff members are all affected by the emergency.

Cardiac arrest survivors should be evaluated for anxiety, depression, posttraumatic stress, and fatigue.[22] Survivors should also be assessed for rehabilitation to treat physical, neurological, cardiopulmonary, and/or cognitive impairments as a result of cardiac arrest and critical illness. Comprehensive discharge care planning is necessary.

CASE STUDY

A 53-year-old patient with a history of hypertension is admitted for chest pain and shortness of breath. Upon entering the room, the patient becomes unresponsive. The nurse, who is ACLS certified, observes VT on the monitor. A palpable carotid pulse and spontaneous respirations are absent.

Questions

1. What is the priority for the nurse in this case scenario?
2. Based on the case presentation, what are potential reasons for cardiac arrest?
3. The patient's family is requesting to come bedside. How should the nursing supervisor proceed?
4. The patient is intubated, and capnography is now being monitored. The code leader notes a slow downward trend in the end-tidal CO_2. How should the code leader interpret this assessment finding and what intervention should be implemented? How will the code leader know that the intervention was effective?

KEY POINTS

- The RRT is a group of multiprofessionals trained in emergency response who are available 24 hours a day, 7 days a week.
- The goal of the RRT is to identify clinical deterioration or a worsening clinical state early and prevent its progression. Once a patient fulfills predefined criteria, such as deterioration in vital signs, mental status, and laboratory values, the RRT is activated, bringing specialized personnel and equipment to the patient's bedside.
- When patients experience cardiac arrest, the rapid initiation of BLS and ACLS improve their outcomes.
- Most hospitals have teams designated to code response, which may consist of a provider, critical care or emergency department nurses, a nursing supervisor, a respiratory therapist, a pharmacist or pharmacy technician, and a chaplain.
- After recognizing a patient is in cardiac arrest, the first responder calls for help and begins life-support measures immediately, while another team member immediately brings the code cart and defibrillator to the patient's bedside. The code cart contains basic emergency equipment and medications used during BLS and ACLS.
- Both BLS and ACLS are intended to support effective circulation, oxygenation, and ventilation until ROSC.
- There are critical actions in the management of the various dysrhythmias with which each critical care nurse should be familiar.
- Electrical therapy consists of defibrillation, AED, cardioversion, and transcutaneous pacing. Each therapy treats specific dysrhythmias and requires either training in BLS, ACLS, or both to be effective.
- Medications that are administered during a code are meant to reestablish and maintain optimal cardiac function, correct hypoxemia and acidosis, and suppress dangerous cardiac ectopic activity. The administration of these medications depends on the patient's stability, cardiac rate and rhythm, provider preference, and patient response.
- After ROSC, the team should debrief to identify opportunities for improvement and evaluate the multiprofessional team's response to the code event.
- Interventions to improve outcomes post–cardiac arrest include advanced airway placement, maintenance of oxygenation and tissue perfusion, advanced neurological monitoring, and the use of TTM.

REFERENCES

1. Institute for Healthcare Improvement. Rapid response teams. Accessed April 13, 2023. http://www.ihi.org/Topics/RapidResponseTeams/Pages/default.aspx.
2. Lyons PG, Edelson DP, Churpek MM. Rapid response systems. *Resuscitation*. 2018;128:191–197. https://doi.org/10.1016/j.resuscitation.2018.05.013.
3. Jones D, Moran J, Winters B, Welch J. The rapid response system and end-of-life care. *Curr Opin Crit Care*. 2013;19(6):616–623. https://doi.org/10.1097/mcc.0b013e3283636be2.
4. Kim JS, Lee MJ, Park MH, Park JY, Kim AJ. Role of the rapid response system in end-of-life care decisions. *Am J Hosp Palliat Care*. 2020;37(11):943–949. https://doi.org/10.1177/1049909120927372.
5. Teuma Custo R, Trapani J. The impact of rapid response systems on mortality and cardiac arrests - a literature review. *Intensive Crit Care Nurs*. 2020;59:102848. https://doi.org/10.1016/j.iccn.2020.102848.
6. Howlett O, Gleeson R, Jackson L, Rowe E, Truscott M, Maggs JA. Family support role in hospital rapid response teams: a scoping review. *JBI Evid Synth*. 2022;20(8):2001–2024. https://doi.org/10.11124/JBIES-21-00189.

7. McGaughey J, Fergusson DA, Van Bogaert P, Rose L. Early warning systems and rapid response systems for the prevention of patient deterioration on acute adult hospital wards. *Cochrane Database Syst Rev*. 2021;11(11):CD005529. https://doi.org/10.1002/14651858.CD005529.pub3.
8. Jones D, Mitchell I, Hillman K, Story D. Defining clinical deterioration. *Resuscitation*. 2013;84(8):1029–1034. https://doi.org/10.1016/j.resuscitation.2013.01.013.
9. Padilla RM, Mayo AM. Clinical deterioration: a concept analysis. *J Clin Nurs*. 2018;27(7–8):1360–1368. https://doi.org/10.1111/jocn.14238.
10. Subbe CP, Bannard-Smith J, Bunch J, et al. Quality metrics for the evaluation of Rapid Response Systems: proceedings from the third international consensus conference on Rapid Response Systems. *Resuscitation*. 2019;141:1–12. https://doi.org/10.1016/j.resuscitation.2019.05.012.
11. Burke JR, Downey C, Almoudaris AM. Failure to rescue deteriorating patients: a systematic review of root causes and improvement strategies. *J Patient Saf*. 2022;18(1):e140–e155. https://doi.org/10.1097/PTS.0000000000000720.
12. Andersen LW, Kim WY, Chase M, et al. The prevalence and significance of abnormal vital signs prior to in-hospital cardiac arrest. *Resuscitation*. 2016;98:112–117. https://doi.org/10.1016/j.resuscitation.2015.08.016.
13. Chua WL, Legido-Quigley H, Ng PY, McKenna L, Hassan NB, Liaw SY. Seeing the whole picture in enrolled and registered nurses' experiences in recognizing clinical deterioration in general ward patients: a qualitative study. *Int J Nurs Stud*. 2019;95:56–64. https://doi.org/10.1016/j.ijnurstu.2019.04.012.
14. Danesh V, Neff D, Jones TL, et al. Can proactive rapid response team rounding improve surveillance and reduce unplanned escalations in care? A controlled before and after study. *Int J Nurs Stud*. 2019;91:128–133. https://doi.org/10.1016/j.ijnurstu.2019.01.004.
15. Tirkkonen J, Tamminen T, Skrifvars MB. Outcome of adult patients attended by rapid response teams: a systematic review of the literature. *Resuscitation*. 2017;112:43–52. https://doi.org/10.1016/j.resuscitation.2016.12.023.
16. Enomoto N, Yamashita T, Furuta M, et al. Effect of maternal positioning during cardiopulmonary resuscitation: a systematic review and meta-analyses. *BMC Pregnancy Childbirth*. 2022;22(1):159. https://doi.org/10.1186/s12884-021-04334-y.
17. American Association of Critical-Care Nurses. AACN Practice Alert: Family Presence During Resuscitation and Invasive Procedures. aacn.org. Published February 2016. Accessed February 19, 2019. https://www.aacn.org/~/media/aacn-website/clincial-resources/practice-alerts/famvisitpafeb2016ccnpages.pdf.
18. Toronto CE, LaRocco SA. Family perception of and experience with family presence during cardiopulmonary resuscitation: an integrative review. *J Clin Nurs*. 2019;28(1–2):32–46. https://doi.org/10.1111/jocn.14649.
19. American Heart Association. *Advanced Cardiovascular Life Support: Instructor Manual*. American Heart Association; 2020.
20. Panchal AR, Bartos JA, Cabañas JG, et al. Part 3: adult basic and advanced life support: 2020 American heart association guidelines for cardiopulmonary resuscitation and emergency cardiovascular care. *Circulation*. 2020;142(16_suppl_2). https://doi.org/10.1161/cir.0000000000000916.
21. Steinberg MF, Olsen JA, Persse D, Souders CM, Wik L. Efficacy of defibrillator pads placement during ventricular arrhythmias, a before and after analysis. *Resuscitation*. 2022;174. https://doi.org/10.1016/j.resuscitation.2022.03.004.
22. Society of Thoracic Surgeons Task Force on Resuscitation After Cardiac Surgery. The Society of Thoracic Surgeons expert consensus for the resuscitation of patients who arrest after cardiac surgery. *Ann Thor Surg*. 2017;103(3):1005–1020.
23. Berg KM, Cheng A, Panchal AR, et al. Part 7: systems of Care: 2020 American Heart Association guidelines for cardiopulmonary resuscitation and emergency cardiovascular care. *Circulation*. 2020;142(16_suppl_2).
24. Panchal AR, Berg KM, Kudenchuk PJ, et al. 2018 American Heart Association focused update on Advanced Cardiovascular Life Support use of antiarrhythmic drugs during and immediately after cardiac arrest: an update to the American Heart Association guidelines for cardiopulmonary resuscitation and emergency cardiovascular care. *Circulation*. 2018;138(23):e740–e749. https://doi.org/10.1161/CIR.0000000000000613.
25. Sawyer KN, Camp-Rogers TR, Kotini-Shah P, et al. Sudden cardiac arrest survivorship: a scientific statement from the American Heart Association. *Circulation*. 2020;141(12). https://doi.org/10.1161/cir.0000000000000747.
26. Lüsebrink E, Binzenhöfer L, Kellnar A, et al. Targeted temperature management in postresuscitation care after incorporating results of the TTM2 Trial. *J Am Heart Assoc*. 2022;11(21):e026539. https://doi.org/10.1161/JAHA.122.026539.
27. Geocadin RG, Callaway CW, Fink EL, et al. Standards for studies of neurological prognostication in comatose survivors of cardiac arrest: a scientific statement from the American Heart Association. *Circulation*. 2019;140(9):e517–e542. https://doi.org/10.1161/CIR.0000000000000702.
28. Fernandez Hernandez S, Barlow B, Pertsovskaya V, Maciel CB. Temperature control after cardiac arrest: a narrative review [published online ahead of print, 2023 Mar 25]. *Adv Ther*. 2023 :10.1007/s12325-023-02494-1. https://doi.org/10.1007/s12325-023-02494-1.
29. Granfeldt A, Holmberg MJ, Nolan JP, Soar J, Andersen LW. International Liaison committee on resuscitation (ILCOR) advanced life support task force. Targeted temperature management in adult cardiac arrest: systematic review and meta-analysis. *Resuscitation*. 2021;167:160–172. https://doi.org/10.1016/j.resuscitation.2021.08.040.
30. Moreda M, Beacham PS, Reese A, Mulkey MA. Increasing the effectiveness of targeted temperature management. *Crit Care Nurse*. 2021;41(5):59–63. https://doi.org/10.4037/ccn2021637.
31. Karcioglu O, Topacoglu H, Dikme O, Dikme O. A systematic review of safety and adverse effects in the practice of therapeutic hypothermia. *Am J Emerg Med*. 2018;36(10):1886–1894. https://doi.org/10.1016/j.ajem.2018.07.024.
32. Chakraborty T, Braksick S, Rabinstein A, Wijdicks E. Status myoclonus with post-cardiac-arrest syndrome: implications for prognostication. *Neurocrit Care*. 2022;36(2):387–394. https://doi.org/10.1007/s12028-021-01344-8.

PART III

Nursing Care During Critical Illness

12

Shock, Sepsis, and Multiple Organ Dysfunction Syndrome

Maureen A. Seckel, APRN, MSN, ACNS-BC, CCNS, CCRN, FCCM, FCNS, FAAN

INTRODUCTION

Shock is a clinical syndrome characterized by inadequate tissue perfusion that results in cellular, metabolic, and hemodynamic derangements. Impaired tissue perfusion occurs when there is an imbalance between cellular oxygen supply and demand. Shock can result from ineffective cardiac function, inadequate blood volume, or inadequate vascular tone.

There are many causes and a variety of clinical manifestations of shock. The effects are not isolated to one organ system; instead, all body systems can be affected. Shock can progress to multiple organ dysfunction syndrome (MODS) and death unless compensatory mechanisms reverse the process or clinical interventions are successfully implemented.[1] Patient response to shock and treatment strategies vary, producing challenges in assessment and management for the multiprofessional healthcare team.

This chapter discusses the various clinical conditions that create the shock state, including hypovolemic shock, cardiogenic shock, distributive shock (i.e., anaphylactic, neurogenic, and septic shock), and obstructive shock. The progression of shock to multiple organ dysfunction syndrome (MODS) is also explained. The pathophysiology, clinical presentation, and definitive and supportive management of each type of shock state are described.

REVIEW OF ANATOMY AND PHYSIOLOGY

The cardiovascular system is a closed, interdependent system composed of the heart, blood, and vascular bed. Arteries, arterioles, capillaries, venules, and veins make up the vascular bed. The microcirculation, the portion of the vascular bed between the arterioles and the venules, is the most significant portion of the circulatory system for cell survival. It delivers oxygen and nutrients to cells, removes the waste products of cellular metabolism, and regulates blood volume. Vessels of the microcirculation constrict or dilate selectively to regulate blood flow to cells in need of oxygen and nutrients.[2]

The structure of the microcirculation is tailored to the function of the tissues and organs it supplies, but all vascular beds have common structural characteristics (Fig. 12.1).[2] As oxygenated blood leaves the left side of the heart and enters the aorta, it flows through progressively smaller arteries until it flows into an arteriole. Arterioles are lined with smooth muscle, which allows the small vessels to change diameter to direct and adjust blood flow to the capillaries. From the arteriole, blood enters a metarteriole, a smaller vessel that branches from the arteriole at right angles. Metarterioles are partially lined with smooth muscle, which allows them to adjust their diameter and regulate blood flow into capillaries.

Blood next enters the capillary network by passing through a muscular precapillary sphincter. Capillaries are narrow, thin-walled vascular networks that branch off the metarterioles. This network configuration increases the surface area, which allows greater fluid and nutrient exchange. It also decreases the velocity of the blood flow to prolong transport time through the capillaries. Capillaries have no contractile ability and are not responsive to vasoactive chemicals, electrical or mechanical stimulation, or pressure across their walls. The precapillary sphincter is the only means of regulating blood flow into a capillary. When the precapillary sphincter constricts, blood flow is diverted away from a capillary bed and directed to one that supplies tissues in need of oxygen and nutrients. The capillary bed lies close to the cells of the body, a position that facilitates the delivery of oxygen and nutrients to the cells.

After nutrients are exchanged for cellular waste products in the capillaries, blood leaves through a venule. These small, muscular vessels are able to dilate and constrict, offering postcapillary resistance for the regulation of blood flow through capillaries. Blood then flows from the venule and enters the larger veins of the venous system. Another component of the microcirculation consists of the arteriovenous anastomoses that connect arterioles directly to venules. These muscular vessels can shunt blood away from the capillary circulation and send it directly to tissues in need of oxygen and nutrients.

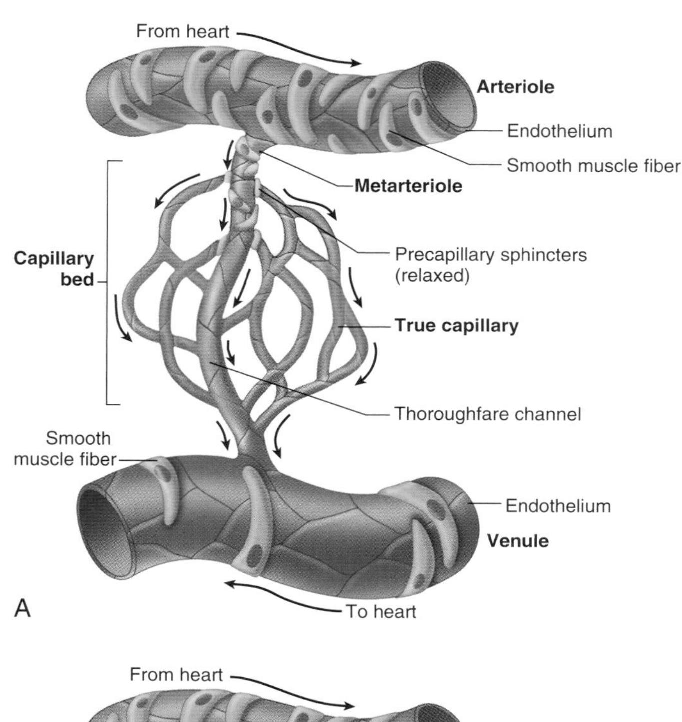

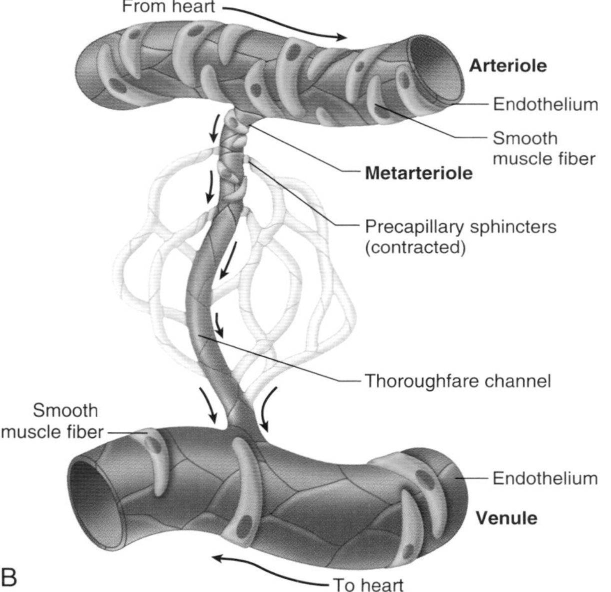

Fig. 12.1 Microcirculation. Control of blood flow through the capillary network is regulated by altering the tone of the precapillary sphincters surrounding arterioles and metarterioles. A, Sphincters are relaxed, permitting blood flow to enter the capillary bed. B, With sphincters contracted, blood flows into the thoroughfare channel, bypassing the capillary bed. (From Patton K, Thibodeau G. *Anatomy & Physiology*. 10th ed. St. Louis, MO: Elsevier; 2019.)

Delivery of oxygen (DO_2) to tissues and cells is required for the production of cellular energy (i.e., adenosine triphosphate [ATP]). DO_2 requires an adequate hemoglobin level to carry oxygen, adequate lung function to oxygenate the blood and saturate the hemoglobin (SaO_2), and adequate cardiac function (i.e., cardiac output [CO]) to transport the oxygenated blood to the cells. Impairment of DO_2 or increased consumption of oxygen by the tissues (VO_2) decreases the oxygen reserve (indicated by the mixed venous oxygen saturation [SvO_2]), which may result in tissue hypoxia, depletion of the supply of ATP, lactic acidosis, organ dysfunction, and death.[2]

TABLE 12.1 Classification of Shock

Type of Shock	Physiological Alteration
Cardiogenic	Inadequate cardiac output due to impaired myocardial function
Distributive (e.g., anaphylactic, neurogenic, septic)	Severe peripheral vasodilation
Hypovolemic (hemorrhagic vs. nonhemorrhagic)	Reduced intravascular volume
Obstructive (e.g., pulmonary embolism, tension pneumothorax, pericardial tamponade)	Obstruction of blood flow from the heart

Adapted from Turner KC, Brashers, VL. Shock, multiple organ dysfunction syndrome and burns in adults. In: McCance KL, Huether SE, eds. *McCance & Huether's Pathophysiology: The Biologic Basis for Disease in Adults and Children*. 9th ed. St. Louis, MO: Elsevier; 2024;48:1557–1590.

Pathophysiology

Diverse events can initiate the shock syndrome. Shock begins when the cardiovascular system fails to function properly because of an alteration in at least one of the four essential circulatory components: blood volume, myocardial contractility, blood flow, or vascular resistance. In healthy circumstances, these components function together to maintain circulatory homeostasis. When one of the components fails, the others compensate. However, as compensatory mechanisms fail, or if more than one of the circulatory components are affected, a state of shock ensues. Shock states are classified according to which component is adversely affected (Table 12.1).

Shock is not a single clinical entity but a life-threatening response to alterations in circulation resulting in impaired tissue perfusion.[1] As the delivery of adequate oxygen and nutrients decreases, impaired cellular metabolism occurs. Cells convert from aerobic to anaerobic metabolism. Less energy in the form of ATP is produced. Lactic acid, a byproduct of anaerobic metabolism, causes tissue acidosis, which further impairs cellular metabolism. Shock is not selective in its effects; all cells, tissues, and organ systems suffer as a result of the physiological response to shock. The end result is multi-organ dysfunction due to decreased blood flow through the capillaries that supply the cells with oxygen and nutrients (Fig. 12.2).[1]

Stages of Shock

The response to shock is highly individualized, and a pattern of stages progresses at unpredictable rates. If each stage of shock is not recognized and treated promptly, progression to the next stage occurs. The pathophysiological events and associated clinical findings for each stage are summarized in Table 12.2.

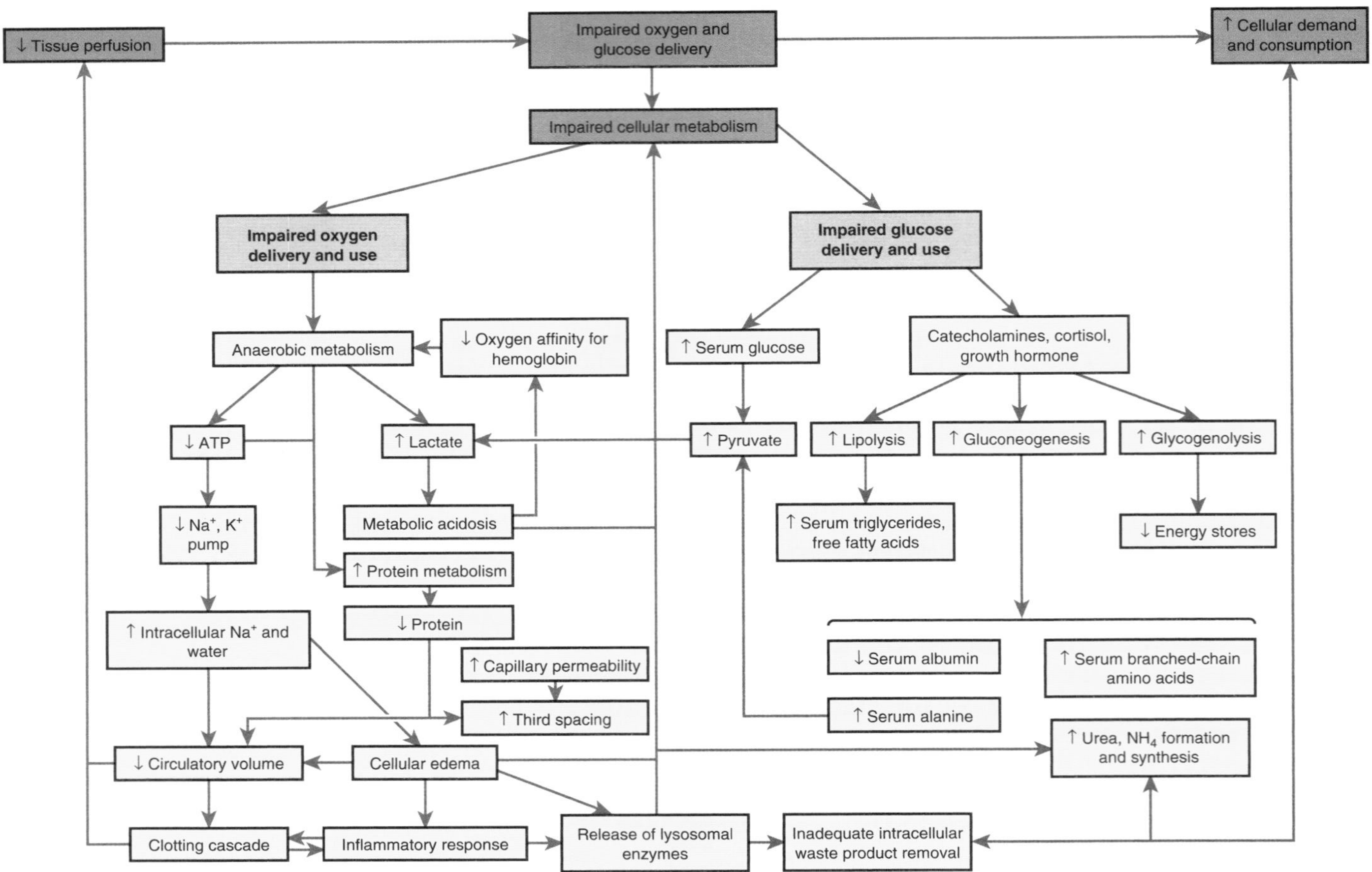

Fig. 12.2 Impairment of cellular metabolism by shock. *ATP,* Adenosine triphosphate; *K^+,* potassium; *Na^+,* sodium; *NH_4,* ammonia. (From Rogers JL. *McCance & Huether's Pathophysiology: The Biologic Basis for Disease in Adults and Children.* 9th ed. St. Louis, MO: Elsevier; 2024.)

Stage I: Initiation. The process of shock is initiated by subclinical hypoperfusion that is caused by inadequate DO_2, inadequate extraction of oxygen, or both.[1] No obvious clinical indications of hypoperfusion are seen in this stage, although hemodynamic alterations, such as an occult decrease in cardiac output, can occur.

Stage II: Compensatory Stage. The sustained reduction in tissue perfusion initiates a set of neural, endocrine, and chemical compensatory mechanisms in an attempt to maintain blood flow to vital organs and to restore homeostasis. During this stage, symptoms become apparent, but shock is potentially reversible with minimal morbidity if appropriate interventions are initiated.

Neural compensation. Baroreceptors (which are sensitive to pressure changes) and chemoreceptors (which are sensitive to chemical changes) located in the carotid sinus and aortic arch detect the reduction in arterial blood pressure. Impulses are relayed to the vasomotor center in the medulla oblongata, stimulating the sympathetic branch of the autonomic nervous system to release the catecholamines epinephrine and norepinephrine from the adrenal medulla.

In response to the catecholamine release, heart rate and myocardial contractility increase to improve cardiac output.[2] Dilation of the coronary arteries increases perfusion to the myocardium to meet the increased demands for oxygen. Systemic vasoconstriction occurs, leading to a redistribution of blood flow. Arterial vasoconstriction improves blood pressure, whereas venous vasoconstriction augments venous return to the heart, increasing preload and therefore cardiac output. Blood is shunted from the kidneys, gastrointestinal tract, and skin to the heart and brain. Bronchial smooth muscles relax, and respiratory rate and depth are increased, improving gas exchange and oxygenation. Blood glucose levels increase as the liver is stimulated to convert glycogen to glucose for energy production.[3] Additional catecholamine effects include pupil dilation as well as cool, moist skin due to increased sweat gland activity.[4]

Endocrine compensation. Overall, endocrine compensation attempts to combat shock by providing glucose for energy and increasing intravascular blood volume to increase blood

TABLE 12.2 Stages of Shock

Stage of Shock	Physiological Events	Clinical Presentation
I. Initiation	**Decreased tissue oxygenation caused by:** ↓ Intravascular volume (hypovolemic shock) ↓ Myocardial contractility (cardiogenic shock) Obstruction of blood flow (obstructive shock) Peripheral vasodilation (distributive shock) Mediator release (septic shock) Histamine release (anaphylactic shock) Suppression of SNS (neurogenic shock)	No observable clinical indications ↓ CO may be assessed with hemodynamic monitoring
II. Compensatory	**Neural compensation by SNS** ↑ Heart rate and contractility Vasoconstriction Redistribution of blood flow to essential organs Bronchodilation **Endocrine compensation** (RAAS, ADH, glucocorticoid release) Renal reabsorption of sodium, chloride, and water Vasoconstriction Glycogenolysis and gluconeogenesis **Chemical compensation** **Hyperventilation** **Cerebral vasoconstriction**	↑ Heart rate (except in neurogenic shock) Narrowed pulse pressure Thirst Cool, moist skin Oliguria Diminished bowel sounds Restlessness progressing to confusion Hyperglycemia ↑ Urine specific gravity and ↓ creatinine clearance Rapid, deep respirations causing respiratory alkalosis
III. Progressive	Progressive tissue hypoperfusion Anaerobic metabolism with lactic acidosis Failure of sodium-potassium pump Cellular edema	Dysrhythmias ↓ Systolic pressure with narrowed pulse pressure Tachypnea Cold, clammy skin Decreased capillary refill Mottling Anuria Absent bowel sounds Lethargy progressing to coma Hyperglycemia resistant to insulin ↑ BUN, creatinine, and potassium Respiratory and metabolic acidosis
IV. Refractory	Severe tissue hypoxia with ischemia and necrosis Worsening acidosis SIRS MODS	Life-threatening dysrhythmias Severe hypotension despite vasopressors Respiratory and metabolic acidosis ARDS DIC Hepatic dysfunction or failure Acute kidney injury Myocardial ischemia, infarction, or failure Cerebral ischemia or infarction

ADH, Antidiuretic hormone; *ARDS*, acute respiratory distress syndrome; *BUN*, blood urea nitrogen; *CO*, cardiac output; *DIC*, disseminated intravascular coagulation; *MODS*, multiple organ dysfunction syndrome; *RAAS*, renin-angiotensin-aldosterone system; *SNS*, sympathetic nervous system.

pressure. In response to the reduction in blood pressure, messages are relayed to the hypothalamus, which stimulates the anterior and posterior pituitary glands. The anterior pituitary gland releases adrenocorticotropic hormone (ACTH). ACTH acts on the adrenal cortex to release glucocorticoids and mineralocorticoids. Glucocorticoids increase blood glucose by stimulating the conversion of glycogen (glycogenolysis), as well as fat and protein (gluconeogenesis) to glucose. Mineralocorticoids act on the renal tubules causing reabsorption of sodium and water, resulting in an increased intravascular volume.[5]

The posterior pituitary gland releases antidiuretic hormone (ADH). ADH is released in response to an increase in plasma osmolality or a decrease in intravascular volume. In response to ADH, water reabsorption increases from the renal distal tubules and collecting ducts, resulting in urine concentration.[5]

In response to decreased renal perfusion, the renin-angiotensin-aldosterone system (Fig. 12.3) is stimulated by

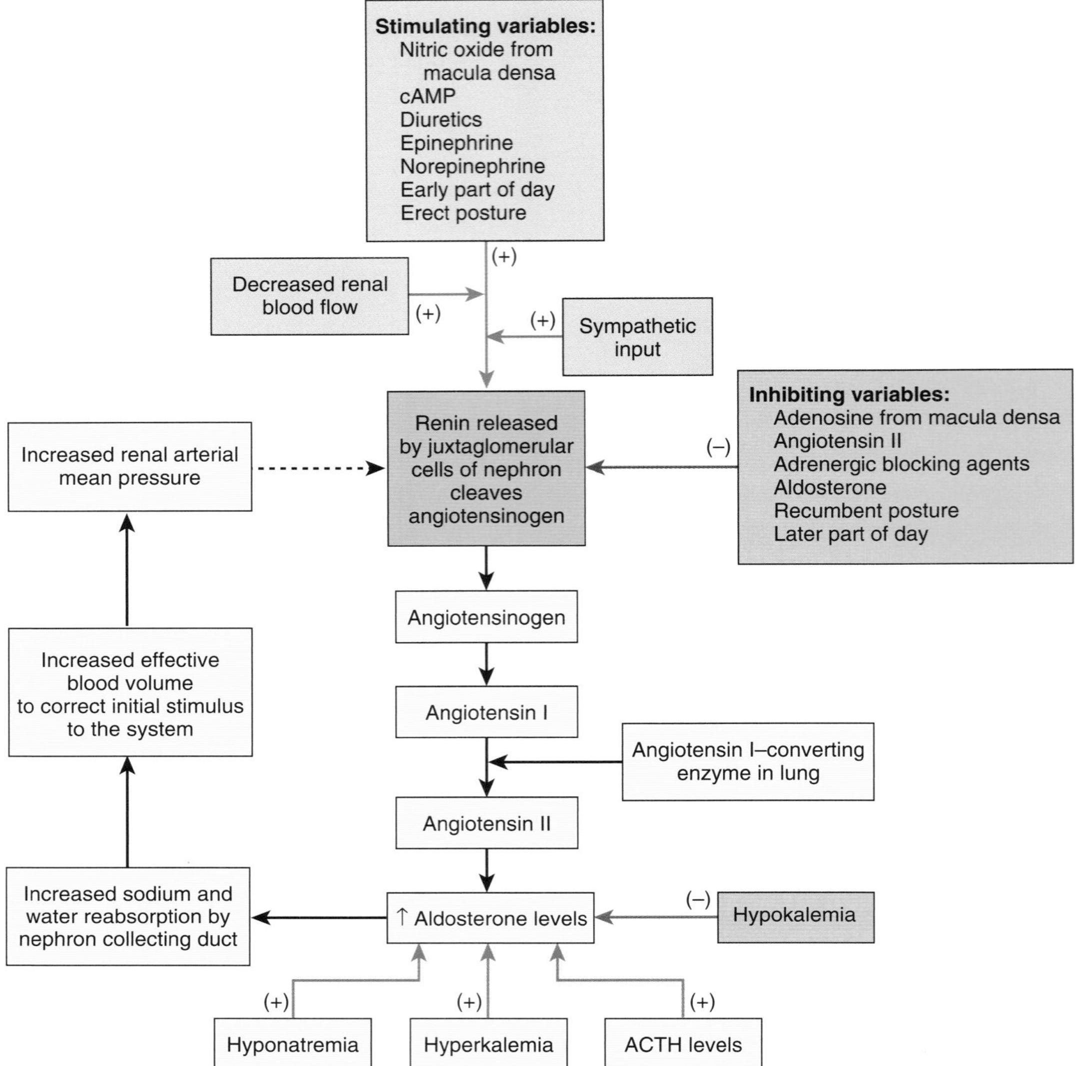

Fig. 12.3 Feedback mechanisms regulating aldosterone secretion. *ACTH,* Adrenocorticotropic hormone; *cAMP,* cyclic adenosine monophosphate. (From Rogers JL. *McCance & Huether's Pathophysiology: The Biologic Basis for Disease in Adults and Children.* 9th ed. St. Louis, MO: Elsevier; 2024.)

the reduction of pressure in the renal arterioles and decrease in sodium levels as sensed by the juxtaglomerular apparatus of the kidney.[6] The juxtaglomerular apparatus releases renin, which circulates in the blood and reacts with angiotensinogen to produce angiotensin I. Angiotensin I circulates through the lungs, where it forms angiotensin II, a potent arterial and venous vasoconstrictor that increases blood pressure and improves venous return to the heart. Angiotensin II also activates the adrenal cortex to release aldosterone (a mineralocorticoid).[6]

Chemical compensation. Chemical compensation attempts to combat shock by increasing oxygen supply; however, cerebral perfusion may decrease as a consequence. As pulmonary blood flow is reduced, ventilation-perfusion imbalances occur.[1] Initially, alveolar ventilation is adequate, but the alveolar capillary bed perfusion is decreased. Aorta and carotid artery chemoreceptors are stimulated in response to low oxygen tension in the blood. Consequently, the rate and depth of respirations increase, resulting in hyperventilation.[7] Hyperventilation causes carbon dioxide excretion, resulting in respiratory alkalosis. The alkalotic state causes vasoconstriction of cerebral blood vessels. Coupled with the reduced oxygen tension, vasoconstriction may lead to cerebral hypoxia and ischemia.

Stage III: Progressive Stage. If the cause of hypoperfusion is not corrected or the compensatory mechanisms continue without reversing the shock, profound hypoperfusion and further deterioration result. Vasoconstriction continues in the systemic circulation. Although this effect shunts blood to vital organs, the decreased blood flow leads to ischemia in the extremities, weak or absent pulses, and altered body defenses. Prolonged vasoconstriction results in decreased capillary blood flow and cellular hypoxia. The cells convert to anaerobic metabolism, producing lactic acid, which leads to metabolic acidosis.[1] Anaerobic metabolism produces less ATP than aerobic metabolism, which reduces the energy available for cellular metabolism. The lack of ATP causes failure of the sodium-potassium pump. Sodium and water accumulate within the cell, resulting in cellular swelling and a further reduction in cellular function.

The microcirculation exerts the opposite effect and dilates to increase the blood supply to meet local tissue needs.[1] Whereas the arterioles remain constricted in an attempt to keep vital organs perfused, the precapillary sphincters relax, allowing blood to flow into the capillary bed. Meanwhile, postcapillary sphincters remain constricted. As a result, blood flows freely into the capillary bed but accumulates in the capillaries as blood flow exiting the capillary bed is impeded. Capillary hydrostatic pressure increases, and fluid is pushed from the capillaries into the interstitial space, causing interstitial edema (i.e., "third-spacing").

This intravascular-to-interstitial fluid shift is further aggravated by the release of histamine and other inflammatory mediators.[1] These mediators increase capillary permeability, causing loss of proteins through enlarged capillary pores, which decreases capillary oncotic pressure. As intravascular blood volume further decreases, the blood becomes more viscous, and blood flow slows. As a result, capillary sludging occurs as red blood cells, platelets, and proteins clump together. The loss of intravascular volume and capillary pooling further reduce venous return to the heart and cardiac output.

Coronary artery perfusion pressure is decreased. The ischemic pancreas releases myocardial depressant factor (MDF), decreasing myocardial contractility. Cardiac output, blood pressure, and tissue perfusion continue to decrease, contributing to worsening cellular hypoxia. At this point, the patient shows classic signs and symptoms of shock. This phase of shock responds poorly to fluid replacement alone, and reversal requires aggressive interventions.

Stage IV: Refractory Stage. Prolonged inadequate tissue perfusion that is unresponsive to therapy ultimately contributes to MODS and death. A large volume of the blood remains pooled in the capillary bed, and the arterial blood pressure is too low to support perfusion of the vital organs.[1]

Dysrhythmias occur because of the failure of the sodium-potassium pump, which results from decreased ATP, hypoxemia, ischemia, and acidosis. Cardiac failure may occur because of ischemia, acidosis, and the effects of MDF.[1]

Endothelial damage in the capillary bed and precapillary arterioles, along with damage to the type II pneumocytes, which make surfactant, leads to acute respiratory distress syndrome (ARDS). Hypoxemia causes vasoconstriction of the pulmonary circulation and pulmonary hypertension. Ventilation-perfusion mismatch occurs because of disturbances in ventilation and perfusion. Pulmonary edema may result from disruption of the alveolar-capillary membrane, ARDS, heart failure, and/or overly aggressive fluid resuscitation.

When cerebral perfusion pressure is significantly impaired, loss of autoregulation occurs, resulting in brain ischemia.[8] Cerebral infarction may occur. Sympathetic nervous system dysfunction results in massive vasodilation, depression of cardiac and respiratory centers (resulting in bradycardia and bradypnea), and loss of normal thermoregulation.

Renal vasoconstriction and hypoperfusion of the kidney decrease the glomerular filtration rate. Prolonged ischemia causes acute kidney injury with acute tubular necrosis. Metabolic acids accumulate in the blood, worsening the metabolic acidosis caused by lactic acid production during anaerobic metabolism.[6]

Hypoperfusion damages the reticuloendothelial cells, which recirculate bacteria and cellular debris, thereby predisposing the patient to bacteremia and sepsis. Damaged hepatocytes impair the liver's ability to detoxify drugs, toxins, and hormones; conjugate bilirubin; or synthesize clotting factors. Hepatic dysfunction decreases its ability to mobilize carbohydrate, protein, and fat stores, resulting in hypoglycemia.[3]

Hyperglycemia may occur because of endogenous and/or exogenous corticosteroids as well as insulin resistance. Hyperglycemia results in dehydration and electrolyte imbalances related to osmotic diuresis. Leukocyte function is impaired, leading to an increased risk of infection and depression of the immune response. A decrease in gastric motility contributes to negative nitrogen balance and decreased wound healing.[1]

Ischemia and increased gastric acid production caused by glucocorticoids increase the risk of stress ulcer development. Prolonged vasoconstriction and ischemia lead to the inability of the intestinal walls to act as intact barriers to prevent the migration of bacteria out of the gastrointestinal tract. This may result in the translocation of bacteria from the gastrointestinal tract into the lymphatic and vascular beds, increasing the risk of infection.[1]

Hypoxia and the release of inflammatory cytokines impair blood flow and result in microvascular thrombosis. Sluggish blood flow, massive tissue trauma, and consumption of clotting factors may cause disseminated intravascular coagulation (DIC). The bone marrow releases white blood cells, causing leukocytosis early in shock, then leukopenia as depletion of white blood cells occurs. Tissue injury caused by widespread ischemia stimulates the development of systemic inflammatory response syndrome (SIRS) with a massive release of mediators of the inflammatory process.[1]

The skin is negatively impacted by impaired blood flow and tissue perfusion. Hypotension activates the sympathetic nervous system, resulting in vasoconstriction and further decreasing blood flow. As blood is shunted from the peripheral circulation, the capillaries close at lower pressures, which may lead to skin failure.[9,10]

Poor renal function, respiratory failure, and impaired cellular function aggravate the existing state of acidosis, which contributes to further fluid shifts, loss of vasomotor tone, and intravascular hypovolemia.[1] Alterations in the cardiovascular system and continued acidosis reduce the heart rate, impair myocardial contractility, and further decrease cardiac output and tissue perfusion. Cerebral ischemia occurs because of the reduction in cerebral blood flow. Consequently, the sympathetic nervous system is stimulated, an effect that aggravates the existing vasoconstriction, increasing afterload and decreasing cardiac output. Prolonged cerebral ischemia eventually causes the loss of sympathetic nervous system response, and vasodilation and bradycardia result. The patient's decreasing blood pressure and heart rate cause a lethal decrease in tissue perfusion, MODS that is unresponsive to therapy, brain death, and cardiopulmonary arrest.

CHECK YOUR UNDERSTANDING

1. The patient arrives at the critical care unit with a diagnosis of pneumonia. He has an increased heart rate, oliguria, and cool, moist skin. A glucose level is obtained, and the patient has hyperglycemia. An accurate history is challenging to obtain, as the patient is restless with intermittent confusion. The patient's clinical presentation indicates which of the following stages of shock?
   A. Initiation
   B. Compensatory
   C. Progressive
   D. Refractory

Systemic Inflammatory Response Syndrome

SIRS is a widespread inflammatory response that can occur in patients with diverse disorders such as ARDS, infection, trauma, shock, pancreatitis, or ischemia.[1,11] It may result from or lead to MODS.

The inflammatory cascade maintains homeostasis through a balance between proinflammatory and antiinflammatory processes. Although inflammation is normally a localized process, SIRS is a systemic response associated with the release of mediators. The mediators increase the permeability of the endothelial wall, shifting fluid from the intravascular space into extravascular spaces, including the interstitial space. Intravascular volume is reduced, resulting in relative hypovolemia. Other mediators cause microvascular clotting, impaired fibrinolysis, and widespread vasodilation.

ASSESSMENT

An understanding of the pathophysiology of shock and identification of patients at risk are essential for the prevention of and timely response to shock. Assessment focuses on three areas: history, clinical presentation, and laboratory studies. Review the patient's history first, and then assess the systems most sensitive to lack of oxygen and nutrients. The patient's history may include an identifiable predisposing factor or cause of the shock state.

Clinical Presentation

Multiple body systems are affected by shock syndrome. The clinical presentation specific to each classification of shock will be discussed herein; however, the patient's age or stage of life may alter the clinical presentation (see Lifespan Considerations box).[12–15]

LIFESPAN CONSIDERATIONS

Older Adults

- Changes in immunological function with age are referred to as immunosenescence. These changes result in impaired immune responses and inflammatory dysregulation, which may affect the aging body's ability to respond to infection.
- As the body ages, the left ventricular wall thickens, ventricular compliance decreases, and calcification and fibrosis of the heart valves occur. Coronary artery blood flow is decreased. The sensitivity of the baroreceptors is decreased, and the heart rate is less responsive to sympathetic nervous system stimulation in the early stage of shock. The aging heart relies on increased preload and stroke volume to increase cardiac output, which increases sensitivity to hypovolemia. Paradoxically, due to changes in cardiac compliance, even a small amount of fluid can precipitate pulmonary edema. Arterial walls lose elasticity, increasing systemic vascular resistance (SVR), which increases the myocardial oxygen demand and decreases the responsiveness of the arterial system to the effects of catecholamines.
- Aging decreases lung elasticity, alveolar perfusion, and alveolar surface area and causes thickening of the alveolar-capillary membrane. These changes limit the body's ability to increase oxygen levels and improve tissue perfusion during shock states. The diaphragm flattens and becomes less efficient, leading to difficulties in ventilator weaning.
- The ability of the kidneys to concentrate urine decreases with age, which limits the body's ability to conserve water when required. Aging is an independent risk factor for acute kidney injury (AKI).
- Skin turgor decreases, making fluid status assessment more difficult. Dehydration is common and may increase the risk for hypovolemia.

Pregnant People

- It is important to note that care of these patients should include obstetricians, neonatologists, critical care specialists, and other members of the multidisciplinary team.
- Factors affecting maternal oxygenation also affect fetal oxygenation. A higher maternal PaO_2 (>75 mm Hg) is needed to protect the fetus.
- Physiological cardiovascular changes during pregnancy include increased heart rate, blood volume, and cardiac output, along with a decreased systemic vascular resistance. Awareness of these normal physiological changes are important when assessing pregnant people in a shock state.
- Consider left lateral positioning to prevent compression of the vena cava. The enlarged uterus may reduce both venous return and cardiac output while in the supine position.
- Assess fetal heart tones; consult obstetrics nurses for assistance.
- Assess pregnant people for signs and symptoms of uterine hemorrhage.

Breastfeeding People

- Establish a plan for continued breastfeeding, expressing milk, or suppressing milk supply, if indicated.
- The multiprofessional team must be aware of the breastfeeding plan so that medications and nutrition are prescribed accordingly.

! CLINICAL ALERT

Shock

Assessment findings in the initial stages of shock include increased heart rate and respiratory rate; decreased urine output; cool, moist skin; decreased capillary refill; and restlessness or confusion. These signs and symptoms are related to the body's attempt to compensate and restore homeostasis. Later signs of shock include hypotension, dysrhythmia(s), respiratory distress, decreased responsiveness, anuria, and skin mottling. These symptoms are the result of decreased organ and tissue perfusion.

Central Nervous System. The central nervous system is the most sensitive to changes in the supply of oxygen and nutrients, and it is the first system affected by changes in cellular perfusion. Initial responses to shock include restlessness, agitation, and anxiety. As the shock state progresses, the patient becomes confused and lethargic, then unresponsive if left untreated.

Cardiovascular System. A major focus of assessment is blood pressure; therefore, it is important to know the patient's baseline blood pressure. During the compensatory stage, innervation of the sympathetic nervous system increases myocardial contractility and vasoconstriction, which results in a normal or slightly elevated systolic pressure, an increased diastolic pressure, and a narrowed pulse pressure. As the shock state progresses, systolic blood pressure decreases, but diastolic pressure remains normal or increased, resulting in a narrowed pulse pressure. The narrowed pulse pressure may precede changes in heart rate or be accompanied by tachycardia.

Although definitions vary, hypotension is generally considered when systolic blood pressure is less than 90 mm Hg or mean arterial pressure is less than 65 mm Hg.[1,16] If the patient has a history of hypertension, a decrease in systolic pressure of 40 mm Hg from the baseline is considered hypotension. Noninvasive, automated blood pressure monitoring in shock is often inaccurate because of peripheral vasoconstriction. Arterial pressure monitoring may be indicated to obtain accurate readings to guide therapy (see Chapter 9, Hemodynamic Monitoring).

Evaluate the rate, quality, and character of major pulses (i.e., carotid, radial, femoral, posterior tibial, and dorsalis pedis). In shock states, the pulse is often weak and thready. The pulse rate is increased, usually greater than 100 beats/min, through stimulation of the sympathetic nervous system as a compensatory response to the decreased cardiac output and increased cellular oxygen demand.

Normal compensatory responses to shock are often altered if the patient is taking certain medications. Negative inotropic agents, such as beta-blocking agents (e.g., propranolol, metoprolol), are widely used in the treatment of angina, hypertension, and dysrhythmias. By blocking the beta effects of the sympathetic nervous system, the body is unable to increase heart rate and cardiac output to compensate for shock.

Assessment of the jugular veins provides information on the volume and pressure in the right side of the heart (see Chapter 9, Hemodynamic Monitoring). It is an indirect method of evaluating the central venous pressure (CVP). Jugular venous distension is noted in patients with obstructive or cardiogenic shock. Neck veins are flat in those with hypovolemic shock.

Capillary refill assesses the ability of the cardiovascular system to maintain perfusion to the periphery. The normal response to pressure on the nail beds is blanching, with color returning to a normal pink hue within 1 to 2 seconds after pressure is released. A delay in the return of color indicates peripheral vasoconstriction. Capillary refill provides a quick assessment of overall cardiovascular and intravascular fluid status, but this assessment is not reliable in a patient who is hypothermic or has peripheral circulatory problems.

Assessment of fluid responsiveness is an important consideration for the management of shock. Only about 50% of patients respond to fluid administration as evidenced by an increase of 10% to 15% or more in their stroke volume or cardiac output.[17,18] It is important to note that measures of positive fluid responsiveness do not always lead to fluid administration but are used as part of the clinical assessment and weighed against the risk of fluid overload.[19] CVP monitoring was traditionally used to assess fluid responsiveness; however, it has been found to be a poor discriminator for predicting fluid responsiveness.[16,20]

Dynamic indicators of fluid responsiveness include either a fluid challenge or a *passive leg raise* (PLR). A fluid challenge is 250–500 mL of a crystalloid solution rapidly infused over 15 to 30 minutes.[18,21] During a *passive leg raise*, the blood volume from the lower body is mobilized to the heart and temporarily mimics an approximate 300 mL fluid challenge. The resultant increase in preload causes an increase in cardiac output, resulting in increased blood pressure. Perform the PLR by placing the patient in a semirecumbent position with the head of the bed at 45 degrees. Record baseline measurements, and then lower the head of the bed and elevate the legs at 45 degrees. Measure blood pressure and indices of stroke volume and/or cardiac output within 30 to 90 seconds after fluid challenge completion or PLR.[19] The patient's response depends on the type of shock. Patients experiencing cardiogenic shock with ventricular dysfunction may demonstrate signs of fluid overload after administration of very small volumes of fluid or PLR, whereas patients with distributive shock will continue to demonstrate vasodilation-associated hypotension.

A pulmonary artery (PA) catheter may be a useful tool for diagnosing and treating the patient in shock. The risks associated with catheter insertion and central line–associated bloodstream infection must be weighed against the clinical information obtained from this invasive diagnostic device.[22] The PA catheter provides information on cardiac dynamics, fluid balance, and effects of vasoactive medications. Preload is used to assess fluid balance and is measured by right atrial pressure (RAP) for the right ventricle and the pulmonary artery occlusion pressure (PAOP) as a surrogate for the left ventricle. Cardiac output and index, afterload, and stroke work indices can also be assessed with a PA catheter (see Chapter 9, Hemodynamic Monitoring). Table 12.3 describes hemodynamic values and alterations in each classification of shock.

The use of PA catheters in the management of shock has decreased as newer, less invasive technology has been introduced. Devices that use pulse contour methods for hemodynamic assessment (see Chapter 9, Hemodynamic Monitoring) provide stroke volume variation (SVV), pulse pressure variation (PPV), continuous cardiac output, and other hemodynamic parameters that better predict fluid responsiveness. Outcomes associated with using these newer devices continue to be evaluated (see Evidence-Based Practice box).

EVIDENCE-BASED PRACTICE

Use of the Passive Leg Raise to Guide Resuscitation in Septic Shock

Problem

The science of measuring fluid responsiveness has evolved, and the use of dynamic measures to identify patients who may benefit from additional fluid resuscitation is now recommended. The use of a passive leg raise (PLR), along with dynamic measures to predict fluid responsiveness, is advocated by both the European Society of Intensive Care Medicine and the Surviving Sepsis Campaign. The use of dynamic indices, such as stroke volume variation, changes in stroke volume or cardiac output, and pulse pressure variation, are better methods of evaluating fluid responsiveness and directing therapy. However, the clinical impact on mortality in septic patients had not been determined previously.

Clinical Question

Does a PLR-guided fluid resuscitation strategy improve mortality in patients with septic shock when compared to the standard of care?

Evidence

A meta-analysis of five randomized controlled trials was conducted analyzing the outcomes of 462 patients who underwent acute volume resuscitation with either standard or PLR-guided care. Standard care included fluid administration without any hemodynamic monitoring in four studies and the use of central venous pressure (CVP) measurement in one study. The PLR-guided group used different modalities to measure fluid responsiveness, including two studies using bioreactance with SV measurement and each utilizing either Doppler ultrasound technology, echocardiography, or pulse contour analysis. The patients all had septic shock and were treated either in the emergency department or the critical care unit. There was no significant difference between the mortality in PLR-guided group and that in the standard care group. While the patient populations were similar, there was a lack of statistically significant heterogeneity, which made it difficult to report secondary outcomes.

Conclusions

The use of PLR-guided fluid resuscitation with measures of change in stroke volume and cardiac output continues to need further research to determine the best measurement modalities for septic shock and effect on outcomes. Previous research had included studies with a variety of shock states requiring fluid resuscitation.

Implications for Nursing

The use of dynamic measures with PLR-guided fluid resuscitation in septic shock is a relatively newer recommendation, and the research is quickly evolving. Understanding the new technology regarding dynamic measures and developing knowledge and skill in interpretation of findings may better guide resuscitation and possibly reduce adverse events (i.e., prolonged ventilation, extended critical care unit length of stay). While the research adds to the body of evidence, it is not recommended to change current practice due to the study limitations.

Level of Evidence

A— Systematic review and meta-analysis

Reference

Azadian M, Win S, Abdipour A, Kim CK, Nguyen HB. Mortality benefit from the passive leg raise maneuver in guiding resuscitation of sepsis shock patients: a systematic review and meta-analysis of randomized trials. *J Intensive Care Med.* 2022;37(5):611–617.

TABLE 12.3 Hemodynamic Alterations in Shock States

Hemodynamic Parameter (Normal Value)	Hypovolemic Shock	Cardiogenic Shock	Obstructive Shock	DISTRIBUTIVE SHOCK Septic Shock	Anaphylactic Shock	Neurogenic Shock
Heart rate (60–100 beats/min)	High	High	High	High	High	Normal to low
Blood pressure (SBP >90 mm Hg, MAP >65 mm Hg)	Normal to low	Normal to low	Normal to low	Normal to low	Normal to low	Normal to low
Cardiac output (4–8 L/min) & Cardiac index (2.5–4.2 L/min/m^2)	Low	Low	Low	High then low	Normal to low	Normal to low
RAP (2–6 mm Hg)	Low	High	High	Low to variable	Low	Low
PAOP (8–12 mm Hg) or PADP (8–15 mm Hg)	Low	High	High if impaired diastolic filling or high LV afterload Low if high RV afterload	Low to variable	Low	Low
SVR (770–1500 dynes/sec/cm^{-5})	High	High	High	Low to variable	Low	Low
SvO_2 (60%–70%) & $ScvO_2$ (65%–85%)	Low	Low	Low	High then low	Low	Low

LV, Left ventricular; *PADP*, pulmonary artery diastolic pressure; *PAOP*, pulmonary artery occlusion pressure; *RAP*, right atrial pressure; *RV*, right ventricular; *$ScvO_2$*, central venous oxygen saturation; *SvO_2*, mixed venous oxygen saturation; *SVR*, systemic vascular resistance.

Critical care management involves optimizing cardiac output and minimizing myocardial oxygen consumption. The SvO_2 obtained from a PA catheter reflects the amount of oxygen bound to hemoglobin brought back to the heart and the balance between DO_2 and VO_2 (see Chapter 9, Hemodynamic Monitoring). If a PA catheter is not used, a central venous oxygen saturation ($ScvO_2$) may be obtained as a surrogate for SvO_2 and is obtained from a central venous catheter (CVC) in the vena cava.

If the SvO_2 is less than 60%, the DO_2 is inadequate or the VO_2 is excessive. The SvO_2 is decreased in all forms of shock except in early septic shock, in which poor oxygen extraction causes the SvO_2 value to be high. SvO_2 is useful in evaluating the effectiveness of treatment.

Respiratory System. In the early stage of shock, respirations are rapid and deep. The respiratory center responds to shock and metabolic acidosis with an increase in respiratory rate to eliminate carbon dioxide. Direct stimulation of the medulla by chemoreceptors alters the respiratory pattern. As the shock state progresses, metabolic wastes accumulate and cause generalized muscle weakness, resulting in shallow breathing with poor gas exchange. Increased capillary permeability leads to interstitial edema and changes in breath sounds (e.g., crackles).[1]

Interpret pulse oximetry values (SpO_2) cautiously because decreased peripheral circulation may result in inaccurate readings. Arterial blood gas (ABG) analysis provides a more accurate assessment of oxygenation and ventilation.

Renal System. Renal hypoperfusion and decreased glomerular filtration rate cause oliguria (urine output <0.5 mL/kg/h). The renin-angiotensin-aldosterone system is activated, which promotes the retention of sodium and reabsorption of water in the kidneys, further decreasing urinary output. This prerenal cause of acute kidney injury is manifested by concentrated urine and an increased blood urea nitrogen level, but the serum creatinine level remains normal. If the decreased perfusion is prolonged, a form of intrarenal failure known as acute tubular necrosis occurs, and creatinine levels increase.

Gastrointestinal System. Hypoperfusion of the gastrointestinal system slows intestinal activity, which results in decreased bowel sounds, increased gastric residual volume, distension, nausea, and constipation.[23] Paralytic ileus and ulceration with bleeding may occur with prolonged hypoperfusion. Hyperpermeability leads to the translocation of organisms into systemic circulation.

Hypoperfusion of the liver leads to decreased function and alterations in liver enzyme levels, such as lactate dehydrogenase (LDH) and aspartate aminotransferase (AST). If decreased perfusion persists, the liver is not able to produce coagulation factors, detoxify drugs, or neutralize invading microorganisms. Clotting disorders, drug toxicity concerns, and increased susceptibility to infection occur. Signs and symptoms of decreased liver function include increased ammonia and bilirubin levels, irritability, ascites, and jaundice. The patient's urine may appear dark, and stools may become light or clay colored.

Hematological System. The interaction between inflammation and coagulation enhances clotting and inhibits fibrinolysis, leading to clotting in the microcirculatory system. Clotting in the microcirculation causes peripheral ischemia manifested by symmetrical cyanosis of the hands, feet, or face and necrosis of digits and extremities. Increased consumption of platelets and clotting factors occurs, causing a consumptive coagulopathy. The inability of the liver to manufacture clotting factors exacerbates the coagulopathy. As the coagulopathy worsens, a decreased platelet count and clotting factors and prolonged clotting times are observed. Petechiae and ecchymosis may occur, along with blood in the urine, stool, gastric aspirate, and tracheal secretions. Leukocytosis frequently occurs, especially in early septic shock. Leukopenia occurs later with the consumption of white blood cells.

Integumentary System. Evaluate skin color, temperature, texture, turgor, and moisture level. Cyanosis may occur, but it is a late and unreliable sign. The patient may exhibit central cyanosis observed in the mucous membranes of the mouth and nose or peripheral cyanosis that is evident in the nails and earlobes. Note that assessment of skin turgor is often an unreliable indicator of hydration in older adults, as they have decreased skin elasticity.

Skin mottling is a common sign of hypoperfusion. Mottling is an irregular, patchy skin discoloration that usually appears around the knees. As hypoperfusion progresses, the mottling extends the length of the leg from the knee toward the groin and toes. It may also be observed in other areas of peripheral circulation such as the fingers and ears.[24] The skin mottling score is a noninvasive bedside tool used to evaluate the severity of mottling and overall tissue perfusion. Scores range from 0 (no mottling) to 5 (extreme mottling of the leg extending into the groin region), with higher scores associated with increased mortality.[25]

Laboratory Studies

Laboratory studies assist in the differential diagnosis of the patient in shock (see Laboratory Alert box). However, by the time many of the laboratory values are abnormal, the patient is in the later stages of shock. The clinical picture is often more useful for early diagnosis and immediate treatment.

An elevated serum lactate level is always considered an abnormal finding and a measure of tissue hypoxia and dysfunction, regardless of the cause. The lactate level is an indicator of inadequate DO_2 to the cells and trends can help determine the adequacy of treatment. Elevated lactate levels produce an acidic environment and decrease arterial pH. The serum lactate level correlates with the degree of hypoperfusion, meaning the higher the lactate level, the more significant the hypoperfusion.

MANAGEMENT

Management of the patient in shock consists of identifying and treating the cause of shock as rapidly as possible. Care is directed toward correcting the altered circulatory component (e.g., blood volume, myocardial contractility, obstruction, vascular resistance) and reversing tissue hypoxia. Fluid, pharmacological, and mechanical therapies are implemented to maintain tissue perfusion and improve DO_2. Interventions include increasing the cardiac output, hemoglobin level, and arterial oxygen saturation while minimizing oxygen consumption. Specific management for each classification of shock is discussed later in this chapter.

In addition to treatment specific to the shock state, it is important to implement basic nursing interventions to prevent complications associated with decreased perfusion, hemodynamic alterations, and immobility. For example, these conditions increase the patient's risk for developing a pressure injury, and therapeutic interventions are warranted.[26,27] Refer to the Plan of Care for the Patient in Shock and the Collaborative Care Plan for the Critically Ill Patient found in Chapter 1, Overview of Critical Care Nursing.

Resuscitation

The goal of resuscitation is to maintain circulating blood volume and an adequate hemoglobin level. Regardless of the cause, shock produces profound alterations in fluid balance. Patients with absolute hypovolemia (hypovolemic shock) or relative hypovolemia (distributive shock) require the administration of blood and/or IV fluids to restore intravascular volume, maintain oxygen-carrying capacity, and establish the hemodynamic stability necessary for optimal tissue perfusion. The choice of blood or fluid, volume, and rate of infusion depends on the type of fluid lost, the patient's hemodynamic status, and coexisting conditions.

! LABORATORY ALERT

Shock

Laboratory Test	Normal Range	Critical Value[a]	Significance
Chemistry Studies			
Glucose	74–106 mg/dL	<54 or >400 mg/dL	**Hyperglycemia:** impairs immune response; may cause osmotic diuresis **Hypoglycemia:** altered level of consciousness
Blood urea nitrogen	10–20 mg/dL	>100 mg/dL	**Elevated:** hypoperfusion (prerenal); gastrointestinal bleeding and catabolism
Creatinine	Female: 0.5–1.1 mg/dL Male: 0.6–1.2 mg/dL	>4 mg/dL If patient has chronic kidney disease: ≥ 0.3 mg/dL from baseline within 48 h, or ≥1.5 times baseline within past 7 days	**Elevated:** acute kidney injury
Sodium	136–145 mEq/L	<120 or >160 mEq/L	**Hypernatremia:** hemoconcentration (fluid loss) **Hyponatremia:** hemodilution (excessive hypotonic fluid)
Chloride	98–106 mEq/L	<80 or >115 mEq/L	**Hyperchloremia:** rapid or large volume resuscitation with 0.9% normal saline
Potassium	3.5–5.0 mEq/L	<2.5 or >6.5 mEq/L	**Hypokalemia:** burns, diuretics, diarrhea, vomiting **Hyperkalemia:** impaired elimination from acute kidney injury
Lactic acid (lactate)	0.6–2.2 mmol/L	>2 mmol/L	**Elevated:** hypoxia leading to anaerobic metabolism
AST	0–35 units/L	N/A	**Elevated:** hepatic impairment
LDH	100–190 units/L	N/A	**Elevated:** may indicate hepatic impairment, renal impairment, intestinal ischemia, or myocardial infarction
Hematology Studies			
WBCs	5000–10,000/mm³	<2500 or >30,000/mm³	**Leukocytosis:** response to stress, infection, or steroid administration **Leukopenia:** late shock due to consumption
Hemoglobin	Male: 14–18 g/dL Female: 12–16 g/dL	<5 g/dL or >20 g/dL	**Decreased:** blood loss, hemodilution
Hematocrit	Male: 42%-52% Female: 37%-47%	<15% or >60%	**Elevated:** dehydration, hemoconcentration **Decreased:** blood loss, hemodilution
Platelets	150,000–400,000/mm³	< 50,000/mm³	**Thrombocytopenia:** acute and chronic infections, hemorrhage, large volume PRBC transfusions without platelet administration, inflammation
aPTT/PTT	aPTT: 30–40 sec PTT: 60–70 sec	aPTT: >70 sec PTT: >100 sec	**Elevated:** Hepatocellular dysfunction, disruption of intrinsic clotting pathway, sepsis
PT/INR	PT: 11–12.5 sec INR: 0.8–1.1 sec	PT: 20 sec INR: >5.5	**Elevated:** Hepatocellular dysfunction, disruption of extrinsic clotting pathway, sepsis
Arterial Blood Gas			
pH	7.35–7.45	<7.25 or >7.55	**Alkalosis:** respiratory alkalosis due to hyperventilation in early shock **Acidosis:** metabolic acidosis due to lactic acidosis and respiratory failure in late shock
$PaCO_2$	35–45 mm Hg	<20 or >60 mm Hg	**Hypocapnia/Hypocarbia:** respiratory alkalosis due to hyperventilation in early shock
PaO_2	80–100 mm Hg	<40 mm Hg	**Hypoxemia:** pulmonary edema, ARDS

Continued

! LABORATORY ALERT—cont'd

HCO_3^-	22–26 mEq/L	<15 or >40 mEq/L	**Decreased:** metabolic acidosis caused by hypoxia, anaerobic metabolism, and lactic acidosis in late shock
Base deficit/excess	0 to +2 mEq/L	−3 or +3 mEq/L	Represents the number of buffering anions in the blood **Base deficit (negative value):** indicates metabolic acidosis (e.g., lactic acidosis) **Base excess (positive value):** indicates metabolic alkalosis or a compensatory response to respiratory acidosis
O_2 saturation	Adult: 95%-100% Elderly: 95%	≤75%	Indicates the percentage of hemoglobin saturated with oxygen **Decreased:** As PaO_2 values decrease below 60 mm Hg, small PaO_2 decreases cause a large decrease in the percentage of hemoglobin saturated with oxygen. At O_2 saturation of 70% or below, the tissues are unable to extract enough oxygen to function

[a]Critical values vary by facility and laboratory.
aPTT, Activated partial thromboplastin time; *ARDS*, acute respiratory distress syndrome; *AST*, aspartate aminotransferase; *HCO_3^-*, bicarbonate; *INR*, international normalized ratio; *LDH*, lactate dehydrogenase; *$PaCO_2$*, partial pressure of arterial carbon dioxide; *PaO_2*, partial pressure of arterial oxygen; *PRBC*, packed red blood cells; *PT*, prothrombin time; *PTT*, partial thromboplastin time; *WBCs*, white blood cells.
Data from Pagana KD, Pagana TJ, Pagana TN. *Mosby's Diagnostic and Laboratory Test Reference.* 16th ed. St. Louis, MO: Elsevier, Inc.; 2023.

CHECK YOUR UNDERSTANDING

2. A patient is admitted with a suspected urinary tract infection. Upon admission, they require intubation due to their altered mental status and hypotension requiring vasopressor support and fluid administration. Which of the following abnormal laboratory results would the nurse expect for this patient based on the assessment findings? What type of shock is this patient experiencing?
   A. Lactic acid 4.5 mmol/L; distributive shock
   B. Hgb 6 g/dL; hypovolemic shock
   C. Base excess 2.5 mEq/L; obstructive shock
   D. Creatinine 2.2 mg/dL; cardiogenic shock

Benefits of IV fluid administration include increased intravascular volume, increased venous return to the right side of the heart, optimal stretching of the ventricles, and increased cardiac output. Most patients in shock require some initial fluid resuscitation; however, the volume administered needs to be continuously assessed and balanced with the risk of overload.[14,28-30] Fluid administration is adjusted based on changes in blood pressure, urine output, hemodynamic values, diagnostic test results, and the clinical picture of the patient's response to treatment. Values obtained from hemodynamic monitoring also assist in evaluating the effects of treatment. Volume replacement usually continues until dynamic measures of fluid responsiveness, static trends (i.e., CVP, RAP, PAOP, lactate levels), and/or assessment findings (i.e., capillary refill) indicate the patient has achieved volume resuscitation.[12] If blood pressure remains inadequate after optimal fluid resuscitation, then vasopressors or inotropes are used to achieve blood pressure and cardiac output goals.

IV Access. Patients in severe shock may require immediate, rapid volume replacement as well as IV medication administration. The patient in shock requires a minimum of two large-gauge IV catheters (i.e., 18- to 20-gauge) as access to provide a route for rapid administration of fluids and medications. Establishing IV routes in a patient in shock is challenging due to peripheral vasoconstriction and venous collapse. Ultrasound may be used to guide peripheral IV insertion but requires additional training.

Intraosseous (IO) access is used during emergent situations if peripheral access is not readily obtainable.[31] An IO needle is most commonly inserted into the proximal tibia but may also be inserted in the distal tibia and proximal humerus.[31] IO access is equivalent to central venous access. Fluids and medications may be given through the device at the same concentrations and rates as a CVC.

A CVC may be inserted for large-volume replacement and/or the infusion of high-dose or escalating vasopressors. However, resuscitation should not be delayed if other access is available.[12] CVCs are typically inserted into the subclavian, internal jugular, or femoral veins. An upper-body insertion site is preferred over the femoral vein due to a decreased risk of infection.[32] Multilumen catheters, which provide multiple access ports, allow the concurrent administration of fluid, medication, and blood products.

Fluids often need to be infused at a rapid rate. Infusion pumps are recommended to administer large volumes of fluids rapidly and accurately but are generally limited to a programmed rate of 999 mL per hour per infusion. Several additional strategies can be used for rapid administration of fluids, including infusion of multiple liters concurrently, use of a pressure bag, large-bore infusion tubing, or a rapid-infusion device (Fig. 12.4).

Types of Fluids. The choice of fluids depends on the cause of the volume deficit and the patient's clinical status. It is important to understand the rationale for the prescribed fluid and the expected effects of therapy. Crystalloids and colloids may be given alone or in combination with blood and blood products to restore intravascular volume. Crystalloid infusions, such as 0.9% normal saline and Lactated Ringer's solution, are a first line to resuscitative therapy in shock.[12,33] Crystalloids are classified by tonicity and balance. Isotonic solutions (e.g., 0.9% normal saline) have approximately the same tonicity as plasma (osmolality of 285 to 295 mOsm/L). In addition to being isotonic, balanced solutions (e.g., Lactated Ringer's solution) have sodium, chloride, and potassium contents similar to those of plasma and are felt to have fewer effects on acid-base balance.[29,34,35] There is evidence to support administration of a balanced solution, such as Lactated Ringer's solution, as a more appropriate first choice for fluid

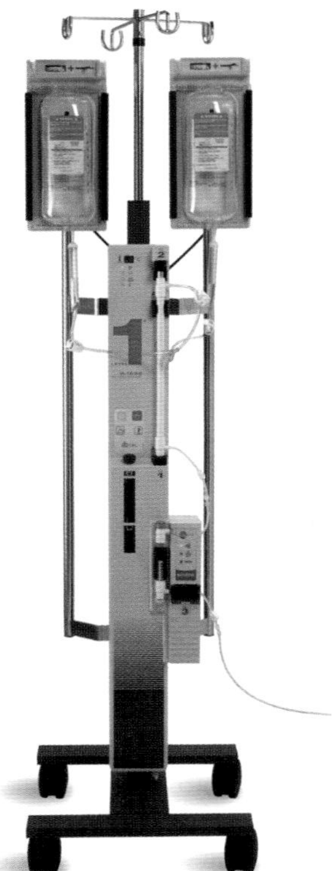

Fig. 12.4 Level 1 rapid infuser. (Courtesy Smiths Medical, Rockland, MA.)

resuscitation compared to 0.9% normal saline.[12,35] Since 0.9% normal saline is not a balanced solution, there are associated side effects, which include hypernatremia, hypokalemia, and hyperchloremic metabolic acidosis.[12,35] Solutions of 5% dextrose in water (D_5W) and 0.45% normal saline are hypotonic and are not used for fluid resuscitation. Hypotonic solutions rapidly leave the intravascular space, causing interstitial and intracellular edema.

When large volumes of crystalloids are infused, the patient is at risk for hemodilution of red blood cells and plasma proteins. Hemodilution of red blood cells impairs DO_2, and the cardiac output cannot increase enough to compensate. Hemodilution after fluid resuscitation for septic shock is associated with longer lengths of stay and increased mortality.[36]

Blood loss should be treated with blood products and hemorrhage control (see Blood Products section of this chapter). If blood products are not readily available and the patient is unstable, crystalloids may be administered using a restrictive volume strategy to maintain hemodynamic stability and avoid fluid overload until blood products are available.[37]

Colloids (e.g., albumin) contain proteins that theoretically increase osmotic pressure. Osmotic pressure pulls in and holds fluid to increase intravascular volume. Because colloids remain in the intravascular space longer than crystalloids, smaller volumes of colloids may be given in shock states. A potential complication of colloid administration is pulmonary edema, due to increased pulmonary capillary permeability or increased capillary hydrostatic pressure in the pulmonary vasculature created by rapid plasma expansion. Administration of colloids has not been shown to reduce mortality and is more costly compared to crystalloids.[12,38]

Albumin is a naturally occurring colloid solution from pooled human plasma that can be infused when the decrease in volume is caused by a loss of plasma rather than blood, such as peritonitis or bowel obstruction. Five percent albumin is considered an adjunct in volume resuscitation and is suggested when large volumes of crystalloids have been given in septic shock.[12] Typing and crossmatching of albumin is not required, but consent for administration may be necessary, as they are derivatives of blood; refer to hospital policy for guidance. Hetastarch (Hespan) is a semisynthetic starch colloid solution that acts as a plasma expander. A recent publication from the U.S. Food and Drug Administration (FDA) recommends that hetastarch not be used if there are adequate alternative treatments available. Resuscitation with starch solutions have been associated with acute kidney injury, coagulopathies, and increased mortality.[39]

Blood Products. Blood products, such as packed red blood cells (PRBCs), fresh frozen plasma (FFP), and platelets, are administered to treat major blood loss. Typing and crossmatching of these products are performed to identify the patient's blood type (A, B, AB, or O) and Rhesus (Rh) factor to ensure compatibility with the donor blood and prevent transfusion reactions.[40] In extreme emergencies, patients are transfused with uncrossmatched Rh-negative or Rh-positive O blood, which is considered universally compatible. Uncrossmatched Rh-negative type O blood should be administered to females of childbearing age in emergency situations to avoid fetal health problems in the event of pregnancy.[40]

Transfusions require an IV access with at least a 20- to 24-gauge catheter. Use a larger bore 18- to 20-gauge catheter when rapid transfusion is needed.[41] Administer only 0.9% normal saline with blood; other solutions cause red blood cells to aggregate, swell, and burst. Never infuse IV medications in the same port with blood. Follow hospital policy to ensure patient and blood identification before starting a transfusion.

Administer transfusions with a blood filter to trap debris and clots. Assess the patient's vital signs frequently during a blood transfusion to monitor for adverse reactions. Signs and symptoms of a transfusion reaction include fever, chills, rash, petechiae, respiratory distress, and hypotension.[42,43] In the event of a reaction, stop the transfusion, disconnect the transfusion tubing from the IV access site, and keep the vein open with an IV infusion of 0.9% normal saline. Continue to assess the patient and notify the provider and blood bank of the reaction. Send all transfusion equipment (i.e., bag, tubing, and remaining solutions) and any blood or urine specimens obtained to the blood bank according to hospital policy. Document the events of the reaction, interventions performed, and patient's response to treatment. Transfusion reactions, presentation, and nursing implications are listed in Table 12.4.

Transfusion administration time varies with the type of blood product used and the patient's condition. During transfusion, document the blood product administered, baseline vital signs, start and completion times of the transfusion, volume of blood and fluid administered, assessment of the patient during the transfusion, and any nursing actions taken.

Packed red blood cells increase the blood volume and provide more oxygen-carrying capability. One unit of PRBCs increases the hematocrit value by about 3% and the hemoglobin value by 1 g/dL.[40] Typing and crossmatching of PRBCs should be obtained in nonemergent situations. PRBCs may be modified based on patient need. Examples include leukocyte reduction to reduce white blood cells, irradiated to reduce lymphocytes, or washed to

TABLE 12.4 Types of Transfusion Reactions

Transfusion Reaction	Clinical Presentation	Nursing Implications
Acute hemolytic transfusion reaction	Chills DIC Dyspnea Fever Hematuria Hypotension Pain Rigors	Stop transfusion and notify provider Provide supportive care by initiating fluid resuscitation to maintain blood pressure Administer diuretics as ordered to maintain urine output
Allergic and anaphylactic transfusion reaction	Angioedema Hypotension Pruritus Respiratory distress Urticaria Wheezing	Stop transfusion and notify provider Provide supportive care based on symptoms (e.g., epinephrine, antihistamines, bronchodilators, and corticosteroids)
Febrile nonhemolytic transfusion reaction	Chills Fever Hypertension Rigor Tachycardia Tachypnea	Stop transfusion and notify provider Provide supportive care including antipyretics and meperidine
Transfusion-related acute lung injury (TRALI)	Chills Dyspnea Fever Hypoxia Tachycardia Tachypnea	Stop transfusion and notify provider Provide supportive care including supplemental oxygen Assist with intubation and monitor mechanical ventilation
Transfusion-associated circulatory overload (TACO)	Chills Dyspnea Fever Hypertension Hypoxemia Jugular venous distention Peripheral edema Tachycardia Tachypnea	Stop transfusion and notify provider Provide supportive care including supplemental oxygen Administer diuretics or initiate hemodialysis as ordered for fluid removal

DIC, Disseminated intravascular coagulation
Harding MM, Kwon J, Hagler D. Rome SI. Chapter 34: Hematologic problems. In: Lewis's Medical-Surgical Nursing: Assessment and management of clinical problems 12th ed. Elsevier, 2022:715–766; Raval JS, Griggs JR, Fleg A. Blood product transfusion in adults: indications, adverse reactions, and modifications. *Am Fam Physician.* 2020;102(1):30–38.

reduce plasma components. Administration of 10 or more units of PRBCs is associated with decreased 2,3-diphosphoglycerate (2,3-DPG) levels, causing a shift of the oxyhemoglobin dissociation curve to the left, which impairs the DO_2 to the tissues. Stored blood is anticoagulated with citrate, which leads to the chelating of calcium.[44,45] Therefore, monitor ionized calcium levels when transfusing large volumes of PRBCs.

FFP is administered to replace all clotting factors except platelets. Typing and crossmatching of FFP are required.

Platelets are given rapidly to help control bleeding caused by low platelet counts (usually <50,000/mm^3). Do not administer platelets under pressure, as this can negatively affect their function. Typing of platelets, but not crossmatching, is required.

Although control of hemorrhage is a treatment priority, transfusions are often needed. In the case of hemorrhagic shock, a massive transfusion protocol (MTP) should be implemented. There are various definitions of MTP, with two common definitions being (1) requiring five units or more of blood within a 3-hour period and (2) transfusion of 10 or more PRBCs in 24 hours.[46,47] MTPs recommend giving a ratio of 1:1:1 (PRBCs, FFP, and platelets).[48] Some centers may administer fresh whole blood, if available, rather than component therapy (see Chapter 20, Trauma and Surgical Management).

CLINICAL JUDGMENT ACTIVITY

What are clinical signs of adequate fluid resuscitation to assess during and after fluid resuscitation? Discuss physical assessment, hemodynamic monitoring, and laboratory values.

Maintain Arterial Oxygen Saturation and Ventilation

Airway maintenance is a priority (see Chapter 10, Ventilatory Assistance). Administer oxygen to increase arterial oxygen tension, thereby improving tissue oxygenation. Oxygen administration methods range from nasal cannula to mechanical ventilation, depending on the patient's condition.

Mechanical ventilation also assists in maintaining adequate ventilation, as reflected by a normal partial pressure of arterial carbon dioxide ($PaCO_2$). Another benefit of mechanical ventilation in a patient with shock is to reduce the work of breathing and the associated increase in oxygen consumption. Strategies to prevent ventilator-induced lung injury, such as low tidal volume ventilation, are implemented if mechanical ventilation is needed.[49] Additional treatment with analgesia or sedation, with or without neuromuscular blockade, may be required to reduce oxygen demand (see Chapter 6, Comfort and Sedation, and Chapter 10, Ventilatory Assistance).

Pharmacological Support

Pharmacological management of shock is based on manipulation of the determinants of cardiac output: heart rate, preload, afterload, and contractility. Fig. 12.5 shows therapies used to manipulate these parameters. Many medications used to treat the symptoms of shock are vesicants and are preferably administered through a CVC. Assess effectiveness of medications through noninvasive and invasive hemodynamic monitoring (see Chapter 9, Hemodynamic Monitoring). Older adults are particularly sensitive to the physiological effect of medications and the deleterious effects of polypharmacy, which requires closer monitoring. Medications commonly administered in shock are listed in Table 12.5.

Cardiac Output. Dysrhythmias, including low or high heart rates, decrease cardiac output. Chronotropic and antidysrhythmic medications are administered as indicated.

Preload. In hypovolemic and distributive shock, fluid administration is the primary treatment to increase preload. In cardiogenic shock, the myofibrils are overstretched, and strategies to reduce the preload are implemented. Medications that reduce preload include venous vasodilators and diuretics.

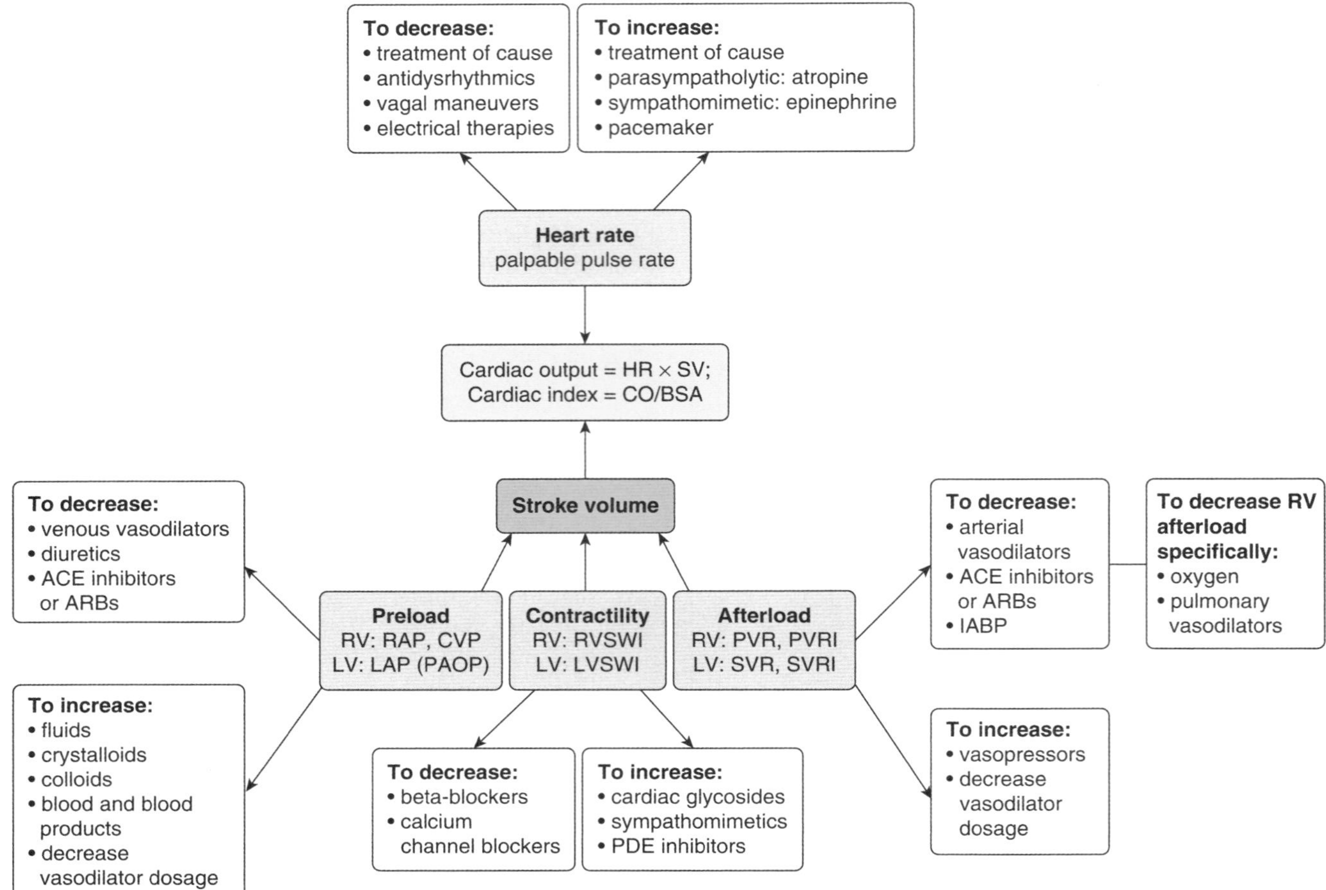

Fig. 12.5 Therapeutic manipulations to optimize cardiac output and/or minimize myocardial oxygen consumption. *ACE,* Angiotensin-converting enzyme; *ARB,* angiotensin receptor blocker; *BSA,* body surface area; *CO,* cardiac output; *CVP,* central venous pressure; *HR,* heart rate; *IABP,* intraaortic balloon pump; *LAP,* left atrial pressure; *LV,* left ventricle; *LVSWI,* left ventricular stroke work index; *PAOP,* pulmonary artery occlusion pressure; *PDE,* phosphodiesterase; *PVR,* pulmonary vascular resistance; *PVRI,* pulmonary vascular resistance index; *RAP,* right atrial pressure; *RV,* right ventricle; *RVSWI,* right ventricular stroke work index; *SV,* stroke volume; *SVR,* systemic vascular resistance; *SVRI,* systemic vascular resistance index. (Modified from Dennison RD. *Pass CCRN!* 5th ed. St. Louis, MO: Mosby; 2019.)

TABLE 12.5 PHARMACOLOGY

Medications Commonly Used for Treating Shock

Inotropic Agents

Medication	Action and Use	Dose and Route[a]	Side Effects	Nursing Implications[b]
Dobutamine (Dobutrex)	Stimulates beta-1 receptors to ↑ contractility and HR (for cardiogenic and distributive shock and acute decompensated heart failure); stimulation of beta-2 can cause vasodilation (no to minimal decrease in systolic pressure)	*Continuous infusion:* Initial, 5 mcg/kg/min IV Maintenance, 2–20 mcg/kg/min IV Titrate based on response	Anxiety Chest pain Dyspnea Headache Hypertension Hypotension Nausea Palpitations Tachyarrhythmias Vomiting	Monitor BP, HR, and ECG. If available, monitor CO/CI, SvO_2, and/or $ScvO_2$. Use cautiously in patients with myocardial ischemia or atrial fibrillation. Treat hypovolemia and electrolytes before initiation of infusion. Central venous catheter preferred.

TABLE 12.5 **PHARMACOLOGY—cont'd**

Medications Commonly Used for Treating Shock

Dopamine (Intropin)	Dose-dependent effect 2–10 mcg/kg/min: stimulates $beta_1$ receptors (↑ contractility and HR) 10–20 mcg/kg/min: stimulates alpha receptors (vasoconstriction to ↑ SVR) May be used for symptomatic bradycardia or refractory distributive shock	*Continuous infusion:* Initial, 5 mcg/kg/min IV Maintenance, 5–20 mcg/kg/min IV Titrate by 5–10 mcg/kg/min q 10 to 30 minutes to clinical end point	Anxiety Chest pain Dyspnea Headache Hypertension Palpitations Piloerection Tachyarrhythmias Vomiting	Monitor HR, BP, and ECG. If available, monitor SVR and CO/CI. Treat hypovolemia before initiation. Dosing >20 mcg/kg/min decreases perfusion to the kidneys. Central venous catheter preferred. Tissue necrosis if extravasation (treat with phentolamine [Regitine]).
Milrinone (Primacor)	Inhibits phosphodiesterase (PDE) resulting in increased contractility and vasodilation (reduces preload and afterload) Used in acute decompensated heart failure	*Continuous infusion:* Initial, 0.125–0.25 mcg/kg/min IV Maintenance, 0.125–0.75 mcg/kg/min IV titrated to clinical end point	Angina Chest pain Headache Hypotension Palpitations Tachyarrhythmias Thrombocytopenia	Monitor BP, HR, and ECG. If SBP drops 30 mm Hg, stop infusion, and notify provider.
Vasopressors				
Epinephrine	Stimulates beta-1 receptors to ↑HR and contractility; stimulates alpha receptors to cause peripheral vasoconstriction Stimulates beta-2 receptors to promote bronchodilation in anaphylactic shock	**Distributive shock** *Continuous infusion:* Initial, 0.01–0.2 mcg/kg/min IV or 1–15 mcg/min Maintenance, titrate q 10–15 min to clinical end point, no true maximum **Anaphylactic shock** *Intramuscular:* 0.5 mg, IM (anterior thigh preferred; can be given through clothing) *Intravenous:* Bolus: 0.1 mg of 0.1 mg/mL IV solution over 5 to 10 minutes *Continuous infusion:* Initial, 2–15 mcg/min IV (with crystalloid administration)	Anxiety Chest pain Dizziness Dyspnea Headache Hypertension Ischemia (peripheral, gastrointestinal) Pallor Palpitations Pulmonary edema Sweating Tachyarrhythmias Vomiting	Monitor HR, BP, and ECG. Invasive BP monitoring recommended. Assess and correct volume depletion before and during administration. Central venous catheter preferred. Tissue necrosis if extravasation (treat with phentolamine [Regitine]).
Norepinephrine (Levophed)	Stimulates alpha receptors causing peripheral vasoconstriction and beta-1 receptors to ↑ contractility and HR Used in any shock state after appropriate volume resuscitation	*Continuous infusion:* 0.05–0.15 mcg/kg/min IV or 5–15 mcg/min Titrate to clinical end point, no true maximum	Anxiety Chest pain Dysrhythmias Headache Hypertension Ischemia (peripheral, gastrointestinal)	Monitor BP, HR, and ECG. Invasive BP monitoring recommended. Central venous catheter preferred. Tissue necrosis if extravasation (treat with phentolamine [Regitine]).
Phenylephrine (Neo-synephrine)	Stimulates alpha causing peripheral vasoconstriction Used in distributive shock	*Continuous infusion:* Initial, 10–35 mcg/min IV Maintenance, titrate to maintain desired BP range; maximum dose, 200 mcg/min	Anxiety Blurred vision Bradycardia Chest pain Headache Ischemia (peripheral, gastrointestinal) Nausea, vomiting Palpitations Restlessness Tremor	Monitor HR, BP, and ECG. Invasive BP monitoring recommended. Treat reflex bradycardia with atropine. Central venous catheter preferred. Tissue necrosis if extravasation (treat with phentolamine [Regitine]).

Continued

TABLE 12.5 PHARMACOLOGY—cont'd

Medications Commonly Used for Treating Shock

Vasopressin (Vasostrict)	Vasoconstriction through smooth muscle contraction of all parts of capillaries, arterioles, and venules Used in vasodilatory states to restore vascular tone	**Septic shock** *Continuous infusion:* 0.03–0.04 units/min IV fixed dose **Postcardiotomy shock** *Continuous infusion:* 0.03 units/min IV and titrate to BP with maximum dose 0.1 units/min IV	Dysrhythmias Hyponatremia Ischemia (cardiac, mesenteric) Thrombocytopenia	Monitor HR, BP, ECG, and urine output.
Synthetic angiotensin II (Giapreza)	Vasoconstriction and increase in aldosterone release Used in septic or other distributive shocks on 2 or more vasopressors with continued hypotension	*Continuous infusion:* First 3 h with target MAP ≥75 mm Hg, 20 ng/kg/min IV, titrate every 5 min to BP, maximum dose 80 ng/kg/min IV Maintenance with target MAP ≥65 mm Hg, maximum dose 40 ng/kg/min IV, doses as low as 1.25 ng/kg/min IV based on BP	Acidosis Delirium Dysrhythmias Fungal infection Hyperglycemia Peripheral ischemia Thrombocytopenia Thromboembolic events (e.g., DVT)	Monitor HR, BP, and ECG. All patients should be on VTE prophylaxis. Invasive BP monitoring recommended.
Vasodilators				
Nitroglycerin	Vasodilation by direct smooth muscle relaxation, predominantly venous Used in cardiogenic shock for preload and/or afterload reduction Dose-dependent effect Arterial dilation only if infusion >1 mcg/kg/min	*Continuous infusion:* Initial, 5 mcg/min IV Maintenance, increase by 5 mcg/min IV q 3–5 min to clinical end point If no response at 20 mcg/min IV, increase by 10–20 mcg/min IV to clinical end point	Abdominal pain Angina Apprehension Dizziness Flushing Headache Hypotension Methemoglobinemia Nausea and vomiting Palpitations Syncope Tachycardia Weakness	Monitor HR, BP, ECG and RAP, PAP, PAOP, SVR, CO, and CI if available. Use cautiously in cases of hypotension. Administer in non-polyvinyl chloride (PVC) plastic or glass bottle with non-PVC tubing.
Nitroprusside (Nipride)	Vasodilation by direct smooth muscle relaxation, predominantly arterial Used in cardiogenic shock for preload and/or afterload reduction	*Continuous infusion:* Initial, 0.3 mcg/kg/min IV Maintenance, titrate by 0.5 mcg/kg/min IV to achieve desired BP; maximum dose, 10 mcg/kg/min IV	Abdominal pain Cyanide toxicity Diaphoresis Dizziness Headache Hypoxemia (from nitroprusside-induced intrapulmonary thiocyanate toxicity) Methemoglobinemia Nausea Palpitations Precipitous hypotension Tachycardia Thrombocytopenia Vomiting	Monitor continuous BP Serum thiocyanate levels are only useful to confirm suspected toxicity in symptomatic patients. Invasive BP monitoring recommended. If cyanide toxicity is suspected, stop infusion immediately; notify provider. Methemoglobinemia is treated with methylene blue. If suspected, stop infusion immediately; notify the provider. Protect from light by wrapping with opaque material. Cyanide toxicity (metabolic acidosis, hypoxemia, bradycardia, AMS) Methemoglobinemia (>10 mcg/kg/min; impaired oxygen delivery despite normal PaO_2 and CO)

[a]All medications are administered by volumetric infusion pump.
[b]All vasoactive and inotropic medications require appropriate fluid resuscitation to ensure adequate intravascular volume prior to administration.
AMS, Altered mental status; *BP,* Blood pressure; *CI,* cardiac index; *CO,* cardiac output; *ECG,* electrocardiogram; *HR,* heart rate; *IM,* intramuscular; *MAP,* mean arterial pressure; *PAOP,* pulmonary artery occlusion pressure; *PAP,* pulmonary artery pressure; *PVC,* premature ventricular contraction; *q,* every; *RAP,* right atrial pressure; *SBP,* systolic blood pressure; *$ScvO_2$,* central venous oxygen saturation; *SvO_2,* mixed venous oxygen saturation; *SVR,* systemic vascular resistance; *VTE,* venous thromboembolism.
From Gahart B, Nazareno A, Ortega MQ, Collins SR. *Elsevier's 2023 Intravenous Medications.* 39th ed. St. Louis, MO: Elsevier, Inc.; 2023; La Jolla. Giaprezza (angiotensin II) injection for intravenous infusion. Available at: prescribing/GIAPREZA.pdf (firebasestorage.googleapis.com). Accessed December 17, 2023.

Afterload. Afterload is low in distributive shock. In this situation, medications that cause vasoconstriction are administered to increase vascular tone (i.e., SVR) and tissue perfusion pressure. Examples of vasoconstrictive medications include phenylephrine, norepinephrine, epinephrine, vasopressin, and synthetic angiotensin II.[50] A negative effect of medications that increase afterload is an increase in myocardial oxygen demand.

Do not administer vasopressor medications to treat hypovolemic shock until hypovolemia is addressed with volume replacement. Administration of vasopressors in hypovolemia causes vasoconstriction and further diminishes tissue perfusion.

In cardiogenic shock, afterload must be reduced. The use of arterial vasodilators to reduce afterload may be limited by the patient's blood pressure. When hypotension prevents the use of arterial vasodilators, an intraaortic balloon pump (IABP) is used to decrease afterload (see Cardiogenic Shock section).

Contractility. Medications that increase contractility, inotropic agents such as dobutamine, milrinone, and digoxin, may be administered in shock.[51,52]

Other Medications. Other medications used to manage shock include sedatives, analgesics, insulin, corticosteroids, and antibiotics. Although respiratory acidosis is treated by improving ventilation, metabolic acidosis caused by lactic acidosis is best treated by improving DO_2, SaO_2, hemoglobin level, and cardiac output. Monitor ABG analysis and serum lactate levels to guide treatment.

Insulin therapy should be initiated when two consecutive blood glucose levels are greater than 180 mg/dL. The goal is to maintain a blood glucose level of 180 mg/dL or less.[12] Low-molecular-weight heparin is often prescribed for venous thromboembolism prophylaxis. Peptic ulcer prophylaxis is often initiated with an H_2-receptor antagonist or proton pump inhibitor.

Nonpharmacological Support

Body Temperature. Monitor the patient's temperature and implement care to maintain a normal body temperature. Fever in critical care is generally defined as a core temperature above 38.3°C.[53,54] Increased body temperature increases oxygen demand and can negatively affect the already stressed cardiovascular system.

Hypothermia is defined as a drop in core body temperature below 35°C.[55] Hypothermia causes dysrhythmias, depresses cardiac contractility, and reduces cardiac output, ultimately decreasing DO_2. The coagulation pathway is altered, and platelet function is impaired in hypothermia, which can result in significant coagulopathies. Anticipate hypothermia when fluids are infused rapidly, and proactively use warming methods (e.g., fluid warmer, heated forced air blankets). Keep the patient warm and comfortable, avoiding hyperthermia.

Nutritional Support. Nutritional support is essential for patient survival. The goals of nutritional support are to initiate enteral feedings as soon as possible and to maintain sufficient caloric intake to assist the healing process. Early administration of enteral nutrition within 48 hours of admission may assist with maintenance of gut integrity, prevent intestinal permeability, and reduce insulin resistance after the initial uncontrolled shock is resolved.[12,56,57] Overfeeding patients in the early phases of shock is associated with adverse outcomes.[58]

Enteral feeding is the preferred method; however, administration of enteral nutrition may be limited by paralytic ileus, gastric dilation, or both, which are common in shock. Total parenteral nutrition is considered if patients are unable to tolerate enteral feeding (see Chapter 7, Nutritional Therapy).

Psychological Support. Nursing interventions focus on identifying the effect of the illness on the patient and the family. Provide information that is essential for the psychological well-being of the patient and family and that may help give them a sense of understanding and control of the situation. Since shock has a high mortality rate, initiate a discussion regarding the patient's goals of care and life-sustaining therapies (see Chapter 2, Patient and Family Response to the Critical Care Experience, Chapter 3, Ethical and Legal Issues in Critical Care Nursing, and Chapter 4, Palliative and End-of-Life Care). Given the high mortality rate, nurses must also prioritize their own psychological well-being (see Nursing Self-Care box).

NURSING SELF-CARE

Expressing Gratitude

Expressing and receiving gratitude can significantly improve health and well-being for self, coworkers, and family.

Gratitude is a feeling that embodies kindness and can lead to connectedness and a strong network of support. The health benefits include better self-care, cardiovascular health, and positive emotions, including hope.

Simple ways to express gratitude can be easily incorporated into personal habits and the work environment. Strategies include but are not limited to:

1. Gratitude "shout out" during shift huddles
2. Gratitude board in the unit for staff to post thanks or other comments
3. Keeping a gratitude journal
4. Creating a habit of writing or thinking about three things to be grateful for that day

Actively focusing on positive thoughts and offering gratitude influences the part of our brain called the reticular activation system (RAS), improving overall health and well-being.

From The American Nurses Association Enterprise. *Well-Being Initiative.* American Nurses Association Enterprise. Accessed January 16, 2023. https://www.nursingworld.org/practice-policy/work-environment/health-safety/disaster-preparedness/coronavirus/what-you-need-to-know/the-well-being-initiative/; Day G, Robert G, Rafferty AM. Gratitude in health care: a meta-narrative review. *Qual Health Res.* 2020;30(14):2303–2315. https://doi.org/10.1177/1049732320951145.

PLAN OF CARE

For the Patient in Shock

Patient Problem

Decreased Multisystem Tissue Perfusion. Risk factors include decreased blood volume (i.e., hypovolemic shock), decreased myocardial contractility (i.e., cardiogenic shock), impaired circulatory blood flow (i.e., obstructive shock), and widespread vasodilation (i.e., distributive shock).

Desired Outcomes

- Vital signs and hemodynamic parameters within normal limits (Table 12.3).
- Oxygen saturation 90% or greater.
- Urine output at least 0.5 mL/kg/h.
- Normal serum and urine laboratory values and ABG results.
- Absence of complications (ARDS, DIC, acute kidney injury, hepatic failure, MODS).
- Normal mentation.

Nursing Assessments/Interventions	Rationales
• Monitor for early symptoms of shock (Table 12.2).	• Initiate early support to improve outcomes and reduce risk of complications, organ dysfunction, and death.
• Establish IV access using large-bore catheters (i.e., 18- to 20-gauge).	• Provide rapid medication and fluid administration.
• Obtain central venous access, if applicable.	• Reduce risk of infiltration and irritation of peripheral IV site.
• Control bleeding through the application of pressure or surgical intervention.	• Prevent blood loss.
• Administer fluids (e.g., crystalloids, colloids) as ordered.	• Maintain tissue perfusion.
• Consider warming fluids before and during infusion.	• Reduce hypothermia
• Replace blood and blood components as indicated; obtain laboratory specimens for type and screen and crossmatch.	• Replace volume loss associated with blood loss; prevent transfusion reaction.
• Evaluate patient's response to fluid challenges and blood product administration such as improved vital signs, level of consciousness, urinary output, hemodynamic values, and serum and urine laboratory values.	• Monitor response to treatment.
• Monitor for clinical indications of fluid overload (↑HR, ↑RR, dyspnea, crackles) when fluids are administered rapidly.	• Assess for signs of volume overload in response to treatment.
• Monitor cardiopulmonary status: ○ HR ○ RR ○ BP/MAP ○ Skin color ○ Temperature ○ Moisture ○ Capillary refill ○ Mottling ○ Hemodynamic values ○ Cardiac rhythm ○ Neck veins ○ Lung sounds	• Monitor response to treatment.
• Monitor level of consciousness.	• Assess perfusion of the central nervous system.
• Monitor gastrointestinal status: ○ Abdominal distension ○ Bowel sounds ○ Vomiting ○ Bowel movements	• Assess perfusion of the gastrointestinal system.
• Monitor fluid balance: ○ I&O ○ Daily weights ○ Amount and type of drainage (i.e., chest tube, nasogastric tube, wounds)	• Evaluate the need for continued fluid volume support. • Alterations in fluid balance may indicate end organ damage (i.e., acute kidney injury).
• Monitor serial serum values: ○ Hct ○ Hgb ○ WBC ○ PT ○ aPTT ○ D-dimer ○ Platelets ○ ABGs ○ Chemistry profile ○ Lactate ○ Cultures	• Evaluate physiological status and response to treatment.
• Administer medications as prescribed and based on the classification of shock (Tables 12.5 and 12.6).	• Improve outcomes and reduce complications.
• Evaluate patient response to interventions and adjust treatments accordingly. • Monitor for complications.	• Monitor patient response to determine need for modification of treatment and/or nursing care.

ABG, Arterial blood gas; *aPTT,* activated partial thromboplastin time; *ARDS,* acute respiratory distress syndrome; *BP,* blood pressure; *DIC,* disseminated intravascular coagulation; *Hct,* hematocrit; *Hgb,* hemoglobin; *HR,* heart rate; *I&O,* intake and output; *MAP,* mean arterial pressure; *MODS,* multiple organ dysfunction syndrome; *PT,* prothrombin time; *RR,* respiratory rate; *WBC,* white blood cell.
Adapted from Snyder J, Sump C. *Swearingen's All-in-One Nursing Care Planning Resource.* 6th ed. Elsevier; 2024.

TABLE 12.6 Classifications of Shock

Classification	Possible Causes	Clinical Presentation	Management
Hypovolemic shock	*External loss of blood:* • GI hemorrhage • Surgery • Trauma *External loss of fluid:* • Diarrhea • Diuresis • Burns *Internal pooling of blood/fluid:* • Hemoperitoneum • Retroperitoneal hemorrhage • Hemothorax • Hemomediastinum • Dissecting aortic aneurysm • Femur or pelvic fracture • Ascites • Pleural effusion	↑ HR ↓ BP Tachypnea Oliguria Cool, pale skin Decreased mentation Flat neck veins ↓ CO/CI, RAP, PAP, PAOP ↑ SVR ↓ $SvO_2/ScvO_2$ ↑ Hematocrit if from nonblood losses ↓ Hematocrit if from blood loss	Eliminate and treat the cause Replace lost volume with appropriate replacement (e.g., crystalloid, blood) Use vasoactive medications if blood pressure does not respond quickly or delay in blood products
Cardiogenic shock	Myocardial infarction Myocardial contusion Cardiomyopathy Myocarditis Severe heart failure Dysrhythmias Valvular dysfunction Ventricular septal rupture	↑ HR Dysrhythmias ↓ BP Chest pain Tachypnea Oliguria Cool, pale skin ↓ Mentation Left ventricular failure Right ventricular failure ↓ CO/CI ↑ RAP, PAP, PAOP, SVR ↓ $SvO_2/ScvO_2$	Improve contractility with inotropic medications Mechanical circulatory support Emergency revascularization Optimize preload Reduce afterload Prevent or treat dysrhythmias
Obstructive shock	*Impaired diastolic filling:* • Cardiac tamponade • Tension pneumothorax • Constrictive pericarditis • Compression of great vein *Increased right ventricular afterload:* • Pulmonary embolism • Severe pulmonary hypertension • Increased intrathoracic pressure *Increased left ventricular afterload:* • Aortic dissection • Systemic embolization • Aortic stenosis • Abdominal hypertension	↑ HR Dysrhythmias ↓ BP Chest pain Dyspnea Oliguria Cool, pale skin Decreased mental status Jugular venous distension Cardiac tamponade: muffled heart sounds, pulsus paradoxus Tension pneumothorax: diminished breath sounds on affected side, tracheal shift away from affected side Pulmonary embolism: right ventricular failure Aortic dissection: ripping chest pain, pulse differences between left and right side, widened mediastinum ↓ CO/CI ↑ or normal RAP, PAP, PAOP ↑ PVR, SVR ↓ $SvO_2/ScvO_2$	Eliminate source of obstruction or compression Pericardiocentesis for cardiac tamponade Fibrinolytics are the first-line treatment in PE associated with obstructive shock Emergency decompression for tension pneumothorax Use vasoactive/inotropic medications to support CO/CI while treating underlying cause

Continued

TABLE 12.6 Classifications of Shock—cont'd

Classification	Possible Causes	Clinical Presentation	Management
Distributive shock – Anaphylactic	*Foods:* fish, shellfish, eggs, milk, wheat, strawberries, peanuts, tree nuts (e.g., pecans, walnuts), food additives *Medications:* antibiotics, ACE inhibitors, aspirin, local anesthetics, narcotics, barbiturates, contrast media, blood and blood products, allergic extracts *Bites or stings:* venomous snakes, wasps, hornets, spiders, jellyfish, stingrays, deer flies, fire ants *Chemicals:* latex, lotions, soap, perfumes, iodine-containing solutions	↑ HR; dysrhythmias ↓ BP Chest pain Tachypnea Dyspnea, cough, stridor, wheezing, dysphagia Urticaria, angioedema, hives Flushed, warm to hot skin Oliguria Restlessness, change in LOC, seizures Nausea, vomiting, abdominal cramping, diarrhea ↓ CO/CI ↓ RAP, PAP, PAOP, SVR ↓ $SvO_2/ScvO_2$ ↑ IgE	Remove/discontinue offending agent or slow absorption (i.e., remove stinger; apply ice to sting or bite; lavage stomach if antigen ingested; flush skin with water) Maintain airway, oxygenation, and ventilation; intubation may be necessary Modify or block the effects of mediators: epinephrine, antihistamines, steroids Use vasoactive medications to maintain MAP
Distributive shock – Neurogenic shock	General or spinal anesthesia Epidural block Spinal cord injury at or above the level of T6 *Medications:* barbiturates, phenothiazines, sympathetic blocking agents	↓ HR ↓ BP Hypothermia Warm, dry, flushed skin Oliguria Neurological deficit ↓ CO/CI ↓ RAP, PAP, PAOP, SVR ↓ $SvO_2/ScvO_2$	Eliminate and treat the cause, if applicable Use vasoactive medications to maintain MAP and HR
Distributive shock – Septic shock	*Immunosuppression:* • Extremes of age • Malnutrition • Alcoholism or drug abuse • Malignancy • History of splenectomy • Chronic health problems • Immunosuppressive therapies *Significant bacteremia:* • Invasive procedures or devices • Wounds or burns • GI infection or untreated disease • Peritonitis • Food poisoning • Prolonged hospitalization	↑ HR ↑ RR ↓ BP Temperature >38.3°C or <36°C WBC >12/mm³ or <4/mm³ Lactate >4 mmol/L or >2 mmol/L after fluid resuscitation Confusion Widened pulse pressure Skin warm, flushed Poor capillary refill Mottling Oliguria ↑ CO, CI ↓ RAP, PAP, PAOP, SVR Early: ↑ $SvO_2/ScvO_2$ Late: ↓ $SvO_2/ScvO_2$	Obtain blood cultures/identify source of infection Administer antibiotics within 1 h of diagnosis Administer fluid bolus (30 mL/kg) in the first 3 h; additional fluid guided by hemodynamic status Administer vasoactive medications if needed to maintain MAP ≥65 mm Hg Avoid NPO status: initiate and maintain enteral nutrition Antibiotics as indicated by culture results

ACE, Angiotensin-converting enzyme; *BP*, blood pressure; *CI*, cardiac index; *CO*, cardiac output; *GI*, gastrointestinal; *HR*, heart rate; *IgE*, immunoglobulin E; *LOC*, level of consciousness; *MAP*, mean arterial pressure; *NPO*, nothing by mouth; *PAOP*, pulmonary artery occlusion pressure; *PAP*, pulmonary artery pressure; *PE*, pulmonary embolism; *PVR*, pulmonary vascular resistance; *RAP*, right atrial pressure; *$ScvO_2$*, systolic blood pressure; *SvO_2*, mixed venous oxygen saturation; *SVR*, systemic vascular resistance; *WBC*, white blood cell.

CLASSIFICATIONS OF SHOCK

Table 12.6 summarizes the classifications of shock.

Hypovolemic Shock

Hypovolemic shock occurs when the circulating blood volume is inadequate to fill the vascular network. Intravascular volume deficits may be caused by external or internal losses of blood or fluid. In these situations, the intravascular blood volume is depleted and unavailable to transport oxygen and nutrients to tissues. The severity of hypovolemic shock depends on the degree of volume loss, the type of fluid lost, and the age and preinjury health status of the patient.

External volume deficits include loss of blood, plasma, or body fluids. The most common cause of hypovolemic shock is hemorrhage. External loss of blood may occur after traumatic injury, surgery, obstetric delivery, or with coagulation alterations (e.g., hemophilia, thrombocytopenia, DIC, anticoagulant medications). External plasma losses may be seen in patients with burn injuries who have significant fluid shifts from the intravascular space to the interstitial space (see Chapter 21, Burns). Excessive external loss of fluid may occur through the gastrointestinal tract because of suctioning, upper gastrointestinal bleeding, vomiting, diarrhea, reduction in oral fluid intake, or fistulas; through the genitourinary tract as a result of excessive diuresis, diabetes mellitus with polyuria, diabetes insipidus, or Addison's disease; or through the skin due to diaphoresis without fluid and electrolyte replacement.

Blood or body fluids may be sequestered, or pooled, within the body outside the vascular bed. For example, blood may sequester secondary to a ruptured spleen or liver, hemothorax, hemorrhagic pancreatitis, fractures of the femur or pelvis, and dissecting aneurysm. Other forms of internal sequestration of body fluids include ascites, peritonitis, and intestinal obstruction (whereby fluid leaks from the intestinal capillaries into the lumen of the intestine).

Assess for both obvious and subtle fluid losses. Assess dressings; measure drainage from chest or nasogastric tubes; monitor potential sites for bleeding, such as surgical wounds or IV or intraarterial catheter sites after removal; and consider insensible losses, such as perspiration. Measure abdominal girth periodically in patients in whom occult bleeding may be suspected or in those with ascites. Obtain daily weights using the same scale with the patient wearing the same clothing at approximately the same time each day. If a bed scale is used, ensure that the equipment and tubing do not touch the bed and have a standard linen protocol for obtaining weights. Evaluate serial hematocrits to help determine whether blood or fluid was lost. In a patient with blood loss, the hematocrit is decreased, whereas in a patient with fluid loss, the hematocrit is increased.

Hypovolemic shock results in a reduction of intravascular volume and a decrease in venous return to the right side of the heart. Ventricular filling pressures (preload) are reduced, resulting in decreased stroke volume and cardiac output. As the cardiac output decreases, blood pressure and tissue perfusion also decrease. Fig. 12.6 summarizes the pathophysiology of hypovolemic shock.

Patients with hypovolemic shock present with signs and symptoms as a result of poor organ perfusion, including altered mentation ranging from lethargy to unresponsiveness; rapid, deep respirations; cool, clammy skin with weak, thready pulses; tachycardia; and oliguria. Hypovolemic shock resulting from hemorrhage is classified according to the volume of blood lost and the resultant effects on the level of consciousness, vital signs, and urine output (Table 12.7).

An increase in abdominal girth may indicate abdominal bleeding or fluid loss into the abdomen. Consider monitoring intraabdominal pressures to assess for abdominal compartment syndrome. Abdominal compartment syndrome can compound hypovolemic shock via obstructive shock, leading to rapid patient deterioration if not emergently decompressed. Ultrasonography is performed to detect abdominal bleeding or fluid loss. Particularly in trauma patients, a focused assessment with sonography for trauma (FAST) exam is used to evaluate the torso for free fluid, which may be indicative of noncompressible torso hemorrhage (see Chapter 20, Trauma and Surgical Management). If fluid is found, computed tomography (CT) may be used to pinpoint sources of bleeding in the hemodynamically stable patient. In the hemodynamically unstable bleeding patient, either interventional radiology or surgical intervention is warranted.

Management of hypovolemic shock focuses on identifying, treating, and eliminating the cause of hypovolemia and replacing lost fluid. Consider the type of fluid lost when determining fluid replacement. Treatment can include surgery, antidiarrheal medication for diarrhea, reversal of anticoagulation, and insulin for hyperglycemia. Fluid and blood administration is not a substitute for definitive bleeding control.[59]

Isotonic crystalloids, such as Lactated Ringer's solution or 0.9% normal saline, are typically used first, although blood and blood products should be administered if the patient is bleeding. Trauma guidelines recommend limiting fluid resuscitation with crystalloids to no more than 1 L in hypovolemic shock resuscitation due to blood loss, and quickly transitioning to the administration of blood products if the patient is unresponsive to fluids.[60] Overresuscitation with crystalloids dilutes the blood and impairs oxygen-carrying capacity and clotting factors, which can lead to decreased tissue perfusion and increased bleeding.[60,61] Consider assessment and treatment of coagulopathies related to not only the potential cause of bleeding but as a sequela of massive transfusion resuscitation.[59] Monitor the patient's response to therapy by assessing oxygenation, blood pressure, pulse, level of consciousness, capillary refill, and urine output.

Cardiogenic Shock

Cardiogenic shock can occur when the heart fails to act as an effective pump. A decrease in myocardial contractility results in decreased cardiac output and impaired tissue perfusion. Cardiogenic shock is one of the most difficult types of shock to treat and carries a hospital mortality rate as high as 51%.[62]

The most common cause of cardiogenic shock is extensive left ventricular myocardial infarction. The degree of myocardial damage correlates with the likelihood of cardiogenic shock. If 40% or more of the left ventricle is damaged, the likelihood of cardiogenic shock increases.[63] Other causes of cardiogenic shock include dysrhythmias, congenital abnormalities, cardiomyopathy, myocarditis, valvular dysfunction, severe heart failure, and structural disorders.[62]

The pathophysiology of cardiogenic shock can be understood by reviewing the dynamics of cardiac output and stroke volume. When damage to the myocardium occurs, contractile force is reduced, and stroke volume decreases. Ventricular filling pressures increase because blood remains in the cardiac chambers. Cardiac output and ejection fraction decrease, causing hypotension. Increased left ventricular end-diastolic pressure creates pulmonary congestion with resultant hypoxia. A progressive decrease in cardiac output leads to further impairment of coronary artery perfusion and tissue perfusion. Neurohormonal mechanisms trigger peripheral vasoconstriction with retention of sodium and water, which in turn increases preload.[30] Fig. 12.7 illustrates the pathophysiology of cardiogenic shock.

Increased demand is placed on the myocardium as it attempts to increase perfusion to the cells. The heart rate increases as a compensatory mechanism, increasing the oxygen demand of an overworked myocardium. Compensatory mechanisms may increase myocardial oxygen requirements, which may further increase infarction size.

The clinical presentation of cardiogenic shock includes manifestations of left ventricular failure (e.g., S_3 heart sound, crackles, dyspnea, hypoxemia, hypotension) and right ventricular failure (e.g., jugular venous distension, peripheral edema, hepatomegaly). Hemodynamic monitoring via a PA catheter or less invasive

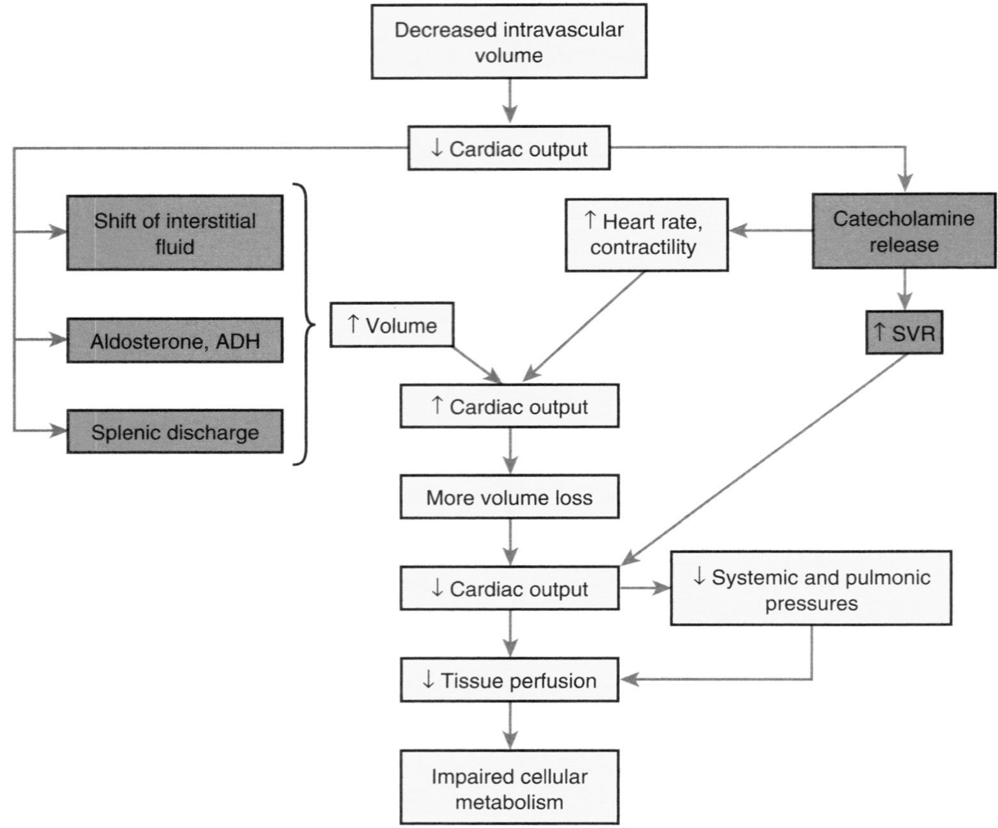

Fig. 12.6 Hypovolemic shock. Hypovolemic shock becomes life-threatening when compensatory mechanisms *(orange boxes)* are overwhelmed by continuous loss of intravascular volume. *ADH,* Antidiuretic hormone; *SVR,* systemic vascular resistance. (From Rogers JL. *McCance & Huether's Pathophysiology: The Biologic Basis for Disease in Adults and Children.* 9th ed. St. Louis, MO: Elsevier; 2024.)

TABLE 12.7 Severity of Hemorrhagic Shock

	CLASS			
Indicators	**I**	**II Mild**	**III Moderate**	**IV Severe**
Blood loss (% blood volume)	<15%	15%–30%	31%–40%	>40%
Heart rate (beats/min)	No change	Mild tachycardia	Tachycardia	Marked tachycardia
Blood pressure	No change	No change	Mild hypotension	Marked hypotension
Respiratory rate (breaths/min)	No change	Mild increase	Mild tachypnea	Tachypnea
Urine output (mL/h)	No change	No change	Decreased	Decreased
Glasgow Coma Scale score	No change	No change	Decreased	Decreased
Base deficit	0 to −2 mEq/L	−2 to −6 mEq/L	−6 to −10 mEq/L	−10 mEq/L or less
Need for blood products	Monitor for need	Possible need	Needed	Massive transfusion protocol

Modified from American College of Surgeons' Committee on Trauma. *Advanced Trauma Life Support (ATLS) Program for Doctors: Student Manual.* 10th ed. Chicago, IL: American College of Surgeons; 2018.

technologies may be useful for assessment and monitoring response to treatment.[30,62,63] In cardiogenic shock, cardiac output and cardiac index decrease; however, RAP, pulmonary artery pressure (PAP), and PAOP increase as pressure and volume back up into the pulmonary circulation and the right side of the heart. A chest radiograph, 12-lead electrocardiogram, and transthoracic or transesophageal echocardiogram may assist in diagnosis of cardiogenic shock.

Treatment of cardiogenic shock focuses on promoting myocardial contractility, decreasing the myocardial oxygen demand, and increasing the oxygen supply to the damaged tissue. Administer oxygen to increase DO_2 to the ischemic muscle and preserve myocardial tissue.

Aggressive management after a myocardial infarction includes percutaneous coronary interventions, with or without intracoronary stent placement; fibrinolytic agents when primary percutaneous coronary intervention is not available; glycoprotein IIb/IIIa inhibitors; and beta-blockers to limit the size of the infarction. Pain relief and rest reduce the workload of the heart and the infarct size.

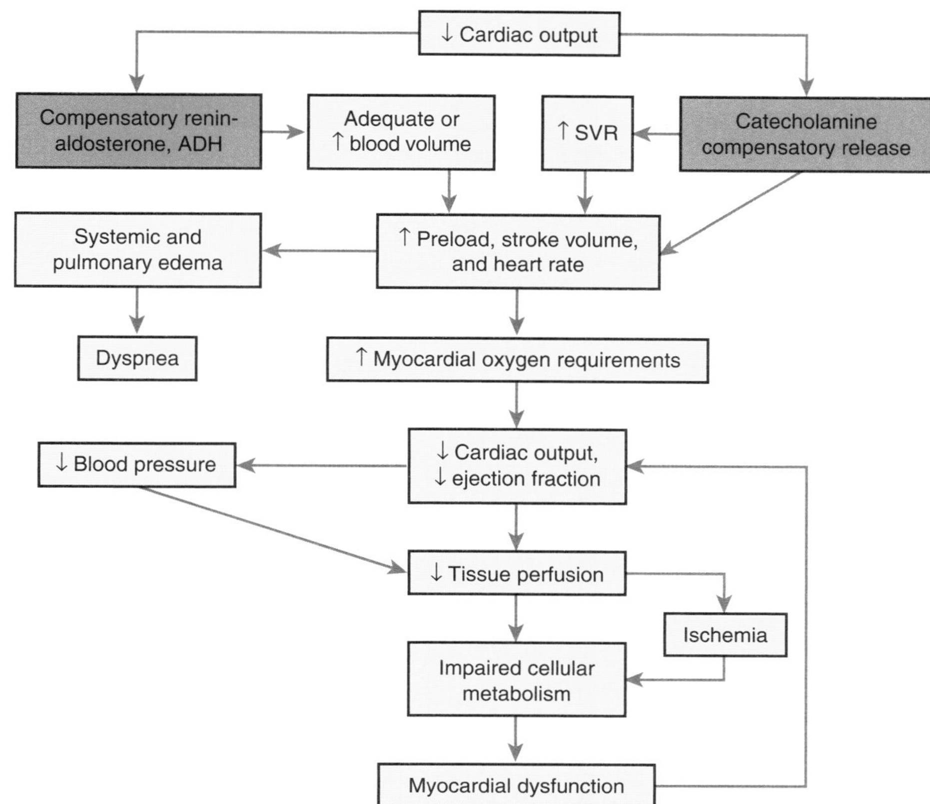

Fig. 12.7 Cardiogenic shock. Cardiogenic shock becomes life-threatening when compensatory mechanisms *(orange boxes)* increase myocardial oxygen requirements. *ADH,* Antidiuretic hormone; *SVR,* systemic vascular resistance. (From Rogers JL. *McCance & Huether's Pathophysiology: The Biologic Basis for Disease in Adults and Children.* 9th ed. St. Louis, MO: Elsevier; 2024.)

Medications are administered to decrease preload (RAP and PAOP), decrease afterload (SVR), increase cardiac index, and increase contractility (Table 12.5). Diuretics (e.g., furosemide) and venous vasodilators (e.g., morphine, nitroglycerin, nitroprusside) reduce preload and venous return to the heart. Nitroglycerin at low doses (<1 mcg/kg/min) causes venous vasodilation to decrease preload. At higher doses (>1 mcg/kg/min), arterial vasodilation decreases afterload. Administer medications cautiously because they may cause hypotension, further contributing to cellular hypoperfusion.

Positive inotropic medications (e.g., milrinone, dobutamine) are given to increase the contractile force of the heart. As contractility increases, ventricular emptying improves, filling pressures decrease (i.e., RAP and PAOP), and stroke volume improves. The improved stroke volume increases cardiac output and improves tissue perfusion. However, positive inotropic medications also increase myocardial oxygen demand and must be used cautiously in patients with myocardial ischemia.

Afterload reduction may be achieved by the cautious administration of arterial vasodilators (e.g., nitroprusside) to decrease SVR, increase stroke volume, and increase cardiac index. Closely monitor blood pressure to keep the mean arterial pressure (MAP) above 65 mm Hg to ensure organ perfusion. Significant hypotension may limit the use of arterial vasodilators because coronary artery perfusion pressure may be reduced and worsen myocardial ischemia. In this situation, afterload reduction is achieved through the insertion of an IABP.

The IABP is a mechanical circulatory support device that provides *counterpulsation therapy* concurrently with pharmacological support. The IABP improves coronary artery perfusion, reduces afterload, and improves perfusion to vital organs. Desired outcomes for a patient in cardiogenic shock with an IABP include decreased SVR, diminished symptoms of myocardial ischemia (i.e., chest pain, ST-segment elevation), and increased stroke volume and cardiac output.

Other mechanical circulatory devices may be required to temporarily support a failing ventricle that has not responded to IABP and pharmacological therapy.[64] The devices are used to treat cardiogenic shock by allowing the ventricle to recover or to support the patient awaiting cardiac transplantation. Examples include the Impella (Abiomed, Danvers, MA), TandemHeart (LivaNova, Houston, TX), or extracorporeal membrane oxygenation (ECMO). These devices can support the left ventricle, the right ventricle, or both ventricles.[65] Additional information about the IABP and other mechanical assist devices is provided in Chapter 13, Cardiovascular Alterations.

Distributive Shock

Distributive shock, also known as vasodilatory shock, describes several types of shock that manifest with widespread vasodilation and decreased SVR, including neurogenic, anaphylactic, and septic shock. Vasodilation increases the vascular capacity, but the blood volume is unchanged, resulting in relative hypovolemia. This causes a decrease in venous return to the right side of the heart and a reduction in ventricular filling pressures. Anaphylactic shock and septic shock are also complicated by an increase in capillary permeability, which decreases intravascular volume, further compromising venous return. In all forms of distributive shock, stroke volume, cardiac output, and blood pressure eventually decrease, resulting in decreased tissue perfusion and tissue hypoxia, leading to impaired cellular metabolism.

Neurogenic Shock. Neurogenic shock occurs when a disturbance in the nervous system affects the vasomotor center in the medulla. In healthy persons, the vasomotor center initiates sympathetic stimulation of nerve fibers that travel down the spinal cord and out to the periphery, where they innervate the smooth muscles of the blood vessels and cause vasoconstriction. In neurogenic shock, there is an interruption of impulse transmission or a blockage of sympathetic outflow that results in vasodilation, inhibition of baroreceptor response, and impaired thermoregulation. These reactions produce vasodilation with decreased SVR, venous return, preload, and cardiac output and a relative hypovolemia. Fig. 12.8 summarizes the pathophysiology of neurogenic shock.

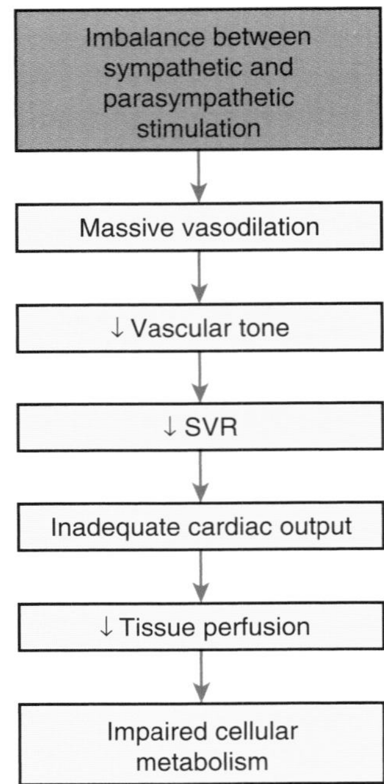

Fig. 12.8 Neurogenic shock. *SVR,* Systemic vascular resistance. (From Rogers JL. *McCance & Huether's Pathophysiology: The Biologic Basis for Disease in Adults and Children.* 9th ed. St. Louis, MO: Elsevier; 2024.)

Causes of neurogenic shock include direct and indirect insults to the nervous system. Spinal cord injuries are the most common cause of neurogenic shock, specifically at or above the level of T6.[5] Neurogenic shock may also result from surgical intervention including anesthesia, cerebral ischemia, Guillain-Barré syndrome, and injury to the medulla or triggered by extreme stress or severe pain.[66–68]

The most profound features of neurogenic shock are bradycardia with hypotension from the decreased sympathetic activity. The skin is frequently warm, dry, and flushed. Hypothermia develops from uncontrolled heat loss. Initiate rewarming slowly because rapid rewarming may cause vasodilation and worsen the patient's hemodynamic status. Venous pooling in the lower extremities promotes the formation of deep vein thrombosis, which increases the risk of a pulmonary embolism.

Management focuses on treating the cause, including reversal of contributing medications. Immobilization of spinal injuries or surgical intervention to stabilize the injury assists in preventing severe neurogenic shock.[68] For patients receiving spinal anesthesia, elevate the head of the bed to prevent the progression of the spinal blockade up the cord. Infuse IV fluids to treat hypotension and reassess volume status to prevent fluid overload and cerebral or spinal cord edema.

Vasopressors are frequently required to restore vascular tone and maintain perfusion. Alpha- and beta-adrenergic medications, such norepinephrine, are preferred. Pure alpha-adrenergic agents, such as phenylephrine, are associated with persistent bradycardia and are avoided.[68] The target MAP for patients with a spinal injury may be as high as 85 to 90 mm Hg in the first 7 days to improve spinal cord perfusion.[69] Atropine is administered for symptomatic bradycardia, but a temporary or permanent pacemaker may be required.

CHECK YOUR UNDERSTANDING

3. A patient is involved in a sports-related injury. The patient is unable to move or feel their upper and lower extremities. The patient is hypotensive and bradycardic. What type of shock is suspected, and what priority interventions should the nurse recommend?
   A. Cardiogenic shock; initiation of intraaortic balloon pump
   B. Anaphylactic shock; administration of epinephrine IV
   C. Neurogenic shock; spinal stabilization, administration of isotonic fluids and norepinephrine
   D. Hypovolemic shock; administration of blood products via massive transfusion

Anaphylactic Shock. A severe allergic reaction can precipitate a distributive shock known as anaphylactic shock. Antigens, which are foreign substances to which someone is sensitive, initiate an antigen-antibody response. Table 12.6 lists some common antigens (e.g., foods, medications, animal bites or stings, chemicals) that cause anaphylaxis.

After an antigen enters the body, the antibodies (i.e., immunoglobulin E [IgE]) produced attach to mast cells and basophils. The greatest concentrations of mast cells are found in the lungs, around blood vessels, in connective tissue, and in the uterus. Mast cells are also found to a lesser extent in the kidneys, heart, skin, liver, spleen, and in the omentum of the gastrointestinal tract. Basophils circulate in the blood. Mast cells and basophils contain histamine and histamine-like substances, which are potent vasodilators.

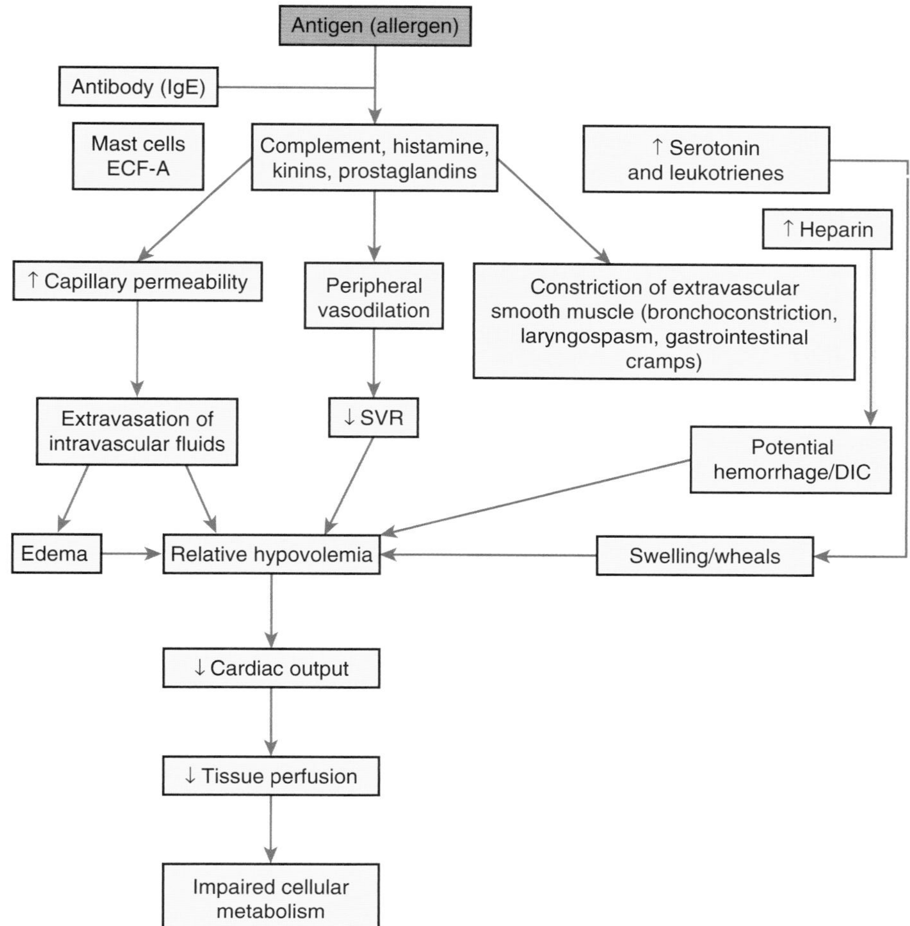

Fig. 12.9 Anaphylactic shock. *DIC,* Disseminated intravascular coagulation; *ECF-A,* eosinophil chemotactic factor of anaphylaxis; *IgE,* immunoglobulin E; *SVR,* systemic vascular resistance. (From Rogers JL. *McCance & Huether's Pathophysiology: The Biologic Basis for Disease in Adults and Children.* 9th ed. St. Louis, MO: Elsevier; 2024.)

The initial exposure (primary immune response) to the antigen does not usually cause harmful effects, but subsequent exposures to the antigen may cause an anaphylactic reaction (secondary immune response). The antigen-antibody reaction causes cellular breakdown and the release of powerful mediators from the mast cells and basophils. The mediators cause bronchoconstriction, excessive mucus secretion, vasodilation, increased capillary permeability, inflammation, gastrointestinal cramping, and cutaneous reactions that stimulate nerve endings, causing itching and pain. Fig. 12.9 summarizes the pathophysiology of anaphylactic shock. The combined effects result in decreased blood pressure, relative hypovolemia caused by vasodilation and fluid shifts, and symptoms of anaphylaxis that primarily affect the dermal, respiratory, and gastrointestinal systems.

Obtain a thorough history of allergies and medication reactions, especially reactions to medications with similar structures. Monitor the response to IV administration of medications, particularly antibiotics. Collaborate with the clinical pharmacist if a medication must be administered to a patient in whom a known or suspected allergy exists. In this situation, a small amount of medication may be given as a test dose or prior to administration of the full dose.[70]

Transfusion of blood or blood products can also result in allergic reactions. Observe the patient receiving any of these products closely for any signs of an allergic reaction (e.g., sudden shortness of breath, hives, tachycardia, hypotension, anxiety). Table 12.4 lists some common reactions and complications.

The clinical presentation of anaphylactic shock includes flushing, pruritus, urticaria, and angioedema (i.e., swelling of eyes, lips, tongue, hands, feet, and genitalia). Cough, runny nose, nasal congestion, hoarseness, dysphonia, and dyspnea are common because of upper airway obstruction from edema of the larynx, epiglottis, or vocal cords. Stridor may occur as a result of laryngeal edema. Lower airway obstruction may result from diffuse bronchoconstriction and cause wheezing and chest tightness. Tachycardia and hypotension occur, and the patient may show signs of pulmonary edema. Gastrointestinal symptoms of nausea, vomiting, cramping, abdominal pain, and diarrhea may also occur. Neurological symptoms include lethargy and decreased consciousness. Elevated levels of IgE are seen on laboratory analysis.

Goals of therapy are to remove the antigen, reverse the effects of the mediators, and promote adequate tissue perfusion. If the anaphylactic reaction results from medications, contrast dye, or blood or blood products, immediately stop the infusion and support airway, ventilation, and circulation. Laryngeal edema may be severe enough to require intubation or cricothyrotomy if swelling is so severe that an endotracheal tube cannot be placed. Administer oxygen, usually by nonrebreather mask, to keep the SpO_2 greater than 90%. Obtain IV access and volume resuscitate with IV fluids. Remove the offending agent; for example, remove a stinger, administer antivenom, stop the medication, or flush the skin to remove a tropical allergen.

Epinephrine is the medication of choice for treating anaphylactic shock.[71–73] Epinephrine is an adrenergic agent that promotes bronchodilation and vasoconstriction. Anaphylaxis is often treated with epinephrine autoinjectors (e.g., EpiPens, Auvi-Q), as many allergic individuals carry this life-saving medication. An epinephrine infusion may be needed for continued refractory analphylaxis.[71] To block histamine release, an H_1-receptor blocker (e.g., diphenhydramine [Benadryl]) or an H_2-receptor blocker (e.g., famotidine [Pepcid]), may decrease some of the cutaneous symptoms of anaphylaxis, but both are considered second-line treatment.[71] Corticosteroids such as methylprednisolone (Solu-Medrol) are used to reduce inflammation. Nebulized bronchodilators may be given for wheezing. Inotropic and vasoactive medications may be required.

CLINICAL JUDGMENT ACTIVITY

Determine the type of shock associated with the following hemodynamic changes:

1. Bradycardia, decreased SVR, decreased SvO_2
2. Tachycardia, decreased SVR, increased SvO_2 (early)
3. Decreased RAP, PAOP, and SvO_2; increased SVR

Septic Shock. Sepsis and septic shock are medical emergencies.[12] *Sepsis* is defined as life-threatening organ dysfunction caused by a dysregulated host response to infection.[74] *Septic shock* is a life-threatening complication of sepsis in which the underlying circulatory and cellular or metabolic abnormalities are profound enough to substantially increase mortality. The definitions and diagnostic criteria are presented in Table 12.8. The criteria provide a tool for recognizing and diagnosing sepsis quickly, prompting the search for an infectious source, and initiating the appropriate therapy.

Invasion of the host by a microorganism or an infection begins the process that may progress to sepsis, followed by

TABLE 12.8 Sepsis Continuum: Definitions, Diagnostic Criteria, and Management

Clinical Condition and Definition	Diagnostic Criteria	Management
Sepsis: Life-threatening organ dysfunction caused by a dysregulated host response to infection	Suspected or known source of infection Organ dysfunction can be identified by Sequential (sepsis-related) Organ Failure Assessment (SOFA), quick SOFA (qSOFA) score ≥2, or other organ dysfunction indicators such as: SBP <90 mm Hg or MAP <65 mm Hg Urine output <0.05 mL/kg/h × 2 h or creatinine >2.0 mg/dL Creatinine >0.5 mg/dL above baseline if history of chronic kidney disease Platelets <100,000 mm³ INR >1.5 or aPTT >60 sec Serum lactate >2 mmol/L New need for noninvasive or invasive ventilation New need for oxygen Change in mental status	Medical emergency and treatment should be prompt Administer antibiotics within 1 h of recognition Use lactate and capillary refill to guide resuscitation Monitor for hypotension Administer at least 30 mL/kg of IV crystalloid fluid within the first 3 h for hypotension or increased lactate ≥4 mmol/L Use dynamic measures to assess response to fluid Maintain adequate ventilation and oxygenation Remove/treat source of infection Monitor and support organ function
Septic shock: Sepsis in which circulatory and cellular or metabolic dysfunction substantially increase mortality	Subset of sepsis characterized by persistent hypotension requiring vasopressors to maintain a MAP ≥65 mm Hg AND a serum lactate >2 mmol/L despite fluid resuscitation	Ensure the above management of sepsis is completed Maximize oxygen delivery; minimize oxygen demand Administer vasopressors to maintain a target MAP >65 mm Hg Administer vasoactive medications Correct acid-base abnormalities Monitor and support organ function

aPTT, Activated partial thromboplastin time; *INR,* international normalized ratio; *MAP,* mean arterial pressure; *SBP,* systolic blood pressure.
Modified from Levy M, Evans L, Rhodes A. The surviving Sepsis Campaign bundle. *Crit Care Med.* 2018;46(6):997–1000; Evans L, Rhodes A, Alhazzani W et al. Surviving Sepsis Campaign. *Crit Care Med.* 2021;49(11):e1063-e1143; Singer M. Deutschman CS, Seymour CW et al. The third international consensus definitions for sepsis and septic shock (Sepsis-3). *JAMA.* 2016;315(8):801–810.

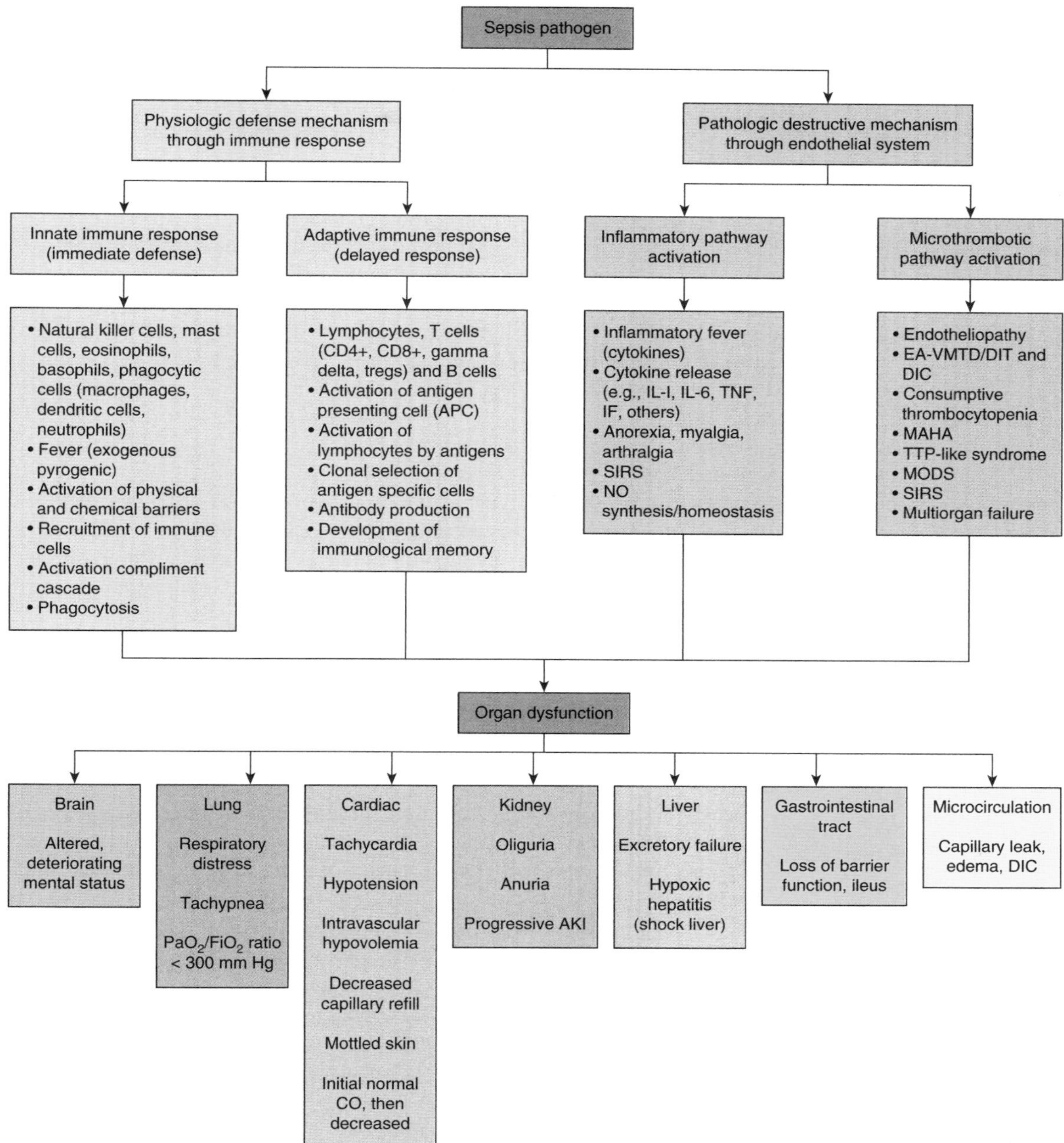

Fig. 12.10 Sepsis pathophysiology and immune response. *AKI*, Acute kidney injury; *CO, cardiac output; DIC*, disseminated intravascular coagulation; *DIT*, disseminated intravascular microthrombosis; *EA-VMTD*, endotheliopathy-associated vascular microthrombotic disease; *FiO_2, fraction of inspired oxygen; MAHA*, microangiopathic hemolytic anemia; *MODS*, multiorgan dysfunction syndrome; *NO;* nitric oxide; *IF*, interferon; *IL*, interleukin; *PaO_2, partial pressure of oxygen, SIRS*, systemic inflammatory response syndrome; *TNF*, tumor necrosis factor; *TTP*, thrombotic thrombocytopenic purpura. (Adapted from Chang JC. Sepsis and septic shock: endothelial molecular pathogenesis associated with vascular microthombotic disease. *Thromb J.* 2019;17:10. https://doi.org/10.1186/s12959-019-0198-4.)

septic shock, which can progress to MODS. After a pathogen (bacteria, virus, parasite) has invaded the host, an inflammatory response is initiated to restore homeostasis. For reasons not completely understood, the inflammatory response may progress to septic shock and MODS (Fig. 12.10).

An infection triggers a complex set of events. The immune response is the body's defense mechanism and consists of a complex array of cellular and chemical mediators. The innate response occurs when a pathogen is recognized from a previous exposure. The immune response is amplified, leading to the clinical and cellular symptoms of sepsis. The response is thought to eradicate damage-associated molecular patterns (DAMPs) and pathogen-associated molecular patterns (PAMPs) but also may become over activated and lead to increasing inflammation.

The adaptive immune response triggers a number of immunoregulatory cells such as T and CD4+ cells in sepsis that experience cell death with an ineffective immune defense and contribute to immunosuppression. The inflammatory response is activated, and cytokines are released. Cytokines are proinflammatory or antiinflammatory. In sepsis, continued activation of proinflammatory cytokines overwhelms the antiinflammatory cytokines, and excessive systemic inflammation results.

A state of enhanced coagulation occurs through stimulation of the microthrombotic pathway. This results in the generation of thrombin and the formation of microemboli that impair blood flow and organ perfusion. Fibrinolysis is activated in response to the activation of the coagulation cascade to promote clot breakdown. However, activation is followed by inhibition, further promoting coagulopathy. This imbalance among inflammation, coagulation, and fibrinolysis results in systemic inflammation, widespread coagulopathy, and microvascular thrombi that impair tissue perfusion, leading to MODS.

As sepsis progresses with its dysregulated host response, producing profound vasodilation and increased capillary permeability, tachycardia, hypotension, and low SVR result. Although norepinephrine and the renin-angiotensin-aldosterone system are activated in response to this clinical state, the molecules are unable to enter the cells, and hypotension and vasodilation persist unless treated.

Sepsis can advance to septic shock with signs of end-organ hypoperfusion.[12,74,75] Symptoms include hypotension, chills, decreased urine output, decreased skin perfusion, poor capillary refill, skin mottling, decreased platelets, petechiae, hyperglycemia, and unexplained changes in mental status.[12,14]

Factors that increase the risk of developing sepsis include immunosuppression or situations that increase the risk of infection (Table 12.6). There are multiple electronic health record (EHR) alert tools available, such as the National Early Warning Score (NEWS), Modified Early Warning Score (MEWS) or EHR, specifically for identifying patients with suspected infection who are at risk for sepsis. The Sequential Organ Failure Assessment (SOFA) evaluates respiratory, coagulation, hepatic, cardiovascular, central nervous, and renal systems in a patient already identified as or suspected of having sepsis.[74,76] The patient's risk of morbidity and mortality increases with the score. The quick Sequential Organ Failure Assessment (qSOFA) tool uses just three criteria—respiratory rate of 22 breaths/min or faster, Glasgow Coma Scale less than 15, and a systolic blood pressure of 100 mm Hg or lower—to identify patients who are likely to have worse outcomes.[74] The SOFA better predicts risk of death for patients with an infection while in the critical care unit. The qSOFA better identifies patients at high risk of death in the hospital.[77]

Infection prevention efforts include proper handwashing, use of aseptic technique, and awareness of at-risk patients. Most critically ill patients are debilitated and have many potential portals of entry for bacterial invasion. Meticulous technique is required during procedures such as suctioning, dressing changes, wound care, and when handling catheters or tubes. Maintain an awareness of patient-specific baseline assessment criteria such as mental status and vital signs. Frequently assess for signs and symptoms of infection, including elevated or decreased temperature, increased heart rate, increased respiratory rate, hypotension, and changes in mentation. Evaluate wounds, as well as IV and device insertion sites, for signs and symptoms of infection. Review laboratory results, including white blood cell count, differential counts, and cultures, for the identification of infection.[78]

CLINICAL JUDGMENT ACTIVITY

Consider factors in the critically ill patient that increase susceptibility to the development of sepsis and septic shock. Discuss nursing interventions to reduce the risk of infection.

Gram-positive bacteria, such as *Staphylococcus aureus* and *Streptococcus* species, can lead to sepsis and septic shock. These bacteria release a potent toxin that exerts its effects within hours. Gram-positive infection has been associated with the use of tampons in menstruating women (toxic shock syndrome), but it is also seen after vaginal and cesarean delivery and in patients with surgical wounds, abscesses, infected burns, abrasions, insect bites, herpes zoster, cellulitis, septic abortion, and osteomyelitis.

Infections caused by Gram-negative organisms are associated with a high financial burden due to antimicrobial resistance and high morbidity and mortality.[79] Common sites of infection for both Gram-positive and Gram-negative organisms include the pulmonary, urinary, and gastrointestinal systems, as well as skin and soft tissue.

Pneumonia is a common trigger for sepsis.[80] Infection-related, ventilator-associated conditions such as pneumonia are significant risk factors for sepsis. Implement nursing interventions for ventilated patients to reduce the risk of ventilator-associated conditions (see Chapter 10, Ventilatory Assistance). For example, provide regular oral care, titrate to the lightest level of sedation, and assess readiness to wean and extubate.[81]

Other causes of sepsis include parasitic, fungal, and viral infections such as influenza or severe acute respiratory syndrome coronavirus-2 (SARS-CoV-2, the virus that causes Coronavirus disease [COVID-19]). While these infections may not require antibiotics, they can lead to sepsis and septic shock. Patients with these types of infections require other sepsis bundle treatment measures and specific treatment related to the causal agent.[82,83]

Timely identification of the causative organism and the initiation of appropriate antibiotics (as indicated) improve survival of patients with sepsis or septic shock.[12] Remove invasive devices (i.e., source control) if they are suspected to be the cause of the infection. Surgery may be required to locate the source of infection, drain an abscess, remove a tunnelled line, or debride necrotic tissue.

Obtain blood cultures and cultures of other suspicious sources before initiating antibiotics. The Surviving Sepsis Campaign international guidelines recommend obtaining these cultures first unless doing so will delay the initial administration of antibiotics by more than 45 minutes.[12] The choice of the initial antibiotic is directed toward the most likely organism. Empiric, broad-spectrum antibiotics are frequently initiated within 1 hour of identification of sepsis.[12,77] The antibiotic regimen is modified, if indicated, after culture and sensitivity results are available.

The application of sepsis bundle measures decreases the mortality rate among patients with sepsis and septic shock,

BOX 12.1 Surviving Sepsis Campaign Bundles

Within 1 hour of sepsis recognition:

- Measure lactate level. Remeasure if initial lactate is >2 mmol/L.
- Obtain blood cultures prior to administration of antibiotics.
- Administer broad-spectrum antibiotics.
- Rapidly administer 30 mL/kg crystalloid for hypotension or initial lactate ≥4 mmol/L.
- Administer vasopressors if patient is hypotensive during or after fluid resuscitation to maintain MAP ≥65 mm Hg.

From Levy MM, Evans LE, Rhodes A. The Surviving Sepsis Campaign bundle: 2018 update. *Crit Care Med.* 2018;46(6):997–1000.
MAP, Mean arterial pressure.

and they should be initiated within the first hour of sepsis recognition (Box 12.1).[12,84,85] The sepsis bundle includes IV fluid resuscitation if MAP is less than 65 mm Hg or lactate level is ≥4 mmol/L.[85]

Isotonic crystalloid solutions are infused for fluid resuscitation, with some evidence suggesting that balanced solutions, such as Lactated Ringer's, are preferred.[12,34,35] Colloids may also be given after the initial crystalloid resuscitation.[12] Administer vasopressors to increase SVR and MAP if hypoperfusion persists despite aggressive fluid resuscitation. Norepinephrine is the first choice for vasopressor support.[12] A low dose of vasopressin may be added to the norepinephrine dose to maintain the MAP ≥65 mm Hg. Low-dose vasopressin causes vasoconstriction without the adverse effects of tachycardia and ventricular ectopy seen with catecholamines such as dopamine or norepinephrine. At higher doses, vasopressin may cause cardiac, digital, and splanchnic ischemia.[12] Adding epinephrine is the next consideration if the required norepinephrine dose continues to escalate to maintain adequate MAP.[12] Dobutamine may be added to increase the myocardial contractility and improve the cardiac index and DO_2 in patients who have persistent hypoperfusion despite adequate fluid resuscitation and ongoing use of vasopressors.[12] Transfusion of PRBC is recommended when hemoglobin is less than 7 g/dL.[12] IV hydrocortisone is recommended for ongoing vasopressor requirements for at least 4 hours.[12]

Hyperglycemia and insulin resistance are common in the patient with sepsis. Although aggressive management of blood glucose is no longer advocated, institute a blood glucose management protocol when two consecutive blood glucose levels are greater than 180 mg/dL.[12]

Pyrogens (polypeptides that produce fever) aid in activation of the immune response. Treatment of fever has no clear effect on mortality but may be considered.[53] Treatment of fever includes administration of antipyretics (acetaminophen, ibuprofen, or aspirin). Avoid overcooling because hypothermia adversely affects DO_2 and may result in shivering, which increases oxygen consumption.

Obstructive Shock

Obstructive shock (extracardiac) occurs when a blockage or compression impairs circulatory blood flow from the heart.

CLINICAL EXEMPLAR

Quality and Safety

The nurse in the critical care unit identified lack of consistent documentation of "time zero" (the time at which sepsis or septic shock is identified) for patients transferred from the emergency department with sepsis. The nurse noted time zero was inconsistently communicated during verbal handoff and documentation was not always located in the same place in the electronic medical record. Lack of a standardized way to communicate time zero often led to confusion and missed opportunities to adhere to the sepsis bundle guidelines. The nurse collaborated with nursing leadership, nursing quality, and nursing informatics to create a standardized area for time zero documentation in the electronic health record. Standardized documentation of time zero led to improved adherence with sepsis bundle guidelines and provided a framework for development of a sepsis tracking tool within the electronic health record.

Causes of obstructive shock include impaired diastolic filling (e.g., cardiac tamponade, tension pneumothorax, constrictive pericarditis, compression of the great veins), increased right ventricular afterload (e.g., pulmonary embolism, severe pulmonary hypertension, increased intrathoracic pressures), and increased left ventricular afterload (e.g., aortic dissection, systemic embolization, aortic stenosis). Obstruction of the heart or great vessels impedes venous return to the right side of the heart or prevents effective pumping action of the heart. This results in decreased cardiac output, hypotension, decreased tissue perfusion, and impaired cellular metabolism (Fig. 12.11).

Common clinical findings in obstructive shock include chest pain, dyspnea, jugular venous distension, and hypoxia. Other findings depend on the cause. Cardiac tamponade manifests with muffled heart sounds, hypotension, and pulsus paradoxus. *Pulsus paradoxus* is a decrease in systolic blood pressure of more than 10 mm Hg during inspiration. Tension pneumothorax is characterized by diminished breath sounds on the affected side and tracheal shift away from the affected side. A massive pulmonary embolism presents with clinical manifestations of right ventricular failure (jugular venous distension, peripheral edema, hepatomegaly). Aortic dissection is characterized by complaints of ripping chest pain that radiates to the back; pulse differences between the left and right side; and a widened mediastinum on the chest radiograph, echocardiogram, or CT scan.

Obstructive shock may be prevented or treated by aggressive interventions to relieve the source of the compression or obstruction. Cardiac tamponade is treated by a *pericardiocentesis,* which is the removal of fluid from the pericardial sac. A tension pneumothorax from blunt or penetrating chest injuries is relieved by a needle *thoracentesis* to remove the accumulated intrathoracic pressure. The risk of pulmonary embolism is reduced by early surgical reduction of long bone fractures, devices to enhance circulation in immobile patients (e.g., intermittent pneumatic compression devices), progressive mobility and prophylactic anticoagulant therapy. Pulmonary embolism is treated based on hemodynamic stability and right heart strain and may include intravenous thrombolysis, interventional or surgical thrombus removal, and anticoagulation.[86,87]

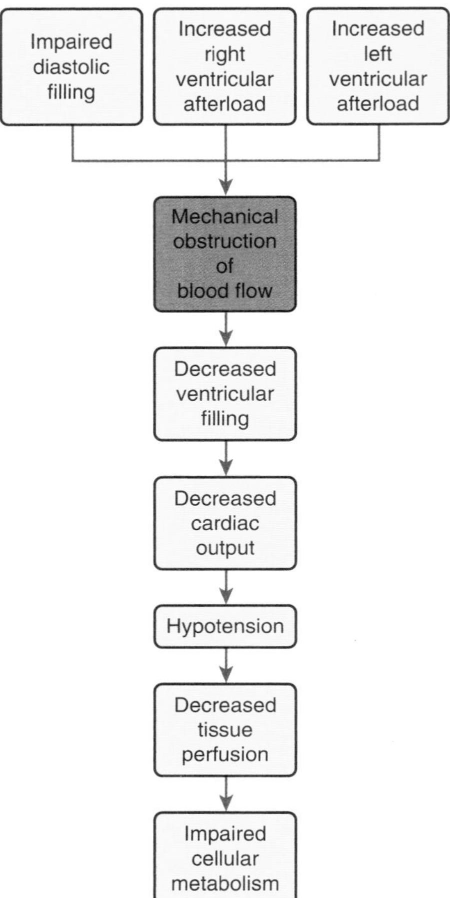

Fig. 12.11 Obstructive shock.

MULTIPLE ORGAN DYSFUNCTION SYNDROME

MODS is the progressive dysfunction of two or more organ systems as a result of an uncontrolled inflammatory response to severe illness or injury.[1] Organ dysfunction can progress to organ failure and death. The most common cause of MODS is septic shock; however, MODS can occur after any severe injury or disease process that activates a massive systemic inflammatory response, which includes any classification of shock. The immune system and the body's response to stress can cause maldistribution of circulating volume, global tissue hypoxia, and metabolic alterations that damage organs. MODS frequently leads to a persistent, prolonged state known as *chronically critically ill*.[88] The risk of death associated with MODS is 54% when two organ systems fail and increases to 100% when five organ systems fail.[1]

Pathophysiology

Damage to organs may be primary or secondary. In *primary MODS*, there is direct injury to an organ from shock, trauma, burn, or infection with impaired perfusion that results in dysfunction. Decreased perfusion may be localized or systemic. The stress and inflammatory responses are activated, with the release of catecholamines and activation of mediators that affect cellular activity (Fig. 12.12).

Secondary MODS is a consequence of widespread systemic inflammation that results in dysfunction of organs not involved with the initial insult. It occurs in response to altered regulation of the acute immune and inflammatory responses. Failure to control the inflammatory response leads to excessive production of inflammatory and biochemical mediators that cause widespread vascular endothelium and organ damage. The interaction of injured organs then leads to self-perpetuating inflammation with maldistribution of blood flow and hypermetabolism.

Maldistribution of blood flow refers to the uneven distribution of flow to various organs and between the large vessels and capillary beds. It is caused by vasodilation, increased capillary permeability, selective vasoconstriction, and impaired microvascular circulation. This impaired blood flow leads to impaired tissue perfusion and decreased oxygen supply to the cells. The organs most severely affected are the lungs, splanchnic bed, liver, and kidneys.

Hypermetabolism with altered carbohydrate, fat, and lipid metabolism is initially compensatory to meet the body's increased demands for energy. Eventually, hypermetabolism becomes detrimental, placing tremendous demands on the heart as cardiac output increases up to twice the normal value. Hyperglycemia occurs as gluconeogenesis by the liver increases and glucose use by the cells decreases.

Decreased DO_2 to the cells from maldistribution of blood flow and increased oxygen needs of the cells from hypermetabolism create an imbalance in oxygen supply and demand. In MODS, the amount of oxygen consumed depends on the amount of oxygen that can be delivered to the cells. Hypoxemia, cellular acidosis, and impaired cellular function result, leading to multiple organ failure.

The clinical picture of MODS is caused by inflammatory mediator damage, tissue hypoxia, and hypermetabolism. Damage to the organs is usually sequential rather than simultaneous. The first system frequently affected is the pulmonary system, with ARDS developing within 12 to 24 hours after the initial insult. Coagulopathy frequently develops, followed by renal, hepatic, and intestinal impairment.[1] Failure of the cardiovascular system or neurological system is frequently fatal. MODS progresses from minor dysfunction of one or more organs to multiple organs requiring support.

Diagnosis

Criteria used in the diagnoses of organ dysfunction are described in Table 12.9. Pulmonary dysfunction manifests with tachypnea, hypoxemia despite high levels of supplemental oxygen, and chest radiographic changes. Hematological dysfunction manifests with petechiae, bleeding, thrombocytopenia, prolonged prothrombin time (PT) and activated partial thromboplastin time (aPTT), increased fibrin split products, and a positive D-dimer. The earliest sign of hepatic dysfunction is hypoglycemia, which is followed by increased levels of liver enzymes and bilirubin (jaundice), prolonged PT, and decreased albumin. The first indication of intestinal dysfunction is frequently intolerance of enteral feedings with abdominal distension and increased residual volumes greater than 500 mL.[57] Renal dysfunction progresses from oliguria to anuria, increased levels of blood urea nitrogen and creatinine, and fluid and electrolyte imbalances. Tachycardia (frequently with dysrhythmias), hypotension, and

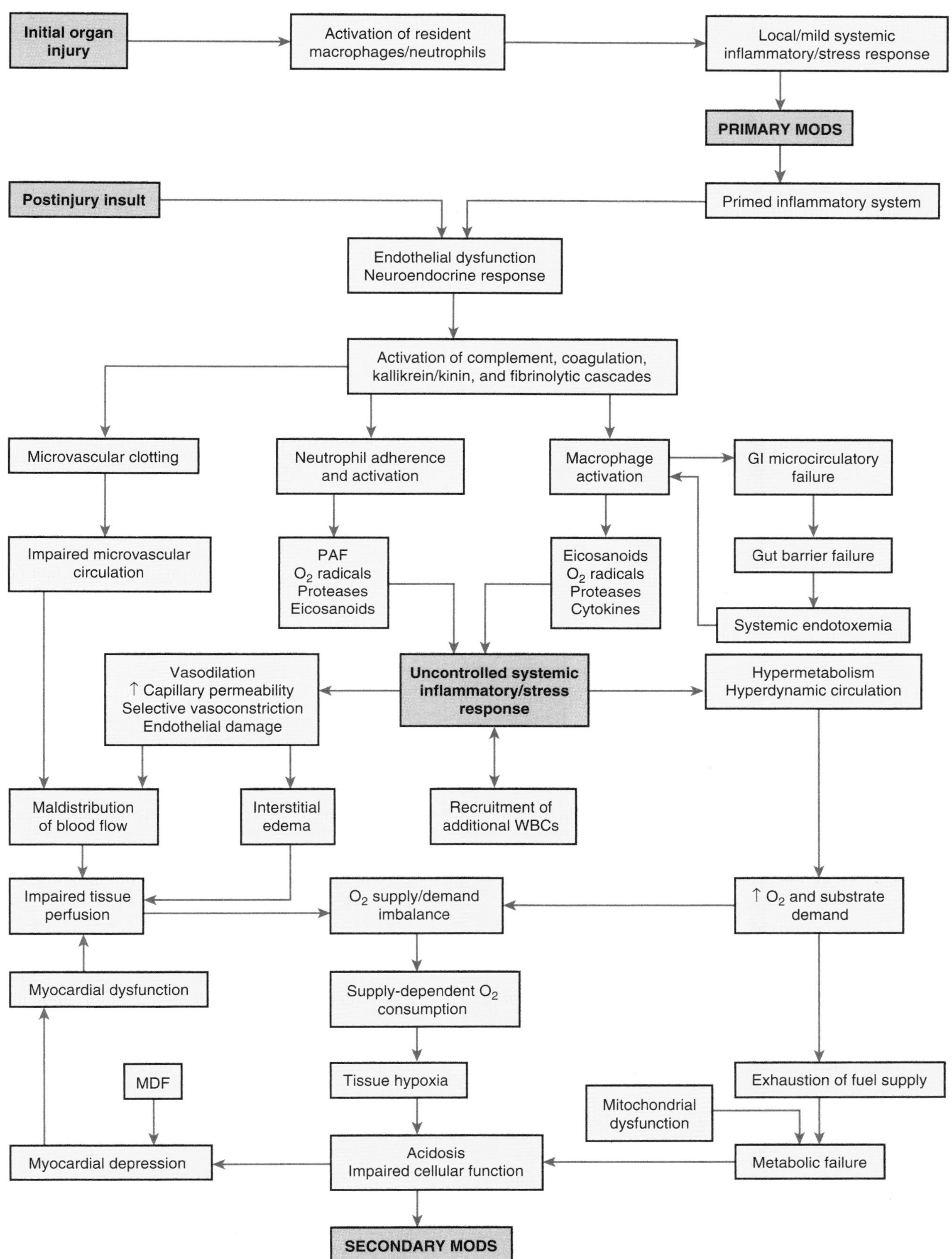

Fig. 12.12 Pathogenesis of multiple organ dysfunction syndrome (MODS). *GI,* Gastrointestinal; *MDF,* myocardial depressant factor; *PAF,* platelet-activating factor; *WBCs,* white blood cells. (From Rogers JL. *McCance & Huether's Pathophysiology: The Biologic Basis for Disease in Adults and Children.* 9th ed. St. Louis, MO: Elsevier; 2024.)

TABLE 12.9 **Multiple Organ Dysfunction Syndrome**

System	Dysfunction	Clinical Presentation
Pulmonary	Acute respiratory distress syndrome (ARDS)*	Predisposing factor such as shock or sepsis Within 1 week of a clinical insult OR new or worsening respiratory symptoms Respiratory failure is not fully explained by fluid overload or cardiac failure Bilateral opacities on chest imaging PaO_2/FiO_2 ratio ≤300 with either PEEP or CPAP ≥5 Dyspnea Tachypnea
Cardiovascular	Hyperdynamic	Increased oxygen consumption Increased cardiac output Tachycardia
	Hypodynamic	Myocardial depression Decreased oxygen consumption Decreased cardiac output
Hematological	Disseminated intravascular coagulation	Fibrin split products >1:40 or D-dimer >2 mg/L Thrombocytopenia Prolonged PT and aPTT INR >1.5 Bleeding Petechiae
Renal	Acute tubular necrosis	Oliguria ↑ Serum creatinine, ↑ BUN Urine sodium >20 mEq/L
Liver	Hepatic dysfunction/failure	↑ Serum bilirubin ↑ AST, ALT, LDH Jaundice Hepatomegaly ↑ Serum ammonia ↓ Serum albumin
CNS	Cerebral ischemia or infarction	Lethargy Altered level of consciousness progressing to unresponsiveness Hyperthermia Hypothermia
Metabolic	Lactic acidosis	↑ Serum lactate level

*Adapted from ARDS Definition Task Force, Ranieri VM, Rubenfeld GD et al. Acute respiratory distress syndrome: the Berlin Definition. *JAMA*. 2012;307(23):2526–2533. https://doi.org/10.1001/jama.2012.5669.

ALT, Alanine transaminase; *aPTT*, activated partial thromboplastin time; *AST*, aspartate transaminase; *BUN*, blood urea nitrogen; *CNS*, central nervous system; CPAP, continuous positive airway pressure; *FiO_2*, fraction of inspired oxygen; *INR*, International Normalized Ratio; *LDH*, lactic dehydrogenase; *PaO_2*, partial pressure of arterial oxygen; PEEP, positive end-expiratory pressure; *PT*, prothrombin time.

hemodynamic alterations indicate cardiovascular dysfunction. Cerebral dysfunction manifests with confusion, a change in the level of consciousness, and focal neurological signs such as hemiparesis. The final response to MODS is hypotension unresponsive to fluids and vasopressors, followed by cardiac arrest.

Management

Management of MODS focuses on prevention, early recognition, and support.[89] Eliminate or control the initial source of inflammation and avoid a secondary insult. Remove potential sources of infection. Medical interventions include debriding necrotic tissue, draining abscesses, reducing the number of invasive procedures performed, and removing hematomas. Goals are to control infection, provide adequate tissue oxygenation, restore intravascular volume, and support organ function. Administer antibiotics or other antiinfectives as indicated. Implement adequate oxygen and assess ABGs and pulse oximetry to improve tissue oxygenation. Initiate aggressive fluid therapy with isotonic crystalloid solutions early during systemic vasodilation to promote DO_2 to the tissues.

Support must be provided for each organ. Respiratory failure is managed with mechanical ventilation with low tidal volumes, high oxygen concentrations, and appropriate positive end-expiratory pressure (PEEP) (see Chapter 10, Ventilatory Assistance, and Chapter 15, Acute Respiratory Failure).[49] Adequate nutrition and metabolic support are provided with enteral feedings (see Chapter 7, Nutritional Therapy). Acute kidney injury is managed with continuous renal replacement therapies or hemodialysis (see Chapter 16, Acute Kidney Injury). Inotropic medications (e.g., dobutamine) or vasopressor medications (e.g., norepinephrine or epinephrine) may be needed to maximize cardiac contractility and peripheral vasoconstriction to maintain cardiac output and blood pressure.

CASE STUDY

A 43-year-old patient had complaints of shortness of breath and tachycardia when evaluated in the emergency department. Medical history was significant for pulmonary sarcoidosis (an autoimmune disease) treated with oral prednisone daily. The patient reported a history of a dog bite to the right arm 7 days earlier, for which the patient did not receive treatment.

Initial assessment in the emergency department revealed the following: weight, 75 kg; temperature, 37.9°C (100.2 °F); blood pressure, 85/54 mm Hg; heart rate, 138 beats/min; respiratory rate, 28 breaths/min; and oxygen saturation, 91% on room air. Blood cultures were obtained. Initial laboratory results included the following: white blood cell count, 31,300/mm^3; hemoglobin, 12.8 g/dL; hematocrit, 38.5%; platelet count, 50,000/mm^3; blood urea nitrogen, 13 mg/dL; creatinine, 2.12 mmol/L; and lactate, 5 mmol/L. Three liters of Lactated Ringer's solution and a broad-spectrum antibiotic were administered.

The patient was admitted to the critical care unit for further treatment. An arterial catheter was placed in the left radial artery, and a central venous catheter (CVC) was placed in the right jugular vein. An infusion of norepinephrine was initiated for persistent hypotension after fluid resuscitation. The patient required endotracheal intubation due to increased work of breathing. The wound on the right arm was irrigated and debrided. When blood cultures were finalized with *Pasteurella multocida*, a common pathogen transmitted by dog bites, antibiotics were streamlined to treat appropriately. Extubation occurred on hospital day 5, and the patient transitioned out of the critical care unit on hospital day 7.

Questions

1. Based on the assessment findings in the emergency department, in what type of shock does the patient present? Discuss the patient's risk factors for this type of shock.
2. Given weight-based recommendations, how much crystalloid infusion was indicated for *initial* resuscitation in this case?
3. After initial resuscitation, what dynamic measures could be used to assess for ongoing fluid resuscitation needs? If resuscitation is no longer indicated based on dynamic measures, what other pharmacological interventions may be indicated?
4. The patient responded positively to the treatment and interventions implemented. What potential assessment findings would indicate the patient was not effectively responding to therapy?

KEY POINTS

- Shock is a life-threatening emergency; early recognition and management can help prevent progression to MODS.
- The clinical presentation of shock varies based by type and stage of shock.
- There are four categories of shock: hypovolemia, cardiogenic, obstructive, and distributive.
  - Hypovolemic shock occurs when the circulating blood volume is inadequate to fill the vascular network, whether from external or internal blood loss or other body-fluid losses.
  - Cardiogenic shock can occur when the heart fails to act as an effective pump.
  - Distributive shock describes several types of shock that manifest with widespread vasodilation and decreased systemic vascular resistance, including neurogenic, anaphylactic, and septic shock.
  - Obstructive shock occurs when a blockage or compression impairs circulatory blood flow from the heart.
- Each shock state requires identification and removal/reversal of the source or cause, as well as appropriate management with adequate resuscitation; maintaining perfusion, oxygenation, and body temperature; and nutritional and psychological support.
- Alterations in fluid balance are common in most shock states requiring resuscitation with crystalloids, albumin, and/or blood.
- MODS can progress to organ failure or death as the number of dysfunctional organ systems continue to increase secondary to an uncontrolled inflammatory response.

REFERENCES

1. Turner KC, Brashers, VL. Chapter 48: shock, multiple organ dysfunction syndrome and burns in adults. In: Rogers JL, ed. *McCance & Huether's Pathophysiology: The Biologic Basis for Disease in Adults and Children*. 9th ed. St. Louis, MO: Elsevier; 2024:1557–1590.
2. Turner KC, Brashers VL. Structure and function of the cardiovascular and lymphatic systems. In: Rogers JL, ed. *McCance & Huether's Pathophysiology: The Biologic Basis for Disease in Adults and Children*. 9th ed. St. Louis, MO: Elsevier; 2024:1020–1058.
3. Turner KC. Structure and function of the digestive system. In: Rogers JL, ed. *McCance & Huether's Pathophysiology: The Biologic Basis for Disease in Adults and Children*. 9th ed. St. Louis, MO: Elsevier; 2024:1285–1317.
4. Takahaski LK. Stress and disease. In: Rogers JL, ed. *McCance & Huether's Pathophysiology: The Biologic Basis for Disease in Adults and Children*. 9th ed. St. Louis, MO: Elsevier; 2024:310–328.
5. Turner KC, Brashers V. Mechanisms of hormonal regulation. In: Rogers JL, ed. *McCance & Huether's Pathophysiology: The Biologic Basis for Disease in Adults and Children*. 9th ed. St. Louis, MO: Elsevier; 2024:662–687.
6. Turner KC. Structure and function of the renal and urologic systems. In: Rogers JL, ed. *McCance & Huether's Pathophysiology: The Biologic Basis for Disease in Adults and Children*. 9th ed. St. Louis, MO: Elsevier; 2024:1211–1232.

7. Winton MB, Brashers VL. Alterations of pulmonary function. In: Rogers JL, ed. *McCance & Huether's Pathophysiology: The Biologic Basis for Disease in Adults and Children*. 9th ed. St. Louis, MO: Elsevier; 2023:1153–1190.
8. Turner KC. Structure and function of the neurologic system. In: Rogers JL, ed. *McCance & Huether's Pathophysiology: The Biologic Basis for Disease in Adults and Children*. 9th ed. St. Louis, MO: Elsevier; 2023:439–473.
9. Cox J. Risk factors for pressure injury development among critical care patients. *Crit Care Nurs Clin N Am*. 2020;32:473–488.
10. Delmore B, Cox J, Smith D, Chu AS, Rolnitzky L. Acute skin failure in the critical care patient. *Adv Skin Wound Care*. 2020;33:192–201.
11. American College of Chest Physicians/Society of Critical Care Medicine Consensus Conference. Definitions for sepsis and organ failure and guidelines for the use of innovative therapies in sepsis. *Crit Care Med*. 1992;20(6):864–874.
12. Darden DB, Moore FA, Brakenridge SC, et al. The effect of aging physiology on critical care. *Crit Care Clin*. 2021;37(1):135–150.
13. Pandya ST, Krishna SJ. Acute respiratory distress syndrome in pregnancy. *Indian J Crit Care Med*. 2021;25(Suppl 3):S241–S247.
14. Yeomans ER, Gilstrap LC. Physiologic changes in pregnancy and their impact on critical care. *Crit Care Med*. 2005;33(Suppl):S256–S258.
15. Crozier T. General care of the pregnant patient in the intensive care unit. *Semin Respir Crit Care Med*. 2017;38(02):208–217.
16. Evans L, Rhodes A, Alhazzani W, et al. Surviving Sepsis Campaign: international guidelines for management of sepsis and septic shock 2021. *Crit Care Med*. 2021;49(11):e1063–e1143.
17. Monnett X. Prediction of fluid responsiveness. What's new? *Ann Intensive Care*. 202212:46. https://doi.org/10.1186/s13613-022-01022-8.
18. Pickett JD, Bridges E, Kritek PA, Whitney JD. Responsiveness: systematic review. *Crit Care Nurs*. 2017;37(2):32–48.
19. Alvarado Sanchez JI, Caicedo Ruiz JD, Diaztagle Fernandez JJ, Amaya Zuniga WF, Ospina-Tascon GA, Cruz Martinez LE. Predictors of fluid responsiveness in critically ill patients mechanically ventilated at low tidal volumes: systematic review and meta-analysis. *Ann Intensive Care*. 2021;11(1):28. https://doi.org/10.1186/s13613-021-00817-5.
20. Bednarczyk JM, Fridfinnson JA, Kumar A, et al. Incorporating dynamic assessment of fluid responsiveness into goal-directed therapy: a systematic review and meta-analysis. *Crit Care Med*. 2017;45(9):1538–1545.
21. Toscani L, Aya HD, Antonakaki D, et al. What is the impact of the fluid challenge technique on diagnosis of fluid responsiveness? A systematic review and meta-analysis. *Critical Care*. 2017;21:207. https://doi.org/10.1186/s13054-017-1796-9.
22. De Backer D, Vincent J. The pulmonary artery catheter: is it still alive? *Curr Opin Crit Care*. 2018;24(3):204–208.
23. Meng M, Klingensmith NJ, Coopersmith CM. New insights into the gut as the driver of critical illness and organ failure. *Curr Opin Crit Care*. 2017;23(2):143–148.
24. Hariri G, Joffre J, Leblanc G, et al. Narrative review: clinical assessment of peripheral tissue perfusion in septic shock. *Ann Intensive Care*. 2019;9:37. https://doi.org/10.1186/s13613-019-0511-1.
25. Jouffroy R, Saade A, Tourtier JP, et al. Skin mottling score and capillary refill time to assess mortality of septic shock since pre-hospital setting. *Am J Emerg Med*. 2019;37(4):664–671.
26. Kayser SA, VanGilder CA, Ayello EA, Lachenbruch C. Prevalence and analysis of medical device-related pressure injuries: results from the International Pressure Ulcer Prevalence Survey. *Adv Skin Wound Care*. 2018;31(6):276–285.
27. National Pressure Ulcer Advisory Panel. *Pressure Ulcer Prevention Points*. https://www.npuap.org/resources/educational-and-clinical-resources/pressure-injury-prevention-points/. Published April 2019.
28. Meyhoff TS, Hjortrup PB, Wetterslev J, et al. Restriction of intravenous fluid in ICU patients with septic shock. *New Eng J Med*. 2022;386(26):2459–2470.
29. Barlow A, Barlow B, Tang N, Shah BM, King AE. Intravenous fluid management in critically ill adults: a review. *Crit Care Nurs*. 2020;40(6):e17–e27.
30. Braile-Sternieri MCVB, Mustafa EM, Ferreira VRR, et al. Main considerations of cardiogenic shock and its predictors: systematic review. *Cardiol Res*. 2018;9(2):75–82.
31. Petitpas F, Guenezan J, Vendeuvre T, et al. Use of intra-osseous access in adults: a systematic review. *Crit Care*. 2016;20(1):102.
32. Buetti N, Maraschall J, Drees M, et al. Strategies to prevent central line-associated bloodstream infections in acute-care hospitals: 2022 update. *Infect Control Hosp Epidemiol*. 2022;43:553–569.
33. Zampieri FG, Machado FR, Biondi RS, et al. Effect of intravenous fluid treatment with a balance solution vs 0.9% saline solution on mortality in critically ill patients. *JAMA*. 2021;326(9):818–829.
34. Brown RM, Wang L, Coston TD, et al. Balanced crystalloids versus saline in sepsis. A secondary analysis of the SMART clinical trial. *Am J Respir Crit Care Med*. 2019;200:1487–1495.
35. Semler MW, Self WH, Wanderer JP, et al. SMART Investigators and the Pragmatic Critical Care Research Group: balanced crystalloids versus saline in critically ill adults. *N Engl J Med*. 2018;378. 829–839 335.
36. Maiden MJ, Finnis ME, Peake S, et al. Haemoglobin concentration and volume of intravenous fluids in septic shock in the ARISE trial. *Crit Care*. 2021;22:118. https://doi.org/10.1186/s13054-018-2029-6.
37. Spahn DR, Bouillon B, Cerny V, et al. The European guideline on the management of major bleeding and coagulopathy following trauma: fifth edition. *Critical Care*. 2019;23:98. https://doi.org/10.1186/s13054-019-2347-3.
38. Martin GS, Bassett P. Crystalloids vs. colloids for fluid resuscitation in the intensive care unit: a systematic review and meta-analysis. *J Critical Care*. 2019;50:144–154.
39. U.S. FoodDrug Administration. Labeling changes on mortality, kidney injury, and excess bleeding with hydroxyethyl starch products. https://www.fda.gov/vaccines-blood-biologics/safety-availability-biologics/labeling-changes-mortality-kidney-injury-and-excess-bleeding-hydroxyethyl-starch-products; 2021. August 28, 2022.
40. American Red Cross. *A Compendium of Transfusion Practice Guidelines*. edition 4.0. 2021. 334401_compendium_v04jan2021_bookmarkedworking_rwv01.pdf. redcross.org. Accessed August 29, 2022.
41. Gorski LA, Hadaway L, Hagle ME, et al. Infusion therapy standards of practice. 8th edition *J Infus Nurs*. 2021;44(1S):S1–S224.
42. Raval JS, Griggs JR, Fleg A. Blood product transfusion in adults: indications, adverse reactions, and modifications. *Am Fam Physician*. 2020;102(1):30–38.
43. Passerini HM. Contemporary transfusion science and challenges. *AACN Adv Crit Care*. 2019;30(2):139–150.
44. Li K, Xu Y. Citrate metabolism in blood transfusions and its relationship due to metabolic alkalosis and respiratory acidosis. *Int J Clin Exp Med*. 2015;8(4):6578–6584.
45. DiFrancesco NR, Gaffney TP, Lashley JL, Hickerson KA. Hypocalcemia and massive blood transfusions: a pilot study in a level 1 trauma center. *J Trauma Nurs*. 2019;26(4):186–192.

46. Thomasson RR, Yazer MH, Gorham JD, et al. International assessment of massive transfusion protocol contents and indications for activation. *Transfusion*. 2019;59(5):1637–1643.
47. McQuilten ZK, Crighton G, Brunskill S, et al. Optimal dose, timing and ratio of blood products in massive transfusion: results from a systematic review. *Trans Med Rev*. 2018;32(1):6–15.
48. Meneses E, Boneva D, McKenney M, Elkbuli A. Massive transfusion protocol in adult trauma population. *J Emerg Med*. 2020;38:2662–2666.
49. Walkey AJ, Goligher EC, Del Sorbo L, et al. Low tidal volume versus non–volume-limited strategies for patients with acute respiratory distress syndrome: a systematic review and meta-analysis. *Ann Am Thorac Soc*. 2017;14(Suppl_4):S271–S279.
50. Collins SR. *Gahart's 2022 Intravenous Medications*. 38th ed. St Louis, MO: Elsevier Health Sciences; 2022.
51. Biswas S, Malik AH, Bandyopadhyay D, et al. Meta-analysis comparing the efficacy of dobutamine versus milrinone in acute decompensated heart failure and cardiogenic shock. *Curr Probl Cardiol*. 2022:101245. https://doi.org/10.1016/j.cpcardiol.2022.101245. Online ahead of print.
52. Liao X, Qian L, Zhang S, Chen X, Lei J. Network meta-analysis of the safety of drug therapy for cardiogenic shock. *J Healthc Eng*. 2020:8862256. https://doi.org/10.1155/2020/8862256.
53. O'Grady NP, Barie PS, Bartlett JG, et al. Guidelines for evaluation of new fever in critically ill adult patients: 2008 update from the American College of Critical Care Medicine and the Infectious Diseases Society of America. *Crit Care Med*. 2008;36(4):1330–1349.
54. Walter EJ, Hanna-Jumma S, Carraretto M, Forni L. The pathophysiological basis and consequences of fever. *Crit Care*. 2016;20(1):200.
55. Morrison G. Management of acute hypothermia. *Medicine*. 2017;45(3):135–138.
56. Ortiz-Reyes L, Patel JJ, Jiang X, et al. Early versus delayed enteral nutrition in mechanically ventilated patients with circulatory shock: a nested cohort analysis of an international multicenter, pragmatic clinical trial. [published correction appears in Crit Care. 2022 Jun 28;26(1):192] *Crit Care*. 2022;26(1):173. https://doi.org/10.1186/s13054-022-04047-4. . Published 2022 Jun 9.
57. Singer P, Blaser AR, Berger MM, et al. ESPEN guideline on clinical nutrition in the intensive care unit. *Clin Nutr*. 2019;38:48–79.
58. Compher C, Bingham AL, McCall M, et al. Guidelines for the provision of nutrition support therapy in the adult critically ill patient: the American Society for Parenteral and Enteral Nutrition. *J Parenter Enteral Nutr*. 2022;46:12–41.
59. American College of Surgeons' Committee on Trauma. *Advanced Trauma Life Support (ATLS) Program for Doctors: Student Manual*. 10th ed. Chicago, IL: American College of Surgeons; 2018.
60. Cannon JW. Hemorrhagic shock. *N Eng J Med*. 2018;378(4):370–379.
61. Claure-Del Granado R, Mehta RL. Fluid overload in the ICU: evaluation and management. *BMC Nephrol*. 2016;17(1):109.
62. Vahdatpour C, Collins D, Goldberg S. Cardiogenic shock. *J Am Heart Assoc*. 2019;8(8):e011991. https://doi.org/10.1161/JAHA.119.011991.
63. Bednarczyk JM, Fridfinnson JA, Kumar A, et al. Incorporating dynamic assessment of fluid responsiveness into goal-directed therapy: a systematic review and meta-analysis. *Crit Care Med*. 2017;45(9):1538–1545.
64. Hajjar LA, Teboul J-L. Mechanical circulatory support devices for cardiogenic shock: state of the art. *Crit Care*. 2019;23(1):76.
65. Asber SR, Shanahan KP, Lussier L, et al. Nursing management of patients requiring acute mechanical circulatory support devices. *Crit Care Nurse*. 2020;40(1):e1–e11.
66. Singhal V, Aggarwal R. Spinal shock. In: Prabhakar H, ed. *Complications in Neuroanesthesia*. London, England: Academic Press; 2016:89–94.
67. Standl T, Annecke T, Cascorbi I, et al. The nomenclature, definition and distinction of types of shock. *Dtsch Arztebl Int*. 2018;115(45):757–768.
68. Stein DM, Knight WA. Emergency neurological life support: traumatic spine injury. *Neurocrit Care*. 2017;27(Suppl 1):170–180.
69. Trauma Quality Program American College of Surgeons. *Best Practice Guidelines: Spine Injury*; 2022. spine_injury_guidelines.pdf. facs.org. Accessed August 16, 2022.
70. Khan DA, Banerji A, Blumenthal KG, et al. Drug allergy: a 2022 practice parameter update. *J Allergy Clin Immunol*. 2022. https://doi.org/10.1016/j.jaci.2022.08.028.
71. Krishnaswamy G. Critical care management of the patient with anaphylaxis: a concise definitive review. *Crit Care Med*. 2021;49(5):838–857.
72. Dodd A, Hughes A, Sargant N, Whyte AF, Soar J, Turner PJ. Evidence update for the treatment of anaphylaxis. *Resuscitation*. 2021;183:86–96.
73. Shaker MS, Wallace DV, Golden DBK, et al. Analphylaxis: a 2020 practice parameter update, systematic review, and grading of recommendations, assessment, development and evaluation (GRADE) analysis. *J Allergy Clin Immunol*. 2021;145(4):1082–1123.
74. Singer M, Deutschman CS, Seymour CW, et al. The third international consensus definitions for sepsis and septic shock (Sepsis-3). *JAMA*. 2016;315(8):801–810.
75. Lester D, Hartjes T, Bennett ACE. A review of the revised sepsis care bundles. *Am J Nurs*. 2018;118(8):40–49.
76. Vincent J-L, de Mendonca A, Cantraine F, et al. Use of the SOFA score to assess the incidence of organ dysfunction/failure in intensive care units: results of a multicenter, prospective study. *Crit Care Med*. 1998;26(11):1793–1800.
77. Schorr CA, Seckel MA, Papathanassoglou E, Kleinpell R. Nursing implication of the updated 2021 surviving sepsis Campaign guidelines. *Am J Crit Care*. 2022;31(4):329–336.
78. Swearingen PL. *All-in-One Nursing Care Planning Resource: Medical-Surgical, Pediatric, Maternity, and Psychiatric-Mental Health*. 5th ed. St. Louis, MO: Elsevier; 2018.
79. MacVane SH. Antimicrobial resistance in the intensive care unit: a focus on gram-negative bacterial infections. *J Intens Care Med*. 2017;32(1):25–37.
80. Rhee C, Jones TM, Harmad Y, et al. Prevalence, underlying causes, and preventability of sepsis-associated mortality in US acute care hospitals. *JAMA Netw Open*. 2019;2(2):e187571. https://doi.org/10.1001/jamanetworkopen.2018.7571.
81. Klompas M, Branson R, Cawcutt K, et al. Strategies to prevent ventilator-associated pneumonia, ventilator-associated events, and nonventilator hospital-acquired pneumonia in acute-care hospitals: 2022 update. *Infect Control Hosp Epidemiol*. 2022;43:687–713.
82. COVID-19 Treatment Guidelines Panel. *Coronavirus Disease 2019 (COVID-19) Treatment Guidelines. National Institutes of Health*. Available at: https://www.covid19treatmentguidelines.nih.gov/. Accessed September 11, 2022.

83. Alhazzani W, Evans L, Fayez A, et al. Surviving Sepsis Campaign guidelines on the management of adults with coronavirus disease 2019 (COVID-19) in the ICU: first update. *Crit Care Med.* 2021;49(3):e219–e231.
84. Townsend SR. Effects of compliance with the early management bundle (SEP-1) on mortality changes among medicare beneficiaries with sepsis: a propensity score matched cohort study. *Chest.* 2022;161(1):392–406.
85. Levy MM, Evans LE, Rhodes A. The surviving sepsis Campaign bundle: 2018 update. *Crit Care Med.* 2018;46(6):997–1000.
86. Konstandinides S, Meyer G, Becattini C, et al. 2019 ESC guidelines for diagnosis and management of acute pulmonary embolism developed in collaboration with the European Respiratory Society (ERS); the task force for the diagnosis and management of acute pulmonary embolism for the European Society of Cardiology (ESC). *Eur Heart J.* 2020;41(4):543–603.
87. Stevens SM, Woller SC, Kreuziger LB, et al. Executive summary: antithrombotic therapy for VTE disease: second update of the CHEST guideline and expert panel report. *Chest.* 2021;160(6):2247–2259.
88. Mira JC, Gentile LF, Mathias BJ, et al. Sepsis pathophysiology, chronic critical illness, and persistent inflammation-immunosuppression and catabolism syndrome. *Crit Care Med.* 2017;45(2):253–262.
89. Gourd NM, Nikitas N. Multiple organ dysfunction syndrome. *J Intensive Care Med.* 2020;35(12):1564–1575.

13

Cardiovascular Alterations

Sarah E. Schroeder, PhD, ACNP-BC, MSN RN, AACC

INTRODUCTION

Care of the patient with decreased cardiac function presents unique challenges because of potential serious hemodynamic changes that can affect the prognosis of the critically ill patient. The critical care nurse needs both theoretic knowledge and practice-related understanding of common cardiac diseases to have the sound clinical judgment necessary for making rapid and accurate decisions and responding with optimal interventions. The purpose of this chapter is to identify and explore common cardiac alterations that are likely to be encountered by the acute and critical care nurse caring for adult patients with compromised cardiac status and to describe the nursing care required to optimize patient outcomes.

NORMAL STRUCTURE AND FUNCTION OF THE HEART

The heart muscle is approximately the size of a person's closed fist and lies within the mediastinal space of the thoracic cavity—between the lungs, directly under the lower half of the sternum, and above the diaphragm (Fig. 13.1). It is covered by the *pericardium,* which has an inner visceral layer and an outer parietal layer. Certain diseases can cause this covering to become inflamed (e.g., pericarditis) and can subsequently diminish the effectiveness of the heart as a pump. Several cubic milliliters of lubricating fluid are present between these layers. Some pathological conditions can increase the amount and the consistency of this fluid, affecting the pumping ability of the heart. The heart muscle itself is composed of three layers. The outer layer, or *epicardium,* covers the surface of the heart and extends to the great vessels; the middle muscular layer, or *myocardium,* is responsible for the heart's pumping action; and the inner endothelial layer, or *endocardium,* covers the heart valves and the small muscles associated with the opening and closing of those valves. These layers may be damaged or destroyed when a patient has a myocardial infarction (MI).

Functionally, the heart is divided into right-sided and left-sided pumps that are separated by a septum. The right side is considered a low-pressure system, whereas the left side is a high-pressure system. Each side has an atrium that receives the blood and a ventricle that pumps the blood out. Blood travels from the atria to the ventricles by means of a pressure gradient between the chambers. The right atrium receives deoxygenated blood from the body through the superior vena cava and the inferior vena cava. The right ventricle pumps the deoxygenated blood to the lungs through the pulmonary artery for oxygen and carbon dioxide exchange. The left atrium receives the newly oxygenated blood by way of the pulmonary veins from the lungs, and the left ventricle pumps the oxygenated blood through the aorta to the systemic circulation (Fig. 13.2). This flow pattern is unique to the heart, as in most other systems, veins carry deoxygenated blood to the lungs, and arteries carry oxygenated blood away from the heart.

The four cardiac valves maintain the unidirectional blood flow through the chambers of the heart. The valves also assist in producing the pressure gradient needed between the chambers for the blood to flow through the heart. There are two types of valves: the atrioventricular (AV) valves, which separate the atria from the ventricles, and the semilunar (SL) valves, which separate the pulmonary artery from the right ventricle and the aorta from the left ventricle (Fig. 13.3). The AV valves are the tricuspid valve, which lies between the right atrium and the right ventricle, and the mitral valve, located between the left atrium and the left ventricle. Each AV valve is anchored by chordae tendineae to the papillary muscles on its ventricular floor. The SL valves are the pulmonic valve, which lies between the right ventricle and the pulmonary artery, and the aortic valve, located between the left ventricle and the aorta. These SL valves are not anchored by chordae tendineae. Instead, their closing is passive and is caused by differences in pressure between the chamber and the respective great vessel.

Autonomic Control

The autonomic nervous system (sympathetic and parasympathetic) exerts control over the cardiovascular system. The sympathetic nervous system releases norepinephrine, which has alpha- and beta-adrenergic effects. Alpha-adrenergic effects cause arterial vasoconstriction. Beta-adrenergic effects increase sinus

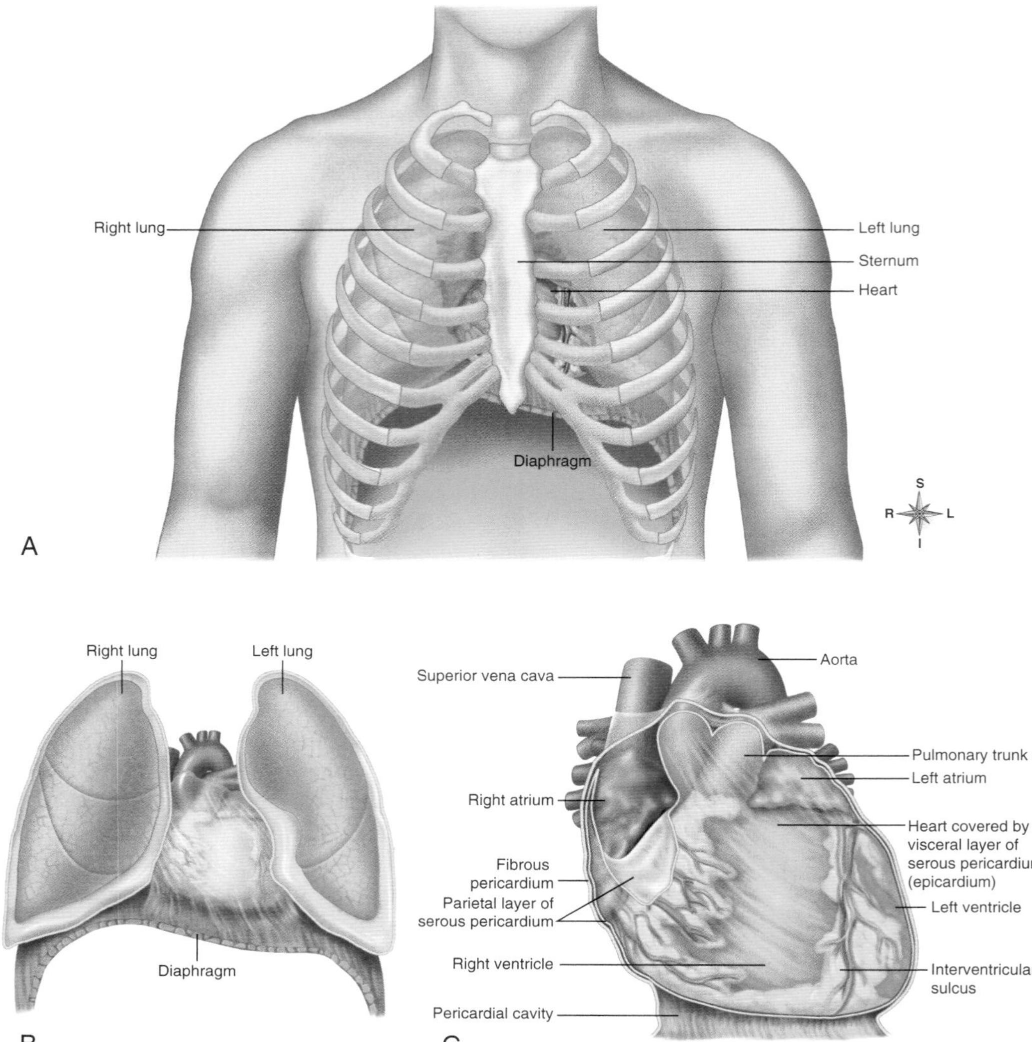

Fig. 13.1 Location of the heart. A, Heart in mediastinum showing relationship to lungs, ribs, sternum, and other thoracic structures. B, Anterior view of isolated heart and lungs. Portions of the parietal pleura and pericardium have been removed. C, Detail of heart resting on diaphragm with pericardial sac opened. (From Patton KT, Thibodeau GA. *Anatomy and Physiology*. 10th ed. St. Louis, MO: Elsevier; 2019.)

node discharge (positive chronotropic effect), increase the force of contraction (positive inotropic effect), and accelerate the AV conduction time (positive dromotropic effect). The parasympathetic nervous system releases acetylcholine through stimulation of the vagus nerve. It causes a decrease in sinus node discharge and slows conduction through the AV node.

In addition to this innervation, receptors help control cardiovascular function. The first group of receptors is the *chemoreceptors,* which are sensitive to changes in partial pressure of arterial oxygen (PaO_2), partial pressure of arterial carbon dioxide ($PaCO_2$), and pH blood levels. Chemoreceptors stimulate the vasomotor center in the medulla; this center controls vasoconstriction, which occurs during conditions of decreased PaO_2 and/or increased $PaCO_2$ and decreased pH, and vasodilation, which occurs when there is an increased PaO_2 and/or decreased $PaCO_2$, and increased pH. The second group of receptors is the *baroreceptors,* which are sensitive to stretch and pressure. If blood pressure (BP) increases, the baroreceptors cause the heart rate to decrease. If BP decreases, the baroreceptors stimulate an increase in heart rate (Fig. 13.4).

CHECK YOUR UNDERSTANDING:

1. A patient with sleep apnea was informed of the risk of cardiovascular disease. What is the nurse's best explanation to the patient?
   A. Sleep apnea causes periods of low PaO_2 and elevated $PaCO_2$, which cause vessels to constrict, increasing the stress on the heart and risk of heart disease.
   B. Sleep apnea causes periods of low $PaCO_2$ and hypoventilation that may lead to stress on the heart by causing vessels to dilate.
   C. Increased heart rate may occur with sleep apnea, increasing the work of the heart and dysfunction.
   D. Sleep apnea reduces circulating oxygen, requiring the heart to beat faster to deliver oxygen to the body, which creates stress on the heart.

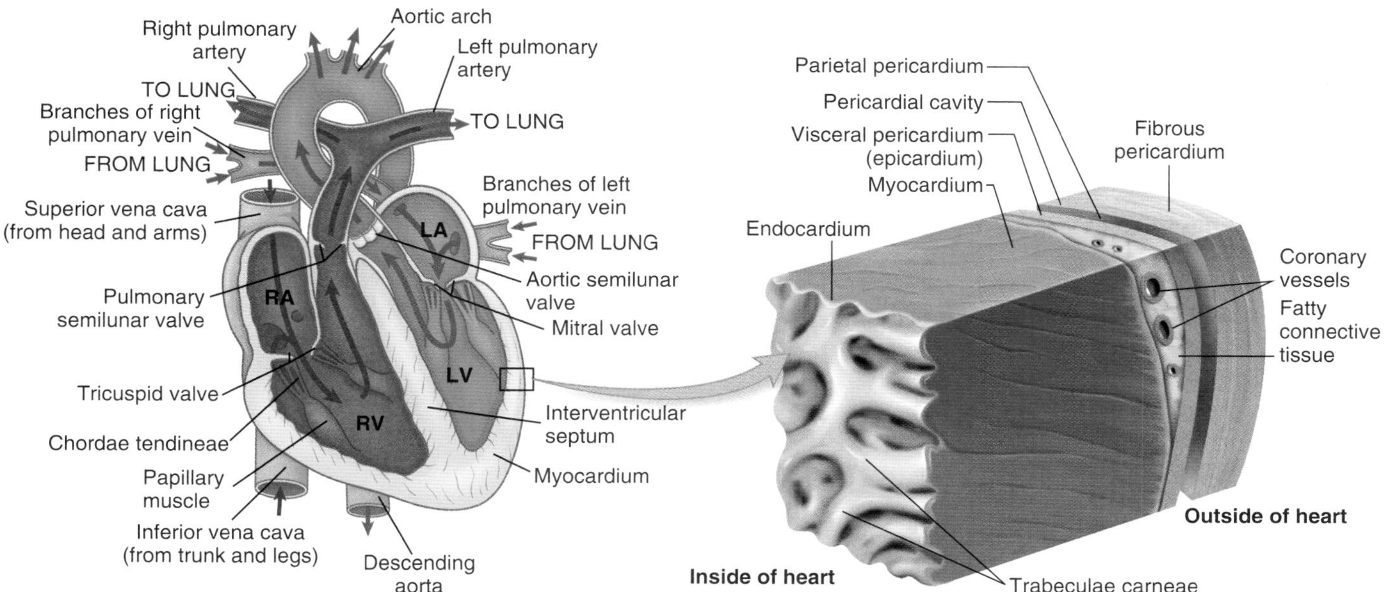

Fig. 13.2 Structures that direct blood flow through the heart. Arrows indicate the path of blood flow through chambers, valves, and major vessels. (From Rogers J. *McCance and Huether's Pathophysiology: The Biologic Basis for Disease in Adults and Children.* 9th ed. St. Louis, MO: Elsevier; 2023:1021.)

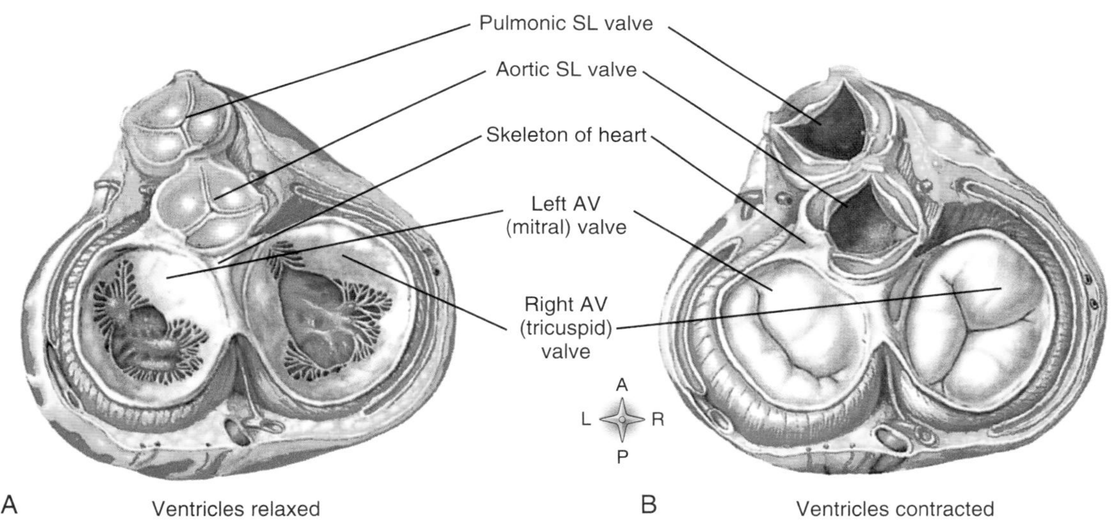

Fig. 13.3 A, The atrioventricular (AV) valves in the open position and the semilunar *(SL)* valves in the closed position. B, The AV valves in the closed position and the SL valves in the open position. (From Patton KT, Thibodeau GA. *Anatomy and Physiology.* 10th ed. St. Louis, MO: Elsevier; 2019.)

Coronary Circulation

Many cardiac problems result from complete or partial occlusion of a coronary artery. The blood supply to the myocardium is derived from the coronary arteries that branch off the aorta immediately above the aortic valve (Fig. 13.5). Two major branches exist: the left coronary artery, which splits into the left anterior descending and left circumflex branches, and the right coronary artery. Knowledge of the portion of the heart that receives its blood supply from a particular coronary artery allows the acute and critical care nurse to anticipate problems related to occlusion of that vessel (Box 13.1). Variations in branching and in the exact placement of the coronary arteries are common.

Blood flow to the coronary arteries occurs during ventricular diastole, when the aortic valve is closed, and the sinuses of Valsalva are filled with blood. Myocardial fibers are relaxed at this time, promoting blood flow through the coronary vessels. The coronary veins return blood from the coronary circulation back into the heart through the coronary sinuses to the right and left atria.

Heart Sounds

The vibrations produced by vascular walls, flowing blood, heart muscle, and heart valves create sound waves known as heart sounds. Auscultation of these sounds with a stethoscope over

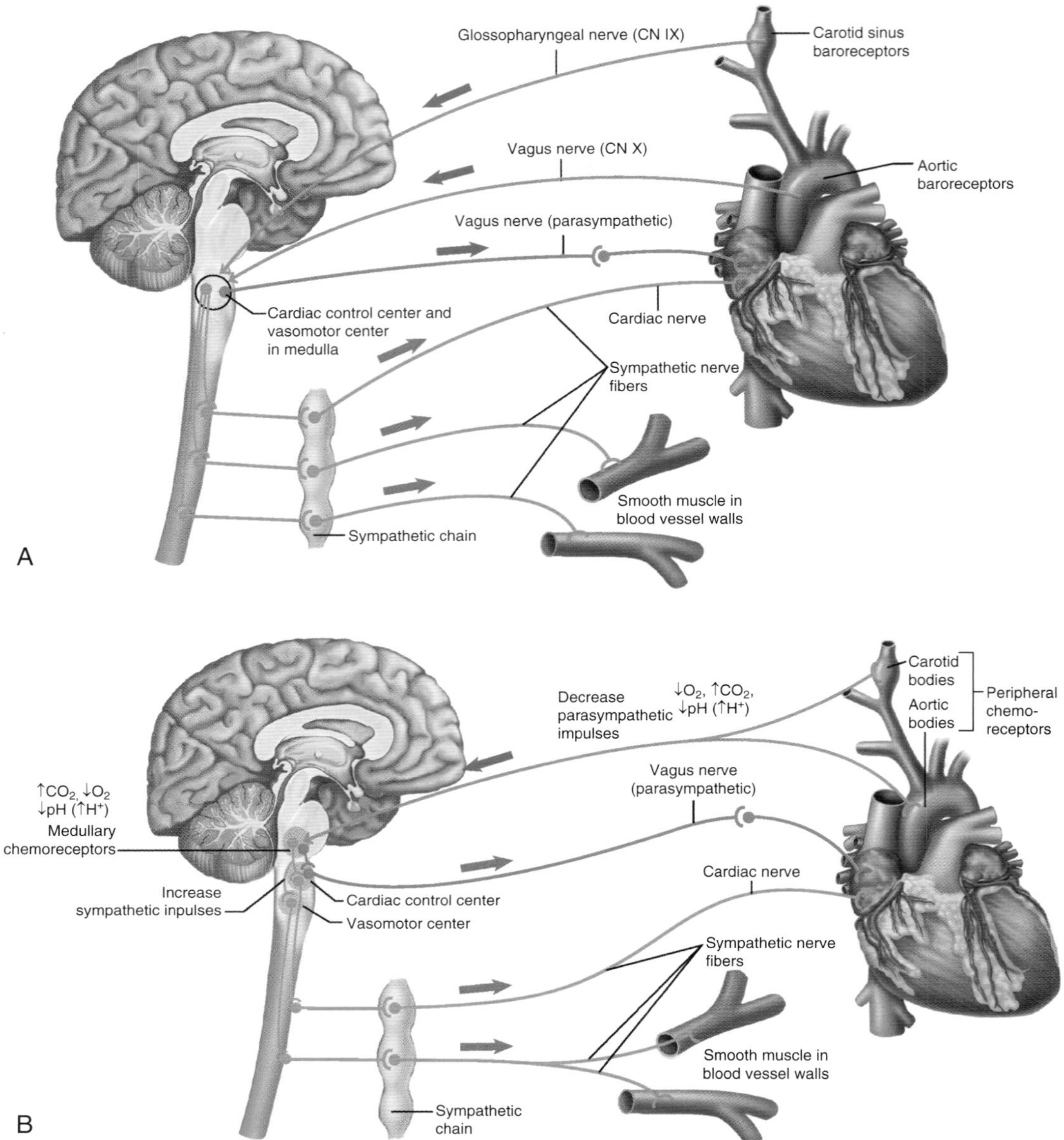

Fig. 13.4 A, Vasomotor pressoreflexes. B, Vasomotor chemoreflexes. (From Patton KT, Thibodeau GA. *Anatomy and Physiology*. 10th ed. St. Louis, MO: Elsevier; 2019.)

the heart provides valuable information about valve and cardiac function (Fig. 13.6). Ventricular systole occurs when the pulmonic and aortic valves open to allow blood to be pumped to the lungs (right ventricle, pulmonic valve) and to the systemic circulation (left ventricle, aortic valve). Ventricular diastole occurs when the tricuspid and mitral valves open to allow the ventricles to fill with blood.

The first heart sound is known as S_1. This sound has been described as "lub." It is caused by closure of the tricuspid and mitral valves. It is best heard at the apex of the heart (fifth intercostal space, left midclavicular line) and represents the beginning of ventricular systole (Fig. 13.6). The second heart sound, or S_2, has been described as "dub." It is caused by closure of the pulmonic and aortic valves. It is best heard at the second intercostal space at the left or right sternal border and represents the beginning of ventricular diastole. The first and second heart sounds are best heard with the diaphragm of the stethoscope. Murmurs are best heard at Erb's point, located at the third intercostal space, left of the sternal border.

A third heart sound, known as S_3 or ventricular gallop, is a normal variant in young adults but usually represents a pathological process in an older adult. The sound is caused by rapid left ventricular filling and may be produced when the heart is already overfilled or poorly compliant. The S_3 sound is low pitched and can best be heard with the bell of the stethoscope at the fifth intercostal space, at the left midclavicular line. It occurs immediately after S_2. Together with S_1 and S_2, S_3 produces a "lub-dubba" or "ken-**tuk**'e" sound. S_3 is often heard in patients with heart failure (HF) or fluid overload. A fourth heart sound, known as S_4 or atrial gallop, is produced from atrial contraction

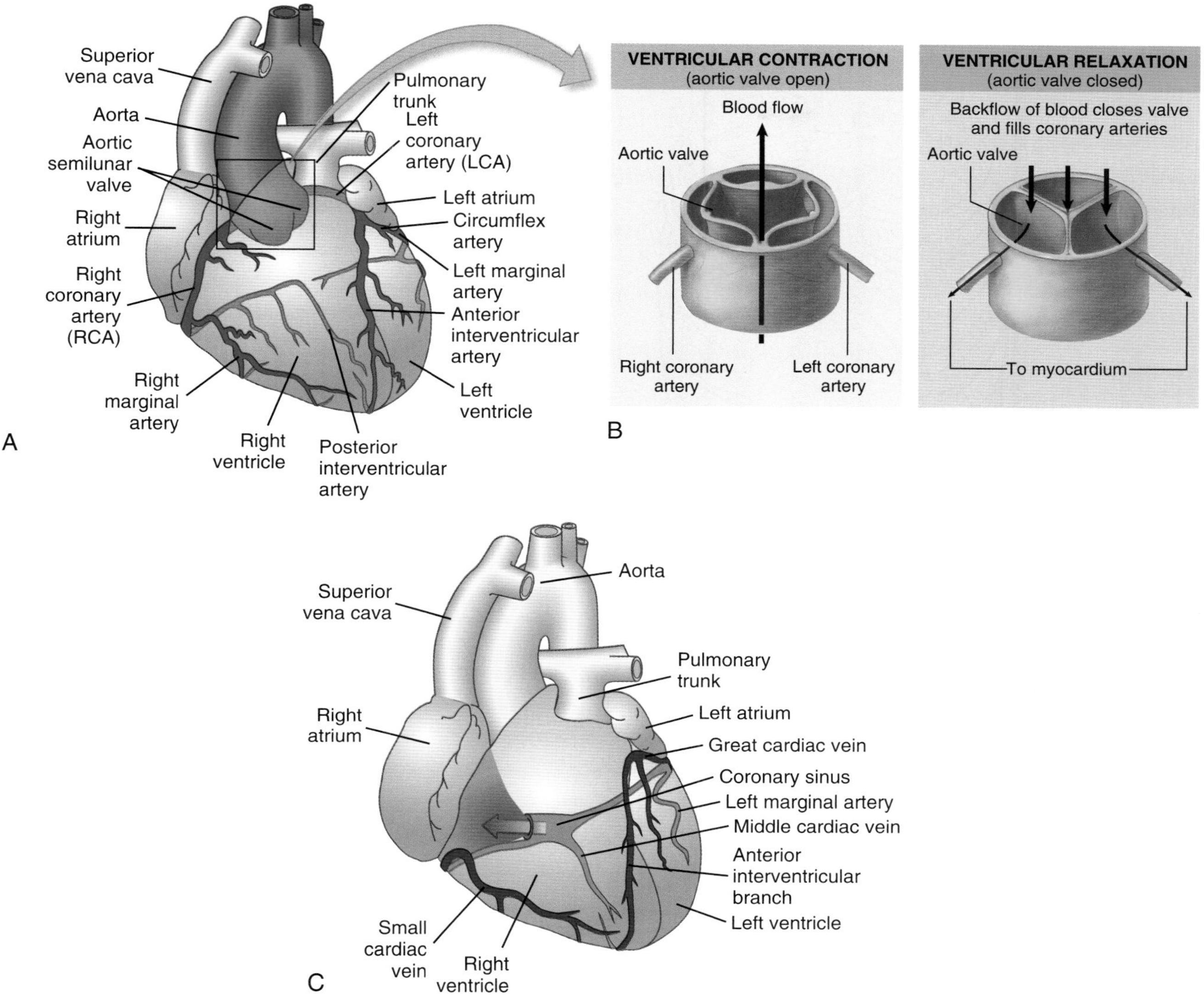

Fig. 13.5 A, Arteries. B, Coronary artery openings from the aorta. Placement of the coronary artery opening behind the leaflets of the aortic valve allows the coronary arteries to fill during ventricular relaxation. C, Veins. Both A and C are anterior views of the heart. Vessels near the anterior surface are more darkly colored than vessels of the posterior surface seen through the heart. (From Patton KT, Thibodeau GA. *The Human Body in Health & Disease*. 8th ed. St. Louis, MO: Elsevier; 2018.)

BOX 13.1 Coronary Artery Distribution

Right Coronary Artery

- Right atrium
- Right ventricle
- Sinoatrial node
- Atrioventricular bundle
- Posterior portion of the left ventricle

Left Anterior Descending Artery

- Anterior two-thirds of the intraventricular septum
- Anterior left ventricle

Circumflex Artery

- Left atrium

that is more forceful than normal. Together with S_1 and S_2, S_4 produces a "te-lubb-dubb" or "**ten**′-ne-see" sound. S_4 can be normal in elderly patients, but it is often heard after an acute MI (AMI), when the atria contract more forcefully against ventricles distended with blood.

In the severely failing heart, all four sounds may be heard, producing a "gallop" rhythm, so named because it sounds like the hoofbeats of a galloping horse. It can best be heard with the bell of the stethoscope at the fifth intercostal space, at the left midclavicular line. It is often documented as S_4, S_1, S_2, S_3 because of the order in which the sounds are heard. A summation gallop occurs when the third and fourth heart sounds are superimposed; it is usually an indication of heart disease.

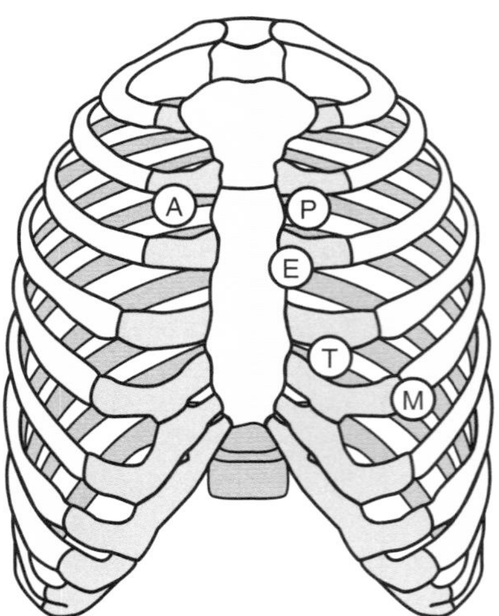

- **A**ortic Valve best heard at right 2nd intercostal space along the right sternal border
- **P**ulmonic Valve best heard at left 2nd intercostal space along the left sternal border
- **E**rb's Point represents the area where murmurs are best heard 3rd intercostal space left of sternal border
- **T**ricuspic Valve best heard at the left lower sternal border near 4th and 5th intercostal space
- **M**itral Valve best heard at the left 5th intercostal space at the left midclavicular line

Fig. 13.6 Chest areas from which each valve sound is best heard.

Heart Murmur

A heart murmur is a sound caused by turbulence of blood flow through the valves of the heart. A murmur is usually a rumbling, blowing, harsh, or musical sound. It is important to determine the sound, anatomical location, loudness, and intensity of a murmur and whether extra heart sounds are heard. Table 13.1 presents a grading of heart murmurs. Murmurs are audible when a septal defect is present, when a valve (usually aortic or mitral) is stenosed, or when the valve leaflets fail to approximate (valve insufficiency). The presence of a new murmur warrants special attention, particularly in a patient with AMI. A papillary muscle may have ruptured, causing the mitral valve to not close correctly, which can be indicative of severe damage and impending complications (e.g., HF and pulmonary edema). Auscultation of heart sounds is a skill developed from practice in listening to many different patients' hearts and correlating the sounds heard with the patients' pathological conditions.

TABLE 13.1 Grading of Heart Murmurs

Intensity of Murmur Graded From I to VI Based on Increasing Loudness

Grade I	Lowest intensity, usually not audible by inexperienced clinicians
Grade II	Low intensity, usually audible by inexperienced clinicians
Grade III	Medium intensity without a thrill
Grade IV	Medium intensity with a thrill
Grade V	Loudest murmur, audible when stethoscope is placed on the chest; associated with a thrill
Grade VI	Loudest intensity, audible when stethoscope is removed from chest; associated with a thrill

CORONARY ARTERY DISEASE

Coronary artery disease (CAD) is a broad term used to refer to the narrowing or occlusion of the coronary arteries. Other terms used to describe CAD include coronary heart disease and atherosclerotic cardiovascular disease (ASCVD).

Pathophysiology

Progressive narrowing of one or more coronary arteries by atherosclerosis is known as CAD, which results in ischemia when the internal diameter of the coronary vessel is reduced by 50% or more (Fig. 13.7).[1] Atherosclerosis is an inflammatory disease that progresses from endothelial injury to fatty streak, plaque, and complex lesion. The process begins with injury to the endothelium caused by cardiac risk factors such as smoking, hypertension, diabetes, and hyperlipidemia (Box 13.2). Once injury occurs, endothelial cells become inflamed, causing release of cytokines. Macrophages adhere to the injured endothelium and release enzymes and toxic oxygen radicals that create oxidative stress, oxidize low-density lipoproteins (LDLs), and further injure the vessel. Inflammation with additional oxidative stress and activation of macrophages occurs. Oxidized LDLs penetrate the arterial wall and are engulfed by macrophages, creating foam cells that release cytokines, tissue factor, reactive oxygen species, metalloproteinases, and growth factor. Cytokines and LDLs stimulate vascular smooth cell proliferation, which leads to vascular remodeling (Fig. 13.8). Accumulation of foam cells leads to fatty streak formation.[2] With age, most individuals develop fatty streaks, accumulations of serum lipoproteins in the intima of the vessel wall, in their coronary arteries. The dysfunctional formation of a fatty streak leads to the presence of fibrotic plaque. Over time, a collagen cap is formed from connective tissue (fibroblasts and macrophages) and LDL[1] (Fig. 13.7C).

Plaques may rupture, causing the contents to interact with blood, producing a thrombus. The thrombus can occlude a coronary artery, with resulting myocardial injury and infarction. Rupture of the plaque starts the coagulation cascade,

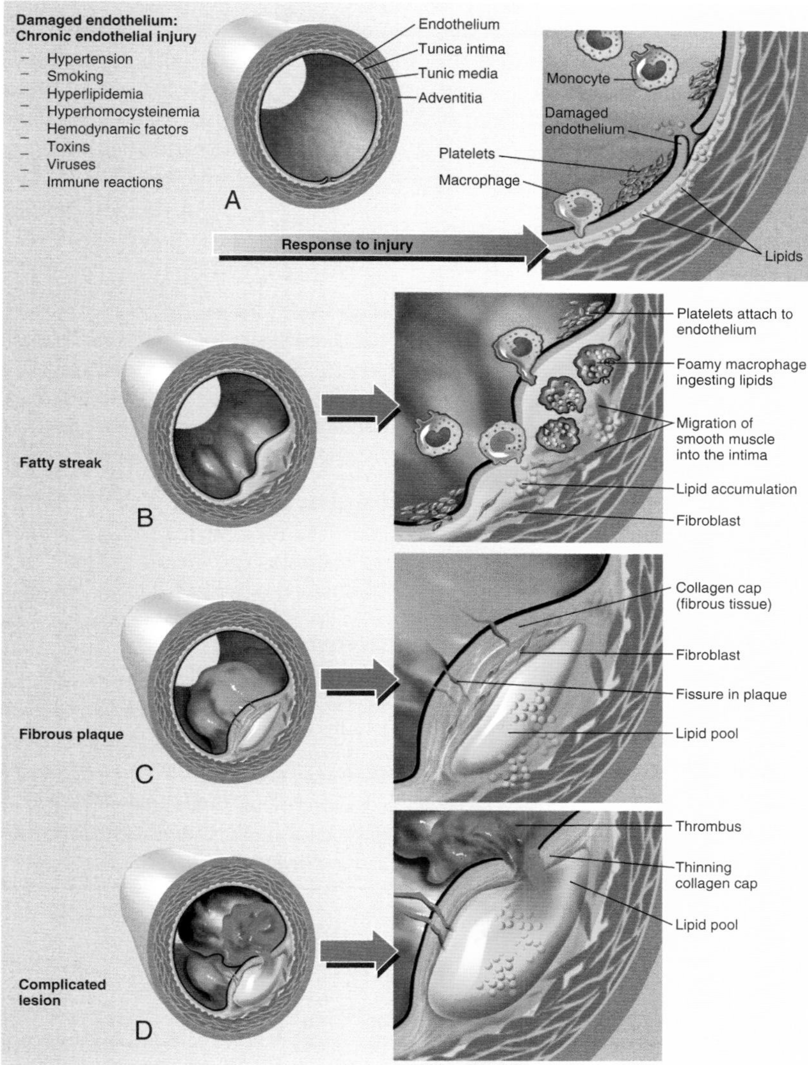

Fig. 13.7 Progression of atherosclerosis. A, Damaged endothelium. B, Fatty streak and lipid core formation. C, Fibrous plaque (raised plaques are visible: some are *yellow*; others are *white*). D, Complicated lesion (thrombus is *red*; collagen is *blue*). (From Rogers J. *McCance and Huether's Pathophysiology: The Biologic Basis for Disease in Adults and Children.* 9th ed. St. Louis, MO: Elsevier; 2023:1070.)

leading to the initiation of thrombin production, conversion of fibrinogen to fibrin, and platelet aggregation at the site. After injury to the endothelium, platelets are exposed to proteins that bind to receptors, causing adhesion of platelets at the site of injury. Next, the platelets are activated and change shape. They release thromboxane A_2, which in turn binds to thromboxane receptors that enhance platelet activation, vasoconstriction, and plaque progression. At the same time, the platelets aggregate with one another. This process of adhesion, activation, and aggregation causes a rapidly growing thrombus that compromises coronary blood flow (e.g., myocardial ischemia and infarction).[1]

Assessment

Patient Assessment. A thorough history and cardiovascular assessment provide data to develop a comprehensive plan of care for the critically ill patient with cardiovascular disease. The history includes subjective data on health history, prior hospitalizations, allergies, and family health history. Several risk factors associated with CAD are also assessed (Box 13.2). Knowledge of prior hospitalizations is also important so that medical records can be obtained for review. Records are especially useful if the patient was hospitalized for a cardiac event or underwent cardiac diagnostic testing. Information on the patient's current medications, both prescription and over the

BOX 13.2 Risk Factors for Coronary Artery Disease

Several risk factors predispose an individual to coronary artery disease (CAD). Some risk factors cannot be changed (e.g., sex, heredity, age). Other risk factors are modifiable, including smoking, high blood cholesterol, high blood pressure (BP), physical inactivity, overweight or obesity, and diabetes.

Gender

Males have a greater risk of CAD and myocardial infarction (MI) than females, and they have MI earlier in life.

Heredity

A family history of early heart disease is an unmodifiable risk for CAD. A positive history is defined as having a first-degree relative (i.e., parent, sister, brother, or child) with CAD diagnosed before 55 years of age in biological male relatives or before 65 years of age in biological female relatives.

Age

Males in their mid-40s or older and females once they reach menopause are considered to be at higher risk for CAD.

Smoking

Smokers have a higher risk of CAD. Smoking increases low-density lipoprotein (LDL) levels and damages the endothelium of coronary vessels. These are predisposing factors for the development of atherosclerosis. Smoking also causes vasoconstriction of coronary vessels, thus decreasing blood flow to the heart muscle itself.

High Blood Cholesterol

Serum cholesterol or lipid levels play a key role in the development of atherosclerosis. An elevated total cholesterol value (>200 mg/dL) is considered a risk factor for CAD. Cholesterol is insoluble in plasma and must be transported by lipoproteins that are soluble. High-density lipoproteins (HDLs) are considered the "good" cholesterol. HDLs assist in transporting cholesterol to the liver for removal. A high HDL level (>40 mg/dL for males and >50 mg/dL for females) may reduce the incidence of CAD, whereas a low HDL level (<40 mg/dL) may be considered a risk factor for developing CAD.

LDLs are considered the "bad" cholesterol. LDLs transport and deposit cholesterol in the arterial vessels, thus facilitating the process of atherosclerosis. Other non-HDL lipoproteins also contribute to the development of CAD. Very-low-density lipoproteins are largely composed of triglycerides and contribute to an increased risk of CAD.

High Blood Pressure

Though there are many hypertension guidelines, most agree that a BP greater than 140/90 mm Hg or taking antihypertensive medication is a risk factor for CAD. Hypertension causes direct injury to the vasculature, leading to the development of CAD. Oxygen demands are also increased. The heart muscle enlarges and weakens over time, thereby increasing the workload of the heart.

Physical Inactivity

Lack of physical activity is a risk factor for CAD. Regular aerobic exercise reduces the incidence of CAD. Exercise also helps control other risk factors such as high BP, diabetes mellitus, and obesity.

Overweight and Obesity

Obesity increases the atherogenic process and predisposes persons to CAD. In addition, obesity is related to hypertension and diabetes, two other major risk factors. The waist-to-hip ratio and body mass index (BMI) are important assessments.

Diabetes Mellitus

Diabetes mellitus is associated with increased levels of LDLs and triglycerides. Glycation associated with mellitus diabetes decreases the uptake of LDLs by the liver and increases the hepatic synthesis of LDLs.

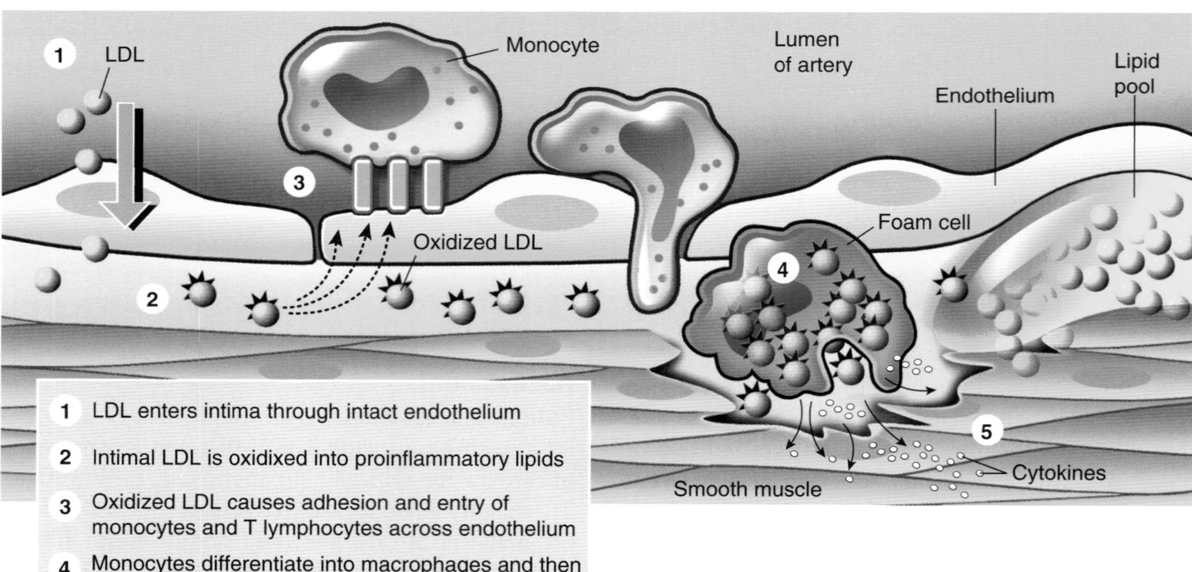

Fig. 13.8 Low-density lipoprotein (LDL) oxidation. (1) LDL enters the arterial intima through an intact endothelium. (2) and (3) Inflammation and oxidized LDL cause endothelial cells to express adhesion molecules that bind monocytes and other inflammatory and immune cells. Monocytes penetrate the vessel wall, becoming macrophages. (4) Lipid-laden macrophages are called "foam cells." (5) Foam cells accumulate and form the fatty streak, and many inflammatory cytokines and enzymes are released that injure the vessel wall. (From Rogers J. *McCance and Huether's Pathophysiology: The Biologic Basis for Disease in Adults and Children.* 9th ed. St. Louis, MO: Elsevier; 2023:1071.)

counter, includes assessment of the patient's understanding and use of these medications. For example, when considering nitroglycerin (NTG) administration, it is necessary to know if the patient also uses phosphodiesterase type 5 inhibitors taken for erectile dysfunction, such as sildenafil (Viagra), tadalafil (Cialis), vardenafil (Levitra), or avanafil (Stendra). These medications potentiate the hypotensive effects of nitrates such as NTG; therefore, the concurrent use is contraindicated because of the significant risk of hypotension with concomitant use. It is also important to determine whether the patient has any food, medication, or environmental allergies. A psychosocial or personal history is important for the planning of the critically ill patient's care. This history includes information related to daily activities such as sleep, diet, and exercise (Box 13.3).

Before beginning the physical examination, determine recent and recurrent symptoms that may be related to the patient's current problems. Such symptoms include the presence or absence of fatigue, fluid retention, dyspnea, irregular heartbeat (palpitations), and chest pain (see Clinical Alert box). There is extreme importance in knowing that chest pain may be described in different ways based upon each individual. For example, females, those who are overweight, diabetics, individuals over 75 years of age, and African Americans may not experience the classic type of chest pain in the center of the chest.[3] Instead, individuals may experience what is called "*anginal equivalent*" chest pain, which may include but is not limited to: shortness of breath, fatigue, or pain in other parts of the body; it may even be asymptomatic, described as feeling "*not quite right.*" Asking focused questions are key in determining whether the symptoms an individual is experiencing are cardiovascular related to avoid a delay in care.

The physical examination itself encompasses all body systems and is not limited to the cardiovascular system. Because all body systems are interrelated and interdependent, it is imperative that a total evaluation be completed regarding the physical status of the patient. Patients whose primary problems are cardiovascular most commonly exhibit alterations in circulation and oxygenation. Therefore, all systems are examined from this perspective.

! CLINICAL ALERT

PQRST Assessment of the Patient With Chest Pain

- P = Provocation
- Q = Quality
- R = Region/Radiation
- S = Severity
- T = Timing (when began) and Treatment

BOX 13.3 Assessment of Daily Activities

- What, if any, is the critically ill patient's exercise routine, including the type, amount, and regularity of the activity?
- What are the critically ill patient's daily food pattern and intake?
- What is the critically ill patient's sleep pattern?
- What are the critically ill patient's habitual social patterns in using tobacco, alcohol, medications, coffee, tea, and caffeinated sodas?

The examination is performed in an orderly, organized manner and involves the techniques of inspection, palpation, percussion, and auscultation. A baseline assessment summary is provided in Table 13.2.

CHECK YOUR UNDERSTANDING:

2. A patient reports chest tightness with strenuous exercise that is increasing in frequency. How does the nurse interpret this symptom as part of the assessment?
   A. Quality
   B. Region/Radiation
   C. Severity
   D. Provocation

Diagnostic Studies. Many diagnostic studies are fundamental for the care and treatment of critically ill patients with CAD. The following paragraphs describe common diagnostic studies the cardiac patient may encounter.

12-Lead electrocardiography (ECG). ECG, a noninvasive test also commonly referred to as an EKG, is usually preliminary to most other tests performed. It is useful for identification of rhythm disturbances; pericarditis; pulmonary diseases; left ventricular hypertrophy; and myocardial ischemia, injury, and infarction. The importance of this basic test should not be underestimated. (See Chapter 8, Dysrhythmia Interpretation and Management.)

Chest radiography. This study is usually performed in the anteroposterior view. Chest radiography is used to detect cardiomegaly, cardiac positioning, degree of fluid infiltrating the pulmonary or pericardial space, and other structural changes that may affect the physical ability of the heart to function in a normal manner.

Holter or event monitors. Though more commonly used in the acute care unit or outpatient environment, Holter or event monitors are used to detect suspected dysrhythmias. The Holter monitor is a small portable recorder (about the size of a large cellular phone) connected to the patient by three to five electrodes. The recorder is worn for 24 to 48 hours. Event monitors come in different models; some models are leadless and can be worn for longer periods. The patient engages in normal daily activities and keeps a log of all activities and symptoms during the monitoring period. The recording is analyzed for abnormalities and correlated with the documented activities and symptoms.

Exercise tolerance test. During an exercise tolerance test, a noninvasive test also known as a stress test, the patient is connected to an ECG machine while exercising. Physical stress causes an increase in myocardial oxygen consumption. If oxygen demand exceeds supply, ischemia may result. The stress test is used to document exercise-induced ischemia and can identify individuals who are prone to cardiac ischemia during activity, even though their resting ECGs are normal. The exercise usually involves pedaling a stationary bike or, more commonly, walking on a treadmill. The exercise tolerance test is complete when 85% of the target heart rate is reached or the individual can no longer continue exercising due to symptoms.[4] The patient is constantly monitored, BP is checked at intervals, and the ECG printout is analyzed at the end of the testing period. Changes in the ST segments of the ECG can indicate ischemia. Beta-blockers are often withheld on the morning of an exercise tolerance test so that an adequate heart rate can be attained during the test. Patients return to their room or go home after the heart rate returns to baseline.

Pharmacological stress testing. If a patient is physically unable to perform the exercise required by an exercise tolerance test, a pharmacological stress test can be done. This test is done in conjunction with radionuclide scintigraphy or echocardiography. Medications such as regadenoson, dipyridamole, or adenosine are used to cause vasodilation of normal coronary arteries. If an area of a blood vessel is stenosed, it does not dilate, and the corresponding muscle displays as hypoperfusion on radionuclide scanning or as hypokinesis on echocardiography. Alternatively, dobutamine can be used to increase heart rate and contractility. Areas that are not perfused well because of blockages are evident when scanned.

Nuclear stress testing. This test can be done with exercise to increase the sensitivity of the test. It is used for patients who have an ECG that precludes accurate interpretation of ST-segment changes, and it is also used in conjunction with medications for patients who cannot walk on a treadmill. Technetium-99m and thallium-201 are radionuclides given intravenously to image the heart at rest and under stress (induced by either exercise or use of a pharmacological agent). The stress images are compared with the resting images. Perfusion defects seen on rest and stress images are evidence of infarct, whereas defects observed on stress images that are normal during the rest study indicate ischemia.

Echocardiography. This is a noninvasive imaging procedure that uses ultrasound to visualize the cardiac structures and the motion and function of cardiac valves and chambers. A transducer placed on the chest wall sends ultrasound waves at short intervals. The reflected sound waves, termed *echoes*, are displayed on a graph for interpretation. Echocardiography is used to assess valvular function, evaluate congenital defects, measure the size of cardiac chambers, evaluate cardiac disease progression, evaluate ventricular function, diagnose myocardial tumors and effusions, and to a lesser degree, measure cardiac output. Ventricular function is evaluated by measuring the left ventricular ejection fraction (LVEF). The LVEF is the percentage of blood ejected from the left ventricle during systole, normally 55% to 60%. There are a few patient considerations that may limit the accuracy of echocardiographic image interpretation. These include mechanical ventilation or lung disease, pleural effusions, the presence of chest bandages, significant breast tissue, body habitus, and arrhythmias.[5–7]

Transesophageal echocardiography (TEE). TEE provides ultrasonic imaging of the heart as viewed from behind the heart. In TEE, an ultrasound probe is fitted on the end of a flexible gastroscope, which is inserted into the posterior pharynx and advanced into the esophagus. This technique provides a clear picture of the heart because the esophagus lies against the back of the heart and parallel to the aorta. TEE is indicated to visualize prosthetic heart valves, mitral

TABLE 13.2 Major Systems Assessment for Cardiovascular Disease

System	Assessment
Neurological	Level of consciousness and orientation to person, place, time, events; presence of hallucinations, depression, withdrawal, restlessness, apprehensiveness, irritability, cooperativeness, response to tactile stimuli; type and location of pain; how pain is relieved; trembling; pupils (size, equality, response); paresthesias; eye movements; hand grips (strength and equality); leg movement
Skin	Color (mottling, cyanosis, pallor), temperature, dryness, turgor, presence of rashes, broken areas, pressure areas, urticaria, incision site, wounds
Cardiovascular	BP (bilaterally); apical heart rate and radial pulses; pulse deficit; monitor leads on patient in correct anatomical placement; regularity of rhythm, presence of ectopy; PR, QRS, and QT intervals; heart sounds; presence of abnormalities (rubs, gallops, clicks); neck vein distension with head of bed at what angle; edema (sacral and dependent); calf pain; varicosities; presence of pulses: bilateral carotid, radial, femoral, posterior tibial, dorsalis pedis; capillary refill in extremities; hemodynamic measurements; temporary pacemaker settings; medications to maintain BP or rhythm
Respiratory	Rate, depth, and quality of respirations; oxygen needs; accessory muscle use; cough; sputum: type, color, suctioning frequency; symmetry of chest expansion and breath sounds, breath sounds (crackles, wheezing); interpretation of ABG results; chest tube with description of drainage, fluctuation in water seal, bubbling, suction applied; tracheostomy or endotracheal tube; ventilator used; ventilator settings; ventilator rate versus patient's own breaths
Gastrointestinal	Abdominal size and softness, bowel sounds, nausea and vomiting, bowel movement, dressing and/or drainage, NG tube with description of drainage, feeding tube: type and frequency of feedings, drains
Genitourinary	Voiding or indwelling urinary catheter, urine color, quality, and quantity; vaginal or urethral drainage
Wounds	Dry or drainage (type, color, amount, odor); hematoma; inflamed; drains; dressing changes; cultures
Intravenous access sites	Volume of fluid, type of solution, rate; IV site condition

ABG, Arterial blood gas; *BP,* blood pressure; *IV,* intravenous; *NG,* nasogastric.

valve function, aortic dissection, vegetative endocarditis, congenital heart defects in adults, cardiac masses and tumors, and embolic phenomena. It is also used intraoperatively to assess left ventricular function. Based on which procedure is to be completed, patients should fast (except for medications) for a minimum of 2 hours before the examination. This recommendation allows clear liquids up to 2 hours before the procedure.[8] During the procedure, vital signs, cardiac rhythm, oxygen saturation, and sedation level are monitored. After the procedure, the patient is unable to eat until the gag reflex returns. A rare complication of TEE is esophageal perforation. The signs of perforation are sore throat, dysphagia, stiff neck, and epigastric or substernal pain that worsens with breathing and movement or pain in the back, abdomen, or shoulder.

Multigated blood acquisition scan (MUGA). MUGA is used to assess left ventricular function. An isotope is injected, and images of the heart are taken during systole and diastole to assess the LVEF of the heart. An LVEF of 55% to 60% and symmetrical contraction of the left ventricle are considered normal test results. This test is not as accurate in patients with irregular heart rhythms.

Cardiac magnetic resonance imaging (MRI). MRI is a noninvasive testing method used to evaluate tissues, structures, and blood flow. The technique uses magnetic resonance to create images of hydrogen ions as they are emitted, picked up, and fed into a computer. The computer reconstructs the image, which can be used to differentiate between healthy and ischemic tissue. MRI is used to diagnose or evaluate CAD, aortic aneurysm, congenital heart disease, left ventricular function, cardiac tumors, thrombus, valvular disease, and pericardial disorders. One of the advantages of MRI is that it does not involve exposure to ionizing radiation. A contrast agent can be used with MRI to enhance results.

MRI cannot be performed on patients with cochlear implants or some types of brain clips (used to treat cerebral aneurysms). It generally cannot be performed on patients with pacemakers or defibrillators. The test can be very stressful for patients who are claustrophobic, and in such situations, open MRI may be indicated. Cardiac monitors that are designed for use in MRI suites have been developed to ensure adequate monitoring of critically ill patients during the procedure.

Cardiac computed tomography (CT). The cardiac CT scan is a noninvasive way to image the heart three-dimensionally. It is used to evaluate for CAD, valvular disease, pericardial disease, and aneurysms and to map the pulmonary veins before ablation. When used with contrast, it is called *CT angiography*.

Positron emission tomography (PET). A PET scan is a noninvasive way to study cardiac tissue perfusion. Radioactive isotopes are injected intravenously to enable the imaging.

Cardiac catheterization and angiography. A cardiac catheterization is an invasive procedure that can be divided into two stages (right-sided and left-sided catheterization). It is used to measure pressures in the chambers of the heart, cardiac output, and blood gas content; to confirm and evaluate the severity of lesions within the coronary arteries; and to assess left ventricular function. (See Chapter 9, Hemodynamic Monitoring.)

Right-sided catheterization is performed by placing a pulmonary artery catheter in the femoral, brachial, or internal jugular vein and then carefully advancing it into the right atrium, right ventricle, and pulmonary artery. The healthcare provider measures pressures in the right atrium, right ventricle, and pulmonary artery, as well as the pulmonary artery occlusion pressure. Oxygen saturations can be measured, if indicated, to detect disease (i.e., valve disease or septal defect). A right-sided cardiac catheterization may be used to gather additional information if HF or pulmonary hypertension is suspected.

Left-sided catheterization is performed to visualize coronary arteries, to determine the area and extent of lesions within native vessel walls, and bypass grafts. It is also used to evaluate angina-related spasms, to locate areas of infarct, and to perform interventions such as percutaneous angioplasty or stent placement. Left-sided catheterization is performed by cannulation of a femoral, brachial, or radial artery. The procedure entails positioning a catheter into the aorta at the proximal end of the coronary arteries. Dye is injected into the arteries, and a radiographic picture is recorded as the dye progresses or fails to progress through the coronary circulation. In addition, dye is injected into the left ventricle, and the amount of dye ejected with the next systole is measured to determine the LVEF.

After the procedure, the catheters are removed. There are numerous vascular closure devices (VCDs) to prevent bleeding from the venous (right-sided catheterization) and arterial (left-sided catheterization) sites. VCDs include a sealing device made of collagen (e.g., Angio-Seal), a clip-mediated device (e.g., StarClose), a suture device (e.g., Perclose), and a hemostatic bandage (e.g., QuikClot). Commercial devices are available to assist in applying pressure to the site. For the radial artery, a compression device (e.g., TR Band) can be used (Fig. 13.9). If a VCD is not used, apply firm pressure to the site for 15 to 30 minutes. Depending on the diagnostic study results and the patient's status, patients are usually discharged within 4 to 8 hours after completion of the test.

Nursing care for a patient undergoing cardiac catheterization involves preprocedure education (the procedure will be performed using local anesthesia, and the patient may feel a warm or hot flush sensation or flutter of the catheter as it moves about) and postprocedure instruction. The postprocedure routine is described in Box 13.4.

Electrophysiology. An electrophysiology study is an invasive procedure that involves the introduction of an electrode catheter percutaneously from a peripheral vein or artery into the cardiac chamber or sinuses and the performance of programmed electrical stimulations of the heart. Electrophysiology studies aid in recording intracardiac ECGs, diagnosing cardiac conduction defects, evaluating the effectiveness of antiarrhythmic medications, determining the proper choice of pacemaker programming, and mapping the cardiac conduction system before ablation.

Laboratory Diagnostics. Other diagnostic measures include the evaluation of serum electrolytes and cardiac enzymes.

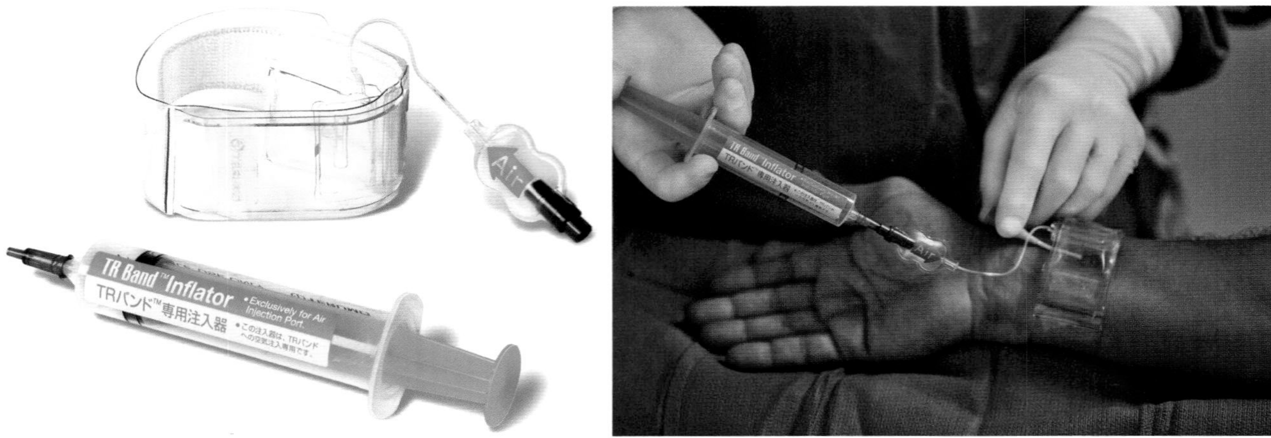

Fig. 13.9 TR Band Radial Compression Device. ()

BOX 13.4 Nursing Care After Cardiac Catheterization and Angiography

- Maintain the patient on bed rest (time varies depending on the size of the catheter used, the access site, and the method for preventing arterial or venous bleeding).
- Keep the extremity used for catheter insertion immobile.
- Observe the insertion site for bleeding or hematoma, especially if the patient is receiving postprocedure anticoagulant therapy.
- Mark a hematoma with a marker around its outer perimeter to aid in assessing for an increase in bleeding.
- Assess for bruits.
- Maintain head of bed elevation no higher than 30 degrees (if femoral access).
- Monitor peripheral pulses, color, and sensation of the extremity distal to insertion site (every 15 min × 4; every 30 min × 4; every 1 hour × 2). In addition, monitor the opposite extremity pulse to assess for presence of equal pulses and bilaterally for color and sensation.
- Observe cardiac rhythm.
- Encourage fluid intake if not contraindicated.
- Monitor intake and output.
- Observe for an adverse reaction to dye (angiography).
- Assess for chest pain, back pain, and shortness of breath. Notify provider if they develop or if the quality of symptoms change.

TABLE 13.3 ECG Changes Associated with Electrolyte Imbalances

Electrolyte Abnormality	ECG Abnormality
Increased calcium	Prolonged PR interval Shortened QT interval
Decreased calcium	Prolonged QT interval
Increased potassium	Narrowed, elevated T waves AV conduction changes Widened QRS complex
Decreased potassium	Prolonged U wave Prolonged QT interval

AV, Atrioventricular; *ECG*, electrocardiography.
From Pagana KD, Pagana TJ, Pagana TN. Cardiac stress testing (exercise stress testing). In: *Mosby's® Diagnostic and Laboratory Test Reference*. 15th ed. Elsevier Health Sciences; 2021.

Because many resources are available for interpretation of the laboratory values, this section presents a brief overview of the more important blood studies that are frequently used to assess the patient with a cardiovascular alteration.

Serum electrolytes. Electrolytes are important in maintaining the function of the cardiac conduction system. Imbalances in sodium, potassium, calcium, and magnesium can result in cardiac dysrhythmias. Therefore, analysis of serum electrolytes is a routine part of the assessment and treatment of the cardiac patient. Table 13.3 reviews ECG changes that may alert the nurse to possible electrolyte abnormalities.

Cardiac enzymes—high sensitivity cardiac troponin, troponin I, and troponin T. Serum troponin levels aid in the early diagnosis of AMI. Levels are normally undetectable in healthy people but become elevated as early as 1 hour after myocardial cell injury. Testing for troponin can be done quickly in the field or in the emergency department. The normal value of troponin I (unique to the heart muscle) is less than 0.04 ng/L, and that of troponin T is less than 0.1 ng/L.[9] The high sensitivity troponin (HS-cTN) is the preferred biomarker to assess cardiac related events and should be utilized to expedite the assessment for acute coronary syndrome (ACS). An HS-cTN value >100 ng/L is strongly suggestive of ACS[10]; however, cardiac troponins may be elevated not only due to a MI, but also noncardiac related situations such as a pulmonary embolism, chronic renal insufficiency, stroke, high intensity exercise, pneumonia, or sepsis.[9]

CHECK YOUR UNDERSTANDING:

3. The patient's echocardiography test showed a 58% left ventricular ejection fraction (LVEF). The nurse understands this result to be:
   A. Abnormally high
   B. Abnormally low
   C. Inconclusive
   D. Within normal limits

LIFESPAN CONSIDERATIONS

Several lifespan factors must be considered for the patient with cardiovascular disease. Cardiovascular issues can occur as a result of pregnancy. Many females are delaying pregnancy, which increases risks. In addition, females with a history of heart defects and cardiovascular disease are choosing to become pregnant. Older adults also need special consideration.

Older Adults

- Exercise caution when administering medications. Older adults have greater sensitivity to medications and may require lower dosages for some medications. Conversely, dosages may have to be increased for medications taken for long periods of time.
- Monitor closely for signs of medication effectiveness, adverse reactions, and possible interactions with other medications.
- Provide information in an easy-to-understand form and reinforce teaching. Consider having a family member or other caregiver present when teaching. Use the teach-back strategy to ensure understanding.
- Careful monitoring and continuous assessment are warranted postprocedure and in the postoperative period. Circulation decreases with aging. In addition, anesthesia and a major surgical procedure contribute to changes in level of consciousness and circulation.
- Always involve family members or close friends in the care of older adults. These individuals can assist the patient as they adjust to changes in treatment, activity, diet, and medications.
- Older adults may need assistance to maintain activities of daily living.
- Rehabilitation may be an important treatment after interventions, AMI, or surgery. Facilitate rehabilitation and encourage older adults to adhere to the set regimen to progress to maximum cardiac and vascular function.

Pregnant People

- Several cardiovascular conditions can occur during pregnancy. Some are more severe than others.
  - Peripartum cardiomyopathy may occur if heart failure (HF) occurs late in pregnancy or in the postpartum period.
  - Pregnancy-induced hypertension occurs in about 6% to 8% of females.
  - Acute myocardial infarction (AMI) is rare but can occur in people with a history of coronary artery disease (CAD) or from a spontaneous clot, since pregnancy increases the risks of blood clots.
  - A heart murmur may be noted secondary to increased blood volume in pregnancy. If noted, a cardiac workup is indicated.
  - Increased heart rate is a physiological response to pregnancy and increased blood volume. Although dysrhythmias may occur, most do not require treatment.
- Females with a history of cardiovascular disease can have a successful pregnancy with close observation during pregnancy, labor, and delivery. It is important to discuss pregnancy plans with the obstetrician and cardiologist prior to pregnancy.
  - If the pregnant person requires antidysrhythmic medications, the effects of the medication on the fetus must be considered.
  - Females with valvular disorders or artificial heart valves need to be monitored closely during pregnancy. The risk for endocarditis is higher. Those with artificial heart valves may need to change anticoagulants during pregnancy.
  - HF can develop or worsen in pregnancy secondary to increased blood volume.
  - Babies of people with a history of a congenital heart defect may have a greater risk of developing a heart defect as well. Prenatal evaluation for defects is indicated.
  - Planning and careful monitoring during delivery and in the immediate postpartum period are essential to reduce stress on the body associated with delivery. Vaginal delivery is often possible.

Patient Problems

Because CAD is a broad diagnostic area, patients may present with several problems. With the complications of CAD, such as angina, MI, and HF, the problems are more specific. Patient problems for those with CAD include the following:

- Acute pain (angina) from decreased oxygen supply to the myocardium
- Fatigue with decreased exercise tolerance because of generalized weakness and imbalance between oxygen supply and demand occurring with tissue ischemia secondary to MI
- Need for health teaching because of unfamiliarity with the disease process and lifestyle implications of CAD

Interventions

Nursing Interventions. Nursing interventions encompass health assessment and patient education. Assessment of the patient's psychosocial status and family support, as well as the history and physical examination findings, are used to guide interventions. Instruct the patient about risk factor modification and signs and symptoms of progression of CAD that warrant medical treatment. See Lifespan Considerations for population specific considerations.

Medical Management. The goal of medical management is to reduce risk factors for progression of CAD. Strategies for risk factor modification include a low-fat, low-cholesterol diet; exercise; weight loss; smoking cessation; and control of other risks such as diabetes and hypertension. The American Heart Association and the American College of Cardiology revised the cholesterol guidelines in 2022 and developed a consensus statement describing referral considerations. Rather than recommending therapy to reach a specific LDL level, statin therapy is now recommended based on a patient history of clinical ASCVD, diabetes mellitus, LDL level, and CAD risk. The focus of these new guidelines was not only to address gaps in lowering the LDL-C based on the status of ASCVD risk factors but also to address specific situations pertaining to appropriate usage of nonstatin therapies (such as ezetimibe, proprotein convertase subtilisin/kexin type 9 [PCSK9] mAb, or a combination of any of these) in certain populations.[11] Clinical ASCVD includes history of AMI, ACS, stable or unstable angina, coronary or other arterial revascularization, stroke, transient ischemic attack (TIA), or peripheral arterial disease presumed to be of atherosclerotic origin. Referral to a lipid specialist should be considered in individuals with ASCVD risk and an LDL-C ≥190 mg/dL.[11] Updated guidelines describe individualizing cholesterol lowering therapies based on LDL-C levels, with or with out ASCVD risk factors, as well as appropriate up-titration of medications to reach acceptable cholesterol levels[11] (Fig. 13.10 and Box 13.5).

Medications to reduce serum lipid levels. Lipid-lowering medications include statins, ezetimibe, niacinamide and a newer class of medications called PCSK9 inhibitors (Table 13.4). The statins are officially classified as 3-hydroxy-3-methylglutaryl-coenzyme A (HMG-CoA) reductase inhibitors. Statin medications lower LDL by slowing the production of cholesterol and increasing the liver's ability to remove LDL from the body and are well tolerated by most individuals. It is recommended that some statins be given as a single dose in the evening because the body makes more cholesterol at night.[12] A disadvantage of statins is that they can cause liver damage; therefore, ensure that the patient has liver enzymes measured periodically. Rarely, the medications cause myopathies; instruct patients to contact their healthcare provider if they develop any muscle aches (myalgia) or join pain (arthralgia). Statins are considered to be the best treatment for cholesterol management. Other medications may be prescribed for patients who are intolerant of statins.[12]

Selective cholesterol-absorption inhibitors (e.g., ezetimibe) work in the digestive tract by blocking the absorption of cholesterol from food. They are often used in conjunction with other cholesterol-reducing medications. A side effect includes liver disease; therefore, liver function tests must be monitored, and the medication is contraindicated in patients with severe hepatic disease. When added to a statin, ezetimibe reduces cardiovascular events.[13]

Antilipemic agents (e.g., niacinamide) reduce total cholesterol, LDL, and triglyceride levels and increase high-density lipoproteins (HDLs). The medication is available over the counter; however, its use in lowering cholesterol must be done under the supervision of a healthcare provider.

BOX 13.5 Intensity of Statin Therapy

High-Intensity Statin Therapy	Moderate-Intensity Statin Therapy	Low-Intensity Statin Therapy
Daily dose lowers LDL-C, on average, by approximately ≥50%	*Daily dose lowers LDL-C, on average, by approximately 30% to 50%*	*Daily dose lowers LDL-C, on average, by <30%*

bid, twice daily; *LDL-C,* Low-density lipoprotein cholesterol.
Modified from Grundy SM, Stone NJ, Bailey AL et al. 2018 AHA/ACC/AACVPR/AAPA/ABC/ACPM/ADA/AGS/APhA/ASPC/NLA/PCNA guideline on the management of blood cholesterol. *J Am Coll Cardiol.* 2019;73(24):3234-3237.

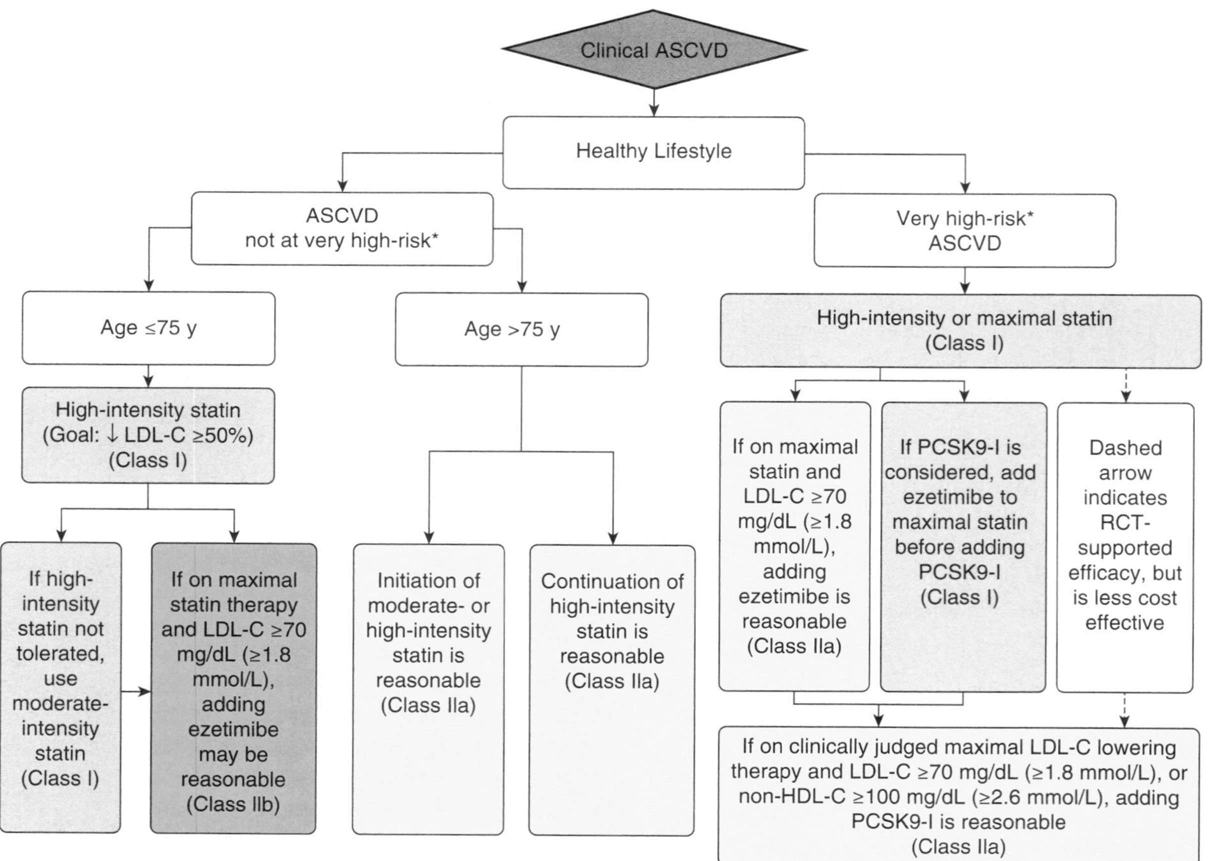

Fig. 13.10 Secondary prevention statin recommendations for the treatment of blood cholesterol. *ASCVD,* atherosclerotic cardiovascular disease; *HDL-C,* high-density lipoprotein cholesterol; *LDL-C,* low-density lipoprotein cholesterol; *PCSK9-I,* proprotein convertase subtilisin/kexin type 9 inhibitor; *RCT,* randomized controlled trial. (From Grundy SM, Stone NJ, Bailey AL, et al. 2018 AHA/ACC/AACVPR/AAPA/ABC/ACPM/ADA/AGS/APhA/ASPC/NLA/PCNA guideline on the management of blood cholesterol. *J Am Coll Cardiol.* 2019;73[24]:3234-3237.)

TABLE 13.4 **PHARMACOLOGY**

Medications (Antilipemic Agents) for Lowering Cholesterol and Triglycerides

Medication	Action/Use	Dose/Route	Side Effects	Nursing Implications
HMG-CoA Reductase Inhibitors				
Lovastatin (Altocor)	Competitively inhibits HMG-CoA reductase, which affects cholesterol biosynthesis; lowers total and LDL-C levels; increases HDL-C; and is used to lower total cholesterol and LDL-C	Immediate release: 40–80 mg daily PO with evening meal Extended release: 40–60 mg daily PO at bedtime	Constipation Dizziness Headache Hepatic dysfunction Increased creatine phosphokinase (CPK) levels Myopathy Rhabdomyolysis	Report severe muscle pain or weakness, which can be signs of rhabdomyolysis. Obtain baseline liver function and lipid profile tests before starting therapy 6 weeks later and periodically or when dose is increased. Do not give in pregnancy.
Atorvastatin (Lipitor)	Same; High-intensity therapy used to help reduce the risk of AMI and stroke	10–80 mg PO daily	Same	Same
Fluvastatin (Lescol XL)	Same	20–80 mg daily PO qhs	Same	Same
Pravastatin (Pravachol)	Same	10–80 mg daily PO qhs	Same	Same
Rosuvastatin (Crestor)	Same; High-intensity therapy used to help reduce the risk of AMI and stroke	5–40 mg daily PO daily	Same	Same
Simvastatin (Zocor)	Same	5–80 mg daily PO qhs	Same	Same The FDA has mandated no more new prescriptions of 80 mg. (Patients who have been stable for >1 year may continue to take 80 mg/day.) Maximum dose of 20 mg for patients taking amiodarone, amlodipine, or ranolazine, and 10 mg for patients taking verapamil or diltiazem. Contraindicated in patients taking gemfibrozil; antifungal medications; antibiotics such as erythromycin, clarithromycin; and HIV protease inhibitors
Niacinamide				
Niacinamide (Niacin)	Inhibits VLDL synthesis Used for adjunctive treatment of hyperlipidemia	*Immediate release:* 250 mg daily PO, increase as tolerated to 1.5–2 g daily (divided in 2–3 doses), may further titrate to max 6 g/day; max 6 g/day *Extended release:* 500 mg daily at qhs PO; titrate in 500-mg intervals (up to 2 g) q4 weeks based on tolerability and efficacy; maintenance, 1 to 2 g PO daily; max 2 g/day	Bloating Flatulence Flushing Headache Hepatic toxicity Nausea	Should be taken after meals. Report persistent GI disturbances or changes in color of urine or stool. May premedicate with aspirin 30 minutes before dose to minimize flushing.
Cholesterol Absorption Inhibitors				
Ezetimibe (Zetia)	Inhibits absorption of cholesterol in the small intestine	*Tablet:* 10 mg daily	Diarrhea Dizziness Headache Hepatotoxicity Joint pain Myalgia Myopathy Runny nose Sneezing Sore throat	Monitor for signs of liver failure.

TABLE 13.4 PHARMACOLOGY—cont'd

Medications (Antilipemic Agents) for Lowering Cholesterol and Triglycerides

Medication	Action/Use	Dose/Route	Side Effects	Nursing Implications
Proprotein Convertase Subtilisin/Kexin Type 9 (PCSK9)				
Alirocumab (Praluent) Evolocumab (Repatha)	Controls number of LDL receptors to regulate cholesterol levels; decreases LDL receptor degradation and increased LDL clearance	Alirocumab 75–150 mg SQ q2 weeks Evolocumab: 140 mg SQ q2 weeks or up to 420 mg SQ q2 weeks to 1 month	Angioedema Bronchitis Cough Diarrhea Dizziness Hypersensitivity Increase in liver enzymes Injection site reaction	Caution use if latex allergy due to cross reaction potential Dosing may need to be adjusted if renal or liver dysfunction.

AMI, Acute myocardial infarction; *bid,* twice daily; *FDA,* U.S. Food and Drug Administration; *GI,* gastrointestinal; *HDL-C,* high-density lipoprotein cholesterol; *HMG-CoA,* 3-hydroxy-3-methylglutaryl-coenzyme A; *LDL-C,* low-density lipoprotein cholesterol; *max,* maximum; *PO,* orally; *q,* every; *qhs,* bedtime; *VLDL,* very–low–density lipoprotein.
From Skidmore-Roth L. *Mosby's 2023 Nursing Drug Reference.* 36th ed. Elsevier; 2023.

If a patient does not respond adequately to single-medication therapy, combined-medication therapy is considered to further lower LDL levels. For example, statins may be combined with bile acid resins or PCSK9 inhibitors. PCSK9 inhibitors are monoclonal antibodies approved by the U.S. Food and Drug Administration (FDA) for treatment of heterozygous familial hypercholesteremia and for those with ASCVD who require additional LDL lowering.[14] PCSK9 regulates cholesterol metabolism; thus, a PCSK9 inhibitor slows cholesterol metabolism and lowers LDL levels. Minimal side effects or drug-to-drug interactions have been reported.[15] Careful monitoring of liver function and blood sugars in patients on two or more lipid-lowering agents are simultaneously performed because of the risk of liver disease and the increased risk of the development of diabetes.[16] If triglyceride levels are elevated, patients may be prescribed agents that specifically lower triglyceride levels.

Medications to prevent platelet adhesion and aggregation. Medications are often prescribed for the patient with CAD to reduce platelet adhesion and aggregation. A single dose of enteric-coated aspirin (81 to 325 mg) is commonly prescribed. To prevent further platelet aggregation, other agents may be prescribed along with aspirin, such as a P2Y12 inhibitor.

Patient Outcomes

Several outcomes are expected after treatment. These include relief of pain; less anxiety related to the disease; adherence to health-behavior modification to reduce cardiovascular risks; and the ability to describe the disease process, causes, factors contributing to the symptoms, and procedures for disease or symptom control.

ANGINA

Angina is chest pain or discomfort caused by myocardial ischemia that is attributed to an imbalance between myocardial oxygen supply and demand. CAD and coronary artery spasms are common causes of angina.

Pathophysiology

Angina (from the Latin word meaning "squeezing") is the chest pain associated with myocardial ischemia. It is transient and does not cause cell death, but it may be a precursor to cell death from MI. The neural pain receptors are stimulated by accelerated metabolism, chemical changes and imbalances, and/or local mechanical stress resulting from abnormal myocardial contractions. The level of oxygen circulating via the vascular system to the myocardial cells decreases, causing ischemia to the tissue and resulting in pain. Angina occurs when oxygen demand is higher than oxygen supply. Box 13.6 shows factors influencing oxygen supply and demand that may result in angina.

Types of Angina

Different types of angina exist: stable angina, unstable angina, and variant (Prinzmetal's) angina. *Stable angina* occurs with exertion and is relieved by rest. It is sometimes called chronic exertional angina. *Unstable angina* is often more severe, may occur at rest, and requires more frequent nitrate therapy. It

BOX 13.6 Factors That Influence Oxygen Supply and Demand

Increased Oxygen Demand

- Increased heart rate: exercise, tachydysrhythmias, fever, anxiety, pain, thyrotoxicosis, medications, ingestion of heavy meals, adapting to extremes in temperature
- Increased preload: volume overload
- Increased afterload: hypertension, aortic stenosis, vasopressors
- Increased contractility: exercise, medications, anxiety

Reduced Oxygen Supply

- Coronary artery disease
- Coronary artery spasms
- Anemia
- Hypoxemia

is sometimes described as crescendo (increasing) in nature. During an unstable episode, the ECG may show ST-segment depression, T-wave inversion, or no changes at all. The patient has an increased risk of MI within 18 months after onset of unstable angina, warranting medical and/or surgical interventions. Patients are often hospitalized for diagnostic workup and treatment. The treatment of unstable angina is discussed more completely in this chapter's section, Acute Coronary Syndrome.

Variant, or *Prinzmetal's*, angina is caused by coronary artery spasms. It often occurs at rest and without other precipitating factors. The ECG shows a marked ST elevation (usually seen only in AMI) during the episode. The ST segment returns to normal after the spasm subsides. AMI can occur with prolonged coronary artery spasm, even in the absence of CAD. Recognizing that not all angina is the same, assessing for anginal equivalents such as shortness of breath, fatigue, or pain in other body parts is very important, especially in women, obese individuals, diabetics, African Americans, and older adults (>75 years of age).

Assessment

Assessment of the patient with actual or suspected angina involves continual observation of the patient and monitoring of signs, symptoms, and diagnostic findings. The patient must be monitored for the type and degree of pain (see Clinical Alert box).

! CLINICAL ALERT

Symptoms of Angina

- Pain is frequently retrosternal, left pectoral, or epigastric. It may radiate to the jaw, left shoulder, or left arm.
- Pain may be associated with fatigue, dyspnea, lightheadedness, or diaphoresis.
- Discomfort may be reported as throat, neck, back, or stomach pain, indigestion, or muscle strain.
- Pain can be described as chest pressure, burning, squeezing, heavy, or smothering.
- Pain usually lasts from 1 to 5 minutes.
- Classic placing of a clenched fist against the chest (sternum) may be seen or may be absent if the sensation is confused with indigestion.
- Pain usually begins with exertion and subsides with rest.

CHECK YOUR UNDERSTANDING:

4. During an assessment of a patient admitted with new-onset angina, the patient suddenly complains of chest pain, and ST-segment elevation is noted on the bedside monitor. The nurse anticipates the patient is experiencing which type of angina?
   A. Exercise-induced
   B. Prinzmetal's
   C. Smoking-induced
   D. Stable

The precipitating factors for anginal pain include physical or emotional stress, exposure to temperature extremes, and ingestion of a heavy meal. It is important to know what factors alleviate the anginal pain, including stopping activity or exercise and taking NTG sublingual tablets or spray.

Diagnostic Studies. Diagnostic studies for angina include the following: history and physical examination, including assessment of pain and precipitating factors; laboratory data, including cardiac enzymes (cardiac troponin I, T, and HS-cTN levels), complete blood count to assess for anemia (hemoglobin and hematocrit values), cholesterol, and triglyceride levels; ECGs during resting periods; stress testing; and coronary angiography. Complications of untreated angina or unstable angina include AMI, HF, dysrhythmias, psychological depression, and sudden death.

Patient Problems

Patients with angina have many problems amenable to nursing interventions. These include the following:

- Acute pain (angina) caused by decreased oxygen supply to the myocardium
- Anxiety caused by actual or perceived threat of death, change in health status, threat to self-concept or role, unfamiliar people and environment, medications, preexisting anxiety disorder, uncertainty
- Need for health teaching because of unfamiliarity with current health status and prescribed therapies

Interventions

Nursing Interventions. Nursing interventions for the patient with angina are aimed at assessing the patient's description of pain; noting exacerbating factors and measures used to relieve the pain; evaluating whether this is a chronic problem (stable angina) or a new presentation; assessing for indications for obtaining an ECG to evaluate ST-segment and T-wave changes; monitoring vital signs during chest pain and after nitrate administration; and monitoring the effectiveness of interventions. Instruct the patient to relax and rest at the first sign of pain or discomfort and to notify the nurse at the onset of any type of chest pain. Nitrates may be used as this time, and oxygen via nasal cannula may be used when oxygen saturations are ≤90%.[17] Offer assurance and emotional support by explaining all treatments and procedures and encouraging questions. Assess the patient's knowledge level regarding the causes of angina, diagnostic procedures, the treatment plan, and risk factors for CAD. For patients who smoke, assess readiness to quit and encourage participation in a smoking cessation program. Refer patients who wish to stop smoking to the American Heart Association, American Lung Association, American Cancer Society, or other organizations for support groups and interventions.

Medical Interventions. The focus of treatment for unstable angina is to improve myocardial perfusion to the coronary arteries as quickly as possible. This may include conservative management, early intervention with percutaneous intervention, or surgical revascularization. Conservative intervention includes the administration of nitrates, beta-adrenergic blocking agents, calcium channel blocking agents, and antiplatelet agents. Additional treatment options may include adding oxygen when oxygen saturations are ≤90% and intravenous heparin (Table 13.5). Angioplasty, stenting, and bypass surgery are interventional approaches to revascularization.

TABLE 13.5 PHARMACOLOGY

Common Medications Used to Treat Common Cardiovascular Problems

Medication	Action/Use	Dose/Route	Side Effects	Nursing Implications
Angiotensin-Converting Enzyme Inhibitors				
Enalapril (Vasotec, Enalaprilat)	Prevents the conversion of AI to AII, resulting in lower levels of AII, which causes an increase in plasma renin activity and a reduction of aldosterone secretion; also inhibits the remodeling process after myocardial injury Used to treat hypertension and heart failure and after MI	*PO:* 2.5–40 mg daily (in 1–2 divided doses) *IV:* 1.25 mg q6h PRN or scheduled	Acute kidney injury Angioedema Cough Dizziness Hyperkalemia Hypotension Orthostatic hypotension	Monitor serum potassium levels. Monitor serum creatinine and BUN. Avoid use of NSAIDs. Contraindicated in pregnancy. Hold therapy and discuss continued therapy with provider in acute kidney injury.
Lisinopril (Prinivil)	Same	*PO:* 5–40 mg daily	Same	Same
Beta-Blockers				
Carvedilol (Coreg, Coreg CR)	Alpha and beta-blocker; decreases vascular resistance acutely and blood pressure; decreases heart rate; may influence the renin-angiotensin system; used for angina, heart failure, acute myocardial infarction, hypertension	*PO:* Immediate release: 3.125–50 mg bid Extended release: 10–80 mg daily PO	Bradyarrhythmias Bronchospasm Fatigue Hypotension Impotence May mask hypoglycemic episodes	Take with meals.
Labetalol (Trandate)	Same as carvedilol	*PO:* 100–400 mg bid to tid (max 2400 mg/day) *IV:* 10–20 mg over 2 min at 10-min intervals (max 300 mg/day)	Same	During IV administration, monitor blood pressure continuously; max effect occurs within 5 min.
Metoprolol (Lopressor, Toprol XL)	Blocks beta-adrenergic receptors, resulting in decreased SNS response such as decreased heart rate, blood pressure, and cardiac contractility; used to treat angina, acute myocardial infarction, dysrhythmias and heart failure, hypertension	*PO:* Immediate release: 25–100 mg bid Extended release: 12.5–200 mg daily *IV:* 5 mg every 2 min for a total of 3 doses	Same	Do not stop abruptly-can exacerbate angina and MI.
Nitrates				
Nitroglycerin (Nitro-Dur, Nitrostat)	Directly relaxes smooth muscle, causing vasodilation of the systemic vascular bed; decreases myocardial oxygen demands; secondary effect is vasodilation of responsive coronary arteries	*SL:* 0.4 mg q5 min for up to 3 doses *Topical:* 0.5–2 in q6 h *Transdermal:* one patch each day *IV:* continuous infusion started at 5 mcg/min and titrated up to a max of 200 mcg/min	Dizziness Flushing Headache Tachycardia Tachyphylaxis with continuous administration Orthostatic hypotension	For topical dosing, patient should have a nitrate-free interval (10–12 h/day) to avoid development of tolerance. Do not take nitrate with medications used to treat erectile dysfunction (e.g., vardenafil, tadalafil, sildenafil).
Isosorbide dinitrate (Isordil) Isosorbide mononitrate (Imdur)	Oral vasodilators (vascular smooth muscle relaxation)	Dinitrate (Isordil): *PO:* Immediate release: 5–40 mg bid to tid Extended release: 40-160 mg/day Mononitrate (Imdur): *PO:* Immediate release: 20 mg BID Extended release: 30–120 mg ER daily in the morning	Bradycardia Dizziness Headaches Hypotension	Dinitrate: Allow for a nitrate-free period between evening and morning dose Mononitrate: Administer immediate release at least 7 hours after morning dose

TABLE 13.5 **PHARMACOLOGY—cont'd**

Common Medications Used to Treat Common Cardiovascular Problems

Medication	Action/Use	Dose/Route	Side Effects	Nursing Implications
Calcium Channel Blockers				
Amlodipine (Norvasc)	Inhibits influx of calcium ions into the vascular smooth muscle to produce peripheral vasodilation reducing peripheral vascular resistance; used to manage blood pressure	*PO:* 5–10 mg daily (max dose 10 mg)	Dizziness Flushing Hypotension Nausea Palpitations Peripheral edema	Monitor pulse and blood pressure.
Diltiazem (Cardizem, Cardizem CD)	Inhibits influx of calcium ions into the vascular smooth muscle and myocardium, producing relaxation of coronary vascular smooth muscle and coronary vasodilation; used for supraventricular tachycardia	*IV:* 0.25 mg/kg x1 bolus, may repeat bolus 0.35 mg/kg x1, follow with continuous infusion: 5–15 mg/h *PO:* 30 mg qid, usual dose 120–380 mg daily *PO sustained release:* 120–360 mg daily, max 480–540 mg	AV block Bradycardia Peripheral edema	IV diltiazem should be avoided in those with acute decompensated heart failure.
Antiplatelet Agents				
Aspirin	Inhibits clotting mechanisms within the clotting cascade to prevent platelet aggregation; used for unstable angina, acute myocardial infarction, and coronary interventions	*PO:* 81–325 mg daily	Bleeding Bruising Epigastric discomfort Gastric ulceration	Instruct patient to take medication with food. Do not crush or chew the enteric-coated forms.
Clopidogrel (Plavix)	Inhibits the binding of adenosine diphosphate (ADP) to the P2Y12 platelet receptor, causing irreversible binding and inhibit platelet aggregation; Used to prevent blood clots in the peripheral vascular system and cerebrovascular system	*PO:* 300-mg loading dose, then 75 mg/day	Bleeding Itching Pancytopenia	Consider holding for a minimum of 5 days prior to surgery. Watch for any signs of bleeding.
Prasugrel (Effient)	Same as clopidogrel	*PO:* 60-mg loading dose, then 10 mg/day	Same	Not recommended for patients >75 years of age, weighing <60 kg, or with history of TIA.
Ticagrelor (Brilinta)	Same as clopidogrel	*PO:* 180-mg (two 90-mg tablets) loading dose (in combination with 325 mg aspirin), then 90 mg/day (with 81 mg aspirin)	Same	Contraindicated in patients with history of intracranial hemorrhage, active pathological bleeding, or severe hepatic impairment. The risk of bleeding is higher with ticagrelor.
Glycoprotein IIb/IIIa Inhibitors				
Tirofiban (Aggrastat)	Binds to the Gp IIb/IIIa receptor site on the surface of the platelet inhibiting platelet aggregation; used in patients with acute coronary syndromes and coronary intervention	*IV:* 0.25 mcg/kg bolus over 3 min, followed by 0.15 mcg/kg/min infusion Reduce loading and maintenance infusion by 50% in patients with CrCl <30 mL/min	Bleeding Bruising Hemorrhage Hypotension Thrombocytopenia	Assess infusion insertion site for bleeding or hematoma formation. Assess puncture site used for coronary intervention frequently. Tirofiban stops working when the infusion is discontinued. Platelet function is restored 4 h after stopping the infusion.

Continued

TABLE 13.5 PHARMACOLOGY—cont'd

Common Medications Used to Treat Common Cardiovascular Problems

Medication	Action/Use	Dose/Route	Side Effects	Nursing Implications
Eptifibatide (Integrilin)	Same	*IV:* 180 mcg/kg loading dose over 2 min, max 22.6 mg, followed by continuous infusion of 2 mcg/kg/min for 18–24 h or until hospital discharge. Reduce maintenance dose by 50% (to 1 mcg/kg/min) in patients with CrCl <50 mL/min; contraindicated if CrCl is <10 mL/min.	Same	Eptifibatide stops working when the infusion is discontinued. Platelet function is restored 4 h after stopping the infusion. Assess infusion insertion site for bleeding or hematoma formation. Assess puncture site used for coronary intervention frequently.
Antithrombin Agents				
Heparin	Enhances inhibitory effects of antithrombin III, preventing conversion of fibrinogen to fibrin and prothrombin to thrombin; used to prevent or delay thrombus formation	*IV:* 60–80 units/kg bolus, followed by infusion of 12–18 units/kg/h, titrated to aPTT/anti-Xa (follow institutional protocol).	Bleeding Bruising Thrombocytopenia	Monitor for signs of bleeding and hematoma formation.
Enoxaparin (Lovenox)	Same	Subcutaneous: 1 mg/kg q12 h. For CrCl <30 mL/min, 1 mg/kg q24 h	Bleeding Bruising Hemorrhage Local site hematomas	Monitor for signs of bleeding and hematoma formation. Do not rub the site after giving the injection. May monitor anti-Xa in special patient populations (e.g., obesity, renal dysfunction).

AI, Angiotensin I; *AII,* angiotensin II; *aPTT,* activated partial thromboplastin time; *AV,* atrioventricular; *bid,* twice daily; *CNS,* central nervous system; *CrCl,* creatine clearance; *Gp,* glycoprotein; *IVP,* intravenous push; *max,* maximum; *MI,* myocardial infarction; *NSAIDs,* nonsteroidal antiinflammatory drugs; *PO,* orally; *q,* every; *qid,* four times daily; *SL,* sublingual; *SNS,* sympathetic nervous system; *TIA,* transient ischemic attack; *tid,* three times daily.
From Skidmore-Roth L. *Mosby's 2023 Nursing Drug Reference.* 36th ed. St. Louis, MO: Elsevier; 2019.

Nitrates are the most common medications used to treat angina. They are direct-acting smooth-muscle relaxants that cause vasodilation of the peripheral or systemic vascular bed. Nitrate therapy is beneficial because it decreases myocardial oxygen demand. The vasodilating effect relieves pain and lowers BP. NTG is available in quick-acting forms such as sublingual tablets or spray or as an IV infusion. Long-acting nitrates are delivered orally or by ointments and skin patches (transdermal). Isosorbide is another oral nitrate that may be used for vasodilatation to treat angina. Side effects of nitrate vasodilators include headache, flushing, tachycardia, dizziness, and orthostatic hypotension. Instructions for NTG therapy are detailed in Box 13.7.

Beta-adrenergic blocking agents may also be used to treat angina. These agents block adrenergic receptors, thereby decreasing heart rate, BP, and cardiac contractility.[1] The side effects of these medications include bradycardia, AV block, asthma attacks, depression, erectile dysfunction, hypotension, memory loss, and masking of hypoglycemic episodes (except for sweating). These medications should be administered as prescribed, do not stop them abruptly, and monitor heart rate and BP at regular intervals. Instruct patients with diabetes to monitor blood glucose levels since hypoglycemic symptoms may be masked.

Calcium channel blockers inhibit the flow of calcium ions across cellular membranes, an effect that causes direct increases in coronary blood flow and myocardial perfusion. In addition to angina, these medications are used to treat tachydysrhythmias, vasospasms, and hypertension. Calcium channel blockers are divided into two categories: dihydropyridines and nondihydropyridines. Dihydropyridines are primarily used to treat hypertension. These medications typically end in the suffix "-pine" (e.g., amlodipine). Nondihydropyridines such as verapamil and diltiazem are more effective for treatment of angina and dysrhythmias. The side effects of calcium channel blockers include dizziness, flushing, headaches, decreased heart rate, and hypotension. Ankle edema is a major side effect of the dihydropyridine-type calcium channel blocker. Monitor the patient's BP for hypotension and heart rate for bradycardia, especially if the agents are taken in combination with nitrates and beta-blockers.

Beta-blockers and calcium channel blockers need to be cautiously used simultaneously in ACS when coexisting with HF, as the HF symptoms may become exacerbated.

BOX 13.7 Instructions Regarding Nitroglycerin

If the patient is discharged on sublingual or buccal nitroglycerin, provide the following education to the patient:

- Have tablets readily available.
- Take a tablet before strenuous activity and in stressful situations.
- Take one tablet when chest pain occurs and another every 5 min up to a maximum total of three times if necessary; obtain emergency medical assistance if pain persists.
- Place the tablet under the tongue or in the buccal pouch and allow it to dissolve thoroughly.
- Store tablets in the tightly capped, original container away from heat and moisture.
- Replace tablets every 6 months or sooner if they do not relieve discomfort.
- Avoid rising to a standing position quickly after taking nitroglycerin.
- Recognize that dizziness, flushing, and mild headache are common side effects.
- Report fainting, persistent or severe headache, blurred vision, or dry mouth.
- Avoid drinking alcoholic beverages.
- Caution against use of medications for erectile dysfunction when taking nitrates because hypotensive effects are exaggerated.
- If nitroglycerin skin patches or paste are prescribed:
  - Provide instructions about correct application, skin care, the need to rotate sites and to remove the old patch, and frequency of change.
  - The patch should be worn no more than 12–14 h/day to prevent development of nitrate tolerance.
  - Caution should be taken not to touch the nitroglycerin paste when applying it to the patient. Gloves will assist in ensuring this does not happen. If the nitroglycerin comes in contact with the skin of the person placing the paste on the patient, hand washing should occur immediately to avoid cross-reaction.

From Skidmore-Roth L. *Mosby's 2023 Nursing Drug Reference*. 36th ed. St. Louis, MO: Mosby; 2023.

Patient Outcomes

The outcomes for patients with angina are as follows: They will verbalize relief of chest discomfort, appear relaxed and comfortable, verbalize an understanding of angina pectoris and its management, describe their own cardiac risk factors and strategies to reduce them, and perform activities within limits of their ischemic disease, as evidenced by absence of chest pain or discomfort and no ECG changes reflecting ischemia.

ACUTE CORONARY SYNDROME

ACS includes the diagnoses of stable angina, unstable angina, and AMI and is defined as myocardial necrosis caused by ischemia.[18,19] Prompt recognition and treatment result in improved outcomes for all patients presenting with ACS.

Pathophysiology

ACS is caused by an imbalance between myocardial oxygen supply and demand. This imbalance is the result of decreased coronary artery perfusion. Most cases of ACS are secondary to atherosclerosis. Other causes include coronary artery spasm, coronary embolism, and blunt trauma. Reduced blood flow to an area of the myocardium causes significant and sustained oxygen deprivation to myocardial cells. Normal functioning is disrupted as ischemia and injury lead to eventual cellular death. Myocardial dysfunction occurs as more cells become involved.

Prolonged ischemia from cessation of blood flow to the cardiac muscle results in infarction and evolves over time. Cardiac cells can withstand ischemic conditions for approximately 20 minutes; after that period, irreversible myocardial cell damage and cellular death begin. The amount of cell death increases, extending from the endocardium to the epicardium as the duration of the occlusion causing the ischemia increases. Contractility in the infarcted area becomes impaired. A nonfunctional zone and a zone of mild ischemia with potentially viable tissue surround the infarct. The ultimate size and extent of cell death determines the size of the infarct, or ischemic zone. Early interventions, such as administration of thrombolytics or minimally invasive coronary angioplasty (e.g., percutaneous coronary intervention [PCI]), can restore perfusion to the ischemic zone and reduce the area of myocardial damage.

Classification of an MI is determined by anatomical causes of the infarction rather than the ECG changes. Type I is a spontaneous MI and occurs because of plaque rupture, leading to occlusion of the artery. Type II is an MI secondary to ischemic imbalance between myocardial oxygen supply and demand. Type II may be caused by coronary endothelial dysfunction, coronary vasospasm, embolism, arrhythmias, anemia, respiratory failure, hypotension, and shock.[20] Most infarcts occur in the left ventricle; however, right ventricular infarction occurs in approximately one-third of patients with inferior wall infarction.[18] While ECG changes are no longer used to classify an MI, the presence or absence of ST elevation on the ECG is used to assess ischemia. ST elevation MI (STEMI) is seen in type II MI events, and non-STEMI (NSTEMI), absence of ST elevation on the ECG, is typically seen in type I events. Both require urgent assessment and interventions to reduce myocardial muscle damage.

The severity of the MI is determined by the success or failure of the treatment and by the degree of collateral circulation present at that particular part of the heart muscle where the ischemic event occurred. The collateral circulation consists of the alternative routes, or channels, that develop in the myocardium in response to chronic ischemia or regional hypoperfusion. Through this small network of extra vessels, blood flow to the threatened myocardium can be improved.

Assessment

Patient assessment includes close observation to identify the classic signs and symptoms of ACS, most notably angina. The skin may be cool, clammy, pale, and diaphoretic; the patient's color may be dusky or ashen, and low-grade fever may be present. The patient may be dyspneic and tachypneic and may feel faint or have intermittent loss of sensorium. Nausea and vomiting commonly occur. Hypotension may be present and is often associated with dysrhythmias, particularly ventricular ectopy, bradycardia, tachycardia, or heart block. The type of dysrhythmia present depends on the area of the MI.

The patient may be anxious or restless or may exhibit certain behavioral responses, including denial, depression, and a sense of impending doom. For females chest pain may not be the most obvious symptom.[21] (See Box 13.8 and the Clinical Alert box.)

! CLINICAL ALERT

Acute Coronary Syndrome in Females

Females are less likely than males to have chest pain in acute coronary syndrome (ACS), and they are more likely to have atypical signs and symptoms such as fatigue, diaphoresis, indigestion, arm or shoulder pain, nausea, and vomiting.

Some individuals have ischemic episodes without knowing it; this is known as a *silent* infarction. Silent infarctions occur with no presenting signs or symptoms and are more common in patients with diabetes secondary to neuropathy. Assessment of a patient experiencing ACS requires evaluation of signs and symptoms interpreted within the context of the patient's history, ACS risk factors, and physical examination.

BOX 13.8 Cardiovascular Disease in Females

Cardiovascular disease is the leading cause of death in females and more females than males die of heart disease.

Risk Factors

- *Age:* Females are at higher risk at age 55, whereas males are at higher risk at age 45.
- *Family history:* Heart disease in a first-degree relative is considered premature if it occurred before age 65 for females or before age 55 for males. Heart disease in a first-degree female relative is a more potent risk factor than heart disease in a male relative.
- *Hypertension:* The risk of heart failure due to hypertension is greater in females.
- *Diabetes:* Diabetes is a greater risk factor for heart disease in females than in males. Risk for fatal heart disease in diabetic females is 3.5 times higher than that in nondiabetic females.
- *Dyslipidemia:* More than half of females in the United States have dyslipidemia, which becomes worse as females age and become menopausal.
- *Smoking:* Female smokers die earlier than male smokers in relation to their nonsmoker counterparts. In addition, the use of oral contraceptives in female smokers increases their risk of acute myocardial infarction.
- *Physical activity:* Females tend to be more sedentary than males.

Symptoms of Ischemia

Females are less likely than males to have chest pain during acute coronary syndrome. They tend to have less severe symptoms and less specific symptoms, such as dyspnea, nausea, vomiting, diaphoresis, syncope, fatigue, and palpitations.

Treatment of Coronary Artery Disease in Females

Although treatment is the same for males and females, females often receive less optimal medical therapy and lifestyle counseling. Females have higher postoperative morbidity and mortality rates, a poorer quality of life postprocedure/postoperatively, and a higher incidence of depression.

Data from Gulati MM, Merz CNB. Cardiovascular disease in women. In: Zipes DP, Libby P, Bonow RO, et al., eds. *Braundwald's Heart Disease: A Textbook of Cardiovascular Medicine.* 11th ed. Philadelphia, PA: Elsevier; 2019:1767-1779.

Diagnostic Studies. Diagnosis of ACS is based on symptoms, analysis of a 12-lead ECG, and cardiac enzyme values. Typical angina, atypical angina, and noncardiac chest pain are described in Table 13.6. Inspect the ECG for ST-segment elevation (>1 mm) in two or more contiguous leads (STEMI). ST-segment depression (≥0.5 mm) and new-onset left bundle branch block also suggest an AMI. The location of AMI is determined by the coronary artery involved and the blood supply to that area (Table 13.7).

Elevated serum cardiac enzyme levels (troponin I, troponin T, and HS-cTN) are used to confirm the diagnosis of AMI. These tests are ordered immediately when a diagnosis of ACS is suspected and periodically (usually every 6 to 8 hours) during the first 24 hours to assess for increasing levels. Emergency cardiac catheterization may be performed in institutions with interventional cardiology services.

Patient Problems

Problems for the patient with ACS are described in the Plan of Care for the Patient with Acute Coronary Syndrome. In addition, many problems and interventions apply from the Collaborative Care Plan found in Chapter 1, Overview of Critical Care Nursing.

Complications of AMI include cardiac dysrhythmias, HF, thromboembolism, ventricular aneurysm, rupture of a portion of the heart (ventricular wall, interventricular septum, or papillary muscle), pericarditis, infarct extension or recurrence, cardiogenic shock, and death (see Chapter 12, Shock, Sepsis, and Multiple Organ Dysfunction Syndrome).

Medical Interventions

Treatment goals for AMI are to establish reperfusion, reduce infarct size, prevent and treat complications, and provide emotional support and education. Medical treatment of AMI is aimed at relieving pain, providing adequate oxygenation to the myocardium, preventing platelet aggregation, and restoring blood flow to the myocardium through thrombolytic therapy or acute interventional therapy (e.g., angioplasty). Hemodynamic monitoring is also used to assess cardiac function and to monitor fluid balance in some patients.

TABLE 13.6 Chest Pain Differences in Angina

Type of Angina	Characteristic of Chest Pain
Typical angina	Pain or discomfort that is (1) retrosternal, (2) provoked by exercise and/or emotion, and (3) relieved by rest and/or nitroglycerin
Atypical angina	Sharp or knifelike, brought on by respiratory movements or coughing; abdominal pain
Nonanginal (or noncardiac) chest pain	Pain that is reproducible with movement or palpation of the chest wall or arms, constant pain that persists for many hours or brief episodes that last a few seconds or less

From Bonaca MP, Sabatine MS. Approach to the patient with chest pain. In: Zipes DP, Libby P, Bonow RO et al., eds. *Braunwald's Heart Disease: A Textbook of Cardiovascular Medicine.* Philadelphia, PA: Elsevier; 2019:1059-1068.

PLAN OF CARE

For the Patient With Acute Coronary Syndrome

Patient Problem

Acute Pain. Risk factors include decreased oxygen supply to the myocardium and reduced circulation.

Desired Outcomes

- Within 30 minutes of pain onset, the patient's perception of pain decreases, as documented by a pain scale.
- Objective indicators, such as grimacing and diaphoresis, are absent or decreased

Nursing Assessments/Interventions	Rationales
• Assess location, character, and severity of the pain. Record severity on a subjective 0 (no pain) to 10 (worst pain) scale.	• Establish baseline and monitor trends in pain and response to treatment.
• Assess HR and BP during episodes of chest pain. Be alert to and report significant findings: increased HR and changes in SBP >20 mm Hg from baseline.	• Assess changes that indicate increased myocardial O_2 demands and need for prompt medical intervention.
• Administer humidified O_2 as prescribed.	• Hypoxia is common because of decreased perfusion and creates additional stress to the compromised myocardium. • Humidity prevents drying of the oral and nasal mucosa.
• Notify the provider if pain is unrelieved.	• Alternative treatments, or additional dosages of medications, may be needed. • Unrelieved pain may indicate the need for additional workup.
• If prescribed or per protocol, increase IV NTG infusion in increments of 10 mcg if pain persists, and monitor SBP. Notify the provider if SBP <90 mm Hg, HR <60 beats/min, or RR <10 breaths/min. Monitor for headache.	• NTG lowers BP. • An SBP ≥90 mm Hg prevents worsening ischemia secondary to hypotension. • Headache is associated with dilation of cerebral blood vessels.
• As prescribed, administer IV morphine sulfate in small increments (2 mg). Monitor HR, RR, and BP.	• Relieve pain. • Decrease HR, BP, RR, and anxiety.
• Obtain ECG per protocol and monitor cardiac rhythm.	• ECG patterns may reveal ischemia: ST- or T-wave changes, new Q waves, or left bundle branch block.
• Stay with the patient and provide reassurance during periods of pain.	• Reduce anxiety and lessen the angina.
• Maintain the patient in a recumbent position with the HOB elevated no higher than 30 degrees during angina and NTG administration.	• Minimize the potential for headache or hypotension by enabling better blood return to the heart and head.
• Emphasize to the patient the importance of immediately reporting chest pain.	• Facilitate prompt treatment to decrease morbidity and mortality.
• Instruct the patient to avoid activities and factors known to cause stress.	• Stress may precipitate angina.
• Implement complementary and alternative strategies: o Relaxation techniques o Soothing music o Biofeedback, meditation o Yoga	• Reduction in stress and anxiety may reduce pain.
• Administer beta-blockers as prescribed. Use with caution in asthmatics because medication antagonizes pulmonary vasodilation.	• Reduce workload of the heart and myocardial O_2 demand, improving myocardial oxygenation.
• Instruct patient to rise slowly from a recumbent or seated position.	• Avoid orthostatic hypotension.
• Administer long-acting nitrates (isosorbide preparations) and/or topical nitrates as prescribed.	• Prevent future angina attacks, lower BP, and decrease O_2 demand.
• Administer ACE inhibitor as prescribed.	• Downregulate the RAAS and reduce BP. • Improve long-term survival.
• Administer calcium channel blockers as prescribed.	• Decrease coronary artery vasospasm, dilate coronary arteries, and increase blood flow to the myocardium.
• Administer thrombolytic agents.	• Reduce platelet aggregation
• Aspirin may also be prescribed.	• Medications increase the risk for bleeding.
• Observe bleeding precautions and review with patient.	
• Administer antihyperlipidemic agents and triglyceride-lowering agents as prescribed.	• Reduce total cholesterol, LDH, and triglyceride levels.
• Administer stool softeners as prescribed.	• Straining at stool or constipation can increase myocardial demand.

ACE, Angiotensin-converting enzyme; *BP,* blood pressure; *ECG,* electrocardiogram; *HOB,* head of bed; *HR,* heart rate; *LDH,* lactate dehydrogenase; *NTG,* nitroglycerin; O_2, oxygen; *RAAS,* renin-angiotensin-aldosterone system; *RR,* respiratory rate; *SBP,* systolic blood pressure.
Adapted from Snyder J, Sump C. *Swearingen's All-in-One Nursing Care Planning Resource,* 6th ed. Elsevier; 2024.

TABLE 13.7 **Myocardial Infarction by Site, Electrocardiographic Changes, and Complications**

Location of MI	Primary Site of Occlusion	Primary ECG Changes	Complications
Inferior MI	RCA (80%–90%) LCX (10%–20%)	II, III, aV_F	First- and second-degree heart block, right ventricular infarction
Inferolateral MI	LCX	II, III, aV_F, V_5, V_6	Third-degree heart block, left HF, cardiomyopathy, left ventricular rupture
Posterior MI	RCA or LCX	No lead truly looks at the posterior surface. Look for reciprocal changes in V_1 and V_2—tall, broad R waves; ST depression; and tall T waves. Posterior leads V_7, V_8, and V_9 may be recorded and evaluated.	First-, second-, and third-degree heart blocks; HF; brady-dysrhythmias
Anterior MI	LAD	V_2–V_4	Third-degree heart block, HF, left bundle branch block
Anterior-septal MI	LAD	V_1–V_3	Second- and third-degree heart block
Lateral MI	LAD or LCX	V_5, V_6, I, aVL	HF
Right ventricular	RCA	V_4R. Right precordial leads V_1R–V_6R may be recorded and evaluated.	Increased RAP, decreased cardiac output, brady-dysrhythmias, heart blocks, hypotension, cardiogenic shock

ECG, Electrocardiographic; *HF,* heart failure; *LAD,* left anterior descending coronary artery; *LCX,* left circumflex artery; *MI,* myocardial infarction; *RAP,* right atrial pressure; *RCA,* right coronary artery.

Pain Relief. The initial pain of AMI may be treated with morphine sulfate administered by the IV route. Observe the patient for hypotension and respiratory depression (Table 13.5). New guidelines suggest there may be drug-to-drug interactions between morphine sulfate and dual antiplatelet therapy with aspirin and one of the P2Y12 inhibitors such as clopidogrel (Plavix), prasugrel (Effient), or ticagrelor (Brilinta). There has been concern regarding the inability to reach a therapeutic drug threshold for effective platelet inhibition after administration of a P2Y12 receptor medication when the patient also receives morphine sulfate.[22]

Nitrates. IV NTG may be given to reduce the ischemic pain of AMI. NTG is a vasodilator and increases coronary perfusion. It is usually titrated until chest pain is absent, systolic BP decreases, or pulmonary artery occlusion pressure decreases. Administer NTG cautiously to patients with inferior or right ventricular infarctions to avoid profound hypotension. Other care requirements for the administration of NTG include use of non–polyvinyl chloride tubing. Do not give nitrates to patients who have used phosphodiesterase inhibitors within the last 24 to 48 hours.[23]

Oxygen. Oxygen has been traditionally administered via nasal cannula at 4 to 6 L/min to treat and prevent hypoxemia in AMI and maintain oxygen saturation at greater than 90%. However, recent guidelines suggest that routine use of supplemental oxygen may not be necessary in patients with uncomplicated ACS without signs of HF or hypoxemia.[18]

Antidysrhythmics. Dysrhythmias are common after AMI. Antidysrhythmic medications are administered when the heart's natural pacemaker develops an abnormal rate or rhythm (see Chapter 8, Dysrhythmia Interpretation and Management).

Prevention of Platelet Aggregation. Alterations in platelet function contribute to occlusion of the coronary arteries. Aspirin (325 mg) is given immediately to all patients with suspected ACS. Aspirin blocks synthesis of thromboxane A_2, thus inhibiting aggregation of platelets. In addition, a P2Y12 receptor inhibitor or a glycoprotein (Gp) IIb/IIIa inhibitor may be added.[23] Heparin or low-molecular-weight heparin may also be administered.

Percutaneous Coronary Intervention. Primary percutaneous coronary intervention (PCI) at a PCI-capable hospital should be performed as part of the management of AMI with ST-segment elevation (i.e., STEMI) within 12 hours after the initiation of ischemic symptoms. PCI should be performed within 90 minutes after first medical contact by emergency department staff. Primary PCI is more effective than thrombolysis in opening acutely occluded arteries when it can be rapidly performed by experienced interventional cardiologists. Placement of bare metal stents or drug-eluting stents is common during PCI. If patients come to a facility without PCI capabilities, they should be transferred to a PCI-capable facility or triaged to receive fibrinolytic therapy at the receiving facility.[18]

Fibrinolytic Therapy. The goals of fibrinolytic therapy are to dissolve the clot that is occluding the coronary artery and to increase blood flow to the myocardium. For treatment to be considered, the patient must have been symptomatic for less than 12 hours, and PCI is not an option. However, the best outcomes occur in patients who are treated within 1 to 2 hours of the onset of symptoms.[18] Table 13.8 lists common thrombolytic agents. Important considerations in the use of thrombolytics include the following:

- Fibrinolysis reduces mortality and salvages myocardium in STEMI or bundle-branch involvement in AMI.
- Fibrinolysis is not effective in the treatment of unstable angina or AMI without ST-segment elevation (i.e., NSTEMI).

TABLE 13.8 PHARMACOLOGY

Thrombolytics

Medication	Dose/Route	Half-Life
Alteplase (tissue plasminogen activator [t-PA])	*Accelerated 90 min infusion:* For adults weighing >67 kg; administer 15-mg bolus IV over 1–2 min, followed by infusion of 50 mg over the first 30 min and 35 mg over next 60 min; total dose not to exceed 100 mg For adults weighing ≤67 kg, 15-mg bolus IV over 1–2 min, followed by infusion of 0.75 mg/kg over the first 30 min (not to exceed 50 mg) and 0.50 mg/kg over next 60 min (not to exceed 35 mg) total dose not to exceed 100 mg *3-h infusion:* For adults weighing ≥65 kg; administer 60 mg over the first hour (6–10 mg as IV bolus over 1–2 min, followed by infusion of remaining dose), 20 mg over second hour, and 20 mg over third hour total dose not to exceed 100 mg For adults weighing <65 kg; administer 0.075 mg/kg as an IV bolus, then 0.675 mg/kg IV infusion for the remainder of the first hour, then 0.25 mg/kg IV infusion the second hour and then 0.25 mg/kg IV the third hour; total dose not to exceed 100 mg	4–5 min
Reteplase (r-PA)	10 units IV bolus over 2 min; repeat 10-unit dose in 30 min. Give through a dedicated IV line. Do not give repeat bolus if serious bleeding occurs after first IV bolus	13–16 min

Data from Skidmore-Roth L. *Mosby's 2023 Nursing Drug Reference*. 36th ed. St. Louis, MO: Elsevier; 2023.

- Thrombolysis should be instituted within 30 to 60 minutes of arrival. The sooner the treatment is initiated, the better the outcome.
- Bleeding from puncture sites commonly occurs.
- The greatest risk associated with fibrinolysis therapy is intracranial hemorrhage.

Nursing care of the patient includes rapid identification of whether the patient is a suitable candidate for IV thrombolytics, screening for contraindications, and prompt administration of thrombolytics. Absolute contraindications for administration of fibrinolytic medications are associated with patient history of recent stroke (ischemic and/or hemorrhagic), head trauma, spinal surgery, and uncontrolled hypertension. Next, secure three vascular access lines and obtain necessary laboratory data. Initiate cardiac monitoring and document rhythm before starting the infusion, at routine intervals throughout the infusion, and at the end of the infusion. Finally, monitor the patient for complications, including reperfusion dysrhythmias (premature ventricular contractions, sinus bradycardia, accelerated idioventricular rhythm, or ventricular tachycardia [VT]), oozing at venipuncture sites, gingival bleeding, reocclusion or reinfarction, and symptoms of hemorrhagic stroke.

Medications. Several medications may be ordered for the patient with ACS. Patients whose chest pain symptoms are suggestive of serious illness need immediate assessment in a monitored unit and early therapy, including an IV line, NTG, aspirin, P2Y12 receptor inhibitors, heparin or low-molecular-weight heparin, beta-blockers, angiotensin-converting enzyme inhibitors, and oxygen.

Beta-blockers. Beta-blockers are used to decrease heart rate, BP, and myocardial oxygen consumption. Morbidity and mortality after AMI have been reduced by the use of beta-blockers. Beta-blockers should be started within 24 hours after ACS begins unless otherwise contraindicated. Carefully assess the patient for hypotension and bradycardia.

Angiotensin-converting enzyme inhibitors. ACS can cause the area of ventricular damage to change shape, or *remodel*. The ventricle becomes thinner and balloons out, thus reducing contractility. Cardiac tissue surrounding the area of infarction undergoes changes that can be categorized as: (1) myocardial stunning (a temporary loss of contractile function that persists for hours to days after perfusion has been restored); (2) hibernating myocardium (tissue that is persistently ischemic and undergoes metabolic adaptation to prolong myocyte survival until perfusion can be restored); and (3) myocardial remodeling (a process mediated by angiotensin II, aldosterone, catecholamines, adenosine, and inflammatory cytokines that causes myocyte hypertrophy and loss of contractile function in areas of the heart distant from the site of infarction). Angiotensin-converting enzyme inhibitors (ACEIs) are usually started within 24 hours to reduce the incidence of ventricular remodeling. The medications may be discontinued if the patient exhibits no signs of ventricular dysfunction (Table 13.5). ACEIs should be prescribed for patients with unstable angina; NSTEMI; STEMI with an LVEF of 40% or less; or a history of hypertension, diabetes, or chronic kidney disease, unless contraindicated. The most common side effect of ACEIs is cough, which is chronic and nonproductive. If side effects occur with an ACEI, angiotensin II receptor blockers (ARBs) should be initiated instead.[23]

Novel Stem Cell Treatment. Autologous bone marrow stem cell therapy is used to prevent ventricular remodeling and improve cardiac function. The stem cells are implanted into mapped areas of dysfunctional and viable myocardium. Research has shown improvement in LVEF in some trials, but more research is needed.[24]

CLINICAL JUDGMENT ACTIVITY

You are taking care of a 58-year-old male patient who was readmitted to the unit after an MI 3 months ago. He is complaining of recurrent chest pain, shortness of breath, and fatigue. Sublingual nitroglycerin (NTG) at home and rest did not relieve the chest pain. Prioritize your nursing assessment, interventions, and actions. What assessment data do you need to obtain? What pertinent information from the patient's history would you want to obtain? What diagnostic tests do you anticipate?

Patient Outcomes

Patient outcomes are generalized to encompass the wide spectrum of patients who have experienced an AMI, uncomplicated or complicated, and have required medical or surgical intervention. Outcomes include adequate cardiac output, ability to tolerate progressive activity, verbalization of relief of pain and fear, and demonstration of positive coping mechanisms.

Interventions for Acute Coronary Syndrome

Interventional Cardiology. Several interventions are used to treat ACS. Primary PCI is recommended for treatment of acute STEMI. The goal is reperfusion of the affected area to reduce ischemia and to prevent further damage to the myocardium. PCI includes percutaneous transluminal coronary angioplasty (PTCA), rotational atherectomy, laser atherectomy, thrombectomy, and intracoronary stenting. An early, invasive PCI procedure is indicated for patients with unstable angina or NSTEMI who are hemodynamically unstable, continue to have angina, or have an elevated risk of clinical events. For the purpose of this book, only PTCA and stenting are discussed. The postprocedure care for all patients who undergo PCI consists of the same interventions.

Percutaneous Transluminal Coronary Angioplasty. The purpose of PTCA is to compress intracoronary plaque to increase blood flow to the myocardium. It is usually the treatment of choice for patients with uncompromised collateral flow, noncalcified lesions, and lesions not present at bifurcations of vessels. PTCA is performed in the cardiac catheterization laboratory. A balloon catheter is inserted into the femoral, brachial, or radial artery, threaded into the occluded coronary artery, and advanced with the use of a guidewire across the lesion. The balloon is inflated under pressure one or several times to compress the lesion (Fig. 13.11). The optimal goal after PTCA is to open and return normal blood flow through the coronary artery (Fig. 13.12). PTCA is rarely done without stenting, but it is usually done to dilate the artery before placement of a bare metal or drug-eluting stent or in the instance of very small vessels.[25]

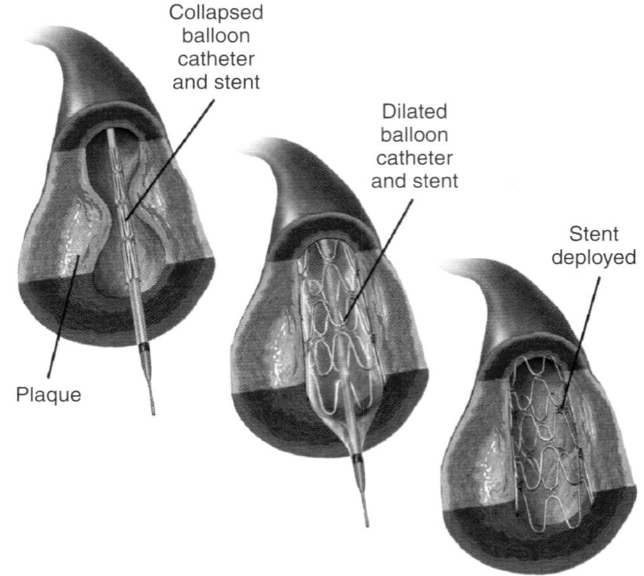

Fig. 13.11 Cardiac stent. (From Good VS, Kirkwood PL. *Advanced Critical Care Nursing*. 2nd ed. St. Louis, MO: Elsevier; 2018.)

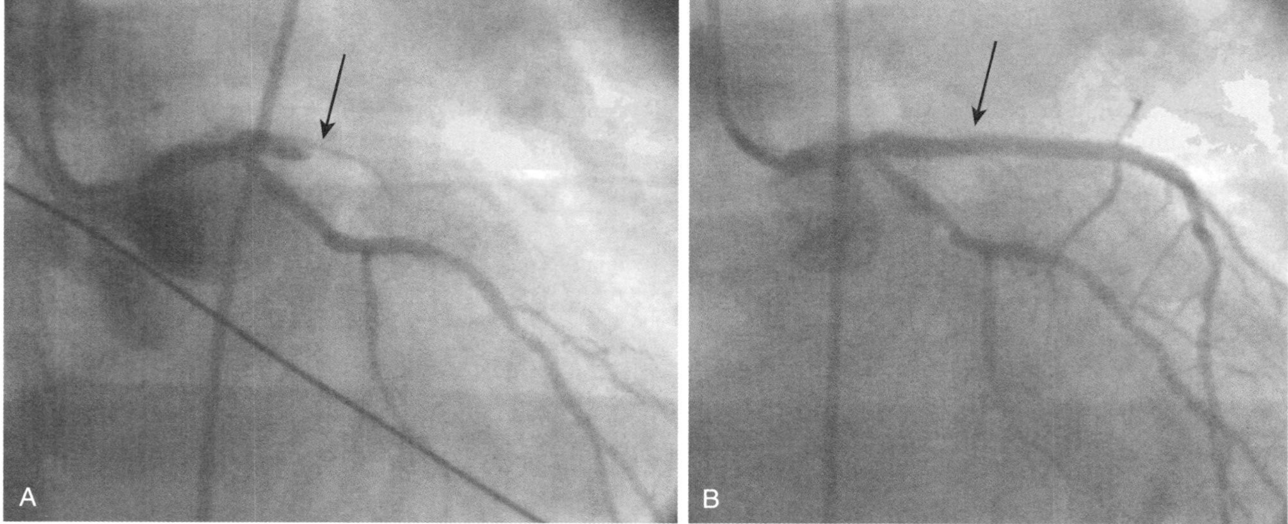

Fig. 13.12 A, 100% thrombotic occlusion of the left anterior descending artery *(arrow)* causing a STEMI. B, After PCI with a drug-coated stent to the left anterior descending artery *(arrow)*. Blood flow is restored to the entire left anterior descending artery. (From Harding MM. *Lewis's Medical Surgical Nursing: Assessment and Management of Clinical Problems*. 12th ed. St. Louis: Elsevier; 2023.)

Complications. Complications of PTCA include hematoma at the catheter insertion site, MI, stroke or TIA, pseudoaneurysm, dysrhythmias, infection, acute kidney injury, and coronary artery dissection. Mortality rates are less than 1% for PTCA.[25]

Coronary stent. Coronary stents are tubes that are implanted at the site of stenosis to widen the arterial lumen by pushing atherosclerotic plaque against the artery's walls (as does PTCA). The stent also keeps the lumen open by providing structural support. Approximately 90% of PCI procedures involve stent placement.[25] Stent designs differ, but most designs have springs, slots, or mesh tubes; some resemble the spiral bindings used in notebooks. Stents are tightly wrapped around a balloon catheter, which is inflated to implant the stent.

The procedure for placing a stent is similar to the procedure in PTCA. The patient first undergoes cardiac angiography for identification of occlusions in coronary arteries. Next, the balloon catheter bearing the stent is inserted into the coronary artery, and the stent is positioned at the desired site. The balloon is inflated, thereby expanding the stent, which pushes the atherosclerotic plaque and intimal flaps against the vessel wall. After the balloon is deflated and removed, the stent remains, holding the plaque and other matter in place and providing structural support to keep the artery from collapsing (Fig. 13.13).

Aggressive anticoagulation therapy before, during, and after the stent procedure is necessary to prevent coagulation. Before sheath removal, monitor peripheral perfusion because the sheath may occlude the artery (femoral or radial approach may be used). Monitor peripheral pulses, skin color, and temperature, and inspect the insertion site for any oozing or bleeding. After sheath removal, maintain hemostasis with manual pressure, a compression device, or an arterial puncture sealing device. Retroperitoneal bleeding or impaired perfusion may occur after sheath removal. Pain management and proper hydration aid in recovery.

Restenosis can occur as a result of neointimal (new intimal cell) growth resulting from the body's natural defense when the inner intimal lining is injured, even slightly, as happens with stent placement. GP IIb/IIIa inhibitors and antithrombotic agents are used after stent placement to prevent acute reocclusion through prevention of platelet aggregation. Therapies in intracoronary stenting have advanced, including drug-eluting stents that are coated with an antiproliferative medication that reduces in-stent thrombosis. The medication is released slowly over time to reduce the risk of neointimal growth.[25] With the use of second-generation stents (e.g., drug-eluting) and dual antiplatelet therapy, restenosis rates have declined to approximately 1% in the first year after stenting.[25]

CHECK YOUR UNDERSTANDING:

5. Discharge medications post coronary stent placement for a male patient included a beta-blocker agent, P2Y12 inhibitor agent, aspirin, and NTG sublingual for chest pain. Which element of the patient's medication history requires further education after coronary stent placement?
   A. Phosphodiesterase type 5 inhibitors for erectile dysfunction
   B. Statin therapy for hyperlipidemia
   C. Acetaminophen for arthritic pain
   D. Nicotine patch for smoking cessation

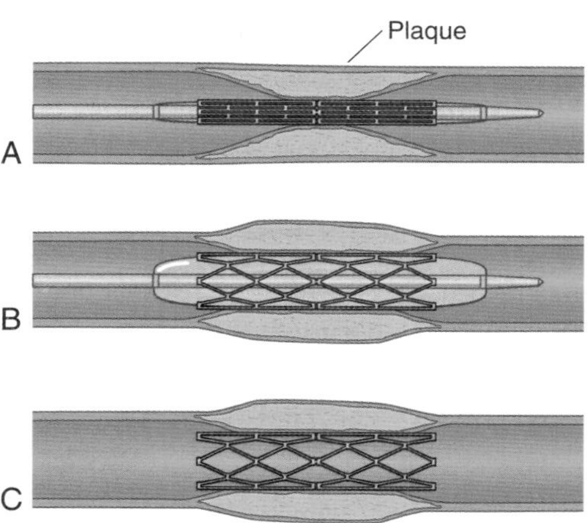

Fig. 13.13 Placement of a coronary artery stent. **A,** The stent is positioned at the site of the lesion. **B,** The balloon is inflated, expanding the stent. The balloon is then deflated and removed. **C,** The implanted stent is left in place. (From Harding MM, Kwong J, Hagler D. *Lewis's Medical-Surgical Nursing: Assessment and Management of Clinical Problems.* 12th ed. St. Louis, MO: Mosby; 2023.)

CLINICAL JUDGMENT ACTIVITY

You are caring for a 63-year-old female who has just returned to the cardiac care unit after placement of a drug-eluting stent in the right coronary artery. The proximal right coronary artery had a 90% occlusive lesion. An occlusive device (TR Band) was in place over the right radial artery. IV NTG and eptifibatide (Integrilin) are infusing.

1. What type of dysrhythmia would you anticipate if the right coronary artery were to reocclude?
2. Prioritize your actions on the patient's arrival to the critical care unit.
3. What type of assessment would you perform regarding the right radial TR Band?

Surgical Revascularization. Surgical approaches used for revascularization include coronary revascularization by coronary artery bypass grafting (CABG), minimally invasive CABG, and transmyocardial revascularization (TMR).

CLINICAL JUDGMENT ACTIVITY

Many patients are admitted into the hospital on the same day that cardiac surgery is performed. Discuss methods for reviewing the patient's understanding of the upcoming cardiac surgery and additional teaching needed (to include immediate postsurgical instruction).

Coronary artery bypass grafting. CABG is a surgical procedure in which the ischemic areas of the myocardium are revascularized by implantation of a graft from the internal mammary artery (IMA) or the coronary occlusion is bypassed with a graft from the saphenous vein or the radial artery. The indications for CABG are chronic stable angina that is refractory to other therapies, significant left main coronary artery occlusion (>50%), triple-vessel CAD, unstable angina pectoris, left ventricular failure, lesions not amenable to PCI, and PCI failure.

CABG is performed in the operating room with the patient intubated and under general anesthesia. One approach is a midsternal, longitudinal incision into the chest cavity. An anterior thoracotomy may also be used. Surgery is done either with cardiopulmonary bypass or without it (e.g., *off-pump*).[26,27] During cardiopulmonary bypass, blood is pumped through an oxygenator, or heart-lung machine, to receive oxygen. Cardioplegia solution is used to stop the heart so that the surgery can be performed.

The coronary arteries are visualized, and a segment of the saphenous vein is grafted or anastomosed distally to the occlusion of the affected vessel, with the proximal end of the graft vessel anastomosed to the aorta (Fig. 13.14). The IMA is often used to create an artery-to-artery graft. IMA revascularization has better long-term patency than saphenous vein grafts. It is the preferred graft for lesions of the left anterior descending coronary artery. Once grafting is completed, the cardiopulmonary bypass (if used) is progressively discontinued, chest and mediastinal tubes are inserted, and the chest is closed. Box 13.9 provides information related to chest and mediastinal tubes.

Minimally invasive coronary artery surgery. Minimally invasive cardiac surgery–coronary artery bypass grafting (MICS CABG) has been evaluated as an alternative to the standard CABG methods. This alternative allows for a thoracotomy approach instead of a sternotomy, resulting in shorter hospital stay and earlier postoperative recovery. It is done without cardiopulmonary bypass. However, no clinical trials have shown improvement in quality of life with MICS CABG. Even so, this is an active area of research.[26] Robotically assisted cardiac surgery, a type of MICS, involves cardiac surgeons using a computer console to control surgical instruments on thin robotic arms. Robotic CABG can be done on-pump or off-pump for single-vessel or multivessel disease and may be the preferred method of cardiac surgery based on patient risk. Robotic cardiac surgery has been associated with lower morbidity and mortality.[27]

Management after cardiac surgery. Patients are usually admitted directly to the critical care unit after cardiac surgery. The patient often has a pulmonary artery catheter, arterial catheter, peripheral IV lines, temporary pacemaker wires, pleural chest tubes, mediastinal tubes, and an indwelling urinary catheter. The patient is usually mechanically ventilated in the immediate postoperative period. Assess the patient often and provide rapid intervention to help the patient recover from anesthesia and to prevent complications. Nursing care for these patients is summarized in Box 13.10.

Complications of cardiac surgery. Closely monitor patients postoperatively for complications such as dysrhythmias (i.e., atrial fibrillation, atrial flutter, VT, ventricular fibrillation), AMI, cardiogenic shock, pericarditis, pericardial effusion, and cardiac tamponade. The critical care nurse caring for a patient who has just undergone CABG must have quick critical thinking and clinical judgment skills to assess the whole clinical picture while prioritizing interventions that must be performed.

Mechanical Therapies

Transmyocardial laser revascularization. In transmyocardial laser revascularization (TMLR), a high-energy laser creates channels from the epicardial surface into the ischemic myocardium of the left ventricular. The purpose of TMLR is to increase perfusion directly to the heart muscle. It is performed on patients in conjunction with CABG or on those who are poor candidates for CABG or PCI and whose symptoms are refractory to medical treatment. To do this procedure, a surgeon makes an

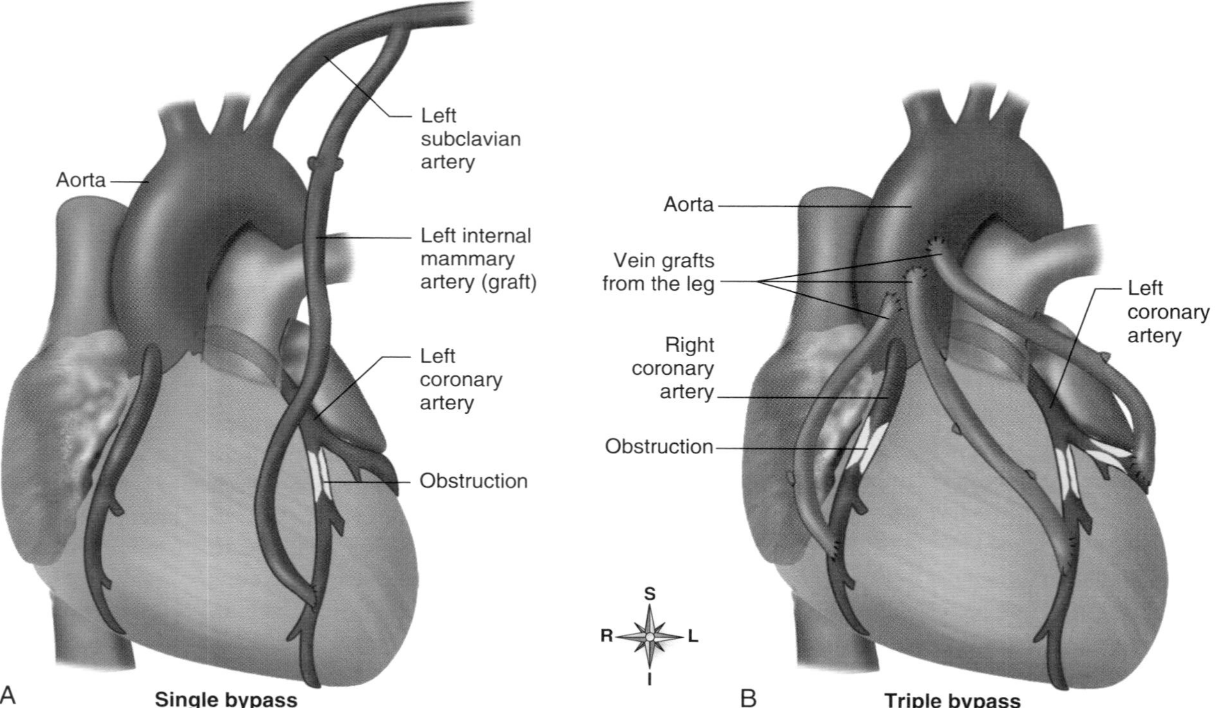

Fig. 13.14 Options for coronary artery bypass surgery. **A,** Internal mammary artery is "rerouted" to bypass the obstruction. **B,** Vessels are "harvested" from other parts of the body and used to construct detours around blocked coronary arteries. Artificial vessels can also be used. (From Patton KT, Thibodeau GA. *Human Body in Health and Disease*. 6th ed. St. Louis, MO: Elsevier; 2018.)

BOX 13.9 Key Points for Maintaining Pleural Chest and Mediastinal Tubes

Definitions

- *Pleural chest tube:* The tube is inserted into the pleural space to maintain the normal negative pressure and to facilitate respiration. It is inserted after cardiac surgery if the pleural space has been opened. It is also inserted as treatment for pneumothorax or hemothorax.
- *Mediastinal tube:* The tube is inserted into the mediastinal space to provide drainage after cardiac surgery.
- *Drainage system:* A water-seal system assists in maintaining negative pressures (chest tube). Some devices are designed to function without water (dry). Suction (up to 20 cm H_2O) is often applied to facilitate drainage.
- *Autotransfusion:* This is defined as reinfusion of autologous drainage from the system back to the patient.

Baseline Assessment

- Ensure that all connections are tight: insertion site to the chest drainage system and suction control chamber to the suction unit.
- Confirm that the dressing over the insertion site is dry and intact.
- Palpate for subcutaneous crepitus around the insertion site and chest wall.
- Auscultate breath sounds bilaterally.
- Observe the color and consistency of fluid in the collecting tubing (a more accurate assessment than fluid in the drainage system); mark the fluid level on the drainage system.
- Assess the drainage system for proper functioning (read instructions for the device being used).
- Check the water in the water-seal chamber; the water level should fluctuate with respirations in chest tubes (not in mediastinal tubes).
- Check suction control and be sure that suction is on, if ordered.
- Check for intermittent bubbling in the water-seal chamber; it indicates an air leak from the pleural space (pleural tube).

Maintaining the Chest Drainage System

- Keep the tubing coiled on the bed near the patient.
- Record drainage in the medical record according to protocol; notify the provider of excessive drainage or acute change in drainage volume and/or color. (The volume to report is determined by unit parameters or written order; it varies depending on the purpose of the tube and the time since insertion.)
- Change the dressing according to unit protocol.
- Splint the insertion site to facilitate coughing and deep breathing.
- Ensure that drainage flows into the drainage system by facilitating gravity drainage; milking or stripping of tubes is not recommended, because these procedures generate high negative pressures in the system.
- If the patient is transported (or ambulated), disconnect the drainage system from suction and keep it upright below the level of the chest. Do not clamp the tube.
- Obtain chest radiographic studies immediately after insertion and, usually, daily thereafter.

Assisting With Removal

- Chest and mediastinal tubes are usually removed by the provider.
- Ensure adequate pain medication before removal.
- Apply an occlusive dressing to the site after removal.
- A chest radiographic study is usually done after removal.

Autotransfusion

- An autotransfusion collection system is attached to the chest drainage device.
- Anticoagulants may be ordered to be added to the autotransfusion system (citrate-phosphate-dextrose, acid-phosphate-dextrose, or heparin); these are not usually necessary with mediastinal drainage.
- Reinfuse drainage within the time frame specified by unit policy. It is recommended that reinfusion begin within 6 hours after initiation of the collection and reinfused to the patient within a 4-hour period.
- Evacuate air from the autotransfusion bag; air embolism may occur unless all air is removed.
- Attach a microaggregate filter and infuse via gravity or a pressure bag.

BOX 13.10 Nursing Interventions After Cardiac Surgery

- Monitor for hypotension; administer fluids and vasopressors as ordered or based on protocol.
- Assess for hypovolemia; monitor and trend output from the pleural chest and mediastinal tubes and urine output.
- Monitor hemodynamic pressures, SvO_2, stroke index, cardiac index, PAOP, and RAP; treat the patient per protocol.
- Rewarm the patient gradually (if applicable).
- Monitor and treat fluid volume status and electrolytes, hemoglobin, hematocrit, renal function, and coagulation studies.
- Provide pain relief.
- Monitor for complications: intraoperative AMI, dysrhythmias, heart failure, cardiac tamponade, thromboembolism, impaired renal function, pneumonia, pneumothorax, pleural effusion, cerebral ischemia, and stroke.
- Wean from mechanical ventilation per protocol; extubate; promote pulmonary hygiene every 1 to 2 hours while the patient is awake.
- Assess wounds and provide incisional care per hospital protocol.
- Gradually increase the patient's activity.
- Provide emotional support to the patient and family.

AMI, Acute myocardial infarction; *PAOP,* pulmonary artery occlusion pressure; *RAP,* right atrial pressure; *SvO_2,* mixed venous oxygen saturation.

incision on the left side of the chest and inserts a laser device into the chest cavity. With the laser, the surgeon makes 1-mm channels through the heart's left ventricle in-between heartbeats. TMLR does not replace CABG or angioplasty as a method of treating CAD. TMLR may be used for patients who are high-risk candidates for a second bypass or angioplasty, such as those whose blockages are too diffuse to be treated with bypass alone.[28]

Enhanced external counterpulsation. Enhanced external counterpulsation (EECP) is a treatment for angina that may be used when the patient is not a candidate for bypass surgery or PCI. Cuffs are wrapped around the patient's legs to increase arterial BP and retrograde aortic blood flow during diastole. Sequential pressure, using compressed air, is applied from the lower legs to the upper thighs. These treatments take place over the course of a few hours per day for several weeks. There are no definitive data showing that EECP reduces ischemia; however, treatment reduces angina and improves quality of life.[29]

CARDIAC DYSRHYTHMIAS

Cardiac dysrhythmias (Chapter 8, Dysrhythmia Interpretation and Management) have many causes, such as CAD, AMI, electrolyte imbalances, and HF. Emergency treatments of dysrhythmias include medications, transcutaneous pacemakers, and cardioversion and defibrillation (Chapter 11, Rapid Response Teams and Code Management). Other medications given to manage dysrhythmias are shown in Table 13.9. Additional surgical and electrical treatments are discussed in the following sections.

Radiofrequency Catheter Ablation

Radiofrequency catheter ablation is a method used to treat dysrhythmias when medications, cardioversion, or both are not effective or not indicated. The objective of catheter ablation is to permanently interrupt electrical conduction or activity in a region of arrhythmogenic cardiac tissue. Indications for radiofrequency catheter ablation include the presence of dysrhythmias such as VT, atrial fibrillation, atrial flutter, and AV nodal reentry tachycardia. The most predominant group are patients with symptomatic paroxysmal atrial fibrillation.

Radiofrequency ablation is performed percutaneously. The procedure begins with a diagnostic electrophysiology study to map the areas to be ablated. A catheter with an electrode is positioned at the accessory (abnormal) pathway, and mild, painless radiofrequency energy (similar to microwave heat) is transmitted to the pathway, causing coagulation and necrosis in the conduction fibers without destroying the surrounding tissue. This stops the area from conducting the extra impulses that cause tachycardia. After each ablation attempt, the patient is retested until there is no recurrence of the tachycardic rhythm.

Current guidelines report that, for patients with atrial fibrillation (AF) and HF with reduced ejection fraction (HFrEF), catheter ablation may be superior to pharmacological management for

TABLE 13.9 PHARMACOLOGY

Medications Used to Treat Dysrhythmias

Medication	Actions/Use	Dose/Route	Side Effects	Nursing Implications
Amiodarone (Cordarone)	Prolongs action potential phase 3; used for atrial fibrillation/flutter, SVT, ventricular dysrhythmias	*IV:* 150 mg IV over 10 min (15 mg/min). Follow with infusion of 360 mg over next 6 hours at 1 mg/min; maintenance infusion of 540 mg over remaining 18 hours (0.5 mg/min) *PO:* For life-threatening dysrhythmias, administer loading dose of 800–1600 mg/day for 1–3 weeks; decrease dose to 600–800 mg/day for 1 month, then decrease to lowest therapeutic dose, usually 400 mg/day	Bradycardia Complete atrioventricular block Hypotension Multiple side effects (thyroid, pulmonary, hepatic, neurological, dermatological) QT prolongation	Has a long half-life. Monitor cardiac rhythm. Obtain baseline pulmonary, liver, and thyroid function tests.
Diltiazem (Cardizem)	Inhibits calcium ion influx into vascular smooth muscle and myocardium; used in atrial fibrillation/flutter, SVT	*IV:* 0.25 mg/kg actual body weight over 2 min; may repeat in 15 min at dose of 0.35 mg/kg actual body weight *Infusion:* 5–15 mg/h	Bradycardia Dizziness Edema Hypotension	Not generally used in heart failure. Observe for dysrhythmias.
Flecainide (Tambocor)	Decreases conduction in all parts of the heart; stabilizes cardiac membrane; used for ventricular dysrhythmias	*PO:* 50–100 mg q 12 h; increase as needed, not to exceed 400 mg/day	Bradycardia Dizziness Heart block Hypotension Respiratory depression Ventricular dysrhythmias Visual disturbances	Interacts with many other medications; check medication guide. Monitor cardiac rhythm. Monitor intake and output. Assess electrolytes. Assess for CNS symptoms. Significant drug interactions
Propafenone (Rythmol)	Stabilizes cardiac membranes; slows conduction velocity; used for ventricular dysrhythmias	*PO:* 150 mg q 8 h; 450–900 mg/day	Altered taste Dizziness Heart failure Nausea/vomiting Ventricular dysrhythmias	Monitor cardiac rhythm. Use in patients without structural heart disease. Significant drug interactions.
Sotalol (Betapace)	Nonselective beta-blocker; used for ventricular dysrhythmias	*PO:* 80 mg bid; increase to 240–320 mg/day Requires renal dose adjustment	Bradycardia Bronchospasm Diarrhea Dizziness Headache Hematological disorders Nausea/vomiting Palpitations QT prolongation Ventricular tachycardia	Monitor BP and heart rate. Check baseline liver and renal function. Monitor hydration. Watch for QT prolongation; requires continuous cardiac monitoring at the initiation of therapy. Teach patient not to decrease medication abruptly.

bid, Twice daily; *BP,* blood pressure; *CNS,* central nervous system; *PO,* orally; *q,* every; *SVT,* supraventricular tachycardia.
From Skidmore-Roth L. *Mosby's 2023 Nursing Drug Reference.* 36th ed. St. Louis, MO: Elsevier; 2023.

quality of life, functional status, and improved ejection fraction (EF). However, another randomized controlled trial showed that ablation was not superior to medication therapy in outcomes such as death, stroke, bleeding, or cardiac arrest.[30,31] Thus, the provider will review risk benefit for this procedure with the patient.

Pacemakers

Temporary pacemakers are used to treat patients with urgent dysrhythmias, postcardiac surgery, and to treat conduction disturbances of the heart. (See Chapter 8, Dysrhythmia Interpretation and Management.) *Cardiac resynchronization therapy (CRT)* is permanent pacing with an additional lead placed in the left ventricle. It is indicated for patients with HF who have a widened QRS complex and an LVEF of 35% or less and have remained symptomatic despite maximum medical therapy.[32] CRT involves biventricular pacing to synchronize contractions of both ventricles. This improves symptoms of HF, decreases mortality, and decreases hospital readmissions. It can be implanted as a pacemaker device or, as is more common, in combination with a defibrillator.

Defibrillators

Implantable cardioverter-defibrillators (ICDs) are placed in patients for primary or secondary prevention of potentially lethal dysrhythmias. In primary prevention, they are indicated for patients who are at risk for sudden cardiac death, such as patients with HF, genetic mutations that put them at risk for ventricular dysrhythmias, and certain congenital and structural heart diseases. In secondary prevention, ICDs are implanted in patients who have survived cardiac arrest or sustained VT. Current indications for ICD therapy are listed in Box 13.11.

BOX 13.11 Class I Indications for an Implantable Cardioverter-Defibrillator

- Cardiac arrest resulting from VT or VF not produced by a transient or reversible cause or in the event of acute MI when revascularization cannot be done.
- Spontaneous sustained VT in association with structural heart disease.
- Syncope of undetermined origin with clinically relevant, hemodynamically significant sustained VT or VF induced during electrophysiological study.
- Nonsustained VT in patients with coronary artery disease, prior MI, left ventricular dysfunction, and sustained VT or inducible VF during electrophysiological study.
- Patients with LVEF of 30% or less at least 40 days after MI and who are in NYHA Class I 3 months after coronary revascularization.
- ICD therapy is indicated in patients with nonischemic dilated cardiomyopathy who have an LVEF of 35% or less and who are in NYHA functional Class II or III.
- ICD therapy is indicated in patients with nonsustained VT due to prior MI, LVEF of 40% or less, and inducible VF or sustained VT at electrophysiological study.

ICD, Implantable cardioverter-defibrillator; *LVEF,* left ventricular ejection fraction; *MI,* myocardial infarction; *NYHA,* New York Health Association; *VF,* ventricular fibrillation; *VT,* ventricular tachycardia.
Modified from Swerdlow CD, Wang PJ, Zipes DP. Pacemakers and implantable cardioverter-defibrillators. In: Zipes DP, Libby P, Bonow RO, et al., eds. *Braunwald's Heart Disease: A Textbook of Cardiovascular Medicine.* 11th ed. Philadelphia, PA: Elsevier; 2019:780-806.

ICDs detect tachydysrhythmias and, when necessary, deliver a shock to the heart to stop the abnormal heart rhythm. ICDs are implanted in the same manner as pacemakers by electrophysiologists (cardiologists who specialize in cardiac rhythms). All ICDs are developed to include pacemaker capabilities in the rare instance the patient needs backup pacing after receiving an ICD shock. Pacemaker and ICD functions are periodically checked in the office and at home using telemonitoring. These checks help to ensure proper functioning of the device and to determine when the battery needs to be replaced. Instruct the patient to carry a wallet identification card at all times. Box 13.12 lists patient and family teaching points. Although newer devices are MRI compatible, patients who have older devices are restricted from undergoing an MRI.

HEART FAILURE

HF is a complex clinical syndrome that results from the heart's inability to pump blood sufficiently to meet the metabolic

BOX 13.12 Patient and Family Teaching for an Implantable Cardioverter-Defibrillator

Preprocedural Teaching

- Device and how it works.
- Lead and generator placement.
- Implantation procedure.
- Educational materials from the manufacturer.

Postprocedural Teaching

- Site care and symptoms of complications.
- Hematoma at the site, most common when the patient takes anticoagulant or antiplatelet medications.
- Restricting activity of the arm on the side of the implant.
- Identification (MedicAlert jewelry and ICD card).
- Diary of an event if the device fires.
- Response if the device fires (varies, ranging from falling, tingling, or discomfort to no awareness of the shock); family members need to help in assessment.
- Safety measures:
  - Avoid strong magnetic fields (no magnetic resonance imaging).
  - Avoid sources of high-power electricity.
  - Keep cellular phones at least 6 inches from the ICD.
  - Inform airline security personnel about the device; avoid the metal detector; the security wand may be used but should not be left over the device.
  - The defibrillator therapy may be turned off for surgical procedures using electrocautery. This final decision is based on the type of surgery to be performed and the discretion of the surgical team.
- Everyday activities:
  - Hair dryers, microwaves, and razors are safe.
  - Sexual activity can be resumed; tachycardia associated with sexual activity may cause the device to fire; rate adjustments may be needed; if shock occurs during sexual activity, it will not harm the partner.
  - Avoid driving for 6 months if there is a history of sudden cardiac arrest.
- Replacement of the device.
- Instruction of family members in cardiopulmonary resuscitation and in how to contact emergency personnel.
- Support groups in the local community.

ICD, Implantable cardioverter-defibrillator.

demands of the body. HF can result from any structural or functional cardiac disorder that impairs the ability of the ventricle to fill or eject blood. CAD is the primary underlying cause of HF; however, several nonischemic causes have been identified, including hypertension, valvular disease, pulmonary hypertension, exposure to myocardial toxins, myocarditis, untreated tachycardia, alcohol abuse, and in 20% to 30% of cases, unidentifiable causes (that result in idiopathic dilated cardiomyopathy).[32]

The cardinal manifestations of HF are dyspnea, fatigue, exercise intolerance, and fluid retention, which may lead to pulmonary and peripheral edema. Signs and symptoms of HF consist of progressive exertional dyspnea, paroxysmal nocturnal dyspnea, orthopnea, fatigue, loss of appetite, abdominal bloating, nausea or vomiting, and eventual organ system dysfunction (particularly the renal system as the HF advances).

The American Heart Association and American College of Cardiology developed a classification system for HF. A patient is classified by stage (A through D) based on the results of a physical examination, diagnostic tests, and clinical symptoms. This terminology helps in understanding that HF is often a progressive condition that worsens over time. HF can be asymptomatic (stages A [pre-HF] and B) or symptomatic (stages C and D). HF also has a classification system based on functional symptoms and limitations. The New York Heart Association (NYHA) Heart Failure Symptom Classification System is used to determine functional limitations and as an indicator of prognosis. The categories range from Class I, which refers to no symptoms with activity, to Class IV, which indicates dyspnea with little or no exertion. The two classification systems can be used together (Table 13.10).[32]

Pathophysiology

HF is defined as impaired cardiac function of one or both ventricles. Patients can have one of four different types of HF: preserved ejection fraction (HFpEF), reduced ejection fraction (HFrEF), mid-range ejection fraction (HFmrEF) and improved ejection fraction (HFimpEF).[33] Patients with HFpEF have an LVEF of 50% or greater, those with HFrEF have an LVEF of less than 40%, patients with HFmrEF have an LVEF between 40% and 49%, and those with HFimpEF had a previous LVEF of 25% but improved their LVEF to greater than 50%.[33,34] Those with LVEF values between 40% and 50% are considered borderline.[34]

In left-sided HF, the left ventricle cannot pump efficiently. The ineffective pumping action causes a decrease in cardiac output, leading to poor perfusion. The volume of blood remaining in the left ventricle increases after each beat. As this volume increases, it backs up into the left atrium, pulmonary veins, and lungs, causing congestion. Eventually, fluid accumulates in the lungs and pleural spaces, causing increased pressure in the lungs. Gas exchange (oxygen and carbon dioxide) in the pulmonary system is impaired. The backflow can continue into the right ventricle and right atrium and into the systemic circulation (right-sided HF). Right-sided dysfunction is usually a consequence of left-sided HF; however, it can be a primary cause of HF after a right ventricular MI, or it may occur secondary to pulmonary pathology.[35] Selected causes of HF are noted in Box 13.13.

When gas exchange is impaired and carbon dioxide levels increase, the respiratory rate increases to help eliminate the excess carbon dioxide. This phenomenon causes the heart rate to increase, pumping more blood to the lungs for gas exchange. The increased heart rate results in the pumping of more blood from the systemic circulation into the cardiopulmonary circulation, which is already dangerously overloaded, and thus a vicious cycle ensues. As the heart begins to fail to meet the body's metabolic demands, several compensatory mechanisms are activated to improve cardiac output and tissue perfusion. The most noteworthy of these neurohormonal systems are the renin-angiotensin-aldosterone system and the adrenergic nervous system. These interrelated systems act in concert to redistribute blood to critical organs in the body by increasing peripheral vascular tone, heart

BOX 13.13 Causes of Heart Failure

- Myocardial infarction
- Coronary artery disease
- Familial cardiomyopathy
- Hypertension
- Valvular heart disease
- Tachydysrhythmias and bradydysrhythmias
- Toxins: cocaine, ethanol, chemotherapy agents
- Viral or infectious agents
- High-output states
- Infiltrative disease: amyloid sarcoid
- Cor pulmonale
- Metabolic disorders
- Nutritional disorders
- Anemia

TABLE 13.10 ACC/AHA/NYHA 2022 Guidelines for Heart Failure Management

ACC/AHA		NYHA	
Category	**Definition**	**Category**	**Definition**
A	At high risk of developing HF but without structural heart disease or symptoms of HF	None	
B	Structural heart disease or symptoms of HF	I	Asymptomatic
C	Structural heart disease with prior or current symptoms of HF	II	Symptomatic with moderate exertion
		III	Symptomatic with minimal exertion
		IV	Symptomatic with rest
D	Refractory HF requiring specialized interventions	IV	Symptomatic with rest

ACC, American College of Cardiology; *AHA,* American Heart Association; *HF,* heart failure; *NYHA,* New York Heart Association.
Modified from Januzzi JL, Mann DL. Approach to the patient with heart failure. In: Zipes DP, Libby P, Bonow RO, et al., eds. *Braunwald's Heart Disease: A Textbook of Cardiovascular Medicine.* 11th ed. Philadelphia, PA: Elsevier; 2019:403-417.

rate, and contractility. The activation of these diverse systems may account for many of the symptoms of HF and may contribute to progression of the syndrome. Although these responses are initially viewed as compensatory, many of them are or become counterregulatory and lead to adverse effects.[36]

The *renin-angiotensin-aldosterone system* plays a major role in the pathogenesis and progression of HF. Angiotensin II is a potent vasoconstrictor and promotes salt and water retention by stimulation of aldosterone release. Sodium reabsorption increases, and this, in turn, increases blood volume. In patients with impaired function, the heart is unable to handle the extra volume effectively, resulting in edema (peripheral, visceral, and hepatic) (Fig. 13.15).

The *adrenergic nervous system* is activated in HF. Although this is initially beneficial in preserving cardiac output and systemic BP, chronic activation is deleterious. Activation (1) produces tachycardia, thereby decreasing preload and contributing to a decrease in stroke volume; (2) causes vasoconstriction, which increases afterload, further decreasing stroke volume; and (3) increases contractility, which increases myocardial oxygen demand, thereby decreasing contractility and possibly decreasing stroke volume.[36] These changes are progressive. In time, the ventricle dilates, hypertrophies, and becomes more spherical. This process of cardiac remodeling generally precedes symptoms by months or even years.

CHECK YOUR UNDERSTANDING:

6. A patient is admitted with exacerbated left-sided HF with reduced ejection fraction (HFrEF). The patient reports increased fatigue, weight gain, and shortness of breath. What priority interventions does the nurse anticipate?
   A. 12-lead ECG and electrolyte laboratory analysis
   B. Troponin and coagulation laboratory analysis
   C. Place the patient in semi-Fowler's position and administer diuretic
   D. Weigh the patient and administer diuretic

Assessment

Patient assessment includes identification of the cause of both right-sided and left-sided HF, the signs and symptoms, precipitating factors, and results of diagnostic studies. Signs and symptoms of HF are presented in Box 13.14.

Diagnostic Studies

In diagnosing HF, it is important to identify the etiology or precipitating factors and to determine whether ventricular dysfunction is present. There is also importance in determining if there is a reversible cause such as alcohol use, tachycardiac-induced HF, or illicit drug use. Therapies differ for different causes. Ischemic cardiac events are the leading cause of HF. Identifying ischemia as a cause of HF is important because most of these patients can benefit from revascularization.

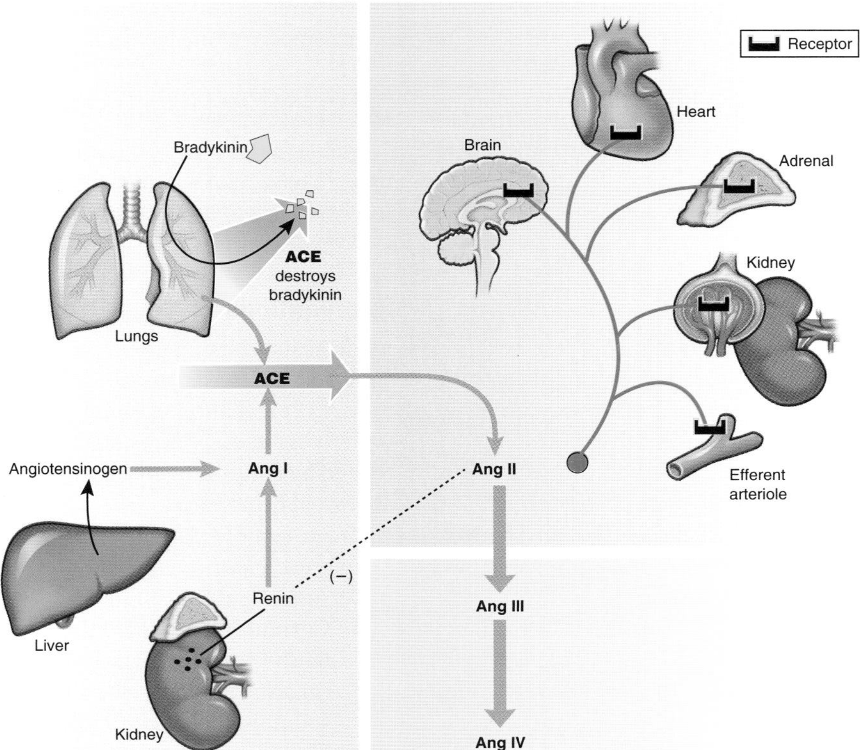

Fig. 13.15 Angiotensins and the organs affected. The shaded blue area is the classical pathway of biosynthesis that generates the renin and angiotensin I *(Ang I)*. Angiotensinogen is synthesized in the liver and released into the blood, where it is cleaved to form Ang I by renin secreted by cells in the kidneys. Angiotensin-converting enzyme *(ACE)* in the lung catalyzes the formation of angiotensin II *(Ang II)* from Ang I and destroys the potent vasodilator, bradykinin. Further cleavage generates the angiotensins III and IV (*Ang III* and *Ang IV*). The reddish shading shows the organs affected by Ang II, including the brain, heart, adrenals, kidneys, and the kidneys' efferent arterioles. The dashed line shows the inhibition of renin by Ang II. (From McCance KL, Huether SE. *Pathophysiology: The Biologic Basis for Disease in Adults and Children*. 8th ed. St. Louis, MO: Elsevier; 2019.)

BOX 13.14 Signs and Symptoms of Heart Failure

Left-Sided Heart Failure: Poor Pump
- Dyspnea or orthopnea
- Cheyne-Stokes respiration
- Paroxysmal nocturnal dyspnea
- Cough (orthopnea equivalent)
- Fatigue or activity intolerance
- Pulmonary crackles
- Weight gain
- Somnolence
- Elevated pulmonary artery occlusion pressure
- S_3 and S_4 gallop
- Tachycardia
- Tachypnea

Right-Sided Heart Failure: Excess Volume
- Jugular venous distention
- Edema
- Loss of appetite, nausea, vomiting
- Increased abdominal girth

Diagnosis of the patient with suspected HF includes the following:

- A complete *history,* including precipitating factors
- *Physical examination,* including assessment of the following:
  - Intravascular volume, with examination of neck veins and presence of hepatojugular reflux
  - Presence or absence of edema
  - Perfusion status, which includes BP, quality of peripheral pulses, capillary refill, and temperature of extremities
  - Lung sounds, which may not be helpful. In many cases, the lung fields are clear when the patient is obviously congested, a reflection of chronicity of the disease and adaptation.
- *Chest radiographic study* to view heart size and configuration and to check the lung fields to determine whether they are clear or opaque (i.e., fluid filled).
- *Hemodynamic monitoring.* Invasive monitoring may be done to assess mixed venous oxygen saturation, stroke index, cardiac index, and pulmonary artery pressures, especially in those who do not respond to conventional therapy. Noninvasive methods of determining hemodynamic parameters may also be used (see Chapter 9, Hemodynamic Monitoring).
- *Noninvasive imaging of cardiac structures.* The single most useful test in evaluating patients with HF is the echocardiogram, which can evaluate ventricular enlargement, wall motion abnormalities, and valvular structures. It can also be used to determine the LVEF.
- *Measurement of arterial blood gases* to assess oxygenation and acid-base status.
- *Serum electrolytes.* Many electrolyte imbalances are seen in patients with HF. A low serum sodium level is a sign of advanced or end-stage disease; a low potassium level is associated with diuresis; a high potassium level is seen in renal impairment; blood urea nitrogen and creatinine levels are elevated in low perfusion states, in renal impairment, or with over diuresis.
- *Complete blood count* to assess for anemia.
- *B-type (brain) natriuretic peptide (BNP).* BNP is a cardiac hormone that is secreted by ventricular myocytes in response to wall stretch. Assays of BNP and its prohormone, proBNP, are useful in the diagnosis of patients with dyspnea of unknown etiology. BNP is a good marker for differentiating between pulmonary and cardiac causes of dyspnea.[34,35] Plasma concentrations of BNP reflect the severity of HF. In decompensated HF, the BNP concentration increases as a response to wall stress or stretch. As the HF is treated, BNP is used to assess the response to therapy. The normal BNP concentration is less than 100 pg/mL. A BNP level greater than 400 pg/mL is highly specific and indicates increased mortality risk.[3] Patients are at increased risk for readmission and death if the BNP concentration remains persistently elevated at the time of discharge. BNP is not a good indicator of HF for patients with chronic renal insufficiency.
- *Liver function studies.* The liver often becomes enlarged with tenderness because of hepatic congestion. Serum transaminase and bilirubin levels are elevated with diminished liver function. Function usually returns once the patient is treated and euvolemic.
- *ECG.* Intraventricular conduction delays are common. Left bundle branch blocks are often associated with structural abnormalities. Patients frequently have premature ventricular contractions, premature atrial contractions, and atrial dysrhythmias. Sinus tachycardia at rest implies substantive cardiac decompensation, and detection of this occurrence is essential.

? CLINICAL JUDGMENT ACTIVITY

A patient has been hospitalized three times in the past 2 months with mid-range ejection fraction HF (HFmrEF). The patient reports being tired of living with limitations on activity and poor quality of life. What person-centered education and resources can you implement to address the patient's concerns?

Interventions

Medical and nursing interventions for the patient with HF consist of a threefold approach: (1) treatment of the existing symptoms, (2) prevention of complications, and (3) treatment of the underlying cause. For example, some patients with HF can be treated by controlling hypertension or by repairing or replacing abnormal heart valves.

Treatment of existing symptoms includes the following:

1. *Improve pump function, fluid removal, and enhanced tissue perfusion* (Tables 13.11 and 13.12).
   a. Current gold standard treatment for HF begins with angiotensin receptor neprilysin inhibitors (ARNIs) and continues with beta-blockers, aldosterone antagonists, and sodium-glucose cotransporter 2 (SGLT2).[37]
   b. First-line medications include diuretics (e.g., furosemide, torsemide, bumetanide, and metolazone) and ARNI agents. If unable to tolerate ARNI for whatever reason, an angiotensin receptor blocker (ARB) or angiotensin converting enzyme-inhibitor (ACE-I) may be substituted.[37]
   c. Additional medication therapies to cautiously consider include digoxin, hydralazine, and nitrates.

TABLE 13.11 Medication Subsets for Heart Failure

Medication	Management of Heart Failure
Aldosterone antagonists	HFrEF (EF ≤ 40%) to improve all cause mortality and HF-related admissions; HFpEF (EF ≥ 50%) with elevated BNP or hospitalized for HF in past 12 months to decrease HF-related admissions
Angiotensin converting enzyme inhibitor (ACEI)	Slow disease progression and remodeling, improve exercise capacity, and decrease hospitalization and mortality
Angiotensin II receptor antagonists (ARB)	Reduce afterload and improve cardiac output; can be used for patients with ACEI cough
Angiotensin receptor neprilysin inhibitor (ARNI)	Gold standard for HF management. Reduces morbidity and mortality in HFrEF and reduces HF-related admission in HFpEF
Beta-blockers (BB)	HFrEF to reduce mortality and combined risk of death or hospitalization
Digoxin	Improve symptoms, exercise tolerance, and quality of life; no effect on mortality
Diuretics	Manage fluid overload
Afterload reducers	Vasodilator; Alternative therapy in HFrEF who cannot tolerate and ARNI, ACEI, and ARB or additional therapy for blood pressure control
Sodium-glucose cotransporter-2 (SGLT2)	Provides mild diuretic effect, reduces preload through decreased sodium reabsorption; decreases afterload through blood pressure reduction effects.

ACEI, Angiotensin-converting enzyme inhibitor; *ANP,* atrial natriuretic peptide; *ARB,* angiotensin II receptor antagonists; *ARNI,* angiotensin receptor neprilysin inhibitor; *BB,* beta-blockers; *BNP,* brain natriuretic peptide; *HF,* heart failure; *HFrEF,* heart failure with reduced EF; *HrpEF,* heart failure with preserved EF; *LV,* left ventricular; *SGLT2,* sodium-glucose cotransporter-2.

TABLE 13.12 PHARMACOLOGY

Specific Medications for Heart Failure

Medication	Action/Use	Dose/Route	Side Effects	Nursing Implications
Afterload Reducers				
Hydralazine	Direct vasodilator, decreasing systemic vascular resistance	Oral: 25 mg TID PO in combination with isosorbide dinitrate; target dose 75–100 mg TID PO	Constipation Diarrhea Flushing Headache Hypotension Loss of appetite Tachycardia	Monitor blood pressure.
Isosorbide dinitrate (Isordil)	Same	Oral: 20 mg TID PO, target dose 40 mg TID PO	Headache Hypotension Rebound hypertension Syncope	Monitor blood pressure; may give patient a headache.
Aldosterone Receptor Antagonists				
Spironolactone (Aldactone)	Competes with aldosterone for receptor sites in distal renal tubules, increasing sodium chloride and water excretion while conserving potassium and hydrogen ions; may block the effect of aldosterone on arterial smooth muscle	Oral: 12.5 mg daily PO, target dose 50 mg daily PO (in 1 or 2 divided doses)	Gynecomastia Hyperkalemia	Monitor serum potassium and renal function; medication is potassium sparing. Do not initiate if eGFR ≤ 30 or serum potassium ≥ 5.0 mEq/L
Eplerenone (Inspra)	Same	Oral: 25 mg daily PO, target dose 50 mg daily PO	Hyperkalemia Increased SCr	Same Use in HF patients with CrCl ≥ 30.
Angiotensin-Converting Enzyme Inhibitors (ACEIs)				
Enalapril (Vasotec)	Prevents the conversion of AI to AII, causing an increase in plasma renin activity and a reduction of aldosterone secretion; also inhibits the remodeling process after myocardial injury	Oral: 2.5 mg BID PO, target dose 10–20 mg BID	Acute kidney injury Angioedema Cough Hypotension Hyperkalemia Orthostatic hypotension	Monitor serum potassium. Avoid use of NSAIDs. Monitor serum creatinine and BUN. Hold in acute kidney injury. Contraindicated in pregnancy.
Lisinopril (Prinivil, Zestril)	Same	Oral: 2.5–5 mg daily PO, target dose 20–40 mg daily PO	Same	Same

Continued

TABLE 13.12 PHARMACOLOGY—cont'd

Specific Medications for Heart Failure

Medication	Action/Use	Dose/Route	Side Effects	Nursing Implications
Angiotensin Receptor Blocker (ARB)				
Valsartan (Diovan)	Selective and competitive AII receptor antagonist; blocks the vasoconstrictor and aldosterone-secreting effects of AII	Oral: 20–40 mg BID PO, target dose 160 mg BID PO	Acute kidney injury Dizziness Hyperkalemia Hypotension Upper respiratory tract infection	Avoid use of NSAIDs. Monitor serum potassium. Monitor serum creatinine and BUN. Hold in acute kidney injury. Contraindicated in pregnancy.
Candesartan (Atacand)	Same	Oral: 4–8 mg daily PO, target dose 32 mg daily PO	Same	Same
Angiotensin Receptor Neprilysin Inhibitor (ARNI)				
Sacubitril/valsartan (Entresto)	Increases peptides, including natriuretic peptides inducing vasodilation and natriuresis	Oral: 24/26 mg tablet BID PO, target dose 97/103 mg tablet BID PO	Acute kidney injury Angioedema Cough Dizziness Hyperkalemia Hypotension Thrombocytopenia	Monitor serum potassium. Monitor serum creatinine and BUN. Hold in acute kidney injury. Contraindicated in pregnancy.
Beta-Blockers (BB)				
Metoprolol succinate (Toprol XL)	Blocks beta-adrenergic receptors with resulting decreased sympathetic nervous system responses such as decreases in HR, BP, and cardiac contractility in heart failure; may improve systolic function over time	Oral: Initial: 12.5–25 mg daily PO Target: 200 mg daily PO	Atrioventricular blocks Bradycardia Fatigue Hypotension Impotence May mask hypoglycemic episodes	Patient should not abruptly stop taking. Start on the lowest dose and titrate to the max tolerated dose.
Carvedilol (Coreg, Coreg CR)	Alpha and beta-blocker; Decreases vascular resistance acutely and blood pressure; Decreases heart rate; May influence the renin-angiotensin system	Oral: Carvedilol IR: 3.125 mg BID PO, target dose 25–50 mg BID PO Carvedilol CR: 10 mg daily PO, target dose 80 mg daily PO	Same	Same
Bisoprolol (Concor)	Same as metoprolol	Oral: 1.25 mg daily PO, target dose 10 mg daily PO	Same	Same
Diuretics				
Furosemide (Lasix)	Loop diuretic, inhibits reabsorption of sodium and chloride in the ascending loop of Henle; used for the management of edema or fluid volume overload	Oral/Intravenous: 20–600 mg daily Typically, IV dosing is half of oral dosing (e.g., furosemide 40 mg PO would equal furosemide 20 mg IV)	Constipation Cramping Diarrhea Gout Hearing impairment Hypokalemia Orthostatic hypotension Tinnitus (rapid IV administration) Vertigo	Monitor laboratory results, especially potassium levels. Monitor cardiovascular and hydration status regularly. In decompensated patients, use IV route until euvolemic status is reached.
Bumetanide (Bumex)	Same	Oral/Intravenous/ Intramuscular: 0.5–10 mg daily	Same	Same
Torsemide (Demadex)	Same	Oral/Intravenous: 10–200 mg daily (max 200 mg daily)	Same	Same
Metolazone (Zaroxolyn)	Thiazide-related diuretic, inhibits sodium transport to the renal tubules, causing decreased sodium reabsorption, and increased sodium, chloride, and water excretion **VERY POTENT when used with additional loop diuretics**	Oral: 2.5–20 mg as directed; not commonly used on a daily basis except in severe heart failure	Same	Increased diuretic effect occurs when given with loop diuretics. Administer 30 min before IV loop diuretic.
Ethacrynic acid (Edecrin)	Loop diuretic	Oral: 25–200 mg daily or q 12 h (in 1 to 2 divided doses), for severe refractory edema may give up to 400 mg/day in 2 divided doses	Same	Used in patients with hypersensitivity reaction to sulfonamide-based loop diuretics

TABLE 13.12 PHARMACOLOGY—cont'd

Specific Medications for Heart Failure

Medication	Action/Use	Dose/Route	Side Effects	Nursing Implications
Inotropes				
Digoxin (Lanoxin)	Augments contractility enhancing tissue perfusion; used to treat persistent symptoms despite optimal guideline-directed medical therapy	Oral/Intravenous: 0.125–0.5 mg daily; requires renal dose adjustments	Asystole Bradycardia Confusion/mental disturbances Diarrhea Heart block Nausea Visual disturbances (blurred or yellowed vision) Vomiting	Monitor serum concentrations; toxicity can be life-threatening. Monitor potassium levels; hypokalemia increases risk of digoxin toxicity. Monitor HR and notify provider if rate is <50 beats/min. Treatment of digoxin toxicity is digoxin immune fab (DigiFab).
Dobutamine (Dobutrex)	Beta-adrenergic agonist increasing contractility and heart rate	Continuous infusion: 2–5 mcg/kg/min IV, titrated to clinical endpoint, max 20 mcg/kg/min	Angina Headache Hypotension Increased HR Local inflammatory changes Nausea Ventricular ectopy	Used inpatient for acute decompensated heart failure. Administer into large vein via infusion device. May be used in outpatient settings in patients with end-stage heart failure. Monitor heart rate and rhythm and BP closely.
Dopamine (Intropin)	Low doses: stimulates the receptors in the renal system leading to vasodilation; Then promotes blood flow to preserve glomerular filtration Mid to high doses: Stimulates the beta-1 receptors on the heart to act as a vasopressor (causing constriction of the blood vessels to raise the blood pressure)	Continuous infusion: 1–50 mcg/kg/min IV titrated to desired response	Angina Extravasation can cause tissue necrosis and sloughing Frequent ventricular ectopy Headache Nausea Tachycardia Vasoconstriction Vomiting	Administer into large vein via infusion device. Monitor heart rate and rhythm and BP closely. Dopamine is frequently used to treat hypotension and is often used with dobutamine, which increases cardiac output. Monitor the IV site frequently.
Milrinone (Primacor)	Phosphodiesterase III inhibitor causing increase in contractility and heart rate	Continuous infusion: 0.125–0.25 mcg/kg/min IV, titrated to clinical endpoint, usual dose range 0.125–0.75 mcg/kg/min	Headaches Hypotension May block platelet aggregation Ventricular arrhythmias leading to cardiac ischemia	Higher risk of ventricular arrhythmias compared to dobutamine. Monitor blood pressures frequently. Use cautiously in those with renal failure.
Nitrates				
Nitroglycerin (Tridil)	Directly relaxes smooth muscle, which causes vasodilation of the peripheral vascular bed; decreases myocardial oxygen demands; used to reduce afterload, elevated systemic vascular resistance	Continuous infusion: 5 mcg/min, titrated to a max of 200 mcg/min	Dizziness Flushing Headache Orthostatic hypotension	Monitor BP closely. Titrate to effect.
Sodium Glucose-Cotransporter-2 (SGLT2)				
Dapagliflozin (Farxiga)	Reduces reabsorption of filtered glucose and promoting urinary excretion of glucose Also reduces sodium reabsorption, increasing delivery of sodium to the distal tubule	Oral: 10 mg daily	Acute kidney injury Constipation Euglycemic ketoacidosis Increased urine output Nausea Significant volume depletion Urinary tract infections	Should not be given in those prone to having urinary tract infections. Should be stopped if urinary tract infections occur. Know that urinalysis will contain a high level of glucose intentionally. Consider holding therapy for at least 3 days prior to surgery. Monitor BUN and creatinine.
Empagliflozin (Jardiance)	Same	Oral: 10 mg daily	Same	Same

AI, Angiotensin I; *AII,* angiotensin 2; *AMI,* acute myocardial infarction; *bid,* twice daily; *BP,* blood pressure; *HR,* heart rate; *IM,* intramuscular; *IVP,* intravenous push; *max,* maximum; *NSAIDs,* nonsteroidal antiinflammatory drugs; *PO,* orally; *q,* every; *tid,* three times daily.

d. Inotropes—dobutamine, dopamine, and milrinone—have failed to demonstrate improved mortality in the treatment of severe decompensated HF, despite increasing cardiac output and cardiac contractility leading to improved end-organ perfusion.[38] Inotropes have been used in palliative medicine for HF when no other reasonable options exist, stabilizing symptoms of HF and allowing for the possibility of patients returning home toward the end-of-life.

2. *Optimize gas exchange through supplemental oxygen and diuresis.*
   a. Evaluate the airway, the degree of respiratory distress, and the need for supplemental oxygenation by pulse oximetry, arterial blood gas measurement, or both. Patients are more comfortable in semi-Fowler's position. Adjust oxygen delivery. Consider noninvasive ventilatory support such as continuous positive airway pressure (CPAP) or intermittent noninvasive positive-pressure ventilation (NPPV). CPAP and NPPV have demonstrated effectiveness in the management of HF and often reduce the need for intubation.[39]
   b. Aggressive diuresis. Administer IV diuretics; furosemide, torsemide, and bumetanide are the preferred agents. Ethacrynic acid is useful if the patient has a serious sulfa allergy. These agents are characterized by quick onset; diuresis is expected 15 to 30 minutes after administration. IV loop diuretic administration is preferred over IV thiazide diuretic administration. The goal is to achieve euvolemia, which may take days. After the patient is euvolemic, oral medications are restarted.
   c. Control of sodium and fluid retention sometimes involves fluid restriction of 2 L/day and sodium restriction of 2 g/day. Sodium restriction alone may provide substantial benefits for patients with HF. Discuss management of fluid balance and the importance of avoiding excess intake of sodium, water, or both. Initiate a consult with a dietitian for dietary management and additional teaching.
   d. Daily weights are a priority in these cases. Ensuring accurate daily weights is a primary intervention strategy for assessing changes in fluid balance and making diuretic dosing adjustments.
   e. Accurate records of intake and output are also crucial in HF management regarding the necessary diuresis efforts.

3. *Reduce cardiac workload and oxygen consumption.*
   a. Ultrafiltration is sometimes used for hospitalized patients with HF to remove sodium and reduce water retention. (See Chapter 16, Acute Kidney Injury.) Access is needed, and the risks may not outweigh the benefits. Results from clinical trials have been mixed.[39]
   b. Biventricular pacing may be used for cardiac resynchronization therapy in patients with chronic HF who exhibit dyssynchronous contraction of the left ventricle resulting from abnormal electrical conduction pathways. Biventricular pacing involves placement of a ventricular lead in the right ventricle and another lead down the coronary sinus to the left ventricle. Both ventricles are stimulated simultaneously, resulting in a synchronized contraction that improves cardiac performance and exercise tolerance and decreases hospitalizations and mortality.
   c. Mechanical circulatory support (MCS) has played an important role in the various stages of HF management. Consideration of MCS and temporary devices such as temporary mechanical circulatory support (tMCS), intraaortic balloon pumps (IABP) (Fig. 13.16), and extracorporeal life support (ECLS) (Fig. 13.17) should be considered to reduce the cardiac workload and increase perfusion to maintain satisfactory end-organ function. The temporary devices assist the failing heart and maintain adequate circulatory pressure. The durable MCS (dMCS) devices attach to the patient's own heart, leaving the patient's heart intact with the potential for removal. Each of these devices are described in more detail herein (Box 13.15 and Table 13.13).
   d. tMCS should be considered during an AMI to maintain adequate BP support and end-organ perfusion; during shock states with patient instability caused by lack of end-organ perfusion; during cardiac surgery when there is inability to wean from the cardiopulmonary bypass machine; and for right ventricular failure following the discovery of a pulmonary embolism or placement of a durable MCS device. These temporary devices, based on the indication for placement, may be inserted through the femoral artery or vein or placed through the internal jugular. Right-sided temporary devices focus on resting the right ventricle; in contrast, the left-sided temporary devices focus on resting the left ventricle, with the overall goal of improvement in functionality.
   e. IABP as a circulatory support device is used to provide short-term reduction of cardiac workload and oxygen consumption by improving preload and reducing afterload of the heart. The balloon is inserted through the femoral artery

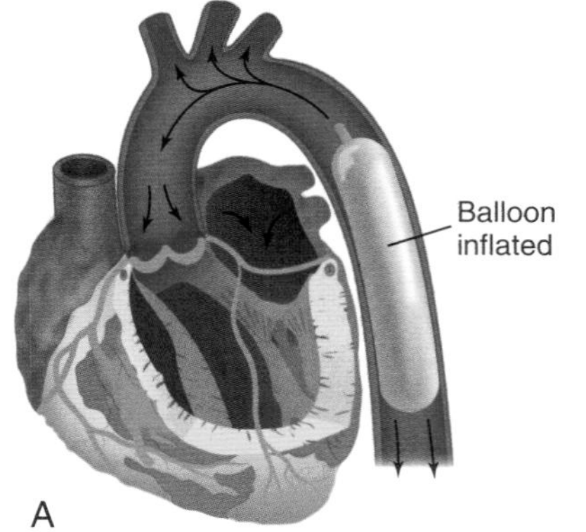

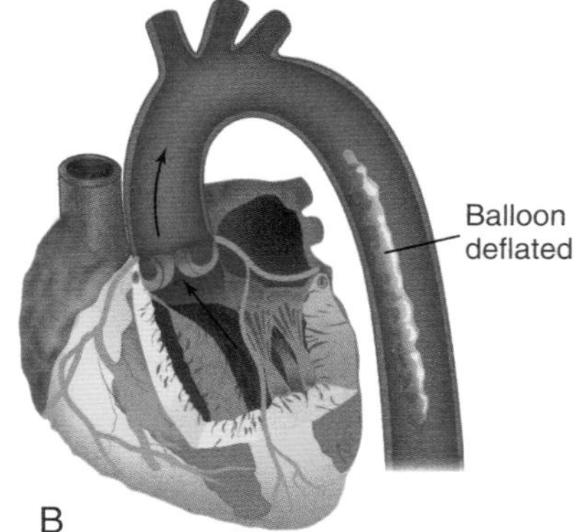

Fig. 13.16 Mechanisms of Action of Intra-aortic Balloon Pump. **A**, Diastolic balloon inflation augments coronary blood flow. **B**, Systolic balloon deflation decreases afterload. (From Urden L, Stacy K, Lough M. *Critical Care Nursing: Diagnosis and Management*. 9th ed. St. Louis: Elsevier; 2022.)

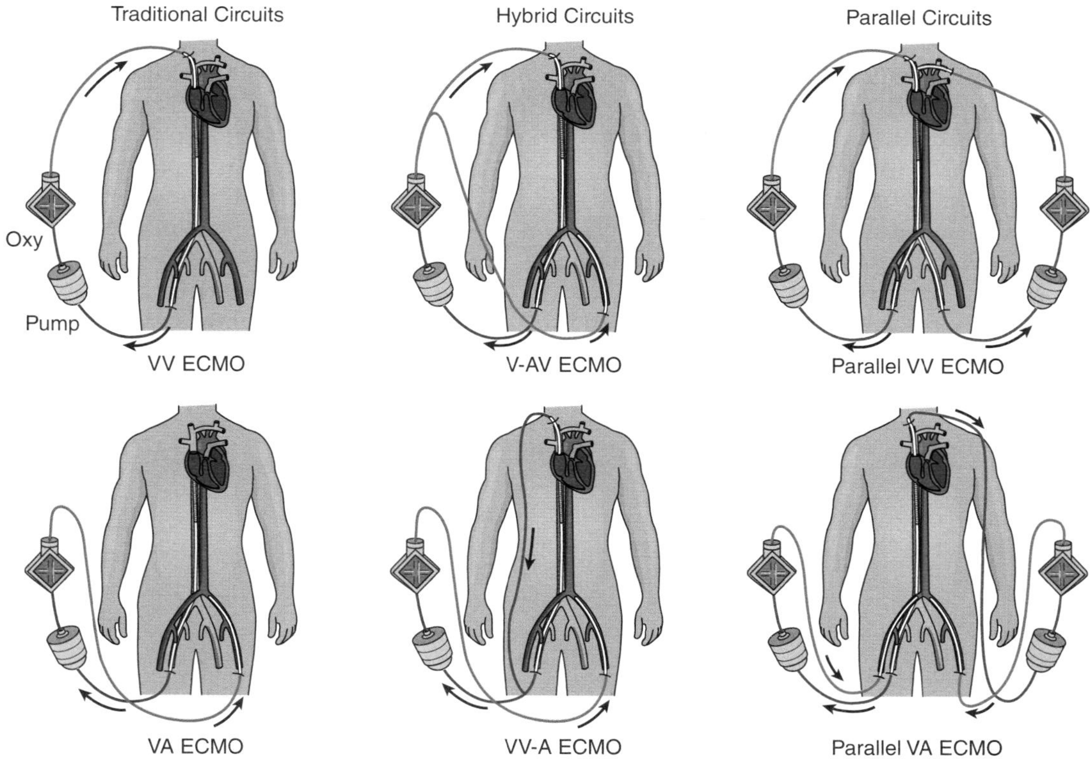

Fig. 13.17 Cannulation types of extracorporeal life support. *ECMO,* Extracorporeal membrane oxygenation; *Parallel ECMO,* parallel is two ECMO circuits running in tandem; *V-AV,* veno-arterial-venous; *VA,* venoarterial; *VV,* veno-venous; *VV-A,* veno-venous-arterial.

BOX 13.15 Mechanical Circulatory Support

Patients with advanced heart failure or cardiogenic shock may require mechanical circulatory support (MCS) to assist ventricular function. MCS therapy is being used to treat not only patients in the hospital, but also long-term outpatients.[1] With the increase in the incidence of heart failure and the shortage of organ donors, demands for MCS have escalated.

Various MCS devices exist that support the left ventricle, right ventricle, or both. MCS devices are indicated as short-term therapy (previously known as a bridge to transplant or bridge to recovery) or long-term therapy (previously known as destination therapy).[2]

Short-term devices, formerly referred to as bridge to recovery (BTR), are used for patients with acute heart failure or cardiogenic shock who have an expectation for recovery but who have failed optimal medical therapy. These devices include the intraaortic balloon pump (IABP; Fig. 13.16), systems such as extracorporeal life support (ECLS), previously known as extracorporeal membrane (ECMO; Fig. 13.17), short-term temporary ventricular assist device (VAD), and, fully implantable VADs (Fig. 13.18).[1] Short-term therapy can last from hours to several days, allowing time for organ recovery or placement of a long-term MCS device.

Another short-term therapy indication, previously referred to as bridge to transplantation (BTT), is used for patients who are unlikely to recover from their cardiogenic shock or decompensated heart failure and who are candidates for heart transplantation. These patients have significant symptoms at rest, often require inotropes, are hemodynamically stable, and do not have significant end-organ damage. They are candidates for a left VAD (LVAD), which may require surgery with cardiopulmonary bypass for implantation.[1]

Long-term therapy, previously known as destination therapy (DT), is used for patients who require long-term support for chronic heart failure that is refractory to medical therapy and who are not candidates for heart transplantation. A long-term LVAD requires major surgery; the patient must be hemodynamically stable, with no significant end-organ damage. An LVAD improves quality of life and decreases mortality despite the significant risk involved (stroke, infection, bleeding, and device malfunction).[1,3]

Patients requiring MCS devices need specialized nursing care.[4] During the early postoperative period, nursing management is focused on avoiding potential complications such as low pump flow, bleeding, infection, organ dysfunction, and cardiac dysrhythmias. Monitor for adequate systemic perfusion (i.e., urine output, mentation, capillary refill) and laboratory values (i.e., electrolytes, mixed venous oxygenation saturation [SvO_2], serum lactate level, white blood cell count, metabolic panel, and coagulation studies). During the late postoperative period, nursing management shifts toward patient and family education and preparation for discharge. Educate patients about infection prevention measures, medication management, nutrition, mobility, and signs and symptoms of complications. Before discharge, patients must demonstrate proper management of their devices, including troubleshooting, battery changes, and emergency responses. The goals of therapy are to optimize functional capacity, improve quality of life, and facilitate integration back into the community.[5]

References

1. Aaronson KD, Pagana FD. Mechanical circulatory support. In: Zipes DP, Libby P, Bonow RO, Mann DL, Tomaselli GF, eds. *Braunwald's Heart Disease: A Textbook of Cardiovascular Medicine.* 11th ed. Philadelphia, PA: Elsevier; 2019:568–579.
2. The Joint Commission. Revision to requirements for advanced certification for ventricular assist device. https://www.jointcommission.org/-/media/tjc/documents/standards/prepublications/vad_prepub.pdf. Accessed December 29, 2023.
3. Mehra MR, Uriel N, Naka Y, et al. A fully magnetically levitated left ventricular assist device-final report. *NEJM.* 2019;380:1618–1627. https://doi.org/10.1056/NEJMoa1900486.
4. Casida JM, Abshire M, Widmar B, Combs P, Freeman R, Baas L. Nurses' competence caring for hospitalized patients with ventricular assist devices. *Dimens Crit Care Nurs.* 2019;38(1):38–49.
5. Peberdy MA, Gluck JA, Ornato JP, et al. Cardiopulmonary resuscitation in adults and children with mechanical circulatory support: a scientific statement from the American Heart Association. *Circulation.* 2017;135(24):e1115–e1134.

and positioned in the thoracic aorta. The device inflates and deflates with the cardiac cycle to reduce the work of the heart. Possible complications if IABP use include bleeding at the insertion site, limb ischemia, systemic thromboembolism, and rarely, death. An IABP should not be used in the settings of *aortic valve insufficiency, aortic dissection, peripheral vascular disease, or aortic aneurysm.*[40]

f. ECLS is also referred to as extracorporeal membranous oxygenation (ECMO) and is used for the acute management of cardiogenic shock or respiratory failure. There are two different ECLS options available based on the needs of the patient: veno-venous (VV) ECLS cannulation (used for hypoxic or hypercapnic respiratory failure, severe pulmonary emboli, or ventilatory support needed for cardiac transplantation) or veno-arterial (VA) ECLS cannulation (most often used with severe cardiogenic shock or cardiac arrest or in settings where cardiopulmonary bypass cannot be weaned off after cardiac surgery).[41,42] ECLS is contraindicated in individuals with irreversible brain injuries, untreatable metastatic cancers, and uncontrolled bleeding and when there are no additional bridging options available, such as cardiac transplantation or placement of a dMCS device.[42,43]

TABLE 13.13 Temporary and Long-Term Mechanical Circulatory Support

Type	Indications	Description
Temporary		
Intraaortic balloon pump (IABP)	Acute cardiogenic shock with hypotension, assistance with high-risk angioplasty; assistance with blood flow follow cardiac bypass surgery	A balloon that is generally placed percutaneously through an artery in the descending aorta to assist the native heart in delivery of oxygenated blood. The balloon inflates when the heart is at rest and deflates when the heart contracts. Aids in maintaining adequate blood flow for end-organ perfusion.
Extracorporeal life support (ECLS)	*Veno-arterial extracorporeal membranous oxygenation* (VA-ECMO)-Used for severe cardiogenic shock *Veno-veno extracorporeal membranous oxygenation* (VV-ECMO)-Used for severe respiratory failure	VA-ECMO: Form of temporary mechanical support where cannulas are placed in a vein and artery. Blood is pulled from the vein, oxygenated through the ECMO machine, and delivered back to the artery, assisting native flow during critical situations such as hemodynamic instability. VV-ECMO: Form of temporary mechanical support where cannulas are placed in two separate veins, providing respiratory support. Blood is typically pulled from the inferior vena cava and returned to the right atrium. An oxygenator is generally involved in this flow pattern. The patient needs to be hemodynamically stable to use this type of temporary support.
CentriMag	Short-term univentricular or biventricular support	Continuous-flow pump that produces blood flow from 0–10 L/min. Blood flow is produced by rotation of a magnetically suspended impeller, eliminating contact between components. Placed either through an open chest or by percutaneous methods.
Left-sided pumps *Impella LP 5.5* *Impella CP* Right-sided pump *Impella RP*	Short-term left or right ventricular support (based on the cannula used)	Continuous-flow pump that has a percutaneously inserted catheter, allowing flow of 2.5 L/min or up to 5.5 L/min based upon which device is used. The catheter is placed retrograde across the aortic valve to pull blood from the left ventricle, which is returned to ascending aorta. The catheter for the Impella RP is placed so that the inlet is positioned in the inferior vena cava, pulling venous blood and expelling it through the outlet located in the pulmonary artery.
LifeSPARC	Short-term left or right ventricular support	Percutaneously inserted device that provides continuous flow up to 6 L/min. LVAD: Inflow is obtained from a catheter positioned in the left atrium (by a transseptal approach), and outflow is through the femoral artery. RVAD: Inflow is obtained from a catheter positioned where the inlet is located in the right atrium, and the outlet is located in the pulmonary artery. Device allows for transport to a center for tertiary care.
Long-Term		
HeartMate II (HM2) (no longer implanted in the US)	Long-term left ventricular support	An electrically driven pump that produces nonpulsatile flow. Previously FDA approved for bridge to transplantation and destination therapy. Smaller size allows for implantation in patients with body surface area <1.5 m^2. Anticoagulation and antiplatelet therapy are required. This pump was left in this list for information, as there are still thousands of patients in the United States that have this pump actively in place.
HeartMate 3 (HM3)	Currently the only approved device for implantation in the United States; long-term left ventricular support for both short- or long-term therapy indications	Magnetically levitated left-sided heart pump that produces centrifugal flow. FDA approved for short-term or long-term therapies. Can be placed via sternotomy or lateral thoracotomy approach. Has an element of pulsatility to allow to this date, no documented pump thrombosis. Anticoagulation and continuous power are required.
HeartWare (HVAD) (no longer implanted as of 2022)	Left ventricular support as long-term or short-term therapy	A continuous flow rotary pump with centrifugal design that produces nonpulsatile flow. FDA approved for bridge to transplant. Its small size allows for placement above the diaphragm in the pericardial space. The pump has no points of mechanical contact, which reduces damage to red blood cells. This pump was left in this list for information, as there are still thousands of patients in the United States that have this pump actively in place.

FDA, U.S. Food and Drug Administration; *LVAD,* left ventricular assist device; *RVAD,* right ventricular assist device.
Data from Mehra MR, Uriel N, Naka Y. et al. A fully magnetically levitated left ventricular assist device-final report. *NEJM.* 2019;380:1618-1627. https://doi.org/10.1056/NEJMoa1900486.

g. dMCS, also referred to as left ventricular assist devices (LVADs), have been used for quite some time to bridge individuals to cardiac transplantation when medications alone are not assisting with HF symptoms (Fig. 13.18). Because of the success in using dMCS support in the HF population, these devices are also approved for individuals who did not meet cardiac transplant criteria but remain in end-stage left-sided HF.

CLINICAL EXEMPLAR

Interprofessional Partnership

According to the World Health Organization, almost 23.6 million people will die of heart disease by the year 2030. The necessity for HF management focusing on intervention is key in decreasing the costs of HF that are estimated to near $70 billion by 2030.[1] Growing evidence supports nurse-led clinics for the management of patients with cardiovascular disease. Research has shown that nurses can intervene in the management of chronic disease by monitoring, managing medications, and providing education and psychological support.

HF is associated with a high readmission rate, with many patients admitted to critical care units. A systematic review and meta-analysis were conducted to evaluate the effects of nurse-led clinics on the morbidity and mortality of patients with cardiovascular disease. The researchers included eight trials that met their inclusion criteria of prospective, randomized controlled trials evaluating the impact of nurse-led clinics for patients with heart disease. Multiple studies showed a 25% reduction in all-cause readmissions when nurse-led clinics were utilized, as well as 13% reduction in all-cause mortality in the nurse-led clinic intervention groups. Overall, the results suggest a positive effect of nurse-led clinics on the morbidity and mortality of patients with cardiovascular disease.[1]

Similarly, Rice[2] and colleagues conducted a systematic review of nurse-led educational topics presented to HF patients prior to discharge and the positive impact on length of stay, quality of life, and hospital readmission.

The acute care nurse practitioners held a journal club on the critical care unit to review patient care transition between outpatient and inpatient practice environments to include nurse-led clinics and nurse-led education prior to discharge. Forming a team of bedside nurses, clinical nurse specialists, nurse leaders of the critical care unit and case management teams, and providers (physicians, physician assistants, and nurse practitioners), a checklist was developed for interprofessional communication and transition of patients out of acute and critical care practice environments. Using a whiteboard in the patient room, a standardized list of essential education that need to be provided to patients with HF and their families was developed. Review of the whiteboard with education completion dates was woven into daily multiprofessional rounds. Patients and family members were also encouraged to post questions on the white board to facilitate care transition.

The acute care nurse practitioners, clinical nurse specialist, and nurse leaders tracked the effectiveness of the white boards, hospital length of stay, communication effectiveness with the nurse-led clinic, and readmissions.

References

1. Son YJ, Choi J, Lee HJ. Effectiveness of nurse-led heart failure self-care education on health outcomes of heart failure patients: a systematic review and meta-analysis. *Int J Environ Res Public Health.* 2020;17(18):6559.
2. Rice H, Say R, Betihavas V. The effect of nurse-led education on hospitalisation, readmission, quality of life and cost in adults with heart failure. A systematic review. *Patient Educ Couns.* 2018;101(3):363–374. https://doi.org/10.1016/j.pec.2017.10.002.

Pulmonary artery (PA) pressure management (CardioMEMS HF System, Abbott, Abbott Park, IL) is an effective way of managing patients with HF from home. A PA sensor is implanted into the distal branch of the descending pulmonary artery, and the patient's PA pressures are monitored remotely. The CHAMPION trial showed a 33% reduction in hospitalization for patients with CardioMEMS.[44] The GUIDE-HF trial randomized NYHA Class II to IV HF patients to either activating the PA hemodynamic monitoring management system or being part of the control group. This trial showed relative risk reduction in African Americans (41%) and women (33%); in addition, we found a 25% reduction in emergency room visits in patients who had the PA sensor implanted.[44]

Cardiac transplantation is a therapeutic option for patients with end-stage HF (see Transplant Considerations box). Patients who have severe cardiac disability refractory to expert management and a poor prognosis for 6-month survival are optimal candidates. For many patients with symptomatic HF and ominous objective findings (LVEF <20%, stroke volume <40 mL, severe ventricular dysrhythmias), timing of the surgery is difficult. Another consideration is quality of life, which is a judgment made between the patient and provider. National standards exist for cardiac transplantation; however, candidacy for cardiac transplantation is determined at the discretion of each multidisciplinary transplant program. This candidacy evaluation is different at each transplant center and may include concerns related to certain cutoff standards for body mass index, time frame free from drug/alcohol/tobacco use, age, or time frame free from malignancy.[45,46]

Once the HF crisis stage has passed and the patient is stabilized, precipitating factors for the complications must be addressed and treated. Treatment consists of surgical or catheter-based interventions, as addressed earlier for a patient with MI, such as CABG, PTCA or stent, and pharmacological therapy (ACEIs, beta-blockers); valve replacement or repair for valvular heart disease; restoration of sinus rhythm if atrial fibrillation or flutter and tachydysrhythmias are present; and management of risk factors such as hypertension, hyperlipidemia, diabetes, and obesity. Compliance

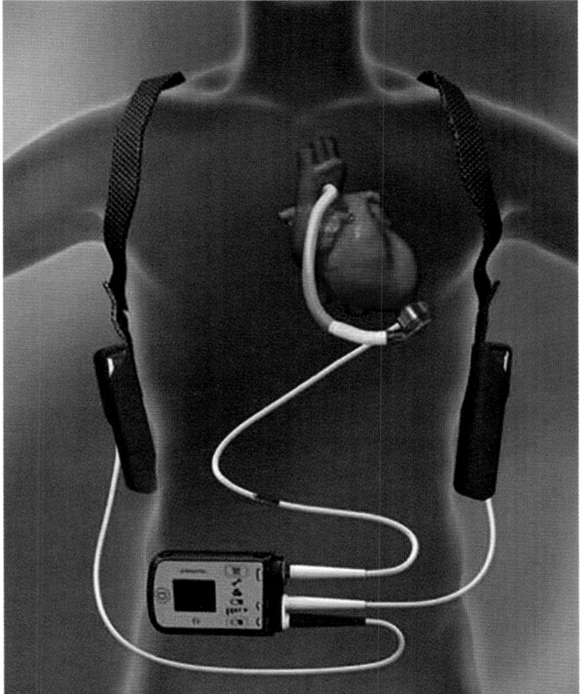

Fig. 13.18 Left ventricular assist device (LVAD) system, including the inflow cannula, pump, outflow graft, driveline cable that exits through the abdomen, power sources, and carrying apparatus. (Courtesy Abbott Corporation.)

with medications and sodium restriction is continually and vigilantly readdressed. Nursing measures that reduce cardiac workload and oxygen consumption include scheduling of rest periods and encouraging patients to modify their activities of daily living. Activity is advanced as tolerated. Patients with HF derive tremendous benefit from formal cardiac rehabilitation to improve activity tolerance and endurance. Nurses make a tremendous impact by teaching and enforcing these concepts throughout the hospital

TRANSPLANT CONSIDERATIONS

Heart Transplantation

Criteria for Transplant Recipients

Indications for cardiac transplantation generally include individuals who are younger than 70 years with end-stage heart disease that is not treatable by other medical or surgical therapies. The Adult Heart Allocation Criteria for Medical Urgency Status is used to classify patients. Scores range from Status 1 (patient has a nondischargeable, surgically implanted, nonendovascular, biventricular support device) to Status 6 (all other active candidates).[1–3] Transplantation is not indicated for those with major systemic disease, including malignancy with metastatic disease, sever neurological deficits, human immunodeficiency virus (HIV) with high viral load, or severe infection or for those who are an active smoker or have a substance use disorder.[2–4]

Several factors considered in determining organ allocation for heart transplant by the United Network for Organ Sharing (UNOS)[3] include:

- Survival benefit
- Donor/recipient immune system compatibility
- Waiting time on the transplantation list
- Distance from the donor hospital
- Pediatric status

Heart allocation through the UNOS was changed October 18, 2018, to prioritize the urgency and need for cardiac transplantation with the primary goal to decrease waitlist mortality. There are now six medical urgency statuses that are used for heart allocation. The statuses are[3,4]:

- Status 1: Includes venoarterial extracorporeal life support (VA ECLS), nondischargeable biventricular cardiac support devices, dMCS with life-threatening arrhythmias
- Status 2: Use of an intra-aortic balloon pump (IABP), nondischargeable durable mechanical circulatory support (dMCS) in place with complications of device malfunction or failure, refractory ventricular arrhythmias, single ventricle patients with a mechanical device in place, endovascular temporary mechanical circulatory support (tMCS) placed percutaneously
- Status 3: Discretionary 30-day period for dischargeable dMCS, use of multiple inotropes with hemodynamic monitoring, dMCS devices with complications
- Status 4: Dischargeable dMCS devices, inotrope therapy, retransplant needs, unrevascularizable ischemic heart disease, hypertrophic or restrictive cardiomyopathy, amyloidosis
- Status 5: Needs multiple organs
- Status 6: Other active candidates

Patient Management

After transplantation, management focuses on optimizing preload, afterload, and contractility. Vasoactive medications and mechanical circulatory support (intraaortic balloon pump, left or right ventricular support) may be indicated.[5]

Immunosuppressive therapy targets different processes in the rejection process: induction, maintenance, and rejection. While there are no standardized guidelines for immunosuppression management, consensus recommendations now exist for immunosuppression following solid organ transplantation.[6] Induction therapy (antithymocyte agents or interleukin-2 receptor blockers) is commonly initiated in the immediate posttransplant period when the risk for rejection is greatest. The primary immunosuppression medications include a calcineurin inhibitor (cyclosporine [Neoral] or tacrolimus [Prograf]), a steroid (methylprednisolone), and an antiproliferative agent (mycophenolate mofetil [CellCept], azathioprine [Imuran]). These medications inhibit T-cell proliferation and differentiation, deplete lymphocytes, and inhibit macrophages.[5,6]

Complications

Infection is the leading cause of morbidity and mortality in the first year after transplantation. In the early postoperative period (within the first month), nosocomial infections predominate, including pneumonia, wound and urinary tract infections, and sepsis.[5–7] Opportunistic infections predominate 1 to 6 months after heart transplantation. Causative organisms include cytomegalovirus (CMV), herpes simplex virus (HSV), varicella zoster (shingles), *Pneumocystis carinii, Aspergillus,* and *Candida.*

After 6 months, most infections are community acquired. Patients are instructed to avoid contact with anyone who is ill, avoid environments high in dust or mold, and use good hand-washing practices. A high index of suspicion must be maintained, as fever can be masked by the effects of the immunosuppressive therapy.[4,37] Complications associated with immunosuppressive therapy include nephrotoxicity, hypertension, diabetes, hyperlipidemia, bone loss, and infection.

Preventing Rejection

Compliance with immunosuppressive medication is essential to reduce the risk of rejection. Hyperacute rejection occurs within minutes or hours of transplantation, is caused by preformed antibodies against the donor, and rarely occurs. Primary graft dysfunction occurs within 24 hours of transplantation. It presents as left and/or right ventricular failure. Aggressive management includes vasoactive medications, mechanical circulatory support, or retransplantation. Acute cellular rejection occurs 3 to 6 months after transplantation and involves the activation and proliferation of T lymphocytes with destruction of cardiac tissue. Humoral or antibody-mediated rejection involves B-cell mediated production of immunoglobulin G antibody against the transplanted organ. Significant hemodynamic compromise and shock can occur, resulting in death.

Rejection is diagnosed by endomyocardial biopsy, initially performed weekly for 4 to 6 weeks and then at increasingly longer intervals based on clinical presentation and cardiac function. Symptoms of rejection may be subtle and include weight gain, shortness of breath, fatigue, abdominal bloating, or fever. Management may include high-dose methylprednisolone; augmenting current maintenance immunosuppression with tacrolimus (Prograf), mycophenolate mofetil (CellCept), rapamycin, or muromonab-CD3 (Orthoclone); and/or plasmapheresis.

Cardiac allograft vasculopathy (CAV), also known in the past as chronic rejection, is an accelerated form of diffuse arteriosclerosis that remains one of the principal limiting factors to long-term survival in cardiac transplant recipients. It can result in myocardial ischemia, infarction, HF, ventricular dysrhythmias, and death.

References

1. Adult heart allocation - OPTN. Organ Procurement and Transplantation Network. https://optn.transplant.hrsa.gov/professionals/by-organ/heart-lung/adult-heart-allocation/. Accessed December 28, 2023.
2. Liu J, Yang BQ, Itoh A, et al. Impact of new UNOS allocation criteria on heart transplantation practices and outcomes. *Transplant Direct.* 2021;7(1):e642.
3. United Network for Organ Sharing (UNOS). How We Match Organs. https://unos.org/transplant/how-we-match-organs/. Accessed December 28, 2023.
4. Mehra MR, Canter CE, Hannan MM, et al. The 2016 International Society for Heart Lung Transplantation listing criteria for heart transplantation: a 10-year update. *J Heart Lung Transplant.* 2016;35(1):1–23. https://doi.org/10.1016/j.healun.2015.10.023.
5. Vega E, Schroder J, Nicoara A. Postoperative management of heart transplantation patients. *Best Pract Res Clin Anaesthesiol.* 2017;31(2):201–213. https://doi.org/10.1016/j.bpa.2017.06.002.
6. Nelson J, Alvey N, Bowman L, et al. Consensus recommendations for use of maintenance immunosuppression in solid organ transplantation: endorsed by the American College of Clinical Pharmacy, American Society of Transplantation, and the International Society for Heart and Lung Transplantation. *ACCP Pharmacotherapy.* 2022;42(8):599–633.
7. Alseed M, Husain S. Infections in heart and lung transplant recipients. *Crit Care Clin.* 2019;35(1):75–93. https://doi.org/10.1016/j.ccc.2018.08.010.

Chelsea Sooy, BSN, RN, CCTC
Melissa A. Kelley, RN, CPTC

stay. Patients may find it easier to continue these habits at discharge if their importance is stressed throughout hospitalization.

Complications

Complications of HF can be devastating. Interventions must be initiated to avoid extending the existing conditions or allowing the development of new, life-threatening complications. Two specific complications for which patients are monitored are pulmonary edema and cardiogenic shock.

Pulmonary Edema. The failing heart is sensitive to increases in afterload. Pulmonary edema develops in some patients with HF when they become hypertensive. The pulmonary vascular system becomes full and engorged. The results are increasing volume and pressure of blood in pulmonary vessels, increasing pressure in pulmonary capillaries, and leaking of fluid into the interstitial spaces of lung tissue. Pulmonary edema greatly reduces the amount of lung tissue space available for gas exchange and results in clinical symptoms of extreme dyspnea, cyanosis, severe anxiety, diaphoresis, pallor, and blood-tinged, frothy sputum. Arterial blood gas results indicate severe respiratory acidosis and hypoxemia.

Patients with persistent volume overload may be candidates for continuous IV diuretics, ultrafiltration, or hemodialysis. Loop diuretics given as an IV bolus are considered along with an IV infusion. Furosemide is the most commonly used loop diuretic, with the dose adjusted upward if the patient is currently receiving oral doses. The diuretic effect occurs in 30 minutes and peaks in 1 to 2 hours. IV torsemide or bumetanide are alternative loop diuretics. Continuous infusion of loop diuretics is considered if the patient does not respond to intermittent dosing. In addition, combinations of diuretics with different mechanisms of action are considered. Thiazide diuretics such as metolazone are often added. Monitor the urinary output hourly to assess the effectiveness of the diuretic therapy. Although diuretic therapy is important, it is also critical to lower the BP and cardiac filling pressures. IV vasodilator such as NTG is administered and titrated until the BP is controlled, resulting in a reduction in both preload and afterload.

Cardiogenic Shock. Cardiogenic shock is the most acute and ominous form of pump failure. Cardiogenic shock can be seen after a severe MI and with dysrhythmias, decompensated HF, pulmonary embolus, cardiac tamponade, and ruptured abdominal aortic aneurysm (AAA). Often, the outcome of cardiogenic shock is death. Cardiogenic shock and its treatment are discussed in depth in Chapter 12, Shock, Sepsis, and Multiple Organ Dysfunction Syndrome. Outcomes for the patient with HF are included in the Plan of Care for the Patient With Heart Failure.

PLAN OF CARE

For the Patient With Heart Failure[a]

Patient Problem

Fluid Overload. Risk factors include compromised regulatory mechanisms occurring with decreased cardiac output.

Desired Outcomes

- Less shortness of breath
- Increased urinary output
- Peripheral edema is decreased
- Weight loss occurs and becomes stable within 2 to 3 days

Nursing Assessments/Interventions	Rationales
• Assess I&O, including insensible losses from diaphoresis and respirations.	• Decreased cardiac output reduces renal blood flow, which may result in decreased urine output.
• Assess daily morning weight; record and report steady losses or gains.	• Identify fluid retention and fluid loss; guide titration of diuretics.
• Assess for dependent edema (legs, ankles, feet, and sacrum).	• Identify fluid retention; guide early treatment, decreasing the potential for rehospitalization.
• Assess lung sounds for signs of fluid retention (i.e., crackles or wheezing).	• Indicate fluid retention.
• Monitor for jugular vein distension and ascites.	• Indicators of fluid overload.
• Monitor for abnormal laboratory results: o Increased urine specific gravity o Decreased Hct and Hgb o Increased urine osmolality o Hyponatremia o Hypokalemia o Hypochloremia	• Indicators of fluid imbalance or side effects of medications.
• Monitor IV flow rate; use an infusion pump for IV fluid administration.	• Prevent volume overload during IV infusion.
• Limit fluid intake per provider orders.	
• Prevent volume overload.	
• Unless contraindicated, provide ice chips or ice pops.	• Provide comfort and reduce thirst while providing minimal amounts of fluid.
• Provide frequent mouth care to reduce dry mucous membranes.	• Small amounts of room-temperature water also relieve thirst.
• Administer diuretics as prescribed and record the patient's response. Use loop diuretics with caution in renal failure or hypokalemia.	• Promote normovolemia by reducing fluid accumulation and blood volume. • Hypokalemia is a common side effect of loop diuretics.
• Administer morphine sulfate if prescribed.	• Induce vasodilation and decrease venous return to the heart; relieve acute anxiety and decrease RR.

PLAN OF CARE—cont'd

***For the Patient With Heart Failure*[a]**

Nursing Assessments/Interventions	Rationales
• A reduced-sodium diet (1–2 g/day) is recommended.	• Hypernatremia can increase fluid retention.
• Teach patients and families about the importance of adhering to a low-sodium diet.	

Patient Problem

Anxiety. Risk factors include an actual or potential life-threatening situation, change in health status, unfamiliar medication, and uncertainty.

Desired Outcomes

- Communicates anxieties and concerns
- Expresses ways to increase physical and psychological comfort

Nursing Assessments/Interventions	Rationales
• Assess for and acknowledge the patient's anxieties and concerns.	• Reduce anxiety.
• Provide opportunities for the patient and significant other to express their feelings.	• Demonstrate support and caring.
• Be reassuring and supportive.	
• Assist the patient in being as comfortable as possible, ensuring prompt pain relief and supportive positioning.	• Promote an overall sense of well-being and positive outcomes.
• Create and maintain a calm and quiet environment.	• Prevent or reduce sensory overload that may cause increased anxiety.
• Explain all treatment modalities, especially those that may be uncomfortable (e.g., O_2 face mask, IV therapy, invasive testing).	• Reduce anxiety and enable a sense of control.

[a]Also refer to the Collaborative Care Plan found in Chapter 1, Overview of Critical Care Nursing.

Hct, hematocrit; *I&O,* intake and output; *O_2,* oxygen; *RR,* respiratory rate.

Snyder J, Sump C. *Swearingen's All-in-One Nursing Care Planning Resource*, 6th ed. Elsevier; 2024.

INFLAMMATORY DISEASES

Pericarditis

Pathophysiology. Pericarditis is acute or chronic inflammation of the pericardium. It may occur as a consequence of AMI or secondary to trauma, infection, radiation therapy, connective tissue diseases, or cancer.[1] The pericardium has an inner layer and an outer layer, with a small amount of lubricating fluid between the layers. When the pericardium becomes inflamed, the amount of fluid between the two layers increases (pericardial effusion). This squeezes the heart, restricting its action, and may result in cardiac tamponade. Chronic inflammation can result in constrictive pericarditis, which leads to scarring. The epicardium may thicken and calcify (Fig. 13.1).

Assessment. The patient with pericarditis usually has precordial pain; this pain may radiate to the shoulder, neck, back, and arm and often mimics the pain associated with an AMI. Other signs and symptoms may include a pericardial friction rub, dyspnea, weakness, fatigue, a persistent temperature elevation, increased white blood cell count, increased sedimentation rate, and increased anxiety.[1] *Pulsus paradoxus* may be noted during auscultation of the BP. Pain due to pericarditis is usually positional and pleuritic (worse with inspiration and cough).

Diagnostic Studies. Detection of a *pericardial friction rub* is the most common method of diagnosing pericarditis. The friction rub is usually heard best on inspiration, when the patient is leaning forward, with the diaphragm of the stethoscope placed over the second, third, or fourth intercostal space at the sternal border. Friction rubs have been described as grating, scraping, squeaking, or scratching sounds. This rubbing sound results from an increase in fibrous exudate between the two irritated pericardial layers.

The ECG is abnormal in 90% of patients with acute pericarditis. On the ECG, diffuse concave ST-segment elevation and PR-segment deviations opposite to P-wave polarity are often seen. T waves progressively flatten and invert, with generalized T-wave inversions present in most or all leads.[1] An echocardiogram is also useful in diagnosis to visualize the effusion. A diagnosis of pericarditis requires at least two of the following four criteria: chest pain characteristic of pericarditis, a pericardial rub, ECG changes characteristic of pericarditis, and new or worsening pericardial effusion.[1]

Interventions. Treatment of patients with pericarditis involves relief of pain (analgesic agents or antiinflammatory agents such as colchicine or ibuprofen) and treatment of other systemic symptoms. Approximately 15 to 50 mL of fluid is normally present in the pericardial space. Excess fluid compresses the heart chambers, limits the filling capacity of the heart, and may result in tamponade. Treatment of cardiac tamponade includes inserting a needle into the pericardial space to remove the fluid (pericardiocentesis). In extreme cases, surgery may be required to remove part of the pericardium (pericardial window).

Endocarditis

Pathophysiology. Infective endocarditis (IE) occurs when microorganisms circulating in the bloodstream attach to an endocardial surface. It is caused by various microbes and frequently involves the heart valves. Endocarditis is increasing in incidence and affects approximately 15 in 100,000 people in the United States. Certain preexisting heart conditions increase the risk for endocarditis, including implantation of an artificial (prosthetic) heart valve, a history of previous endocarditis, and heart valves damaged by conditions such as rheumatic fever, congenital heart defects, or valve defects. Increasing use of implantable cardiac devices and prevalence of drug use have resulted in increased prevalence of IE. *Staphylococcus aureus* accounts for 40% of IE cases.[47]

Infectious lesions, referred to as *vegetations,* form on the heart valves or other implantable device components such as pacemaker leads or inflow cannulas associated with an implantable LVAD. These infectious lesions have irregular edges, creating a cauliflower-like appearance. The mitral valve is the most commonly affected valve. The vegetative processes can grow to involve the chordae tendineae, papillary muscles, and conduction system, causing dysrhythmias or acute HF. The concerns for vegetation on the native valves or artificially implanted pacemaker leads are threefold: (1) systemic infection risk; (2) portions of the vegetation may break off, causing thrombotic-like events including strokes; and (3) impedance of blood flow through the cardiac system.

Assessment. The clinical presentation of patients with acute infectious endocarditis includes high fever, shaking chills, general malaise, and fatigue. Other manifestations include night sweats, cough, weight loss, headache, musculoskeletal complaints, new murmurs, and dyspnea. Abnormal physical findings associated with septic emboli may also be seen, including Janeway lesions (lesions on the palms and soles that are often hemorrhagic), Osler nodes (red-purple lesions on fingers or toes), splinter hemorrhages, and Roth spots (retinal hemorrhages). Skin lesions are referred to as the peripheral stigmata of endocarditis.[48]

Interventions. Treatment of endocarditis involves diagnosing the infective organism through blood cultures and treating with the appropriate IV antibiotics for 2 to 6 weeks. Valve replacement surgery may be indicated in severe cases.[50] Prevention is important. Provide focused education to patients at risk of endocarditis that includes information regarding taking prophylactic antibiotics before dental care, seeking medical care for wounds that are healing poorly, avoidance of tattooing and body piercing, and knowledge of risks associated with IV drug use. Antibiotic prophylaxis is recommended for high-risk patients before procedures are undertaken.[49]

EVIDENCE-BASED PRACTICE

Transcatheter Aortic Valve Replacement for Treatment of Aortic Stenosis

Problem

Traditionally, surgical repair of the aortic valve was the only treatment for severe aortic stenosis in symptomatic patients. Transcatheter aortic valve replacement (TAVR) is an option for patients considered at high risk for surgical aortic valve replacement (SAVR). Novel treatment options are needed to treat patients who need repair of their aortic valve and are at intermediate risk for SAVR.

Clinical Question

Is TAVR a safe alternative for patients at intermediate risk for SAVR?

Evidence

Makkar and colleagues conducted a study to follow outcomes 5-years post TAVR versus those 5-years post SAVR. The TAVR population was stratified to the type of access (transfemoral or transthoracic access), and this population was randomly assigned. At the 5-year mark, there were no significant differences in death or disabling strokes between the populations. However, the authors found death to be higher in the TAVR population when transthoracic access was used. Rehospitalizations were more common after TAVR than after SAVR. Health status in both cohorts was also similar at 5-years, concluding TAVR is an appropriate option for aortic valve replacement if patients meet particular criteria.[1]

Similarly, a systematic review and meta-analysis was completed looking at 1-year survival, paravalvular leaks, and periprocedural complications in those undergoing TAVR with a bicuspid versus a tricuspid aortic valve. Success of the device and 1-year survival rates were similar in the bicuspid and tricuspid aortic valve groups (94% vs. 97% and 90.8% vs. 91.3%, respectively). There were higher periprocedural complications in those undergoing a TAVR with a bicuspid aortic valve. Those also undergoing a TAVR with a bicuspid aortic valve trended toward an increase in moderate to severe paravalvular leaks, cerebral ischemic events, and annular ruptures.[2]

Implications for Nursing

Patients with severe aortic stenosis who are symptomatic have a poor prognosis. TAVR offers an option for those who are deemed to be at intermediate risk for SAVR. It is important for nurses to be aware of novel therapies that might benefit their patients. Care of the patient who has undergone TAVR is similar to that of any postoperative surgical patient and involves evaluation of the patient for any hemodynamic changes and complications. Common postoperative complications of TAVR include stroke, bleeding, acute kidney failure, and dysrhythmias.[40]

Level of Evidence

A—Meta-analysis

References

1. Makkar RR, Thourani VH, Mack MJ, et al. Five-year outcomes of transcatheter or surgical aortic-valve replacement. *N Engl J Med.* 2020;382(9):799–809. https://doi.org/10.1056/NEJMoa1910555.
2. Montalto C, Sticchi A, Crimi G, et al. Outcomes after transcatheter aortic valve replacement in bicuspid versus tricuspid anatomy: a systematic review and meta-analysis. *J Am Coll Cardiol Intv.* 2021;14(19):2144–2155.

VALVULAR HEART DISEASE

Valvular heart disease (VHD) affects approximately 2.5% of the population, with the largest percentage of patients older than 65 years of age. The most common type of VHD is aortic stenosis, followed by mitral regurgitation, aortic regurgitation, and mitral stenosis. Causes include degenerative changes, congenital defects, rheumatic heart disease, ischemic heart disease, and endocarditis. VHD can be initially identified on physical examination by the presence of a murmur on auscultation. Research has revealed that physical examination is not reliable in diagnosing the severity of VHD.[50] An echocardiogram is done to confirm the diagnosis and denote severity. Treatment of VHD consists of surgery to repair or replace the valve.

VASCULAR ALTERATIONS

The aorta is the largest blood vessel in the body in both length and diameter. Shaped like a walking cane, the aorta is an artery that carries blood from the heart. It extends from the aortic valve to the abdomen. Its many branches supply blood to all other areas of the body. The aorta is divided into the thoracic aorta and the abdominal aorta[51] (Fig. 13.19).

The thoracic aorta is divided into the ascending aorta, the aortic arch, and the descending aorta. The thoracic aorta begins at the aortic root, which supports the bases of the three aortic valve leaflets.[2] The rounded segment (cane handle) includes the ascending aorta and the aortic arch. Branches of the ascending aorta include the right and left coronary arteries, which feed the myocardium. The arch vessels include the innominate artery, which branches into the right subclavian artery, the right common carotid artery, the left common carotid, and the left subclavian arteries. These branches send blood to the head and upper extremities. The descending thoracic aorta (the long segment of the cane) lies to the left of midline in the chest. Branches of the descending aorta are the intercostal arteries, which provide the major blood supply to the distal spinal cord. The abdominal aorta begins at the level of the diaphragm. At the umbilicus, it bifurcates into the two iliac arteries. Abdominal branches include the celiac artery, the superior and inferior mesenteric arteries, and the renal arteries.[2]

Aortic Aneurysms

The word *aneurysm* comes from the Greek word *aneurysma*, which means "widening." An aneurysm is a diseased area of an artery causing dilation and thinning of the wall. An aneurysm may be classified as a false (pseudoaneurysm) or a

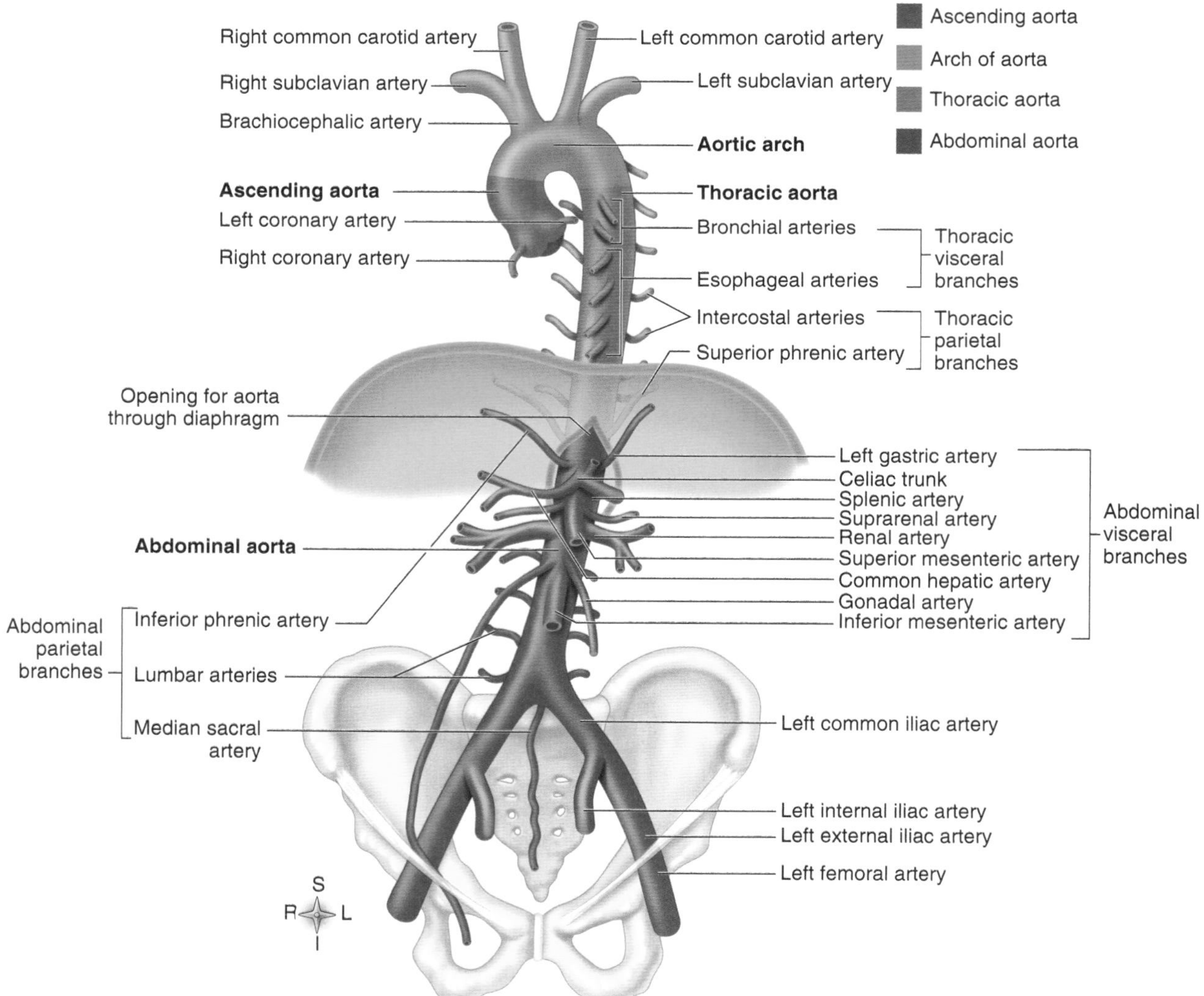

Fig. 13.19 Anatomy of the aorta and its major branches. (From Patton KT, Thibodeau GA. *Anatomy and Physiology*. 10th ed. St. Louis, MO: Elsevier; 2019.)

true aneurysm (Fig. 13.20). A false aneurysm results from a complete tear in the arterial wall (Fig. 13.20C). Blood leaks from the artery to form a clot. Connective tissue is then laid down around this cavity. One example of a false aneurysm is an arterial wall tear resulting from an arterial puncture in the groin area. Anastomotic aneurysms are false aneurysms found at any graft-host artery anastomosis. True aneurysms include fusiform (Fig. 13.20A), saccular (Fig. 13.20B), and dissecting (Fig. 13.20D) aneurysms. Fusiform or spindle-shaped aneurysms are usually found in the abdominal aorta and are the most common type. A saccular aneurysm is a bulbous pouching of the artery and is usually found in the thoracic aorta. Aortic aneurysms are divided into thoracic aortic, thoracoabdominal aortic, and abdominal aortic types.[2]

Atherosclerosis and degeneration of elastin and collagen are the underlying causes in most cases. Aneurysms are also associated with certain connective tissue disorders such as Marfan syndrome (see Genetics box) or Ehlers-Danlos syndrome. Aneurysms are frequently hereditary, with predominance in men. Risk factors for atherosclerosis, such as age, smoking, hyperlipidemia, hypertension, and diabetes, are also risk factors for aortic aneurysms.[2]

Most aneurysms are asymptomatic and are found on routine physical examination or during testing for another disease entity. Back or abdominal pain may be seen with AAAs. The goal of treatment is avoidance of rupture, which is dramatic and often fatal. Risk of rupture is related to the size of the aneurysm, with aneurysms larger than 6 cm carrying the greatest risk. Patients should be monitored closely for changes in size of the aneurysm.

Treatment of an aneurysm is based on the patient's symptoms and the size of the aneurysm. Thoracic aortic or thoracoabdominal aortic aneurysms larger than 5.5 to 6.0 cm and AAAs 5.0 cm or larger are usually surgically repaired. Patients with smaller aneurysms are followed up diagnostically for any change in size. For patients with small AAAs, smoking cessation is emphasized because smokers have a fivefold increase in risk compared with nonsmokers.[2]

Aortic Dissection. Aortic dissection is a life-threatening emergency that requires immediate medical attention. Dissection is a tear in the intimal layer of the vessel that creates a "false lumen," causing blood flow diversion into the false lumen. Sudden, severe chest pain is the most common presenting symptom of aortic dissection. Dissections are classified by the Stanford and DeBakey categories. Stanford categories include type A (proximal) and type B (distal). Type A involves the ascending aorta; it is the more concerning type because dissection can extend into the coronary and arch vessels. It usually manifests as severe anterior chest pain. Type B is confined to the descending thoracic and abdominal aorta and is often associated with pain between the scapulae. DeBakey categories include types I, II, and III. Type I dissections begin in the ascending aorta and may extend all the way to the iliac arteries. Type II dissections involve only the ascending aorta. Type III dissections start in the descending aorta and continue downward to just above (type IIIA) or just below (type IIIB) the diaphragm.[2]

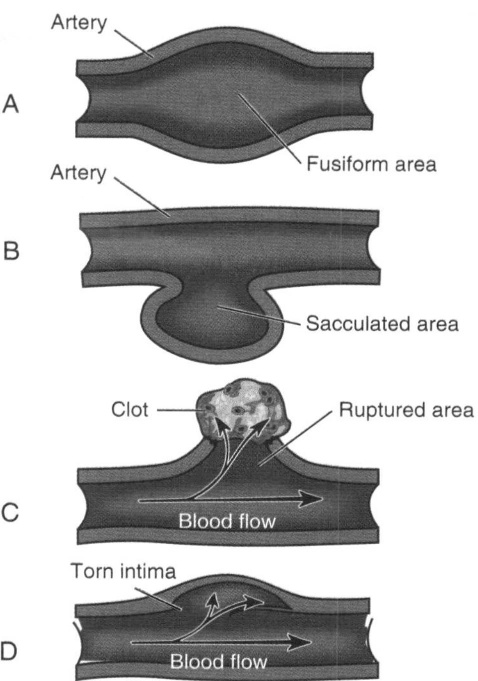

Fig. 13.20 **A**, True fusiform abdominal aortic aneurysm. **B**, True saccular aortic aneurysm. **C**, False aneurysm (pseudoaneurysm). **D**, Aortic dissection. (From Harding MM, Kwon J, Hagler D. *Lewis's Medical-Surgical Nursing: Assessment and Management of Clinical Problems.* 12th ed. Elsevier; 2023.)

Ascending dissections are more common in younger patients, especially those with Marfan syndrome. Immediate treatment is directed at controlling systolic BP to 100 to 120 mm Hg and decreasing the force and rate of contraction of the heart to reduce stress against the vessel wall. Therefore, beta-blockers are the initial pharmacological treatment of choice. Emergency surgery is warranted to prevent death. Once rupture occurs, the overall mortality rate is high.[2]

Assessment

Knowledge of anatomy is the key factor in the treatment and care of patients with aortic aneurysms. Presentation of symptoms, intraoperative risk, and postoperative care are often location dependent. Blood flow to the aortic branches may be hindered by the aneurysm itself, or embolization of the thrombus may cause signs and symptoms such as chest pain, TIAs, arm paresthesia with arch location, transient paralysis with descending aorta involvement, or abdominal or flank pain with AAA. In addition, systolic BP may be different in each arm if the dissection occludes one of the subclavian arteries. A murmur may be auscultated if the dissection results in aortic regurgitation.[2]

Diagnostic Studies

The patient presentation and history are key elements for diagnosis of aortic aneurism and rupture. When performing the *physical examination*, a disparity in BP measurements may be observed between the right and left arms or between the arms

Marfan Syndrome

Marfan syndrome (MFS) is one of the most common inherited disorders affecting connective tissue. Variations or mutations within *FBN1* cause MFS in an autosomal dominant pattern (i.e., 75% of cases) or as a de novo variation (i.e., 25% of cases).[1] In less than 10% of patients with MFS, no mutation of *FBN1* is identified. Note that genes, like *FBN1*, are conventionally written in italics.

FBN1 encodes the synthesis of fibrillin-1, an extracellular protein that is the main component of elastic fibers. Fibrillin provides a matrix to build threadlike microfibril filaments. Microfibrils form elastic fibers that allow skin, ligaments, and blood vessels to stretch and bones to elongate. Microfibrils also support rigid tissues such as heart valves, bones, and the lens of the eye.

MFS has a wide range of symptom onset and disease severity. It is an example of a genetic disorder with a high (but not complete) clinical penetrance and variable expression.[2] *Penetrance* refers to the proportion of individuals with a specific gene who exhibit signs and symptoms of the disorder. *Variable expression* refers to the range of signs and symptoms in individuals with the same gene variation. Researchers have identified more than 1300 *FBN1* polymorphisms, but not all mutations are associated with phenotypic MFS.[3]

Genetic studies have progressed from gene identification in MFS to understanding how fibrillin-1 variations contribute to pathophysiology and tissue fragility. *Proteomics* involves the study of protein structure and function. One example of proteomics in MFS is the interaction between fibrillin-1 and the transforming growth factor (TGF) pathway.[1] The reduced amount and quality of extracellular fibrillin-1 alter TGF bioavailability, leading to inflammation, fibrosis, and activation of enzymes that break down proteins in the affected organ. This interaction, combined with decreased collagen, reduces structural integrity. Aortic dilation and other vascular remodeling occur.

The diagnosis of MFS is based on positive family history and the Ghent Nosology criteria.[4] MFS manifestations, or *phenotype*, include cardiovascular, musculoskeletal, integumentary, ocular, and pulmonary abnormalities. Although genetic testing is sensitive to MFS, it is not specific, because *FBN1* variations are associated with other hereditary connective tissue disorders such as bicuspid aortic valve and Ehlers-Danlos syndrome.

MFS results in vascular necrosis, fibrosis, and loss of smooth muscle cells. An aortic aneurysm is the most concerning manifestation associated with MFS. Typically, the root of the aorta, which connects to the left ventricle, is dilated.

Patients with MFS have characteristic skeletal features. Tall stature and joint hypermobility are common. Other skeletal manifestations include scoliosis, flat feet, or a protruding or indented sternum.

Eye manifestations occur in about 9% of patients with MFS.[1,2] The most common eye symptom is severe myopia from the connective tissue changes in the eye. Dislocation of the eye lens or early cataracts may occur.

Other manifestations of MFS are enlargement of the dural membrane surrounding the lower spine or brainstem (i.e., dural ectasia) that can cause pain from traction on spinal nerve roots. Individuals can also develop emphysema-like changes in the lung, with possible spontaneous pneumothorax. Inguinal or incisional hernias and skin stretch marks (i.e., striae) reflect collagen fragility.

Clinicians tailor the management of MFS to each individual's disease manifestation. For those with aortic manifestations of MFS, beta-blockers and angiotensin-converting enzyme inhibitors or selective angiotensin-2 receptor blockers control blood pressure (BP) and slow the progression of widening in the aorta.[1] Clinicians also advise patients to restrict contact sports and weightlifting, although aerobic exercise like swimming is encouraged. The definitive treatment for aortic dilation consists of surgical intervention to prevent aortic dissection. Clinicians may refer patients with MFS and their family members for genetic testing and counseling, including psychosocial support. A diagnosis confirmed with genetics can affect the timing of the recommended surgical intervention for aortic abnormalities.[5]

Genetic terms: *autosomal dominant, de novo mutation, polymorphism, phenotype, penetrance, variable expression, proteomics.*

References

1. Salik I, Rawla P. Marfan syndrome. In: *StatPearls*. StatPearls Publishing; 2022. https://www.ncbi.nlm.nih.gov/pubmed/30726024. Accessed December 29, 2023.
2. National Institutes of Health. What are reduced penetrance and variable expressivity? https://medlineplus.gov/genetics/understanding/inheritance/penetranceexpressivity/. Updated April 19, 2021. Accessed December 29, 2023.
3. National Institutes of Health. *Marfan Syndrome*. https://www.genome.gov/Genetic-Disorders/Marfan-Syndrome. Published Updated May 30, 2017. Accessed December 29, 2023.
4. von Kodolitsch Y, De Backer J, Schuler H, et al. Perspectives on the revised Ghent criteria for the diagnosis of Marfan syndrome. *Appl Clin Genet.* 2015;8:137–155. https://doi.org/10.2147/TACG.S60472.
5. Musunuru K, Hershberger RE, Day SM, et al. Genetic testing for inherited cardiovascular diseases: a scientific statement from the American Heart Association. *Circ Genom Precis Med.* 2020;13(4):e000067. https://doi.org/10.1161/HCG.0000000000000067.

Chris Winkelman, PhD, ACNP-BC, CCRN, CNE, FAANP, FCCM

and legs, or a diminished pulse may be found in one of the limbs. Palpation reveals decreased or absent peripheral pulses. The patient may have a history of paresthesia, TIAs, lower extremity or buttock claudication, and/or back or abdominal pain. *Imaging studies* will be completed to confirm the diagnosis and size of the aneurysm. *The imaging studies most often ordered include:* abdominal ultrasound, computed tomography, angiography, TEE, and MRI, all of which are accurate diagnostic tools for AAA.

Interventions

Open surgical or endovascular repair is the treatment for large aortic aneurysms, especially acute type A aortic dissections. The open or conventional repair of an aortic aneurysm is the endovascular aneurysm repair (Fig. 13.21). This surgery generally requires a median sternotomy approach.[2]

Uncomplicated type B aortic dissections are often treated medically because of the high mortality rates associated with surgical repair. Complicated acute type B aortic dissections are more likely to be treated with endovascular aneurysm repair.[2] This method is less invasive than open repair; it involves percutaneous stent placement in the descending thoracic or thoracoabdominal aorta. Through a small opening in the exposed femoral artery, an intraluminal sheathed stent is introduced, placed, and deployed with fluoroscopic guidance. Care of the vascular surgery patient is detailed in Box 13.16.

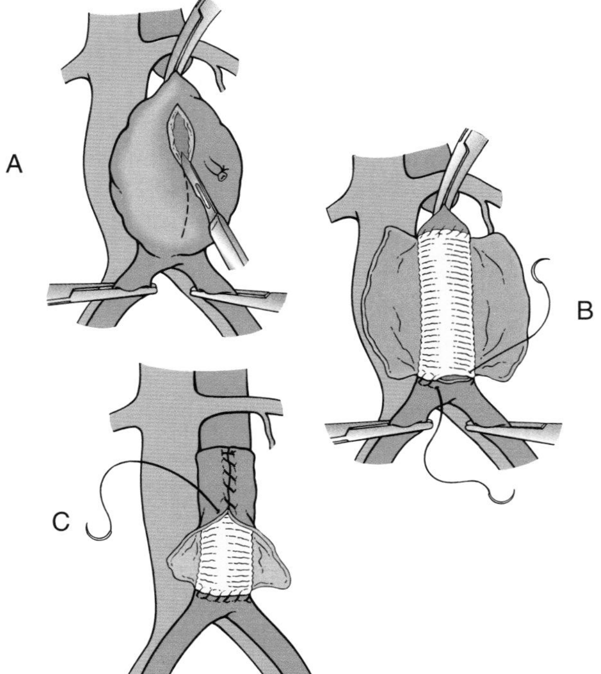

Fig. 13.21 Surgical repair of an abdominal aortic aneurysm. **A**, The aneurysmal sac is incised. **B**, The synthetic graft is inserted. **C**, The native aortic wall is sutured over the synthetic graft. (Harding MM, Kwon J, Hagler D. *Lewis's Medical-Surgical Nursing: Assessment and Management of Clinical Problems.* 12th ed. Elsevier; 2023.)

BOX 13.16 Nursing Interventions After Aortic Surgery

- Monitor vital signs every hour (postrecovery stage); assess for tachycardia and irregular rhythms.
- Blood pressure: Keep the patient normotensive. Hypertension causes bleeding; give vasodilators per protocol. Hypotension causes organ ischemia; give fluids and vasoconstrictors.
- Monitor hemodynamic pressures: SvO_2, cardiac index, PAOP, and RAP; treat per protocols.
- Assess for hypovolemia: Monitor output from chest tubes and drains and urine output every hour.
- Assess for hypothermia; rewarm the patient per protocol.
- Monitor fluid and electrolytes, hemoglobin, hematocrit, renal function, and coagulation studies.
- Monitor the radial, dorsalis pedis, and posterior tibial pulses every hour; use Doppler studies as needed. Assess the ankle-brachial index every 2 hours or as ordered.
- Monitor for complications: Intraoperative AMI, dysrhythmias, heart failure, cardiac tamponade, thromboembolism, impaired renal function, pneumonia, pneumothorax, pleural effusion, cerebral ischemia, stroke.
- Implement ventilator bundle of care (Chapter 10, Ventilatory Assistance); wean from mechanical ventilation and extubate as soon as possible; promote pulmonary hygiene.
- Assess wounds and provide incisional care per protocol.
- Organize nursing care; control environmental stimuli.
- Gradually increase the patient's activity.
- Provide emotional support to the patient and family; assess the family's level of understanding; discuss the postoperative course.
- For abdominal aneurysm, assess for ischemic colitis.

AMI, Acute myocardial infarction; *PAOP,* pulmonary artery occlusion pressure; *RAP,* right atrial pressure; *SvO_2,* mixed venous oxygen saturation.

CASE STUDY

Mr. P. presented to the local critical access emergency department with the complaint of sudden onset of substernal chest pain while he was mowing his lawn. This pain started 3 hours ago. He took aspirin and three sublingual nitroglycerin (NTG) tablets every 5 minutes en route. Mr. P. states that his pain has gone from a 7 to a 3 on a scale from 0 to 10 and continues to be substernal in nature with mild radiation to his left jaw and left shoulder. He is diaphoretic as well.

The cardiac monitor shows he is in a sinus rhythm. His BP is 150/88 mm Hg, his pulse is 96 beats/min, and his respiratory rate is 24 breaths/min and nonlabored. His temperature is 97.4°F (36.3°C). His oxygen saturation is 89% on room air. The nurse starts two IV lines, gives Mr. P. another NTG tablet, places him on oxygen at 2 L/min, and proceeds to obtain a brief history.

Mr. P. is a 68-year-old White male who weighs 220 lb and has a history of hypertension and diabetes. He smokes 1½ packs of cigarettes per day. He is allergic to penicillin.

The monitor alarms, the nurse identifies the rhythm as ventricular fibrillation, and he is without a pulse. Mr. P loses consciousness. The nurse activates a code and begins cardiopulmonary resuscitation. Mr. P. is defibrillated with one 200 J shock using the biphasic defibrillator. After defibrillation, circulation is restored, and his rhythm is regular sinus with frequent premature ventricular contractions. He received a total of 2 minutes of compressions. His BP is 92/56 mm Hg. His pupils are 4 mm, equal, and reactive. His respiratory rate is 16 breaths/min, and his oxygen saturation is 92%. He is not fully awake at this time, but he is moving all of his extremities and breathing on his own. A 150-mg IV bolus of amiodarone is given over 10 minutes, and an infusion is started at 1 mg/min. Laboratory tests and arterial blood gas measurements are ordered, along with a 12-lead electrocardiogram (ECG). Consultation with the cardiologist is urgently requested; however, they are 3 hours away from the cardiac catheterization lab.

Mr. P.'s cardiac enzyme results return as follows:

High sensitivity cardiac specific troponin (HS-cTN)	127 ng/ml
Troponin I	0.5 ng/mL
Troponin T	0.4 ng/mL

His electrolyte values are as follows:

Sodium	143 mEq/L
Potassium	3.4 mEq/L
Chloride	109 mEq/L
Carbon dioxide	34 mEq/L
Glucose	354 mg/dL
Magnesium	1.5 mEq/L

Arterial blood gas values are as follows:

pH	7.32
$PaCO_2$	49 mm Hg
PaO_2	77 mm Hg
Bicarbonate	24 mEq/L
SaO_2	92%

A 12-lead ECG shows ST elevation in leads V_2, V_3, and V_4. Mr. P. is diagnosed with an acute anterior myocardial infarction. His oxygen is increased to 6 L/min by nasal cannula. Based on these assessment and study results and after further instructions from the cardiologist, who is 3 hours away, tissue plasminogen activator (t-PA) is administered.

Questions

1. Identify which assessment data and laboratory analysis suggest the patient is experiencing a cardiac event.
2. Describe nursing care considerations and potential complications that should be anticipated related to the infusion of t-PA. What parameters would the nurse need to monitor?
3. List evaluation criteria that would demonstrate effectiveness of the t-PA infusion administration.
4. Review risk factors for coronary artery disease that should be addressed before the patient is discharged to reduce his risk of another myocardial infarction.

KEY POINTS

- Performing a holistic cardiovascular assessment includes a physical, psychosocial, and emotional-spiritual review with the patient and family.
- It is essential to understanding cardiac physiology to detect abnormal heart sounds, electrolyte abnormalities, and perfusion abnormalities that may lead to cardiac dysrhythmias and ischemic events.
- Women and non-White men may present with signs and symptoms of angina.
- Patients with cardiovascular alterations may be on multiple medications for which the nurse much understand the therapeutic indication, route for safe administration, and potential adverse reactions or side effects.
- Knowledge of STEMI-NSTEMI MI is required to facilitate appropriate urgent and emergent treatment.
- Patients with HF require medical management, knowledge of medications, and diet and exercise guidance.
- Temporary and long-term mechanical circulatory support devices may be necessary for individuals with HF.
- Cardiac transplantation may be an option for some individuals with end-stage heart disease.

REFERENCES

1. Brashers VL. Alterations in cardiovascular function. In: Rogers JL. *McCance & Huether's Pathophysiology: The Biologic Basis for Disease in Adults and Children*, 9th ed. Eslevier 2-24 :1059–1127.
2. Braverman ACS M. Diseases of the aorta. In: Zipes DP, Libby P, Bonow RO, Mann DL, Tomaselli GF, eds. *Braunwald's Heart Disease: Textbook of Cardiovascular Medicine*. 11th ed. Philadelphia, PA: Elsevier; 2019:1295–1327.
3. Gulati M, Levy PD, Mukherjee D, et al. 2021 AHA/ACC/ASE/CHEST/SAEM/SCCT/SCMR guideline for the evaluation and diagnosis of chest pain: a report of the American College of Cardiology/American Heart Association Joint Committee on clinical practice guidelines. *Circulation*. 2021;144:e368–e454.
4. Pagana K, et al. Cardiac stress testing (Exercise stress testing). In: *Mosby's® Diagnostic and Laboratory Test Reference. Available from: Pageburstls*. 15th ed. Elsevier Health Sciences (US); 2021:221.
5. Mavrogeni SI, Bacopoulou F, Markousis-Mavrogenis G, et al. Cardiovascular imaging in obesity. *Nutrients*. 2021;13(3):744.
6. Duarte OJ, Hemu H, Yakupovich A, et al. Influence of breast reconstruction on technical aspects of echocardiographic image acquisition compared with physician-assessed image quality. *Cardiooncology*. 2019;5:17.
7. Papadopoulos CH, Oikonomidis D, Lazaris E, et al. Echocardiography and cardiac arrhythmias. *Hellenic Journal of Cardiology*. 2018;59(3):140–149.
8. American Society of Anesthesiologists. Practice guidelines for preoperative fasting and the use of pharmacologic agents to reduce the risk of pulmonary aspiration: application to healthy patients undergoing elective procedures: an updated report by the American Society of Anesthesiologists task force on preoperative fasting and the use of pharmacologic agents to reduce the risk of pulmonary aspiration. *Anesthesiology*. 2017;126:376–393.
9. Sandoval Y, Apple FS, Mahler SA, Body R, Collinson PO, Jaffe AS. High-sensitivity cardiac troponin and the 2021 AHA/ACC/ASE/CHEST/SAEM/SCCT/SCMR guidelines for the evaluation and diagnosis of acute chest pain. *Circulation*. 2022;146(7):569–581. https://doi.org/10.1161/CIRCULATIONAHA.122.059678.
10. Vasile VC, Jaffe AS. *High-sensitivity Cardiac Troponin in the Evaluation of Possible AMI*. ACC.; 2018. Retrieved March 4th, 2023, from https://www.acc.org/latest-in-cardiology/articles/2018/07/16/09/17/high-sensitivity-cardiac-troponin-in-the-evaluation-of-possible-ami.
11. Lloyd-Jones DM, Morris PB, Ballantyne CM, et al. 2022 ACC Expert consensus decision pathway on the role of nonstatin therapies for LDL-cholesterol lowering in the management of atherosclerotic cardiovascular disease risk: a report of the American College of Cardiology solution set oversight committee. *JACC*. 2022;80(14):1366–1418.
12. Grundy SM, Stone NJ, Bailey AL, et al. 2018 AHA/ACC/AACVPR/AAPA/ABC/ACPM/ADA/AGS/APhA/ASPC/NLA/PCNA guideline on the management of blood cholesterol. *J Am Coll Cardiol*. 2019;73(24):3168–3209.
13. Giugliano RP, Cannon CP, Blazing MA, et al. Benefit of adding ezetimibe to statin therapy on cardiovascular outcomes and safety in patients with versus without diabetes mellitus: results from IMPROVE-IT (Improved Reduction of Outcomes: vytorin Efficacy International Trial). *Circulation*. 2018;137(15):1571–1582.
14. Rosenson RS, Hegele RA, Fazio S, et al. The evolving future of PCSK9 inhibitors. *J Am Coll Cardiol*. 2018;72(3):314–329.
15. Pokhrel B, Yuet WC, Levine SN. PCSK9 inhibitors. In: *StatPearls*. Treasure Island (FL): StatPearls Publishing; January 2022. [Internet].
16. Kosmas CE, Skavdis A, Sourlas A, et al. Safety and tolerability of PCSK9 inhibitors: current insights. *Clin Pharmacol*. 2020;12:191–202.
17. Gibbs LM, Pham K, Langston S. Supplemental oxygen therapy for nonhypoxemic patients with acute coronary syndrome. *Am Fam Physician*. 2020;101(11):687–688.
18. Bohula EAM, David A. ST-elevation myocardial infarction: management. In: Zipes DP, Libby P, Bonow RO, Mann DL, Tomaselli GF, eds. *Braunwald's Heart Disease: A Textbook of Cardiovascular Medicine*. 11th ed. Philadelphia, PA: Elsevier; 2019:1483–1509.
19. Scirica BML P, Morrow DA. ST-elevation myocardial infarction: pathophysiology and clinical evolution. In: Zipes DP, Libby P, Bonow RO, Mann DL, Tomaselli GF, eds. *Braunwald's Heart Disease: A Textbook of Cardiovascular Medicine*. 11th ed. Philadelphia, PA: Elsevier; 2019:1095–1122.
20. Goyal A, Gluckman TJ, Levy A, et al. Translating the fourth universal definition of myocardial infarction into clinical documentation: ten pearls for frontline clinicians. *Cardiol Mag*. 2018;47(11):34–36.
21. Gulati MM CNB. Cardiovascular disease in women. In: Zipes DP, Libby P, Bonow RO, Mann DL, Tomaselli GF, eds. *Braundwald's Heart Disease: A Textbook of Cardiovascular Medicine*. 11th ed. Philadelphia, PA: Elsevier; 2019:1767–1779.
22. Ostroska M, Gorog D. Does morphine remain a standard of care in acute myocardial infarction?. *Via Medica*. 2020;5(1):46–49.

23. Amsterdam EA, Wenger NK. The 2014 American College of Cardiology ACC/American Heart Association guideline for the management of patients with non-ST-elevation acute coronary syndromes: ten contemporary recommendations to aid clinicians in optimizing patient outcomes. *Clin Cardiol.* 2015;38(2):121–123.
24. Carbone RG, Monselise A, Bottino G, Negrini S, Puppo F. Stem cells therapy in acute myocardial infarction: a new era? *Clinical and Experimental Medicine.* 2021;21:231–237. https://doi.org/10.1007/s10238-021-00682-3.
25. Mauri LB, Deepak L. Percutaneous coronary intervention. In: Zipes DP, Libby P, Bonow RO, Mann DL, Tomaselli GF, eds. *Braunwald's Heart Disease: A Textbook of Cardiovascular Medicine.* 11th ed. Philadelphia, PA: Elsevier; 2019:49–69.
26. Guo MH, Wells GA, Glineur D, et al. Minimally Invasive coronary surgery compared to STernotomy coronary artery bypass grafting: the MIST trial. *Contemp Clin Trials.* 2019;78:140–145.
27. Riberio IBG, J .B., Fortier JH, et al. Off pump coronary artery bypass grafting. In: Selke F, Ruel M, eds. *Atlas of Cardiac Surgical Techniques.* 2nd ed. Philadelphia, PA: Elsevier; 2019:49–69.
28. Konstanty-Kalandyk J, Piatek J, Kedziora A, et al. Ten-year follow-up after combined coronary artery bypass grafting and transmyocardial laser revascularization in patients with disseminated coronary atherosclerosis. *Lasers Med Sci.* 2018;33(7):1527–1535.
29. Morrow DA, de Lemos J. Stable ischemic heart disease. In: Zipes DP, Libby P, Bonow RO, Mann DL, Tomaselli GF, eds. *Braunwald's Heart Disease: A Textbook of Cardiovascular Medicine.* 11th ed. Philadelphia, PA: Elsevier; 2019:1209–1270.
30. January CT, Wann LS, Calkins H, et al. 2019 AHA/ACC/HRS focused update of the 2014 AHA/ACC/HRS guideline for the management of patients with atrial fibrillation: a report of the American College of cardiology/American heart association task force on clinical practice guidelines and the heart rhythm society. *Heart Rhythm.* 2019.
31. Kusumoto FM, Schoenfeld MH, Barrett C, et al. 2018 ACC/AHA/HRS guideline on the evaluation and management of patients with bradycardia and cardiac conduction delay: executive summary: a report of the American College of cardiology/American heart association task force on clinical practice guidelines, and the heart rhythm society. *J Am Coll Cardiol.* 2019;74(7):932–987.
32. Mann D. Management of heart failure patients with reduced ejection fraction. In: Zipes DP, Libby P, Bonow RO, Mann DL, Tomaselli GF, eds. *Braunwald's Heart Disease: A Textbook of Cardiovascular Medicine.* 11th ed. Philadelphia, PA: Elsevier; 2019:490–522.
33. Simmonds SJ, Cuijpers I, Heymans S, Jones EAV. Cellular and molecular differences between HFpEF and HFrEF: a step ahead in an improved pathological understanding. *Cells.* 2020;9(10):242. https://doi.org/10.3390/cells9010242.
34. Januzzi JLM DL. Approach to the patient with heart failure. In: Zipes DPL P, Bonow RO, Mann DL, Tomasello GF, Braunwald E, eds. *Braunwald's Heart Disease: A Textbook of Cardiovascular Medicine.* 11 ed. 16. Philadelphia, PA: Elsevier; 2019 (8):e66-e93.
35. Konstam MA, Kiernan MS, Bernstein D, et al. Evaluation and management of right-sided heart failure: a scientific statement from the American Heart Association. *Circulation.* 2018;137(20):e578–e622.
36. Hasenfuss GM DL. Pathophysiology of heart failure. In: Zipes DP, Libby P, Bonow RO, Mann DL, Tomaselli GF, eds. *Braundwald's Heart Disease: A Textbook of Cardiovascular Medicine.* 11th ed. Philadelphia, PA: Elsevier; 2019:442–461.
37. Heidenreich PA, Bozkurt B, Aguilar D, Allen LA, et al. 2022 AHA/ACC/HFSA guideline for the management of heart failure: a report of the American College of Cardiology/American Heart Association joint committee on clinical practice guidelines. *Circulation.* 2022;145(18):e895–e1032. https://doi.org/10.1161/CIR.0000000000001063.
38. VanValkinburgh D, Kerndt CC, Hashmi MF. Inotropes and vasopressors[Updated 2022 Aug 18] In: *StatPearls.* Treasure Island (FL): StatPearls Publishing; 2022. [Internet] https://www.ncbi.nlm.nih.gov/books/NBK482411/.
39. Felker GMT JR. Diagnosis and management of acute heart failure. In: Zipes DP, Libby P, Bonow RO, Mann DL, Tomaselli GF, eds. *Braunwald's Heart Disease: A Textbook of Cardiovascular Medicine.* 11th ed. ; 2019:462–489. Philadelphia, PA.
40. Huu AL, Shum-Tim D. Intra-aortic balloon pump: current evidence & future perspectives. *Future Cardiol.* 2018;14(4):319–328. https://doi.org/10.2217/fca-2017-0070.
41. Manaker S. *Extracorporeal Membrane Oxygenation (ECMO) in Adults*UpToDate ; 2022. Retrieved March 3rd, 2023, from https://www.uptodate.com/contents/extracorporeal-membrane-oxygenation-ecmo-in-adults.
42. Lorusso R, Whitman G, Milojevic M, et al. 2020 EACTS/ELSO/STS/AATS expert consensus on post-cardiotomy extracorporeal life support in adult patients. *Ann Thorac Surg.* 2021;111(1):327–369. https://doi.org/10.1016/j.athoracsur.2020.07.009.
43. Chen YC, Tsai FC, Fang JT, et al. Acute kidney injury in adults receiving extracorporeal membrane oxygenation. *Journal of the Formosan Medical Association.* 2014;113:778–785.
44. Lindenfeld J, Zile MR, Desai AS, et al. Haemodynamic-guided management of heart failure (GUIDE-HF): a randomized controlled trial. *Lancet.* 2021;398(10304):991–1001. https://doi.org/10.1016/S0140-6736(21)01754-2.
45. Vega E, Schroder J, Nicoara A. Postoperative management of the heart transplantation patients. *Best Pract Res Clin Anaesthesiol.* 2017;31(2):201–213.
46. Koomalsingh K, Kobashigawa JA. The future of cardiac transplantation. *Ann Cardiothorac Surg.* 2018;7(1):135–142.
47. Wang A, Gaca JG, Chu VH. Management considerations in infective endocarditis: a review. *JAMA.* 2018;320(1):72–83.
48. Lazkani M, Singh N, Howe C, et al. An updated meta-analysis of TAVR in patients at intermediate risk for SAVR. *Cardiovasc Revasc Med.* 2019;20(1):57–69.
49. Pettersson GB, Hussain ST. Current AATS guidelines on surgical treatment of infective endocarditis. *Ann Cardiothorac Surg.* 2019;8(6):630–644.
50. Otto CMB RO. Approach to the patient with valvular heart disease. In: Zipes DP, Libby P, Bonow RO, Mann DL, Tomaselli GF, eds. *Braunwald's Heart Disease: A Textbook of Cardiovascular Medicine.* 11th ed. Philadelphia, PA: Elsevier; 2019:1383–1388.
51. Baddour LMF WK, Suri RM, et al. Cardiovascular infections. In: Zipes DP, Libby P, Bonow RO, Mann DL, Tomaselli GF, eds. *Braunwald's Heart Disease: A Textbook of Cardiovascular Medicine.* 11th ed. Philadelphia, PA: Elsevier; 2019:442–461.

14

Nervous System Alterations

Catherine D. Robbins, DNP, APRN-BC, CCRN, CNRN,
Erica Ochoa, DNP, APRN, FNP-BC, CNRN

INTRODUCTION

The central and peripheral nervous systems are responsible for producing consciousness and higher mental functions, movement, sensation, and reflex activity. If these structures are damaged, a person's ability to provide self-care and interact with the environment may be greatly altered. This chapter discusses the pathophysiology and clinical assessment of neurological injury, as well as the nursing and medical management related to common neurological problems such as increased intracranial pressure (ICP), traumatic brain injury (TBI), cerebrovascular diseases, status epilepticus (SE), central nervous system (CNS) infections, and spinal cord injury (SCI).

Psychological support is essential for patients and families, as neurological insults usually occur without warning and may be severe. This places the family in a state of shock and disbelief. In addition, the patient has suffered an insult to the nervous system and may respond inappropriately or uncharacteristically or may not be able to respond to the family at all. Neurological insults cause uncertainty regarding the patient's physical and mental outcomes. The associated personality and mental changes can be devastating to the family. One of the best ways to support families is by providing information and psychosocial support to reduce their anxiety.

ANATOMY AND PHYSIOLOGY OF THE NERVOUS SYSTEM

Cells of the Nervous System

The nervous system is composed of two types of cells: neurons and neuroglia. The *neuron,* or nerve cell, is the basic functional unit of the nervous system and transmits nerve impulses (Fig. 14.1). Each neuron is unique in character, and neuronal features are determined by specific function. During nerve transmission, *dendrites* receive an electrical impulse from other neurons. The electrical impulse is then transmitted along the *axon* of the neuron to the *synaptic knobs,* which release neurotransmitters into the synapse. Once in the synapse, the neurotransmitters bind to available receptor sites, usually on a nerve or muscle cell.

Neurotransmitter binding propagates receptor membrane depolarization and the continuation of impulse transmission. Postsynaptic responses may be excitation or inhibition, depending on the type of neurotransmitter released. Acetylcholine, norepinephrine, dopamine, serotonin, glutamate, gamma-aminobutyric acid (GABA), substance P, and endorphins are common neurotransmitters released. In general, neurons are believed to release only one type of neurotransmitter at its nerve terminals.[1] Degeneration of neurons, or the failure of neurons to release or take up neurotransmitters, can be associated with nervous system dysfunction.

Some axons are surrounded by a white protein-lipid complex, *myelin,* that is formed by Schwann cells in the peripheral nervous system (PNS) and by oligodendrocytes in the CNS. Periodic constrictions along the axon lack myelin; these areas, known as nodes of Ranvier, facilitate fast and efficient impulse conduction (Fig. 14.1). The speed of impulse conduction depends on both the thickness of the myelin and the distance between nodes. Loss of myelin (i.e., demyelination) slows or alters neuronal function and is characteristic of diseases such as multiple sclerosis.

Neuroglial cells (glia) constitute the supportive tissue of the CNS. Most primary CNS tumors originate from glial cells and are thus termed *gliomas.* Four types of glial cells exist, each with specific functions. *Microglia* act as phagocytic scavenger cells when nervous tissue is damaged. *Astrocytes* are star-shaped cells that play a critical role in transport of nutrients, gases, and waste products among neurons, the vascular system, and cerebrospinal fluid (CSF); in the formation of scar tissue in the brain; and in the function of the blood-brain barrier. *Oligodendrocytes* are responsible for myelin formation. *Ependymal* cells produce specialized glial tissue that forms the lining of the ventricles of the brain and the central canal of the spinal cord; they also play a role in production of CSF.

Cerebral Circulation

The brain receives approximately 750 mL of blood per minute, or 15% to 20% of the total resting cardiac output.[1] The cerebral circulation must provide sufficient blood to supply oxygen, glucose, and nutrients to the cerebral tissues. The brain does not have any energy stores and is dependent on aerobic metabolism. Therefore, even a brief interruption in blood supply may result in significant ischemic tissue damage.

The blood supply of the brain arises from two major sets of arteries, the carotid arteries (anterior circulation) and the vertebral arteries (posterior circulation). Specifically, the left common carotid artery originates from the aortic arch, and the right common carotid artery originates from the innominate artery. The common carotid arteries then branch to form the external and internal carotid arteries. The external carotid artery supplies the face, scalp, and other extracranial structures. Each internal carotid artery terminates by dividing into anterior cerebral (ACA) and middle cerebral arteries (MCA). The anterior cerebral artery and its branches supply the medial aspects of the motor cortex and the frontal lobes. The MCA comprises the principal blood supply of the frontal, temporal, and parietal lobes. Most strokes involve the MCA due to size, location, and the amount of blood supply provided by the MCA vessel.[1]

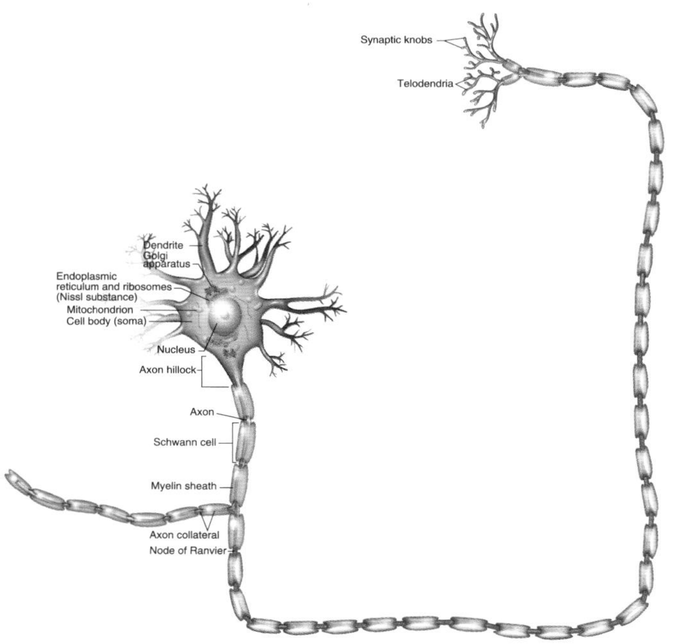

Fig. 14.1 Structure of a typical neuron. (From Patton KT, Bell F, Thompson T, Williamson P. *Anatomy and Physiology*. 11th ed. St. Louis, MO: Elsevier; 2022.)

The paired vertebral arteries originate from the subclavian arteries and enter the skull through the foramen magnum. The vertebral arteries and their branches supply the upper spinal cord, medulla, and cerebellum before joining at the pons to form the basilar artery. The basilar artery sends branches to the cerebellum, medulla, pons, and internal ear. Then the basilar artery bifurcates and terminates as the posterior cerebral arteries, which serve the medial portions of the occipital and inferior temporal lobes.

These two arterial systems interconnect at the base of the brain via communicating arteries. The posterior communicating artery connects the internal carotid artery to the posterior cerebral artery, and the anterior communicating artery connects the two anterior cerebral arteries. This interconnection is known as the cerebral arterial circle (i.e., circle of Willis) at the base of the brain (Fig. 14.2).

Cerebral veins, which do not have a muscle layer or valves, empty blood into venous sinuses located throughout the cranium. Because the venous sinuses play a role in absorption of

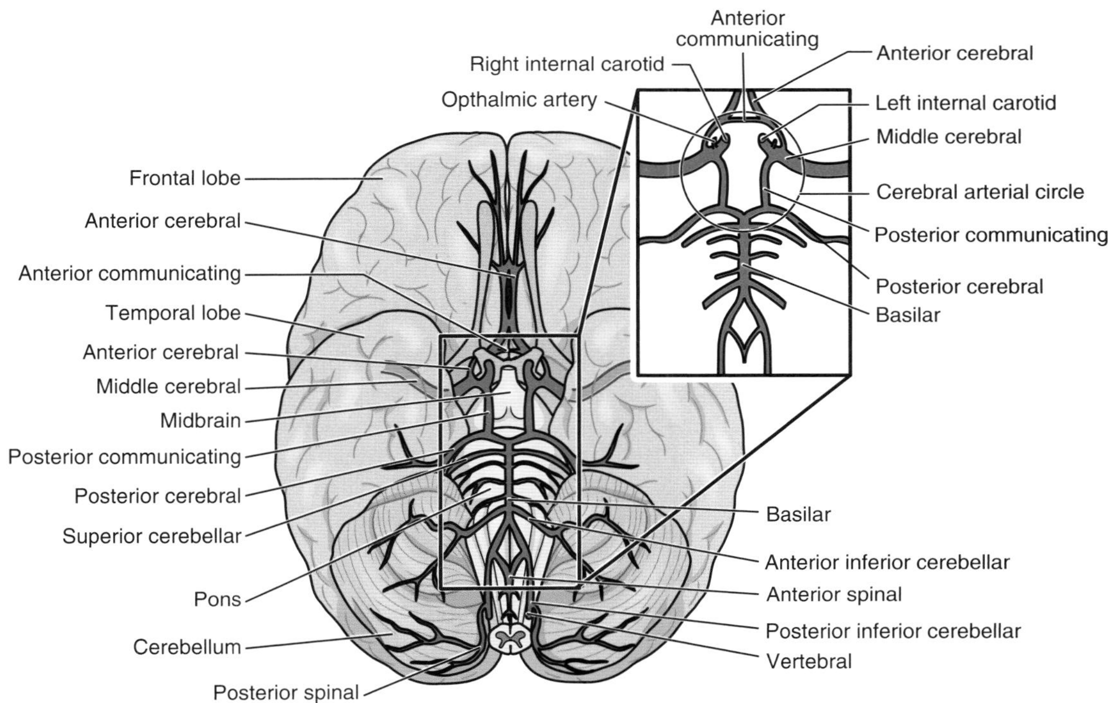

Fig. 14.2 Arterial blood supply of the brain. The cerebral arterial circle (i.e., circle of Willis) is formed by the anterior communicating artery, which joins together the two anterior cerebral arteries, and the posterior communicating arteries, which arise from the internal carotid arteries and connect to the posterior cerebral arteries.

CSF, they parallel the ventricular system, rather than the arterial system as in most other organs.[1] The venous blood is emptied into the internal jugular vein and, ultimately, into the superior vena cava, which returns the blood to the heart.

Cerebral Metabolism

Glucose is the brain's sole source of energy for cellular function. The brain is unable to store glucose, and thus requires a continuous glucose supply to maintain normal brain metabolism. If the cerebral glucose level drops below 70 mg/dL, confusion may develop. Seizures and decreased responsiveness may occur if the glucose level continues to decrease. Cellular damage develops when the brain glucose level drops to less than 20 mg/dL.[1]

Aerobic metabolism is used to meet cerebral energy demands because anaerobic metabolism produces only a minimal amount of adenosine triphosphate (ATP). If the brain is deprived of oxygen, even for a few minutes, metabolism changes from aerobic to the less efficient anaerobic cellular metabolism, resulting in energy failure and neurological deficits (i.e., anoxic brain injury).

Maintaining a constant *cerebral blood flow (CBF)* is essential to sustain normal cerebral metabolism. In the absence of adequate blood flow, cell membrane integrity is lost. This allows extracellular fluid to flow into the cell, causing edema within the cell. The extracellular environment becomes acidotic from lactic acid production, leading to anaerobic metabolism and further cell damage. Prolonged anoxia can lead to the destruction of cerebral neurons, which are unable to regenerate.

A process called autoregulation ensures continuous CBF, regardless of the mean arterial pressure (MAP). *Autoregulation* is defined as the ability of cerebral blood vessels to adjust their diameter to arterial pressure changes within the brain.[2] If a rapid increase in MAP occurs, the cerebral vessels constrict to prevent excessive distension of the cerebral arteries. Conversely, if the MAP drops, the cerebral blood vessels dilate to maintain normal CBF and to prevent cerebral ischemia.

The cerebral vessels are also sensitive to the chemical regulators that maintain CBF, such as the partial pressure of arterial carbon dioxide ($PaCO_2$) or oxygen (PaO_2) and the hydrogen ion (H^+) concentration. Carbon dioxide is the most potent agent influencing CBF.[1] When $PaCO_2$ is greater than 45 mm Hg, cerebral blood vessels vasodilate, increasing CBF. A low $PaCO_2$ causes the cerebral arteries to constrict, leading to decreased CBF and decreased tissue perfusion. Cerebral arteries are less sensitive to changes in PaO_2. When PaO_2 is less than 50 mm Hg, cerebral vessels dilate to increase CBF and oxygen delivery. If the PaO_2 is not raised, anaerobic metabolism begins, resulting in lactic acid accumulation. An increased hydrogen ion concentration further increases vasodilation to facilitate the removal of acidic end products from cerebral tissue.

Blood-Brain Barrier System

The *blood-brain barrier system* protects the brain from toxic elements and disease-causing organisms that may circulate within the blood. The blood-brain barrier operates on the concept of tight junctions between adjacent cells and selective permeability that prevents the free movement of materials from the vascular bed into the brain. Typically, large molecules do not cross the blood-brain barrier, whereas small molecules cross easily. Water, carbon dioxide, oxygen, and glucose freely cross the cerebral capillaries. The movement of other substances into the brain is dependent on their chemical dissociation, lipid solubility, and protein-binding potential.[1] Infections, tumors, and certain other disease states may also alter the blood-brain barrier.

Ventricular System and Cerebrospinal Fluid

The four *ventricles* of the adult brain are hollow spaces lined by ependymal cells. Specialized epithelium in the ventricular wall, called the *choroid plexus,* produces CSF. A smaller amount of CSF is secreted from the ependymal cells that line the ventricles. CSF is continually secreted from these surfaces at a rate of about 500 mL/day, or about 20 mL/hour.[2] On average, 150 mL of CSF is contained in the ventricles and subarachnoid space. The CSF plays a role in metabolic function of the brain and provides a cushioning effect during head movement.

CSF flows from the two lateral ventricles into the third ventricle through the foramen of Monro. From the third ventricle, CSF flows through the aqueduct of Sylvius into the fourth ventricle. From there, the CSF flow is directed through the foramina of Luschka and Magendie into the cisterna and the subarachnoid space (Fig. 14.3). After circulating around the brain and spinal cord, CSF is reabsorbed into the venous sinuses of the brain through the arachnoid villi, which are dural projections from the arachnoid space.[1] If flow out of the ventricular system is blocked, obstructive hydrocephalus occurs. Scarring or inflammation of the arachnoid villi prevents CSF resorption, causing communicating hydrocephalus.

FUNCTIONAL AND STRUCTURAL DIVISIONS OF THE CENTRAL NERVOUS SYSTEM

Meninges

Meninges cover the brain and spinal cord and consist of three layers: dura mater, arachnoid mater, and pia mater. The *dura mater* is the outermost covering and has two layers. The outer surface adheres to the skull, and the inner layer produces prominent folds (i.e., falx cerebri, tentorium cerebelli, falx cerebelli) that subdivide the interior cranial cavity to support and protect the brain. The inner dura mater also covers the spinal cord. The *arachnoid mater* is located inside the dura mater. It is a delicate, avascular layer that loosely encloses the brain and spinal cord. The *pia mater* closely adheres to the brain's outer surface and contains a network of blood vessels. The pia mater surrounding the spinal cord is less vascular.

Actual or potential spaces exist between the meningeal layers. The epidural space is a potential space between the skull and the outer dura mater. The subdural space lies between the dura mater and the arachnoid mater and is filled with a small amount of lubricating fluid. The subarachnoid space, a considerable area between the arachnoid mater and the pia mater, contains circulating CSF. In addition, the subarachnoid space has a vast network of arteries traveling through it.[1]

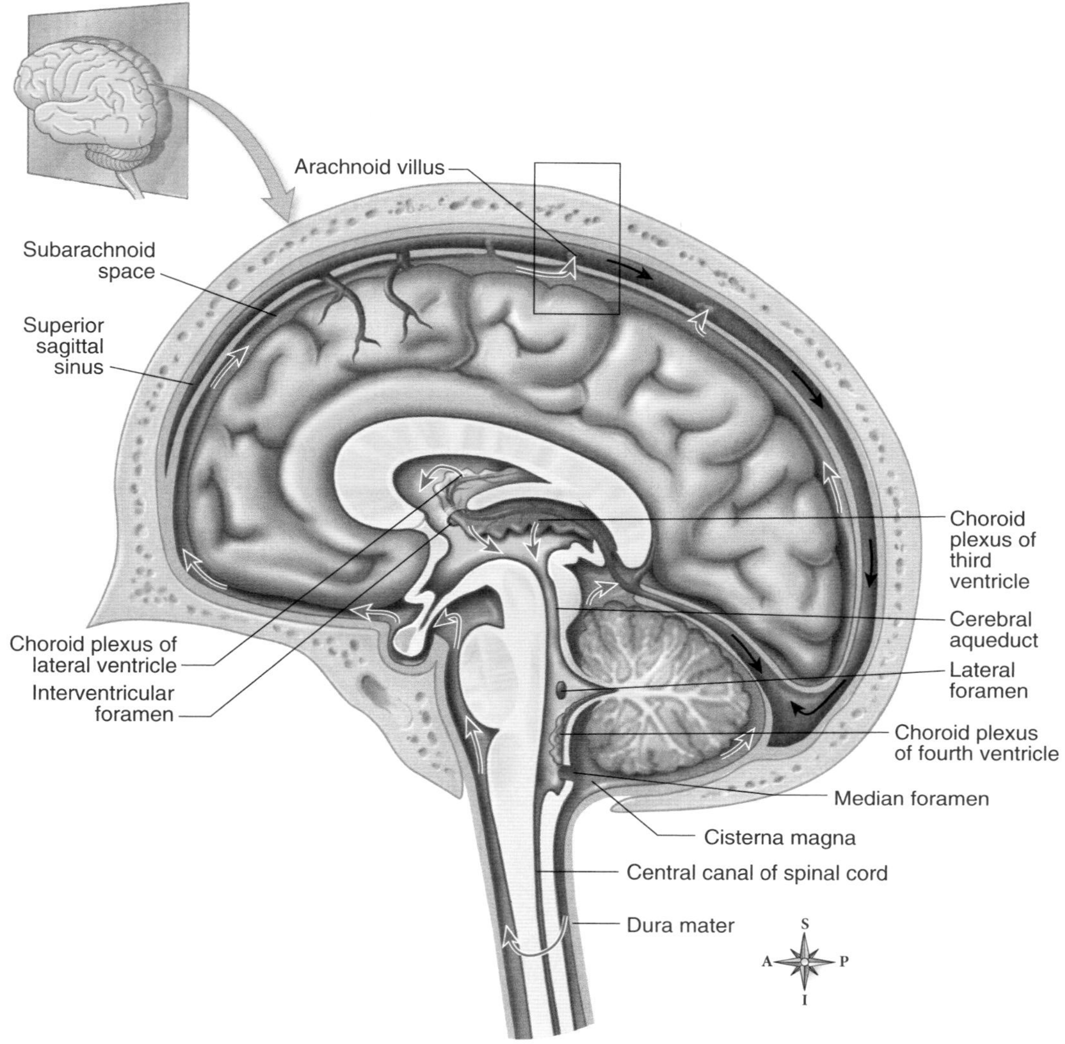

Fig. 14.3 Flow pattern of cerebrospinal fluid within the ventricles of the brain and the surrounding subarachnoid space. (From Patton KT, Bell F, Thompson T, Williamson P. *Anatomy and Physiology*. 11th ed. St. Louis, MO: Elsevier; 2022.)

Brain (Encephalon)

The brain is approximately 2% of the total body weight. Brain weight and size decrease with aging, primarily because of neuronal loss. The brain is divided into three major areas: the cerebrum, the brainstem, and the cerebellum.

Cerebrum. The *cerebrum* is composed of the right and left cerebral hemispheres, basal ganglia, and diencephalon. The cerebrum is also the origin of the first two cranial nerves, the olfactory and optic nerves, respectively (Table 14.1).

Cerebral hemispheres. The left hemisphere dominates language, as well as skilled and gesturing hand movements for most individuals. The right hemisphere specializes in the perception of certain nonverbal auditory stimuli, such as music. Processing visual information and determining spatial relationships are also functions of the right hemisphere; each person has a dominant hemisphere. The cerebral hemispheres are separated by a deep longitudinal fissure, known as the *corpus callosum*, which consists of fibers that travel from one hemisphere to the other, providing intricate connections between the two hemispheres.[3]

The surface of each hemisphere appears wrinkled because of the numerous raised areas called *gyri* (Fig. 14.4). Each gyrus folds into another, causing the convoluted appearance and substantially increasing the surface area of the brain. The surface of the cerebral hemisphere is approximately six cells deep and is called the *cerebral cortex,* or gray matter. Beneath the cortex is a layer of white matter, consisting of mostly myelinated axons, which serve as association and projection pathways.

A *fissure,* or *sulcus,* is a separation in the cerebral hemisphere. The fissures serve as important divisions or landmarks (Fig. 14.4). The longitudinal fissure separates the cerebral hemispheres into left and right sections. The lateral, or Sylvian, fissure divides the frontal and temporal lobes of the cerebrum. The central, or Rolandic, fissure separates the frontal and parietal lobes. The parieto-occipital fissure separates the occipital lobe from the parietal and temporal lobes.[1]

Each lobe of the cerebrum has a specific function. Knowledge of the functions of each lobe (Table 14.2) guides assessment and facilitates localization of the patient's problem. Understand that each region of the brain serves to send impulses and relay information to the sections surrounding, constantly providing information throughout the nervous system.

Basal ganglia. The basal ganglia system is the major subcortical nuclei composed of the caudate nucleus, putamen, and globus pallidus. This system is responsible for emotional, cognitive, and voluntary functions. The basal ganglia are considered a part of the extrapyramidal system given its direct and indirect connections to other parts of the brain, including but not limited to the thalamus and spinal cord. A part of the motor control system, the extrapyramidal system is responsible for involuntary reflexes, stabilization of motor control, and coordinated movement.[1]

Diencephalon. The *diencephalon,* located on the inferior surface of the cerebral cortex and between the two hemispheres, connects the brainstem to the cerebrum and the midbrain. It is divided into four paired regions: thalamus, hypothalamus, subthalamus, and epithalamus. The *thalamus* is the largest structure within the diencephalon; it integrates all bodily sensations except smell. The thalamus assists in recognizing pain, touch, and temperature and relays sensory information

TABLE 14.1 The Cranial Nerves and Their Assessment in the Critically Ill Patient

Nerve	Major Functions	Assessment
I—Olfactory (S)	Smell	Evaluate ability to identify familiar smells. Important to assess with basilar skull fracture or surgery on the skull base.
II—Optic (S)	Visual acuity	Assess gross ability to see and field of peripheral vision.
III—Oculomotor (M)	Movement of eyes; pupillary constriction and accommodation	Evaluate pupil size (mm), shape, and equality with bright penlight or pupillometer in dimly lit room. Assess for direct and consensual reaction to light; rate as brisk, sluggish, or nonreactive.
IV—Trochlear (M)	Movement of eyes	Evaluate voluntary movement of eyes together—up, down, laterally, and diagonally (tests CNs III, IV, and VI). In unconscious patients with stable cervical spine, assess *oculocephalic reflex* (doll's eye): turn the patient's head quickly from side to side while holding the eyes open. Note movement of eyes. The doll's eye reflex is present and cranial nerve intact if the eyes move bilaterally in the opposite direction of the head movement. Do not check if neck is unstable. Assess for nystagmus.
V—Trigeminal (S/M)	Chewing; sensation of scalp, face, teeth	Assess corneal reflex; observe for bilateral blink.
VI—Abducens (M)	Movement of eyes	Similar functions as CN IV associated with eye movement.
VII—Facial (M)	Facial expression; lacrimation, salivation; taste anterior tongue	Assess facial muscles for symmetry; if possible, ask patient to open eyes, arch eyebrows, smile, frown, and puff cheeks.
VIII—Auditory (S)	Hearing (cochlear)	Assess response to verbalization (gross hearing ability).
	Equilibrium (vestibular)	In the unconscious patient, the caloric irrigation test is done to assess the *oculovestibular reflex* (may be more sensitive than the doll's eye): elevate the head of bed to 30 degrees to assess for intact tympanic membrane; irrigate the ear canal with cold water. Bilateral eye movement toward the irrigated ear indicates an intact reflex.
IX—Glossopharyngeal (S/M)	Swallowing; taste posterior tongue; general sensation pharynx	CNs IX and X are evaluated together. Evaluate cough and gag reflex in response to suctioning the endotracheal tube and pharynx. Assess ability to manage oral secretions by swallowing.
X—Vagus (S/M)	Swallowing and laryngeal control; parasympathetic function	See CN IX.
XI—Spinal accessory (M)	Movement of head and shoulders	Assess ability to move and shrug shoulders and turn head.
XII—Hypoglossal (M)	Movement of tongue	If patient is able to follow commands, assess ability to protrude and/or move tongue from side to side.

CN, Cranial nerve; *M,* motor; *S,* sensory; *S/M,* sensory and motor.

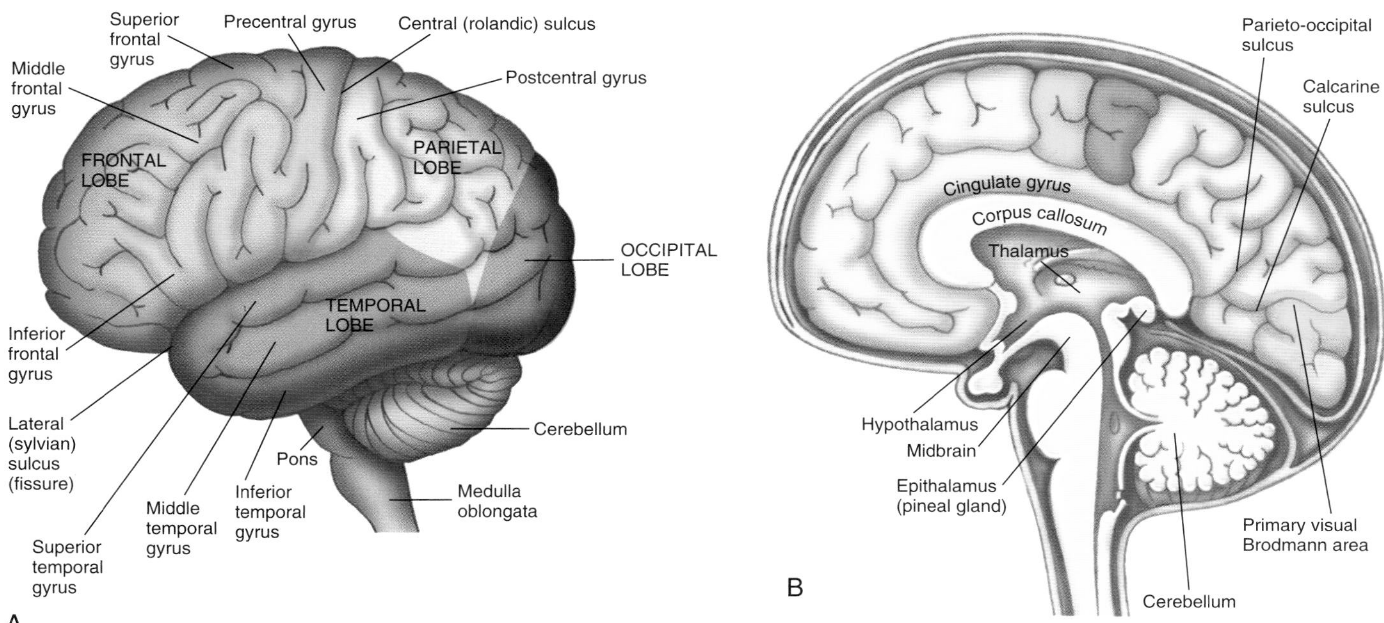

Fig. 14.4 Cerebral hemispheres and structures of the brain. A, Lateral external view. B, Midsagittal view. (From Patton KT, Thibodeau GA. *Anthony's Textbook of Anatomy and Physiology*. 20th ed. St. Louis, MO: Mosby, 2013.)

TABLE 14.2 Functions of the Cerebral Lobes

Structure	Function
Frontal lobes	Conscious thought, abstract thinking, judgment, voluntary movement on opposite side of the body; prefrontal areas are responsible for affect, memory, and concentration; motor expression of language in Broca's area on the left side in most individuals.
Parietal lobes	Processing, association, and interpretation of sensory information from the opposite side of the body.
Temporal lobes	Processing, association, and interpretation of auditory information; comprehension of language in Wernicke's area on the left side in most individuals; medial portion is responsible for memory and social behavior.
Occipital lobes	Visual processing and interpretation.
Basal ganglia	Motor control of fine body movements.

to the cerebrum. It also plays a role in emotions, arousal and alertness, and complex reflexes. The *hypothalamus* acts as a regulatory center for the autonomic nervous system (ANS). The general functions of the hypothalamus include temperature control, water balance, control of appetite and thirst, cardiovascular regulation, sleep-wake cycle, circadian rhythms, and sexual activity. The hypothalamus also controls the release of hormones from the pituitary gland.[1]

Brainstem. The *brainstem* is at the central core of the brain and controls vital functions. The major divisions of the brainstem are the midbrain, pons, and medulla (Fig. 14.4). The *midbrain,* also known as the mesencephalon, is a short segment of brainstem lying between the diencephalon and the pons. It contains nuclei of cranial nerves III (oculomotor) and IV (trochlear). The midbrain relays impulses to and from the cerebrum and lower brainstem. It also serves as the center for auditory and visual reflexes.

The *pons* is seated between the midbrain and the medulla. It contains nuclei of cranial nerves V (trigeminal), VI (abducens), VII (facial), and VIII (vestibulocochlear), and it connects the cerebellum to the brainstem. In conjunction with the medulla, the pons controls the rate and duration of respirations. The *medulla oblongata* is situated between the pons and the spinal cord. It contains nuclei of cranial nerves IX (glossopharyngeal), X (vagus), XI (accessory), and XII (hypoglossal). A summary of the functions of the cranial nerves and their assessment in the critically ill patient is provided in Table 14.1.

The medulla regulates the basic rhythm of respiration, rate and strength of the pulse, and vasomotor activity. In addition, neurons within the medulla regulate certain reflexes, including sneezing, swallowing, coughing, and vomiting.[1]

Cerebellum. The *cerebellum* is located posterior to the brainstem (Fig. 14.4). It is connected to the brainstem at the pons by three paired cerebellar peduncles. The peduncles receive input from the spinal cord and brainstem and send it to the cerebellar cortex. The functions of equilibrium, fine movement, muscle tone, balance, and coordination are mediated by the cerebellum. Unlike the cerebral cortex, the cerebellum controls the ipsilateral side of the body (same side).[1]

Specialized Systems Within the Central Nervous System

The *limbic system* provides primitive control of emotional responses and arousal. Structures of the limbic system include the amygdala (reward and fear stimuli), hippocampus (long-term memory), cingulate gyrus (attention and cognition), and connections to the hypothalamus and thalamus.

The *reticular activating system* (RAS) consists of diffuse fibers that begin in the lower brainstem and connect to various locations in the cerebral cortex. The RAS controls arousal, the sleep-wake cycle, selective attention, and perceptual awareness. If the RAS is intact, a person is aware and attentive. When the RAS is impaired, the person experiences inattention, alterations in the sleep-wake cycle, or decreased arousal, which is manifested as coma.[1]

Spinal Cord

The *spinal cord* is surrounded by the vertebral column and meninges. It begins as an extension from the medulla at the base of the brain and ends at the first or second lumbar vertebra. The end of the spinal cord consists of a bundle of nerves known as the cauda equina. The dura and arachnoid layers of the meninges surround the spinal cord and contain CSF.[1]

The *spinal cord* has 31 segments: 8 cervical, 12 thoracic, 5 lumbar, 5 sacral, and 1 coccygeal (Fig. 14.5). The spinal nerves, originating at each segment of the spinal cord, are part of the PNS. They transmit information to and from the periphery and the spinal cord. These nerves innervate the skin and musculature of most of the body. Each spinal nerve consists of a *ventral root* (anterior) and *a dorsal root* (posterior). The ventral roots carry efferent impulses (muscle signals) from the spinal cord to specific areas of the body known as *myotomes*.[1] The dorsal roots convey afferent impulses (sensory input) into the spinal cord from skin segments that represent specific areas of the body known as *dermatomes*. A dermatome chart traces the spinal nerves to their point of skin innervation and provides anatomical clues about level of injury or dysfunction (Fig. 14.6).

The spinal nerves interconnect in four areas called plexuses: cervical, brachial, lumbar, and sacral; however, the lumbar and sacral are often combined into the lumbosacral plexus. The *cervical plexus* includes spinal nerves C1 to C4 and innervates the muscles of the neck and shoulders. The phrenic nerve originates in this plexus and supplies the diaphragm. The *brachial plexus* comprises spinal nerves C5 to C8 and T1 and innervates the arms via the radial and ulnar nerves. The *lumbosacral plexus* is formed by spinal nerves L1 to L5 and S1 to S3. The femoral nerve arises from the lumbar plexus and the sciatic nerve from the sacral plexus; both nerves innervate the legs.

The cross-sectional size of the spinal cord varies by level, but structures remain the same at all levels. The H-shaped gray matter comprises the center of the cord. The anterior gray matter contains *sensory fibers* that convey sensory impulses from organs and muscles to the spinal cord. The posterior gray matter relays motor impulses from the spinal cord to skeletal muscles.

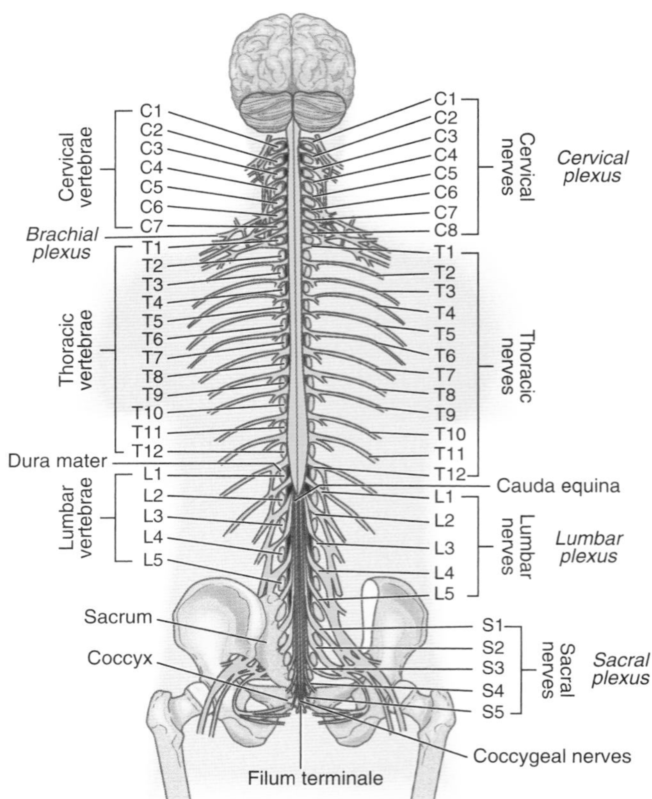

Fig. 14.5 Spinal nerves and nerve plexuses as they relate to vertebral level.

The white matter of the cord consists of fibers that connect with gray matter; together, they comprise the ascending (sensory) and descending (motor) pathways.[1]

Peripheral Nervous System

The PNS comprises the 12 paired cranial nerves, 31 paired spinal nerves, and the ANS. The 12 pairs of *cranial nerves* originate in the brain and brainstem and exit from the cranial cavity. Cranial nerves have sensory or motor functions, or both. These nerves are primarily responsible for the innervation of structures in the head and neck (Table 14.1).

The ANS comprises motor nerves that innervate visceral effectors: cardiac muscle; smooth muscle; adrenal medulla; and various glands, including salivary, gastric, and sweat glands. The ANS controls visceral activities at an unconscious level. The ANS consists of two parallel systems, known as the *sympathetic nervous system* and the *parasympathetic nervous system*. These two systems act to regulate visceral organs in opposing ways—one system stimulates effectors and the other inhibits—to maintain homeostasis.[1]

The *sympathetic nervous system* is also known as the thoracolumbar system because the nerve fibers originate in the thoracic and lumbar regions of the spinal cord. This system contains a chain of ganglia located on each side of the vertebrae. The sympathetic nervous system is sometimes called the *fight-or-flight* system because it is activated and dominates during stressful periods, releasing norepinephrine. Most sympathetic neurons release the neurotransmitter norepinephrine at the visceral effector. Sympathetic impulses cause vasoconstriction in the skin and viscera, vasodilation in the skeletal muscles, and an increase in the heart rate and force of contraction. Sympathetic impulses also cause an increase in blood pressure (BP), dilation of the bronchioles, an increase in sweat gland activity, dilation of the pupils, a decrease in peristalsis, and contraction of the pilomotor muscles (i.e., gooseflesh).[1]

The *parasympathetic nervous system* is also known as the craniosacral system because the preganglionic fibers originate at certain cranial nerves and in the sacral spinal cord. The axons are long, and ganglia are situated adjacent to or within specific organs. The parasympathetic system is dominant in non-stressful situations, stimulating visceral activities associated with maintenance of normal functions. The effects of parasympathetic nervous system stimulation induce the return of systems to a normal state of functioning. All neurons within the parasympathetic nervous system release the neurotransmitter acetylcholine at the visceral effector.[1]

CHECK YOUR UNDERSTANDING

1. The nurse assesses the patient, noting the patient is breathing over the ventilator, is coughing during suctioning, has pupillary reaction to light, and turns when the nurse calls the patient's name. These assessment findings indicate which specific structure of the CNS remains intact?
   A. Brainstem
   B. Cerebellum
   C. Cerebrum
   D. Spinal cord

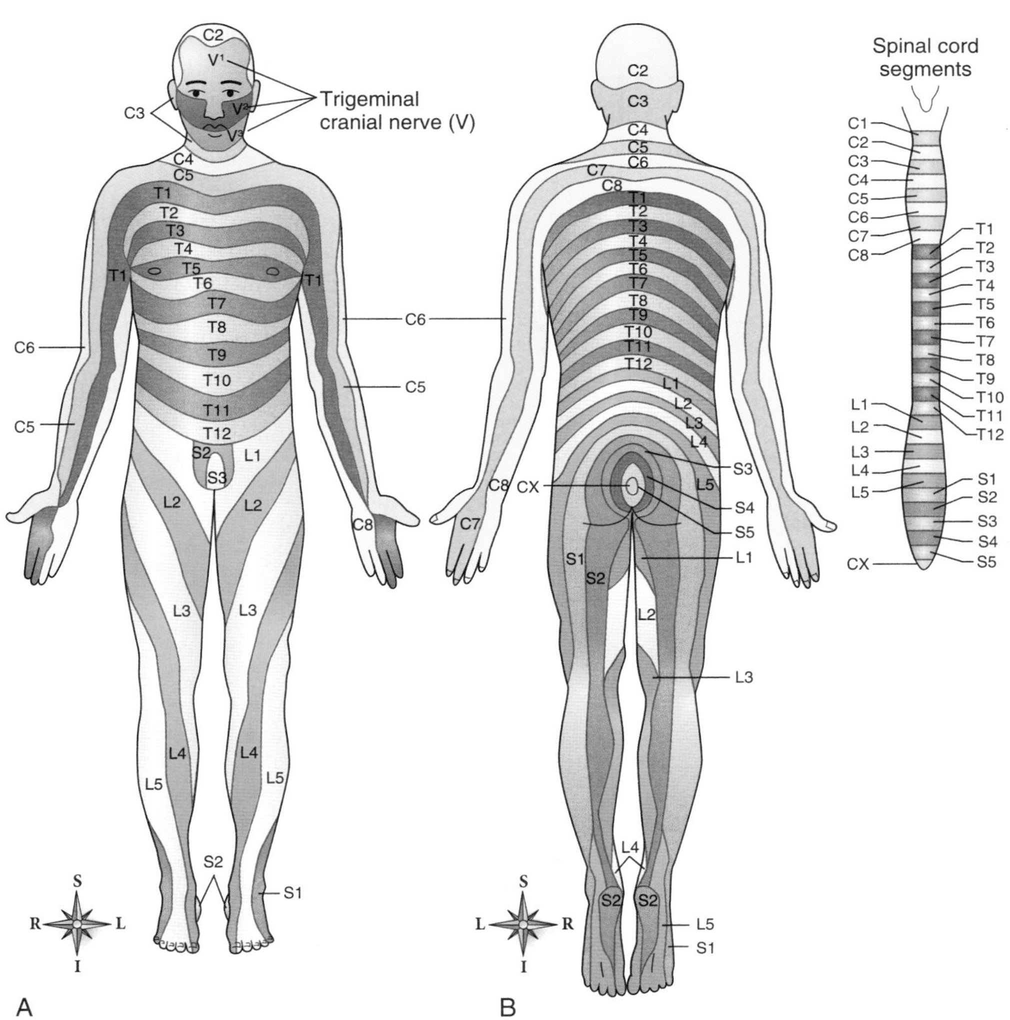

Fig. 14.6 Dermatome distribution of the spinal nerves. A, Distribution in the front. B, Distribution in the back. (Patton KT, Bell F, Thompson T, Williamson P. *Anatomy and Physiology.* 11th ed. St. Louis, MO: Elsevier; 2022.)

ASSESSMENT OF THE NERVOUS SYSTEM

A thorough history provides information about the patient's condition and potential events occurring prior to hospitalization that could have contributed to their diagnosis. Ideally, the patient is the primary source of the historical data. If the patient is unable to give a history, obtain information from family or friends about symptoms, onset, progression, and chronology of the event; comorbidities must also be considered. If pain is a presenting symptom, obtain information about the location, onset, type, and duration, the presence of other symptoms, and what makes the pain better or worse. Some physical and social changes occur with aging that may impact the assessment findings (see Lifespan Considerations box).[4,5]

An initial baseline neurological assessment, along with ongoing assessments, assists in monitoring the patient's condition and the response to treatments and nursing interventions. When performing a neurological assessment, focus on mental status; level of consciousness (LOC); and cranial nerve, motor, and sensory function. The best neurological assessment is completed in the absence of sedation or using minimal sedation; attempt to observe the patient's spontaneous movement without stimulation. Many neurological changes represent life-threatening conditions that require emergent treatment; immediately report changing or evolving assessment findings to the provider.

LIFESPAN CONSIDERATIONS

Effects of Age on the Nervous System

Older Adults

- Comorbidities, such as dementia, cognitive decline, or hearing and vision deficits, can confound the neurological exam. It is important to determine the patient's baseline neurological status.
- In older adults, the effects of certain medications used to decrease intracranial pressure (e.g., osmotic diuretics, barbiturates) are closely monitored because of a decreased ability to absorb, metabolize, and/or excrete these medications.
- Assess for preexisting renal insufficiency and diuretic use because diuretics may place older adults at risk for hypokalemia or hyponatremia when used to reduce intracranial pressure.
- In the older adult, elevating the head of the bed to decrease intracranial pressure may compromise an already diminished cerebral blood flow. Continuous assessment of neurological function and/or cerebral perfusion pressure is necessary to prevent decreasing blood flow to the brain.
- Central cord syndrome is more common in older adults and may result from hyperextension of an osteoarthritic spine.
- Subdural hematomas are more common in older adults because, as the brain atrophies with aging, it shrinks away from the dura and stretches bridging veins, which may easily tear. A large amount of blood can accumulate in the subdural space before the patient demonstrates overt signs and symptoms. Subtle mental status changes are often the first finding and are easily misinterpreted as signs of normal aging.

CLINICAL JUDGMENT ACTIVITY

A patient with prolonged unconsciousness has a strong family support system. The nurse would like to engage the family in the care and rehabilitation of the patient. Who from the multiprofessional team should the nurse engage and what interventions could the nurse implement?

Mental Status

When assessing a patient's mental status, assess consciousness (i.e., awareness of self and the environment), cognition (i.e., the ability to produce a response, including expressive and receptive language), and memory.

The *Glasgow Coma Scale* (GCS) is a commonly used standardized tool that assesses consciousness and cognition (Fig. 14.7). Evaluate the patient's ability to speak, open eyes, and produce a motor response to verbal commands or noxious stimuli. A noxious stimulus may include firm pressure applied to the nail bed, a trapezium squeeze, supraorbital pressure, or sternal pressure. Apply noxious stimuli only if the patient fails to respond to verbal stimuli. Care is taken to avoid injury when applying noxious stimuli.

The best response in each of the three categories of eye opening, verbal response, and motor response is scored, and the three scores are summed. GCS scores range from 3 (deep coma) to 15 (normal functioning). A GCS of 8 or less is consistent with coma. Several conditions limit application of the GCS, including concurrent injuries, like an SCI, treatments such as sedation and neuromuscular blockade, as well as intubation. In patients with either an endotracheal tube or tracheostomy, the GCS can still be scored, but the verbal component is to be documented as "Not Tested." The motor and eye components of the exam can still be calculated and trended as useful assessments.[6] The GCS is a measure of consciousness and cognition; it does not replace neurological assessment of specific brain function.

Additional scales used to monitor overall status in critical care settings have been gaining acceptance. The *Full Outline of UnResponsiveness* (FOUR) score, which evaluates eye response, motor response, breathing pattern, and brainstem reflexes, is one scale in use.[7] Scoring on this scale ranges from 0 to 16, with lower scores indicating a lower level of responsiveness. The FOUR score may be more reliable than the GCS in lower levels of responsiveness and is predictive of in-hospital mortality and poor functional outcomes.[7] Although additional scales, such as the AVPU (alert, responds to voice and pain, unresponsive) scale, are used in some settings, they have not been as widely studied and may not be as accurate at predicting mortality.[8]

CLINICAL ALERT

Neurological Assessment

Perform the neurological assessment with the nurse who just cared for the patient as part of the hand-off report. This ensures complete understanding of the prior documented assessment by the receiving nurse and quick recognition of neurological changes.

Glasgow Coma Scale			
Eyes	Open	Spontaneously	**4**
		To verbal command	**3**
		To pain	**2**
		No response	**1**
Best motor response	To verbal command	Obeys	**6**
	To painful stimulus	Localizes pain	**5**
		Flexion-withdrawal	**4**
		Flexion-abnormal (Decorticate rigidity)	**3**
		Extension (Decerebrate rigidity)	**2**
		No response	**1**
Best verbal response		Oriented and converses	**5**
		Disoriented and converses	**4**
		Inappropriate words	**3**
		Incomprehensible sounds	**2**
		No response	**1**
Total			**3-15**

Fig. 14.7 The Glasgow Coma Scale is a measure of consciousness based on eye opening, movement, and verbal responses. Each response is given a number, and the three scores are summed. Scores range from 3 to 15.

Language

Assess fluency and spontaneity of speech, word-finding ability, and comprehension. If the patient is intubated and responsive, ask the patient to perform simple verbal commands such as pointing to the clock, blinking their eyes, or raising an arm. Language skills may also be evaluated by asking the patient to write responses.

Language deficits are common in neurological disorders. *Expressive aphasia,* also known as Broca's aphasia, is a deficit in language output or speech production caused by a dysfunction in the dominant frontal lobe. It varies from mild word-finding difficulty to complete loss of both verbal and written communication skills. The inability to comprehend language and follow commands is called *receptive aphasia,* also known as Wernicke's aphasia, indicating dysfunction in the dominant temporal lobe. A patient with receptive problems can speak spontaneously, but the verbal response does not follow the context of the conversation. An intubated patient with receptive aphasia may appear to be responsive but is unable to follow simple verbal commands.

Memory

Evaluate both short- and long-term memory. To assess *short-term memory,* ask the patient to recall the names of three common words or objects (e.g., chair, clock, blue) after a 3-minute interval. Test *long-term memory* by asking the patient questions about the distant past (e.g., birthplace, year of birth, year of graduation from school). If intubated, responsive, and following commands, the patient can write the answers.

Cranial Nerve Function

On initial baseline neurological assessment, assess all cranial nerves. Focused cranial nerve assessments may be conducted depending on the anatomy involved. Table 14.1 presents assessments that can be done in patients who are critically ill, who often have a decreased LOC.

Pupil examination is the most critical component of the cranial nerve assessment. Assess pupils for size, shape, equality, and direct and consensual response to light. Normal pupil diameter ranges from 1.5 to 6 mm. Measurement with a millimeter scale is the most reliable method of determining size and equality. A pupillometer may provide a more objective measure than manual testing.[9] Unequal pupils *(anisocoria)* occur normally in some people; otherwise, inequality of pupils is a sign of a pathological process. A change in pupil reaction to light in one or both eyes is an important sign that may indicate increasing ICP or neurological deterioration; expect a concomitant change in mental status if the patient was previously alert. Other conditions that may affect pupillary size and reactivity to light, as well as mental status, include hypoxia and medications (e.g., atropine, sedation); therefore, these should be evaluated as part of the patient's differential diagnosis.

Motor Function

Assess all extremity movement, muscle strength, muscle tone and posture, and coordination. Assess muscle groups for bilateral symmetry (right vs. left) and complete a more comprehensive assessment if the patient is able to follow commands. If the patient does not follow commands, assess motor response to noxious stimuli. Ask the patient to move the extremities on command or observe the patient's ability to move around in bed. Grade muscle strength of the extremities on a five-point scale (Table 14.3). The grading is based on the ability to move muscle groups, hold a position against gravity, and maintain that position against resistance.

Assessing the strength of each limb is important to evaluate for possible differences between the right and left sides and between the upper and lower extremities. In persons with SCI, individual muscle function by myotome (Table 14.4) is assessed to identify the level of injury. *Hemiplegia* exists when one side of the patient's body is affected. *Paraplegia* exists when two of the same extremities are paralyzed. *Quadriplegia* or *tetraplegia* exists when all four extremities are paralyzed.

In a conscious patient, check for *arm drift* to detect subtle weakness. Ask the patient to close their eyes and stretch out their arms with palms up for 20 to 30 seconds. In a brain-injured patient, a downward drift of the arm (towards the ground), or pronation of the palm, indicates subtle weakness in the involved extremity and should be reported to the provider.

Assess muscle tone by taking each extremity through passive range of motion. Normal muscle tone shows slight resistance to

TABLE 14.3 Grading Scale for Motor Responses

Numerical Rating	Motor Response
0	Unable to lift the arm or leg to command or in response to painful stimuli
1	Flicker of movement is felt or seen in the muscle(s) of the limb
2	Moves the limb but unable to raise the extremity off the bed
3	Able to lift the extremity off the bed briefly but does not have the strength to maintain the lift
4	Able to lift the extremity off the bed but has difficulty resisting the examiner ("I am going to push your right arm/leg down, so try to prevent me from doing that.")
5	Able to lift the extremity off the bed and maintain the position against resistance

TABLE 14.4 Spinal Nerve Innervation (Myotomes) of Major Muscle Groups

Spinal Nerve	Muscle Group Movement	Assessment Technique
C4–C5	Shoulder abduction	Shoulders shrugged against downward pressure of examiner's hands
C5	Elbow flexion (biceps)	Arm pulled up from resting position against resistance
C7	Elbow extension (triceps)	From the flexed position, arm straightened out against resistance
	Thumb–index finger pinch	Index finger held firmly to thumb against resistance to pull apart
C8	Hand grasp	Hand grasp strength evaluated
L2	Hip flexion	Leg lifted from bed against resistance
L3	Knee extension	From flexed position, knee extended against resistance
L4	Foot dorsiflexion	Foot pulled up toward nose against resistance
S1	Foot plantar flexion	Foot pushed down (stepping on the gas) against resistance

range of motion. Flaccid muscles have diminished muscle tone, with no resistance to movement. Increased muscle tone is manifested as spasticity or rigidity.

Coordination of movement is under cerebellar control. Ask the patient to perform rapid alternating movements, such as touching the finger to the nose or running the heel down the shin bilaterally. These tests require the patient to be able to follow verbal commands. Incoordination (dysmetria) or exaggerated movements (ataxia) may indicate cerebellar injury.

Abnormal posturing may be observed in unconscious patients with brain damage. These include flexor (decorticate) or extensor (decerebrate) posturing (Fig. 14.8). *Flexor posturing* involves rigid flexion and adduction of the arms, wrist flexion with clenched fists, and extension and internal rotation of the legs. It usually occurs secondary to damage of the corticospinal tract, a key neuronal pathway sending motor signals from the brain down the spinal cord. *Extensor posturing* is the result of a midbrain or pons lesion. In this posture, the arms and legs are rigidly extended, and the feet are in plantar extension. The forearms may be pronated and abducted, and the wrists and fingers are flexed. Abnormal posturing can occur in response to noxious stimuli, such as suctioning or pain, or it may be spontaneous. Different posturing may be noted on each side of the body. Development of abnormal posturing should be reported to the provider.

Reflexes

There are three types of reflexes: deep tendon, superficial, and pathological. *Deep tendon reflexes (DTRs)* are obtained by a brisk tap of a reflex hammer on the tendons of a muscle group to elicit a motor response. The biceps reflex assesses spinal nerve roots, C5-C6; brachioradialis, C5-C6; triceps, C7-C8; patellar, L2-L4; and Achilles tendon, S1-S2. DTRs are graded according to the response elicited: 0, no reflex; 1+, hypoactive; 2+, normal; 3+, hyperactive; 4+, very brisk, clonus. Alterations in DTRs may indicate damage of the spinal cord or brain. In spinal shock, DTRs are absent below the level of injury initially; return of DTRs signals resolution of spinal shock. Aging and metabolic factors, such as thyroid dysfunction or electrolyte abnormalities, may diminish DTRs.

Superficial reflexes are elicited by touching or stroking a specific area and observing the motor response. The corneal reflex is a superficial reflex, as are the palpebral, gag, abdominal, cremasteric, and anal reflexes.

Pathological reflexes are typically present at birth, disappear with maturing of the nervous system, then may reappear with impaired neurological function. The most common pathological reflex is the *Babinski reflex*. When the sole of the patient's foot is lightly stroked, the normal response is plantar flexion of the toes. A Babinski reflex is present when dorsiflexion of the great toe with fanning of the other toes is observed with stimulation. In an adult, the presence of a Babinski reflex is a sign of an upper motor neuron lesion and damage to the corticospinal tract. Other pathological reflexes include the suck (sucking motions in response to touching the lips), snout (lip pursing in response to touching the lips), palmar (grasp in response to stroking the palm), and palmomental (contraction of the facial muscle in response to stimulating the base of the thumb) reflexes in adults.

Sensory Function

Sensory assessment evaluates the patient's ability to discriminate a sharp stimulus (such as a pinprick), position sense, and temperature. Sensory function in the skin is supplied by a single spinal nerve or sensory dermatome (Fig. 14.6). For example, the ability to sense a superficial pinprick on the lateral forearm, thumb, and index finger tests innervation of the C6 dermatome. To assess position sense (proprioception), instruct the patient to close the eyes. Move the patient's thumb or big toe up or down, or leave it in a neutral position, and ask the patient to identify the pattern of movement. To discriminate temperature, ask the patient to identify the sensation when a hot or cold container is touched to the skin. Sensation cannot be assessed in coma but is implied if the patient responds to painful stimulation.

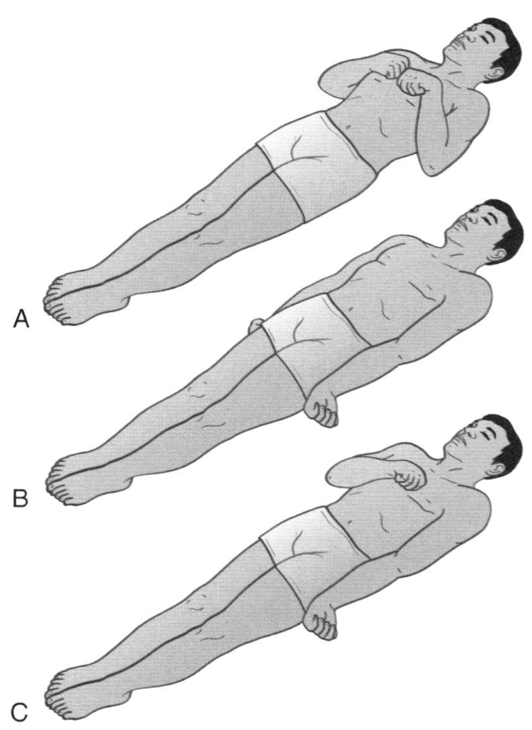

Fig. 14.8 Abnormal motor responses. A, Flexor posturing (decorticate). B, Extensor posturing (decerebrate). C, Flexor posturing on right side and extensor posturing on left side.

Respiratory Assessment

Assess the respiratory pattern and rate as part of the neurological assessment. Changes in the respiratory pattern can indicate neurological deterioration. Table 14.5 describes abnormal respiratory patterns observed in neurological disorders. These patterns may be obscured in mechanically ventilated patients.

Hourly Assessment

Neurological parameters are assessed based on the ordered frequency (often hourly) and the severity of the patient's condition. Reassessment is also done if changes are noted. Table 14.6 contains the components of an hourly neurological assessment for patients with increased ICP, head injury, or acute stroke. Focused assessments are performed based on the patient's specific condition. Complete all neurological assessments as ordered and document all findings per unit protocol. Report abnormal findings to the provider immediately. Additional assessments of brainstem or cranial nerve function may be considered if there is a change in the hourly neurological assessment.

INCREASED INTRACRANIAL PRESSURE

A commonly encountered problem in the critical care setting is increased ICP. Many neurological problems are associated with increased ICP, such as brain injury and stroke. Sustained increases in ICP compound the extent of brain injury and can be life-threatening; therefore, it is important to assess and maintain ICP within normal limits.

Pathophysiology

The rigid cranial vault contains three types of noncompressible contents: brain tissue, blood, and CSF. The pressure exerted by the combined volumes of these three components is ICP. If the volume of any one of these components increases,

TABLE 14.5 Abnormal Respiratory Patterns in Neurological Disorders

Abnormal Respiration	Description	Pattern	Anatomical Correlate
Cheyne-Stokes respiration	Cyclical episodes of hyperventilation and apnea		Bilateral deep cerebral lesion or some cerebellar lesions
Central neurogenic hyperventilation	Deep and rapid respirations (RR >25)		Lesions of the midbrain and upper pons
Apneustic	Deep, regular inspirations with inadequate expiration		Lesions of the middle to lower pons
Cluster (Biot) breathing	Breaths are clustered, then followed by a period of apnea with variable duration		Lesions of the lower pons or upper medulla
Ataxic respirations	Breaths at a low rate; completely irregular depth and pattern with prolonged periods of apnea		Lesions of the medulla

RR, Respiratory rate.
Images from Roy K, Huether SE. Alterations in cognitive systems, cerebral hemodynamics, and motor function. In: Rogers J, ed. *McCance and Huether's Pathophysiology: The Biologic Basis for Disease in Adults and Children*. 9th ed. St. Louis, MO: Elsevier; 2024:509-569.

TABLE 14.6 Components of the Hourly Neurological Assessment for Patients With Increased Intracranial Pressure, Head Injury, or Acute Stroke

Mental Status	Focal Motor	Pupils
Glasgow Coma Scale • Assesses level of consciousness • Language ability (unless intubated or altered consciousness) • Ability to follow commands	Move all extremities Strength and sensation of all extremities (compare right and left sides) Motor response in the patient with altered consciousness	Size Shape (regular or irregular) Reaction to light (direct)

the volume of one or both of the other compartments must decrease proportionally, or an increase in ICP occurs *(Monro-Kellie doctrine)*.

Compensatory change within the brain is called *compliance*. With adequate compliance, an increase in intracranial volume is compensated by displacement of CSF into the spinal subarachnoid space, displacement of blood into the venous sinuses, or both. The ICP remains normal, despite increases in volume. As compensatory mechanisms are exhausted, a small increase in volume leads to a large increase in ICP and a reduction in CBF. When CBF decreases, the brain becomes hypoxic, carbon dioxide levels increase, and acidosis occurs. In response to these changes, the cerebral blood vessels dilate to increase CBF. This compensatory response further increases intracranial volume, creating a vicious cycle that can be life-threatening (Fig. 14.9).

Normal ICP ranges from 0 to 15 mm Hg. Increased ICP is defined as a pressure of 20 mm Hg or greater persisting for 5 minutes or longer; it is a life-threatening event.[9] Sustained increases in ICP can lead to *herniation*, which is caused by shifting of brain tissue from an area of high pressure to one of lower pressure. Herniation syndromes are classified as supratentorial (cingulate, central, transcalvarial, and uncal herniation) or infratentorial (cerebellar tonsil herniation and upward herniation of the cerebellum). These herniation syndromes are described in Table 14.7 and shown in Fig. 14.10.

Along with MAP, the ICP determines cerebral perfusion pressure (CPP), which is the pressure required to perfuse the brain. CPP is calculated as the difference between MAP and ICP (CPP = MAP − ICP). The normal CPP in an adult is between 60 and 100 mm Hg. Typically, CPP is maintained at 60 to 70 mm Hg in those with brain pathology.[9] The CPP goal varies based on the mechanism of injury and the guidelines referenced and may be patient dependent.[10]

Any factor that decreases MAP and/or increases ICP decreases the CPP. CPP determines CBF; therefore, ischemia or infarction can occur if the CPP is inadequate. Measures to promote adequate CPP include lowering of increased ICP or, if this is not possible, increasing MAP to offset the effects of ICP on CPP. Often, MAP will rise in the presence of increased ICP; lowering MAP in this circumstance may decrease CPP and should be prevented.[11]

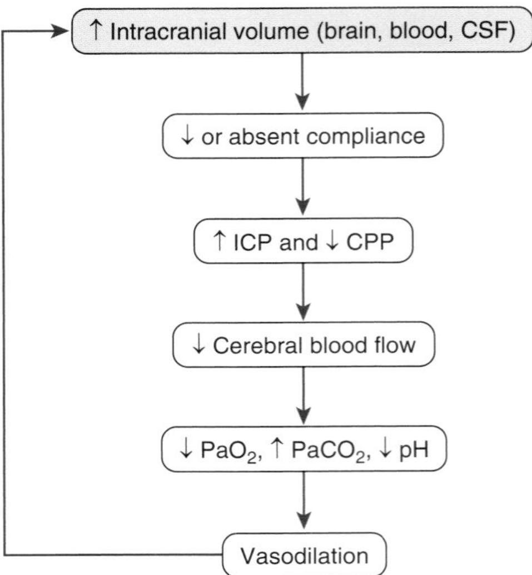

Fig. 14.9 Pathophysiology flow diagram for increased intracranial pressure. *CPP,* Cerebral perfusion pressure; *CSF,* cerebrospinal fluid; *ICP,* intracranial pressure; *$PaCO_2$,* partial pressure of arterial carbon dioxide; *PaO_2,* partial pressure of arterial oxygen.

Causes of Increased Intracranial Pressure

Factors that increase ICP are associated with increased brain volume, increased cerebral blood volume (CBV), and increased CSF.

Increased Brain Volume. A common cause of increased brain volume is cerebral edema, which is an increase in the water content of the brain tissue. Cytotoxic edema and vasogenic edema are two categories of cerebral edema; they may occur independently or together. *Cytotoxic cerebral edema* is characterized by intracellular swelling of neurons, most often because of hypoxia and hypoosmolality. Hypoxia causes decreased ATP production, leading to failure of the sodium-potassium pump in the cellular membrane. This allows sodium, chloride, and water to enter the cell while potassium exits. Cytotoxic edema is associated with brain ischemia or hypoxic events such as stroke or cardiac arrest. It is also seen with hypoosmolar conditions, including water intoxication and hyponatremia. *Vasogenic cerebral edema* occurs because of increased capillary permeability.

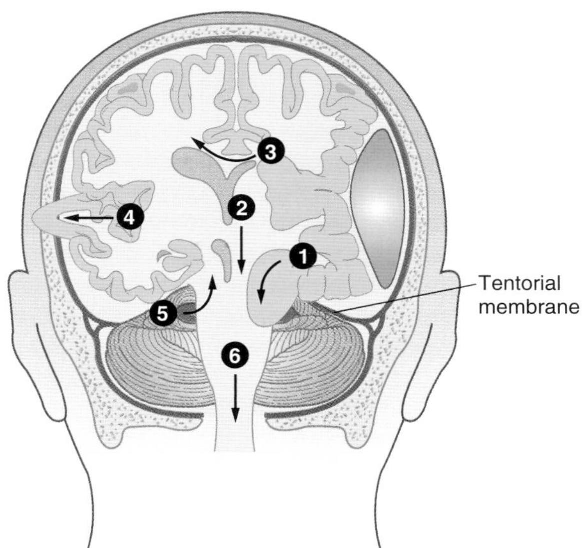

Fig. 14.10 Types of brain herniation. Herniation can occur above and below the tentorial membrane. Supratentorial: 1, uncal (transtentorial); 2, central; 3, cingulate; 4, transcalvarial (external herniation through an opening in the skull). Infratentorial: 5, upward herniation of cerebellum; 6, cerebellar tonsillar moves down through the foramen magnum. (From Rogers J. *McCance and Huether's Pathophysiology: The Biologic Basis for Disease in Adults and Children.* 9th ed. St. Louis, MO: Elsevier; 2024.)

With increased permeability, osmotically active substances (proteins) leak into the brain interstitium and draw water from the vascular system, leading to an increase in fluid in the extracellular space and, consequently, an increase in ICP. Brain injuries, brain tumors, meningitis, and brain abscesses are common causes of vasogenic cerebral edema. It is important to distinguish between the two types of edema when possible, as treatments may differ.

Increased Cerebral Blood Volume. Several mechanisms increase CBV, including loss of autoregulation, physiological responses to decreased cerebral oxygenation, increased metabolic demand, and obstruction of venous outflow.

Within normal limits, the cerebral vasculature exhibits pressure and chemical autoregulation. Autoregulation provides a constant CBV and CPP over a wide range of MAPs. Pathological states such as head injury or hypertension often lead to a loss of autoregulation. Without autoregulation, hyperemia may occur, leading to increased ICP.[1]

Decreased cerebral oxygenation causes cerebral vasodilation in an attempt to improve oxygen delivery. Hypercapnia also causes vasodilation in the brain. Any factor that results in hypoxemia or hypercapnia, such as ineffective ventilation, airway obstruction, or endotracheal suctioning, can contribute to an increase in ICP.

CBF may increase to augment oxygen supply in response to increased metabolic demands. Several factors increase oxygen demands, including fever, physical activity, pain, shivering, and seizures.[9] Grouping nursing activities together (e.g., bathing, suctioning, turning) may also increase metabolic demands. Although sleep and rest are important, oxygen demands are higher during rapid eye movement (REM) sleep. Increases in ICP may be noted during any of these situations.

Obstruction of venous outflow results in increased CBV and ICP. Hyperflexion, hyperextension, rotation of the neck, or tightly applied rigid cervical collars or tracheostomy or endotracheal tube ties may compress the jugular vein, which inhibits venous return and causes central venous engorgement. A tumor or abscess can compress the venous structures, causing an outflow obstruction. Mechanisms that increase intrathoracic or intraabdominal pressure also impair venous return (e.g., coughing, vomiting, posturing, isometric exercise, Valsalva maneuver, positive end-expiratory pressure, hip flexion).

Increased Cerebrospinal Fluid. Hydrocephalus, an increase in CSF, can also increase ICP. Hydrocephalus may occur in any circumstance in which CSF flow is obstructed, such as with a tumor of the third ventricle; when CSF absorption is blocked due to subarachnoid hemorrhage (SAH) or infection (e.g., meningitis, encephalitis); or when excess CSF is produced.

Assessment

Assess vital signs and perform a thorough neurological examination with emphasis on LOC and motor and cranial nerve function. Early signs of increasing ICP include increasing BP, nausea, vomiting, headache, restlessness, and drowsiness. Hypertension represents a compensatory mechanism to augment CPP in these early stages of increasing ICP.[2] Cushing's triad is a late sign of increased ICP and consists of systolic hypertension with a widening pulse pressure, bradycardia, and irregular respirations. It often signifies irreversible damage. Although a late sign of elevated ICP, pupillary changes often correlate with ICP changes and are the most critical cranial nerve assessment.

Monitoring Techniques. Invasive monitoring of ICP, cerebral oxygenation, and other physiological parameters may be used to augment the clinical assessment.

Intracranial pressure monitoring. ICP monitoring is used to correlate objective data with the clinical picture and to determine cerebral perfusion. Monitoring is indicated for patients who have a GCS score between 3 and 8 due to a severe brain insult.[9] It is used to assess response to therapy (e.g., after administration of osmolar diuretic) or to augment the neurological assessment in the intubated patient.

ICP monitoring systems are classified by location of device or type of transducer system. Devices can be placed in one of the ventricles; in the parenchyma; or in the subarachnoid, epidural, or subdural spaces (Fig. 14.11). Each site has advantages and disadvantages (Table 14.8). External ventricular drains

TABLE 14.7 Herniation Syndromes

Tentorial Location	Syndrome	Definition	Symptoms
Supratentorial	Cingulate	Shift of brain tissue from one cerebral hemisphere under the falx cerebri to the other hemisphere	No specific symptoms; may have focal motor deficit; herniation may compromise cerebral blood flow
Supratentorial	Central	Downward shift of cerebral hemispheres, basal ganglia, and diencephalon through the tentorial notch that compresses the brainstem	**Early** • Decrease in LOC • Motor weakness • Cheyne-Stokes respiration • Small, reactive pupils **Late** • Coma • Pupils dilated and fixed • Abnormal flexor posturing, progressing to abnormal extensor posturing • Unstable vital signs progressing to cardiopulmonary arrest
Supratentorial	Transcalvarial	Brain shifts through an opening in the skull (i.e., craniectomy); potentially increases the risk of hemorrhagic infarction	Vary; disproportionate when compared to the area of the brain affected; may present with delayed neurological deterioration
Supratentorial	Uncal	Unilateral lesion forces uncus of temporal lobe to displace through the tentorial notch, compressing the midbrain Symptoms can progress rapidly	**Early** • Decreased LOC • Increased muscle tone • Positive Babinski reflex • Cheyne-Stokes respiration, progressing to central neurogenic hyperventilation • Ipsilateral dilated pupil • Weakness **Late** • Pupils dilated and fixed • Paralyzed eye movements • Contralateral hemiplegia • Abnormal flexor posturing, progressing to abnormal extensor posturing • Unstable vital signs progressing to cardiopulmonary arrest
Infratentorial	Cerebellar tonsil	Displacement of cerebellar tonsils through foramen magnum, compressing the pons and medulla	Alterations in respiratory and cardiopulmonary function, rapidly progressing to cardiopulmonary arrest
Infratentorial	Upward herniation of the cerebellum	A cerebellar tonsil or the lower brainstem is forced upward, which may compress the ascending arousal system, cerebral aqueduct, or superior cerebellar artery	Alterations in respiratory and cardiopulmonary function, rapidly progressing to cardiopulmonary arrest

LOC, Level of consciousness.

(EVDs) are the most commonly used devices for monitoring because they also allow therapeutic interventions, such as CSF and blood drainage, as well as medication instillation (e.g., antibiotics). An EVD, also known as a *ventriculostomy*, may be connected to a drainage bag to drain CSF in a controlled manner to relieve increased ICP, divert the flow of CSF after surgery, or to remove blood products after subarachnoid or intraventricular hemorrhage. The ventricular catheter system allows continuous monitoring only, continuous CSF drainage only, or both monitoring and CSF drainage, depending on patient need and the system used.

The transducer system may be a microchip sensor device, a fiberoptic catheter, or a fluid-filled system. The fluid-filled system is most often used for ICP monitoring. This system is similar to that used for hemodynamic monitoring, with a few exceptions. Prime the pressure tubing with sterile 0.9% normal saline *without* preservatives (because preservatives may damage brain tissue). Once primed, *do not use* pressurized fluid or flush the system while the system is attached to the patient; this may increase ICP and harm the patient. Zero reference the air-fluid interface at the level of the foramen of Monro (anatomically at the tragus of the outer ear); at this level, ICP is believed to be most accurate. Observe the ICP waveform on a channel on the bedside monitor and record the mean ICP.

Catheters with internal microchip sensors and fiberoptic catheters have the transducer built into the tip of the catheter. These devices only need to be zero referenced before insertion. They are connected via a cable to a stand-alone monitor provided by the manufacturer. Some devices can be connected to the bedside monitor for an additional display of ICP and waveforms. Other advantages of connecting to the bedside monitor include enabling alarm and waveform monitoring at a central station, automatic calculation of CPP, and documentation of the ICP measurement in the electronic health record (EHR).

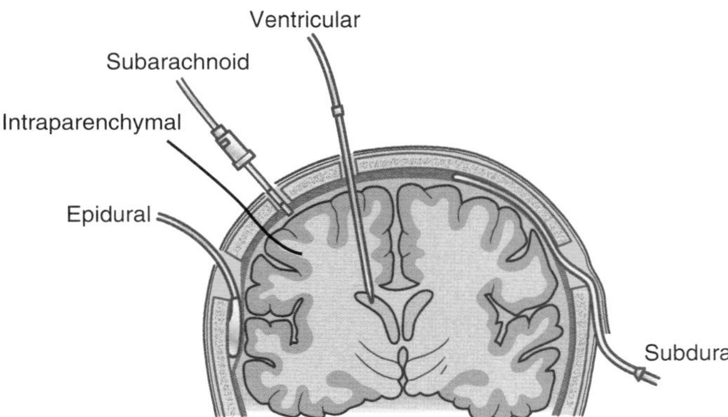

Fig. 14.11 Intracranial pressure monitoring sites. (From Harding MM, Kwong J, Hagler D, Reinisch C. *Medical Surgical Nursing: Assessment and Management of Clinical Problems*. 12th ed. St. Louis, MO: Mosby; 2022.)

ICP monitoring systems allow nurses to observe an ICP waveform pattern. The normal intracranial pulse waveform has three defined peaks of *decreasing* height that correlate with the arterial pulse waveform and are identified as P_1, P_2, and P_3 (Fig. 14.12). P_1 (percussion wave) is fairly consistent in shape and amplitude; it represents the blood being ejected from the heart and correlates with cardiac systole. Extremes in blood pressure produce changes in P_1. The second wave, P_2 (tidal wave), represents brain compliance and is variable in shape. Decreased compliance exists when P_2 is equal to or higher than P_1. It also is helpful in predicting the risk for increases in ICP. P_3 (dicrotic wave) follows the dicrotic notch and represents closure of the aortic valve, correlating with cardiac diastole. Smaller peaks that follow the three main peaks vary among individual patients.[12]

Cerebral oxygenation monitoring. CBF and brain oxygen use may be monitored by *jugular vein oxygen saturation* (SjO_2), although this monitoring approach is not used routinely in facilities. The technology is similar to that for measurement of mixed venous oxygen saturation (SvO_2) in the pulmonary artery. SjO_2 is monitored via a fiberoptic catheter inserted retrogradely (toward the brain) through the internal jugular vein into the jugular venous bulb. Placement of the catheter is verified by a neck radiograph. Oxygen saturation of venous blood is measured as it leaves the brain and provides a global measure of cerebral oxygenation. The normal value is 60% to 70%. Values less than 50% suggest cerebral ischemia. However, because the jugular vein drains only a portion of the brain,

TABLE 14.8 Intracranial Pressure Monitoring Devices

Device	Location	Advantages	Disadvantages
Intraventricular catheter (i.e., ventriculostomy, external ventricular device) or fiberoptic transducer	Lateral ventricle of nondominant hemisphere; may be tunneled or bolted	Therapeutic or diagnostic removal of CSF to control ICP Good ICP waveform quality Accurate and reliable	Highest risk for infection Consistency in zero leveling Risk of hemorrhage Longer insertion time Rapid CSF drainage may result in collapsed ventricle CSF leakage around insertion site
Subarachnoid bolt or screw	Subarachnoid space	Inserted quickly Does not penetrate brain	Bolt can become damaged during insertion Only provides the local ICP, which may be misleading CSF leakage may occur CSF drainage not possible
Epidural sensor or transducer	Between the skull and the dura	Least invasive Low risk of infection Low risk of hemorrhage Recommended in patients at risk for meningitis or other CNS infections	Indirect measure of ICP Less accurate and reliable CSF drainage not possible
Parenchymal fiberoptic catheter	1 cm into brain tissue	Inserted quickly Accurate and reliable Good ICP waveform quality	CSF drainage not possible Catheter relatively fragile Expensive

CNS, Central nervous system; *CSF,* cerebrospinal fluid; *ICP,* intracranial pressure.

Data from Evensen KB, Eide PK. Measuring intracranial pressure by invasive, less invasive or non-invasive means: limitations and avenues for improvement. *Fluids Barriers CNS.* 2020;17(1):34. https://doi.org/10.1186/s12987-020-00195-3; Nag DS, Sahu S, Swain A, Kant S. Intracranial pressure monitoring: gold standard and recent innovations. *World J Clin Cases.* 2019;7(13):1535-1553. https://doi.org/10.12998/wjcc.v7.i13.1535.

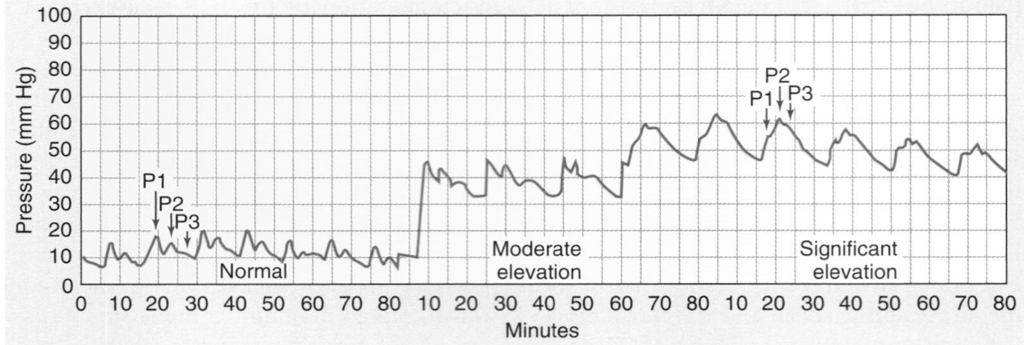

Fig. 14.12 Intracranial pressure (ICP) monitoring can be used to continuously measure ICP. The ICP tracing shows normal, elevated, and plateau waves. At high ICP, the P2 peak is higher than the P1 peak, and the peaks become less distinct and plateau. (From Harding MM, Kwong J, Hagler D, Reinisch C. *Medical Surgical Nursing: Assessment and Management of Clinical Problems.* 12th ed. St. Louis, MO: Mosby; 2022.)

CLINICAL EXEMPLAR

Quality and Safety

A nurse notices that stopcock covers on the external ventricular drainage (EVD) system are the same red color as those used on the arterial pressure and IV lines, making it difficult to distinguish lines and contributing to potential for inadvertent injection of medications into the EVD system. The nurse recognizes that inadvertent injection of medications into the EVD system could contribute to severe neurotoxicities and increased intracranial pressures. The nurse brings the issue to a staff meeting for discussion and learns that several staff members have experienced a near-miss event related to challenges with line identification. The nurse works with the unit manager to develop a task force to identify options that would facilitate a clearer system for line identification. One task force member identified additional stopcock color options; another investigated options for different EVD systems; and a third nurse surveyed other institutions in the area for additional solutions. Staff nurses were encouraged to provide suggestions. Options were reviewed with the supply management team to determine availability and cost. Two potential solutions were identified: line labels specifying line type, and stopcock covers of different colors for different types of lines. The two options were presented by the task force to the entire critical care team, and staff nurses voted on the choice they believed to be most appropriate. Different-colored stopcock covers were ultimately used for each line type. Signs were made and posted above each patient bed providing a legend for stopcock cover colors. The nurse worked with the staff educator to inform nurses about the change in stopcock cover color. The nurse worked with the clinical nurse specialist to conduct episodic audits of appropriate stopcock cover use and any additional near-miss events.

normal values do not ensure adequate perfusion to all brain areas.[11]

The partial pressure of oxygen within brain tissue ($PbtO_2$) can be measured by placing a monitoring probe directly into the brain white matter and attaching it to a stand-alone monitor. The probe may be inserted into the damaged portion of the brain to measure regional oxygenation, or it may be inserted into an undamaged portion of the brain to measure global oxygenation. In a patient with a TBI, the goal of therapy is to maintain an adequate $PbtO_2$. Current studies recommend a $PbtO_2$ greater than 20 mm Hg. However, the science of brain tissue oxygenation is evolving, and target values may change. Values may also be device specific; therefore, it is important to review the manufacturer's recommendations. Management of low $PbtO_2$ is directed at treating the underlying cause. Though future research is needed, studies have not found an association between $PbtO_2$ and improved neurological outcomes, but there may be a survival benefit with $PbtO_2$ directed therapy.[11]

Other physiological monitoring. Hemodynamic monitoring may be used to monitor fluid status and to assist in maintaining adequate cerebral perfusion (see Chapter 9, Hemodynamic Monitoring). Continuous monitoring of arterial oxygen saturation via pulse oximetry (SpO_2) and of end-tidal carbon dioxide levels is useful to ensure adequate gas exchange in the neurological patient. Periodic arterial blood gas samples may also be obtained. The bispectral index (BIS) is used by anesthesia providers to monitor the effect of anesthetic agents on the brain and CNS by use of a single or series of electrode(s) placed on the forehead. The BIS is recommended for monitoring the critically ill patient receiving deep sedation with or without neuromuscular blockade to assist with titrating analgesics and sedatives; these pharmacological interventions may be required to effectively manage elevated ICP.[13]

Diagnostic Testing

The initial baseline and ongoing laboratory tests obtained in a patient with increased ICP include the following:

- Arterial blood gas, SpO_2, end-tidal carbon dioxide
- Complete blood count, with an emphasis on hematocrit, hemoglobin, and platelets
- Coagulation profile, including prothrombin time, international normalized ratio (INR), and activated partial thromboplastin time (aPTT) because a brain injury may induce a coagulopathy
- Electrolytes (in particular sodium), blood urea nitrogen, creatinine, liver function, and serum osmolality; these

patients may also require urine osmolality and urine specific gravity to evaluate for diabetes insipidus (see Chapter 19, Endocrine Alterations).

Radiological studies and other diagnostic tests that may be performed on a patient with increased ICP include the following:[14–16]

- Computed tomography (CT) scan (usually without contrast) to assess the potential for a worsening intracranial mass effect.
- Magnetic resonance imaging (MRI) to provide anatomical detail of pathology contributing to increased ICP.
- Continuous bedside electroencephalography (EEG) monitoring provides a recording of electrical activity in the brain. A continuous EEG may be obtained to identify seizure activity, including subclinical (not present on physical exam) seizure activity; lack of electrical activity, which may be consistent with brain death; and the etiology of indeterminable altered mental status. It can also be used to monitor brain activity in patients who are in a pharmacologically induced coma, particularly with the use of pentobarbital in patients with increased ICP.[16]

Patient Problems

Refer to this chapter's Plan of Care for the Patient with Traumatic Brain Injury, Increased Intracranial Pressure, or Acute Stroke for a detailed description of patient problems, specific nursing interventions, and selected rationales. Other interventions are discussed in the Collaborative Care Plan found in Chapter 1, Overview of Critical Care Nursing.

PLAN OF CARE

For the Patient With Traumatic Brain Injury, Increased Intracranial Pressure, or Acute Stroke

Patient Problem

Potential for Increased Intracranial Pressure (ICP). Risk factors include underlying brain injury, volume overload, fever, pain, seizures, positional factors, or increased intrathoracic or intraabdominal pressure.

Desired Outcomes

- Prevention of increased ICP (ICP <20 mm Hg).
- Neurological status stable or improved from baseline.
- Stable VS.
- Optimal fluid balance.
- Absence of seizures.

Nursing Assessments/Interventions	Rationales
• Assess neurological status hourly, including level of consciousness, pupillary function (other cranial nerve functions as indicated), strength and equality in bilateral extremity movements, and sensory function, where appropriate.	• Detect changes indicative of increased ICP.
• Monitor ICP and CPP; notify provider if ICP >20 mm Hg sustained for more than 5 min or if CPP <60 to 70 mm Hg.	• Ensure adequate cerebral perfusion (CPP >60–70 mm Hg).
• Maintain airway; monitor SpO_2 and $ETCO_2$, or ABG, for evidence of hypoxemia/hypercapnia; hyperoxygenate the patient before and after suctioning.	• Ensure adequate cerebral perfusion; prevent cerebral vasodilation.
• Monitor VS; be alert to changes in respiratory pattern, fluctuations in BP, bradycardia, widening pulse pressure.	• Detect responses to increased ICP; however, these signs occur very late.
• Maintain patient's head in a neutral position; maintain HOB elevation that keeps ICP and CPP within normal ranges.	• Facilitate cerebral venous drainage and prevent increased ICP.
• Monitor fluid volume status by measuring I&O, skin turgor, daily weight, breath sounds, and invasive and noninvasive hemodynamic monitoring, as appropriate; ensure precise delivery of IV fluids; administer osmotic diuretics as ordered.	• Prevent fluid volume excess or deficit, both of which can affect ICP. • Fluid monitoring can also assess for diabetes insipidus in the patient with brain injury.
• Evaluate patient's response to nursing interventions; space activities to avoid increases in ICP.	• Prevent sustained elevations in ICP; ICP should return to normal values within 5 min after completion of activities.
• Prevent increases in intrathoracic and intraabdominal pressure through proper positioning, avoiding coughing and Valsalva maneuver.	• Facilitate cerebral venous drainage and prevent increased ICP.
• If patient is hyperthermic, administer treatments to reduce temperature to normal.	• Reduce cerebral metabolic demands.
• Administer antiepileptic medications as ordered to prevent seizures; if seizures occur, treat promptly.	• Seizures increase CBF and can increase ICP.
• Administer medications as needed for pain.	• Pain may contribute to increased ICP.

PLAN OF CARE—cont'd

For the Patient With Traumatic Brain Injury, Increased Intracranial Pressure, or Acute Stroke

Nursing Assessments/Interventions	Rationales
• Weigh daily. • Monitor I&O hourly. • Monitor laboratory results (electrolytes, serum, and urine osmolality). • Assess skin and mucous membranes.	• Monitor fluid volume status (all interventions).

Patient Problem

Potential for Decreased Cerebral Tissue Perfusion. Risk factors include increased ICP and decreased cerebral blood flow.

Desired Outcomes

- VS within normal limits.
- Improved cerebral perfusion.
- Neurological status within normal limits.

Nursing Assessments/Interventions	Rationales
• Assess neurological status hourly using GCS, FOUR score, or NIHSS; monitor VS.	• Assess for alterations in ICP.
• Assess for restlessness, anxiety, or mental status changes as early indicators of altered cerebral tissue perfusion. Institute safety precautions as needed.	• Mental status changes are often the earliest indicators of altered tissue perfusion. • Mental status changes may predispose the patient to injury.
• Perform interventions to prevent and treat increased ICP. • Maintain head in a midline position. • Elevate HOB >30 degrees. • Assess and treat pain.	• Ensure adequate cerebral tissue perfusion.
• Maintain BP within desired range with prescribed medications; maintain IV fluid therapy.	• Decreases in BP and hypovolemia may decrease CPP.

ABG, Arterial blood gas; *BP*, blood pressure; *CBF*, cerebral blood flow; *CPP*, cerebral perfusion pressure; *$ETCO_2$*, end-tidal carbon dioxide; *FOUR*, full outline of unresponsiveness; *GCS*, Glasgow Coma Scale; *HOB*, head of bed; *ICP*, intracranial pressure; *I&O*, intake & output; *NIHSS*, National Institutes of Health Stroke Scale; *SpO_2*, arterial oxygen saturation via pulse oximetry; *VS*, vital signs.
Adapted from Swearingen PL, Wright JD. *All-in-One Nursing Care Planning Resource*. 5th ed. St. Louis, MO: Elsevier; 2019.

Medical and Nursing Interventions

The goal of management is to maintain an ICP of less than 20 mm Hg while maintaining the CPP between 60 and 70 mm Hg.[9] The first task is to prevent an increase in ICP. If the ICP is elevated, therapy is instituted to decrease ICP and then identify the cause of increased ICP. Once the cause is discovered, management is centered on permanently decreasing the high ICP, maintaining CPP, maintaining the airway, providing ventilation and oxygenation, and decreasing the metabolic demands placed on the injured brain.

Nursing Interventions to Manage Intracranial Pressure. Patient positioning is a key nursing intervention that may minimize ICP and maximize CPP. Elevate the head of the bed to 30 degrees and keep the head and neck in a neutral midline position, which facilitates venous drainage and decreases the risk of venous obstruction. Elevated ICPs are not a reason to avoid repositioning. Rather, it is imperative for the nurse to monitor and document the patient's individualized cerebral and hemodynamic response during any position or head of bed changes.[17] If the ICP and CPP do not return to their baseline values within 5 minutes after the position change, reposition the patient to the position that maximized CPP and minimized ICP.

Because endotracheal suctioning is associated with hypoxemia, suction the patient only when necessary. Preoxygenate the patient with 100% oxygen before and between suction attempts and for 1 minute after the procedure. Limit each suction pass to less than 10 seconds, with no more than two suction passes. Maintain the head in a neutral position during the suctioning procedure.

Several nursing activities are associated with increases in ICP, including the previously mentioned interventions, as well as hygiene measures. Elevated ICP resulting from nursing care is usually temporary, and the ICP should return to the resting baseline value within a few minutes. Sustained increases in ICP lasting longer than 5 minutes should be prevented. Spacing nursing care activities allows for rest between activities. If ICP pressure monitoring is available, monitor the ICP in response to care and other interventions.

Family presence has been shown to decrease ICP (e.g., handholding, speaking softly to the patient).[18] However, caution family members to avoid excess stimulation of the patient or unpleasant conversations in the patient's room that may emotionally stimulate the patient (e.g., prognosis, condition, deficits, restraints) because this can cause an elevation in ICP. Assess the patient's physiological response to visitors and intervene accordingly.

CLINICAL JUDGMENT ACTIVITY

You are caring for a patient who has sustained a traumatic brain injury from a motor vehicle collision and is presenting with a Glasgow Coma Scale score of 6. The patient has an external ventricular drain for continuous measurement of intracranial pressure (ICP). The ICP has been stable at 13 mm Hg for the past 4 hours. The alarm on the monitor sounds because the ICP is now 20 mm Hg. What are your priority assessments and interventions?

Medical Management. Medical management of increased ICP includes the following: adequate oxygenation and ventilation; cautious, limited use of hyperventilation; osmotic diuretics; euvolemic fluid administration; maintenance of BP; and reduction of metabolic demands. Corticosteroids are useful for reducing cerebral edema associated with brain tumors and meningitis, but studies do not support administration of corticosteroids to reduce ICP associated with other intracranial conditions.[19]

Adequate oxygenation. Maintain the PaO_2 above 80 mm Hg to ensure that oxygen delivery to the brain exceeds oxygen consumption. The goal PaO_2 varies based on the underlying disease process and cause of elevated ICP.[20] A PaO_2 below 50 mm Hg can precipitate increased ICP. For many patients with increased ICP, short-term management of the airway is accomplished by an endotracheal tube and mechanical ventilation. Positive end-expiratory pressure (PEEP) may be added to facilitate oxygenation; however, it must be used with extreme caution because it may prevent venous outflow and further increase ICP. The use of higher levels of PEEP should be assessed based on the patient's ICP stability and sensitivity to PEEP increases.[21] A tracheostomy tube may be required for long-term ventilatory management, though the optimal timing of insertion may vary based on etiology. In addition, adequate hematocrit and hemoglobin levels are maintained to promote oxygenation.

Management of carbon dioxide. Hyperventilation decreases $PaCO_2$, which causes vasoconstriction of the cerebral arteries and a reduction of CBF. In the past, hyperventilation was commonly used to manage ICP, but hyperventilation may cause neurological damage by decreasing cerebral perfusion and oxygenation.[22,23] For this reason, the routine use of hyperventilation is not recommended for the management of elevated ICP.[22,23] Hyperventilation is used to decrease ICP for short periods when acute neurological deterioration is occurring (i.e., herniation) and other methods to reduce ICP have failed. If the $PaCO_2$ level is purposefully lowered to less than 35 mm Hg for an extended period, oxygen delivery at the cellular level should be evaluated with the use of a jugular venous bulb or cerebral tissue oxygen monitor.[11] Given the current evidence, $PaCO_2$ should be kept within a normal range, 35 to 45 mm Hg, except in rare situations. Hyperventilation should also be avoided when providing manual ventilation via a bag-valve-mask device.

Hyperosmolar therapy. Hyperosmolar agents are administered to reduce CBV by removing fluid from the brain's extracellular compartment. Hypertonic saline (in solutions ranging from 3% to 23% normal saline) and mannitol, an *osmotic diuretic,* draw water from the extracellular space to the plasma by creating an osmotic gradient, thereby decreasing ICP (Table 14.9). The effects

TABLE 14.9 PHARMACOLOGY

Frequently Used Medications in Nervous System Alterations

Medication	Actions/Use	Dose/Route	Side Effects	Nursing Implications
Hyperosmolar Agents				
Hypertonic Saline (3%, 23.4%)	Osmotic agent Pulls water from brain interstitium into plasma Used to treat ↑ ICP	Concentration % leads dosing *Intravenous*: Bolus, 3%, 2.5–5 mL/kg IV over 5–20 min or 250 mL IV over 30 min 23.4%, 30 mL IV over 10–20 min	Electrolyte disturbances Extravasation Osmotic demyelination syndrome	Neurological assessment every hour Monitor ICP, CPP, electrolytes (particularly sodium and chloride), Hold administration in patients with Na >155 mEq/L Central venous catheter preferred with higher concentrations and infusion rates
Mannitol	Osmotic diuretic Pulls water from brain interstitium into plasma Used to treat ↑ ICP	*Intravenous:* Bolus, 0.5–1.5 g/kg IV over 5–20 min q 4–6 h	Dehydration Electrolyte disturbances Extravasation Hypotension Nephrotoxicity Rebound cerebral edema/ increased ICP when used for an extended period Tachycardia	Neurological assessment every hour Monitor ICP, CPP, serum osmolality, electrolytes May crystalize at room temperature Use an in-line filter to administer

Continued

TABLE 14.9 PHARMACOLOGY—cont'd

Frequently Used Medications in Nervous System Alterations

Medication	Actions/Use	Dose/Route	Side Effects	Nursing Implications
Barbiturate Therapy				
Pentobarbital sodium (Nembutal)	Sedative, hypnotic agent Used to treat increased ICP	*Continuous infusion:* 10 mg/kg over 30 min, followed by 5 mg/kg/h x 3 h, then 1 mg/kg/h, titrate up to 4 mg/kg/h to maintain burst suppression	Hypotension Ileus Myocardial and respiratory depression Thrombocytopenia purpura	Monitor ICP, CPP, and hemodynamic responses Monitor pentobarbital levels when clinically indicated (e.g., prior to determining neuroprognostication) Continuous EEG monitoring is needed for continuous infusion titration
Antihypertensives				
Labetalol (Normodyne, Trandate)	Nonselective beta-blocker used to ↓ BP	*Intravenous:* IV Push, 10–20 mg IV over 2 min May repeat with 40–80 mg IV at 10-min intervals until desired BP is achieved *Continuous:* 2–8 mg/min IV Do not exceed 300 mg IV per 24 h	Bradycardia Bronchospasm Diaphoresis Flushing Hypoglycemia Hypotension Orthostatic hypotension Somnolence Weakness/fatigue	Monitor BP, HR May potentiate with calcium channel blockers
Nicardipine (Cardene)	Calcium channel blocker Used to decrease BP	*Continuous infusion:* Maintenance, 2.5–5 mg/h IV, titrate, max 15 mg/h IV	Confusion Flushing Headache Hypotension Nausea/vomiting Tachycardia	Monitor BP continuously Lower doses and slower titration required for persons with HF or impaired hepatic or renal function Administer through large peripheral vein or central line (venous irritant)
Calcium Channel Blocker for Vasospasm Prevention				
Nimodipine	Calcium channel blocker given to prevent vasospasm; reduces neurological deficits after aSAH	*Oral/Enteral:* 60 mg PO or via NG/OG tube q 4 h for 21 days; start within 96 h of aSAH	Bradycardia Headache Hypotension Nausea	Monitor VS
Benzodiazepines				
Diazepam (Valium)	Antiepileptic, sedative-hypnotic Anxiolytic	**Status epilepticus** *Intravenous:* 5–10 mg IV, may repeat in 3–5 min (alternative agent to lorazepam) *Rectal:* 0.2–0.5 mg/kg, max 20 mg PR (when IV access not present)	Drowsiness Hypotension Lethargy Respiratory depression	Monitor respiratory status, BP, HR Assess IV site for phlebitis Vesicant, do not administer through small veins
Lorazepam (Ativan)	Antiepileptic Sedative-hypnotic Anxiolytic	**Status epilepticus** *Intravenous:* Bolus, 0.1 mg/kg, administer 2 mg/min, maximum 4 mg May repeat in 3–5 min	Bradycardia Confusion Excessive drowsiness Hypotension Respiratory depression Somnolence	Monitor resp status, BP, HR

TABLE 14.9 **PHARMACOLOGY—cont'd**

Frequently Used Medications in Nervous System Alterations

Medication	Actions/Use	Dose/Route	Side Effects	Nursing Implications
Antiepileptics				
Fosphenytoin (Cerebyx)	Depresses seizure activity by altering ion transport in motor cortex	**Status epilepticus** *Intravenous:* Bolus, 10–20 mg PE/kg IV Administer each 100–150 mg PE over a minimum of 1 min	Drowsiness/fatigue Hypotension Nausea/vomiting Nystagmus/ataxia Rash Severe cardiovascular effects (e.g., bradycardia, heart block, ventricular tachycardia or fibrillation)	Slow infusion rate for bradycardia, hypotension, burning, itching, numbness, or pain along injection site Monitor ECG, BP, and pulse Monitor renal, hepatic, and hematological status Interacts with many medications
Levetiracetam (Keppra)	Depresses seizure activity Mechanism of action unknown May inhibit intracellular sodium influx in motor cortex	**Status epilepticus** *Intravenous:* Bolus, 60 mg/kg IV, maximum 4500 mg Maintenance, 500–1500 mg IV bid	CNS depression (e.g., drowsiness, fatigue, dizziness) Delayed hypersensitivity reactions Pancytopenia Psychosis Suicidal ideation	Adjust dose with acute kidney injury Monitor CBC Monitor for adverse changes in mental status
Phenytoin (Dilantin)	Depresses seizure activity by altering ion transport in motor cortex	**Status epilepticus** *Intravenous:* Initial, 10–20 mg/kg IV administer over 20–30 min Do not exceed a total dose of 2 g Maintenance, 100 mg IV over 2 min q 6–8 h	Blood dyscrasias Drowsiness/fatigue Gingival hyperplasia Hypotension Lymphadenopathy Nausea Nystagmus/ataxia Rash Severe cardiovascular effects (e.g., bradycardia, heart block, ventricular tachycardia or fibrillation) Stevens-Johnson syndrome	Slow infusion rate if bradycardia, hypotension, or cardiac dysrhythmias occur Monitor plasma phenytoin levels Monitor ECG, BP, pulse Monitor renal, hepatic, and hematological status Interacts with many medications

ABG, Arterial blood gas; *BP,* blood pressure; *CBC,* complete blood count; *CNS,* central nervous system; *CPP,* cerebral perfusion pressure; *ECG,* electrocardiogram; *EEG,* electroencephalogram; *HR,* heart rate; *I&O,* intake & output; *ICP,* intracranial pressure; *Na,* sodium; *NG,* nasogastric; *PE,* phenytoin equivalent; *OG,* orogastric; *PO,* orally; *q,* every; *RBCs,* red blood cells; a*SAH,* aneurysmal subarachnoid hemorrhage; *VS,* vital signs.
Adapted from Oh S, Delic JJ. Hyperosmolar therapy in the management of intracranial hypertension. *AACN Adv Crit Care.* 2022;33(1):5-10. https://doi.org/10.4037/aacnacc2022743; Collins SR. *Elsevier's 2023 Intravenous Medications.* 39th ed. St. Louis, MO: Elsevier; 2023; Kim D, Kim JM, Cho YW et al. Antiepileptic drug therapy for status epilepticus. *J Clin Neurol.* 2021;17(1):11-19. https://doi.org/10.3988/jcn.2021.17.1.11.

of decreasing ICP and increasing CPP occur within 15 to 30 minutes of administration. By increasing the serum osmolarity, osmotic diuretics rapidly expand the intravascular volume, then swiftly remove intravascular volume via their diuretic effects. This places the patient at risk for both volume overload and subsequent hypovolemia and hypotension. This fluctuation increases the risk for acute kidney injury as well as electrolyte imbalances. Another troubling side effect, more common with mannitol, is rebound elevation in ICP; avoiding prolonged therapy can mitigate this risk. Due to the mechanism of action for hyperosmolar agents, vital signs, volume status, electrolytes, renal function, and in the case of mannitol, serum osmolarity should be monitored closely.[14,24]

Optimal fluid administration. Fluid administration is provided to optimize MAP, maintain intravascular volume, and normalize CPP. Isotonic solution, 0.9% normal saline is recommended for volume resuscitation in TBI.[25] Hypotonic solutions, glucose-containing solutions and colloids are avoided to prevent an increase in cerebral edema.[26] Strict measurement of intake and output while monitoring serum sodium, potassium, and osmolarity is required. The goal is to keep serum osmolality at less than 320 mOsm/L. If needed, blood products are administered to restore volume and maintain adequate hematocrit and hemoglobin levels.[26] Hemodynamic monitoring may be used to optimize fluid administration.

Blood pressure management. BP must be carefully controlled in a patient with increased ICP. The MAP is usually kept between 70 and 90 mm Hg; however, it is critical to monitor the ICP and MAP collectively to sustain an adequate CPP of at least 60 to 70 mm Hg.[9] Hypotension decreases CBF, which leads to cerebral ischemia. When hypotension occurs or ICP cannot be reduced, manipulating the systolic BP with fluids and vasopressor medications may be necessary to achieve an adequate CPP. The goal is to reduce the risk of brain ischemia and tissue death; however, the risk versus benefit of maintaining tissue perfusion must be assessed. For example, a patient with an ICP of 30 mm Hg would need a MAP of at least 90 mm Hg to maintain a CPP of at least 60 mm Hg; this may not always be feasible or safe to achieve, depending on the patient's clinical condition and comorbidities. Multiprofessional collaboration is vital in such situations to determine appropriate and patient-specific cerebral hemodynamic goals.

Hypertension (>160 mm Hg systolic) can worsen cerebral edema by increasing microvascular pressure (ischemia or hemorrhage). However, hypertension may be necessary for adequate cerebral perfusion and appropriateness should be determined by the multiprofessional team. If CPP is not a concern, systolic BP can be lowered with antihypertensive medications (e.g., beta-blockers such as labetalol). Beta-blockers decrease the sympathetic response and catecholamine release associated with neurological injury. Some antihypertensive medications (e.g., nitroprusside, nitroglycerin) and some calcium channel blockers (e.g., verapamil, nifedipine) cause cerebral vasodilation, which increases CBF and causes increased ICP. Administration of these medications is avoided in patients with poor intracranial compliance. Nicardipine is a calcium channel blocker medication that does not affect cerebral vasculature; it is very effective in providing faster and tighter control of BP than other antihypertensive medications (Table 14.9).

Reducing metabolic demands. Several therapies may be required to reduce metabolic demands. These include temperature control, seizure prophylaxis, analgesia and sedation, and barbiturate therapy.

Temperature management. Fever increases oxygen demands, CBF, and ICP, which may lead to secondary brain damage. Therefore, it is vital to promptly recognize and treat fever in an effort to maintain normothermia in patients with neurological injuries. Pharmacological interventions such as antipyretics can be used to treat hyperthermia in this population.[27,28]

Targeted temperature management (TTM) is a treatment modality used to manage fever, maintain normothermia or induce therapeutic hypothermia. Body temperature may be controlled noninvasively with the use of a cooling blanket or skin pads placed in direct contact with the skin (external cooling) or invasively by using a catheter placed in a large vein (intravascular cooling). In the patient population with elevated ICP, TTM can be used to manage fever and maintain normothermia, especially when traditional therapies such as antipyretics are contraindicated or ineffective. The risks of shivering, which increases metabolic demands, must be considered.

Hypothermia decreases the cerebral metabolic rate and oxygen consumption and lowers the levels of glutamate and interleukin-1 (IL-1), therefore decreasing ICP and increasing CPP. In theory, therapeutic hypothermia would protect the brain; however, evidence does not support the use of hypothermia, as outcomes did not improve when compared to standard care or maintenance of normothermia. Further research is needed but may hold promise for patients with very elevated ICPs (≥30 mm Hg). Therapeutic hypothermia, also known as prophylactic hypothermia, increases the risk of cardiac dysrhythmias, hypokalemia, pneumonia, and coagulopathy[27,28]

Seizure prophylaxis. Patients with a brain disorder or injury are prone to seizures, which increase metabolic demands. Typically, seizure prophylaxis is initiated based on mechanism of injury, disease process, and the risk of developing seizures, as adverse effects can occur from prophylactic medications (i.e., phenytoin can impair cognition; carbamazepine can decrease sodium level and white blood cell count). Patients with elevated ICPs secondary to TBI or SAH may benefit the most from a short course of antiepileptic drug therapy.[29]

Analgesia and sedation. Administering analgesics and sedatives decreases ICP by reducing cerebral metabolic demand, pain, agitation, restlessness, and resistance to mechanical ventilation. Both analgesics and sedatives can be administered in frequent IV boluses or as a continuous infusion, based on the patient's needs. Common sedatives administered are benzodiazepines and propofol. Benzodiazepines do not affect CBF or ICP. Propofol, a sedative-hypnotic medication, reduces cerebral metabolism and ICP. Propofol is an ideal sedative, as it is short-acting with a rapid onset and rapid clearance, which allows for an improved neurological assessment. Use of propofol can cause a secondary effect of epileptic suppression.[29,30]

Though these are common medications used in this population, the pain and sedation regimen must be tailored to the patient based on their history and physical assessment. For example, liver or kidney injury may alter the regimen based on medication metabolism. Refer to Chapter 6, Comfort and Sedation for further information. BP must be closely monitored when analgesics and sedatives are used, as hypotension may be a side effect.

Neuromuscular blockade. Due to insufficient evidence, guidelines specific to sustained neuromuscular blockade (NMB) do not make recommendations for patients with acute brain injury with elevated ICP as to whether this intervention is beneficial to this population.[31] In patients with an elevated ICP secondary to TBI, administration of an NMB bolus "test dose" is recommended only when other interventions have failed (i.e., hyperosmolar therapy, analgesia, sedation, CSF drainage). If the patient's ICP responds to the bolus of NMB, then a continuous infusion may be considered.[32]

Barbiturate therapy. Through suppression of the cerebral metabolism, barbiturate therapy (i.e., pentobarbital) can improve ICP and reduce CBV. Though effective at lower ICPs, there is no evidence to support that barbiturate therapy improves outcomes. In fact, the BP lowering side effect of barbiturate therapy may offset any ICP benefit in one in four patients.[33] Even with the lack of demonstrated benefit, barbiturate therapy is still recommended as salvage therapy for elevated ICP secondary to TBI (Table 14.9).[32] If this therapy is used, continuous bedside EEG should be initiated to monitor and titrate barbiturate therapy based on a burst suppression goal established by the multiprofessional team. Burst suppression is an EEG waveform that vacillates between high-power, broad spectrum oscillations and isoelectricity.

Surgical Interventions

Surgical intervention may be required to remove a mass or lesion that is causing the increased ICP. Surgery may involve the removal of infarcted areas or hematomas (epidural, subdural, or intracerebral). Decompressive hemicraniectomy is occasionally performed for severe brain injury or large-volume stroke. The cranial bone is removed, and the dura is opened to create more space for edematous tissue. Protection of the patient's brain from trauma during repositioning, hygiene activities, and out-of-bed mobility is imperative when there is missing bone.

CHECK YOUR UNDERSTANDING

2. The nurse is caring for a patient with an ICP of 23 mm Hg, sustained for 7 minutes. Which of the following interventions should the nurse initiate first?
   A. Continue to wait, as this is not a sustained ICP elevation.
   B. Elevate the head of bed to 30 degrees and ensure the head and neck are midline.
   C. Administer an intermittent IV push of analgesic.
   D. Administer 3% hypertonic saline, as ordered.

TRAUMATIC BRAIN INJURY

TBI is a common occurrence in the United States. TBIs resulted in 69,473 deaths in 2021 and hospitalization of 214,110 individuals in 2020. Males are about three times as likely as females to die from a TBI. The highest incidences of TBI occur in persons aged 75 years and older. Survival after TBI is dependent on prompt emergency treatment and focused management of primary and secondary injuries.[34] The severity of traumatic brain injury is classified by the patient's GCS score, duration of loss of consciousness, and any associated signs and symptoms (Table 14.10).

Pathophysiology

Traumatic injury can result in damage to the scalp, skull, meninges, and brain, including neuronal pathways, cranial nerves, and intracranial vessels. The extent of TBI can range from mild to severe. Injuries may be open or closed. With an open injury, the scalp is torn, bone may be exposed, and the fracture can extend into the sinuses or middle ear. The meninges can also be penetrated, presenting as pneumocephalus or a CSF leak, increasing the risk of infection.[35]

A closed TBI occurs when there is no break in the scalp. Acceleration-deceleration is a common mechanism for TBI. With this injury, the movement of the head follows a straight line, and the moving head (acceleration) hits a stationary object (deceleration). Rotation or a twisting of the brain within the cranial vault adds to the insult and often leads to the development of a diffuse axonal injury (DAI).[35] Genetics may play a role in both injury and recovery (see Genetics box).

Skull Fractures. The skull has high compressive strength and is somewhat elastic. After impact, there is an in-bending of the skull at the point of impact and an out-bending at the vertex. The area of out-bending creates a fracture line that moves toward the base of the skull. There are several types of skull fractures—linear, depressed, and comminuted—and various locations of the fractures (Fig. 14.13).

Linear skull fracture. A linear fracture is the most common type of skull fracture. This fracture usually does not lead to significant complications unless there is an extension of the fracture to the orbit, to the sinus, or across a vessel. If there is extension of the fracture, the patient is admitted for observation of signs of intracranial bleeding and epidural hematoma, as well as follow-up imaging.

Linear fractures at the skull base are termed *basilar fractures*. This type of fracture is difficult to confirm on a skull radiographic study and is diagnosed clinically. Battle sign (bruising behind the ear) and the presence of "raccoon eyes" (bilateral periorbital edema and bruising) may be indicative of a basilar skull fracture (Fig. 14.14). Dural tears are very common with a basilar skull fracture and may lead to meningitis. Drainage of CSF from the nose (rhinorrhea), postnasal drainage, or drainage of CSF from the ear (otorrhea) may indicate a dural tear. With otorrhea, patients may complain of decreased hearing. Blood encircled by a yellowish stain on a dressing or bed linens, called the *halo sign*, usually indicates CSF. If CSF is suspected in the drainage, a sample of the drainage is sent to the laboratory for analysis (i.e., beta-2 transferrin). In the event of a CSF leak, it is important to allow the CSF to flow freely. Nothing should be placed in

TABLE 14.10 Traumatic Brain Injury Severity

Severity of TBI	Mild	Moderate	Severe
GCS	13–15	9–12	3–8
Signs/symptoms	Disorientation Amnesia Transient loss of consciousness	Confusion Somnolence Focal neurological deficits (i.e., hemiparesis)	Coma Unable to follow commands

TBI, Traumatic brain injury; *GCS*, Glasgow Coma Scale.
Adapted from Greenberg MS. *Handbook of Neurosurgery*. 9th ed. New York, NY: Thieme Medical Publishers; 2020.

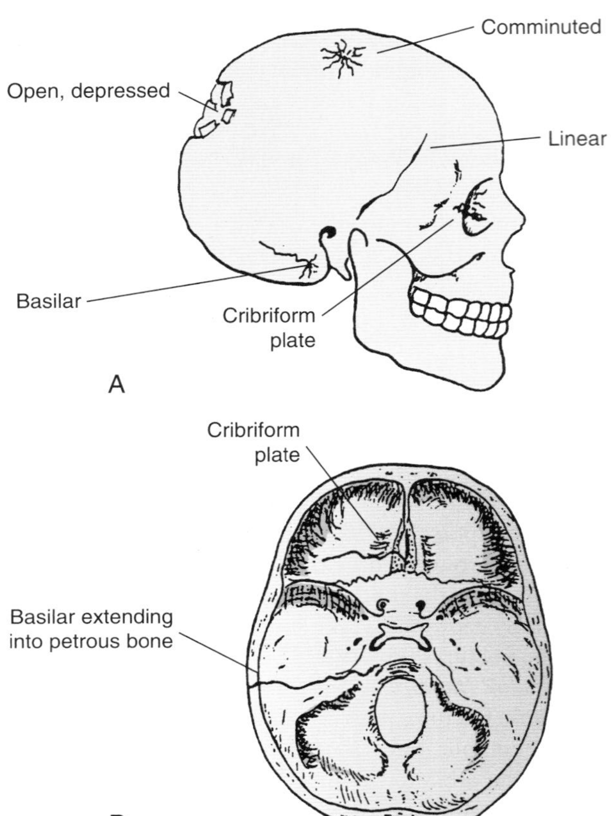

Fig. 14.13 Types of skull fractures. A, Linear; open, depressed; basilar; and comminuted fractures. B, View of the base of skull with fractures. (From Barker E. *Neuroscience Nursing: A Spectrum of Care*. 3rd ed. St. Louis, MO: Mosby; 2008.)

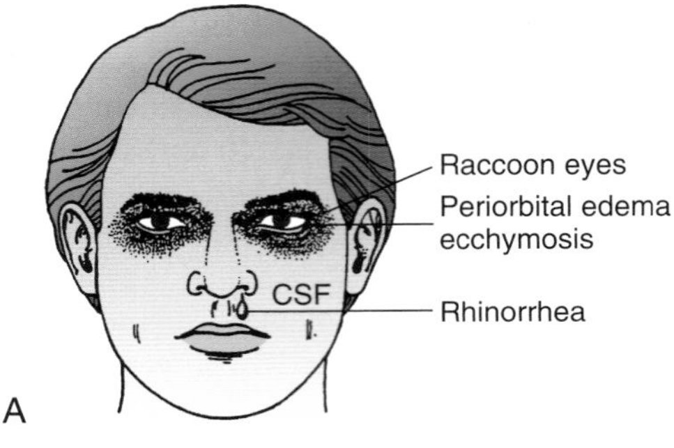

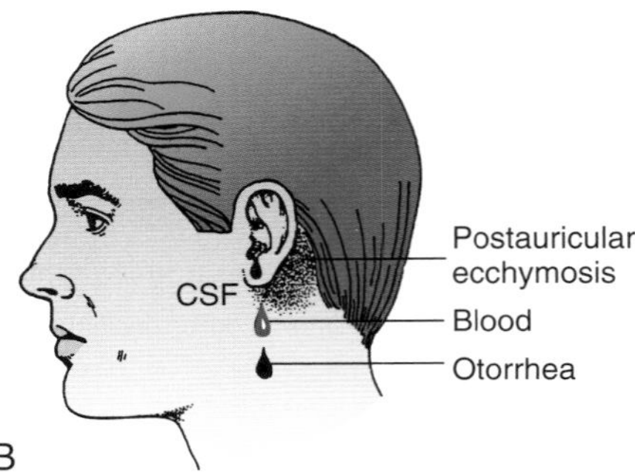

Fig. 14.14 A, Raccoon eyes, rhinorrhea. B, Battle sign with otorrhea. *CSF,* Cerebrospinal fluid. (From Barker E. *Neuroscience Nursing: A Spectrum of Care*. 3rd ed. St. Louis, MO: Mosby; 2008.)

the nose or ear, although small bandages under the nose or around the ear can be used to collect the drainage. Instruct the patient to avoid blowing their nose. Insert tubes (e.g., gastric tubes, suction catheters, endotracheal tubes) through the mouth rather than through the nose to avoid penetrating the brain through the dural tear.

Depressed skull fracture. A depressed skull fracture occurs when the outer table of the skull is depressed below the inner table of the surrounding intact skull. The dura may be intact, bruised, or torn. If the scalp is lacerated, and the dura is torn, there is direct communication between the brain and the environment, and meningitis can occur. In addition, the compressed and bruised brain beneath the depressed bone, or bone lodged in brain parenchyma, can be the source of focal neurological deficits.

Comminuted skull fracture. A comminuted skull fracture occurs when there are multiple linear fractures with a depressed area at the site of impact. The fracture radiates away from the impact site. A comminuted skull fracture is referred to as an "eggshell fracture" because of the appearance of the skull. Risks are similar to those occurring with a depressed fracture.

Brain Injury. TBI is classified as primary or secondary. Primary brain injury can be further divided into focal lesions (i.e., concussions, contusions, hematomas, penetrating injuries) and diffuse lesions (i.e., DAI).

Primary brain injury. Primary brain injury is a direct injury that occurs to the brain from an impact. With impact, the semisolid brain moves around inside the skull. The area under the direct impact is injured *(coup injury).* Injury distal to the site of impact can occur as the brain moves inside the skull *(contrecoup injury).* The stretching, shearing, rotational, and tearing forces that result from impact interrupt normal neuronal pathways. Concussion, contusion, penetrating injuries, DAI, and hematomas are all types of primary brain injury. Secondary brain injury may occur because of biochemical consequences of the primary injury (Fig. 14.15).

Concussion. Concussion occurs when a mechanical force of short duration is applied to the skull. This injury results in the temporary failure of impulse conduction. The neurological deficits are reversible and are generally mild. Patients may lose consciousness for a few seconds at the time of injury, but lasting effects are not common. Concussions are not diagnosed from imaging alone, but rather based on suspicion from clinical exam. Signs and symptoms can include amnesia, confusion, disorientation, personality changes, nausea and vomiting, headache, photophobia, sensitivity to sound, and fatigue.[35]

Contusion. Contusion is the result of coup and contrecoup injuries accompanied by bruising and bleeding into brain tissue. Lacerations of the cortical (outer) surface associated with contrecoup injuries may be greater than those seen

GENETICS

Traumatic Brain Injury

A condition is referred to as a *multifactorial* disorder when there is a complex interaction of genes with the environment and lifestyle or behaviors. One example of a multifactorial disorder is traumatic brain injury (TBI). For example, a concussion is a mild brain injury that manifests in various symptoms with a trajectory of recovery that is variable and unpredictable.[1] Individual disease manifestation and recovery differences are not explained by injury severity or type, patient characteristics like age and ethnicity, or the biochemical alterations that occur immediately postinjury. *Precision medicine* looks globally at gene-gene, gene-environment, gene-lifestyle, and gene-environment-lifestyle interactions to build knowledge around TBI pathophysiology and treatment.[2] For example, *single nucleotide polymorphisms (SNP)* in genes for neurotransmitter production and metabolism in the CNS may contribute to patient outcomes, including neuropsychiatric outcomes and behaviors, following TBI.[3]

Neuroregenerative genetic variations affect the repair and plasticity or growth of neurons. Apolipoprotein E (APOE) is the most studied variant in this category. Patients with an *APOE-4* allele are more likely to have an unfavorable outcome after severe TBI. Patients who are *homozygous* for *APOE-4* have the greatest disability following TBI.[2] The *APOE-4* allele is associated with prolonged complications from repeated mild brain injuries resulting in chronic traumatic encephalopathy.[2]

Brain-derived neurotrophic factor (BDNF) promotes neuronal survival and axon regeneration. Variations in BDNF synthesis by glial cells may modulate neuronal damage and the subsequent cognitive and mental health recovery following TBI.[3] This type of genetic finding illustrates the importance of glial cells in brain injury and recovery.

Mitochondrial DNA (mtDNA) may also contribute to TBI severity and recovery.[4] Mitochondria generate cell energy, regulate the cell cycle and differentiation, support and provide cell signaling and calcium storage, and signal apoptosis. Disturbance in the mitochondrial network is implicated in many neurodegenerative diseases. It may be that the changes in energy substrates—small molecules produced by mitochondria and other cells—mitigate or enhance secondary brain injury after trauma.[4]

Proteomic studies in patients with TBI have contributed to diagnostic investigations.[5] For example, SB-100 is recognized as a biomarker associated with TBI severity.[6] The pathological disruption of the blood-brain barrier following injury allows proteins in the cerebrospinal fluid to transfer into the plasma. Additional serum biomarkers for moderate and severe TBI may provide new opportunities to evaluate treatment, predict health outcomes, and establish precision medicine for this multifactorial condition.

References

1. Center for Disease Control and Prevention. *CDC Heads Up*. https://www.cdc.gov/headsup/index.html. [Updated Feb 25, 2022]. Accessed December 18, 2023.
2. Reddi S, Thakker-Varia S, Alder J, Giarratana AO. Status of precision medicine approaches to traumatic brain injury. *Neural Regen Res*. 2022;17(10):2166–2171. https://doi.org/10.4103/1673-5374.335824.
3. Zeiler FA, McFadyen C, Newcombe VFJ, et al. Genetic influences on patient-oriented outcomes in traumatic brain injury: a living systematic review of non-apolipoprotein E single-nucleotide polymorphisms. *J Neurotrauma*. 2021;38(8):1107–1123. https://doi.org/10.1089/neu.2017.5583.
4. Singh LN, Kao SH, Wallace DC. Unlocking the complexity of mitochondrial DNA: a key to understanding neurodegenerative disease caused by injury. *Cells*. 2021;10(12):3460. https://doi.org/10.3390/cells10123460.
5. O'Connell GC, Smothers CG, Gandhi SA. Newly-identified blood biomarkers of neurological damage are correlated with infarct volume in patients with acute ischemic stroke. *J Clin Neurosci*. 2021;94:107–113. https://doi.org/10.1016/j.jocn.2021.10.015.
6. Habli Z, Kobeissy F, Khraiche ML. Advances in point-of-care platforms for traumatic brain injury: recent developments in diagnostics. *Rev Neurosci*. 2022;33(3):327–345. https://doi.org/10.1515/revneuro-2021-0103.

Chris Winkelman, PhD, ACNP-BC, CCRN, CNE, FAANP, FCCM

Genetic terms: *precision medicine, single nucleotide polymorphism (SNP), mitochondrial DNA (mtDNA), allele, proteomics, metabolomics, precision medicine, multifactorial.*

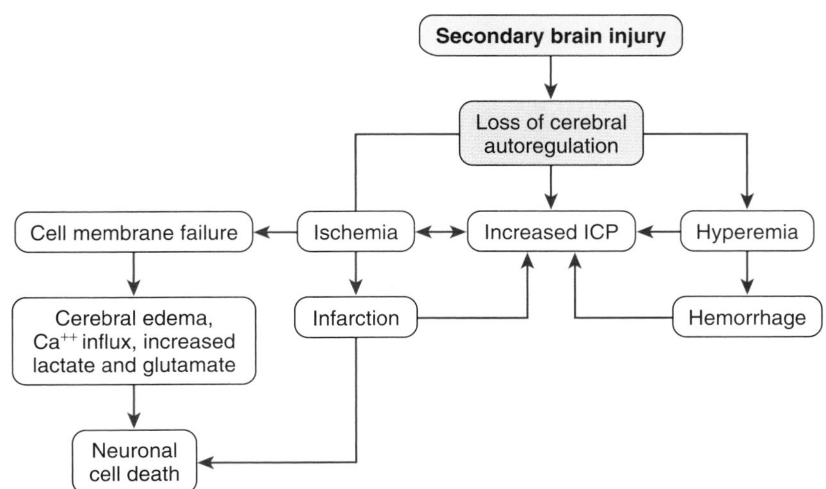

Fig. 14.15 Pathophysiology of secondary brain injury. *Ca^{++}*, Calcium; *ICP*, intracranial pressure.

directly under the point of impact (scalp). Signs and symptoms are variable, depending on the location and extent of bleeding. Contusions require close radiographic monitoring and frequent neurological assessments. These injuries may also require ICP monitoring due to the likelihood of an abnormal neurological exam, use of mechanical ventilation requiring sedation, and swelling from the secondary injury that can occur days after the initial trauma.[9]

Diffuse axonal injury. A more global brain injury is DAI. With this injury, widespread white matter axonal damage occurs secondary to rotational and shearing forces. This type of injury is associated with disruption of axons

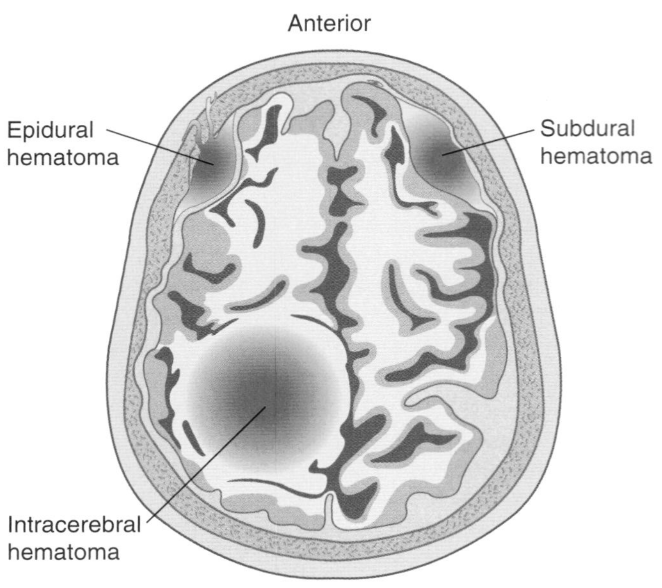

Fig. 14.16 Types of hematomas. (From Rogers J. *McCance and Huether's Pathophysiology: The Biologic Basis for Disease in Adults and Children.* 9th ed. St. Louis, MO: Elsevier; 2024.)

in the cerebral hemispheres, diencephalon, and brainstem. This injury results in vasodilation and increased CBV that precipitates increased ICP. Signs and symptoms are variable, and prognosis is poor.

Penetrating injury. Penetrating injuries are the result of low- or high-velocity forces such as those from gunshots, knives, or sharp objects. With this type of injury, there is a deep laceration of brain tissue and possible damage to the ventricular system. A low-velocity (stabbing) injury is limited to the tract of entry, and the greatest concern is bleeding and infection. A high-velocity (gunshot) injury causes extensive damage because of the entry of bone fragments at the site. In addition, because bullets spin irregularly, they create many paths and shock waves that cause extensive brain damage.

Hematoma. Acute hematomas can be life-threatening. There are three types of hematomas: epidural, subdural, and intracerebral (Fig. 14.16).

Epidural hematoma. Collection of blood in the potential space between the inner table of the skull and the dura causes an *epidural hematoma.* This hematoma is typically associated with a linear fracture of the temporal bone and results from tearing of the middle meningeal artery. Arterial blood accumulates rapidly in this space. The patient typically experiences a brief loss of consciousness followed by a lucid period before neurological deterioration. The lucid period can last for a few hours to 48 hours. As the patient's condition deteriorates, the LOC decreases, contralateral deficits appear, and the pupil on the side of the lesion *(ipsilateral)* becomes fixed and dilated.

Subdural hematoma. Collection of blood in the subdural space causes a *subdural hematoma.* It occurs when a surface vein is torn around the cerebral cortex. There are three kinds of subdural hematomas: acute, subacute, and chronic. *Acute subdural hematoma* occurs within 48 hours of an injury. Symptoms can begin with headache, restlessness, and confusion, then progress to loss of consciousness, changes in respiratory pattern, and pupillary dilation as the ICP increases and CPP decreases.[35] It is almost always seen with cortical or brainstem injury and represents a mass (space-occupying) lesion. The risk of death is high because of injury to brain tissue and the mass effect caused by an expanding hematoma within a short time frame. Surgical intervention occurring within 4 hours after the injury improves the mortality risk.[9] Symptoms of a *subacute subdural hematoma* occur anywhere from 48 hours to 2 weeks after an injury. The onset of symptoms is later because the hematoma grows slowly. A *chronic subdural hematoma* occurs as a result of a low-velocity impact. Symptoms occur from 2 weeks to several months after an injury. A higher incidence of chronic subdural hematomas is seen in the elderly, those with chronic alcohol use disorder, and those taking anticoagulants, aspirin, or antiplatelet medications. The patient may complain of a headache and appear to have progressive dementia.[35] Because symptoms are often subtle, the diagnosis of chronic subdural hematoma is frequently missed.

Intracerebral hematoma. A traumatic intracerebral hematoma is a hemorrhage into brain tissue that creates a mass lesion. This lesion can occur anywhere in the brain. It can be caused by penetrating injuries, deep depressed skull fractures, or extension of a contusion. Signs and symptoms vary according to the location of the lesion and extent of hemorrhage.

Secondary brain injury. Secondary brain injury occurs as a consequence of the initial head trauma. It is characterized by an inflammatory response and release of cytokines from macrophages, causing increased vascular permeability of the blood vessel wall, which leads to vasogenic cerebral edema. A series of events also contribute to the overproduction of oxygen radicals that disrupt the cellular membrane, impair cellular metabolism, and cause neuronal deterioration (Fig. 14.15). Decreased cerebral perfusion from hypoxia, infection, and/or fluid and electrolyte imbalances contribute to secondary brain injury. These insults add to the degree and extent of cellular dysfunction after TBI, increase the extent of brain damage, and affect functional recovery. Proper management minimizes the effects of secondary brain injury, as even a single episode of hypoxia or hypotension can negatively impact patient outcomes.

Assessment

The GCS (Fig. 14.7) is used as a guide in assessing a patient with a TBI. The assessment is supplemented with a thorough neurological examination specific to the area of the brain involved. Assessment of airway and oxygenation status is essential to ensure adequate oxygenation and CBF. Patients may not be able to safely clear their airway in the setting of brain insult or injury, increasing the risk of aspiration. Report and document abnormal respiratory patterns because pattern changes usually indicate deterioration in neurological status. Additional assessment data include ICP, CPP, and hemodynamic monitoring. A patient with a TBI requires the same laboratory and diagnostic studies as a patient with increased ICP.

Patient Problems

The same collaborative care plan for a patient with increased ICP is applicable for a patient with TBI (see Plan of Care for the Patient with Traumatic Brain Injury, Increased Intracranial Pressure, or Acute Stroke earlier in this chapter and the Collaborative Care Plan found in Chapter 1, Overview of Critical Care Nursing). These patient problems cover both primary and secondary head injuries. Additional patient problems include dysphagia and potential for aspiration, fever, headache, constipation, fluid imbalance, altered functional ability, malnutrition, and communication barriers.

Medical and Nursing Interventions

The treatment of a patient with a TBI is the same as for a patient with increased ICP. The emphasis is on reducing ICP and preventing secondary brain injury by maintaining the airway, providing adequate oxygenation, maintaining cerebral perfusion, and reducing metabolic demands. Additional priorities include special considerations for nutrition, as well as specific guidelines for venous thromboembolism (VTE) and seizure prophylaxis.

Nutrition. Nutritional support after TBI is essential. Hypermetabolism, accelerated catabolism, and excess nitrogen losses are responses to TBI. These responses result in depletion of energy stores, loss of lean muscle mass, reduced protein synthesis, loss of gastrointestinal mucosal integrity, and immune compromise. Nutritional support decreases susceptibility to infections, promotes wound healing, and facilitates weaning from mechanical ventilation.[36]

Venous Thromboembolism Prophylaxis. Patients with severe TBI are at high risk for the development of VTE due to their hypercoagulable state and immobility.[37] Early initiation of mechanical prophylaxis is appropriate for the majority of patients; however, chemoprophylaxis is preferred, given the reduction in VTE risk.[37] Low-molecular-weight heparin is safe to initiate after 24 to 72 hours if the head injury is considered stable and the risks of hematoma expansion are sufficiently low.[32]

Seizure Prophylaxis. Seizure prophylaxis with antiepilepic medication is typically initiated within 7 days of injury to decrease the incidence of early posttraumatic seizures (PTS). Risk factors for PTS include loss of consciousness for more than 30 minutes, patients older than 65 years of age, chronic alcohol use, skull fractures, and patients with penetrating brain injury.[9] Phenytoin is the most commonly used antiepilepic medication and the one most extensively studied for patients with TBI.[38] Levetiracetam is a newer antiepilepic medication with fewer side effects and drug interactions when compared to phenytoin and a similar efficacy. Current guidelines do not recommend one medication over another.[9]

Surgical Interventions

Various surgical procedures exist to treat TBI. A depressed skull fracture may require surgery to elevate and repair or remove bone fragments. Craniotomy is used to evacuate epidural and acute subdural hematomas to prevent herniation. Burr holes are an alternative to craniotomy used for acute subdural hematomas to relieve pressure on the brain. Penetrating wounds to the skull and brain may necessitate a craniotomy to explore the pathway of the missile, repair lacerations of intracranial vessels and brain tissue, remove bone fragments, or retrieve a foreign body such as a bullet. There will be times when surgery is not feasible due to the location of the injury or because the risk of further harm is greater than the ability to reduce the trauma.

Postoperative goals include sustaining normal ICP and CPP, maintaining the airway and ventilation, preventing fluid and electrolyte imbalances, preventing complications of immobility, avoiding nutritional deficits, and reducing the incidence of infection.

The craniotomy dressing is assessed for drainage color, odor, and amount. Once the dressing is removed, assess the incision for swelling, redness, drainage, and tenderness. Persistent CSF drainage from the wound after surgery may indicate a dural tear. If a tear is present, a lumbar drain or ventriculostomy may be required for several days to decrease pressure at the surgical site and to aid in healing. A craniotomy may be necessary to repair the dura if leakage persists. Patients with penetrating wounds to the brain are at high risk for the development of infections and brain abscesses.

CLINICAL JUDGMENT ACTIVITY

The family of a patient with a severe TBI is preparing to visit the patient for the first time. How can the nurse prepare the family for a successful visit with the patient? Discuss what assessments can assist the nurse in evaluating the patient's tolerance of visitation.

ACUTE STROKE

Stroke is a major public health problem and a leading cause of death and disability in the United States. Although many strokes are preventable by controlling major risk factors, such as hypertension, more than 610,000 new strokes and 185,000 recurrent strokes occur each year in the United States. The cost of hospitalization, rehabilitation, long-term care, and lost wages from stroke is estimated at $53 billion annually.[39] Stroke results in infarction of a focal area of the brain. Early recognition of the signs and symptoms (i.e., facial droop, arm weakness, speech difficulties) is essential to preserve blood flow to the brain. A stroke should be assessed and treated as a life-threatening emergency, because optimal early treatment improves long-term outcomes.[40]

Stroke occurs when the blood supply to the brain is disturbed by occlusion (ischemia) or hemorrhage. The hallmark of stroke is the sudden onset of focal neurological symptoms associated with changes in blood flow to the brain resulting from either a blockage of flow or hemorrhage. Stroke can manifest with maximal focal neurological deficits or as stroke in evolution, in which symptoms evolve over several hours. The definition of stroke includes neurological deficits lasting 24 hours or longer. Although symptoms may completely resolve, CT or MRI will show evidence of permanent damage to the cerebral tissue.

Early identification of a stroke is vital so that rapid treatment can be initiated. The public must be educated on the symptoms of a stroke because early intervention can minimize stroke deficits. Patients at high risk of stroke are taught risk reduction, the signs and symptoms of stroke, and to seek medical attention immediately (Clinical Alert box). Specialized stroke centers improve patient outcomes. The stroke center concept is designed to expedite evaluation and management of suspected ischemic stroke, transient ischemic attack (TIA), and intracerebral hemorrhage (ICH). A stroke center is equipped with an emergency department; a stroke team of physicians, nurses, and allied professionals with stroke-specific training; treatment protocols; emergent neuroradiology services; and access to neurosurgical services.[40]

! CLINICAL ALERT

- Weakness or numbness of one side of the body (i.e., face, arm, leg, or any combination of these)
- Slurred speech or an inability to comprehend what is being said
- Visual disturbance, such as transient loss of vision in one or both eyes, double vision, or a visual field deficit
- Dizziness, incoordination, ataxia, or vertigo
- Sudden-onset, severe headache (e.g., "worst headache of my life")

Assessment

The neurological examination includes evaluation of mental status (i.e., LOC, arousal, orientation), cranial nerve function, motor strength, sensory function, neglect, coordination, and deep tendon reflexes. The full baseline neurological examination may be obtained by the provider to help locate where the stroke originated in the brain; however, the nurse also obtains a neurological exam for the purposes of stroke scoring. The National Institutes of Health Stroke Scale (NIHSS) is used to assess the severity of the presenting signs and symptoms, especially in the patient with an ischemic stroke who may be a candidate for thrombolytic therapy (Table 14.11).[40] Assessment and stabilization of the airway, breathing, and circulation are a priority, as with all acute neurological conditions. Fluctuations in the respiratory pattern can indicate that the stroke is extending and more neurological damage is occurring; this would include irregular breathing and snoring. Cardiac assessment, including the presence of cardiac dysrhythmias (i.e., consistent or transient irregularities, specifically atrial fibrillation), is important to determine whether the stroke was potentially caused by a cardioembolic event. Of priority, IV access is obtained, and a 0.9% normal saline infusion is started. Obtain a serum glucose level because many patients who present with stroke are hyperglycemic, and approximately 30% of patients with stroke are diabetic.[41]

Older adult patients presenting with stroke are often dehydrated secondary to an age-related decreased thirst perception causing inadequate water intake, drowsiness, dysphagia, possible infection, diuretic use, or uncontrolled diabetes. Dehydration after a stroke can cause an increased hematocrit and a reduced BP that can worsen the ischemic process.[1]

TABLE 14.11 National Institutes of Health Stroke Scale

Instructions	Scale	Definition
1a. **Level of Consciousness (LOC):** The investigator must choose a response if a full evaluation is prevented by such obstacles as an endotracheal tube, language barrier, or orotracheal trauma or bandages.	0	**Alert;** keenly responsive
	1	**Not alert** but arousable by minor stimulation
	2	**Not alert;** requires repeated stimulation to attend
	3	**Responds** only with reflex motor or autonomic effects, or totally unresponsive, flaccid, and areflexic
1b. **LOC Questions:** The patient is asked the month and his or her age. The answer must be correct—there is no partial credit for being close.	0	**Answers** both questions correctly
	1	**Answers** one question correctly
	2	**Answers** neither question correctly
1c. **LOC Commands:** The patient is asked to open and close the eyes and then to grip and release the nonparetic hand. Substitute another one-step command if the hands cannot be used.	0	**Performs** both tasks correctly
	1	**Performs** one task correctly
	2	**Performs** neither task correctly
2. **Best Gaze:** Only horizontal eye movements are tested. Voluntary or reflexive (oculocephalic) eye movements are scored, but caloric testing is not done.	0	**Normal**
	1	**Partial gaze palsy;** gaze is abnormal in one or both eyes
	2	**Forced deviation,** or total gaze paresis not overcome by the oculocephalic maneuver
3. **Visual:** Visual fields (upper and lower quadrants) are tested by confrontation, using finger counting or visual threat as appropriate.	0	**No visual loss**
	1	**Partial hemianopia**
	2	**Complete hemianopia**
	3	**Bilateral hemianopia** (blind)

Continued

TABLE 14.11 National Institutes of Health Stroke Scale—cont'd

Instructions	Scale	Definition
4. **Facial Palsy:** Ask—or use pantomime to encourage—the patient to show teeth or raise eyebrows and close eyes.	0	**Normal** symmetric movements
	1	**Minor paralysis** (asymmetry on smiling)
	2	**Partial paralysis** (total or near-total paralysis of lower face)
	3	**Complete paralysis** of one or both sides
5. **Motor Arm:** The limb is placed in the appropriate position: extend the arms (palms down) 90 degrees if sitting or 45 degrees if supine. Drift is scored if the arm falls before 10 seconds. 5a. Left arm 5b. Right arm	0	**No drift;** limb holds position for 10 seconds
	1	**Drift;** limb holds position but drifts down before full 10 seconds
	2	**Some effort against gravity;** limb cannot get to or maintain position, drifts down to bed, has some effort against gravity
	3	**No effort against gravity;** limb falls
	4	**No movement**
	UN	**Amputation** or joint fusion
6. **Motor Leg:** The limb is placed in the appropriate position: hold the leg at 30 degrees (always tested supine). Drift is scored if the leg falls before 5 seconds. 6a. Left leg 6b. Right leg	0	**No drift;** leg holds position for full 5 seconds
	1	**Drift;** leg falls by the end of the 5-sec period but does not hit bed
	2	**Some effort against gravity;** leg falls to bed. By 5 seconds, has some effort against gravity
	3	**No effort against gravity;** leg falls to bed immediately
	4	**No movement**
	UN	**Amputation** or joint fusion
7. **Limb Ataxia:** The finger-nose-finger and heel-shin tests are performed on both sides with eyes open.	0	**Absent**
	1	**Present in one limb**
	2	**Present in two limbs**
	UN	**Amputation** or joint fusion
8. **Sensory:** Sensation or grimace to pinprick when tested or withdrawal from noxious stimulus in the obtunded or aphasic patient	0	**Normal;** no sensory loss
	1	**Mild to moderate sensory loss;** feels that pinprick is less sharp or is dull on the affected side, or there is a loss of superficial pain with pinprick but awareness of being touched
	2	**Severe to total sensory loss;** patient is not aware of being touched in the face, arm, or leg
9. **Best Language:** Using items from the published scale, patient is asked to describe what is happening in a picture, to name the items on a naming sheet list, and to read from a set of sentences. Comprehension is judged from responses as well as responses to all of the commands in the preceding general neurological examination.	0	**No aphasia;** normal
	1	**Mild to moderate aphasia;** some obvious loss of fluency or facility of comprehension, without significant limitation on ideas
	2	**Severe aphasia;** all communication is through fragmentary expression; great need for inference, questioning, and guessing by the listener
	3	**Mute, global aphasia;** no usable speech or auditory comprehension
10. **Dysarthria:** An adequate sample of speech must be obtained by asking the patient to read or repeat words from the published list.	0	**Normal**
	1	**Mild to moderate dysarthria;** patient slurs some words; can be understood with some difficulty
	2	**Severe dysarthria;** patient's speech is so slurred as to be unintelligible; or patient is mute/anarthric
	UN	**Intubated** or other physical barrier
11. **Extinction and Inattention (Formerly Neglect):** Sufficient information to identify neglect may have been obtained during prior testing. If the patient has a severe visual loss preventing visual bilateral simultaneous stimulation and the cutaneous stimuli are normal, the score is normal.	0	No abnormality
	1	**Visual, tactile, auditory, spatial, or personal inattention** or extinction to bilateral simultaneous stimulation in one of the sensory modalities
	2	**Profound hemi-inattention or extinction to more than one modality;** does not recognize own hand or orients to only one side of space

LOC, Level of consciousness.
From National Institute of Neurological Disorders and Stroke, National Institutes of Health. NIH Stroke Scale. http://www.nihstrokescale.org/. Published 1999. Accessed December 18, 2023.

Once the patient has been transferred to the critical care unit, neurological assessments are compared with the baseline assessments performed upon identification of the stroke symptoms. If changes are noted, follow-up imaging is warranted. Hemodynamic instability is common in acute stroke because of cardiac disorders and the sympathetic response caused by the brain insult; therefore, assessment of the airway, vital signs, cardiac function, and fluid and electrolyte status continues to be a priority. Ongoing assessments of patients with acute stroke are similar to those of patients with increased ICP.

Diagnostic Tests

Diagnostic tests are performed to differentiate ischemic from hemorrhagic stroke and to establish baseline parameters to monitor the effects of treatment.[2] Common diagnostic tests are summarized in Box 14.1.

BOX 14.1 Diagnostic Testing for Stroke

Initial Diagnostic Testing

- Emergency head CT scan without contrast
- 12-Lead electrocardiogram
- Review the time of onset and inclusion criteria for patients eligible for rt-PA, including NIHSS assessment
- **Complete blood count:** red blood cells, hemoglobin, hematocrit, platelet count
- **Coagulation studies:** PT/INR, aPTT
- Serum electrolytes and glucose
- Urinalysis
- Troponin and cardiac enzymes, to rule out myocardial infarction

Additional Diagnostic Testing

- **Arteriography (diagnostic cerebral angiogram):** detects shallow ulcerated plaques, thrombus, aneurysms, dissections, multiple lesions, AVM, and collateral blood flow
- **CT perfusion images:** detects altered CBF and CBV
- **CT angiography images:** detects carotid occlusion and intracranial stenosis or occlusions
- **Digital subtraction angiography:** detects carotid occlusion and intracranial stenoses or occlusions
- **Doppler carotid ultrasound:** detects stenosis or occlusions of the carotid arteries
- **MRA images:** detects carotid occlusion and intracranial stenosis or occlusions
- **MRI with diffusion and perfusion images:** detects ischemia, altered CBF, and CBV
- **Transcranial Doppler ultrasound:** detects stenosis or occlusion of the circle of Willis, vertebral arteries, and basilar artery
- **Transthoracic echocardiography:** detects cardioembolic abnormalities
- **Transesophageal echocardiography:** detects cardioembolic abnormalities; more sensitive than transthoracic echocardiography

aPTT, Activated partial thromboplastin time; *AVM,* arteriovenous malformation; *CBF,* cerebral blood flow; *CBV,* cerebral blood volume; *CT,* computed tomography; *INR,* international normalized ratio; *MRA,* magnetic resonance angiography; *MRI,* magnetic resonance imaging; *NIHSS,* National Institutes of Health Stroke Scale; *PT,* prothrombin time; *rt-PA,* recombinant tissue plasminogen activator.

Patient Problems

A patient with stroke has a collaborative care plan similar to those of patients with increased ICP and TBI. Refer to this chapter's Plan of Care for the Patient with Traumatic Brain Injury, Increased Intracranial Pressure, or Acute Stroke.

Stroke Types

Stroke etiology presents as either ischemic or hemorrhagic, meaning either occlusion of a blood vessel perfusing the brain or a mass lesion caused by a bleeding blood vessel within the brain, respectively. Though there can be similarities in assessment and presentation, treatments can be vastly different. Ischemic and hemorrhagic strokes is discussed herein, as well as their subtypes.

Ischemic Stroke

Pathophysiology. Approximately 87% of all strokes in the United States are ischemic.[39] *Ischemic stroke* is caused by large artery atherosclerosis, cardioembolic events (Fig. 14.17), or small artery occlusive disease (lacunar stroke); in some cases, the cause is unknown (cryptogenic stroke). Brain cells survive only about 3 to 4 minutes when deprived of blood and oxygen. Normal CBF is 50 mL/100 g of brain tissue/min. When CBF drops to 25 mL/100 g/min, neurons become electrically silent but remain potentially viable for several hours. The region of brain with this level of CBF is known as the *ischemic penumbra* (Fig. 14.18). If CBF falls to less than the critical level of 10 mL/100 g/min or reperfusion of the penumbra does not occur, irreversible damage occurs. A cascade of metabolic disturbances follows, including lactic acidosis, glutamate release, depletion of ATP, and entry of sodium and

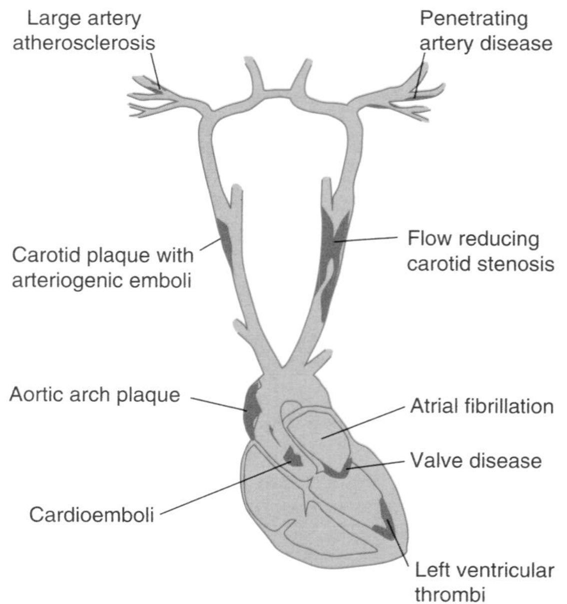

Fig. 14.17 Common arterial and cardiac abnormalities causing ischemic stroke. (From Albers GW, Easton JD, Sacco RL et al. Antithrombotic and thrombolytic therapy for ischemic stroke. *Chest.* 1998;114[Suppl 5]:683S-698S.)

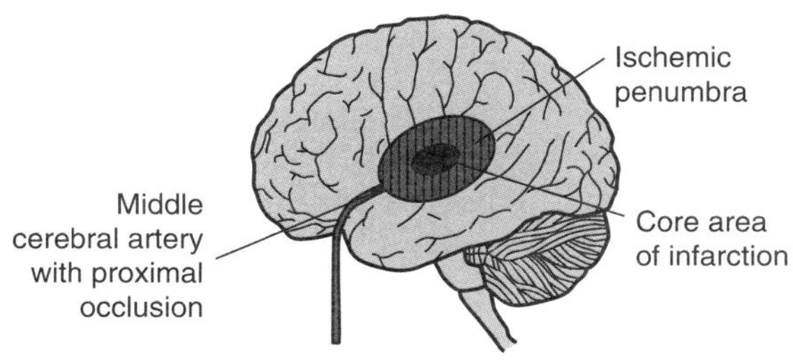

Fig. 14.18 Proximal occlusion of left middle cerebral artery with infarction. Ischemic penumbra represents regional blood flow at about 25 mL/100 g/min. Ischemic penumbra is the area where acute therapies for stroke are targeted.

calcium into the cells, leading to cytotoxic cerebral edema and mitochondrial failure.

Large artery atherosclerosis. *Large artery atherosclerosis* is the result of stenosis in the large arteries of the head and neck; it is caused by a cholesterol plaque or a thrombus superimposed on plaque. Blood flow may be greatly reduced (stenosis), causing ischemia, or occluded completely, causing a stroke. Hypertension, diabetes, smoking, obesity, birth control pills, and hyperlipidemia are risk factors for this type of stroke.

Cardioembolic stroke. Low-flow states or stasis of blood within the cardiac chambers may result in blood clot formation. An embolism occurs when a blood clot or plaque fractures from the heart, breaks off, and travels to the brain. The most common causes of *cardioembolic stroke* are atrial fibrillation, rheumatic heart disease, acute myocardial infarction, endocarditis, mitral valve stenosis, and prosthetic heart valves. Because a cardiac abnormality is the source of the cerebral emboli, it is important to identify and treat the underlying cardiac problem as well as the neurological problem.

Lacunar stroke. *Lacunar stroke* (small vessel occlusive disease) is caused by chronic hypertension, hyperlipidemia, obesity, and diabetes. These disease states cause lipid material to coat the small cerebral arteries within deep structures of the brain. This process leads to a thickening of the arterial walls, decreased blood flow, and ultimately, a stroke. The characteristic locations of lacunar infarcts are the basal ganglia, subcortical white matter, thalamus, cerebellum, and brainstem. The recurrence rate of lacunar strokes is about 10- to 12-fold compared with other types of stroke. A lacunar stroke causes not only physical impairment but also cognitive impairment, such as vascular dementia. Patients can have pure motor, pure sensory, or both motor and sensory features of stroke.

Cryptogenic stroke. The *cryptogenic* subtype refers to a stroke of unknown origin.

Medical and nursing interventions.

Blood pressure management. The goal for ischemic stroke is to keep systolic BP less than 220 mm Hg and diastolic BP less than 120 mm Hg. If the BP is greater than these parameters, it is reasonable to initially lower BP by 15%. Hypotension and hypovolemia should be avoided and rapidly corrected in an effort to support end-organ function.[42] Higher BP parameters are often indicated to maintain CPP in damaged brain tissue caused by decreased blood flow (stroke) to maintain adequate blood perfusion to damaged areas until further treatment can be given, if indicated. The BP goals may change based on the interventions initiated (e.g., intravenous fibrinolytic therapy, mechanical thrombectomy).

Candidates for thrombolysis. Early thrombolysis is recommended and can be provided only at primary or comprehensive stroke centers due to the specialty services required to offer the intervention.[40,43] Thrombolysis, provided as recombinant tissue plasminogen activator (IV alteplase), is the first medication approved by the U.S. Food and Drug Administration for acute ischemic stroke and must be given within 4.5 hours after symptom onset.[40,44] Administration after 4.5 hours has not been shown to be beneficial and increases the risk of hemorrhagic transformation of the infarct (bleeding into the stroke). More recently, tenecteplase, a modified version of IV alteplase studied in the cardiac population, has been used in place of IV alteplase due to cost, availability, and improved reperfusion rates.[45] Tenecteplase is administered as a single IV bolus, which may prove to be more appealing and decrease the complexity of administration compared to IV alteplase. Only about 5% of eligible patients actually receive IV alteplase due to presentation time and other exclusion criteria (e.g., head trauma or spine surgery within 3 months or active internal bleeding at any site).[40,43] Thrombolytic medication does not affect the infarcted area; however, by lysing the clot, it revitalizes the ischemic penumbra and improves overall neurological function. Careful assessment of patients who are potentially eligible for thrombolytic therapy is necessary to ensure safe administration and improved patient outcomes (Box 14.2).

Before the administration of IV alteplase, insert two peripheral IV lines—one for the administration of IV alteplase and one for fluids. If possible, place any catheters that are needed (e.g., urinary catheters, nasogastric tubes) before IV alteplase is administered to reduce the risk of bleeding. After the administration of IV alteplase, invasive procedures may be performed, but the risk of bleeding is higher for 24 to 36 hours post administration.[46] Anticoagulants, such as heparin or warfarin, and antiplatelet aggregates, such as aspirin, are withheld for 24 hours after administration of IV alteplase due to the increased risk of bleeding.[47]

Ischemic strokes have the propensity to bleed due to altered coagulation and blood flow; therefore, symptomatic hemorrhage is the most common complication after IV alteplase administration, with an incidence of 6.4%.[46,48] The highest risk of hemorrhage is within the first 36 hours after administration. Bleeding into the area of infarct, or hemorrhage transformation, is one of the common locations of post-thrombolysis bleeding and the greatest-feared complication. If bleeding occurs, the ischemic stroke is then classified as an ICH. The incidence of hemorrhagic transformation may be reduced by ensuring IV alteplase is given within 4.5 hours after symptom onset and by maintaining the systolic BP less than 180 mm Hg and the diastolic BP less than 105 mm Hg.[48] Antihypertensive agents are administered as needed to control the BP.

Signs and symptoms of ICH manifest as neurological deterioration, increased ICP, or cerebral herniation. If ICH is

BOX 14.2 Administration of Tissue Plasminogen Activator for Acute Ischemic Stroke

Inclusion Criteria

- Onset of stroke symptoms less than 4.5 hours
- Clinical diagnosis of ischemic stroke with a measurable deficit using the NIHSS
- Older than 18 years of age
- CT scan consistent with ischemic stroke and without evidence of hemorrhage

Exclusion Criteria

- Stroke symptoms more than 4.5 hours after symptom onset
- History of or current intracranial hemorrhage
- Subarachnoid hemorrhage
- Active internal bleeding
- Recent (within 3 months):
  - Intracranial or intraspinal surgery
  - Serious head trauma
  - Ischemic stroke
- Presence of conditions that may increase the risk of harm or bleeding (e.g., some cranial neoplasms, aortic arch dissection, infective endocarditis)
- GI malignancy or bleeding within 21 days
- Coagulopathy
- Current use of anticoagulants:
  - Full dose LMWH within 24 hours
  - Direct thrombin inhibitors or direct factor Xa inhibitors within 48 hours (administration may be considered if laboratory coagulation studies are normal)

Administration

- IV alteplase dosing: 0.9 mg/kg IV up to maximum of 90 mg
- Give bolus of 10% of total calculated dose IV over 1 minute
- Administer the remaining 90% over the next 60 minutes

Modified from Powers WJ, Rabinstein AA, Ackerson T et al. Guidelines for the early management of patients with acute ischemic stroke: 2019 update to the 2018 guidelines for the early management of acute ischemic stroke: a guideline for healthcare professionals from the American Heart Association/American Stroke Association [published correction appears in *Stroke*. 2019;50(12):e440-e441]. *Stroke*. 2019;50(12):e344-e418. https://doi.org/10.1161/STR.0000000000000211.

AVM, Arteriovenous malformation; *LMWH,* low-molecular-weight heparin; *NIHSS,* National Institutes of Health Stroke Scale; *CT,* computed tomography; *GI,* gastrointestinal.

suspected, the IV alteplase infusion is stopped, and an emergency noncontrast CT scan of the head is obtained. The nurse should obtain a complete blood count, coagulation studies, and a type and crossmatch. Administer cryoprecipitate and tranexamic acid as ordered if hemorrhagic conversion is noted on the CT scan of the head.[48] Neurosurgery should be consulted and supportive care provided via blood pressure management, stabilization of cerebral hemodynamics, and temperature and glucose control.[48]

Systemic bleeding can also occur; signs and symptoms include hypotension, tachycardia, pallor, restlessness, or lower back pain. Monitor stool, urine, and gastric secretions for the presence of blood. Assess IV sites and gums for signs of bleeding. Compare baseline hemoglobin, hematocrit, and coagulation studies with current studies and notify the provider of any significant changes.

One additional and life-threatening adverse event from IV alteplase administration is angioedema, which may occur up to 2 hours after administration.[49] If this occurs, priority interventions include maintaining the airway and discontinuing the IV alteplase, as well as holding any angiotensin-converting enzyme inhibitors. Administer methylprednisolone, diphenhydramine, and a histamine-2 blocker as ordered. If the angioedema continues to progress, epinephrine should be administered subcutaneously or via nebulizer.[46] Once stabilized, the nurse will continue to provide supportive care.

Given the aforementioned risks and potential complications of administering IV alteplase, perform neurological assessment (LOC; language, motor, and sensory testing; pupillary response) and assess vital signs every 15 minutes for the first 2 hours, every 30 minutes for the next 6 hours, and every hour for 16 hours (24 hours in total).[46] Monitor strict intake and output to assess fluid balance and renal function. Continuous cardiac monitoring is done throughout the hyperacute phase (i.e., first 24–72 hours). Administer oxygen to maintain the SpO_2 at 94%.[46] Pneumonia is a common complication after stroke due to an altered ability to clear the airway; therefore, frequent patient repositioning and nebulizer therapy may be indicated.

Mechanical thrombectomy. For a patient with stroke who is not a candidate for thrombolytic therapy, mechanical thrombectomy via stent retriever or direct aspiration should be considered within 24 hours of symptom onset for patients with specific advanced imaging criteria (i.e., stroke location). Of note, some patients who receive IV alteplase may still be considered for mechanical thrombectomy. Stent retrievers extract blood clots via a wire cage device that is deployed around the clot which is then seized and removed. Direct aspiration involves threading a catheter to the clot and then removing the clot via forceful suction. If mechanical thrombectomy is performed, maintain the systolic BP less than 180 mm Hg and the diastolic BP less than 105 mm Hg for 24 hours.[50]

Patients without intervention. Perform neurologic, respiratory, and cardiac assessments and obtain vital signs every 1 to 2 hours during the first 24 hours after stroke. Control BP to prevent bleeding while maintaining an adequate CPP. BP is managed carefully with IV medications such as labetalol or nicardipine. Rapid drops in BP can cause further neurological deterioration by decreasing cerebral perfusion and extending the area of cerebral ischemia.

Other interventions are implemented to decrease ICP (see Increased Intracranial Pressure subsection) and improve or maintain hemodynamic stability. The incidence of cerebral herniation peaks at about 72 hours after the stroke.[50] Hyponatremia due to cerebral salt wasting may occur; sodium and fluid replacement are necessary to maintain a normal sodium level. Because hyperglycemia may exacerbate the extent of neurological injury, glycemic control is advocated (see Chapter 19, Endocrine Alterations).[50]

Anticoagulants, such as warfarin, low-molecular-weight heparin, or factor Xa inhibitors (i.e., rivaroxaban), are not recommended for the prevention of recurrent ischemic stroke.[51] Antiplatelet aggregates, such as aspirin or a combination of aspirin and clopidogrel, may be given for prevention of recurrent ischemic stroke within 24 to 48 hours after onset.[50]

Maintain adequate fluid balance to ensure proper hydration and normothermia to reduce the metabolic needs of the brain. Direct injury to the hypothalamus may alter the hypothalamic set point that regulates body temperature, resulting in hyperthermia. Systemic infection or drug reactions may result in fever due to pyrogens increasing body temperature above the hypothalamic set point.

Implement aspiration precautions, including elevating the head of the bed greater than 30 degrees and maintaining nothing-by-mouth status until a swallow screening or formal study rules out dysphagia. Often, a speech pathologist completes the initial dysphagia screening.[50]

Hemorrhagic Stroke. While ischemic strokes contribute to 87% of stroke cases, *hemorrhagic strokes* account for the remaining 13% in the United States.[39] Hemorrhagic stroke occurs when there is bleeding into the brain tissue (intracerebral) or subarachnoid space (on the surface of the brain or into the ventricle) or a combination of the two. Each hemorrhagic stroke has specific pathophysiology, as well as medical and nursing interventions; therefore, each is discussed in its entirety herein prior to the introduction of the next hemorrhagic stroke type.

Intracerebral hemorrhage.

Pathophysiology. The most common cause of ICH is uncontrolled hypertension.[52] Another less common cause of ICH is cerebral amyloid angiopathy. Generally seen in the older population, this condition is the result of abnormal amyloid protein deposits in the cerebral blood vessels over time. As a result, the cerebral blood vessels become friable and prone to spontaneous rupture, even in patients without hypertension.[52] When a blood vessel ruptures, the escaped blood forms a mass that displaces and compresses brain tissue. The severity of the symptoms depends on the location and amount of the hemorrhage. If the hemorrhage is large enough, herniation may result. Additional causes of ICH include excessive anticoagulation, inappropriate use of thrombolytics (i.e., IV alteplase), vasopressor medications, substance use disorder (e.g., cocaine), and coagulopathies. A sudden and often severe motor deficit, paired with or without nausea and vomiting and changes in consciousness, is observed with ICH, although a small ICH may manifest as a headache only. Patients with ICH may continue to bleed; therefore, close neurological monitoring is necessary.

Medical and nursing interventions. Patients with an ICH may develop elevated ICP, and the management of this sequela is outlined in the Increased ICP section. As with other neurological events, glucose and temperature should be well controlled to ensure normal ranges.[52] Mechanical VTE prophylaxis should be initiated at the time of admission with intermittent pneumatic compression devices. Initiation of VTE chemoprophylaxis with low-molecular-weight heparin (i.e., enoxaparin) or unfractionated heparin within 24 to 48 hours of ICH onset is reasonable.[52]

Blood pressure management. Control of BP is important to prevent hematoma expansion. The optimal systolic BP target is 140 mm Hg, with a goal range of 130 to 150 mm Hg. Lowering the systolic BP below 130 mm Hg in spontaneous ICH is potentially harmful and should be avoided.[52] If treatment is required, BP is lowered cautiously, avoiding large fluctuations to prevent a sudden decrease in cerebral perfusion.

Anticoagulant reversal. Discontinue anticoagulant therapy immediately. The administration of reversal agents should not be delayed by pending laboratory studies. Anticoagulant reversals, as appropriate based on type and reversal availability, should be administered expeditiously.[52]

Surgical intervention. Assessment focuses on determining the size and location of the ICH and whether it is amenable to surgical intervention. Small bleeds usually resolve without surgery. In these instances, more aggressive BP management may be indicated. Minimally invasive surgery (MIS), such as endoscopic aspiration of the hematoma, may be a useful intervention for reducing mortality in patients with a GCS of 5 to 12 and an ICH between 20 and 30 mL in volume. MIS may be preferred over traditional craniotomy and improve functional outcomes, though the mortality benefit is uncertain and more research is needed. A limitation of MIS implementation is the availability of skilled surgeons and centers to provide the intervention.[52]

Hemorrhagic stroke due to ruptured cerebral aneurysm.

Pathophysiology. *Cerebral aneurysm* is a localized dilation of the cerebral artery wall that causes the artery to weaken and become susceptible to rupture. Most aneurysms develop at the bifurcation of large arteries at the base of the brain (circle of Willis).[2] Not all aneurysms rupture; some aneurysms are found incidentally when imaging is done for unrelated reasons. Patients with cerebral aneurysms are asymptomatic before the rupture unless they experience a warning "leak" or sentinel bleeding.[2] Aneurysms most commonly rupture into the subarachnoid space at the basal cisterns (i.e., aneurysmal SAH [aSAH]), which is the focus of the following discussion. Less commonly, an aneurysm can rupture into the brain parenchyma or ventricle, or a combination of these locations. Bleeding into the subarachnoid space can cause increased ICP, impaired cerebral autoregulation, reduced CBF, blockage of the reabsorption of CSF, and irritation of the meninges.[2] The bleeding generally stops through the formation of a fibrin plug and platelet aggregation within the ruptured artery. The Hunt and Hess grading scale (Table 14.12) is used to classify the severity of subarachnoid hemorrhage.[2] This scale is based on the patient's clinical condition and is also used to predict mortality. The higher the grade, the lower the chance of survival.

Early diagnosis of the cause of aSAH helps to guide treatment. Although a CT scan helps differentiate an aneurysm from an arteriovenous malformation (AVM), definitive diagnosis of an aneurysm is determined by digital subtraction (intraarterial procedure) or CT angiography.[53]

After an aneurysm rupture, the patient can develop cardiac dysrhythmias, rebleeding, hydrocephalus, seizures, and cerebral vasospasm. Cardiac dysrhythmias occur as a result of

TABLE 14.12 Hunt and Hess Classification of Subarachnoid Hemorrhage

Grade	Clinical Findings
1	Asymptomatic or mild headache and minimal nuchal rigidity
2	Moderate to severe headache, nuchal rigidity, cranial nerve palsy
3	Mild focal neurological deficits, lethargy, or confusion
4	Stuporous, moderate to severe hemiparesis
5	Comatose, decerebrate rigidity, moribund appearance
Add one grade for serious comorbidities (e.g., hypertension, diabetes mellitus, severe atherosclerosis, chronic obstructive pulmonary disease) or severe vasospasm seen on angiogram.	

Adapted from Greenberg MS. *Handbook of Neurosurgery*. 9th ed. New York, NY: Thieme Medical Publishers; 2020.

sympathetic nervous system stimulation. Increased sympathetic tone can cause elevated T waves, prolonged QT intervals, and ST abnormalities. Rebleeding after the initial aneurysm rupture may occur before the aneurysm is secured. The mechanism causing the rebleeding is increased tension on the artery from hypertension or normal breakdown of the clot, which occurs 7 to 10 days after the initial hemorrhage.[2]

Cerebral vasospasm is a narrowing of arteries adjacent to the aneurysm that results in delayed cerebral ischemia (DCI) and infarction of brain tissue if either untreated or refractory to treatment. Vasospasm and DCI are the leading causes of death after aneurysmal rupture and aSAH.[54] The usual period for vasospasm to occur is between 3 and 14 days after the rupture but as far out as 21 days. The exact mechanism for vasospasm is unknown, but some factors that contribute to vasospasm are structural changes in the adjacent cerebral arteries, denervation of adjacent arteries, generation of oxygen radicals, and release of vasoactive substances (i.e., serotonin, catecholamines, prostaglandins) that initiate vasospasm, the inflammatory response, and calcium influx.[2] Signs and symptoms of vasospasm may include difficulty speaking, confusion, and weakness on one side of the body.

Medical and nursing interventions. Assess neurological status frequently by using the GCS and monitoring for focal deficits and pupillary changes. Monitor temperature because persons with aSAH often have a fever, which is associated with a worse neurological outcome.[53–54] An enteral feeding tube may be required for nutritional support (see Chapter 7, Nutritional Therapy). Initiate measures for VTE prevention, including mechanical prophylaxis and then chemoprophylaxis with unfractionated heparin 24 hours after the aneurysm has been secured.[55] Monitor hemoglobin to assure adequate oxygen carrying capacity. Other important interventions include providing analgesia and bed rest.

Increased intracranial pressure. *Hydrocephalus* can occur after aSAH through two mechanisms. Bleeding into the intraventricular space can block the flow of CSF and cause acute obstructive hydrocephalus. As blood enters the subarachnoid space, an inflammatory response is triggered that causes fibrosis and thickening of the arachnoid villi, thereby preventing CSF reabsorption and producing communicating hydrocephalus. The management of this sequela is outlined in the Increased Intracranial Pressure section. Patients with severe neurological compromise after a ruptured aneurysm may benefit from emergency ventriculostomy. The ventriculostomy assists in treating the hydrocephalus as a result of bleeding into the intraventricular space. The EVD also allows the clinician to monitor ICP and remove CSF to lower ICP, if needed (see Increased Intracranial Pressure section). If appropriate, ventriculostomy placement is not performed until after the aneurysm has been secured, because changing the ICP can contribute to rebleeding due to the fluctuation in pressures within the brain. If waiting for aneurysm securement is not possible, a ventriculostomy can be ordered to drain less aggressively, as to not cause a sudden drop in ICP.

Blood pressure management. BP control is a key component of aSAH management. Administer medications to reduce BP before the aneurysm is secured to prevent rebleeding with a goal of systolic less than 160 mm Hg. After the aneurysm is secured, BP is allowed to rise to prevent vasospasm. If vasospasm occurs, BP may be purposely increased with fluids and medications to augment CBF. When appropriate, systolic BP is maintained greater than 160 mm Hg (and sometimes higher), but available data does not suggest a specific BP parameter; however, cardiovascular comorbidities should be taken into consideration. The increase in volume and BP forces blood through the vasospastic area at a higher pressure, maintaining arterial dilation. If the patient's BP cannot be maintained at the increased level required, vasoactive medications such as phenylephrine may be warranted. Conversely, patients with a significant cardiac history may not tolerate increases in BP.[56,57]

Prevention of vasospasm. Nimodipine, a neurospecific calcium channel blocker, should be administered to all patients with an aSAH. This medication has been found to reduce the incidence and severity of deficits, morbidity, and mortality associated with aSAH and is the most effective in reducing vasospasm compared to placebo (see Evidence-Based Practice box).[53,56]

Monitor for signs of vasospasm (change in neurological status, motor strength), because early intervention results in better patient outcomes. Signs of vasospasm can be difficult to assess in high-grade aSAH due to poor neurological status, for which diagnostic studies become paramount. During the 14-day

EVIDENCE-BASED PRACTICE

Prophylactic Therapies for Morbidity and Mortality After Aneurysmal Subarachnoid Hemorrhage

Problem

Aneurysmal subarachnoid hemorrhage (aSAH) is associated with a high morbidity and mortality. More than 30% of patients die within the first few days to weeks after the initial hemorrhage, and the survivors experience both long-term disabilities and impairments. Vasospasm is a common complication, occurring among 70% of patients with somewhere between 17% to 40% of patients with aSAH developing delayed cerebral ischemia (DCI). There are multiple pharmacological interventions, and the comparative therapeutic benefits are unknown.

Clinical Question

What are the relative benefits of pharmacological prophylactic treatments in patients with aSAH?

Evidence

A search of Medline, Web of Science, Embase, Scopus, ProQuest, and Cochrane Central was completed, including randomized controlled trials published on or before February 2020. A total of 53 trials enrolling 10,415 patients were included that compared the prophylactic effects of any oral or intravenous medications or intracranial drug-eluting implants to either placebo or another medication or standard of care in adult hospitalized patients with aSAH. The most effective treatment based on either moderate or high certainty evidence was nimodipine showing benefit in reducing all-cause mortality, DCI, and cerebral vasospasm and improving function.

Implications for Nursing

Most guidelines recommend the use of nimodipine for calcium channel blockade, and the meta-analysis supports its ongoing use in the aSAH population. Nurses should advocate to initiate nimodipine in patients with an aSAH to reduce vasospasm and the risk of DCI, while improving morbidity and mortality. Future research is needed to clarify the role of other therapeutics in the management of aSAH.

Level of Evidence

A – Meta-analysis

Reference

Dayyani M, Sadeghirad B, Grotta JC et al. Prophylactic therapies for morbidity and mortality after aneurysmal subarachnoid hemorrhage: a systematic review and network meta-analysis of randomized trials. *Stroke.* 2022;53(6):1993-2005. https://doi.org/10.1161/STROKEAHA.121.035699.

monitoring period, transcranial Doppler studies are completed daily or every other day to evaluate the velocities of intracranial arteries to monitor for vasospasm; the higher the velocity, the more likely the presence of vasospasm. The modified Fisher Grading Scale (Table 14.13) is used to classify the appearance of aSAH on CT scan and the risk of vasospasm.

Triple H therapy (i.e., hypervolemia, hemodilution, hypertension) was traditionally referred to as the treatment approach for vasospasm prevention and management; however, vasospasm management is now focused on euvolemic hypertension.[56,57]

If euvolemic hypertension fails, the treatment of symptomatic vasospasm includes intraarterial vasodilators (i.e., nicardipine, verapamil) via angioplasty or cerebral balloon angioplasty.[53] Risks of angioplasty include perforation or rupture, cerebral artery thrombosis, recurrent vasospasm, and transient neurological deficits. Both intraarterial vasodilators and cerebral balloon angioplasty attempt to reduce vasospasm by dilating the spasmodic vessels.[53,56]

Seizure prophylaxis. *Seizures* can occur at aSAH onset because of meningeal irritation by the hemorrhage or within the first 12 hours after rupture due to increased ICP or rebleeding of the aneurysm. Seizures are also more likely to happen with more diffuse subarachnoid bleeding, classified by a worse Hunt and Hess score. Seizures occurring later are more likely due to ischemic damage secondary to vasospasm. Prophylactic antiepileptic medications have not been found to significantly reduce the risk of seizure in aSAH. Long-term use of seizure prophylaxis should be considered if the patient has a known risk for delayed seizure disorder (i.e., history of seizures, ICH, intractable hypertension, aneurysm to the middle cerebral artery, or infraction), but should not be routinely initiated.[53]

Surgical intervention. The ideal timing of surgical and/or endovascular intervention is unclear; however, the guidelines recommend repair as soon as possible to prevent rebleeding and vasospasm. Surgical clipping is a procedure involving an open craniotomy. The surgery involves occluding the neck of the aneurysm with a metal clip; reinforcing the sac by wrapping it with muscle, fibrin foam, or solidifying polymer; or proximally ligating a feeding vessel. If the neck of the aneurysm is narrow and accessible, use of a metal clip is desirable. If the neck of the aneurysm is too broad, reinforcing the aneurysmal sac to prevent rebleeding is the goal of surgery. Proximal ligation may be preferred if the aneurysm is directly fed by the internal carotid artery. The disadvantage of this procedure is the potential for stroke, should collateral circulation fail.[53,56]

Endovascular therapy with coils, stents, or a combination of the two may be used to occlude the aneurysm. This therapy consists of navigating a microcatheter through the femoral artery to the aneurysm and placing either platinum coils into the aneurysm sac or a stent to cover the opening of the aneurysm. Both interventions cause a thrombosis, occluding the aneurysm from the feeder vessel. If endovascular attempts fail to obliterate the aneurysm, surgical clipping may be required. Incomplete surgical obliteration may require additional endovascular treatment to continue to reduce the risk of rebleeding.

Hemorrhagic stroke due to arteriovenous malformation.

Pathophysiology. An AVM is a congenital anomaly that forms an abnormal communication network between the arterial and venous systems in the brain. Arterial blood under pressure is directly shunted into the venous system without a capillary network. This predisposes the vessels to rupture into the ventricular system or subarachnoid space, causing a SAH, or into the brain parenchyma, causing an ICH.[2] Hemorrhage from an AVM is usually low-pressure venous bleeding, and initial rate of hemorrhage is about 2% to 4%; rebleeding after initial AVM hemorrhage is about 6% but generally similar to initial rupture rates.[39] The rebleeding rate is also much lower than for an aneurysm, and for that reason, surgical intervention is less time sensitive than a ruptured aneurysm causing aSAH. Timing of surgical intervention for an AVM can be delayed up to 4 weeks, whereas timing for a ruptured intracranial aneurysm is ideally 0 to 3 days. Impaired perfusion

TABLE 14.13 Modified Fisher Grading Scale

Modified Fisher Scale Group	Blood on CT scan	Symptomatic Vasospasm
0	No SAH or IVH	
1	Focal or diffuse thin SAH, no IVH	24%
2	Focal or diffuse thin SAH with IVH	33%
3	Focal or diffuse thick SAH, no IVH	33%
4	Focal or diffuse thick SAH with IVH	40%

CT, Computed tomography; *IVH*, intraventricular hemorrhage; *SAH*, subarachnoid hemorrhage.
Adapted from Greenberg MS. *Handbook of Neurosurgery*. 9th ed. New York, NY: Thieme Medical Publishers; 2020.

of the cerebral tissue adjacent to the AVM also occurs. Some AVMs do not hemorrhage but rather cause varying degrees of ischemia, scarring of brain tissue with seizures, abnormal tissue development, compression, or hydrocephalus. AVMs are more prevalent in males and are commonly diagnosed after the patient has had a seizure. Headache is another common manifestation of AVM. AVMs may also cause symptoms due to ischemia or act as a space-occupying lesion, similar to a tumor.[50,58,59]

Medical and surgical interventions. Treatment interventions for an AVM include embolization, surgery, radiotherapy, or a combination of all three. Embolization is not a curative approach to most AVMs; rather, it is used in preparation for surgery to reduce blood flow to the AVM. Embolization may occur in a single setting or may be staged in several procedures over days to weeks. Radiotherapy may be performed alone or for residual AVM after surgery, and results are manifested over years. Surgery for removal of an AVM is done as a single step or in multiple stages, pending risk of rebleeding, location of the AVM, neurological status of the patient, and size of the malformation. Postoperatively, the major problem is breakthrough bleeding from cauterized vessels. Rapid increases in BP during recovery from anesthesia are avoided, and BP must be tightly controlled during the first 48 hours after resection to prevent bleeding.[50,58,59]

POSTOPERATIVE NEUROSURGICAL CARE FOR INTRACRANIAL SURGERY

Assessment and Management

The postoperative care of a patient who has undergone a neurosurgical procedure involves frequent and ongoing BP, respiratory, metabolic, and neurological assessments, which are most-often supported in a critical care unit. Most postoperative intracranial patients will require a higher acuity level of care due to the multitude of potential postoperative complications until deemed stable for less-frequent examinations, which is patient-dependent. The most common postoperative complications are infection, ICH, increased ICP, hydrocephalus, and seizures.

Complications

ICH is detected by a decline in neurological status, signs of increasing ICP, and new or worsening focal deficits (i.e., hemiparesis/hemiplegia, aphasia); hemorrhage is confirmed by CT scan. Treatment depends on CT findings and may require emergency intervention. Oxygenation and tissue perfusion are monitored. Chest radiographs, CT scans, EEGs, and other diagnostic tests may be necessary to monitor progress. The head of the bed should generally be elevated greater than 30 degrees to prevent aspiration, unless it is contraindicated or there is a provider's order not to elevate the head of bed based on the patient's condition.[60]

Hydrocephalus can develop at any time during the postoperative course as a result of developing edema from tumor occurrence or bleeding into the subarachnoid space. Signs and symptoms of hydrocephalus include headaches, nausea, vomiting, vision changes, drowsiness, irritability, decreased mentation, loss of bladder control, balance problems, and poor coordination. Treatment may include placement of a ventriculostomy to drain CSF temporarily. If the hydrocephalus does not resolve within a few days, a surgical shunting procedure, known as ventriculoperitoneal (VP) shunt, may be indicated to relieve the brain of excessive CSF.

Seizures can occur at any time but are most common within the first 7 days after surgery. Focal seizures in the form of twitching of selected muscles, particularly of the face and hand, are often seen. Patients may receive postoperative antiepileptic medications such as, levetiracetam (Keppra), or phenytoin (Dilantin) if concern for seizures is high. If a patient is receiving phenytoin, serum phenytoin levels are monitored to maintain a therapeutic range.

CHECK YOUR UNDERSTANDING

3. The nurse caring for a patient presenting with an acute ischemic stroke anticipates:
   A. Holding blood pressure medications to promote cerebral perfusion so that blood pressure can increase to greater than 200 mm Hg
   B. Planning for inducing hypothermia to protect ischemic brain
   C. Preparing the patient for emergency surgery
   D. Identifying the precise time of stroke symptom onset when possible

TRANSIENT ISCHEMIC ATTACKS

Pathophysiology

A transient ischemic attack (TIA) is defined as the sudden onset of a temporary focal neurological deficit caused by a vascular event. During a TIA, a transient decrease in CBF occurs, but the patient does not experience any permanent deficits.

Assessment

A TIA is commonly caused by stenosis of the carotid arteries; therefore, a common presentation includes amaurosis fugax (monocular blindness) due to transient occlusion of the central retinal artery. Although symptoms of a TIA mimic those of stroke, by definition, TIA symptoms last for 24 hours or less.[49]

Medical and Nursing Interventions

In general, patients with symptoms of TIA should receive a complete stroke workup to determine the cause of TIA. Patients may be managed with antiplatelet or dual antiplatelet therapy depending on the etiology of the symptoms.[51] It is important that preventative measures be initiated for people with TIAs, as the risk of stroke is significantly increased after experiencing a TIA.[61]

A common cause of TIA is carotid artery stenosis. Patients experiencing TIAs with carotid stenosis are evaluated for carotid endarterectomy or carotid angioplasty and stenting. If a patient has carotid stenosis greater than 69% on the symptomatic side, carotid endarterectomy is recommended. Carotid angioplasty with stenting is also an accepted method of treating carotid stenosis for select patients.[51]

SEIZURES AND STATUS EPILEPTICUS

A seizure is an abnormal electrical discharge in the brain that can be caused by a variety of neurological disorders, systemic diseases, and metabolic disorders. Seizures consist of repetitive depolarization of hyperactive, hypersensitive cells that cause an altered state of brain function. In 2017, the International League Against Epilepsy (ILAE) revised its classification of seizures (Table 14.14). The new classification system is based on three key features: where seizures begin in the brain, level of awareness during a seizure, and other features of seizures.[62]

TABLE 14.14 Classification of Seizures

Location of Seizure	
Focal	Starts in an area on one side of brain *Focal motor:* twitching, jerking, stiffening, rubbing hands, walking, running *Focal nonmotor:* changes in sensorium, emotions, or thinking occur first *Auras:* symptoms felt at start of seizure
Generalized	Involves an area on both sides of the brain at the onset *Generalized motor:* stiffening (tonic) and jerking (clonic) *Generalized nonmotor:* brief periods of awareness, staring, repeated movements (lip-smacking)
Unknown onset	Onset of seizure unknown
Focal to bilateral	Starts on one side of brain and spreads to both sides
Level of Awareness	
Focal aware	Awareness remains intact even if person is unable to talk or respond
Focal impaired awareness	Awareness impaired
Awareness unknown	Unknown if person is aware or not if person lives alone or has seizures only at night

Adapted from Fisher RS. The new classification of seizures by the International League Against Epilepsy. *Curr Neurol Neurosci Rep.* 2017;17(6):48-53.

Pathophysiology

When seizures occur in close proximity to each other, they have the potential to lead to a life-threatening medical emergency known as *status epilepticus (SE)*. SE is more likely to occur with tonic-clonic seizures that have a specific causative factor than with idiopathic seizures. The most frequent precipitating factors for SE are irregular intake of antiepileptic drugs, withdrawal from habitual use of alcohol or sedative drugs, electrolyte imbalance, azotemia, head trauma, infection, and brain tumor.[63]

Physiological changes that occur during SE are divided into two phases. Phase one is the time at which seizures no longer stop spontaneously; therefore, treatment should be initiated. In tonic-clonic seizures, this is at 5 minutes, 10 minutes for focal status with or without impairment of consciousness and absences.[63] During *phase one,* cerebral metabolism is increased and compensatory mechanisms (i.e., increased CBF and catecholamine release) prevent cerebral damage from hypoxia or metabolic injury; however, these compensatory mechanisms can lead to other problems. Hyperglycemia occurs from release of epinephrine and activation of hepatic gluconeogenesis. Hypertension occurs due to increased CBF. Hyperpyrexia results from excessive muscle activity and catecholamine release. Lactic acidosis occurs from anaerobic metabolism. Elevated epinephrine and norepinephrine levels and acidosis contribute to cardiac dysrhythmias. Autonomic dysfunction manifested as tachycardia, diaphoresis, hyperventilation, and hypertension can cause cardiac arrest due to the sympathetic stimulation associated.

Phase two begins at 30 minutes for tonic-clonic SE and 60 minutes for focal status.[63] Decompensation occurs because the increased metabolic demands cannot be met. This causes decreased CBF, systemic hypotension, increased ICP, and failure of cerebral autoregulation. The patient develops metabolic and respiratory acidosis from hypoxemia and hypoglycemia from depleted energy stores. The lack of oxygen and glucose results in cellular injury. Pulmonary edema is common, and aspiration can occur from decreased laryngeal reflex sensitivity. Cardiac dysrhythmias and heart failure result from hypoxemia, hyperkalemia (caused by increased muscle activity), and metabolic acidosis. Acute kidney injury may result from post-status rhabdomyolysis and acute myoglobinuria (Acute Kidney Injury, Chapter 16). Myoglobin is released secondary to excessive muscle activity and exhaustion from prolonged skeletal muscle contraction and traumatic injury during the seizure.

Death from SE is more likely to occur when an underlying disease is responsible for the seizure or from the acute illness that precipitated the seizure. Generalized seizures that last for 30 to 45 minutes can result in neuronal necrosis and permanent neurological deficits. Prompt diagnosis and treatment are important because seizure duration is an important prognostic factor in mortality associated with SE.[63]

Assessment

Assessment during SE incorporates the neurologic, respiratory, and cardiovascular systems. Identify characteristics of the seizure and the neurological state before, between, and after seizures. Collect information, including precipitating factors, regarding preceding aura, type of movement observed, automatisms, changes in size of pupils or eye deviation, responsiveness to auditory or tactile stimuli, LOC throughout the seizure, urinary or bowel incontinence, behavior after the seizure, weakness or paralysis of extremities after the seizure, injuries caused by the seizure, and duration of the seizure. Additionally, assess respiratory status and SpO_2 to ensure adequate oxygenation. Because decompensation can result in pulmonary edema, observe for the onset of fine basilar crackles and have suction equipment and oxygen readily available. Cardiac monitoring is necessary to assess for dysrhythmias. Assess blood glucose because hypoglycemia is an important cause of SE.

Diagnostic Tests

Laboratory studies for a patient with SE include serum electrolytes, liver function studies, serum medication levels, and blood and urine toxicology screens. Measurements of cardiac enzymes and arterial blood gases assist in assessing the effect of the seizure on other body systems. Patient monitoring includes electrocardiogram (ECG), continuous EEG, noninvasive BP, and pulse oximetry.

Radiological studies are performed to rule out pathology that may be responsible for the episode of SE. These may include CT or MRI, with or without contrast. Additional studies may be done as needed.

Patient Problems

In addition to the patient problems stated in the Collaborative Care Plan found in Chapter 1, Overview of Critical Care Nursing, other patient problems relevant to the patient experiencing SE include impaired tissue perfusion (cerebral and cardiopulmonary), decreased gas exchange, potential for airway compromise, and need for health teaching,

Medical and Nursing Interventions

Management during SE includes maintaining a patent airway, providing adequate oxygenation, obtaining and maintaining vascular access for the administration of medications and fluids, administering appropriate medications, maintaining patient safety, and maintaining seizure precautions. Facilitate a patent airway by positioning the patient appropriately; use of an oral or nasal airway or endotracheal tube may be necessary. Do not force the mouth open or place padded tongue blades between the clenched teeth of a patient undergoing a seizure; patients have inadvertently been injured from aspirating teeth that were loosened during forceful attempts to insert a padded tongue blade between their teeth. Suction as needed to remove secretions that collect in the oropharynx. Administer supplemental oxygen to improve oxygenation. NMB may be used to facilitate intubation but will not be effective in halting neuronal firing; attention to seizure control is necessary, even if the patient is paralyzed. Never administer NMB without first providing analgesia and sedation. A nasogastric tube with intermittent suction may be needed to reduce the risk of aspiration.

Maintain vascular access to provide a route for the administration of medications. If IV access cannot be established, some antiepileptic medications can be administered rectally. The specific medication given to arrest the seizure depends on its type and duration. Monitoring BP and administering volume replacement and vasoactive medications as needed is essential. IV dextrose is administered unless the blood glucose level is known to be normal or high. Administer thiamine prior to glucose if Wernicke's encephalopathy is suspected. Wernicke's encephalopathy is caused by thiamine deficiency and presents with a classic triad of confusion, ataxia, and weakness of the eye muscles (ophthalmoparesis).

Seizure precautions are continued during SE. Precautions include padding the side rails on the patient's bed and ensuring the bed has full-length side rails. Keep the bed in a low position with side rails up except when providing direct nursing care. If the patient is in a chair when a seizure begins, lower the patient to the floor and place a soft object under the patient's head. Remove the patient's restrictive clothing and jewelry while always maintaining the patient's privacy. During the seizure, remove any items surrounding the patient that may cause harm. Do not restrain the patient, because forceful tonic-clonic movements can injure the patient.

SE must be treated immediately. Ensure a patent airway and maintain breathing and circulation. Administer medications with a sequential approach that progressively uses more potent medications to control the seizure. The first-line medication is a benzodiazepine, usually IV diazepam (Valium) or IV lorazepam (Ativan). If the benzodiazepine fails to stop seizure activity within 10 minutes, or if intermittent seizures persist for longer than 20 minutes, levetiracetam (Keppra), phenytoin (Dilantin), or fosphenytoin (Cerebyx) may be administered (Table 14.9).[63] If SE continues after administration of one benzodiazepine and one antiepileptic agent, it is considered refractory, and initiation of a continuous anesthetic should be started within 30 to 60 minutes to prevent neuronal damage.[2] Typically, midazolam (Versed) is the first line for continuous anesthetic; however, if the patient continues to experience SE, other common anesthetics added are propofol (Diprivan), pentobarbital, thiopental, and ketamine, so long as they are used at high enough doses to be anesthetic. Patients require intubation and mechanical ventilation if continuous anesthetics are administered. Continuous EEG is to be applied to monitor seizure activity and effect of the treatment regimen.[63]

? CLINICAL JUDGMENT ACTIVITY

An 18-year-old patient is admitted in status epilepticus. Describe the appropriate nursing and medical interventions.

CENTRAL NERVOUS SYSTEM INFECTIONS

The brain and spinal cord are relatively well protected from infective agents by the bones of the skull and vertebral column, the meninges, and the blood-brain barrier. However, infective

BOX 14.3 Causes of Meningitis

Bacterial
- *Streptococcus pneumoniae* (pneumococcus)
- *Neisseria meningitidis* (meningococcus)
- *Haemophilus influenzae* type B (Hib)
- *Staphylococci* (*Staphylococcus aureus*)
- Gram-negative bacilli (*Escherichia coli, Enterobacter, Serratia*)

Viral
- Echovirus
- Coxsackievirus
- Mumps virus
- Herpes simplex virus types 1 and 2
- St. Louis encephalitis virus
- Colorado tick fever virus
- Epstein-Barr virus
- West Nile virus
- Influenza virus types A and B

Fungal
- Histoplasma
- Candida
- Aspergillus

agents can enter the CNS through the air sinuses, the middle ear, or blood. Injuries and treatments that disrupt the dura (e.g., basilar skull fractures, missile injuries, neurosurgical procedures) also increase the risk for infection. *Meningitis* (infection of the meninges) may be caused by bacteria, viruses, fungi, parasites, or other toxins. These infections are classified as acute, subacute, or chronic. Box 14.3 lists common organisms that cause meningitis. The pathophysiology, clinical presentation, and management differ for each type of microorganism.

Patient Problems

The following problems may be applicable to a patient with a CNS infection: fever, potential for injury from seizures, potential for decreased cerebral perfusion, and acute pain.

Bacterial Meningitis

Bacterial meningitis is a neurological emergency that can lead to substantial morbidity and mortality as bacteria travels through the blood to the meninges, causing inflammation of the membranes that cover the CNS. More than 300,000 people die worldwide of bacterial meningitis, with a significant fatality rate among adolescents. Meningitis particularly affects the very young, the very old, and immunosuppressed individuals. Because of its high mortality rate, vaccination against bacterial meningitis is recommended.[64]

Pathophysiology. Bacterial meningitis is an infection of the pia mater and arachnoid layers of the meninges, along with the CSF in the subarachnoid space.[2] Bacteria gain access in one of three ways: (1) via the blood or through the spread of nearby infection, such as sinusitis; (2) by CSF contamination through surgical procedures or catheters; or (3) through the skull. Airborne droplets can be passed from infected individuals through sneezing, coughing, or kissing, and droplets can be passed through saliva and transmitted via drinks, cigarettes, or utensils.[2] Bacteria enter through the choroid plexuses, multiply in the subarachnoid space, and irritate the meninges. An exudate forms that thickens the CSF and alters CSF flow through and around the brain and spinal cord, resulting in obstruction, interstitial edema, and further inflammation.[2]

Assessment. A thorough history and neurological assessment are completed for patients with bacterial meningitis. Patients often are seen in the emergency department with an acute onset of symptoms (e.g., headache, fever, stiff neck, vomiting) that developed over 1 to 2 days. There may be a recent history of infection (ear, sinus, or upper respiratory tract), foreign travel, or illicit drug use. The clinical presentation often reveals signs of systemic infection, including fever (temperature as high as 39.5 °C), tachycardia, chills, and petechial rash. Initially, the rash may be macular, but it progresses to petechiae and purpura, mainly on the trunk and extremities. Meningeal irritation produces a throbbing headache, photophobia, vomiting, and nuchal rigidity. A positive *Kernig sign* (pain in the neck when the thigh is flexed 90 degrees and the leg extended at the knee) and a positive *Brudzinski sign* (involuntary flexion of the hips when the neck is flexed toward the chest) may be present. The patient's condition can quickly deteriorate to hypotension, shock, and sepsis.[2]

Assess the patient's LOC, motor response, and cranial nerves. Confusion and decreasing LOC are evidence of cortical involvement. Focal neurological deficits may be seen, including hemiparesis, hemiplegia, and ataxia, as well as seizure activity and projectile vomiting. Irritation and damage to cranial nerves occur as a result of inflamed sheaths. As ICP increases, unconsciousness may occur.[2]

Diagnostic Tests. The gold standard for the diagnosis of meningitis is examination of the CSF. A sample may be obtained by lumbar puncture or by aspiration from a ventricular catheter. Diagnosis can also be based on a nasopharyngeal smear and antigen tests. Blood and urine cultures are obtained before antibiotics are started. A CT scan, MRI study, or both may be beneficial in diagnosing bacterial meningitis to exclude other neurological pathological conditions such as cerebral edema, hydrocephalus, fractures, inner ear infection, or mastoiditis. Do not delay the lumbar puncture procedure to obtain scans if the patient has significant neurological deficits.[64]

Medical and Nursing Management. Antibiotics are started as soon as possible once the diagnosis is suspected because of the rapid progression of the disease process.[64] After administration of antibiotic therapy, the search begins for the offending organism based on patient history, physical examination, CSF cultures, and blood cultures. Droplet isolation is maintained for 24 hours after the initiation of antibiotic therapy. Unusual bacteria and other microorganisms are increasingly responsible for meningitis. Identification of the offending organism or organisms may take time, and final culture results may redirect treatment.

Place the patient in a private room and dim the lighting. Implement seizure precautions. Assess temperature and manage fever with antipyretics and cooling devices. As the acute inflammatory period subsides, monitor the patient closely to prevent secondary complications. These include seizures, increased ICP, syndrome of inappropriate antidiuretic hormone secretion (SIADH), cerebral infarction, gastric bleeding, venous thromboembolism, pressure injuries, pneumonia, and sepsis. The Clinical Alert box outlines additional care considerations.

! CLINICAL ALERT

Meningitis Care and Precautions

Haemophilus influenzae type B and *Neisseria meningitidis* are common bacteria that cause meningitis. These bacteria are easily spread by droplets generated by coughing, sneezing, or talking and during invasive respiratory procedures. Any patient with suspected meningitis should be placed on droplet precautions. Once these bacteria have been ruled out as the source of infection or after effective antibiotic therapy has been instituted for 24 hours, droplet precautions may be discontinued.

During the acute phase of bacterial meningitis, the patient requires close monitoring. Increased intracranial pressure may occur, requiring administration of mannitol or hypertonic saline, placement of a ventriculostomy catheter to drain cerebrospinal fluid, or both. Maintain bed rest with the head of the bed elevated 30 to 40 degrees. Continue IV antibiotic therapy to treat the specific organism identified. Corticosteroids adminstered IV may reduce hearing loss, and neurological sequelae by decreasing meningeal inflammation.[64,65] Current evidence supports the administration of dexamethasone (Decadron) 10 mg before or with the first dose of antibiotics and then every 6 hours for 4 days in adult patients with suspected bacterial meningitis.[65]

CHECK YOUR UNDERSTANDING

4. A patient is admitted to the critical care unit with a diagnosis of possible meningitis. Actions the nurse anticipates include all of the following except:
   A. Placing the patient on contact precautions
   B. Obtaining blood and urine cultures
   C. Administering antibiotics as soon as possible
   D. Preparing the patient for lumbar puncture

SPINAL CORD INJURY

About 250-450,000 people in the United States are living with SCI. Each year, there are approximately 55 per million new SCI cases in the United States. The average age range at time of injury is 16-30 years, and 80% of new SCI injuries are in males.[66] The most common causes of SCI are motor vehicle crashes in young patients, followed by falls in the elderly; other contributing causes are violence, firearms, and sports-related injuries.[66] Providing emergency intervention at the scene by skilled providers, decreasing transport time to the hospital, and implementing evidence-based SCI guidelines improve a patient's outcome.

Pathophysiology

SCI occurs with or without associated vertebral injury and results in complex and multifaceted biochemical changes in the spinal cord. An inflammatory reaction creates spinal cord edema, which compresses tissue and blood vessels. Cord edema can ascend or descend from the level of injury; vascular changes also occur. Microscopic hemorrhages occur in the central gray matter of the spinal cord, with extension into surrounding white matter. Hemorrhage exacerbates edema and further decreases blood flow, resulting in ischemia. If the ischemia is not reversed, axonal degeneration and conduction failure of the neurons occur. Eventually, cell death occurs, with permanent loss of function (Fig. 14.19).[2]

SCI produces two types of shock. *Spinal shock* is an electrical silence of the cord below the level of injury that causes complete loss of motor, sensory, and reflex activity. It begins within minutes after an injury, can progress for several hours, and can last for 2 to 3 days. Often, the permanence of injury is not known until spinal shock resolves. Resolution is signaled by the return of deep tendon reflexes; rarely, motor or sensory function may return. *Neurogenic shock* occurs from disruption of autonomic pathways at or above the level of T6; it results in temporary loss of autonomic function below the level of the injury. Sympathetic input is lost, causing vasodilation and distributive shock, which manifests as hypotension, bradycardia, and hypothermia (see Chapter 12, Shock, Sepsis, and Multiple Organ Dysfunction Syndrome). The venous stasis caused by neurogenic shock, the loss of vasomotor tone, and paralysis increase the risk of VTE. Duration of neurogenic shock is variable; resolution is signaled by return of sympathetic tone.[2]

SCI can result in a complete or incomplete lesion (Fig. 14.20). A *complete lesion* causes total, permanent loss of motor and sensory function below the level of injury. An incomplete lesion is more common and results in the sparing of some motor and sensory function below the level of injury. The three types of *incomplete lesions* are the *central cord, anterior cord,* and *Brown-Séquard* syndromes. The clinical presentation of each syndrome is based on damage to spinal cord organization and crossing of tracts. Many patients present with a picture of a complete lesion until spinal shock resolves; those with an incomplete lesion show a mixed pattern of motor and sensory function and have a potential for at least partial recovery.[2]

Assessment

Neurological. All components of the neurological examination are performed for the patient with a SCI, with an emphasis on motor, reflex, and sensory responses. An assessment of the major muscle groups (Table 14.4) and sensory level (Fig. 14.6) is completed to determine the level of injury. The *American Spinal Injury Association's* (ASIA) *International Standards for Neurological Classification of Spinal Cord Injury* (ISNCSCI) is the gold standard for assessing the level and severity of spinal cord injury.[66] The tool provides a guide for identifying the motor and sensory level of injury, in addition to whether the SCI is complete (meaning no sensory or motor function preserved) or incomplete (a portion of sensory or motor function is preserved below the level of injury). The test may be referred to as the ASIA assessment or ASIA Impairment Scale. Please refer to the ASIA website for learning resources and the latest version of the ISNCSCI assessment (https://asia-spinalinjury.org/international-standards-neurological-classification-sci-isncsci-worksheet/).

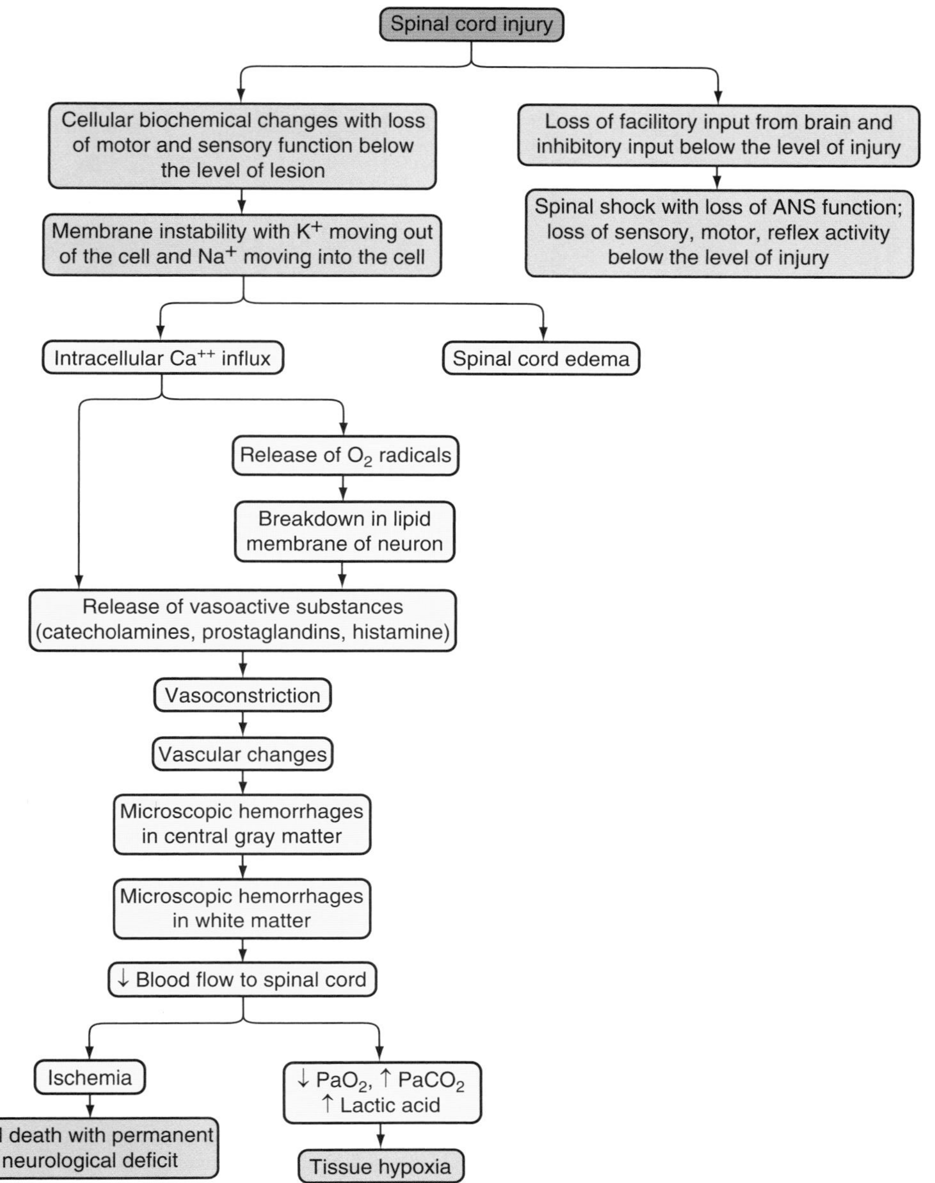

Fig. 14.19 Pathophysiology flow diagram for spinal cord injury. *ANS,* Autonomic nervous system; *Ca^{++},* calcium; *K^+,* potassium; *Na^+,* sodium; *O_2,* oxygen; *$PaCO_2$,* partial pressure of arterial carbon dioxide; *PaO_2,* partial pressure of arterial oxygen.

Airway and Respiratory. The respiratory status depends upon the neurological level of injury. Respiratory problems are common with cervical and thoracic SCI. Ineffective breathing patterns are caused by paralysis of the diaphragm, the intercostal muscles, or both. Baseline arterial blood gas measurements are obtained on admission. Ongoing assessment of the adequacy of the airway and ventilation, including continuous monitoring of SpO_2, is essential. Emergent treatment, including endotracheal intubation and mechanical ventilation, may be needed. Early tracheostomy (open or percutaneous) is recommended for patients with cervical SCI after stabilization, as it improves patient outcomes, decreases hospital length of stay, and decreases morbidity and mortality.[65]

Respiratory impairment varies with the level and type of injury (complete or incomplete). Complete lesions are associated with the following:[2]

- C1-C3: ventilator dependency
- C4-C5: phrenic nerve impairment that may be treated with a phrenic nerve pacemaker
- C6-T6: intact diaphragmatic breathing, with varying impairment of intercostal and abdominal muscle function

Those with incomplete spinal cord lesions present with varying degrees of respiratory impairment, depending on the level of the lesion and whether the respiratory muscles are involved.

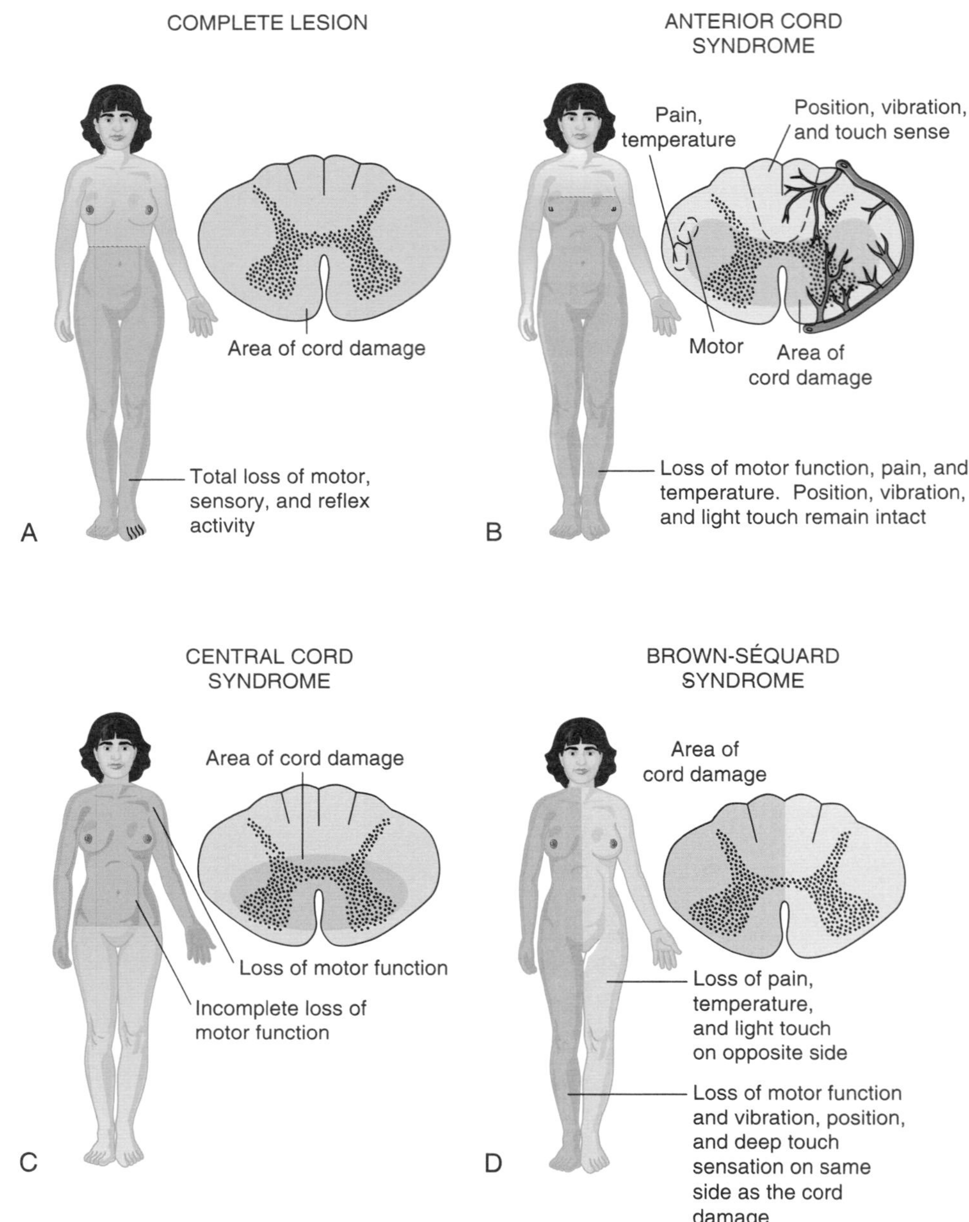

Fig. 14.20 Common spinal cord syndromes. **A**, Complete lesion. **B**, Anterior cord syndrome. **C**, Central cord syndrome. **D**, Brown-Séquard syndrome. (Modified from Ignatavicius DD, Workman ML. *Medical-Surgical Nursing: Patient-Centered Collaborative Care*. 7th ed. Philadelphia, PA: Saunders; 2013.)

Hemodynamic. Avoiding hypotension in the patient with acute SCI is vital.[66] If the patient's level of injury is T6 or higher, they are at risk for developing neurogenic shock, which presents as hypotension and bradycardia (see Chapter 12, Shock, Sepsis, and Multiple Organ Dysfunction Syndrome). Decreases in heart rate may also be associated with hypothermia and hypoxemia. Patients with SCI require cardiac and hemodynamic monitoring; BP monitoring may need to be invasive via an arterial line, depending on hemodynamic stability.

Temperature. A patient with neurogenic shock (injury at T6 and higher) is unable to regulate body temperature; body temperature accommodates to the environmental temperature. The inability to adequately autoregulate body temperature is called *poikilothermia*. Closely monitor temperature, regulate the room temperature to avoid hypothermia, and keep the patient warm with blankets, as needed. Hyperthermia can occur quickly if the patient is excessively warmed and should also be avoided, as the goal is normothermia.

Bowel and Bladder Function. Spinal shock results in atony of the bowel and bladder. The bladder does not contract, and the detrusor muscle does not open. Urinary retention occurs, and an indwelling urinary catheter is required during the acute phase to prevent damage to the bladder wall and to monitor urinary output. Patients who have a known or suspected ureteral abnormality may need a suprapubic catheter.[66]

Loss of peristaltic movement increases the risk of paralytic ileus and prolonged colonic transit times. Neurogenic bowel may lead to constipation, incontinence, and abdominal distention.[66] The pathophysiology of a SCI requires close monitoring of gastrointestinal function and nutrition tolerance (see Chapter 7, Nutritional Therapy). Patients with a SCI often require initiation of a bowel program to achieve future continence and improve their quality of life.

Skin. Because of impaired circulation and immobility, the patient with a SCI is at risk for skin breakdown. A complete assessment of all skin surfaces is done every 4 hours. If halo traction or cervical tongs are used to stabilize a cervical fracture, carefully inspect the skin around pin sites and under traction devices. Observe the site for redness, swelling, drainage, and pain. If a cervical collar is in place, assess skin integrity with an emphasis on pressure points (occipital, chin, and sternal regions).

Psychological. A psychological assessment is important during the acute phase of SCI. Initially, the patient is concerned with surviving the injury and does not realize the extent of injury or disability. The patient's perceptions are also impaired by medications and the physiological effects of injury. Patients often experience denial, anger, and depression. As the patient gains insight into the situation, include the patient in care planning and give the patient choices because feelings of powerlessness are common.

Family members also go through a similar experience. First, they experience shock related to the injury itself and the seriousness of the patient's condition. During that time, family members need support and answers to their questions. Consultation with a psychiatric or mental health provider may be indicated.[66] Involve the patient and family early in plans for rehabilitation.

Diagnostic Studies

Baseline laboratory studies include electrolytes, complete blood count, prothrombin time, aPTT, platelet count, and arterial blood gases. Common diagnostic studies to confirm the extent of vertebral and cord injury include anteroposterior and lateral spine radiographic studies, chest radiographic studies, CT, MRI, and myelography. Myelography is typically reserved for when patients are unable to undergo an MRI due to retained metal fragments or noncompatible pacemaker. Somatosensory-cortical evoked potentials may be performed to determine whether sensory pathways between the site of stimulation and the site of recording are intact; these are typically completed in the operating room.

Patient Problems

Patient problems relevant for this population are outlined in this chapter's Plan of Care for the Patient with Spinal Cord Injury and Collaborative Care Plan found in Chapter 1, Overview of Critical Care Nursing). Once neurogenic shock has resolved, the patient with a complete SCI above T6 must be observed for autonomic dysreflexia (see Clinical Alert box).

PLAN OF CARE

For the Patient with Spinal Cord Injury

Patient Problem

Decreased Functional Ability. Risk factors include muscle weakness or paralysis and spinal motion restriction.

Desired Outcomes

- Consequences of immobility minimized (i.e., pressure injury, VTE, pneumonia).
- Maintenance of vertebral alignment.
- Absence of progressive neurological dysfunction.
- Improved sensory, motor, and reflex function.

Nursing Assessments/Interventions	Rationales
• Perform neurological assessments (motor, reflex, and sensory).	• Assess subtle changes indicating neurological deterioration or improvement.
• Report progression of deficits from baseline (e.g., difficulty with swallowing or coughing, respiratory stridor, sternal retraction, bradycardia, fluctuating BP, and motor and sensory loss at a higher level than the initial findings).	• Detect worsening of symptoms that indicate need for interventions (e.g., airway management and ventilation).
• Institute measures to prevent consequences of immobility: frequent repositioning, use of heel and elbow protectors, and passive range of motion.	• Promote blood flow to lungs and ventilation efforts; improve pulmonary function; minimize risk for skin breakdown; prevent muscle breakdown and promote venous return from lower extremities.
• Assess for signs and symptoms of VTE and address initiation of VTE chemoprophylaxis on multiprofessional rounds daily.	• Not all VTEs are preventable; therefore, frequent assessment and monitoring allows for early identification and mitigation. • Addressing VTE chemoprophylaxis on rounds daily assists with earlier initiation.
• Maintain halo, tong traction, or rigid cervical collar for spinal motion restriction.	• Maintain alignment and prevent complications.
• Perform tong insertion site care (pin care) as ordered or per policy.	• Prevent infection at the pin site.
• Evaluate pin sites for redness, pain, or drainage suggestive of possible infection.	
• If skeletal traction slips or is accidentally removed, maintain the patient's head in a neutral position.	• Maintain alignment and prevent further damage.
• Turn, lift, and transfer the patient using at least three people, with one at the head of the bed to stabilize neck and to coordinate the move (log roll).	• Maintain the spinal cord in alignment to prevent further trauma to the spinal cord.

Continued

PLAN OF CARE—cont'd

For the Patient with Spinal Cord Injury

Patient Problem

Potential for Impaired Temperature Regulation. Risk factors include the body's inability to adapt to environmental temperature changes and the absence of sweating below the level of injury.

Desired Outcomes

- Normothermia within 2 to 4 hours of diagnosis.
- Normothermia maintained.

Nursing Assessments/Interventions	Rationales
• Monitor temperature at least every 4 hours.	• Assess need for intervention.
• Assess for signs of ineffective thermoregulation (e.g., skin warm above level of injury or cool below; complaints of being too cold or warm, pilomotor erection).	• Identify need for intervention to maintain normothermia.
• Implement measures to attain normothermia (i.e., warm or cool as indicated; adjust ambient room temperature).	• Maintain normothermia; prevent complications.

Patient Problem

Decreased Tissue Perfusion (cerebral and cardiac). A risk factor is the loss of vasomotor tone and subsequent hypovolemia.

Desired Outcomes

- Adequate cardiac output.
- Orientation to name, place, time.
- SBP >90 mm Hg or within 20 mm Hg of baseline.
- MAP > 85–90 mm Hg for first 7 days after injury to promote spinal cord perfusion.
- HR 60 to 100 beats/min, ECG shows NSR.

Nursing Assessments/Interventions	Rationales
• Monitor symptoms of low CO: hypotension, lightheadedness, confusion.	• Identify low CO to provide prompt interventions.
• Monitor hemodynamic measurements; administer fluids.	• Provide objective data to guide and monitor treatment.
• Continuously assess the ECG.	• Identify dysrhythmias associated with low CO.
• Implement measures to prevent orthostatic hypotension: change position slowly; apply antiembolic hose; apply abdominal binder.	• Prevent orthostatic hypotension.

Patient Problem

Potential for Infection and Pressure Injury. Risk factors include immobilization, surgical intervention, and presence of invasive devices.

Desired Outcomes

- Absence of skin breakdown and pressure injury.
- Absence of infection at tong insertion site, surgical incision sites, or from an IV or urinary catheter.

Nursing Assessments/Interventions	Rationales
• Assess insertion sites and incisions for signs of infection.	• Identify risk and signs of infection.
• Perform tong insertion site care (pin care).	• Prevent infection.
• Reposition frequently, avoiding pressure on bony prominences.	• Decrease risk for pressure injury.
• Assess all skin surfaces every 4 hours.	• Early identification of skin alterations and implementation of corrective measures.

Patient Problem

Constipation. Risk factors include immobility, atonic bowel, and loss of sensation and voluntary sphincter.

Desired Outcome

- Soft, formed bowel movement within 48 hours of initiating a bowel program.

Nursing Assessments/Interventions	Rationales
• Monitor for nausea, vomiting, abdominal distension, malaise, and the presence of a hard fecal mass on digital examination.	• Assess constipation and fecal impaction.
• Monitor the patient's bowel sounds.	• Assess bowel function.
• Administer stool softeners.	• Promote adequate bowel movement.
• Document the patient's bowel movements.	• Assess effectiveness of bowel management program.

BP, Blood pressure; *CO,* cardiac output; *ECG,* electrocardiogram; *HR,* heart rate; *IV,* intravenous; *NSR,* normal sinus rhythm; *SBP,* systolic blood pressure; *SCI,* spinal cord injury; *VTE,* venous thromboembolism; *WBC,* white blood cell count.

Adapted from Swearingen PL, Wright J. *All-in-One Nursing Care Planning Resource.* 5th ed. St. Louis: Elsevier; 2019.

! CLINICAL ALERT

Autonomic Dysreflexia

Medical Emergency: Can Result in Stroke, Seizures, or Other Complications

- Occurs with injury at T6 or above, after spinal shock has resolved
- Characterized by exaggerated response of the sympathetic nervous system

Triggered by a Variety of Stimuli

- Bladder—kinked indwelling catheter, distension, infection, calculi, cystoscopy
- Bowel—fecal impaction, rectal examination, insertion of suppository
- Skin—tight clothing, irritation from bed linens, temperature extremes

Common Signs and Symptoms

- Sudden, severe, pounding headache
- Elevated, uncontrolled blood pressure
- Bradycardia
- Nasal congestion
- Blurred vision
- Profuse diaphoresis above the level of injury
- Flushing above the level of injury
- Pallor, chills, and pilomotor erection below the level of the injury
- Anxiety

Treatment

- Find and remove the cause of stimulation
- Elevate the head of bed
- Remain calm and supportive
- If symptoms persist, give vasodilators as ordered to decrease blood pressure
- Teach patient to recognize and report symptoms

Medical and Nursing Interventions

Airway. Maintaining a patent airway and respiratory function is a priority. Endotracheal intubation and mechanical ventilation are often required, especially in high cervical spine injuries. Care must be taken to prevent neck hyperextension during endotracheal intubation.

Spinal Motion Restriction. Prehospital spinal motion restriction is achieved with a cervical collar to prevent further injury. A long spine board (backboard), scoop stretcher, and/or vacuum splint may be used when extricating or transporting the patient. These devices are removed once the patient is placed on a stretcher. Once the patient has been hospitalized, *external* stabilization of a fracture or dislocation is often accomplished by use of a cervical collar, skeletal traction (cervical tongs), a halo vest, or a brace (Fig. 14.21).[66] Surgical stabilization of vertebral instability may be required, and studies support surgical intervention within 24 hours of the injury due to increased risk of secondary complications from prolonged best rest. Conversely, the patient's hemodynamic stability, clinical status, and other orthopedic injuries will need to be assessed to determine the appropriate timing of surgical intervention.[66]

Blood Pressure Management. Maintaining perfusion to the spinal cord is crucial. Hypotension contributes to secondary injury by decreasing spinal cord blood flow and perfusion, leading to ischemia and neurological deficit. Current guidelines recommend patients with acute SCI maintain a MAP between 85 and 90 mm Hg for the first 7 days after injury to ensure adequate spinal cord perfusion.[67] The use of vasopressors after appropriate resuscitation may be required to maintain the MAP at this goal range; therefore, the risks and benefits of increasing the BP to achieve this goal must be weighed by the multiprofessional team.[67] If bradycardia is related to neurogenic shock, treatment with a medication that has both alpha- and beta-adrenergic properties is recommended to improve both heart rate and BP (e.g., norepinephrine).[66] Vasopressor response can vary widely because of autonomic instability.

Pressure Injury and Infection Prevention. Always keep the skin clean and dry. Various skin protection devices may be required, including therapeutic beds, mattress overlays, boots, and skin barrier creams.

Bowel and Bladder Management. Insert an indwelling urinary catheter immediately on admission to prevent bladder distension. Initiate a bladder program once spinal shock has resolved. The patient's urinary output, level of injury, and functional recovery must be taken into consideration when developing the bladder program. Intermittent straight catheterization is the ideal bladder management intervention and should be adjusted from four to six times every 24 hours to achieve a urine output less than 400 mL. The goal of intermittent straight catheterization is to avoid bladder distention and reduce the risk of urinary tract infection (UTI).[66]

Bowel programs often include oral medications such as laxatives, stool softeners, prokinetic medications to stimulate the gastrointestinal tract, proper diet and fluid intake, and assisted defecation (i.e., disimpaction, digital stimulation).[66] The type of bowel program initiated is dependent upon the level and completeness of injury. It is essential to implement early bowel and bladder interventions to reduce the risk of secondary complications such as UTI, ileus, autonomic dysreflexia, and skin breakdown.[66] Involve both physical and occupational therapy as appropriate and available.

Venous Thromboembolism Prophylaxis. Because of the limited mobility of patients with SCI, measures to prevent VTE are started immediately on admission, typically starting with mechanical prophylaxis.[66] Chemoprophylaxis should be started within 72 hours of injury; however, there is not an evidence-based standard for initiation in this population.[66] If the patient is not a candidate for VTE chemoprophylaxis within 72 hours of injury, surveillance duplex ultrasounds to exclude deep vein thrombosis may be considered and continued until therapy can be initiated.[66]

Management of Spasticity. After SCI, spasticity or an increase in muscle tone can occur. This upper motor neuron syndrome can interfere with activities of daily living, cause pain and muscle spasms, and interfere with movement. Involve physical therapy to prevent contractures and sustain range of motion. Although there is limited evidence of its effectiveness, antispasmodic agents such as baclofen can be used in conjunction with physical therapy treatments.[66]

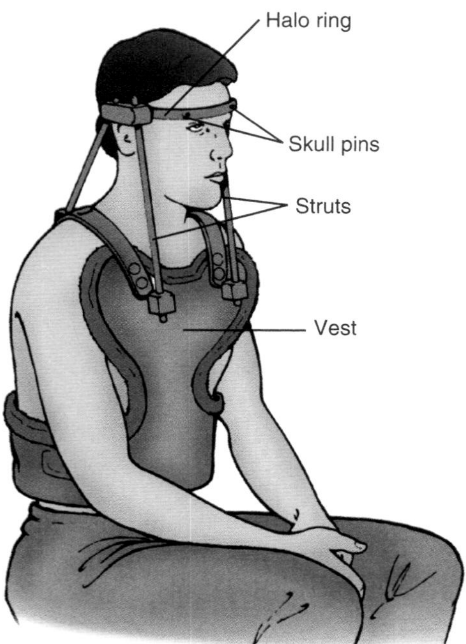

Fig. 14.21 Bremer halo vest. (From Urden LD, Stacy KM, Lough ME. *Priorities in Critical Care Nursing*. 9th ed. St. Louis: Elsevier; 2024.)

Surgical Intervention

SCIs may require surgical intervention to achieve greater neurological recovery and restore spinal stability. Surgery is indicated for neurological deterioration, unstable fractures, cord compression in the presence of an incomplete injury and gross spinal misalignment. Surgery may involve the placement of plates or rods and a bone graft to fuse the spine. Depending on the injury, bone fragments may be removed, or the spine may need to be realigned. The issue of when surgery should be performed is controversial.[66] External immobilization devices, such as cervical traction or a halo vest, may also be used (Fig. 14.21).

CHECK YOUR UNDERSTANDING

5. A patient is admitted after a fall from 15 feet in which the patient landed on their head. The patient is hypotensive and bradycardiac after initial fluid resuscitation. Though the room and fluids are warmed, the patient remains hypothermic. What type of shock is the patient most likely experiencing?
   - **A.** Septic shock
   - **B.** Hypovolemic shock
   - **C.** Neurogenic shock
   - **D.** Cardiogenic shock

CASE STUDY

A 45-year-old patient with a subarachnoid hemorrhage underwent clipping of an aneurysm 5 days ago. At present, the patient is receiving mechanical ventilation and has an arterial catheter and ventriculostomy in place. Nimodipine was started on admission. The patient is lightly sedated, responding to voice and following commands intermittently in all four extremities. Glasgow Coma Scale (GCS) score is 9 (verbal not tested). The current vital signs are heart rate of 80 beats/min, respirations 16 breaths/min at a set rate, blood pressure of 138/80 mm Hg, mean arterial pressure of 99 mm Hg, and ICP 10 mm Hg.

Questions

1. What assessments are a priority for this patient?
2. Explain the purpose of a ventriculostomy in this patient.
3. Based on the patient's presentation and recent aneurysmal clipping, what interventions should the nurse expect?
4. The patient's neurological status is beginning to decline, and the patient is becoming difficult to arouse. The patient is localizing to pain with notably less movement on the left side. GCS score is 7 (verbal not tested). Transcranial Dopplers are completed in the morning and indicate the patient is experiencing cerebral vasospasm. The nurse notifies the provider, who wants to begin hypervolemia, hypertension, and hemodilution therapy. How should the nurse respond?
5. After initiation of the appropriate vasospasm management, how would the nurse evaluate that therapy was effective?

KEY POINTS

- The brain receives 750 mL of blood per minute, 15% to 20% of the total resting cardiac output. The body produces about 500 mL of spinal fluid per day or 20 mL per hour.
- Carbon dioxide is the most potent agent influencing cerebral blood flow (CBF). High levels cause cerebral vasodilation and increased CBF, whereas low levels cause cerebral vasoconstriction and decreased CBF.
- Having a baseline neurological exam is key for identifying changes during follow-up assessments.
- The development of abnormal posturing may indicate a neurological emergency and should be reported to the provider immediately.
- The most commonly used device for monitoring intracranial pressure (ICP) is an external ventriculostomy drain (EVD), which can monitor ICP and be used for therapeutic interventions (i.e., cerebrospinal fluid [CSF] and blood drainage and medication instillation). Conversely, an ICP monitor, also known as a bolt, is used only for monitoring ICP.
- Medical management of increased ICP consists of maintaining the ICP less than 20 mm Hg and cerebral perfusion pressure (CPP) greater than 60 to 70 mm Hg. Interventions to reduce ICP and increase CPP may include: head of bed elevation greater than 30 degrees; neutral neck alignment; administration of hyperosmolar therapies, analgesics, sedatives, neuromuscular blockade, and/or barbiturates; maintaining normothermia; and blood pressure management.
- Concussion, contusion, penetrating injuries, diffuse axonal injury (DAI), and hematomas are all types of primary brain injury. Secondary brain injury may occur because of biochemical consequences of the primary injury.
- Blood pressure parameters differ between ischemic and hemorrhagic stroke. Ischemic stroke systolic blood pressure parameters are typically higher to encourage cerebral perfusion in the infarcted or near-infarcted areas of cerebral tissues. Conversely, blood pressure parameters for hemorrhagic stroke are aimed at reducing systolic blood pressure to decrease the risk of bleeding.

- A common complication of aneurysmal subarachnoid hemorrhage (aSAH) is vasospasm. Prevention with nimodipine is preferred; however, if this fails, euvolemic hypertension is recommended. If symptomatic vasospasm continues, treatment includes intraarterial (via angioplasty) vasodilator administration or cerebral balloon angioplasty. Prognosis for subarachnoid patients is measured with the Hunt and Hess scale and Fisher scale.
- All patients with symptoms of transient ischemic attack (TIA) should receive a complete stroke workup to determine the cause of TIA and a treatment plan to avoid stroke in the future.
- Nursing management for patients in status epilepticus includes maintaining a patent airway, providing adequate oxygenation, administration of medications and fluids, maintaining patient safety, and maintaining seizure precautions.
- The gold standard for the diagnosis of meningitis is examination of the CSF.
- Patients with an acute spinal cord injury (SCI) must maintain a MAP between 85 and 90 mm Hg for the first 7 days after injury to ensure adequate spinal cord perfusion.

REFERENCES

1. Turner KC. Chapter 15: structure and function of the neurologic system. In: Rogers J. *McCance and Huether's Pathophysiology: The Biologic Basis for Disease in Adults and Children*. 9th ed. St. Louis, MO: Elsevier; 2024: 441b-473.
2. Roy K, Huether SE. Chapter 17: alterations in cognitive systems, cerebral hemodynamics, and motor function. In: Rogers J. *McCance and Huether's Pathophysiology: The Biologic Basis for Disease in Adults and Children*. 9th ed. St. Louis, MO: Elsevier; 2024: 509-569.
3. Patton KT, Bell F, Thompson T, Williamson P. *Anatomy and Physiology*. 11th ed. St. Louis, MO: Elsevier; 2022.
4. Seraji-Bzorgzad N, Paulson H, Heidebrink J. Neurologic examination in the elderly. *Handb Clin Neurol*. 2019;167:73–88. https://doi.org/10.1016/B978-0-12-804766-8.00005-4.
5. Segal DN, Grabel ZJ, Heller JG, et al. Epidemiology and treatment of central cord syndrome in the United States. *J Spine Surg*. 2018;4(4):712–716. https://doi.org/10.21037/jss.2018.11.02.
6. The Glasgow Structured Approach to assessment of the Glasgow Coma Scale. FAQ: Glasgow Coma Scale. https://www.glasgowcomascale.org/faq/. Accessed April 27, 2023.
7. Foo CC, Loan JJM, Brennan PM. The relationship of the FOUR Score to patient outcome: a systematic review. *J Neurotrauma*. 2019;36(17):2469–2483. https://doi.org/10.1089/neu.2018.6243.
8. Zadravecz FJ, Tien L, Robertson-Dick BJ, et al. Comparison of mental-status scales for predicting mortality on the general wards. *J Hosp Med*. 2015;10(10):658–663. https://doi.org/10.1002/jhm.2415.
9. Carney N, Totten AM, O'Reilly C, et al. Guidelines for the management of severe traumatic brain injury, fourth edition. *Neurosurgery*. 2018;80(1):6–15.
10. Donnelly J, Czosnyka M, Adams H, et al. Individualizing thresholds of cerebral perfusion pressure using estimated limits of autoregulation. *Crit Care Med*. 2017;45(9):1464–1471. https://doi.org/10.1097/CCM.0000000000002575.
11. Hays LMC, Udy A, Adamides AA, et al. Effects of brain tissue oxygen ($PbtO_2$) guided management on patient outcomes following severe traumatic brain injury: a systematic review and meta-analysis. *J Clin Neurosci*. 2022;99:349–358. https://doi.org/10.1016/j.jocn.2022.03.017.
12. Rivera LL, Püttgen HA. Multimodality monitoring in the neurocritical care unit. *Continuum*. 2018;24(6):1776–1788.
13. Devlin JW, Skrobik Y, Gélinas C, et al. Clinical practice guidelines for the prevention and management of pain, agitation/sedation, delirium, immobility, and sleep disruption in adult patients in the ICU. *Crit Care Med*. 2018;46(9):e825–e873. https://doi.org/10.1097/CCM.0000000000003299.
14. Sacco TL, Davis JG. Management of intracranial pressure part I: pharmacologic interventions. *Dimen Crit Care Nurs*. 2018;37(3):120–129.
15. Topbaş E. Diagnosis and monitoring of neurological changes in intensive care. *Emerg Med Crit Care*. 2018;2(1):10–19.
16. Herman ST, Abend NS, Bleck TP, et al. Consensus statement on continuous EEG in critically ill adults and children, part I: indications. *J Clin Neurophysiol*. 2015;32(2):87–95. https://doi.org/10.1097/WNP.0000000000000166.
17. Ledwith MB, Bloom S, Maloney-Wilensky E, et al. Effect of body position on cerebral oxygenation and physiologic parameters in patients with acute neurological conditions. *J Neurosci Nurs*. 2010;42(5):280–287.
18. Hendrickson SL. Intracranial pressure changes and family presence. *J Neurosci Nurs*. 1987;19(1):14–17. https://doi.org/10.1097/01376517-198702000-00003.
19. Cook AM, Morgan Jones G, Hawryluk GWJ, et al. Guidelines for the acute treatment of cerebral edema in neurocritical care patients. *Neurocrit Care*. 2020;32(3):647–666. https://doi.org/10.1007/s12028-020-00959-7.
20. Demiselle J, Calzia E, Hartmann C, et al. Target arterial PO_2 according to the underlying pathology: a mini-review of the available data in mechanically ventilated patients. *Ann Intensive Care*. 2021;11(1):88. https://doi.org/10.1186/s13613-021-00872-y.
21. Robba C, Poole D, McNett M, et al. Mechanical ventilation in patients with acute brain injury: recommendations of the European Society of Intensive Care Medicine consensus. *Intensive Care Med*. 2020;46(12):2397–2410. https://doi.org/10.1007/s00134-020-06283-0.
22. Zhang Z, Guo Q, Wang E. Hyperventilation in neurological patients: from physiology to outcome evidence. *Curr Opin Anaesthesiol*. 2019;32(5):568–573. https://doi.org/10.1097/ACO.0000000000000764.
23. Gouvea Bogossian E, Peluso L, Creteur J, Taccone FS. Hyperventilation in adult TBI patients: how to approach it? *Front Neurol*. 2021;11:580859.
24. Oh S, Delic JJ. Hyperosmolar therapy in the management of intracranial hypertension. *AACN Adv Crit Care*. 2022;33(1):5–10. https://doi.org/10.4037/aacnacc2022743.
25. Lombardo S, Smith MC, Semler MW, et al. Balanced crystalloid versus saline in adults with traumatic brain injury: secondary analysis of a clinical trial. *J Neurotrauma*. 2022;39(17–18):1159–1167. https://doi.org/10.1089/neu.2021.0465.

26. SAFET trial, Rossi S, Picetti E, Zoerle T, et al. Fluid management in acute brain injury. *Curr Neurol Neurosci Rep*. 2018;18:74. https://doi.org/10.1007/s11910-018-0885-8.
27. Birg T, Ortolano F, Wiegers EJA, et al. Brain temperature influences intracranial pressure and cerebral perfusion pressure after traumatic brain injury: a CENTER-TBI study. *Neurocrit Care*. 2021;35(3):651–661. https://doi.org/10.1007/s12028-021-01294-1.
28. Kim J, Lee S-H, Hur JW, et al. Current prophylactic hypothermia for intracranial hypertension after traumatic brain injury. *Journal of Neurointensive Care*. 2020;3(2):29–32. https://doi.org/10.32587/jnic.2020.00311.
29. Schizodimos T, Soulountsi V, Iasonidou C, et al. An overview of management of intracranial hypertension in the intensive care unit. *J Anesth*. 2020;34:741–757.
30. Oddo M, Crippa IA, Mehta S, et al. Optimizing sedation in patients with acute brain injury. *Crit Care*. 2016;20(1):128. https://doi.org/10.1186/s13054-016-1294-5.
31. Murray MJ, DeBlock H, Erstad B, et al. Clinical practice guidelines for sustained neuromuscular blockade in the adult critically ill patient. *Crit Care Med*. 2016;44(11):2079–2103. https://doi.org/10.1097/CCM.0000000000002027.
32. American College of Surgeons Committee on Trauma. ACS Trauma Quality Improvement Program: best practice for the management of traumatic brain injury. Accessed January 5, 2023. https://www.facs.org/media/mkej5u3b/tbi_guidelines.pdf.
33. Roberts I, Sydenham E. Barbiturates for acute traumatic brain injury. *Cochrane Database Syst Rev*. 2012;12(12):CD000033. https://doi.org/10.1002/14651858.CD000033.pub2.
34. TBI data. Centers for Disease Control and Prevention. https://www.cdc.gov/traumaticbraininjury/data/index.html. Published September 7, 2023. Accessed December 27, 2023.
35. Powers J, Hubner KE. Chapter 18: alterations of the brain, spinal cord, and peripheral nerves. In: Rogers J, ed. *McCance and Huether's Pathophysiology : The Biologic Basis for Disease in Adults and Children*. 9th ed. St. Louis, MO: Elsevier; 2024: 570-617.
36. Abdelmalik PA, Draghic N, Ling GSF. Management of moderate and severe traumatic brain injury. *Transfusion*. 2019;59(S2):1529–1538. https://doi.org/10.1111/trf.15171.
37. Rappold JF, Sheppard FR, Carmichael Ii SP, et al. Venous thromboembolism prophylaxis in the trauma intensive care unit: an American association for the surgery of trauma critical care committee clinical consensus document. *Trauma Surg Acute Care Open*. 2021;6(1):e000643. https://doi.org/10.1136/tsaco-2020-000643. Published 2021 Feb 24.
38. Wat R, Mammi M, Paredes J, et al. The effectiveness of antiepileptic medications as prophylaxis of early seizure in patients with traumatic brain injury compared with placebo or no treatment: a systematic review and meta-analysis. *World Neurosurg*. 2019;122:433–440. https://doi.org/10.1016/j.wneu.2018.11.076.
39. Centers for Disease Control and Prevention. *Stroke Facts*. https://www.cdc.gov/stroke/facts.htm. Reviewed Octoberber 14, 2022. Accessed February 10, 2023.
40. Powers WJ, Rabinstein AA, Ackerson T, et al. Guidelines for the early management of patients with acute ischemic stroke: 2019 update to the 2018 guidelines for the early management of acute ischemic stroke: a guideline for healthcare professionals from the American Heart Association/American Stroke Association. *Stroke*. 2019;50(12):e344–e418. https://doi.org/10.1161/str.0000000000000211.
41. Kernan WN, Forman R, Inzucchi SE. Caring for patients with diabetes in stroke neurology. *Stroke*. 2023;54(3):894–904. https://doi.org/10.1161/STROKEAHA.122.038163.
42. Gorelick PB, Whelton PK, Sorond F, Carey RM. Blood pressure management in stroke. *Hypertension*. 2020;76(6):1688–1695. https://doi.org/10.1161/HYPERTENSIONAHA.120.14653.
43. Herpich F, Rincon F. Management of acute ischemic stroke. *Critical Care Medicine*. 2020;48(11):1654–1663. https://doi.org/10.1097/ccm.0000000000004597.
44. Activase (alteplase) for Injection - Food and Drug Administration. https://www.accessdata.fda.gov/drugsatfda_docs/label/2015/103172s5203lbl.pdf. Accessed February 13, 2023.
45. Potla N, Ganti L. Tenecteplase vs. Alteplase for acute ischemic stroke: a systematic review. *Int J Emerg Med*. 2022;15(1):1–6. https://doi.org/10.1186/s12245-021-00399-w.
46. O'Carroll CB, Aguilar MI. Management of postthrombolysis hemorrhagic and orolingual angioedema complications. *Neurohospitalist*. 2015;5(3):133–141. https://doi.org/10.1177/1941874415587680.
47. Wang X, Ouyang M, Yang J, Song L, Yang M, Anderson CS. Anticoagulants for acute ischaemic stroke. *Cochrane Database of Syst Rev*. 2021;10:CD000024. https://doi.org/10.1002/14651858.CD000024.pub5.
48. Yaghi S, Willey JZ, Cucchiara B, et al. Treatment and outcome of hemorrhagic transformation after intravenous alteplase in acute ischemic stroke: a scientific statement for healthcare professionals from the American Heart Association/American Stroke Association. *Stroke*. 2017;48(12):e343–e361. https://doi.org/10.1161/str.0000000000000152.
49. Easton JD, Saver JL, Albers GW, et al. Definition and evaluation of transient ischemic attack: a scientific statement for healthcare professionals from the American heart association/American stroke association stroke council; council on cardiovascular surgery and anesthesia; council on cardiovascular radiology and intervention; council on cardiovascular nursing; and the interdisciplinary council on peripheral vascular disease. The American academy of neurology affirms the value of this statement as an educational tool for neurologists. *Stroke*. 2009;40(6):2276–2293. https://doi.org/10.1161/STROKEAHA.108.192218.
50. Derdeyn CP, Zipfel GJ, Albuquerque FC, et al. Management of brain arteriovenous malformations: a scientific statement for healthcare professionals from the American Heart Association/American Stroke Association. *Stroke*. 2017;48(8):e200–e224. https://doi.org/10.1161/str.0000000000000134.
51. Kleindorfer DO, Towfighi A, Chaturvedi S, et al. 2021 Guideline for the prevention of stroke in patients with stroke and transient ischemic attack: a guideline from the American Heart Association/American Stroke Association. *Stroke*. 2021;52(7):e364–e467. https://doi.org/10.1161/STR.0000000000000375. [published correction appears in Stroke. 2021 Jul;52(7):e483-e484].
52. Greenberg SM, Ziai WC, Cordonnier C, et al. 2022 Guideline for the management of patients with spontaneous intracerebral hemorrhage: a guideline from the American Heart Association/American Stroke Association. *Stroke*. 2022;53(7):e282–e361. https://doi.org/10.1161/STR.0000000000000407.
53. Connolly ES, Rabinstein AA, Carhuapoma JR, et al. Guidelines for the management of aneurysmal subarachnoid hemorrhage. *Stroke*. 2012;43(6):1711–1737. https://doi.org/10.1161/str.0b013e3182587839.
54. Burns SK, Brewer KJ, Jenkins C, et al. Aneurysmal subarachnoid hemorrhage and vasospasm. *AACN Adv Crit Care*. 2018;29(2):163–174.
55. Nyquist P, Bautista C, Jichici D, et al. Prophylaxis of venous thrombosis in neurocritical care patients: an evidence-based

guideline: a statement for healthcare professionals from the Neurocritical Care Society. *Neurocrit Care*. 2016;24(1):47–60. https://doi.org/10.1007/s12028-015-0221-y.

56. Maher M, Schweizer TA, Macdonald RL. Treatment of spontaneous subarachnoid hemorrhage: guidelines and gaps. *Stroke*. 2020;51(4):1326–1332. https://doi.org/10.1161/STROKEAHA.119.025997.
57. Kim SM, Woo HG, Kim YJ, Kim BJ. Blood pressure management in stroke patients. *Journal of Neurocritical Care*. 2020;13(2):69–79. https://doi.org/10.18700/jnc.200028.
58. A. Malformations. AANS. https://www.aans.org/en/Patients/Neurosurgical-Conditions-and-Treatments/Arteriovenous-Malformations. Accessed February 12, 2023.
59. Chauhan R, Bloria SD, Luthra A. Management of postoperative neurosurgical patients. *Indian Journal of Neurosurgery*. 2019;08(03):179–184. https://doi.org/10.1055/s-0039-1698001.
60. Siegemund M, Steiner LA. Postoperative care of the neurosurgical patient. *Current Opinion in Anaesthesiology*. 2015;28(5):487–493. https://doi.org/10.1097/aco.0000000000000229.
61. Lioutas VA, Ivan CS, Himali JJ, et al. Incidence of transient ischemic attack and association with long-term risk of stroke. *JAMA*. 2021;325(4):373–381. https://doi.org/10.1001/jama.2020.25071.
62. Fisher RS. The new classification of seizures by the International League against Epilepsy. *Curr Neurol Neurosci Rep*. 2017;17(6):48–53.
63. Trinka E, Leitinger M. Management of status epilepticus, refractory status epilepticus, and super-refractory status epilepticus. *Continuum (Minneap Minn)*. 2022;28(2):559–602. https://doi.org/10.1212/CON.0000000000001103.
64. Marcus R, Walter K. Bacterial meningitis. *JAMA*. 2022;328(21):2170. https://doi.org/10.1001/jama.2022.21603.
65. Brouwer MC, McIntyre P, Prasad K, van de Beek D. Corticosteroids for acute bacterial meningitis. *Cochrane Database Syst Rev*. 2015;2015(9):CD004405.
66. American College of Surgeons Committee on Trauma. ACS Trauma Quality Improvement Program: Best practice guidelines: spine injury. Accessed January 8, 2023. https://www.facs.org/media/k45gikqv/spine_injury_guidelines.pdf.
67. Evaniew N, Mazlouman SJ, Belley-Côté EP, Jacobs WB, Kwon BK. Interventions to optimize spinal cord perfusion in patients with acute traumatic spinal cord injuries: a systematic review. *J Neurotrauma*. 2020;37(9):1127–1139. https://doi.org/10.1089/neu.2019.6844.

15

Acute Respiratory Failure

Jenny Lynn Sauls, PhD, MSN, RN, CNE

INTRODUCTION

Acute respiratory failure (ARF) is one of the most common admitting diagnoses in critical care units, resulting in significant cost and in-hospital mortality.[1] It may occur as the primary problem or secondary to other conditions. Mechanical ventilation is the most commonly used support required by 20% to 40% of patients admitted to critical care units in the United States.[2] This chapter includes a review of the pathophysiology, as well as common causes, symptoms, medical management, and nursing care involved in the treatment of patients with ARF.

ACUTE RESPIRATORY FAILURE

Definition

ARF is defined as an inability of the respiratory system to provide oxygenation and/or to remove carbon dioxide from the body. ARF is classified as oxygenation failure resulting in hypoxemia without a rise in carbon dioxide levels or ventilation failure resulting in hypercapnia and hypoxemia. Oxygenation failure, also known as hypoxemic or type 1 ARF, is characterized by a partial pressure of arterial oxygen (PaO_2) lower than 60 mm Hg with normal to decreased levels of carbon dioxide. Ventilation failure, also known as hypercapnic or type 2 ARF, is characterized by a partial pressure of arterial carbon dioxide ($PaCO_2$) greater than 50 mm Hg. These values are based on arterial blood levels with the patient breathing room air. ARF differs from chronic respiratory failure in that it evolves rapidly over minutes to hours, providing little time for physiological compensation. Chronic respiratory failure develops over time and allows the body's compensatory mechanisms to activate. ARF and chronic respiratory failure are not mutually exclusive. ARF may occur when a person who has chronic respiratory failure develops a respiratory infection or is exposed to other types of stressors, creating an increased demand or decreased supply of oxygen (O_2) that overwhelms the already compromised respiratory system. This is referred to as acute-on-chronic respiratory failure.

Pathophysiology

Failure of Oxygenation. Oxygenation failure occurs when the PaO_2 cannot be adequately maintained; it is the most common type of ARF observed in the clinical setting. Five generally accepted mechanisms that reduce PaO_2 and create a state of hypoxemia are hypoventilation, intrapulmonary shunting, ventilation-perfusion ($\dot{V}/\dot{Q}$) mismatching, diffusion defects, and decreased barometric pressure (Fig. 15.1). Decreased barometric pressure, which occurs at high altitudes, is not addressed in this text. Nonpulmonary conditions such as decreased cardiac output and low hemoglobin levels may also result in tissue hypoxia.

Hypoventilation. Alveolar ventilation refers to the amount of gas that enters the alveoli per minute. In the normal lung, the partial pressure of alveolar oxygen (PAO_2) is approximately equal to the PaO_2. If the alveolar ventilation is reduced because of hypoventilation, the PAO_2 and the PaO_2 are both reduced. Factors that can lead to hypoventilation include any condition that causes central nervous system (CNS) depression (e.g., drug overdose, metabolic encephalopathy), neurological disorders that decrease the rate or depth of respirations, and abdominal or thoracic surgery leading to shallow breathing patterns associated with pain on inspiration. Hypoventilation also produces an increase in the alveolar carbon dioxide (CO_2) level because the CO_2 that is produced in the tissues is delivered to the lungs but is not released from the body.

Intrapulmonary shunting. In normally functioning lungs, a small amount of blood returns to the left side of the heart without engaging in alveolar gas exchange. This is referred to as the *physiological shunt*. If, however, a larger amount of blood returns to the left side of the heart without participating in gas exchange, the shunt becomes pathological, and a decrease in the PaO_2 occurs. A pathological shunt exists when areas of the lung that are inadequately ventilated but are adequately perfused (Fig. 15.1), causing the blood to shunt past the lung and return unoxygenated to the left side of the heart. Common causes of shunting leading to hypoxemia include atelectasis, pneumonia, and pulmonary edema.

As the shunt worsens, the PaO_2 continues to decrease. This cause of hypoxemia cannot be treated effectively solely by increasing the fraction of inspired oxygen (FiO_2) because the increased O_2 is unable to reach the alveoli. Treatment is directed toward interventions that open the alveoli and improve ventilation.

Ventilation-perfusion mismatch. Gas exchange in the lungs is dependent on the balance between ventilated areas of the lung (ventilation) receiving blood flow (perfusion). The rate of ventilation ($\dot{V}$) usually equals the rate of perfusion ($\dot{Q}$), resulting in a $\dot{V}/\dot{Q}$ ratio of 1.0. If ventilation exceeds blood

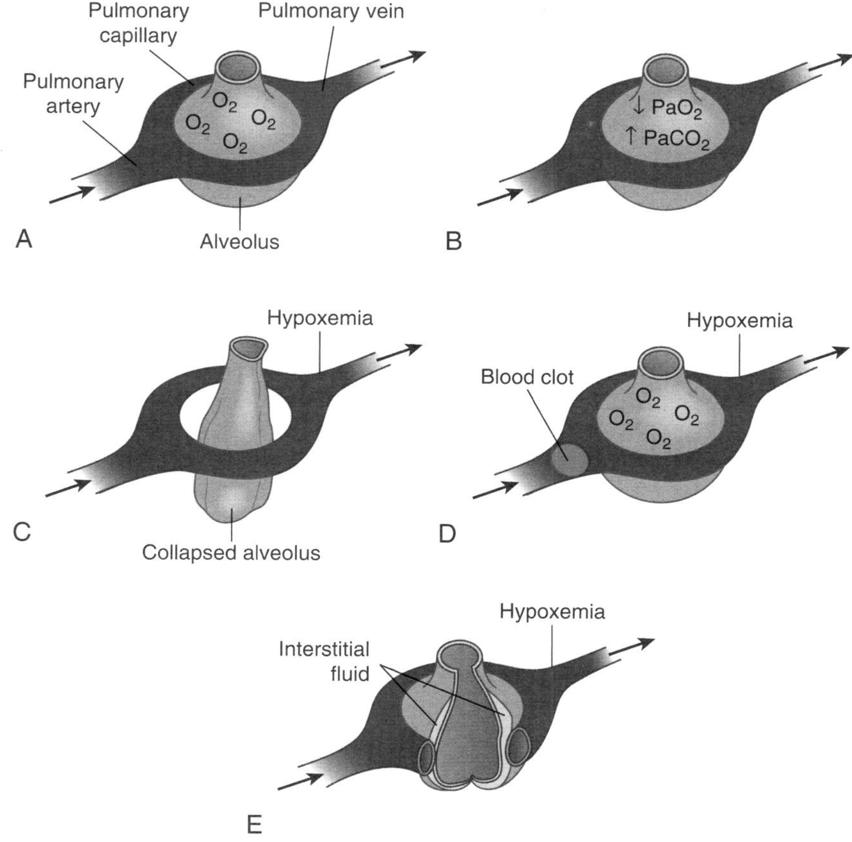

Fig. 15.1 Pulmonary causes of hypoxemia. A, Normal alveolar-capillary unit. B, Hypoventilation causes an increased partial pressure of carbon dioxide ($PaCO_2$) and a decreased partial pressure of arterial oxygen (PaO_2). C, Shunt. D, Ventilation-perfusion mismatch resulting from pulmonary embolus. E, Diffusion defect due to increased interstitial fluid. *O_2*, Oxygen.

flow, the $\dot{V}/\dot{Q}$ ratio is greater than 1.0; if ventilation is less than blood flow, the $\dot{V}/\dot{Q}$ ratio is less than 1.0. $\dot{V}/\dot{Q}$ mismatch can occur in conditions such as pneumonia or pulmonary edema, when obstructed airways inhibit ventilation (and perfusion is normal), or in the case of pulmonary embolism, when a clot in the pulmonary circulation obstructs perfusion.

Diffusion defects. Diffusion is the movement of gas from an area of high concentration to an area of lower concentration. In the lungs, O_2 and CO_2 move between the alveoli and the blood by diffusing across the alveolar-capillary membrane. The alveolar-capillary membrane has six barriers to the diffusion of O_2 and CO_2: surfactant, alveolar epithelium, interstitial fluid, capillary endothelium, plasma, and the red blood cell membrane. Under normal circumstances, O_2 and CO_2 diffuse across the alveolar-capillary membrane in 0.25 seconds. The distance between an alveolus and a pulmonary capillary is usually only one or two cells thick. This narrowness of space facilitates efficient diffusion of O_2 and CO_2 across the cell membrane.

In respiratory failure, the distance between the alveoli and the capillaries may be increased by accumulation of fluid in the interstitial space (Fig. 15.1). Changes in capillary perfusion pressure, leakage of plasma proteins into the interstitial space, and destruction of the capillary membrane contribute to the buildup of fluids around the alveolus. Fibrotic changes in the lung tissue itself, such as those seen in chronic obstructive pulmonary disease (COPD), can also contribute to a reduction in the diffusion capacity of the lungs. As diffusion capacity is reduced, reductions in PaO_2 occur first, resulting in hypoxemia. Because CO_2 is more readily diffusible than O_2, hypercapnia is a late sign of diffusion defects.

Low cardiac output. Adequate tissue oxygenation depends on a balance between O_2 supply and demand. The mechanism for delivering O_2 to the tissues is cardiac output. A normal cardiac output results in the delivery of 600 to 1000 mL/min of O_2, which generally exceeds the normal amount of O_2 needed by the tissues. If the cardiac output decreases, less oxygenated blood is delivered. To maintain normal aerobic metabolism in low cardiac output states, the tissues must extract increasing amounts of O_2 from the blood. When this increase in extraction can no longer compensate for the decreased cardiac output, the cells convert to anaerobic metabolism. This results in the production of lactic acid, which depresses the function of the myocardium and further lowers cardiac output.

Low hemoglobin level. Between 96% and 100% of the body's O_2 is transported to the tissues bound to hemoglobin. When all O_2 binding sites are filled, each gram of hemoglobin can carry 1.34 mL of O_2. Arterial oxygen saturation (SaO_2) refers to the percentage of O_2 binding sites on each hemoglobin molecule that are filled with O_2 (normally 96% to 100%). If a patient's hemoglobin level is lower than normal, O_2 supply to the tissues may be impaired, and tissue hypoxia can occur. An alteration in hemoglobin function (e.g., carbon monoxide poisoning, sickle cell disease) can also decrease O_2 delivery to the tissues.

Tissue hypoxia. The final step in oxygenation is the use of O_2 by the tissues. Anaerobic metabolism occurs when the tissues cannot obtain adequate O_2 to meet metabolic needs. Anaerobic metabolism is inefficient and results in the accumulation of lactic acid. The point at which anaerobic metabolism begins to occur is not known and may vary for each organ system. The effects of tissue hypoxia are dependent upon the severity of hypoxia but may result in cellular death and subsequent organ failure.

Failure of Ventilation. $PaCO_2$ is the variable used to evaluate ventilation. When ventilation is reduced, $PaCO_2$ is increased (hypercapnia). When ventilation is increased, $PaCO_2$ is reduced (hypocapnia). Hypoventilation and $\dot{V}/\dot{Q}$ mismatching are the two mechanisms responsible for hypercapnia. Hypercapnia induces cerebral vasodilation, which significantly increases cerebral blood flow, causing the patient to appear restless and disoriented. As intracranial pressure rises, the level of consciousness (LOC) decreases, progressing to coma if effective treatment does not occur.

Hypoventilation. Hypoventilation is the cause of respiratory failure that occurs in patients with CNS abnormalities, neuromuscular disorders, overdoses (e.g., alcohol, benzodiazepines, opioids), and chest wall abnormalities (Fig. 15.1). In hypoventilation, CO_2 accumulates in the alveoli and is not exhaled. Respiratory acidosis occurs rapidly, before renal compensation can occur. Mechanical ventilation may be necessary to support the patient until the initial cause of the hypoventilation can be corrected.

Ventilation-perfusion mismatch. Because the upper and lower airways do not participate in gas exchange, the volume of inspired gas that fills these structures is referred to as physiological dead space. This dead space normally accounts for 25% to 30% of the inspired volume. A major mechanism for the elevation of $PaCO_2$ is an increase in the volume of dead space in relation to the total tidal volume (V_T). Dead space increases when an area that is well ventilated has reduced perfusion and no longer participates in gas exchange, as is created in shock or pulmonary embolism.

Assessment

Respiratory assessment and evaluation of gas exchange are discussed in depth in Chapter 10, Ventilatory Assistance. Changes in mental status resulting from hypoxemia and hypercapnia begin with anxiety, restlessness, and confusion and may deteriorate to lethargy, severe somnolence, and coma if respiratory failure is not resolved.

Observe the rate, depth, and pattern of respiration. In response to hypoxemia, compensatory mechanisms produce tachypnea and an increase in V_T (hyperventilation). As these compensatory mechanisms fail, respirations become shallow, however bradypnea is an ominous sign. Use of accessory muscles and intercostal retractions are also cause for concern because they indicate respiratory muscle fatigue. By auscultation, assess the adequacy of airflow and the presence of adventitious breath sounds. Also note the presence of a cough and the amount and characteristics of any sputum production.

A thorough cardiac assessment provides information about the heart's ability to deliver O_2 to the tissues and cells. Monitor for changes in blood pressure (BP), heart rate, and cardiac rhythm. ARF initially causes tachycardia and increased BP. Worsening of ARF can result in dysrhythmias, angina, hypotension, and cardiac arrest. Evaluate peripheral perfusion by palpating pulses for strength and bilateral equality and assess the skin for a decrease in temperature and the presence of mottling, cyanosis, or pallor.

Nutritional status is an important factor in maintaining respiratory muscle strength. Assess for recent weight loss, muscle wasting, nausea, vomiting, abdominal distension, and skin turgor quality.

The psychosocial status of the patient can also affect outcomes; therefore, identify the patient's significant others and their roles in the family structure. An understanding of the patient's educational level, socioeconomic background, spiritual beliefs, and cultural or ethnic practices are important in determining an educational plan for discharge and future self-care.

Serial chest radiographs and pulmonary function tests provide important assessment information. Laboratory studies that are essential for the patient with respiratory failure include: electrolytes, which determine adequate muscle function; hemoglobin and hematocrit, to evaluate the blood's O_2 carrying capacity; and arterial blood gas (ABG) measurements, to assess gas exchange and acid-base balance. Noninvasive monitoring of oxygenation, such as pulse oximetry (SpO_2), provides information about the patient's oxygenation, whereas continuous end-tidal CO_2 monitoring provides information about the patient's ventilation.

Physiological changes with aging may make identifying the signs and symptoms of ARF more difficult in older adults. The most common early sign of hypoxemia in the older adult is a change in mental status, such as confusion or agitation. These changes are often mistaken for dementia or a normal sign of advancing age. See the Lifespan Considerations box for additional information.[3-4]

CLINICAL JUDGMENT ACTIVITY

A 66-year-old patient who has smoked 1.5 packs of cigarettes per day for 40 years (60 pack-years) is admitted with an acute exacerbation of COPD. A baseline ABG is unavailable. In the critical care unit, the patient has coarse crackles in his left posterior lower lung and a mild expiratory wheeze bilaterally. The patient's cough is productive, with thick yellow sputum. Skin turgor is poor; the patient is febrile, tachycardic, and tachypneic. The most recent ABG while receiving O_2 at 2 L/min via a nasal cannula is as follows: pH, 7.32; $PaCO_2$, 64 mm Hg; PaO_2, 50 mm Hg; HCO_3, 30 mEq/L; SaO_2, 86%. Interpret the ABG findings. What is the probable cause of the patient's COPD exacerbation, and what treatment is indicated at this time?

LIFESPAN CONSIDERATIONS

Older Adults

- Rib ossification results in decreased compliance of the thorax.
- Decreased vital capacity and ventilator reserve as well as an increased residual volume are associated with decreased chest wall mobility.
- Loss of alveolar wall tissue and capillaries decreases surface area for gas exchange, resulting in decreased PaO_2, which reduces exercise tolerance.
- Decline in muscle mass contributes to respiratory muscle fatigue and decreased endurance.
- Decreased effectiveness of the immune system increases susceptibility to infection.
- Chemoreceptor and CNS function declines, causing:
  - A lower ventilatory response to hypoxia and hypercapnia.
  - Less of a compensatory increase in heart rate, stroke volume, and cardiac output to hypoxia.
  - An increased risk for respiratory depression caused by medications.
- Feelings of dyspnea remain intact and may be enhanced despite the decline in the compensatory response.
- Slower response to O_2 therapy.
- PaO_2 levels decrease with age, but aging does not produce significant alterations in pH or $PaCO_2$. For this reason, hypercapnia and a falling pH are causes for concern.

Pregnant People

- Advanced stages of pregnancy challenge pulmonary mechanics through elevation of the diaphragm and altered thoracic configuration, resulting in increased negative pleural pressures, reduced functional residual capacity (FRC) and expiratory reserve volume (ERV), and a shortened chest height.
- O_2 consumption and basal metabolic rate (BMR) increase, which lowers O_2 reserve.
- Dyspnea and breathlessness are commonly reported by healthy pregnant people starting from the first trimester.
- Due to physiological changes in pregnancy, monitor ventilation and oxygenation frequently.

Interventions

The goals for treating patients with ARF include maintaining a patent airway, optimizing O_2 delivery, minimizing O_2 demand, treating the cause of ARF, and preventing complications.

Maintain a Patent Airway. Some causes of ARF, such as COPD, cardiogenic pulmonary edema, pulmonary infiltrates in immunocompromised patients, and palliation in the terminally ill, may be effectively treated with noninvasive positive-pressure ventilation (NPPV).[5-7] However, if a patient is unable to maintain a patent airway or if NPPV does not improve ventilation or oxygenation, intubation and mechanical ventilation may be indicated. (Refer to Chapter 10, Ventilatory Assistance, for nursing care related to NPPV and mechanical ventilation.)

Optimize Oxygen Delivery. Strategies for optimizing O_2 delivery depend on the needs of the patient. Initially, provide supplemental O_2 via nasal cannula or face mask to maintain the PaO_2 higher than 60 mm Hg. The optimal SaO_2 and SpO_2 goals are unknown. Evidence suggests maintaining saturations between 94% to 96% may reduce the risk of harm in the critically ill patient; however, additional research is needed, and the saturation goal may vary based on the patient's clinical condition.[8-10]

If supplemental O_2 is ineffective in raising PaO_2 levels, high-flow nasal cannula[11] or noninvasive mechanical ventilation may be considered.[12] Invasive mechanical ventilation is the next step (see Clinical Alert box).

Patients are positioned for ease of breathing and to enhance $\dot{V}/\dot{Q}$ matching. Other methods to optimize O_2 delivery include red blood cell transfusion to ensure adequate hemoglobin levels for transport of O_2 and enhancing cardiac output and BP to deliver sufficient O_2 to the tissues. Refer to the Plan of Care for the Patient With Acute Respiratory Failure for detailed interventions and rationales for optimizing oxygenation.

Minimize Oxygen Demand. Decreasing the patient's O_2 demand begins with providing adequate rest. Avoid unnecessary physical activity. Agitation, restlessness, pain, fever, infection, and patient-ventilator dyssynchrony must be addressed because they all contribute to increased O_2 demand and consumption.

Treat the Cause of Acute Respiratory Failure. While the patient is being treated for hypoxemia and/or hypercapnia, efforts must be made to identify and reverse the cause of ARF. Specific interventions for acute respiratory distress syndrome (ARDS), COPD, asthma, pneumonia, and pulmonary embolism are detailed in this chapter.

CLINICAL ALERT

Acute Respiratory Failure

Concern	Symptoms	Nursing Actions
Respiratory muscle fatigue	Diaphoresis Nasal flaring Tachycardia Abdominal paradox Muscle retractions • Intercostal • Suprasternal • Supraclavicular Central cyanosis	**Improve oxygen (O_2) delivery:** • Administer O_2 • Ensure adequate cardiac output and blood pressure • Correct low hemoglobin • Administer bronchodilators **Decrease O_2 demand:** • Provide rest • Reduce fever • Relieve pain and anxiety • Position patient for optimum gas exchange and perfusion • Prepare for possible intubation and mechanical ventilation
Cerebral hypoxia and carbon dioxide (CO_2) narcosis from increased CO_2 retention	Lethargy Somnolence Coma Respiratory acidosis	**Maintain airway patency** • Prepare for possible intubation and mechanical ventilation

Prevent Complications. Finally, be alert to the potential complications that the patient with ARF may encounter. Implement measures to prevent immobility, adverse effects from medications, fluid and electrolyte imbalances, development of gastric ulcers, and hazards of mechanical ventilation.

Early mobility may be an important nursing intervention for all patients with ARF. Physical therapy for critically ill patients while in the critical care unit can improve mobility and strength and decrease length of stay (LOS),[13] but use of a physical therapist (PT) to provide therapy is infrequent.[14] The critical care nurse can have a positive impact on in-hospital outcomes by initiating progressive mobility early in the patient's stay and collaborating with the provider to consult physical therapy based on the patient's needs.

Patient Problems

Several problems are considered in the care of a patient with ARF (see Plan of Care for the Patient With Acute Respiratory Failure box), depending on the etiology and other comorbidities. Expected outcomes include adequate organ and tissue oxygenation, effective breathing, and adequate gas exchange.

PLAN OF CARE

For the Patient With Acute Respiratory Failure[a]

Patient Problem

Decreased gas exchange. Risk factors include ventilation-perfusion ($\dot{V}/\dot{Q}$) mismatch, diffusion abnormality, alveolar-capillary membrane changes, decreased hemoglobin-carrying capacity, and decreased cardiac output.

Desired Outcomes

- PaO_2 80 to 100 mm Hg.
- $PaCO_2$ 35 to 45 mm Hg or within patient's expected range.
- SaO_2 or SpO_2 > 93% or within patient's expected range.
- Alert and oriented to person, place, and time or no further decline in LOC.
- Pink skin color or absence of cyanosis.
- Heart rate < 100 beats/min.
- RR ≤ 24 breaths/min.

Nursing Assessments/Interventions	Rationales
• Monitor SpO_2 continuously and report values ≤93%.	• Assess response to oxygen therapy. • Values ≤93% can indicate need for increase in supplemental O_2.
• Review ABG levels when available. Report abnormal values to the provider (e.g., pH <7.35 or >7.45; PaO_2 <80 mm Hg; and/or $PaCO_2$ >45 mm Hg).	• Assess values indicative of respiratory failure and response to treatment.
• Monitor heart rate.	• Tachycardia indicates a compensatory mechanism for hypoxemia.
• Monitor for signs and symptoms of respiratory distress and report promptly: restlessness, anxiety, change in mental status, shortness of breath, tachypnea, and use of accessory muscles.	• Allows for early identification and treatment.
• Position patient to facilitate comfort and respiratory excursion (usually semi-Fowler's).	• Promote comfort and diaphragmatic descent; maximize inhalation; decrease WOB; and promote ventilation-perfusion matching.
• Administer supplemental oxygen to achieve oxygen saturation >93%. Begin with lower concentrations of FiO_2; if SpO_2 does not rise above 93%, increase FiO_2 in small increments while monitoring SpO_2 or ABG values; notify provider promptly of the need for significant increases in FiO_2.	• Support perfusion of tissues and organs.
• Prepare for use of NPPV or intubation and mechanical ventilation.	• NPPV may prevent the need for intubation; mechanical ventilation may be indicated to achieve oxygenation and ventilation goals.

Patient Problem

Dyspnea. Risk factors include ineffective inspiration and expiration.

Desired Outcomes

- Absence of dyspnea or use of accessory muscles.
- Symmetrical chest wall movement with midline trachea.
- Respirations unlabored at a rate of 12 to 16 breaths/min.
- Patient verbalizes ability to breathe comfortably.

Nursing Assessments/Interventions	Rationales
• Assess respiratory status every 2 to 4 hours based on patient's condition: rate, rhythm, and depth; use of accessory muscles; intercostal retractions; nasal flaring.	• Guide early identification of respiratory distress and initiate immediate intervention.
• Assess position assumed for breathing.	• Three-point position for breathing (bending forward with hands on knees) indicates increasing respiratory distress.
• Consider prone positioning if unable to optimize oxygenation.	• May improve oxygenation in ARDS for patients on mechanical ventilation when used for periods >12 hours/day.
• Encourage slow, deep breathing and/or teach pursed-lip breathing technique to achieve an I:E ratio of 1:2 or 1:3.	• Facilitate controlled breathing pattern and maintain a positive pressure in the airways.

PLAN OF CARE—cont'd

For the Patient With Acute Respiratory Failure[a]

Nursing Assessments/Interventions	Rationales
• Provide pain relief.	• Prevent splinting and hypoventilation.
• If patient has lung pathology, position for maximal gas exchange.	• Increase perfusion to the lungs and facilitate gas exchange.
• Assist with and pace activities; provide patient with periods of rest.	• Reduce oxygen consumption and demands.
• Administer beta-2-agonist drugs by metered-dose inhaler or nebulizer to increase airflow as prescribed; evaluate their effectiveness.	• Decrease airway resistance secondary to bronchoconstriction.
• Administer corticosteroids as indicated based on diagnosis and clinical condition.	• Decrease inflammation and edema to improve airflow in narrowed airways.
• Prepare for chest tube insertion for pneumothorax, hemothorax, or flail chest; connect to drainage system.	• Remove air or blood from pleural space and promote reexpansion of lung.
• Anticipate the need for intubation and mechanical ventilation.	• Early intubation and ventilation can prevent deterioration of respiratory function or respiratory arrest.
• If patient is mechanically ventilated, sedate according to goals for patient; avoid oversedation.	• Facilitate gas exchange and mechanical ventilation; promote earlier weaning and extubation.

Patient Problem

Insufficient airway clearance. Risk factors include the inability to cough, presence of endotracheal tube, and thick secretions.

Desired Outcomes

- Ability to cough effectively to clear secretions.
- Tolerates suctioning to clear secretions while maintaining an $SpO_2 > 93\%$.
- Breath sounds clear after cough or suctioning.

Nursing Assessments/Interventions	Rationales
• Auscultate anterior and posterior bilateral breath sounds every 1-2 hours, after coughing or suctioning, and otherwise as needed.	• Presence of crackles or rhonchi indicates fluid accumulation; presence of wheezes indicates bronchoconstriction. • Fine crackles should clear with deep breathing. • Coarse crackles require deep cough and/or suctioning.
• Assess sputum characteristics: amount, color, consistency, odor. Document findings and culture as appropriate.	• Provide assessment data about the cause of respiratory failure: colored sputum, infection; thick tenacious sputum, dehydration; frothy sputum, pulmonary edema.
• Change patient's position every 2 hours.	• Mobilize secretions.
• Encourage patient to cough and deep breathe at least every 2 hours.	• Improve lung capacity, clear secretions, and facilitate gas exchange.
• Assess the need for hyperinflation therapy. Encourage patient to slowly and deeply inhale approximately twice the normal VT, hold the breath for 5 seconds, and exhale; repeat 10 times every hour.	• Inability to take deep breaths indicates a need for hyperinflation therapy to maximize alveolar expansion and mobilize secretions.
• Suction (nasotracheal or endotracheal) as determined by patient assessment.	• Prevent unnecessary suctioning and reduce complications associated with suctioning.
• Provide adequate humidification with supplemental oxygen or mechanical ventilation.	• Prevent drying of secretions and facilitate secretion removal.
• When not contraindicated, encourage fluid intake of at least 2.5 L/day.	• Reduce viscosity of secretions and promote expectoration.

[a] Refer to the Collaborative Care Plan found in Chapter 1, Overview of Critical Care Nursing, and the Plan of Care for the Mechanically Ventilated Patient found in Chapter 10, Ventilatory Assistance.

Adapted from Swearingen PL, Wright JD. *All-in-One Nursing Care Planning Resource*. 5th ed. St. Louis, MO: Elsevier; 2019.

ABG, Arterial blood gas; *ARDS*, acute respiratory distress syndrome; *I:E ratio*, inspiratory-to-expiratory ratio; FiO_2, fraction of inspired oxygen; *LOC*, level of consciousness; *NPPV*, noninvasive positive-pressure ventilation; O_2, oxygen; $PaCO_2$, partial pressure of arterial carbon dioxide; PaO_2, partial pressure of arterial oxygen; *RR*, respiratory rate; SaO_2, arterial oxygen saturation; SpO_2, pulse oximetry; $\dot{V}/\dot{Q}$, ventilation/perfusion; *VT*, total tidal volume; *WOB*, work of breathing.

RESPIRATORY FAILURE IN ACUTE RESPIRATORY DISTRESS SYNDROME

Definition

ARDS, the most severe form of ARF, was originally described in 1967 as an acute illness manifested by dyspnea, tachypnea, decreased lung compliance, and diffuse alveolar infiltrates on chest radiographic studies. The syndrome was observed after trauma in young adult patients who developed shock, required excessive fluid administration, or both. Autopsy results revealed that pathological heart and lung findings were similar to those described in infant respiratory distress syndrome.

Although mortality attributed to ARDS has trended downward over the past several decades, death rates vary depending on etiology, disease severity, age, body mass index (BMI), geographical location, race, sex, and season.[15-17] As an example, those who did not survive coronavirus disease (COVID-19) had an ARDS incidence of 90% with a mortality rate of 45%

(see Clinical Alert box).[18-26] The average annual in-hospital case mortality has been reported at 47% using a nationwide sample.[27]

! CLINICAL ALERT

Acute Respiratory Failure Resulting From COVID-19

The COVID-19 pandemic resulted in hospitalizations in excess of 5 million and more than 1 million deaths nationwide from August 2020 to August 2022, draining resources and creating a global healthcare crisis. At its peak, 34.3% of patients hospitalized with COVID-19 were admitted to critical care, 27.3% of the cases required invasive mechanical ventilation, and the mortality rate was 21.7% among intubated patients.

Of those who survived critical care admission, long-term ventilation was often required, with approximately 70% of these patients successfully weaning. Functional challenges following discharge of survivors included physical disabilities, altered pulmonary function, and frailty, leading to poor health requiring long-term follow up for this population.

Pandemics will occur again with varying levels of severity, as has occurred historically with SARS-CoV-2, influenza, and Ebola viruses. Recognize and support nurses who provide care to these patients and their families. Adequate supplies, including personal protective equipment, appropriate staffing, administrative and emotional support are essential to prevent moral distress, burnout, and feelings of isolation and depression.

The current definition of ARDS, known as the Berlin criteria, was revised in 2012. Criteria for ARDS include: (1) acute onset within 1 week after clinical insult; (2) bilateral pulmonary opacities not explained by other conditions; (3) respiratory failure without a cardiac origin of edema (i.e., cardiac failure, fluid overload); and (4) altered PaO_2/FiO_2 ratio. Severity is determined by the PaO_2/FiO_2 ratio when the patient is treated with positive end-expiratory pressure (PEEP) or continuous positive airway pressure (CPAP) of 5 cm H_2O or higher: mild ARDS, 201 to 300 mm Hg; moderate ARDS, 101 to 200 mm Hg; and severe ARDS, 100 mm Hg or less.[28]

Etiology

Several possible causes of ARDS are listed in Box 15.1; they are categorized into direct and indirect factors. However, certain risk factors such as pneumonia, sepsis, aspiration, and trauma have a higher associated frequency of ARDS, and the presence of two or more factors increases the risk.[17,29]

As more individuals survive ARDS, prevention of long-term disabilities is a priority of care. Survivors report ongoing concerns regarding physical well-being, as well as mental and social health, all of which have a tremendous effect on quality of life and are often impacted by prehospital health status.[30] Reports of weakness, mobility issues, breathing problems, nausea, swallowing difficulties, fatigue, problems with memory, anxiety, and depression are commonly reported.[31,32] Fifty-nine percent of survivors experience some combination of general anxiety, depression, and posttraumatic stress for as long as 2 years. For those who undergo mechanical ventilation, many do not survive past 5 years and, during that time, experience impairments related to activities of daily living that impact quality of life.[33]

BOX 15.1 Possible Causes of Acute Respiratory Distress Syndrome

Direct Causes

- Aspiration of gastric contents
- Fat embolism
- Inhalation of toxic gases
- Multisystem trauma (chest and/or lung injury)
- Near-drowning
- Pneumonia
- Coronavirus disease (COVID-19)

Indirect Causes

- Burns
- Cardiopulmonary bypass
- Drug overdose
- Fractures, especially of the pelvis or long bones
- Multiple transfusions
- Multisystem trauma (without chest and/or lung injury)
- Pancreatitis
- Sepsis

Greater strength at discharge can improve long-term survival and quality of life, and early, progressive mobility may be a nursing intervention that could limit this sequela.[31]

It is important to educate the patient and family about what to expect after discharge and to help them develop coping strategies to manage these stressors. The critical care nurse can prepare the patient and family for discharge by providing information on community resources, support groups, and respite care.

? CLINICAL JUDGMENT ACTIVITY

A 41-year-old patient was admitted to the critical care unit and required mechanical ventilation for acute asthma. The patient was extubated and will transfer out of the critical care unit in 24 hours. What are the important points the nurse must cover in providing patient education?

Pathophysiology

ARDS is characterized by acute and diffuse injury to the lungs, leading to respiratory failure. A cell-mediated, overly aggressive immune response results in alveolar-capillary membrane damage and massive fluid leakage throughout the body, producing edema. Alveolar flooding leads to noncardiogenic pulmonary edema, shunting, $\dot{V}/\dot{Q}$ mismatch, decreased compliance, and hypoxemia. ARDS occurs in three overlapping phases: the exudative or inflammatory phase, the proliferative phase, and the fibrotic phase.[34]

The *exudative phase* occurs within 72 hours of lung insult.[34] This phase is characterized by uncontrolled inflammation, which produces excessive amounts of inflammatory mediators that damage the pulmonary capillary endothelium, activating massive aggregation of platelets and formation of intravascular thrombi. The platelets release serotonin and a substance that activates neutrophils. Other inflammatory factors, such as endotoxin, tumor necrosis factor, and interleukin-1, are also activated. Neutrophil activation causes release of inflammatory mediators such as proteolytic enzymes, toxic O_2 products, arachidonic acid metabolites, and platelet-activating factors. These mediators damage the alveolar-capillary membrane, which leads to increased capillary membrane permeability. Fluids, protein, and blood cells leak from the capillary beds into the alveoli, resulting in pulmonary edema. Pulmonary hypertension occurs secondary to vasoconstriction caused by the inflammatory mediators. The pulmonary hypertension and pulmonary edema lead to $\dot{V}/\dot{Q}$ mismatching. The production of surfactant is stopped, and the surfactant that is present is inactivated, which contributes to the decrease in lung compliance.[34]

During the exudative phase of ARDS, damage to the alveolar epithelium and the vascular endothelium occurs. The damaged cells become susceptible to bacterial infection and pneumonia. The lungs become less compliant, resulting in decreased ventilation. A right-to-left shunt of pulmonary blood develops, and hypoxemia refractory to O_2 supplementation becomes profound. The work of breathing increases.[34]

The *proliferative phase* of ARDS occurs within 1 to 3 weeks after lung insult. During this phase, pulmonary edema resolves, and a fibrin matrix (hyaline membrane) forms, resulting in progressive hypoxemia.[34]

The final phase of ARDS, the *fibrotic phase*, occurs 2 to 3 weeks after the initial insult. During this phase, fibrosis obliterates the alveoli, bronchioles, and interstitium. The lungs become fibrotic, with decreased functional residual capacity and severe right-to-left shunting. The inflammation and edema become worse with narrowing of the airways. Resistance to airflow and atelectasis increase.[34]

The inflammatory mediators responsible for alveolar-capillary membrane damage cause similar damage to capillaries throughout the body, resulting in widespread edema and multiple organ dysfunction syndrome (MODS; see Chapter 12, Shock, Sepsis, and Multiple Organ Dysfunction Syndrome). Cause of death may not be related to ARF but more likely to MODS related to ARDS.[34] The pathophysiology of ARDS is outlined in Fig. 15.2.

Assessment

Assessment of a patient with ARDS is collaborative. A key clinical finding of ARDS is respiratory distress with dyspnea, tachypnea, and hypoxemia that does not respond to supplemental O_2 therapy (refractory hypoxemia). Hypoxemia triggers hyperventilation, resulting in respiratory alkalosis. Initial signs of ARDS may also include fine crackles, restlessness, disorientation, and change in LOC. Pulse and temperature may be increased. Chest radiographic studies show interstitial and alveolar infiltrates over the first 24 to 48 hours after onset.[34]

As ARDS progresses and the PaO_2 decreases, dyspnea becomes severe. Intercostal and suprasternal retractions are often present, with a significant increase in work of breathing. Other signs may include tachycardia and central cyanosis. As pulmonary edema develops, the lungs become noncompliant, making ventilation increasingly difficult, resulting in hypoventilation and respiratory acidosis. For patients who are already intubated, peak inspiratory pressures will be elevated as an indicator of decreased static lung compliance. Patients developing ARDS frequently require noninvasive supplemental O_2 at the maximum level, with little effect on the PaO_2. Metabolic acidosis caused by lactic acid buildup often results and is confirmed by serum lactate levels.

Once ARDS is diagnosed, important assessment data used to guide treatment include hemodynamic measurements, ABG levels, mixed venous blood gas levels, serial chest radiographic studies, computed tomography (CT), echocardiography, and bronchoscopy. Nutritional needs and psychosocial needs of the patient and family must also be assessed.

CHECK YOUR UNDERSTANDING

1. A patient is admitted with new-onset pneumonia. The chest x-ray from the emergency department reveals bilateral opacities. The patient is intubated, with a PEEP of 10, FiO_2 of 60%, and ABG results as follows: pH, 7.35; $PaCO_2$, 47 mm Hg; PaO_2, 58 mm Hg; and HCO_3, 25 mEq/L. Would the patient meet the Berlin criteria for ARDS, and if so, what severity?
   - A. No, the patient is just experiencing acute respiratory failure secondary to pneumonia
   - B. Yes, mild ARDS
   - C. Yes, moderate ARDS
   - D. Yes, severe ARDS

Interventions

Achieving adequate oxygenation is the primary goal in the treatment of ARDS. This can be accomplished with the use of NPPV in some patients,[35] but many patients require endotracheal intubation and mechanical ventilation.[36] Early recognition of the need for intubation is essential in preventing increased morbidity and mortality.[16,37] Lung-protective ventilation strategies, including lower tidal volumes, appropriate PEEP, and permissive hypoxemia, have proven to be effective. Other treatments currently being researched are extracorporeal membrane oxygenation (ECMO), corticosteroid therapy, prone positioning, and therapeutic hypothermia. Other treatments are primarily supportive, providing an opportunity for the body to heal itself.

Oxygenation. Patients with ARDS usually require intubation and mechanical ventilation to meet oxygenation demands. Selection of ventilator settings is based on lung-protective strategies that attempt to achieve adequate oxygenation while minimizing the risk of ventilator-associated complications such as oxygen toxicity, barotrauma, and volutrauma. Lung-protective strategies consist of low V_T (4–8 mL/kg of predicted ideal body weight [IBW]), low end-inspiratory plateau pressure (<30 cm H_2O), FiO_2 at nontoxic levels (<0.50), and PEEP. Actual body weight should not be used to calculate V_T. The body weight may change secondary to accumulation of body fluid, but the size of the lungs does not change. Large clinical trials have shown reduced mortality and complications with the use of low V_T and low plateau pressure.[38-40] These lower volumes and plateau pressures prevent the alveoli from overdistending and minimize shearing.

Ventilatory support for patients with ARDS typically includes PEEP to restore functional residual capacity, open collapsed alveoli, preventing collapse of unstable alveoli, and

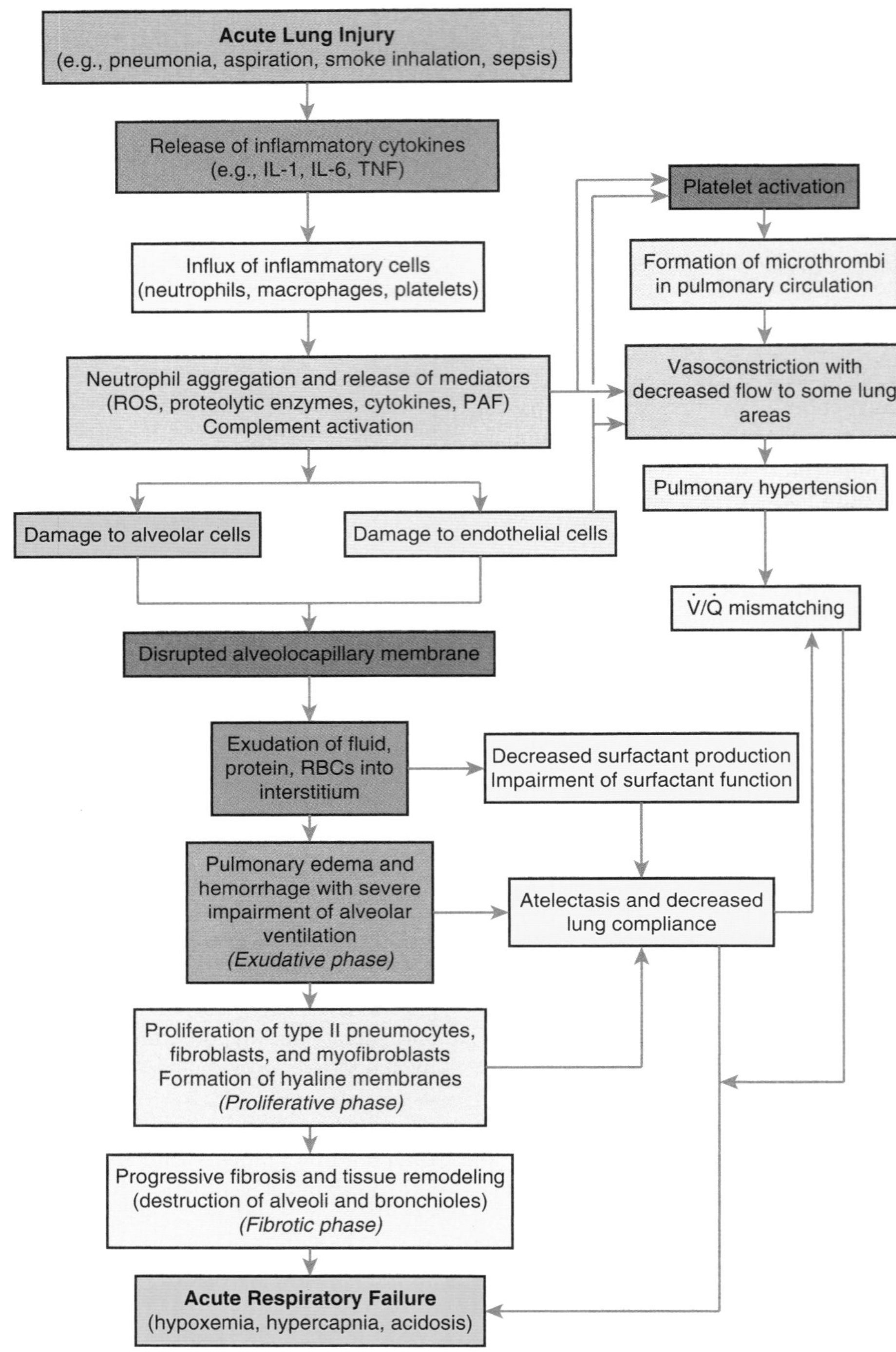

Fig. 15.2 Pathogenesis of acute respiratory distress syndrome (ARDS). *IL*, Interleukin; *PAF*, platelet-activating factor; *RBCs*, red blood cells; *ROS*, reactive oxygen species; *TNF*, tumor necrosis factor; *V̇/Q̇*, ventilation/perfusion. (From Rogers JL. *McCance & Huether's Pathophysiology: The Biologic Basis for Disease in Adults and Children*. 9th ed. Elsevier; 2024.)

improving arterial oxygenation. A meta-analysis indicated that low versus high levels of PEEP makes no significant difference in critical care, hospital, or 28-day mortality.[41] The optimal PEEP to treat ARDS and improve outcomes needs further study, although current clinical guidelines include the use of higher levels of PEEP for patients with moderate to severe disease.[38] When using high levels of PEEP, assess for potential adverse effects (see Chapter 10, Ventilatory Assistance). PEEP increases intrathoracic pressure, potentially decreasing cardiac output. Excessive pressure in stiff lungs increases peak inspiratory and plateau pressures, which may result in barotrauma and pneumothorax. Treatment of a pneumothorax requires prompt insertion of a chest tube. Monitor patients receiving high levels of PEEP therapy every 2 to 4 hours and after every adjustment in the PEEP setting for changes in respiratory status such as increased respiratory rate, worsening adventitious breath sounds, decreased or absent breath sounds, decreased SpO_2, and increasing dyspnea.

Patients with ARDS require significant support to achieve and maintain arterial oxygenation. High levels of FiO_2 may be required for short periods while aggressive efforts are made to reduce the FiO_2 to the lowest level that maintains the PaO_2 above 60 mm Hg. To prevent O_2 toxicity and increased mortality, the goal is to maintain the PaO_2 with levels of FiO_2 at or below 0.50.[38,42]

Nontraditional modes of mechanical life support may be used in some patients to treat ARDS with hypoxemia refractory to standard modes. These include ECMO and pressure-controlled, inverse-ratio ventilation. These modes may offer improved alveolar ventilation and arterial oxygenation while decreasing the risk of lung injury in select patients (see Chapter 10, Ventilatory Assistance).[38,43-44] Ongoing studies on the use of ECMO show promise, but evidence is currently inconclusive (see Evidence-Based Practice box).

EVIDENCE-BASED PRACTICE

Extracorporeal Membrane Oxygenation in Acute Respiratory Distress Syndrome

Problem

Patients with acute respiratory distress syndrome (ARDS) require mechanical ventilation and other support to ensure adequate oxygenation and ventilation.

Clinical Question

What is best practice for extracorporeal membrane oxygenation (ECMO) in patients with ARDS?

Evidence

In this systematic review and meta-analysis, the authors analyzed 11 studies. They compared mortality rates of ECMO with conventional mechanical ventilation. Findings indicated that, although 30-day and 90-day mortality were lower in the ECMO group, there was no significant difference for in-hospital or critical care mortality, and critical care length of stay (LOS) was longer in the ECMO group. However, the strength of the evidence was limited, as relatively few studies met the inclusion criteria. Although ECMO offers promise in mortality reduction, more studies are needed to determine the role of ECMO as a strategy for the treatment of ARDS.

Implications for Nursing

Nurses must collaborate with respiratory therapists and intensivists to provide the safest and most effective management strategy for each patient. Protocols that include nontraditional modes of mechanical support such as ECMO may be effective for improving outcomes for select patients with ARDS. Assessment for tolerance, improvement in oxygenation, and adverse effects is essential for optimal outcomes.

Level of Evidence

A—Meta-analysis

Reference

Sedhai, YR, Shrestha, D, Budhathoki, P et al. Extracorporeal membrane oxygenation in ARDS: a systematic review and meta-analysis. *Crit Care Med.* 2022;50(1):573. https://doi.org/10.1097/01.ccm.0000810920.05539.66.

Pharmacological Treatment. Despite clinical studies of various medications, no pharmacological agents are considered standard therapy for ARDS. The use of corticosteroid therapy for the treatment of ARDS has been debated for many years. Research has failed to produce strong enough results to use these medications as standard of care,[45-46] although there is ongoing research in this area that suggests improved outcomes for certain subsets of patients with ARDS.[46-49]

Sedation and Comfort. Patients with ARDS routinely receive sedation to promote comfort, alleviate anxiety, prevent self-extubation or harm, and enhance ventilator synchrony. Dyssynchrony between the patient and the ventilator causes inadequate gas exchange and increases the risk for ventilator-induced lung injury.[50] Adapting ventilator settings to the patient's respiratory efforts can be effective in alleviating dyssynchrony.

The amount of sedation used must be monitored carefully with validated sedation scales to achieve predetermined end points or goals for each individual patient situation (see Chapter 6, Comfort and Sedation).[51-53] Oversedation can lead to long-term sequelae, such as delirium, resulting in an increase in ventilator days, prolonged LOS, and increased mortality. Light sedation with both sedatives and analgesics can be safely administered to promote comfort, decrease agitation associated with mechanical ventilation, and control dyssynchrony.[51,53] Depending on the patient's ARDS severity and oxygenation needs, deep sedation may be needed. If neuromuscular blocking (NMB) agents are administered, a deep level of sedation is required.

Therapeutic paralysis with an NMB agent may be required to reduce the work of breathing and improve ventilator synchrony. The use of 48 hours of NMB therapy in early moderate to severe ARDS has been found to improve oxygenation, reduce the risk of barotrauma, and decrease 21- to 28-day mortality but does not improve 90-day mortality.[54] Initial sedation prior to administration of any NMB agent is essential to protect the patient from mental awareness during muscle paralysis. Incidence of awareness during paralysis seems to be higher in mechanically ventilated patients in critical care units than in the operating room.[55] Mitigate this risk by providing adequate analgesia and sedation prior to and during NMB therapy.

Prone Positioning. Placing the patient in the prone position for more than 12 hours in a 24-hour period in conjunction with lower V_T ventilation has been shown to decrease mortality in those with moderate to severe ARDS.[38] Turning the patient to the prone position (proning) alters the $\dot{V}/\dot{Q}$ ratio by maintaining posterior perfusion while allowing optimal ventilation in the larger, dorsal portion of the lungs. Placing the patient prone removes the weight of the heart and abdomen from the lungs, facilitates removal of secretions, improves oxygenation, and enhances recruitment of airways.[56]

The use of prone positioning for nonintubated patients who are awake is indicated for those suffering from hypoxemic respiratory failure and results in improved oxygenation, lower rates of intubation,[57] and improved 28-day survival when used within 24 hours of high-flow nasal cannula (HFNC) initiation.[58]

Turning the patient to the prone position is a procedure that requires several multiprofessional team members, one of whom should be a respiratory therapist. Adequate staffing to turn the patient ensures both patient and team member safety. Care must be taken to avoid dislodging the endotracheal tube (ETT), as well as other tubes and lines. Several commercial devices and pronation beds are available to assist in turning the patient. Potential complications from the prone position are accidental dislodgement of tubes and lines, vomiting, brachial plexus injury, pressure injuries to nontraditional areas, corneal ulceration, increased intraocular pressure, facial edema, and agitation. Continue gastric enteral nutrition as tolerated. Administer promotility agents if the patient demonstrates signs and symptoms of gastrointestinal intolerance. Postpyloric enteral access should only be considered if enteral intolerance persists after initiating promotility agents. Maintain proper body alignment while the patient is in the prone position to decrease the risk of nerve damage. Use pillows and foam support equipment to prevent overextension or flexion of the spine or shoulders and reduce weight bearing on bony prominences. Place prophylactic silicone dressings on the chest, pelvis, elbows, extremities, and other anatomical locations at risk for pressure during prone positioning to maintain skin integrity. To avoid peripheral nerve injury and contractures of the shoulders, position the arms carefully and reposition them often via the swimmer's position. Reposition the head every two hours to reduce facial edema, pressure injury risk, and ocular pressure. Provide frequent oral care and suctioning as needed. Apply moisture barrier to the patient's entire face to protect the skin from the massive amount of drainage from the mouth and nose. Every 4 hours, clean the eyes with saline-soaked gauze, then lubricate the eyes and tape eyelids closed horizontally to prevent corneal drying and abrasions. Assess the patient frequently for tolerance of proning. Patient and family education regarding the use of prone positioning is essential in decreasing anxiety (see Clinical Exemplar box).[59]

CLINICAL EXEMPLAR

Communication and Interprofessional Collaboration

When reviewing recent incident reports, the manager of a critical care unit noted an increase in endotracheal tube (ETT), orogastric tube, and vascular access dislodgments during manual prone positioning. The manager engaged the clinical nurse specialist (CNS), and the two began observing when patients were placed prone or supine. They observed that the patients' nurses were directing the turn versus the respiratory therapist, who was protecting and controlling the airway. In addition, a countdown to the turn was not occuring. These observations were discussed during the next unit-based council meeting involving the multiprofessional team. The multiprofessional team identified the following practice to prevent future dislodgments and ensure patient safety when placing the patient prone or supine:

The respiratory therapist is located at the head of the patient's bed, securing the airway. Prior to turning, all team members will perform a visual check of all lines, tubes, and drains to validate readiness for turning. The respiratory therapist will then ask, "All ready?" Once all team members respond with "yes," the respiratory therapist will state, "On three. One. Two. Three." At which point the patient is turned on their side. The process is repeated, starting with the visual check of all lines, tubes, and drains, until the patient is placed prone/supine. Any member of the team is encouraged to stop the process if there is a concern regarding the patient's safety.

After implementing the practice change, the team monitored line, tube, and drain dislodgments, observing and sustaining a dramatic reduction in the prone patient population.

Fluids and Electrolytes. Fluid therapy is highly individualized and dependent on the patient's clinical condition; however, the goal is to maintain adequate tissue perfusion without causing fluid overload.[60] A cumulative positive fluid balance is associated with an increased risk for ventilator-associated events and increased mortality for those with acute respiratory failure, sepsis, and acute kidney injury.[61] Chapter 9, Hemodynamic Monitoring, and Chapter 12, Shock, Sepsis, and Multiple Organ Dysfunction Syndrome, provide best practices for pressure monitoring and fluid resuscitation.

Nutrition. The goal of nutritional support is to provide adequate nutrition that is tolerated to meet the patient's level of metabolism and reduce morbidity (see Chapter 7, Nutritional Therapy). It is generally recommended to begin early enteral nutrition (within 24 hours) in critically ill patients; however, delivering a higher number of calories to those with ARDS results in an increased likelihood of mortality.[62] Current opinion supports withholding enteral nutrition for patients with ARDS in the most acute phase of the illness. Feeding intolerance in critically ill, mechanically ventilated patients occurs frequently, interfering with nutrition delivery, and is associated with less favorable clinical outcomes[63]; this suggests prevention, early identification, and management lead to improved outcomes.

Psychosocial Support. The onset of ARDS and its long recovery phase result in stress and anxiety for both the patient and the family. The patient may also experience feelings of isolation and dependence because of impaired communication and potential separation during the recovery phase. Always remember to provide a warm, nurturing environment in which the patient and family can feel safe. Providing a therapeutic environment includes taking the time to explain procedures, equipment, changes in the patient's condition, and outcomes to the patient and family members. Encourage family presence and allow the patient and family to participate in the planning of care and to verbalize fears and questions.

CHECK YOUR UNDERSTANDING

2. A patient is admitted to the critical care unit with a diagnosis of ARDS. Collaboration among the multiprofessional team identifies the need to initiate which ventilator strategies to improve patient outcomes?
   A. VT calculated according to current patient weight
   B. VT at 4 to 8 mL/kg predicted ideal body weight
   C. Consistent use of 100% FiO_2
   D. PEEP levels of 30 cm H_2O for 8 hours each day

ACUTE RESPIRATORY FAILURE IN CHRONIC OBSTRUCTIVE PULMONARY DISEASE

Pathophysiology

COPD is a progressive, yet preventable disease characterized by airflow limitations that are not fully reversible. These airflow limitations are associated with an abnormal inflammatory response to noxious particles or gases. COPD is a disease of the small airways and the lung parenchyma that results in chronic bronchitis and emphysema. The incidence and effect on chronic morbidity and mortality are increasing. COPD is the sixth leading cause of death in the United States. The primary cause of COPD is tobacco smoke, and smoking cessation is the most effective intervention to reduce the risk of developing COPD and stop disease progression. Other contributing factors to the development of COPD include air pollution, occupational exposure to dust or chemicals, low socioeconomic status, and the genetic abnormality alpha$_1$-antitrypsin deficiency.[34,64]

The primary pathogenic mechanism in COPD is chronic inflammation, which may directly injure the airway and lead to systemic effects. Exposure to inhaled particles leads to airway inflammation and injury. The body repairs this injury through the process of airway remodeling, which causes scarring, narrowing, and obstruction of the airways. Destruction of alveolar walls and connective tissue results in permanent enlargement of air spaces. Increased mucus production results from enlargement of mucus-secreting glands and an increase in the number of goblet cells. Areas of cilia are destroyed, contributing to the patient's inability to clear thick, tenacious mucus. Structural changes in the pulmonary capillaries thicken the vascular walls and inhibit gas exchange. Systemic inflammation also causes direct effects on peripheral blood vessels and may be a concomitant factor in the association of cardiovascular disease with COPD.[64] Table 15.1 outlines the physiological changes that result from COPD.

ARF can occur at any time in a patient with COPD. These patients normally have little respiratory reserve, and any condition that increases the work of breathing worsens $\dot{V}/\dot{Q}$ mismatching. Common causes of ARF in patients with COPD are acute exacerbations, heart failure, dysrhythmias, pulmonary edema, pneumonia, dehydration, and electrolyte imbalances.

Assessment

The hallmark symptoms of COPD are progressive dyspnea, chronic cough, and sputum production. The diagnosis is confirmed by post bronchodilator spirometry that documents irreversible airflow limitations. These pulmonary function tests show an increase in total lung capacity and a reduction in forced expiratory volume over 1 second (FEV_1) with an FEV_1/forced vital capacity (FVC) ratio less than 0.70.[64] Functional residual capacity is increased as a result of air trapping.

TABLE 15.1 Pathological and Physiological Changes in Chronic Obstructive Pulmonary Disease

Pathological Changes	Physiological Changes
Mucus hypersecretion	Sputum production
Ciliary dysfunction	Retained secretions Chronic cough
Chronic airway inflammation	Expiratory airflow limitation
Airway remodeling	Terminal airway collapse Air trapping Lung hyperinflation
Thickening of pulmonary vessels	Poor gas exchange with hypoxemia and hypercapnia Pulmonary hypertension Cor pulmonale (right ventricular enlargement and heart failure)

CLINICAL JUDGMENT ACTIVITY

A patient has just been intubated for ARF. Currently, the patient is agitated and very restless. What contributing factors may be associated with the patient's agitation? What nursing actions are indicated in this situation?

By the time the characteristic physical findings of COPD are evident on physical examination, a significant decline in lung function has occurred. The chest is often overexpanded or barrel shaped because the anterior-posterior diameter increases in size. Assess for use of accessory muscles and pursed-lip breathing. Clubbing of the fingers indicates long-term hypoxemia. Lung auscultation usually reveals diminished breath sounds, prolonged exhalation, wheezing, and crackles. ABG results show mild hypoxemia in the early stages of the disease and worsening hypoxemia and hypercapnia as the disease progresses. Over time, as a compensatory mechanism, the kidneys increase bicarbonate production and retention in an attempt to keep the pH within normal limits.

Exacerbation of COPD often results in a change in the patient's baseline dyspnea and an increase in sputum volume. Assess for changes in the character of the sputum, which may signal the development of a respiratory infection. Assess for additional symptoms, which may include anxiety, wheezing, chest tightness, tachypnea, tachycardia, fatigue, malaise, confusion, fever, and sleeping difficulties. Wheezing indicates narrowing of the airways. Retraction of intercostal muscles may occur with inspiration, and exhalation is prolonged through pursed lips. The patient is typically more comfortable in the upright position. Tachycardia and hypotension may result from reduced cardiac output.

Life-threatening ARF is indicated by tachypnea of more than 30 breaths/min, accessory muscle use, acute decline in mental status, $PaCO_2$ greater than 60 mm Hg, pH less than 7.25, or hypoxemia that does not improve with supplemental oxygen via Venturi mask with FiO_2 greater than 40%.[64]

If possible to obtain, the patient's baseline ABG values assist in detecting changes that indicate ARF. At baseline, the patient with COPD usually has ABG results that show a normal pH, a moderately low PaO_2 in the range of 60 to 65 mm Hg, and an elevated $PaCO_2$ in the range of 50 to 60 mm Hg (compensated respiratory acidosis).

Interventions

The care of patients with stable COPD is outlined in Box 15.2. These interventions are individualized to reduce risk factors, manage symptoms, limit complications, and enhance quality of life. When a patient has an acute exacerbation, the goals of therapy are to provide support during the episode of acute failure, treat the triggering event, and return the patient to the previous level of functioning.

Oxygen. The most important intervention for an acute exacerbation of COPD is to correct hypoxemia. Oxygen is administered to achieve an SaO_2 of 88% to 92%. A Venturi mask delivers more precise oxygen concentrations than nasal prongs but may not be tolerated as well. High-flow oxygen therapy by nasal cannula may be better tolerated and has been shown to effectively oxygenate some patients with COPD experiencing ARF. When delivering high concentrations of O_2, be aware of the possibility that it can blunt the hypoxic drive of the patient with COPD, which can diminish respiratory efforts and further increase CO_2 retention. Titrate oxygen slowly and incrementally and reevaluate ABG results frequently after the initiation of therapy to monitor both O_2 and CO_2 levels.[64]

Bronchodilator Therapy. The use of short-acting inhaled beta-2-agonists with or without short-acting anticholinergics is recommended for treating an acute exacerbation.[64] Table 15.2 lists commonly administered bronchodilator agents. Short-acting, inhaled beta-2-agonists cause bronchial smooth muscle relaxation that reverses bronchoconstriction. They are primarily administered via a nebulizer or a metered-dose inhaler with a spacer. The dosage and frequency vary, depending on the delivery method and the severity of bronchoconstriction. Adverse effects are dosage related and are more common with oral or IV administration than with inhalation. Adverse effects include tachycardia, dysrhythmias, tremors, hypokalemia, anxiety, bronchospasm, and dyspnea.

BOX 15.2 Treatment of Stable Chronic Obstructive Pulmonary Disease

- Reduce exposure to airway irritants
- Counseling or treatment for smoking cessation
- Remain in an air-conditioned environment during times of high air pollution
- Influenza and pneumococcal vaccinations
- Inhaled bronchodilators (short-acting, long-acting, or combination)
- Inhaled glucocorticosteroids for severe disease and repeated exacerbations
- Pulmonary rehabilitation program with exercise training
- Long-term administration of oxygen for more than 15 hours/day for severe disease

Corticosteroids. Administration of systemic corticosteroids improves lung function, recovery time, oxygenation, and LOS. Commonly a course of prednisone is prescribed. Nebulizer treatment with budesonide alone can be an effective alternative to oral prednisone for some patients.[64] Common adverse effects of steroid therapy include hyperglycemia and an increased risk of infection.

Antibiotics. Administration of antibiotics to patients with COPD exacerbation improves survival for those who are moderately or severely ill. Antibiotic therapy, preferably by the oral route, is recommended in patients with increased dyspnea and increased sputum volume and purulence or if mechanical ventilation is required. Antibiotic selection should be based on local bacterial resistance patterns; however, initial therapy often begins with an aminopenicillin alone or in conjunction with a clavulanic acid, macrolide, or tetracycline antibiotic. For patients with severe disease or frequent exacerbations, sputum cultures are advised, as gram-negative or resistant pathogens may not be sensitive to commonly prescribed antibiotics.[64]

Ventilatory Assistance. Patients with ARF from COPD exacerbation may require positive-pressure ventilation with or without intubation. Early treatment with NPPV improves outcomes in 85% of patients, resulting in decreased mortality and

TABLE 15.2 PHARMACOLOGY

Bronchodilators

Medication	Action/Use	Dose/Route	Side Effects	Nursing Implications
Beta-2-agonists (short-acting) Albuterol Levalbuterol	Bronchial smooth muscle relaxation; used to treat or prevent bronchospasm	Inhalation; refer to drug guide for specific information related to each medication	Anxiety Bronchospasm Dyspnea Hypertension Hypokalemia Palpitations Paradoxical bronchospasm Refractory asthma Tachycardia Throat irritation Tremor	Assess respiratory and cardiac status. Monitor response to treatment within 1 hour. Teach correct use of inhaler and spacer (specific to metered-dose inhaler medications). Teach proper use of medication for acute exacerbations and prevention.
Anticholinergics Ipratropium bromide (SAMA) Tiotropium bromide (LAMA)	Inhibit action of acetylcholine, causing bronchial smooth muscle relaxation; used to treat or prevent bronchospasm	Inhalation: refer to drug guide for specific information related to each medication	Bitter taste Dizziness Dry mouth Palpitations	Monitor respiratory status and response to treatment. Avoid contact with eyes, and report changes in vision. Provide relief of dry mouth (hard candy, liquids, sugarless gum).

COPD, Chronic obstructive pulmonary disease; *LAMA*, long-acting muscarinic antagonist; *SAMA*, short-acting muscarinic antagonist.

a reduced intubation rate.[6] See the Clinical Alert box for indications for NPPV, which assists the patient's respiratory efforts by delivering positive airway pressure through a nasal, oronasal, or full-face mask (see Chapter 10, Ventilatory Assistance).[64]

! CLINICAL ALERT

Indications of Impending Acute Respiratory Failure in Chronic Obstructive Pulmonary Disease Requiring Noninvasive Ventilation

- Severe dyspnea with respiratory muscle fatigue and/or increased work of breathing (WOB)
- Hypoxemia not responsive to supplemental oxygen
- Respiratory acidosis (pH <7.35)

Intubation and invasive mechanical ventilation are indicated in those patients for whom trials of NPPV have failed. Other indications include persistent or worsening hypoxemia, respiratory or cardiac arrest, decreased LOC, aspiration, inability to remove secretions, hemodynamic instability, or life-threatening ventricular dysrhythmias [64] Long-term morbidity for patients with COPD requiring intermittent mandatory ventilation (IMV) is significant, especially for those with cancer or higher severity of illness.[65]

In the late stages of severe COPD, patients often report that their quality of life deteriorates because of severe activity limitations and comorbid conditions. Decisions regarding intubation, mechanical ventilation, cardiopulmonary resuscitation, and other forms of life support should be made by the patient in conjunction with the patient's family and proivder before ARF occurs. Critical care nurses are in an ideal position to facilitate discussions about advance directives (see Chapter 3, Ethical and Legal Issues in Critical Care Nursing, and Chapter 4, Palliative and End-of-Life Care).

CHECK YOUR UNDERSTANDING

3. A patient is admitted for ARF with COPD. Depending on the patient's clinical condition and disease progression, what possible interventions could the nurse recommend to optimize the patient's outcomes?
   A. Noninvasive ventilation
   B. Bronchodilators
   C. Corticosteroids
   D. All the above

ACUTE RESPIRATORY FAILURE IN ASTHMA

Pathophysiology

Asthma is a chronic inflammatory disorder of the airways. The inflammation causes the airways to become hyperresponsive when the patient inhales allergens, viruses, or other irritants (Box 15.3). Episodic airflow obstruction results because these irritants cause bronchoconstriction, airway edema, mucus plugging, and airway remodeling (Fig. 15.3). Air trapping, prolonged exhalation, and $\dot{V}/\dot{Q}$ mismatching with an increased intrapulmonary shunt occur. The airflow limitations in asthma are largely reversible. When asthma is controlled, symptoms and exacerbations should be infrequent.[34]

BOX 15.3 Asthma Triggers

Inhalant Allergens
- Animals
- Cockroaches
- House-dust mites
- Indoor fungi
- Outdoor allergens
- Occupational exposures
- Chemical agents
- Fumes
- Organic and inorganic dusts

Irritants
- Fumes: perfumes, cleaning agents, sprays
- Indoor or outdoor pollution
- Tobacco smoke

Other Factors Influencing Asthma Severity
- Exercise
- Gastroesophageal reflux disease
- Rhinitis and sinusitis
- Sensitivity: aspirin, other nonsteroidal antiinflammatory drugs, sulfites
- Topical and systemic beta-blockers
- Viral respiratory infections

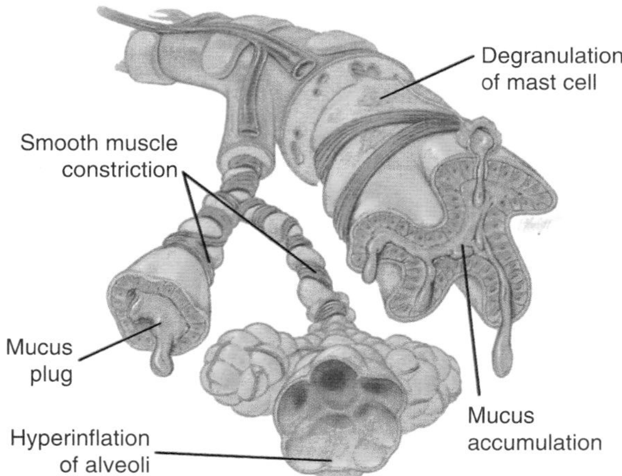

Fig. 15.3 Airway obstruction caused by asthma. Thick mucus, mucosal edema, and smooth muscle spasm cause obstruction of small airways in bronchial asthma. (Modified from Des Jardins T, Burton GC. *Clinical Manifestations and Assessment of Respiratory Disease.* 9th ed. St. Louis, MO: Mosby; 2024.)

Assessment

Initial clinical manifestations of asthma exacerbation include expiratory wheezing, dyspnea, chest tightness, prolonged expiration, tachycardia, tachypnea, and nonproductive cough. The patient initially hyperventilates, producing respiratory alkalosis. As the airways continue to narrow, it becomes more difficult for the patient to exhale. Peak expiratory flow (PEF) readings will be less than 50% of the patient's normal values. The patient may exhibit inspiratory and expiratory wheezing, agitation, use of accessory muscles, and suprasternal retractions.

A severe asthma exacerbation, status asthmaticus, occurs when the bronchoconstriction does not respond to bronchodilator therapy, and ARF ensues, resulting in respiratory acidosis and severe hypoxemia. Auscultation of a "silent" chest, indicating complete absence of air movement, is an ominous sign indicating impending medical emergency requiring prompt intervention to preserve life (see Clinical Alert box).

! CLINICAL ALERT

Asthma

Signs of impending ARF requiring intubation and ventilation in asthma exacerbation:

- "Silent" chest
- Breathlessness at rest and the need to sit hunched forward
- Single-word responses
- Agitation, confusion, drowsiness
- Respiratory rate > 30 breaths/min; heart rate >120 beats/min; $SpO_2 < 90\%$
- PEF 50% or less than predicted or personal best

Interventions

Mild exacerbations of asthma can be managed by the patient at home with the use of inhaled short-acting beta-2-agonists to treat bronchoconstriction and inhaled low-dose corticosteroids for inflammation (Table 15.2). Treatment of acute, severe exacerbations of asthma requires O_2 therapy to maintain SpO_2 of 93% to 95%, repeated administration of rapid-acting inhaled bronchodilators, and systemic steroid administration (Table 15.3).[66]

Most patients respond well to treatment, but some may need intubation and mechanical ventilation. Precise management of mechanical ventilation is required to enhance outcomes and prevent complications. In cases that are refractory to standard treatment, oxygenation may be improved by delivering a mixture of helium and O_2 (heliox) to the lungs. Because helium is less dense than O_2, it enhances gas flow through the constricted airways and may improve oxygenation.[66]

During a patient's recovery from a severe asthmatic event, focus efforts on teaching the patient asthma management techniques to achieve control. Teach the patient to implement environmental controls to prevent symptoms, understand the differences between medications that relieve and those that control symptoms, properly use inhaler devices, monitor the level of asthma control, and schedule a follow-up visit with the healthcare provider within 1 week. A written action plan and goals of treatment mutually determined by the patient and the healthcare provider help patients achieve asthma control and assists with early identification and treatment of exacerbations.[66]

ACUTE RESPIRATORY FAILURE RESULTING FROM PNEUMONIA

Definition and Etiology

Pneumonia is responsible for more than 45,000 deaths each year in the United States and a common cause of ARF. Pneumonia is a lower respiratory tract infection with a variety of risk factors, with older adults being particularly vulnerable, as incidence and mortality are high in this population. Other risk factors include those with compromised immunity, COPD, alcohol use disorder, altered LOC, impaired swallowing, malnutrition, endotracheal intubation, immobilization, heart disease, and liver disease. Nursing home residents and smokers are also at an increased risk for developing pneumonia.[34]

Pathophysiology

For pneumonia to occur, enough organisms must accumulate in the lower respiratory tract to overwhelm the patient's defense mechanisms. The lower respiratory tract is usually a sterile environment. It is protected by the warming and filtering of air as it passes through the upper airway, closure of the epiglottis, cough and sneezing reflexes, mucociliary clearance, and alveolar macrophages. The major routes of entry for these organisms are aspiration of gastric or oropharyngeal secretions (most common), inhalation of aerosols or particles, and hematogenous spread from another infected site into the lungs. The normal bronchomucociliary clearance mechanism is overwhelmed by the infective organism, causing a large influx of phagocytic cells and exudate into the airways and alveoli. This inflammatory response leads to a $\dot{V}/\dot{Q}$ mismatch, resulting in dyspnea, hypoxemia, fever, and leukocytosis.[29]

The pathogens responsible for pneumonia vary depending on the type (community vs. hospital acquired) and on the environmental factor or cause (Table 15.4). The pathogens include viruses, fungi, protozoa, parasites, and bacteria, including multidrug-resistant organisms such as methicillin-resistant

TABLE 15.3 Emergency Treatment of Severe Asthma

Therapy	Purpose	Goals
Oxygen via nasal cannula or face mask	Correct hypoxemia	Maintain SpO_2 at 93%–95%
Inhaled rapid-acting beta-2-agonists via nebulizer (continuous), followed by intermittent on-demand therapy	Relieve airway obstruction caused by bronchoconstriction	Achieve PEF >60% of predicted or personal best; normalize or improve ABG; respiratory rate <30 breaths/min without use of accessory muscles
Inhaled anticholinergics (added to beta-2-agonist therapy)	Relieve bronchoconstriction	Relieve sensation of dyspnea; patient able to complete full sentences without breathlessness
Systemic corticosteroids within 1 hour	Reverse airway inflammation	Improve lung sounds; prevent intubation

ABG, Arterial blood gas; *PEF*, peak expiratory flow; *SpO_2*, arterial oxygen saturation.

TABLE 15.4 Pneumonia Definitions and Common Infectious Causes

Type	Criteria	Infectious Causes
Community-acquired pneumonia (CAP)	Pneumonia that develops outside a healthcare facility	*Streptococcus pneumoniae* *Haemophilus influenza* *Staphylococcus aureus* *Mycoplasma pneumoniae* *Chlamydophila pneumonia* *Moraxella catarrhalis* *Legionella pneumophila* Influenza Rhinovirus Coronavirus
Healthcare–associated pneumonia (HCAP); Hospital acquired pneumonia (HAP); Ventilator-associated pneumonia (VAP)	Pneumonia that develops in individuals with recent hospitalization, nursing home or extended care stays, home infusion therapy, long-term dialysis, or home wound care, as well as those who are nonambulatory, those with tube feedings, or those taking gastric acid reducing agents	*Staphylococcus aureus* *Pseudomonas aeruginosa* *Enterobacter species* *Klebsiella pneumoniae*

From Winton MB, Brashers VL. Alterations of pulmonary function. In: Rogers J, ed. *Pathophysiology: The Biologic Basis for Disease in Adults and Children*. 9th ed. St. Louis, MO: Elsevier; 2024.

Staphylococcus aureus (MRSA). Fungal causes of pneumonia are uncommon, unless the patient is immunocompromised.[34]

Prevention of pneumonia is a priority. The most common bacterial cause of community-acquired pneumonia is streptococcal or pneumococcal infection, in which the risk may be mitigated by receiving the pneumococcal vaccination (Box 15.4). The Centers for Disease Control and Prevention (CDC) recommends that adults 65 years of age or older receive a pneumococcal polysaccharide vaccine (PPSV23), which protects against 23 types of pneumococcal bacteria. Depending on the patient's risk factors and the initial pneumococcal vaccination received, an additional vaccine may be necessary.[67] Influenza is a common cause of viral pneumonia. An annual influenza vaccine is recommended for all persons of at least 6 months of age (with rare exceptions), pregnant people, those with chronic health conditions, and those at high risk for complications of influenza.[68]

Assessment

The clinical presentation for pneumonia commonly begins with fever, cough (often productive), and dyspnea. Other symptoms may include chills, malaise, and pleuritic chest pain. Older adult patients may present with nonspecific symptoms, such as changes in mental status with hypothermia. Physical findings may include crackles, increased tactile fremitus, egophony, and whispered pectoriloquy. Recommended diagnostic studies include a chest radiograph, which may show local or diffuse infiltrates depending on the severity and distribution of the infection, and white blood cell count. Obtain blood and sputum cultures before antibiotic administration without delaying implementation of antibiotic therapy. Abnormal laboratory results include an elevated white blood cell count and ABG results demonstrating hypoxemia and hypocapnia.[34]

Interventions

Initial management of pneumonia requires establishing adequate ventilation and oxygenation, adequate hydration, pulmonary hygiene, and prompt antibiotic administration. Hospitalized patients with viral pneumonia should receive antiviral medication.[34]

BOX 15.4 Pneumococcal Vaccine Recommendations

- **Pneumococcal conjugate vaccine (PCV15 and PCV20)** is recommended for all adults 65 years of age or older as well as adults 19 through 64 years of age with certain risk factors (i.e., chronic heart disease, chronic lung disease, diabetes, CSF leaks, cochlear implants, sickle cell disease, congenital or acquired asplenia or splenic dysfunction, HIV infection, chronic renal failure or nephrotic syndrome, and diseases treated with immunosuppressive medications or radiation such as malignant neoplasm, leukemia, lymphoma, Hodgkin's disease, and solid organ transplantation).
- **Pneumococcal polysaccharide vaccine (PPSV23)** is recommended for all adults 65 years of age or older. People 2 through 64 years of age who are at high risk of pneumococcal disease or those who smoke should also receive PPSV23. Patients at high risk of pneumococcal disease include those with long-term health problems such as heart disease, lung disease, sickle cell disease, diabetes, alcohol use disorder, cirrhosis, CSF leaks, or cochlear implant. Vaccination is also recommended for those with increased risk of infection such as those with Hodgkin's disease, lymphoma or leukemia, kidney failure, multiple myeloma, nephrotic syndrome, HIV infection or AIDS, or damaged or no spleen, as well as those who are organ transplant recipients and those taking immunosuppressant medications.

AIDS, Acquired immunodeficiency syndrome; *CSF*, cerebrospinal fluid; *HIV*, human immunodeficiency virus.
From Centers for Disease Control and Prevention. Pneumococcal Vaccination: Summary of Who and When to Vaccinate. https://www.cdc.gov/vaccines/vpd/pneumo/hcp/who-when-to-vaccinate.html. Reviewed September 22, 2023. Accessed December 28, 2023.

VENTILATOR-ASSOCIATED PNEUMONIA AND EVENTS

One of the complications of mechanical ventilation is ventilator-associated pneumonia (VAP), which significantly increases ventilator time, LOS, cost of care, and ultimately, mortality. VAP is defined as pneumonia that develops in a patient who is intubated and ventilated at the time of or within 48 hours prior to the onset of the event. The National Healthcare Safety Network now includes VAP as one of several problems of oxygenation in the broad category of ventilator-associated events (VAEs).[69] Because limited research has been completed to validate this recent classification, most of the literature still refers to the condition as VAP. VAP is a preventable hospital-acquired infection affecting an average of 25% to 85% of critically ill individuals, depending on the cause,[70-72] and it complicates the course of illness for these patients. The longer the requirement for mechanical ventilation, the greater the likelihood that the patient will develop VAP. The crude mortality rate for VAP ranges from 14% to 59%,[70,73] with bacterial pneumonia resulting in the highest mortality and greatest cost.[74]

Pathophysiology

The pathogenesis of VAP is depicted in Fig. 15.4. Patients with an ETT are at increased risk for aspiration of oral and gastric secretions.[34] The ETT is inserted into the trachea past the vocal cords, thereby holding the glottis in the open position and compromising its ability to prevent aspiration. Sources of exogenous pathogens include contamination from healthcare personnel, ventilator and respiratory equipment, and the biofilm coating on the ETT.

Assessment

VAP has traditionally been diagnosed with clinical criteria, including a new or progressive pulmonary infiltrate along with fever, leukocytosis, and purulent tracheobronchial secretions. However, these criteria lack objectivity, specificity, and sensitivity, making surveillance for VAP a long-standing challenge that has implications for prevention and outcomes for mechanically ventilated individuals.[69] Mini bronchoalveolar lavage fluid amylase levels show promise as a diagnostic tool for VAP.[70,75]

In 2011, the CDC convened a workgroup of experts who developed a new approach for monitoring VAEs, including VAP. The VAE surveillance standards (Fig. 15.5) are based on objective criteria for several complications that can occur in patients who require mechanical ventilation.

Interventions

The interventions for VAP are aimed at prevention and treatment. Because VAP has been identified as the most prevalent infection acquired by critically ill patients requiring mechanical ventilation, prevention of VAP is a major focus. The Institute for Healthcare Improvement endorses a "bundle of care" to improve overall care of mechanically ventilated patients. Bundles are evidence-based interventions that are grouped together to improve outcomes. Current recommendations for preventing VAP and VAEs include several evidence-based strategies that may decrease the duration of intubation, LOS, cost, and mortality. These recommendations include the following: (1) avoid intubation and prevent reintubation using HFNC when possible; (2) use a protocol to minimize sedation, avoiding benzodiazepines, and implement a ventilator liberation protocol; (3) elevate the head of the bed 30 to 45 degrees; (4) facilitate progressive mobility; (5) provide oral care with toothbrushing; (6) provide early enteral nutrition; and (7) change ventilator circuitry only when soiled or malfunctioning per manufacturer's recommendations.[76]

Additional evidence-based interventions that may improve outcomes in some populations but increase risk in other populations include the following: (1) use selective oral or digestive decontamination where there is low risk of antibiotic-resistant microorganisms; (2) use ETT with subglottic drainage ports in patients who may require more than 48 to 72 hours of mechanical ventilation; (3) consider early tracheotomy; and (4) consider

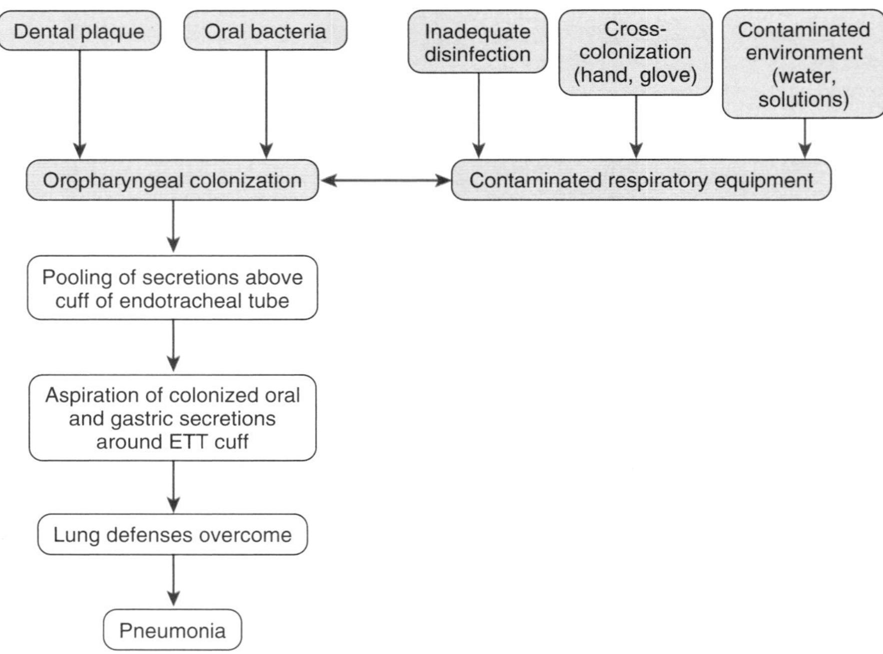

Fig. 15.4 Pathogenesis of ventilator-associated pneumonia. *ETT*, Endotracheal tube.

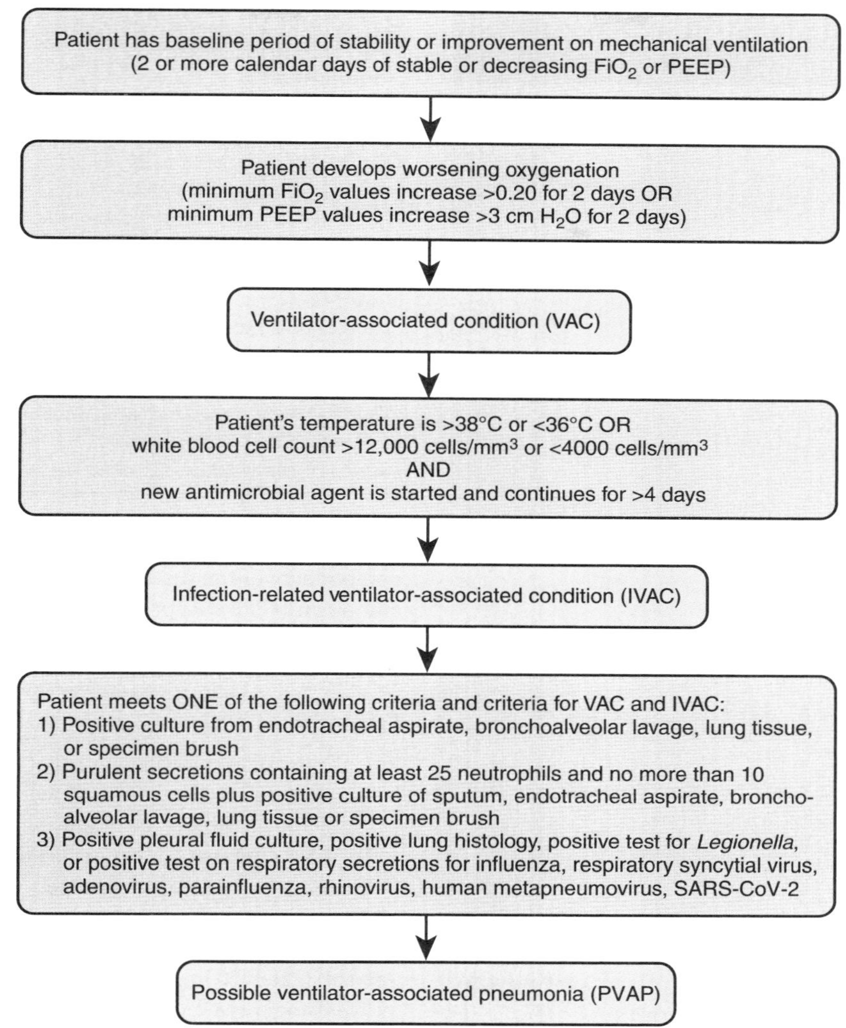

Fig. 15.5 National Healthcare Safety Network (NHSN) surveillance algorithm for ventilator-associated events. *FiO_2*, Fraction of inspired oxygen; *PEEP*, positive end-expiratory pressure; *SARS-CoV-2*, severe acute respiratory syndrome coronavirus-2. (Modified from Centers for Disease Control and Prevention. Device-Associated Module VAE. http://www.cdc.gov/nhsn/PDFs/pscManual/10-VAE_FINAL.pdf. Published January 2024. Accessed January 2, 2024.)

postpyloric feedings for those with gastric intolerance or those at high risk for aspiration.[76]

Interventions not recommended to prevent VAEs or VAP in adults include oral care with chlorhexidine; probiotics; ultra-thin polyurethane ETT cuffs; tapered ETT cuffs; ETTs with automated control of cuff pressure; silver-coated ETTs; kinetic or continuous lateral rotation therapy beds; prone positioning; chlorhexidine bathing; stress ulcer prophylaxis; monitoring gastric residual volumes; and early parenteral nutrition. There is no recommendation related to closed ETT suctioning, as there appears to be no impact on VAP rates or other outcomes, and the impact on cost is unclear.[76]

The critical care nurse is primarily responsible for providing these preventative interventions. Nurses are more likely to adhere to established guidelines if they understand and support the standards. For this reason, it is important that the critical care nurse be involved in the development and implementation of guidelines and standards of care for managing mechanically ventilated patients, working collaboratively with providers and other healthcare personnel to prevent VAP and VAEs.[77] Strategies for prevention of VAP are summarized in Box 15.5, and an example of an oral care protocol is described in Box 15.6.

CHECK YOUR UNDERSTANDING

4. The nurse admits a newly intubated patient to the critical care unit; what are important aspects of the patient's infection prevention plan of care?
   A. Head of bed flat, with patient supine
   B. Spontaneous breathing trials every other day
   C. Provide oral care with toothbrushing without chlorhexidine
   D. Delay enteral nutrition until the patient is extubated

Treatment. VAP is associated with a high risk of mortality and a significant increase in ventilator days and LOS.[70-74] Current guidelines recommend that hospitals develop antibiograms that target their usual pneumonia population to assist in correct antibiotic selection, prevent exposure to unnecessary antibiotics, and decrease the occurrence of antibiotic-resistant organisms.[76]

BOX 15.5 Prevention of Ventilator-Associated Pneumonia

1. Implement effective infection control measures, including staff education and hand hygiene
2. Conduct surveillance of VAE
3. Implement the ventilator-associated pneumonia prevention bundle per the SHEA guidelines:
   - Maintain head-of-bed elevation 30–45 degrees
   - Minimize sedation using a protocol
   - Use a protocol to guide a daily spontaneous breathing trial
   - Avoid intubation and prevent reintubation
   - Daily oral care with toothbrushing
   - Maintain and improve physical conditioning
   - Provide early enteral nutrition
   - Change ventilator circuitry only when visibly soiled or malfunctioning
4. Prevent transmission of microorganisms:
   - Use sterile water in, and for cleaning of, respiratory equipment
   - Drain condensate in ventilator circuits away from the patient
   - Do not instill 0.9% normal saline into the ETT
5. Modify host risk for infections:
   - Use noninvasive ventilation, if possible
   - Intubate patients orally
   - Control cuff pressures at 25 cm H_2O or higher
   - Use orogastric tubes
   - If available, use an ETT that allows for continuous aspiration of subglottic secretions
   - Oropharyngeal/GI decontamination with colistin, tobramycin, and nystatin for those likely to be intubated for at least 48 hours
   - Two to three doses of antibiotics during intubation of those with previously decreased LOC
6. Other prevention strategies:
   - Administer IV fluids judiciously to avoid fluid overload; monitor intake and output
   - Administer analgesics and sedatives using protocols and sedation scales
   - Use lung-protective strategies for mechanical ventilation
   - Discontinue mechanical ventilation as soon as possible

ETT, Endotracheal tube; *GI*, gastrointestinal; *LOC*, level of consciousness; *SHEA*, Society for Healthcare Epidemiology of America; *VAE*, ventilator-associated event.

Data from Klompas M, Branson R, Cawcutt K, et al. Strategies to prevent ventilator-associated pneumonia, ventilator-associated events, and nonventilator hospital-acquired pneumonia in acute-care hospitals: 2022 update. *Infect Control Hosp Epidemiol.* 2022;43:687-703; Rawat N, Yang T, Ali K, et al. Two-state collaborative study of a multifaceted intervention to decrease ventilator-associated events. *Crit Care Med.* 2017;45(7):1208-1215.

ACUTE RESPIRATORY FAILURE RESULTING FROM PULMONARY EMBOLISM

Definition and Classification

An embolus is a clot or plug of material that travels from one blood vessel to another, smaller vessel. The clot lodges in the smaller vessel and obstructs blood flow. When an embolus lodges in the pulmonary vasculature, it is called a pulmonary embolism (PE). The embolus may be a clot that has broken off from a deep vein thrombosis (DVT), a globule of fat from a long bone fracture, septic vegetation, or an iatrogenic catheter fragment. In pregnancy, amniotic fluid can be the cause of a PE. Most PEs originate from a DVT of the lower extremity.[34] PE and DVT are the two components of the disease process known as venous thromboembolism (VTE). Approximately half of all DVTs travel to the lungs, causing a PE. Prognosis depends on the size of the PE, prompt diagnosis and treatment, and underlying disease.[78]

BOX 15.6 Example of an Oral Care Protocol

Equipment

1. Oral suction catheter
2. Soft toothbrush or suction toothbrush
3. Oral swab, or suction swab
4. Mouth rinse or toothpaste
5. Water-based mouth moisturizer
6. Suction source and tubing

Interventions

1. Assess intubated patients every 2 hours. Before repositioning or deflating the endotracheal tube, determine the need for removal of oropharyngeal secretions. Suction as needed.
2. Brush teeth, gums, and tongue twice a day using a soft toothbrush with toothpaste or cleaning solution.
3. Apply moisturizer to oral mucosa and lips every 2 to 4 hours.

Etiology

The three main mechanisms that favor the development of VTE, often referred to as Virchow's triad, are (1) venous stasis, (2) hypercoagulability of blood, and (3) damage to the vessel walls.[34] Specific risk factors for VTE are listed in Box 15.7.

PE is present in approximately 50% of patients who have DVT, but it goes undetected in many cases because approximately half of these patients present without signs or symptoms. Approximately 1 in 1000 individuals develop DVT each year, and half of these cases are complicated by PE.[78] Critically ill patients are at high risk for VTE, and chemoprophylaxis is considered a standard of care for these patients.[79]

Pathophysiology

The pulmonary circulation has an enormous capacity to compensate for a PE. This compensatory mechanism results from the lung vasculature that is necessary to accommodate increased blood flow during exercise, and it is the reason many patients do not initially decompensate from a massive PE. An embolus that lodges in the pulmonary vasculature completely or partially occludes a pulmonary artery or one of its branches, impeding the forward flow of blood. Blood flow to the alveoli beyond the occlusion is eliminated.[34] The result is a lack of perfusion to ventilated alveoli, an increase in dead space, a $\dot{V}/\dot{Q}$ mismatch, and a decrease in CO_2 tension in the embolized lung zone. Gas exchange cannot occur (Fig. 15.1).[34]

Reaction to the mechanical obstruction causes the release of several inflammatory mediators such as prostaglandins, serotonin, and histamine. The ensuing inflammation causes constriction of bronchi and widespread vasoconstriction, resulting in poor pulmonary perfusion and increased dead space. The lack of blood flow to the lung also contributes to inadequate production of surfactant, resulting in atelectasis, which contributes further to hypoxemia. Pulmonary artery constriction

BOX 15.7 Risk Factors for Venous Thromboembolism

Hereditary
- Antithrombin deficiency
- Factor V Leiden
- Protein C deficiency
- Protein S deficiency
- Prothrombin mutations

Acquired
- Acute infectious disease
- Acute myocardial infarction
- Age older than 75 years
- Burns
- Cancer
- Heart failure
- Heparin-induced thrombocytopenia
- History of previous venous thromboembolism
- Immobility for longer than 3 days
- Intravenous (IV) drug use disorder
- Lower extremity fractures
- Major surgery in previous 4 weeks
- Multiple trauma
- Nephrotic syndrome
- Oral contraceptives
- Plane or car trip longer than 4 hours in previous 4 weeks
- Pregnancy/postpartum period
- Sepsis
- Spinal cord injury
- Stroke
- Systemic lupus erythematosus (SLE)
- Ulcerative colitis

leads to increased right ventricular afterload and may eventually cause right ventricular failure.[34]

Approximately 20% of patients treated for PE die within 90 days; however, the PE is not usually the cause of death, as it often occurs as a result of other serious conditions such as sepsis, cancer, or surgery. Prognosis for the patient with a PE depends on the size of the PE, prior underlying disease, and prompt diagnosis and treatment.[78]

Assessment

Because the presenting signs and symptoms for PE are relatively vague, it is important for the critical care nurse to recognize those who have an increased risk. Classic presentation includes sudden onset of pleuritic chest pain, shortness of breath, and hypoxemia. Suspect a PE in any patient who has respiratory distress that cannot be explained by another diagnosis. Assess for the following physical findings that are present in about half of those with PE: tachypnea, crackles, accentuated S2 heart sound, tachycardia, and fever. Less common potential findings include diaphoresis, heart murmur, S3 or S4 gallop heart sounds, evidence of thrombophlebitis, edema of the lower extremities, and cyanosis.[34]

Diagnosis

D-dimer Assay. D-dimers are fibrin degradation products or fragments produced during fibrinolysis. A positive test indicates thrombus formation. A positive D-dimer assay also can occur in many other conditions, such as infection, cancer, surgery, pregnancy, heart failure, and kidney failure. Because D-dimer is nonspecific, it is not recommended for use in diagnosing PE but may be safely used to rule out PE in young, healthy individuals.[34]

Ventilation-Perfusion Scan. A V/Q scan is a noninvasive nuclear medicine procedure that calculates pulmonary airflow and blood flow. A $\dot{V}/\dot{Q}$ scan may detect dead space from impaired perfusion of ventilated alveoli. Results of $\dot{V}/\dot{Q}$ scans are reported as low, medium, or high probability; however, results are not confirmatory. $\dot{V}/\dot{Q}$ scanning may be used if a contrast CT scan is unavailable or contraindicated (i.e., contrast allergy, acute renal failure).[34]

Duplex Ultrasonography (Compression Ultrasound). Duplex ultrasonography is a noninvasive imaging study that is useful in detecting lower-extremity DVT. When evaluating for DVT, the blood flow is assessed as the vessel is compressed. It has a high sensitivity and specificity for DVT in the leg above the knee, but it is not accurate in detecting DVT in pelvic vessels or small vessels in the calf.[34]

High-Resolution Multidetector Computed Tomography Angiography. High-resolution multidetector CT angiography (MDCTA), also called spiral CT, is the preferred tool for detecting a PE. It is highly accurate for direct visualization of large emboli in the main and lobar pulmonary arteries. MDCTA does not always visualize small emboli in distal vessels, but a pulmonary angiogram has the same limitation.[34]

Pulmonary Angiography. Pulmonary angiography provides direct anatomical visualization of the pulmonary vasculature and provides close to 100% certainty of an obstruction when performed correctly, but it is an invasive procedure and difficult to perform. For these reasons, this diagnostic procedure is recommended only if CT scanning is unavailable. MDCTA is now replacing pulmonary angiography as the standard of care because it is noninvasive, less expensive, widely available, and has a high level of sensitivity and specificity.[34] The use of both diagnostic tests may be contraindicated in patients with renal disorders, as contrast injection is required, which could negatively impact a patient's renal function.

CLINICAL JUDGMENT ACTIVITY

A 19-year old patient with no past medical history was hospitalized 5 days ago with bilateral lower extremity fractures after a skiing accident. The patient just transferred to the critical care unit requiring intubation and mechanical ventilation. What is the most likely cause of this patient's acute respiratory failure? What actions should the nurse take to decrease the patient's risk of developing ventilator-associated pneumonia (VAP)?

Interventions

Prevention. The best therapy for VTEs is prevention. A thorough nursing assessment assists in identifying critically ill patients who are at risk for the development of VTEs. Once the patient's risk is assessed, the nurse can tailor interventions to decrease the occurrence of VTE (Box 15.8).[79]

Treatment. For hospitalized critically ill patients, anticoagulation therapy with heparin begins immediately for the initial management of acute PE with low-molecular-weight heparin (LMWH) or IV unfractionated heparin (UFH). An oral anticoagulant, such as warfarin, is started at the time of PE diagnosis and continued for at least 3 months. Direct thrombin inhibitors such as dabigatran or factor Xa inhibitors such as apixaban may be used as an alternative to warfarin for prophylaxis and treatment of PE. LMWH or UFH is continued until international normalized ratio (INR) levels remain at 2.0 for 24 hours but is not discontinued sooner than 5 days after initiation of therapy.[78,80] Anticoagulants work with the body's inherent fibrinolytic system to prevent further clotting and relieve the thromboembolic burden.

While the patient is on anticoagulant therapy, regularly monitor the laboratory values and assess the patient for any signs or symptoms of bleeding or heparin-induced thrombocytopenia (HIT). HIT is a complication of LMWH and UFH caused by the development of antibodies against heparin and platelet factor 4 that activate platelets, leading to thrombocytopenia. HIT syndrome, sometimes referred to as heparin-induced thrombocytopenia and thrombosis (HITT), results in thromboembolisms such as DVT or PE. To detect this problem, observe the patient for a decreasing platelet count, skin lesions at the injection site, and systemic reactions such as fever and chills. The presence of HIT requires the discontinuation of heparin products. Argatroban, bivalirudin, danaparoid, fondaparinux, or a direct oral anticoagulant are alternatives for patients who have developed or have a history of HIT.[81]

Use of thrombolytic medication is based on severity of the PE, risk of bleeding, and prognosis. Thrombolytic therapy is indicated for the treatment of acute PE accompanied by hypotension (systolic BP <90 mm Hg) in the absence of a high risk of bleeding. It may also be considered for those patients receiving anticoagulation who are at risk of developing hypotension and have a low risk of bleeding. Because of the increased risk of major bleeding and lack of demonstration of sustained benefits of reducing mortality when compared to anticoagulation therapy alone, thrombolysis is not recommended for most patients.[78,80,82]

Surgical embolectomy or catheter embolectomy involves manual removal of the thrombus from the pulmonary artery; it is an option for adult patients with massive PE and those who have contraindications for fibrinolytic therapy or who do not respond favorably to those medications. Vena cava filters may be placed in the inferior vena cava to prevent recurrence of PE by capturing clots that are migrating from the lower extremities. Both permanent filters and temporary retrievable filters are available. Permanent vena cava filters are rarely used and have many associated complications. Temporary retrievable vena cava filters are used to prevent PE in patients who have contraindications for anticoagulation therapy, major bleeding during anticoagulation therapy, or recurring PE. These devices can be removed by a minimally invasive technique under fluoroscopy. The routine use of these filters is not recommended, as serious complications can occur.[83]

Other treatments focus on maintaining the airway, breathing, and circulation. Supplemental oxygen may be administered to maintain SpO_2 at greater than 90%. Analgesics are given to alleviate pain and anxiety. If the patient is hemodynamically unstable, inotropic or vasopressor support may be required. ECMO shows promise in reducing mortality in the presence of massive PE-related cardiac arrest.[84]

BOX 15.8 Nursing Interventions to Prevent Venous Thromboembolism

1. Assess patient on admission to unit for VTE risk and anticipate prophylaxis orders.
2. Review daily with healthcare team:
   - Current VTE risk factors
   - Necessity for central venous catheter
   - Current VTE prophylaxis
   - Risk of bleeding
   - Response to treatment
3. Implement prescribed prophylactic regimen:
   - Pharmacological prophylaxis (also known as chemoprophylaxis)*
     - Suggested over mechanical prophylaxis
     - LMWH is more effective at reducing the incidence of DVT than that of UFH
   - Nonpharmacological (mechanical) prophylaxis for patients not receiving pharmacological prophylaxis
     - Intermittent pneumatic compression devices are preferred
     - Graduated compression stockings have not been demonstrated to decrease the incidence of DVT in critically ill patients
   - Efficacy and safety of combing pharmacological and nonpharmacological therapy is unclear
4. Document implementation, tolerance, and complications of prophylaxis.
5. Assess extremities on a regular basis:
   - Pain or tenderness
   - Unilateral edema
   - Erythema
   - Warmth
6. Implement a mobility program.
7. Monitor for low-grade fever.
8. Encourage fluids to prevent dehydration:
   - Administer IV fluids as prescribed
   - Maintain accurate intake and output records
9. Avoid adjusting the knee section of the bed or using pillows under knees.
10. Provide patient education regarding prevention.

* Recommendations on dosing and timing of initiation may vary based on specialty population.

DVT, Deep vein thrombosis; *LMWH*, low–molecular-weight heparin; *UFH*, unfractionated heparin; *VTE*, venous thromboembolism.

CHECK YOUR UNDERSTANDING

5. Determine which of the following patients would be at greatest risk for developing DVT:
   A. 77-year-old male status post motor vehicle collision with a severe traumatic brain injury and bilateral lower extremity fractures
   B. 50-year-old female with atrial fibrillation who was bridged from a heparin drip to oral anticoagulation with therapeutic anticoagulation levels throughout hospitalization
   C. 20-year-old male status post appendectomy who is mobilizing the hallway 4 hours after surgery
   D. 33-year-old female with acute respiratory failure secondary to asthma exacerbation who is out of bed to chair, weaning mechanical ventilation, and receiving pharmacological venous thromboembolism prophylaxis

ACUTE RESPIRATORY FAILURE IN ADULT PATIENTS WITH CYSTIC FIBROSIS

Definition

Cystic fibrosis (CF) is a genetic disorder (see Genetics box) that results from defective chloride ion transport, which leads to the formation of thick mucus. The thick, sticky mucus obstructs glands of the lungs, pancreas, liver, salivary glands, and testes, causing organ dysfunction. Although CF is a multisystem disease, it has its greatest effect on the lungs, with respiratory failure being the primary cause of death. The thick mucus narrows the airways and reduces airflow. The constant presence of thick mucus provides an excellent breeding ground for bacteria, leading to chronic lower respiratory tract infections. The mucus-producing cells in the lungs increase in number and size over time, resulting in mucus plugging. Respiratory complications of CF include pneumothorax, arterial erosion, hemorrhage, chronic bacterial infection, and respiratory failure.[85] Respiratory or cardiorespiratory events cause slightly more than half the deaths associated with CF. The mortality rate, which has experienced a steady decline in the past 3 decades, is 0.8 deaths per 100 persons. This statistic shows promise in that the median age of individuals with CF increased from 12.3 years in 1990 to 20.8 years in 2020.[86]

Etiology

CF affects people of all ethnic and racial groups. For many years, CF was considered a disease of children. Because of significant improvements in care, currently more than half of those with CF are adults older than 18 years of age.[85] The median predicted survival of those born between 2016 and 2020 was 50 years, meaning half of these persons will live to that age or beyond. Survival of individuals with CF has steadily increased over the past 3 decades.[86]

Most children now undergo newborn screening for CF, so the diagnosis is typically made early in life (75% by 2 years of age), but a few patients are diagnosed as adults. Diagnostic testing is a multiple-step process that includes a sweat chloride test (gold standard), a genetic or carrier test, and clinical evaluation at a center accredited by the Cystic Fibrosis Foundation. Sweat test levels of 60 mmol/L or greater indicate CF is likely. Levels between 30 and 59 mmol/L indicate additional testing is in order. Being tested as a carrier is a personal preference, but the American College of Obstetricians and Gynecologists suggests anyone considering having a child be offered the testing opportunity.[85]

Assessment

Individuals with CF may experience a variety of symptoms, including salty-tasting skin, persistent cough (productive at times), frequent lung infections, wheezing, shortness of breath, poor growth despite eating well, fatty and bulky stools, difficulty eliminating, nasal polyps, chronic sinus infections, clubbing of fingers and toes, rectal prolapse, and infertility in males. Assessment of respiratory status, nutritional status, and elimination are routine.[85]

Interventions

Because CF is a complicated and chronic disease, outcomes are best when patients with CF are cared for by experts in an environment in which efforts are comprehensive and coordinated in partnership with CF care teams. As the disease process progresses, patients develop increased ventilator requirements, air trapping, and respiratory muscle weakness. These conditions are complicated by chronic bacterial infections that can quickly become overwhelming. In the past, mechanical ventilation was not considered a treatment option, because patient outcomes were poor. ARF in people with CF is continuously revisited because of improved ventilator modalities, more aggressive pharmacological therapy, and the option of lung transplantation. Lung transplantation provides the opportunity for a tremendous improvement in the quality of life, but acute exacerbations of respiratory failure must be overcome while waiting for a transplant (see Transplant Considerations box).

The goals of care for a patient with CF focus on nutrition and fitness, airway clearance, antibiotic therapy, pancreatic enzyme supplements, *CFTR* modulator therapies, and ventilation support.[85] For those suffering an exacerbation that requires admission to a critical care unit, a multidisciplinary approach includes a PT who specializes in CF to evaluate airway clearance and adjust regimens as appropriate, a dietitian to evaluate caloric needs and any needed adjustments in nutritional requirements, and a pharmacist as well as an infectious disease specialist to evaluate antibiotic selection.[87] The critical care nurse must be aware of potential complications, provide vigilant monitoring, and respond quickly to emergent needs.

GENETICS

Cystic Fibrosis

Cystic fibrosis (CF) is a chronic disease of exocrine dysfunction. It is inherited in an *autosomal recessive* pattern. As with all autosomal recessive conditions, each child, when both parents are carriers of the genetic variation, has a 25% chance of inheriting CF.[1] The disease is most common among Whites of northern European descent, Latinos, and Pueblo and Zuni American natives. Newborn screening for CF uses a combination of biochemical markers and genetic assays and occurs in all 50 United States.[1]

A defect in the chloride ion channel from a variant *cystic fibrosis transmembrane conductance regulator (CFTR)* gene causes CF. Genes are conventionally identified in italics, so the gene that codes the *CFTR* channel is identified as *CFTR*. This gene has more than 2000 *polymorphisms*, but not all variations result in symptomatic CF. *Single gene* variations that cause disease are divided into five classes[2]:

1. Defective protein synthesis
2. Defective protein processing
3. Disordered regulation
4. Defective chloride conductance
5. Accelerated channel turnover

An example of defective protein processing is a genetic variation that prevents the *CFTR* protein from folding properly so that the chloride channel does not reach the cell surface. A different genetic polymorphism, resulting in defective chloride conductance, causes a "sticky" but functional channel gate, slowing chloride entry into the cell and resulting in milder symptoms.

The defects in transporting chloride into and out of cells result in thick mucus that is difficult to clear, particularly in the lungs, the gastrointestinal (GI) tract, and the pancreas. This defect gives the skin a characteristic salty taste in many patients with CF. Thick mucus production in the lungs interferes with gas exchange, leading to chronic hypoxemia. Lung disease from CF can lead to chronic respiratory insufficiency that results in morbidity and erodes the quality of life. Thick mucus production in the GI tract blocks intestinal fluids, causing GI obstruction and impaired absorption of nutrients. The pancreas is unable to excrete digestive enzymes. Thick mucus is more likely to colonize microorganisms, contributing to infection and inflammation with subsequent adverse and irreversible changes in these organs.

Signs and symptoms are typically seen when *CFTR* function is less than 10%.[2] Patients with the most severe symptoms have less than 1% *CFTR* activity and manifest the full spectrum of disease involvement, including recurrent, severe pulmonary infections; GI obstruction; pancreatic insufficiency; and congenital absence of the vas deferens.

New medications target the defective chloride channel, particularly in the pulmonary system.[3] The *CFTR*-modulating medications can be given as a single drug or in combinations to improve the function of the faulty *CFTR* protein. Other drugs are given to thin secretions, reduce inflammation, and manage symptoms. Other interventions include devices to clear pulmonary mucus, nutritional strategies to maintain health, and infection prevention.

People with one copy of the *CFTR* mutation are *heterozygous carriers*. Because more than 10 million individuals in the United States are estimated to have a single gene for CF (i.e., a *single gene trait*), *genetic testing* is recommended for all couples at high risk for carrier status because of their ethnicity or family history. Initially, testing is performed on one future parent. If that person is a *carrier* (i.e., has a single gene or allele with a CF-related variant), the other future parent is tested. Knowing the *CFTR alleles* of both parents allows geneticists to calculate the risk that the children of those two parents will have CF. It is impossible to test for all variations of the *CFTR* gene in a single genetic test; testing typically identifies 90 common mutations. Therefore a negative screen does not guarantee that an individual does not have a *CFTR* mutation that causes CF symptoms.

The clinician individualizes interventions to manage CF based on genotype. For example, some medications to correct the *CFTR* channel defect are not useful in all CF genotypes.[4] Different combinations of *CFTR* modulators may be used depending on gene variants. While most of these drugs have been developed to manage pulmonary symptoms, they improve GI and pancreatic function for some genotypes.[3] In the past 10 years, *CFTR* modulators have improved the life expectancy and quality of life for individuals with CF.

The Cystic Fibrosis Foundation has links to information and support groups for families in which CF is a potential or actual condition.[5] Refer individuals to *genetic counseling* by an expert clinician before genetic testing to help them understand the risk of inheriting CF and the nuances around CF as a chronic condition. Genetic counselors are experts who can facilitate testing and interpretation and help integrate genetic information into treatment options.

References

1. National Institutes of Health *What is Cystic Fibrosis?* https://www.nhlbi.nih.gov/health/cystic-fibrosis. Updated November 21, 2023; Accessed December 26, 2023.
2. Yu E, Sharma S. Cystic Fibrosis. In: *StatPearls*. Stat Pearls; 2022. Publishing. https://www.ncbi.nlm.nih.gov/pubmed/29630258. Accessed December 26, 2023.
3. Ramsey ML, Li SS, Lara LF, et al. Cystic fibrosis transmembrane conductance regulator modulators and the exocrine pancreas: a scoping review. *J Cyst Fibros*. 2022. https://doi.org/10.1016/j.jcf.2022.08.008.
4. Bierlaagh MC, Muilwijk D, Beekman JM, van der Ent CK. A new era for people with cystic fibrosis. *Eur J Pediatr*. 2021;180(9):2731–2739. https://doi.org/10.1007/s00431-021-04168-y.
5. Cystic Fibrosis Foundation. Support. https://www.cff.org/. Accessed February 19, 2023.

Chris Winkelman, PhD, ACNP-BC, CCRN, CNE, FAANP, FCCM

Genetic terms: *single gene trait, autosomal recessive, genetic testing, carrier, heterozygous, genetic counseling*

TRANSPLANT CONSIDERATIONS

Lung Transplantation

Criteria for Transplant Recipients

Criteria for placement on the lung transplant waiting list include patients who have >50% risk of death from lung disease within 2 years and >80% likelihood of 5-year posttransplant survival.[1] Multiple data are evaluated to determine priority status for transplantation: (1) waiting list survival probability during the next year, (2) waitlist urgency measure, (3) survival probability during the first posttransplant year, and (4) estimated posttransplant survival. The Lung Allocation Score (LAS) calculator is a tool that can be used to estimate each lung candidate's medical urgency and expected posttransplant survival rate relative to other patients on the waiting list for a lung transplant.[2] Contraindications for lung transplantation include malignancy with a high risk of recurrence, active substance use or dependence, recent myocardial infarction within 30 days, significant kidney or liver disease, human immunodeficiency virus (HIV) with a high viral load, septic shock, limited functional status, recent stroke, repeated episodes of nonadherence, and progressive cognitive decline.[3]

Patient Management

Postoperative management focuses on maintaining BP, optimizing end-organ perfusion, and proper ventilator management to avoid respiratory acidosis and maintain adequate oxygenation. Minimizing ventilator time can help avoid pulmonary infection and graft dysfunction.[3]

Immunosuppression therapy is needed after organ transplantation and consists of triple therapy: a calcineurin inhibitor (tacrolimus [Prograf] or cyclosporine [Neoral]), a corticosteroid (prednisone), and mycophenolate mofetil (CellCept). These medications inhibit T-cell proliferation and differentiation, deplete lymphocytes, and inhibit macrophages.

Complications

Primary graft dysfunction is a major cause of morbidity and mortality and is comparable to ARDS. Patients present with malaise, increased work of breathing, activity intolerance, and oxygen desaturation. Management includes supplemental oxygen, positive-pressure ventilation, and aggressive pulmonary hygiene. Mechanical ventilation, inhaled nitric oxide, or ECMO may be indicated. Large-airway and vascular anastomosis complications may occur, potentially requiring reanastomosis or stenting if granulomatous tissue threatens airway obstruction. Urgent relisting for lung transplantation may be required.

Infection is a significant cause of morbidity and mortality after lung transplantation. Bacterial and fungal infections occur most frequently in the first few months; viral infections, especially cytomegalovirus (CMV), are more prevalent in the months after transplantation.

Other complications include inadequate bronchial anastomosis, pneumothorax, pleural effusions, gastroesophageal reflux disease (GERD), and those associated with immunosuppression therapy.[1] Complications associated with immunosuppression therapy include nephrotoxicity, hypertension, hyperlipidemia, bone loss, new-onset diabetes mellitus, and infection.[1]

Preventing Rejection

Compliance with immunosuppressive medication is essential to avoid or decrease the incidence of rejection episodes. *Acute* or *cellular-mediated rejection* usually occurs within the first 12 weeks after transplantation. Symptoms include fatigue, dyspnea, fever, hypoxemia, pulmonary infiltrates, or pleural effusions. This can result in acute graft dysfunction and long-term failure.[1] To differentiate rejection from infection, a biopsy may be indicated. Management includes high-dose corticosteroids and optimizing maintenance immunosuppression therapy.

Recurrent acute rejection has been associated with the development of *chronic rejection* or *bronchiolitis obliterans syndrome (BOS)*, in which inflammation and fibrosis of small airways occur. More than 50% of lung transplant recipients develop BOS within 5 years of transplantation.[1] Symptoms include progressive shortness of breath, decreased exercise tolerance, airflow limitation, and progressive decline in pulmonary function. Management is individualized and includes aggressively managing acute rejection and infection and optimizing the immunosuppression regimen.[3]

Reference

1. Costa J, Benvenuto LJ, Sonett JR. Long-term outcomes and management of lung transplant recipients. *Best Pract Res Clin Anaesthesiol.* 2017;31(2):285-297. https://doi.org/10.1016/j.bpa.2017.05.006.
2. Learn about LAS - OPTN. Organ Procurement and Transplantation Network. https://optn.transplant.hrsa.gov/data/allocation-calculators/las-calculator/learn-about-las/. Accessed December 26, 2023.
3. Potestio C, Jordan D, Kachulis B. Acute postoperative management after lung transplantation. *Best Pract Res Clin Anaesthesiol.* 2017;31(2):273-284. https://doi.org/10.1016/j.bpa.2017.07.004.

Chelsea Sooy, BSN, RN, CCTC
Melissa A. Kelley, RN, CPTC

CASE STUDY

A 57-year-old patient was admitted to the critical care unit after a motor vehicle collision. The patient sustained multiple long bone fractures and a chest contusion. While in the emergency department, the patient experienced an episode of hypotension responsive to 500 mL of warmed isotonic crystalloid and 2 units of emergency release blood. Within 12 hours, the patient became short of breath, with an increase in respiratory rate requiring high levels of supplemental oxygen. The patient was intubated and placed on volume-control mechanical ventilation with a PEEP of 5 cm H_2O. Continuous IV analgesia and sedation infusions were started. The goal was to achieve pain control and light sedation per the validated pain and sedation tools. During the next 8 hours, the patient's SpO_2 steadily deteriorated, and the high-pressure alarms on the ventilator activated frequently. The nurse noted steadily rising peak airway pressures. The FiO_2 had to be increased to 0.80 (80%), and the PEEP increased to 14 cm H_2O to maintain the patient's PaO_2 at 60 mm Hg. A chest radiograph showed bilateral infiltrates with normal heart size. The patient's cardiac markers were negative, and the patient remains hemodynamically stable with tachycardia (110 beats/min).The sedation infusion required frequent upward titrations to maintain the desired goal of light sedation. ARDS was diagnosed based on the Berlin definition.

During the next 6 hours, the patient steadily became more hypoxemic. The PEEP was increased to 20 cm H_2O and the FiO_2 to 1.0 (100%) to maintain a PaO_2 greater than 60 mm Hg. The patient was extremely restless, with tachycardia, diaphoresis, and a labile SaO_2. Deep sedation with continuous analgesia and sedation was ordered based on the validated sedation scale, which improved ventilator synchrony. Given the inability to achieve adequate PaO_2 with increasing ventilator settings, the multiprofessional team altered the plan of care to include prone positioning to improve oxygenation. An hour after the patient was turned to the prone position, the patient's SpO_2 began to slowly rise. After 2 hours in the prone position, the patient's SpO_2 stabilized at 93%. Slowly, the FiO_2 was decreased to 0.60, with a stable SpO_2 of 96%. After 16 hours, the patient was returned to the supine position. The patient's SpO_2 decreased to 94% and remained stable. The sedation goal was modified to light sedation. The patient was weaned from sedatives and analgesia as assessed based on validated pain and sedation tools.

The patient slowly improved over the next week. Ventilator settings continued to be weaned, with PEEP decreased to a physiological level. The sedation was interrupted daily to coincide with spontaneous breathing trials. The patient was extubated on the 7th day and transferred on day 8 to the trauma stepdown unit on 4 L of oxygen per nasal cannula.

Questions

1. Identify the risk factors the patient had for the development of ARDS.
2. According to the case study, the patient was diagnosed with ARDS based on the Berlin definition. What diagnostic and assessment findings support this diagnosis?
3. Explain the use of the high PEEP level and the nursing monitoring responsibilities.
4. Explain the rationale for treating patients with moderate to severe ARDS with prone positioning. Discuss nursing interventions to reduce complications associated with prone positioning.
5. What immediate assessment findings indicate the combination of prone positioning, deep sedation to achieve ventilator synchrony, and high PEEP were effective for this patient?

KEY POINTS

- Prompt and thorough respiratory assessment is essential in early detection and treatment of acute respiratory failure.
- Treatment includes maintaining the airway, optimizing oxygen delivery, minimizing demand, and identifying and treating the cause.
- Be alert for signs of impending respiratory failure: severe dyspnea with respiratory muscle fatigue and increased work of breathing, hypoxemia not responsive to supplemental oxygen, and respiratory acidosis.
- Specific management of ARDS includes mechanical ventilation with low tidal volume, low end-inspiratory plateau pressure, $FiO_2 \leq 0.50$, and PEEP.
- Supplemental oxygen to achieve an SaO_2 of 88% to 92% is the most important intervention for an acute exacerbation of COPD.
- Intubation and invasive mechanical ventilation are indicated for ARF in COPD for patients who fail a trial of NPPV.
- A "silent chest" in an acute asthma attack is an ominous sign requiring immediate action.
- Prevention of pneumonia in the older population and possible ARF can best be achieved by pneumococcal and influenza vaccinations.
- Prevention of VAP is best accomplished using the Society for Healthcare Epidemiology of America (SHEA) guidelines (Box 15.5).
- Critically ill patients are prone to developing VTE, which is best prevented by thorough nursing assessment and administration of chemoprophylaxis.
- Adult patients with CF exacerbations have improved outcomes when cared for by a multidisciplinary team including a PT who specializes in CF to evaluate airway clearance, a dietitian to evaluate caloric needs, and a pharmacist and infectious disease specialist to evaluate antibiotic selection.

REFERENCES

1. Parcha V, Kalra R, Bhatt SP, Berra L, Arora G, Arora P. Trends and geographic variation in acute respiratory failure and ARDS mortality in the United States. *Chest*. 2020;159(4):1460–1472.
2. Society of Critical Care Medicine. Critical care statistics. www.sccm.org/Communications/Critical-Care-Statistics. Accessed August 10, 2022.
3. Turner, KC, Brashers VL. Structure and function of the pulmonary system. In: McCance KL, Huether SE. *Pathophysiology: The Biologic Basis for Disease in Adults and Children*. 9th ed. St. Louis, MO: Elsevier; 2024:1131–1148.
4. LoMauro A, Aliverti A, Frykholm P, et al. Adaptation of lung, chest wall, and respiratory muscles during pregnancy: preparing for birth. *J Appl Physiol*. 2019;127:1640–1650.
5. Bhavani MR, Sushm J, Prathyusha M, et al. Effectiveness of noninvasive positive pressure ventilation for acute exacerbation of chronic obstructive pulmonary disease. *IJCT*. 2018;5(2):102–106.
6. Stefan MS, Pekow PS, Shieh MS, et al. Hospital volume and outcomes of noninvasive ventilation in patients hospitalized with an acute exacerbation of chronic obstructive pulmonary disease. *Crit Care Med*. 2017;45(1):20–27.
7. Wilson ME, Majzoub AM, Dobler CC, et al. Noninvasive ventilator in patients with Do-Not-Intubate and Comfort-Measures-Only orders: a systematic review and meta-analysis. *Crit Care Med*. 2018;46(8):1209–1216.
8. van den Boom W, Hoy M, Sankaran J, et al. The search for optimal oxygen saturation targets in critically ill patients: observational data from large ICU databases. *Chest*. 2020;157(3):566–573. https://doi.org/10.1016/j.chest.2019.09.015.
9. Barrot L, Asfar P, Mauny F, et al. Liberal or conservative oxygen therapy for acute respiratory distress syndrome. *N Engl J Med*. 2020;382(11):999–1008.
10. Chu DK, Kim LH, Young PJ, et al. Mortality and morbidity in acutely ill adults treated with liberal versus conservative oxygen therapy (IOTA): a systematic review and meta-analysis. *Lancet*. 2018;391(10131):1693–1705.
11. Delorme M, Bouchard PA, Simon M, et al. Effects of high-flow nasal cannula on the work of breathing in patients recovering from acute respiratory failure. *Crit Care Med*. 2017;45(12):1981–1988.
12. Johnny JD. Risk stratification in noninvasive respiratory support failure: a narrative review. *Crit Care Nurse*. 2022;42(3):62–68.
13. Wang YT, Lang JK, Haines KJ, Skinner EH, Haines TP. Physical rehabilitation in the ICU: a systematic review and meta-analysis. *Crit Care Med*. 2022;50(3):375–388.
14. Jolley SE, Moss M, Needham DM, et al. Point prevalence study of mobilization practices for acute respiratory failure patients in the United States. *Crit Care Med*. 2017;45(2):205–215.
15. Cochi SH, Kempker JA, Annangi S, Kramer MR, Martin GS. Mortality trends of acute respiratory distress syndrome in the United States from 1999-2013. *Ann Am Thorac Soc*. 2016;13(10):1742–1751.
16. Ni YN, Luo J, Yu H, et al. Can body mass index predict clinical outcomes for patients with acute lung injury/acute respiratory distress syndrome? *Crit Care*. 2017;21(36).
17. Villar J, Ambros A, Soler JA, et al. Age, PaO_2/FiO_2, and plateau pressure score: a proposal for a simple outcome score in patients with the acute respiratory distress syndrome. *Crit Care Med*. 2016;44(7):1361–1369.
18. Tzotzos SJ, Fischer B, Fischer H, et al. Incidence of ARDS and outcomes in hospitalized patients with COVID-19: a global literature survey. *Crit Care*. 2020;516(24):1–4.
19. Centers for Disease Control and Prevention: COVID Data Tracker. https://covid.cdc.gov/covid-data-tracker/#new-hospital-admissions. Updated September 20, 2022. Accessed August 31, 2022.
20. Centers for Disease Control and Prevention: COVID Data Tracker. Disease severity among hospitalized patients. https://covid.cdc.gov/covid-data-tracker/#hospitalizations-severity. Accessed August 31, 2022.
21. Saad M, Laghi FA, Brofman J, et al. Long-term acute care hospital outcomes of mechanically ventilated patients with coronavirus disease 2019. *Crit Care Med*. 2022;50(2):256–262.
22. Martillo MA, Dangayach NS, Tabacof L. Postintensive care syndrome in survivors of critical illness related to coronavirus disease 2019: cohort study from a New York City critical care recovery clinic. *Crit Care Med*. 2021;49(9):1427–1438.

23. Taniguchi LU, Avelino-Silva TJ, Dias MB, et al. Patient-centered outcomes following covid-19: frailty and disability transitions in critical care survivors. *Crit Care Med.* 2022;50(6):955–962.
24. Van Gassel RJJ, Bels J, Remij L, et al. Functional outcomes and their association with physical performance in mechanically ventilated coronavirus disease 2019 survivors at 3 months following hospital discharge: a cohort study. *Crit Care Med.* 2021;49(10):1726–1738.
25. Gast S, Barroso J, Blanchard FA, et al. Critical care nurses' experiences of caring for patients with covid-19: results of a thematic analysis. *AJCC.* 2022;31(4):275–282.
26. Kleinpell R, Ferraro DM, Maves RC, et al. Coronavirus disease 2019 pandemic measures: reports from a national survey of 9,120 ICU clinicians. *Crit Care Med.* 2020;15(7):1–10.
27. Ike JD, Kempker JA, Kramer MR, et al. The association between acute respiratory distress syndrome hospital case volume and mortality in a US cohort, 2002–2011. *Crit Care Med.* 2018;46(5):764–773. 15.
28. ARDS Definition Task Force, Ranieri VM, Rubenfeld GD, et al. Acute respiratory distress syndrome: the Berlin Definition. *JAMA.* 2012;307(23):2526–2533. https://doi.org/10.1001/jama.2012.5669.
29. Villar J, Martin-Rodriquez C, Dominguez-Berrot AM, et al. A quantile analysis of plateau and driving pressures: effects on mortality in patients with acute respiratory distress syndrome receiving lung-protective ventilation. *Crit Care Med.* 2017;45(5):843–850.
30. Geense WW, Boogaard MVD, Peters MAA, et al. Physical, mental, and cognitive health status of ICU survivors before ICU admission: a cohort study. *Crit Care Med.* 2020;48(9):1271–1278.
31. Dinglas VD, Friedman LA, Colantuoni E, et al. Muscle weakness and 5-year survival in acute respiratory distress syndrome survivors. *Crit Care Med.* 2017;45(3):446–453.
32. Eakin MN, Patel Y, Mendez-Tellez P, et al. Patients' outcomes after acute respiratory failure: a qualitative study with the PROMIS framework. *AJCC.* 2017;26(6):456–465.
33. Wilson ME, Barwise A, Heise KJ, et al. Long-Term return to functional baseline after mechanical ventilation in the ICU. *CCM Journal.* 2018;46(4):562–568.
34. Winton, MB, Brashers, VL. Alterations of pulmonary function. In: Rogers, JL. *McCance & Huether's Pathophysiology: The Biologic Basis for Disease in Adults and Children.* 9th ed. St. Louis, MO: Elsevier; 2024:1153–1190.
35. Patel BK, Wolfe KS, MacKenzie EL, et al. One-year outcomes in patients with acute respiratory distress syndrome enrolled in a randomized clinical trial of helmet versus facemask noninvasive ventilation. *Crit Care Med.* 2018;46(7):1078–1084.
36. Bellani G, Laffey JG, Pham T, Investigators LUNGSAFE, ESICM Trial Group, et al. Noninvasive ventilation of patients with acute respiratory distress syndrome: insights from the LUNG SAFE study. *Am J Respir Crit Care Med.* 2017;195:67–77.
37. Frat JP, Ragot S, Coudroy R, et al. Predictors of intubation in patients with acute hypoxemic respiratory failure treated with a noninvasive oxygenation strategy. *Crit Care Med.* 2018;46(2):208–215.
38. Fan E, Del Sorbo L, Goligher EC, et al. An official American thoracic society/European society of intensive care medicine/society of critical care medicine clinical practice guideline: mechanical ventilation in adult patients with acute respiratory distress syndrome. *Am J Respir Crit Care Med.* 2017;195(9):1253–1263.
39. Fuller BM, Ferguson IT, Mohr NM, et al. A quasi-experimental, before-after trial examining the impact of an emergency department mechanical ventilator protocol on clinical outcomes and lung-protective ventilation in acute respiratory distress syndrome. *Crit Care Med.* 2017;45(4):645–652.
40. De Monnin K, Terian E, Yaegar LH, et al. Low tidal volume ventilation for emergency department patients: a systemic review and meta-analysis on practice patterns and clinical impact. *Crit Care Med.* 2022;50(6):986–998.
41. Liang M, Chen X. Differential prognostic analysis of higher and lower PEEP in ARDS patients: systematic review and meta-analysis. *J Healthc Eng.* 2022:8. https://doi.org/10.1155/2022/539941642. Article ID 5399416.
42. Aggarwal NR, Brower RG, Hager DN, et al. Oxygen exposure resulting in arterial oxygen tensions above protocol goal was associated with worse clinical outcomes in acute respiratory distress syndrome. *Crit Care Med.* 2018;48(4):517–524.
43. Abrams D, Brodie D. Extracorporeal membrane oxygenation is first-line therapy for acute respiratory distress syndrome. *Crit Care Med.* 2017;45(12):2070–2076.
44. Sahetya S, Brower RG, Stephens S. Survival of patients with severe acute respiratory distress syndrome treated without extracorporeal membrane oxygenation. *AJCC.* 2018;27(3):220–227.
45. Kido T, Muramatsu K, Asakawa T, et al. The relationship between high-dose corticosteroid treatment and mortality in acute respiratory distress syndrome. *BMC Pulm Med.* 2018;18(1):28.
46. Annane D, Pastores SM, Arlt W, et al. Critical illness–related corticosteroid insufficiency (CIRCI): a narrative review from a multispecialty task force of the Society of Critical Care Medicine (SCCM) and the European Society of Intensive Care Medicine (ESICM). *Crit Care Med.* 2017;45(12):2089–2098.
47. Medura GU, Bridges L, Siemienuik RAC, et al. An exploratory reanalysis of the randomized trial on efficacy of corticosteroids as rescue therapy for the late phase of acute respiratory distress syndrome. *Crit Care Med.* 2018;46(6):884–899. 46.
48. Yoshihiro S, Hongo T, Ohki S, et al. Steroid treatment in patients with acute respiratory distress syndrome: a systematic review and network meta-analysis. *J Anesth.* 2022;36(1):107–121. https://doi.org/10.1007/s00540-021-03016-5.
49. Villar J, Ferrando C, Martínez D, et al. Dexamethasone treatment for the acute respiratory distress syndrome: a multicentre, randomised controlled trial. *Lancet Respir Med.* 2020;8(3):267–276. https://doi.org/10.1016/S2213-2600(19)30417-5.
50. Sousa MLA, Magrans R, Hayashi FK, et al. Clusters of double triggering impact clinical outcomes: insights from the EPIdemiology of patient-ventilator aSYNChrony (EPISYNC) cohort study. *CCM Journal.* 2021;49(9):1460–1469.
51. Devlin JW, Yoanna S, Celine G, et al. Clinical practice guidelines for the prevention and management of pain, agitation/sedation, delirium, immobility, and sleep disruption in adult patients in the ICU. *Crit Care Med.* 2018;46(9):1–45.
52. Wongtangman K, Santer P, Wachtendorf LJ, et al. Association of sedation, coma, and in-hospital mortality in mechanically ventilated patients with coronavirus disease 2019- Related acute respiratory distress syndrome: a retrospective cohort study. *Neuro Crit Care.* 2021;49(9):1524–1534.
53. Kallet RH, Zhuo H, Yip V, et al. Spontaneous breathing trials and conservative sedation practices reduce mechanical ventilation duration in subjects with ARDS. *Resp Care.* 2018;63(1):1–10.
54. Torbic H, Krishnan S, Harnegie MP, Duggal A. Neuromuscular blocking agents for ARDS: a systematic review and meta-analysis. *Respir Care.* 2021;66(1):120–128. https://doi.org/10.4187/respcare.07849.

55. Pappal RD, Roberts BW, Winkler W, et al. Awareness with paralysis in mechanically ventilated patients in the emergency department and ICU. *Crit Care Med.* 2021;49(3):e304–e314. https://doi.org/10.1097/CCM.0000000000004824.
56. Munshi L, Del Sorbo L, Adhikari NKJ, et al. Prone position for acute respiratory distress syndrome: a systematic review and meta-analysis. *Ann Am Thorac Soc.* 2017;14(suppl 4):S280–S288.
57. Thompson AE, Ranard BL, Wei Y, Jelic S. Prone positioning in awake, nonintubated patients with covid-19 hypoxemic respiratory failure. *JAMA Inter Med.* 2020;180(11):1537–1540.
58. Kaur R, Vines DL, Mirza S, et al. Early versus late awake prone positioning in non-intubated patients with covid-19. *Crit Care.* 2021;25(340):1–9.
59. Morata L, Vollman K, Rechter J, Cox J. Manual prone positioning in adults: reducing the risk of harm through evidence-based practices. *Crit Care Nurse.* 2023;43(1):59–66. https://doi.org/10.4037/ccn2023174. [published correction appears in Crit Care Nurse. 2023 Apr 1;43(2):7].
60. Ravikumar N, McGee WT. How much fluid should I give to my patient on a ventilator? *Crit Care Med.* 2022;50(2):349–350.
61. Wang W, Zhu S, He Q, Wang M, Kang Y, et al. Fluid balance and ventilator-associated events among patients admitted to ICUs in China: a nested case-control study. *Crit Care Med.* 2022;50(2):307–316.
62. Peterson SJ, Lateef OB, Freels S, et al. Early exposure to recommended calorie delivery in the intensive care unit is associated with increased mortality in patients with acute respiratory distress syndrome. *J Parenter Enteral Nutr.* 2018;42(4):739–747.
63. Heyland D, Ortiz A, Stoppe C, et al. Incidence risk factors and clinical consequences of enteral feeding intolerance in the mechanically ventilated critically ill: an analysis of a multicenter, multiyear database. *Crit Care Med.* 2021;49(1):49–58.
64. Global Initiative for Chronic Obstructive Lung Disease (GOLD). Global strategy for the diagnosis, management, and prevention of Chronic Obstructive Pulmonary Disease, 2022 report. http://www.goldcopd.org/recent-gold-publications/#2022. Accessed September 23, 2022.
65. Gadre SK, Duggal A, Mireles-Cabodevila E, et al. Acute respiratory failure requiring mechanical ventilation in severe chronic obstructive pulmonary disease (COPD). *Medicine.* 2018;97(17):1–5.
66. Global Initiative for Asthma (GINA). Global strategy for asthma management and prevention, Updated 2022. http://www.ginasthma.org/. Published 2022. Accessed September 23, 2022.
67. Centers for Disease Control and Prevention. Pneumococcal Vaccination: What Everyone Should Know. https://www.cdc.gov/vaccines/vpd/pneumo/public/index.html. Reviewed January 24, 2022. Accessed September 23, 2022.
68. Centers for Disease Control and Prevention: key facts about seasonal flu vaccine https://www.cdc.gov/flu/prevent/keyfacts.htm. Updated August 25, 2022. Accessed September 23, 2022.
69. Centers for Disease Control and Prevention. Device-Associated Module PNEU. http://www.cdc.gov/nhsn/PDFs/pscManual/6pscVAPcurrent.pdf. Published January 2022. Accessed September 25, 2022.
70. Samanta S, Poddar B, Azim A, et al. Significance of mini bronchoalveolar lavage fluid amylase level in ventilator-associated pneumonia: a prospective observational study. *Crit Care Med.* 2018;46(1):71–78.
71. Vacheron CH, Lepape A, Savey A, et al. Increased incidence of ventilator-acquired pneumonia in coronavirus disease 2019 patients: a multicentric cohort study. *Crit Care Med.* 2022;50(3):449–458.
72. Wicky PH, d'Humieres C, Timsit JF. How common is ventilator-associated pneumonia after coronavirus disease 2019? *Current Opinion.* 2022;35(2):170–175.
73. Boyd S, Nseir S, Rodriguez A, et al. Ventilator-associated pneumonia in critically ill patients with covid-19 infection: a narrative review. *ERJ Open Res.* 2022;8. https://doi.org/10.1183/23120541.00046-2022. 00046-02022.
74. Zilberberg MD, Nathanson BH, Puzniak LA, et al. Descriptive epidemiology and outcomes of nonventilated hospital-acquired, and ventilator-associated bacterial pneumonia in the United States, 2012-2019. *Crit Care Med.* 2022;50(3):460–468.
75. Sukhen S, Poddar B, Azim A, et al. Significance of mini bronchoalveolar lavage fluid amylase level in ventilator-associated pneumonia: a prospective observational study. *Crit Care Med.* 2018;46(1):71–78.
76. Klompas M, Branson R, Cawcutt K, et al. Strategies to prevent ventilator-associated pneumonia, ventilator-associated events, and nonventilator hospital-acquired pneumonia in acute-care hospitals: 2022 Update. *Inf Control and Hosp Epidem.* 2022;43:687–713.
77. Sherburne LM, Poehler JL, Tietz JM. Reducing ventilator-associated events: a quality improvement project. *Crit Care Nurse.* 2022;42(2):63–70.
78. Kahn SR, deWit K. Pulmonary embolism. *N Engl J Med.* 2022;387:45–57. https://doi.org/10.1056/NEJMcp2116489. . Accessed February 21, 2023. Accessed.
79. Fernando SM, Tran A, Cheng W, et al. VTE prophylaxis in critically ill adults: a systematic review and network meta-analysis. *Chest.* 2022;161(2):418–428. https://doi.org/10.1016/j.chest.2021.08.050.
80. Schunemann HJ, Cushman M, Burnett AE, et al. American Society of Hematology 2018 guidelines for management of venous thromboembolism: prophylaxis for hospitalized and nonhospitalized medical patients. *Blood Adv.* 2018;2(22):3198–3225.
81. Arepally GM, Padmanabhan A. Heparin-induced thrombocytopenia: a focus on thrombosis. *Ateriosclerosis, Thrombosis, & Vascular Biol.* 2021;41:141–152.
82. Aggarwal V, Nicolais CD, Lee A, et al. *Acute Management of Pulmonary Embolism –American College of Cardiology*; 2017. Retrieved from: https://www.acc.org/latest-in. cardiology/articles/2017/10/23/12/12/acute-management-of-pulmonary-embolism.
83. Bikdeli B, Wang Y, Jimenez D, et al. Association of inferior vena cava filter use with mortalitiy rates in older adults with acute pulmonary embolism. *JAMA Intern Med.* 2019;179(2):263–265.
84. Scott JH, Gordon M, Vender R, et al. Venoarterial extracorporeal membrane oxygenation in massive pulmonary embolism-related cardiac arrest: a systematic review. *CCM Journal.* 2021;49(5):760–769.
85. Cystic Fibrosis Foundation. About Cystic Fibrosis. https://www.cff.org/intro-cf/about-cystic-fibrosis. Accessed September 25, 2022.
86. Cystic Fibrosis Foundation. 2020 Patient Registry: Annual Data Report. https://www.cff.org/Patient-Registry-Annual-Data-Report.pdf. Accessed September 25, 2022.
87. Castellani C, Duff AJA, Bell SC, et al. ECFS best practice guidelines: the 2018 revision. *J Cystic Fibro.* 2018;17:153–178.

16

Acute Kidney Injury

Roberta Kaplow, APRN-CCNS, PhD, AOCNS, CCRN, FAAN

INTRODUCTION

The roles of the kidney in maintaining homeostasis include removal of fluid and metabolic waste, maintenance of acid-base balance, regulation of blood pressure, and concentration of electrolytes (e.g., sodium, potassium, calcium, and phosphorus).[1,2] The kidneys receive 20% to 25% of cardiac output. This translates into 1000 to 1200 mL of blood per minute entering into the glomerulus, allowing for reabsorption and filtration and supporting fluid balance and elimination of wastes in urine.[3,4]

Acute kidney injury (AKI), formerly known as *acute renal failure,* is one of the most perilous problems in patients who are critically ill.[5] There are several definitions of AKI. One example is a precipitous increase in serum creatinine levels, a decrease in urinary output, or both,[6–8] although both of these indices are not specific for this syndrome.[6] Another definition includes a decrease in glomerular filtration rate (GFR), which results in a buildup of metabolic waste and incapacity to maintain fluid and electrolyte balance.[5] While a definitive definition of AKI remains to be validated,[6] the condition encompasses an individual's abrupt decrease in kidney function.

The incidence of AKI has increased in past decades[9,10] and ranges from 5% to 20%, with a reported prevalence of 50% or higher in the critical care unit setting.[6,11] The average mortality rate of AKI ranges from 5% to 10%.[9] However, critically ill patients who develop AKI are at higher risk for increased morbidity and mortality,[12,13] with reported mortality rates of 50% or higher.[9] In addition, AKI is associated with the development of cardiovascular events and chronic kidney disease.[14] Nurses play a pivotal role in promoting positive outcomes in patients with AKI. Recognition of high-risk patients, preventive measures, sharp assessment skills, and supportive nursing care are essential to ensure delivery of high-quality care to these challenging and complex patients. This chapter discusses the pathophysiology, assessment, and collaborative management of AKI.

REVIEW OF ANATOMY AND PHYSIOLOGY

The kidneys are a pair of highly vascularized, bean-shaped organs that are located retroperitoneal on each side of the vertebral column, adjacent to the first and second lumbar vertebrae. The right kidney sits slightly lower than the left kidney because the liver lies above it. An adrenal gland sits on top of each kidney and is responsible for the production of aldosterone, a hormone that influences sodium and water balance. Each kidney is divided into two regions: an outer region called the *cortex* and an inner region called the *medulla.*[15]

The *nephron* is the basic functional unit of the kidney. A nephron is composed of a renal corpuscle (glomerulus and Bowman's capsule) and a tubular structure, as depicted in Fig. 16.1. Approximately 1 million nephrons exist in each kidney, and approximately 85% of these nephrons are found in the cortex of the kidney and have short loops of Henle.[15] The remaining 15% of nephrons are called *juxtamedullary nephrons* because of their location just outside the medulla. Juxtamedullary nephrons have long loops of Henle and, along with the vasa recta (long capillary loops), are primarily responsible for concentration of urine. The number of functioning nephrons decreases with age, and after the age of 40 years, the number of functioning nephrons declines by 10% with each decade of life.[15] Nephrons cannot be regenerated, so injured nephrons will not be replaced.

Blood enters the kidneys through the renal artery, travels through a series of arterial branches, and reaches the glomerulus by way of the afferent arteriole (*afferent* meaning "to carry toward"). The glomerulus is a tuft of capillaries that filter blood

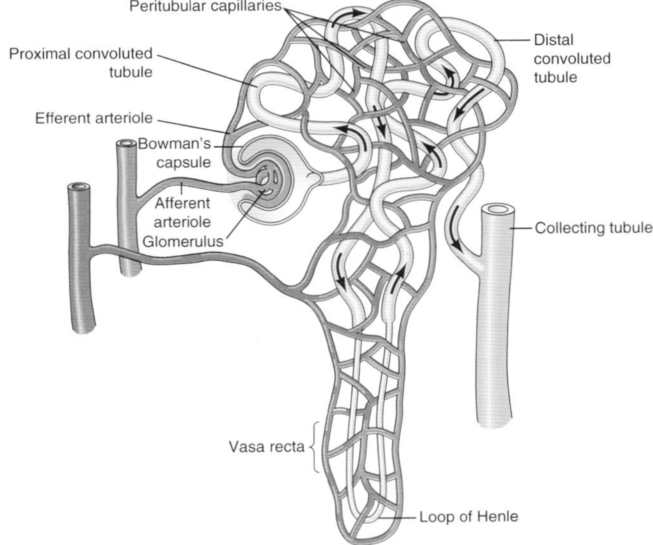

Fig. 16.1 Anatomy of the nephron, the functional unit of the kidney. (From Banasik J. Renal function. In: Banasik J, Copstead L, eds. *Pathophysiology.* 6th ed. Philadelphia, PA: Elsevier; 2019.)

by using the hydrostatic pressure created by the afferent and efferent arterioles. This hydrostatic pressure pushes filtrate into the tubular system. In the tubular region of the nephron, selective absorption and secretion occur. Blood leaves the glomerulus through the efferent arteriole (*efferent* meaning "to carry away from"), which divides into two extensive capillary networks called the *peritubular capillaries* and the *vasa recta*. These capillaries then rejoin to form venous branches by which blood eventually exits the kidney via the renal vein.[15]

The kidneys perform numerous functions that are essential for the maintenance of a stable internal environment. Box 16.1 lists functions of the kidney. The following section provides a brief overview of central roles the kidneys perform in maintaining homeostasis.

Regulation of Fluid and Electrolytes and Excretion of Waste Products

As blood flows through each glomerulus, water, electrolytes, and waste products are filtered out of the blood across the glomerular membrane and into Bowman's capsule, to form what is known as *filtrate*. The glomerular capillary membrane is approximately 100 times more permeable than other capillaries. It acts as a high-efficiency sieve and normally allows only substances below a certain molecular weight to cross. Normal glomerular filtrate is essentially protein-free and contains electrolytes and nitrogenous waste products, such as creatinine, urea, and uric acid, in amounts similar to those in plasma.[2] Red blood cells, albumin, and globulin are too large to pass through a healthy glomerular membrane.

Glomerular filtration occurs as the result of a pressure gradient, which is the difference between the forces that favor filtration and the pressures that oppose filtration. The capillary hydrostatic pressure favors glomerular filtration, whereas the colloid osmotic pressure and the hydrostatic pressure in Bowman's capsule oppose filtration. Under normal conditions, the capillary hydrostatic pressure is greater than the two opposing forces, and glomerular filtration occurs (Fig. 16.2). A mean arterial pressure of at least 60 mm Hg is necessary to maintain capillary hydrostatic pressure.[15] If capillary hydrostatic pressure decreases, glomerular filtration will decrease.

At a normal GFR of 80 to 125 mL/min, the kidneys produce 180 L/day of filtrate. As the filtrate passes through the various components of the nephron's tubules, 99% is reabsorbed into the peritubular capillaries or vasa recta. *Reabsorption* is the movement of substances from the filtrate back into the capillaries. A second process that occurs in the tubules is *secretion*, or the movement of substances from the peritubular capillaries into the tubular network. Various electrolytes are reabsorbed or secreted at numerous points along the tubules, thus helping to regulate the electrolyte composition of urine.

Aldosterone and antidiuretic hormone (ADH) are involved in water reabsorption in the distal convoluted tubule and collecting duct. Aldosterone also plays a role in sodium reabsorption and promotes the excretion of potassium. Eventually the remaining filtrate (1% of the original 180 L/day) is excreted as urine, for an average urine output of 1 to 2 L/day.

BOX 16.1 Functions of the Kidney

- Regulation
  - fluid volume
  - electrolyte balance
  - acid-based balance
  - blood pressure
  - erythropoiesis
- Metabolism of vitamin D
- Excretion of nitrogenous wastes

CHECK YOUR UNDERSTANDING

1. Which statement by a patient demonstrates understanding of monitoring GFR?
   A. "I have diabetes, so I should have a glomerular filtration rate test done."
   B. "Since I have high blood pressure, my kidneys are getting good blood supply. I don't need to test my glomerular filtration rate."
   C. "I already know I have early kidney disease. I don't need a glomerular filtration test to tell me something I already know."
   D. "Even though there is kidney disease in my family, I don't have symptoms, so I don't need to get a glomerular filtration test."

Regulation of Acid-Base Balance

The kidneys help maintain acid-base equilibrium in three ways: (1) reabsorbing filtered bicarbonate in the proximal and distal tubules, (2) producing new bicarbonate, and (3) excreting lesser amounts of hydrogen ions (acid) buffered by phosphates and ammonia.[2] The tubular cells can generate ammonia to help with excretion of hydrogen ions. This ability of the kidney to assist with ammonia production and excretion of hydrogen ions (in exchange for sodium) is the predominant adaptive response by the kidney during acidosis. When an alkalosis is present, increased amounts of bicarbonate are excreted in the urine and cause the serum pH to return toward normal.

Regulation of Blood Pressure

Specialized cells in the afferent and efferent arterioles and the distal tubule are collectively known as the *juxtaglomerular apparatus*. These cells are responsible for the production of a hormone called *renin*, which plays a role in blood pressure regulation. Renin

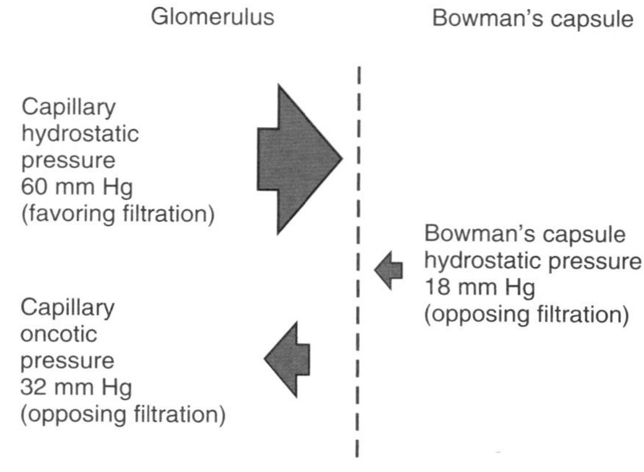

Fig. 16.2 Average pressures involved in filtration from the glomerular capillaries.

is released whenever blood flow through the afferent and efferent arterioles decreases. A decrease in sodium ion concentration of the blood flowing past these specialized cells (e.g., hypovolemia) also stimulates the release of renin. Renin activates the renin-angiotensin-aldosterone cascade (see Fig. 16.3), which ultimately results in the production of angiotensin II, which increases sodium and water reabsorption in the distal tubule and collecting ducts.[2] Angiotensin II also causes vasoconstriction and release of aldosterone from the adrenal glands, thereby raising blood pressure.

Regulation of Erythrocyte Production

Erythropoietin is secreted by the kidneys to stimulate production of red blood cells in the bone marrow. A reduction in production of erythropoietin causes a shortening of the life of red blood cells.[2] Severe anemia can develop in persons with advanced kidney disease as a consequence of reduced erythropoietin production.

Regulation of Vitamin D_3 Production

The kidneys produce the active form of vitamin D known as *calcitriol*. Calcitriol is important for calcium and phosphate regulation, influencing calcium deposition in the bone and reabsorption in the gastrointestinal (GI) tract.[2]

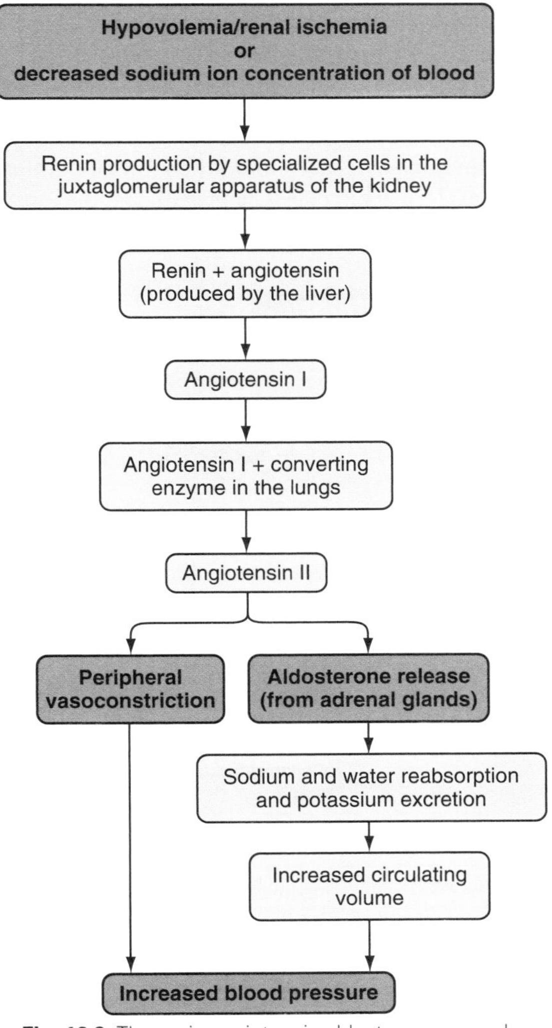

Fig. 16.3 The renin-angiotensin-aldosterone cascade.

CHECK YOUR UNDERSTANDING

2. Which arterial blood gas result should be anticipated in a patient with AKI?

	pH	$PaCO_2$	HCO_3
A.	7.32	48	24
B.	7.46	31	22
C.	7.32	40	18
D.	7.48	47	29

PATHOPHYSIOLOGY OF ACUTE KIDNEY INJURY

Definition

The Kidney Disease Improving Global Outcomes (KDIGO) is an international work group of the National Kidney Foundation. In 2012, the KDIGO *Clinical Practice Guidelines for Acute Kidney Injury* were published, focusing on the prevention, recognition, and management of AKI.[16] These guidelines define AKI as a sudden decline in kidney function that causes disturbances in fluid, electrolyte, and acid-base balances because of a loss in small solute clearance and decreased GFR.[16] The cardinal features of AKI are azotemia and oliguria. *Azotemia* refers to increases in blood urea nitrogen (BUN) and serum creatinine. *Oliguria* is defined as urine output of less than 0.5 mL/kg/h. These guidelines define three stages of AKI, which reflect changes in serum creatinine and urine output and provide a model for early recognition and stage-based management of AKI (Table 16.1).[2,5,14]

Risk Factors for Development of AKI

Long standing data suggests that seven conditions, if present, increase the risk of development of AKI. These conditions are age (over 65 years), infection on admission to the critical care unit, cardiovascular failure, cirrhosis, respiratory failure, chronic heart failure, and leukemia or lymphoma.[17] More recent data

TABLE 16.1 Kidney Disease Improving Global Outcomes (KDIGO) Criteria for the Diagnosis of Acute Kidney Injury

Stage	Serum Creatinine	Urine Output Criteria
1	1.5-1.9 times baseline OR ≥0.3 mg/dL (≥26.5 μmol/L) increase	<0.5 mL/kg/h for 6-12 h
2	2.0-2.9 times baseline	<0.5 mL/kg/h for ≥12 h
3	3.0 times baseline OR Increase in serum creatinine to ≥4.0 mg/dL (≥353.6 μmol/L) OR Initiation of renal replacement therapy OR In patients <18 yr, decrease in eGFR to <35 mL/min/1.73 m^2	<0.3 mL/kg/h for ≥24 h OR Anuria for ≥12 h

eGFR, Estimated glomerular filtration rate.
From Kidney Disease Improving Global Outcomes (KDIGO). Acute Kidney Injury Work Group: KDIGO clinical practice guidelines for acute kidney injury. *Kidney Int Suppl*. 2012;2(1):1-138.

corroborated these findings, and nonmodifiable and modifiable risk factors have been identified. Additional risk factors that are not modifiable include acquired immunodeficiency syndrome (AIDS), chronic kidney disease, diabetes mellitus, peripheral vascular disease, previous kidney surgery, and renal artery stenosis. Modifiable risk factors identified include anemia, hypertension, elevated cholesterol levels, low albumin levels, mechanical ventilation, administration of nephrotoxic drugs, rhabdomyolysis, and sepsis.[14] Most recently, chronic obstructive pulmonary disease was added as a risk factor.[18]

Patients who undergo cardiac surgery are at risk for the development of AKI, although the risk is lower than in the past.[6] Factors felt to be related to the development of postoperative AKI are low cardiac output, presence of preoperative risk factors (e.g., chronic kidney disease, diabetes mellitus), cardiopulmonary bypass–induced hypoperfusion and decreased oxygen delivery, levels of plasma free hemoglobin, transfusion of packed red blood cells, and systemic inflammation.[6,19]

CHECK YOUR UNDERSTANDING

3. Presence of which lab value should alert the nurse to the patient being at risk for the development of AKI?
   A. Hematocrit 38%
   B. Total cholesterol 185 mg/dL
   C. Serum albumin 3.8 g/dL
   D. HbA1c 7.4%

Etiology

The pathophysiology of AKI is divided into three categories—prerenal, intrarenal, and postrenal. A number of causes exist for each of these categories. The causes of AKI are categorized by *where* the precipitating factor exerts a pathophysiological effect on the formation of urine. The formation of urine proceeds in three steps: (1) delivery of blood for ultrafiltration (prerenal); (2) processing of ultrafiltrate by tubular secretion and reabsorption (intrarenal); and (3) excretion of kidney waste products through the ureters, bladder, and urethra (postrenal). Three mechanisms contribute to the development of AKI (Fig. 16.4): (1) alterations in renal blood flow (prerenal), (2) renal tubular injury (intrarenal), and (3) bilateral obstruction to urine flow (postrenal).[5,7,14]

Prerenal Causes of Acute Kidney Injury. Conditions that result in AKI by interfering with renal perfusion are classified as *prerenal.* A mean arterial pressure of at least 60 to 65 mm Hg is required to maintain glomerular filtration.[20] Most prerenal causes of AKI are related to conditions that reduce blood flow to the glomerulus, including severe burns, intravascular volume depletion from hemorrhage or hypovolemia, excessive gastrointestinal loss (e.g., from vomiting, diarrhea, or high ostomy output), decreased cardiac output (e.g., from cardiogenic shock, massive pulmonary embolism, or acute coronary syndrome), systemic vasodilation (e.g., from septic shock, anaphylaxis, hepatorenal syndrome, administration of anesthesia), renal vasoconstriction, or pharmacological agents (e.g., nonsteroidal antiinflammatory drugs [NSAIDs], iodinated contrast, calcineurin inhibitors) that impair autoregulation and GFR (Box 16.2).[14,20] For example, major abdominal surgery can cause hypoperfusion of the kidney because of blood loss during surgery or excessive vomiting or nasogastric suction during the postoperative period.

Abdominal compartment syndrome, an intraabdominal pressure of 20 mm Hg or greater (see Chapter 20, Trauma and Surgical Management), is another prerenal cause of AKI. Primary causes

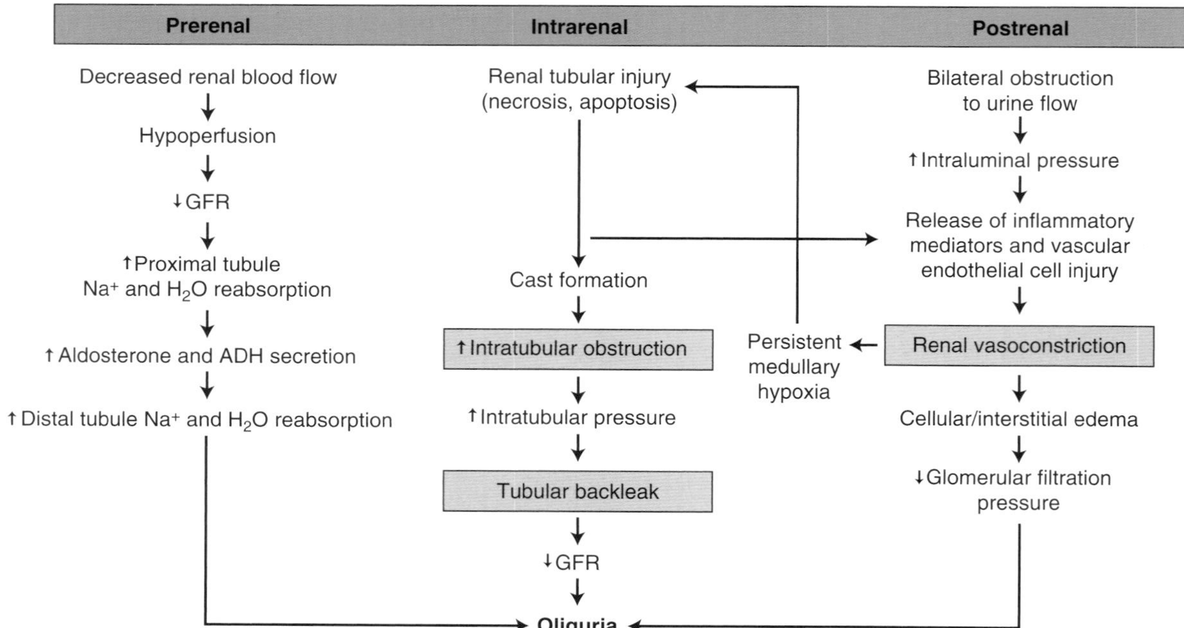

Fig. 16.4 Mechanisms that contribute to oliguria. *ADH,* Antidiuretic hormone; *GFR,* glomerular filtration rate. (From Rogers JL. *McCance & Huether's Pathophysiology: The Biologic Basis for Disease in Adults and Children.* 9th ed. St. Louis, MO: Elsevier; 2024:1256.)

of abdominal compartment syndrome include blunt or penetrating trauma to the abdomen, hemorrhage, and intestinal obstruction. Secondary causes of abdominal compartment syndrome include ileus, ascites, pregnancy, and volume replacement exceeding 3 L.[20] As abdominal pressure increases, there is compression on the renal vasculature, activation of the sympathetic and renin-angiotensin systems, and reduced cardiac output leading to reduced kidney perfusion and the development of AKI.

In prerenal AKI, the body attempts to normalize renal perfusion by reabsorbing sodium and water. If adequate blood flow is restored to the kidney, normal renal function resumes. Most forms of prerenal AKI can be reversed by treating the cause. However, if the prerenal situation is prolonged or severe, it can progress to intrarenal damage, acute tubular necrosis (ATN), or acute cortical necrosis.[21] Implementation of preventive measures, recognition of the condition, and prompt treatment of prerenal conditions are extremely important in preventing the progression to ATN.

BOX 16.2 Prerenal Causes of Acute Kidney Injury

Intravascular Volume Depletion
- Hemorrhage
- Trauma
- Surgery
- Intraabdominal compartment syndrome
- Gastrointestinal loss
- Renal loss
- Diuretics
- Osmotic diuresis
- Diabetes insipidus
- Volume shifts
- Vomiting
- Dehydration
- Heart failure
- Cirrhosis
- Burns

Vasodilation
- Sepsis
- Anaphylaxis
- Medications (e.g., antihypertensives, afterload-reducing agents)
- Anesthesia

Decreased Cardiac Output
- Heart failure
- Myocardial infarction
- Cardiogenic shock
- Dysrhythmias
- Pulmonary embolism
- Pulmonary hypertension
- Positive-pressure ventilation
- Pericardial tamponade

Medications That Impair Autoregulation and Glomerular Filtration
- Angiotensin-converting enzyme (ACE) inhibitors in renal artery stenosis
- Inhibition of prostaglandins by nonsteroidal antiinflammatory medication use during renal hypoperfusion
- Norepinephrine
- Ergotamine
- Hypercalcemia

Intrarenal Causes of Acute Kidney Injury. The causes of *intrarenal* AKI are classified based on the location of the kidney injury (i.e., the glomerulus, vasculature, interstitium, or tubule). The most common intrarenal condition is ATN.[22] This condition may occur after prolonged ischemia (prerenal), exposure to nephrotoxic substances, or a combination of these. Contrast media and heme pigment substances are also considered nephrotoxic.

Ischemic ATN usually occurs when perfusion to the kidney is considerably reduced. The renal ischemia overwhelms the normal autoregulatory defenses of the kidneys, thereby initiating cell injury that may lead to cell death. Some patients have ATN after only several minutes of hypotension or hypovolemia, whereas others can tolerate hours of renal ischemia without any apparent tubular damage.

Nephrotoxic medications (particularly aminoglycosides and radiographic contrast media) damage the tubular epithelium by direct drug toxicity, intrarenal vasoconstriction, and intratubular obstruction. AKI does not occur in all patients who receive nephrotoxic medications; however, predisposing factors such as advanced age, female sex, preexisting renal or hepatic disease, and shock enhance susceptibility to intrinsic damage.[22] Other intrarenal causes of AKI are listed in Box 16.3.

BOX 16.3 Intrarenal Causes of Acute Kidney Injury

Glomerular, Vascular, or Hematological Problems
- Glomerulonephritis (poststreptococcal)
- Vasculitis
- Malignant hypertension
- Systemic lupus erythematosus
- Hemolytic uremic syndrome
- Disseminated intravascular coagulation
- Scleroderma
- Bacterial endocarditis
- Hypertension of pregnancy
- Thrombosis of renal artery or vein

Tubular Problems (Acute Tubular Necrosis or Acute Interstitial Nephritis)
- Ischemia
- Hypotension from any cause
- Hypovolemia from any cause
- Obstetrical complications (hemorrhage, abruptio placentae, placenta previa)
- Medications (see Box 16.5)
- Radiocontrast media (large volume; multiple procedures)
- Transfusion reaction causing hemoglobinuria
- Tumor lysis syndrome
- Rhabdomyolysis
- Preexisting renal impairment
- Diabetes mellitus
- Hypertension
- Volume depletion
- Severe heart failure
- Advanced age
- Miscellaneous: heavy metals (mercury, arsenic), paraquat, snakebites, organic solvents (ethylene glycol, toluene, carbon tetrachloride), pesticides, fungicides

Multiple mechanisms are involved in the pathophysiology of ATN. Fig. 16.5 is a detailed diagram showing some of the mechanisms that play a role in the ATN cascade resulting in reduced GFR. Mechanisms include alterations in renal hemodynamics, tubular function, and tubular cellular metabolism. Decreases in cardiac output, intravascular volume, or renal blood flow activate the renin-angiotensin-aldosterone cascade. Angiotensin II causes further renal vasoconstriction and decreased glomerular capillary pressure, resulting in a decreased GFR. The decreased GFR and renal blood flow lead to tubular dysfunction. In addition, administration of medications that cause vasoconstriction of the renal vessels, including NSAIDs, angiotensin-converting enzyme (ACE) inhibitors, angiotensin II receptor blockers (ARBs), cyclosporine, and tacrolimus, can precipitate ATN.[22] The renal tubules in the medulla are very susceptible to ischemia. The medulla receives only 20% of the renal blood flow but is very sensitive to any reduction in blood flow. When the tubules are damaged, necrotic endothelial cells and other cellular debris accumulate and can obstruct the lumen of the tubule. This intratubular obstruction increases intratubular pressure, which decreases the GFR and leads to tubular dysfunction. In addition, tubular damage often produces alterations in the tubular structure that permit the glomerular filtrate to leak out of the tubular lumen and back into the plasma, resulting in oliguria.[21]

Ischemic episodes result in decreased energy supplies, including adenosine triphosphate (ATP). Oxygen deprivation results in a rapid breakdown of ATP. The proximal tubule is very dependent on ATP, which explains why it is the most commonly injured portion of the renal tubule. Without ATP, the sodium-potassium ATPase pump of the cell membrane is not able to effectively transport electrolytes across the membrane. This leads to increased intracellular calcium levels, free

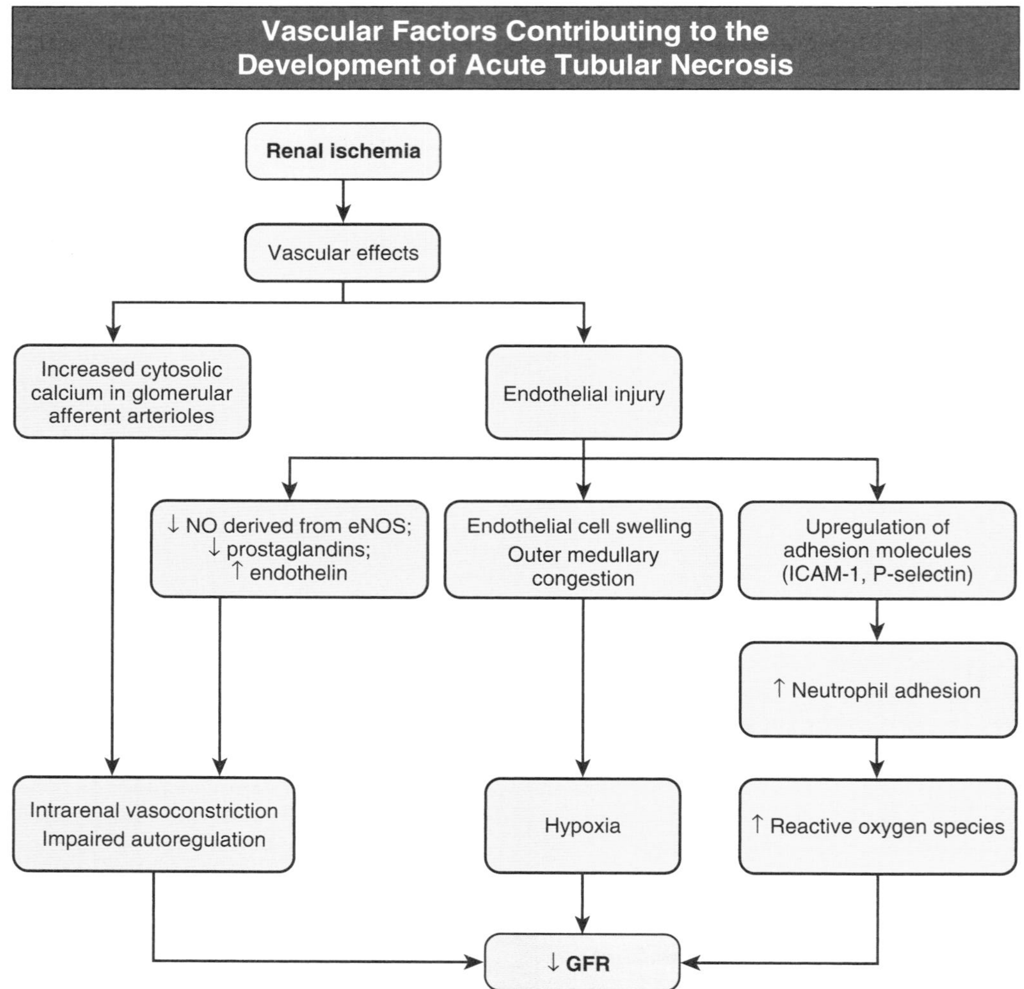

Fig. 16.5 Factors contributing to the development of acute tubular necrosis. Renal vasoconstriction and endothelial injury promote renal ischemia and tubular injury. *eNOS,* Endothelial nitric oxide synthase; *GFR,* glomerular filtration rate; *ICAM-1,* intercellular adhesion molecule 1; *NO,* nitric oxide. (From Haseley L, Jefferson JA. Pathophysiology and etiology of acute kidney injury. In: Feehally J, Floege J, Tonelli M, Johnson R, eds. *Comprehensive Clinical Nephrology.* 6th ed. St. Louis, MO: Elsevier; 2019.)

radical formation, and breakdown of cell structures. Cellular edema occurs, which further decreases renal blood flow, damages the tubules, and ultimately leads to tubular dysfunction and oliguria.[21]

Contrast-induced nephropathy. Contrast-induced nephropathy (CIN), which may also be called *contrast-associated AKI,* manifests with an increase in serum creatinine levels by 25% from baseline or 0.5 mg/dL increase that occurs within 48 to 72 hours following administration of intravenous contrast.[23] Although the administration of contrast media is generally considered safe for individuals with normal kidney function, CIN is the third-leading cause of AKI in the hospitalized patient.[24] Critically ill patients are at increased risk for CIN because of hemodynamic instability, volume depletion, multiple organ dysfunction, and the administration of nephrotoxic medications. While this condition is typically mild and reversible, it is possible for patients to develop irreversible kidney damage and require renal replacement therapy.[24]

Two pathological mechanisms contribute to the development of CIN. The first mechanism is the direct toxic effect of the contrast media on the cells lining the renal tubule. The second mechanism of injury is the result of reduced medullary blood flow.[21] Contrast agents are suspected to initiate vasodilation of renal blood vessels, followed by an intense and persistent vasoconstriction.[21] Oxygen delivery to the renal cells is reduced, precipitating cell injury. In addition, contrast agents stimulate the influx of extracellular calcium, which may lead to a loss of medullary autoregulation and may also have a direct toxic effect on the renal tubules.[11] Patients with chronic renal insufficiency are at the greatest risk for developing CIN. Other risk factors include diabetes mellitus, dehydration, advanced age (greater than 75 years), anemia, use of an intraaortic balloon pump, congestive heart failure, ongoing treatment with nephrotoxic medications, and vascular disease.[24] Many studies have been conducted to evaluate interventions to prevent CIN. Hydration is the intervention that has consistently demonstrated benefit in randomized controlled trials. Other preventive strategies include the use of sodium bicarbonate, *N*-acetylcysteine (NAC), statins, ascorbic acid, theophylline, aminophylline, vasodilators, forced diuresis, renal replacement therapy, and prostaglandin E1.[23] Meta-analysis data reveal that NAC at low doses with 0.9% normal saline and those receiving statins with NAC and 0.9% normal saline achieved some benefit in reducing CIN risk.[14,25] The KDIGO guidelines recommend intravascular volume expansion with 0.9% normal saline or bicarbonate solutions before administration of contrast.[16]

Heme pigment–induced kidney injury. Heme pigment–induced injury occurs in the renal tubules because of the degradation of myoglobin and hemoglobin. The heme pigment, which is a product of degradation, is toxic to the lining of the tubules. Under normal conditions, the kidney can handle the amount of heme pigment that is produced by the body. However, in situations where the heme pigment load is great, such as in rhabdomyolysis or hemolytic transfusion reaction, the risk of tubular injury is increased.

Rhabdomyolysis is a syndrome that occurs with the breakdown of skeletal muscle. Muscle injury can be related to trauma, burns, or compression. Involuntary muscle activity such as rigors, shivering, and seizure activity can produce skeletal muscle breakdown, precipitating rhabdomyolysis. Illicit use of serotonergic drugs such as cocaine and methamphetamines can trigger hypertonicity, seizure activity, and agitation, leading to muscle breakdown. Rhabdomyolysis may be seen with voluntary muscle activity such as running or physical training but is usually associated with concurrent dehydration. A markedly elevated serum creatine kinase level and the presence of tea-colored urine are findings suggestive of rhabdomyolysis.[26]

Postrenal Causes of Acute Kidney Injury. AKI resulting from obstruction of the flow of urine is classified as *postrenal* or obstructive renal injury. Obstruction can occur at any point along the urinary system (Box 16.4). With postrenal conditions, increased intratubular pressure results in a decrease in the GFR and abnormal nephron function. The presence of hydronephrosis on renal ultrasonography or a postvoid residual volume greater than 100 mL suggests postrenal obstruction. Causes of postrenal AKI are either renal or extrarenal in origin. Examples of extrarenal causes of AKI include prostate disease, malignancy of the pelvis, and retroperitoneal conditions. Intrarenal causes include ethylene glycol ingestion or tumor lysis syndrome, both of which cause crystal deposits.[5] The location of the obstruction in the urinary tract determines the method by which the obstruction is treated. Treatment may include bladder catheterization, ureteral stenting, or placement of nephrostomy tubes.

Infection-related acute kidney injury. Infections can cause an obstructive AKI due to formation of white blood cell casts or invasion of the organisms into the epithelia of renal tubules. Such microorganisms include cytomegalovirus, influenza, severe acute respiratory syndrome coronavirus-2 (SARS-CoV-2), and adenovirus.[27]

Course of Acute Kidney Injury

The patient with AKI progresses through three phases of the disease process: the initiation phase, the oliguric phase, and

BOX 16.4 Postrenal Causes of Acute Kidney Injury

- Benign prostatic hypertrophy
- Blood clots
- Renal stones or crystals
- Tumors
- Postoperative edema
- Medications
- Tricyclic antidepressants
- Ganglionic blocking agents
- Urinary catheter obstruction
- Ligation of ureter during surgery

the recovery-diuretic phase.[21] The majority of cases of AKI will resolve in 7 days.[6]

Initiation Phase. The initiation phase is the period that elapses from the occurrence of the precipitating event to the beginning of the change in urine output. In addition to a decrease in urine output, there is an increase in serum BUN and creatinine. This phase spans several hours to 2 days, during which time the normal renal processes begin to deteriorate, but kidney cell death has not yet occurred. The patient is unable to compensate for the diminished renal function and exhibits clinical signs and symptoms of AKI. Kidney injury is potentially reversible during the initiation phase.

Oliguric Phase. During the oliguric phase, intrinsic renal damage is established, and the GFR stabilizes at approximately 5 to 10 mL/min. Urine volume is usually at its lowest point during the oliguric phase; however, the patient may have urine output greater than 400 mL in 24 hours. This phase usually lasts 8 to 14 days but may last up to 11 months. The longer a patient remains in this stage, the slower the recovery and the greater the chance of permanent renal damage. Complications resulting from uremia, including hyperkalemia and infection, occur during this phase. Often, patients require some form of renal replacement therapy.

Recovery-Diuretic Phase. The recovery phase is the period during which the renal tissue recovers and repairs itself. A gradual increase in urine output and an improvement in laboratory values occur. Some patients experience diuresis during this phase. This diuresis reflects excretion of salt and water accumulated during the maintenance phase, the osmotic diuresis induced by filtered urea and other solutes, and the administration of diuretics to enhance salt and water elimination. However, with early and aggressive use of dialysis, many patients are maintained in a relative "dry" or volume-depleted state and do not have a large post-ATN diuresis. Recovery may take as long as 4 to 6 months.

LIFESPAN CONSIDERATIONS

Older Adults

- The most important renal physiological change that occurs with aging is a decrease in the glomerular filtration rate (GFR). Atherosclerosis and hypertension can impair autoregulation and limit the kidneys' capacity to maintain GFR. With advancing age, there is also a decrease in renal mass, the number of glomeruli, and peritubular density.[21,28] Serum creatinine levels may remain the same in the older adult patient even with a declining GFR because of decreased muscle mass, which leads to decreased creatinine production.
- The ability to concentrate and dilute urine is impaired because of an inability of the renal tubules to maintain the osmotic gradient in the medullary portion of the kidney. This tubular change affects the countercurrent mechanism and significantly alters sodium conservation, especially if a salt-restricted diet is being followed. There is a diminished ability to excrete medications, including radiocontrast dyes used in diagnostic testing and antibiotics, which necessitates a decrease in medication dosing to prevent nephrotoxicity.[28]
- Age-related changes in renin and aldosterone levels can lead to fluid and electrolyte abnormalities. Renin levels are decreased in older adults, resulting in less angiotensin II production and lower aldosterone levels.[28]
- Older adults are prone to development of volume depletion (prerenal conditions) because of a decreased ability to concentrate urine and conserve sodium. Volume status is difficult to assess because of altered skin turgor and decreased skin elasticity, decreased baroreceptor reflexes, and mouth dryness. Urinary indices are of limited value in assessment of older adults because of impaired ability to concentrate urine.
- Patients of advanced age tend to exhibit uremic symptoms at lower levels of serum blood urea nitrogen (BUN) and creatinine than do younger patients. The typical signs and symptoms of AKI may be attributed to other disorders associated with aging, delaying prompt diagnosis and treatment. Atypical signs and symptoms of uremia may be seen, such as an unexplained exacerbation of well-controlled heart failure, unexplained mental status changes, or personality changes.[21]

Morbid Obesity

- Morbid obesity is defined as a body mass index (BMI) greater than 40 kg/m^2.[29] The increase in body mass can result in functional and structural nephron changes, including glomerular hyperfiltration, glomerulomegaly, and glomerulosclerosis.[29]
- Detection of acute kidney injury (AKI) is complicated because weight-based formulas for creatinine clearance have not been validated for this population. Whereas the incidence of AKI among morbidly obese patients is unknown, the comorbidities associated with obesity include chronic kidney disease, diabetes mellitus, sleep-disordered breathing, heart failure, and hypertension.[30]
- In morbidly obese patients, medication dosing based on actual weight may result in nephrotoxicity. The use of adjusted body weight (ABW) is recommended for lipophilic nephrotoxic medications, including aminoglycosides.[31] Pharmacists use multiple adjusted and ideal weight formulas based on a medication's pharmacokinetics to calculate ideal dosages.

Pregnant People

- Although the incidence of pregnancy-related AKI is low, it is associated with maternal and fetal mortality. Data suggest that the incidence of pregnancy-related AKI is increasing.[32] Risk factors for the development of AKI include intravascular volume depletion related to nausea and vomiting and urinary tract infection. The kidneys enlarge and the urine collection system dilates to accommodate an increased vascular volume during pregnancy. These changes can lead to the development of hydronephrosis and increased risk for urinary tract infection.[32]
- Additional conditions associated with the development of pregnancy-related AKI include a type of severe preeclampsia known as the HELLP syndrome (*h*emolysis, *e*levated *l*iver enzymes, and *l*ow *p*latelets), as well as septic abortion and sepsis.[32]
- Early detection of pregnancy-related AKI can be challenging because the GFR increases by 50% during pregnancy. However, pregnant individuals may also have a decrease in GFR by 30% to 40% without an associated increase in serum creatinine. This normal renal response facilitates the elimination of metabolic wastes, including creatinine, and should be considered when laboratory parameters are used in the diagnosis of pregnancy-related AKI.[32]

ASSESSMENT

Patient History

It is important to obtain a thorough patient history. Kidney-related symptoms provide valuable clues to assist the clinician in focusing the assessment. For example, dysuria, increased frequency, incontinence, nocturia, pyuria, or hematuria can be indicative of urinary tract infection. The history provides clues about comorbidities that predispose the patient to AKI, including diabetes mellitus, hypertension, immunological diseases, and any hereditary disorders such as polycystic disease. Review the medical record to identify additional risk factors, such as recent transfusions, surgery, or radiographic procedures or exposure to potential nephrotoxic agents.

Risk factors for development of aminoglycoside nephrotoxicity include volume depletion, prolonged use of the drug (>10 days), hypokalemia, sepsis, preexisting renal disease, high trough concentrations, concurrent use of other nephrotoxic drugs, and older age[33] (see Lifespan Considerations box). Symptoms of AKI are usually seen about 1 to 2 weeks after exposure. In addition, a history of over-the-counter medication use, including NSAIDs, is important. Box 16.5 lists medications that are associated with AKI. Recreational drug use (e.g., cocaine, methamphetamines, "bath salts") has been associated with the development of rhabdomyolysis and subsequent AKI. Patients with kidney disease may not have any presenting signs or symptoms, including pain, aside from obstruction of the urinary tract. They may present with an illness risk factor, such as sepsis, that is associated with the development of AKI.[6]

BOX 16.5 Common Nephrotoxic Medications

- Aminoglycosides
- Amphotericin B
- Acyclovir
- Allopurinol
- Angiotensin-converting enzyme (ACE) inhibitors
- Angiotensin receptor blockers (ARBs)
- Adefovir
- Beta-lactam antibiotics
- Cephalosporins
- Cyclosporine
- Cisplatin
- Daptomycin
- Everolimus
- Fluorouracil (5-FU)
- Fluoroquinolones
- Famotidine
- Foscarnet
- Ifosfamide
- Interferon
- Indinavir
- Methotrexate
- Nonsteroidal antiinflammatory drugs (NSAIDs)
- Penicillin
- Pentamidine
- Proton pump inhibitors
- Rifampin
- Ritonavir
- Sulfa drugs
- Tacrolimus
- Temsirolimus
- Tenofovir
- Vancomycin
- Zoledronic acid

EVIDENCE-BASED PRACTICE

Prevention of Acute Kidney Injury (AKI) Following Cardiac Surgery

Problem

AKI is a recognized complication associated with cardiac surgery. It may be related to the use of cardiopulmonary bypass but may also be related to intraoperative and postoperative management.

Clinical Question

Does implementation of the Kidney Disease: Improving Global Outcomes (KDIGO) bundle, which includes optimizing hemodynamic and fluid status, hemodynamic monitoring, avoiding administration of nephrotoxic agents, and mitigating episodes of hyperglycemia in patients who are at high risk, mitigate the development of AKI following cardiac surgery?

Evidence

This multinational, randomized controlled trial evaluated adherence to the KDIGO bundle in 278 cardiac surgery patients to determine if adherence affected development of AKI. Patients in the intervention group received all bundle components as compared to the control group. While there were no statistically significant differences between the two groups, the incidence of moderate and severe AKI was significantly lower in the group that received all components of the bundle.

Implications for Nursing

For nurses caring for preoperative and postoperative cardiac surgery patients, adherence to all aspects of the KDIGO bundle (i.e., optimizing hemodynamic and fluid status, hemodynamic monitoring, avoiding administration of nephrotoxic agents, and mitigating episodes of hyperglycemia) can help mitigate the development of moderate and severe AKI.

Level of Evidence

B—Randomized Controlled Study

Reference

Zarbock A, Küllmar M, Ostermann M et al. Prevention of cardiac surgery-associated acute kidney injury by implementing the KDIGO guidelines in high-risk patients identified by biomarkers: the PrevAKI-multicenter randomized controlled trial. *Anesth Analg.* 2021;133(2):292-302.

Vital Signs

Changes in blood pressure are common in individuals with AKI. Patients with kidney injury from prerenal causes may become hypotensive and experience tachycardia because of volume deficits. ATN, particularly if associated with oliguria, often causes hypertension. Patients may hyperventilate as the lungs attempt to compensate for the metabolic acidosis often seen in AKI. Body temperature may be decreased because of the antipyretic effect of the uremic toxins, normal, or increased because of infection.

Physical Assessment

Assess the patient's general appearance for signs of *uremia* (retention of nitrogenous substances normally excreted by the kidneys), such as malaise, fatigue, disorientation, and drowsiness. Assess the skin for color, texture, bruising, petechiae, and edema. Assess the patient's hydration status. Evaluate current and admission body weight and intake and output information. Skin turgor, mucous membranes, breath sounds, presence of edema, neck vein distension, and vital signs (blood pressure and heart rate) are all key indicators of fluid balance. An oliguric patient with weight loss, tachycardia, hypotension, dry mucous membranes, flat neck veins, and poor skin turgor may be volume depleted (prerenal cause). Weight gain, edema, distended neck veins, and hypertension in the presence of oliguria suggest an intrarenal cause. Table 16.2 summarizes the systemic manifestations of AKI according to body system and lists the pathophysiological mechanisms involved.

Evaluation of Laboratory Values

Creatinine is a byproduct of muscle metabolism and is produced at a relatively constant rate. When kidney function is decreased, creatinine levels rise rapidly, indicating a decline in function or a decrease in the GFR. Serial changes in serum creatinine and urine output are markers for the identification of AKI. However, the value of serum creatinine in predicting kidney cell injury is limited because serum creatinine levels are influenced by muscle mass, age, sex, race, protein catabolic rate, hydration status, and medications.[14] A healthy patient may have up to a 50% decrease in GFR before there will be a noticeable change in serum creatinine. These levels may not change for several days after an insult (see Clinical Alert box).[27] Further, urine output is not a specific indicator of renal function. Patients with acute interstitial nephritis, for example, may have associated polyuria.[6]

! CLINICAL ALERT

Serum Creatinine

The same serum creatinine level can reflect very different glomerular filtration rates (GFRs) in patients because of differences in muscle mass. For example, a 25-year-old man weighing 220 lb (99.8 kg) with a serum creatinine level of 1.2 mg/dL has an estimated GFR of 133 mL/h (normal), whereas a 75-year-old female weighing 121 lb (54.9 kg) with the same serum creatinine level of 1.2 mg/dL has an estimated GFR of 35 mL/h (markedly decreased).

BUN is a blood test associated with kidney function but is not considered a reliable indicator of kidney function. Urea is a byproduct of protein metabolism. Extrarenal factors, including dehydration, a high-protein diet, starvation, and blood in the gastrointestinal tract, can elevate the BUN level. For example, with gastrointestinal bleeding, the blood in the gut breaks down, resulting in an increased protein load and an elevated BUN level.

The BUN-to-creatinine ratio can be useful in differentiating the type of AKI. The normal BUN-to-creatinine ratio ranges from 10:1 to 20:1 (e.g., BUN is 20 mg/dL and creatinine is 1.0 mg/dL). If the ratio is greater than 20:1 (e.g., BUN is 60 mg/dL and creatinine level is 1.0 mg/dL), problems other than kidney injury should be suspected. In prerenal conditions, an increased BUN-to-creatinine ratio is typically noted. There is a decrease in the GFR and a reduction in urine flow through the renal tubules. This allows more time for urea to be reabsorbed from the renal tubules back into the blood. Creatinine is not readily reabsorbed; therefore, the serum BUN level rises out of proportion to the serum creatinine level. A normal BUN-to-creatinine ratio is present in ATN, where there is actual injury to the renal tubules and a rapid decline in the GFR; urea and creatinine levels both rise proportionally from increased reabsorption and decreased clearance.[34]

Historically, the measurement of creatinine clearance over 24 hours has been considered a reliable estimate of GFR.[14] Timed urine collections are cumbersome, and they are susceptible to multiple errors in collection.[6] To measure creatinine clearance accurately, a precise collection procedure is required:

1. The bladder is emptied, the exact time is recorded, and the specimen is discarded.
2. All urine for the next 24 hours is saved in a container and stored in a refrigerator.
3. Exactly 24 hours after the start of the procedure, the patient voids again, and the specimen is saved.
4. The serum creatinine level is assessed at the end of 24 hours.
5. The 24-hour urine collection is sent to the laboratory for testing. (Urine can also be obtained from an indwelling urinary catheter.)

If a reliable 24-hour urine collection is not possible, an estimate of GFR can be made using a serum creatinine value in an evidence-based equation for GFR estimation. Three common equations are the Cockcroft-Gault, Modification of Diet in Renal Disease (MDRD), and Chronic Kidney Disease Epidemiology Collaboration (CKD-EPI) equations. Each of these equations uses serum creatinine values, but they apply different correction factors to address the effects of nutritional state, age, sex, and muscle mass on serum creatinine values.

Several urinary and serum proteins may be used for early detection of AKI.[6] Serum cystatin C is a protein marker of kidney function that is less influenced by muscle mass and diet.[6] It is filtered by the glomerulus and catabolized in the tubules. Serum levels can be used as an alternative measurement of GFR, and the presence of urinary cystatin C in the tubules is a marker for tubular injury.[6] Cystatin C levels are minimally affected by race and muscle mass.[4] Because of inconclusive trials comparing serum cystatin C with serum creatinine in the detection of AKI and differences among assays to measure cystatin C, serum creatinine measurement is recommended by the KDIGO guidelines to evaluate kidney function.[16]

Another laboratory test includes neutrophil gelatinase-associated lipocalin (NGAL, lipocalin-2), a small protein that can be measured in blood or urine samples. Levels rise within 2 hours of injury. NGAL has been studied as a biomarker for AKI in patients after cardiac surgery and in pediatric patients on mechanical ventilation. The NGAL level in urine is reportedly a good biomarker for AKI that has lasted more than 48

TABLE 16.2 Systemic Manifestations of Acute Kidney Injury

System	Manifestation	Pathophysiological Mechanism
Cardiovascular	Heart failure	Fluid overload and hypertension
	Pulmonary edema	↑ Pulmonary capillary permeability Fluid overload Left ventricular dysfunction
	Dysrhythmias	Electrolyte imbalances (especially hyperkalemia and hypocalcemia)
	Peripheral edema	Fluid overload Right ventricular dysfunction
	Hypertension	Fluid overload ↑ Sodium retention
Hematological	Anemia	↓ Erythropoietin secretion Loss of RBCs through gastrointestinal tract, mucous membranes, or dialysis ↓ RBC survival time Uremic toxin interference with folic acid secretion
Electrolyte imbalances	Alterations in coagulation	Platelet dysfunction
	Susceptibility to infection	↓ Neutrophil phagocytosis
	Metabolic acidosis	↓ Hydrogen ion excretion ↓ Bicarbonate ion reabsorption and generation ↓ Excretion of phosphate salts or titratable acids ↓ Ammonia synthesis and ammonium excretion
Respiratory	Pneumonia	Thick, tenacious sputum from ↓ oral intake Depressed cough reflex ↓ Pulmonary macrophage activity
	Pulmonary edema	Fluid overload Left ventricular dysfunction ↑ Pulmonary capillary permeability
Gastrointestinal	Anorexia, nausea, and vomiting	Uremic toxins Decomposition of urea, releasing ammonia that irritates mucosa
	Stomatitis and uremic halitosis	Uremic toxins Decomposition of urea, releasing ammonia that irritates oral mucosa
	Gastritis and bleeding	Uremic toxins Decomposition of urea, releasing ammonia that irritates mucosa, causing ulcerations and increased capillary fragility
Neuromuscular	Drowsiness, confusion, irritability, and coma	Uremic toxins produce encephalopathy Metabolic acidosis Electrolyte imbalances
	Tremors, twitching, and convulsions	Uremic toxins produce encephalopathy ↓ Nerve conduction from uremic toxins
Psychosocial	Decreased mentation, decreased concentration, and altered perceptions	Uremic toxins produce encephalopathy Electrolyte imbalances Metabolic acidosis Tendency to develop cerebral edema
Integumentary	Pallor	Anemia
	Yellowness	Retained urochrome pigment
	Dryness	↓ Secretions from oil and sweat glands
	Pruritus	Dry skin Calcium and/or phosphate deposits in skin Uremic toxins' effect on nerve endings
	Purpura	↑ Capillary fragility Platelet dysfunction
	Uremic frost (rarely seen)	Urea or urate crystal excretion
Endocrine	Glucose intolerance (usually not clinically significant)	Peripheral insensitivity to insulin Prolonged insulin half-life from ↓ renal metabolism
Skeletal	Hypocalcemia	Hyperphosphatemia from ↓ excretion of phosphates ↓ Gastrointestinal absorption of vitamin D Deposition of calcium phosphate crystals in soft tissues

RBCs, Red blood cells.

hours but is not a good biomarker to identify the severity of AKI if the patient's serum creatinine level has already risen. NGAL does have high sensitivity and specificity levels to predict AKI development.[11]

Interleukin-18 is a proinflammatory mediator. Urinary levels have been studied as a biomarker of AKI. Levels increase within 6 hours in adult and pediatric patients following cardiopulmonary bypass procedures. Early data suggest that interleukin-18 demonstrates ability to predict early AKI development in patients in the critical care unit.[11]

Tissue inhibitor of metalloproteinase-2 (TIMP-2) and insulin-like growth factor–binding protein 7 (IGFBP7) are cell cycle arrest markers. Their presence in urine is indicative of tubular injury.[11] Table 16.3 summarizes these tests.

The use of biomarkers for diagnosis of AKI has not yet translated into clinical practice and has been limited to the research setting. This is due to the lack of specificity to kidney disease. One biomarker, myo-inositol oxygenase, has shown early promise in identifying damage to the proximal tubule; further investigation is needed.[27]

Analyses of urinary sediment and electrolyte levels are helpful in distinguishing among the various causes of AKI. Inspect the urine for the presence of cells, casts, and crystals. In prerenal conditions, the urine typically has no cells but may contain hyaline casts. Casts are cylindrical bodies that form when proteins precipitate in the distal tubules and collecting ducts. Red blood cell casts indicate bleeding into the tubules or red blood cells passing through the glomerulus. White blood cell casts indicate an inflammatory process. Coarse, muddy-brown, granular casts are classic findings in ATN. Postrenal conditions may manifest with stones, crystals, sediment, bacteria, or clots from obstruction.

Urine electrolyte levels help discriminate between prerenal causes and ATN. Obtain urine samples (often called *spot urine levels*) for electrolyte determinations before diuretics are administered because these medications alter the urine results for up to 24 hours. Urinary sodium concentrations of less than 10 mEq/L are seen in prerenal conditions because the kidneys attempt to conserve sodium and water to compensate for the hypoperfusion state. Urine sodium concentrations are greater than 40 mEq/L in ATN because of impaired reabsorption in the diseased tubules. Urine electrolytes (i.e., the fractional excretion of sodium or urea) can be used to diagnose prerenal azotemia. There are online tools available to assist the clinician in calculating these data, including https://www.mdcalc.com/calc/62/fractional-excretion-urea-feurea.[14] The fractional excretion of sodium (FE_{Na}) is a useful test for assessing how well the kidney can concentrate urine and conserve sodium. In prerenal conditions, the FE_{Na} is less than 1%, whereas ATN presents with an FE_{Na} greater than 1%.[14]

Urine specific gravity and osmolality have a limited role in the diagnosis of AKI, especially in older adults, because the body's ability to concentrate urine decreases with age.[35] In general, prerenal conditions cause concentrated urine (high specific gravity and osmolality), whereas intrinsic azotemia causes dilute urine (low specific gravity and osmolality). The volume of urine output is also not a good indicator of renal function. Although patients with nonoliguric AKI excrete large volumes of fluid with little solute, they still have renal

TABLE 16.3 Acute Kidney Injury: Selected Laboratory Findings

Laboratory Test	Normal Range	Critical Value[a]	Significance
Creatinine	Male: 0.6-1.2 mg/dL Female: 0.5-1.1 mg/dL	>4 mg/dL	Released by muscle Eliminated by glomerular filtration and is therefore considered a GFR marker
Creatinine clearance	Male: 107-139 mL/min Female: 87-107 mL/min Values decrease 6.5 mL/min with each decade of life past 40 years of age	A decrease in creatinine clearance after correction for age represents decline in kidney function	Measure of GFR
Blood urea nitrogen (BUN)	10-20 mg/dL	>100 mg/dL	Urea is product of protein metabolism Elevation can indicate renal impairment
Serum cystatin C	Investigational use only	Investigational use only	GFR marker
Urine cystatin C	Not present	Indicative of tubule injury	Tubular injury marker
Neutrophil gelatinase-associated lipocalin (NGAL, lipocalin-2)	No rise in NGAL from baseline; results vary according to testing methods	Rise from baseline indicative of renal tubular injury	Tubular injury marker
Tissue inhibitor of metalloproteinase-2 (TIMP-2)	Not present in urine	Presence in urine	Cell cycle arrest marker Appears in urine after kidney injury
Insulin-like growth factor–binding protein 7 (IGFBP7)	Not present in urine	Presence in urine	Cell cycle arrest marker Appears in urine after kidney injury

[a]Critical value may vary depending on the laboratory performing the test.
GFR, Glomerular filtration rate.
Data from Chen LX, Koyner JL. Biomarkers in acute kidney injury. *Crit Care Clin.* 2015;31(4):633-647; Pagana K. Pagana T. *Mosby's Diagnostic & Laboratory Test Reference.* 16th ed. St. Louis: Elsevier; 2023.

dysfunction and azotemia. Table 16.4 summarizes laboratory data that are useful in differentiating among the three categories of AKI.

CHECK YOUR UNDERSTANDING

4. Which finding should indicate the presence of AKI to the nurse?
   A. Specific gravity of urine 1.025
   B. BUN 24 mg/dL
   C. Serum creatinine 1.1 mg/dL
   D. Creatinine clearance 25 mL/min

DIAGNOSTIC PROCEDURES

Various diagnostic procedures are used to evaluate renal function. Noninvasive procedures are usually performed before any invasive procedures are conducted. Noninvasive diagnostic procedures that assess the renal system include radiography of the kidneys, ureters, and bladder (KUB); renal ultrasonography; and magnetic resonance imaging (MRI). KUB radiography delineates the size, shape, and position of the kidneys. It may also detect abnormalities such as calculi, hydronephrosis (dilation of the renal pelvis), cysts, or tumors. Renal ultrasonography is helpful in evaluating for obstruction, which is manifested by hydronephrosis or hydroureter (dilation of the ureters). Ultrasound studies can also document the size of the kidneys, which may be helpful in differentiating acute and chronic renal conditions. The kidneys are often small in chronic kidney disease. Real-time ultrasound is used during renal biopsy and during placement of percutaneous nephrostomy tubes (which are often placed for hydronephrosis). MRI provides anatomical information about renal structures. Invasive diagnostic procedures for assessing the renal system include renal angiography and renal biopsy. Diagnostic procedures are summarized in Table 16.5.

As with all diagnostic procedures, instruct the patient, assist with the procedure, and monitor the patient after the procedure. When evaluation for AKI is performed, it is important to assess for allergies to contrast media and to provide appropriate fluids to the patient to maintain hydration before and after the procedure. Urinary output is closely monitored after the procedure.

CRITICAL JUDGMENT ACTIVITY

Determine two strategies that the critical care nurse can implement independently to help prevent acute kidney injury (AKI).

PATIENT PROBLEMS AND NURSING INTERVENTIONS

Patient Problems

Nursing care of the patient with AKI is complex. The Plan of Care for the Patient With Acute Kidney Injury addresses patient problems, nursing interventions, and expected outcomes. See also the Collaborative Plan of Care for the Critically Ill Patient in Chapter 1, Overview of Critical Care Nursing.

TABLE 16.4 Urine Findings Useful in Differentiating Causes of Acute Kidney Injury

Type of Injury	Specific Gravity	Urine Osmolality	Urine Sodium	Microscopic Examination	BUN/CR Ratio	FENa
Prerenal	>1.020	>500 mOsm/L	<10 mEq/L	Few hyaline casts possible	Elevated	<1%
Intrarenal	1.010	<350 mOsm/L	>20 mEq/L	Epithelial casts, red blood cell casts, pigmented granular casts	Normal	>1%
Postrenal	Normal to 1.010	Variable	Normal to 40 mEq/L	May have stones, crystals, sediment, clots, or bacteria	Normal	>1%

BUN, Blood urea nitrogen; *CR,* creatinine; *FENa,* fractional excretion of sodium.

TABLE 16.5 Diagnostic Procedures for Assessing the Renal System

Procedure	Purpose	Potential Problems
Renal ultrasonography	To obtain information on size, shape, and position of the kidneys	Minimal risk, noninvasive without contrast media
Computed tomography	To visualize the renal parenchyma to obtain data on the size, shape, and presence of lesions, cysts, masses, calculi, obstructions, congenital anomalies, and abnormal accumulation of fluid	Hypersensitivity reaction to contrast media (if used)
Renal angiography	To visualize the arterial tree, capillaries, and venous drainage of the kidneys to obtain data on the presence of tumors, cysts, stenosis infarction, aneurysms, hematomas, lacerations, and abscesses	Hypersensitivity reaction to contrast media Hemorrhage or hematoma at the catheter insertion site Acute kidney injury
Magnetic resonance imaging (MRI)	To visualize renal anatomy	Minimal risk, noninvasive, without contrast media
Renal biopsy	To obtain data for making a histological diagnosis to determine the extent of pathology, appropriate therapy, and possible prognosis	Hemorrhage Postbiopsy hematoma

PLAN OF CARE

For the Patient With Acute Kidney Injury

Patient Problem

Potential for Fluid, Electrolyte, and Acid Imbalance. A risk factor is the kidney's inability to maintain biochemical homeostasis.

Desired Outcomes

- Body weight within patient's normal range.
- Breath sounds clear.
- Hemodynamic parameters within normal limits.
- Electrolytes within normal limits.
- Absence of peripheral edema.

Nursing Assessments/Interventions	Rationales
• Weigh patient daily and report weight gain of 0.5-1.0 kg in 24 h.	• Weight change from the previous 24 h is a sensitive indicator of fluid loss or gain.
• Measure intake and output hourly during critical phase. Report new onset of urine output less than 0.5 mL/kg/h.	• Provide early indication of fluid imbalances.
• Monitor respiratory status for development of adventitious breath sounds, tachypnea, and increased work of breathing.	• The lungs are one of the first organs to be affected by fluid overload; increased work of breathing and tachypnea are early signs of fluid overload.
• Assess hemodynamic response to fluid management interventions.	• Guide fluid management strategies for AKI. • Postural hypotension, tachycardia, and hypotension indicate low preload, whereas jugular vein distension, elevated central venous pressures, and hypertension indicate volume overload.
• Monitor cardiac rhythm.	• Altered levels of potassium, sodium, calcium, and magnesium occur in AKI and are associated with cardiac rhythm disturbances.
• Monitor electrolyte values, especially potassium level.	• Hyperkalemia can cause life-threatening cardiac rhythm disturbances; elevated T waves and widening QRS complexes indicate elevated potassium levels.
• Assess patient for signs and symptoms of uremia: confusion and increased bleeding.	• Assess indicators of uremia.
• Institute safety measures.	• Prevent infection, falls, and pressure ulcers associated with elevated levels of uremic waste.

AKI, Acute kidney injury.
Adapted from Snyder J, Sump C. *Swearingen's All-in-One Nursing Care Planning Resource*. 6th ed. St. Louis: Elsevier; 2024.

Nursing Interventions

Accurate measurement of intake and output and daily weights are two vital nursing interventions. A urine meter or other type of accurate measuring device is essential for recording urinary output. Normal urine output is 0.5 to 1 mL/kg/h. Oral fluid intake must also be carefully monitored. Fluid intake levels are often restricted to the amount of urine output in a 24-hour period plus insensible loss (approximately 600 to 1000 mL/day). Administer IV fluids as prescribed before procedures in which radiocontrast media will be used.

Assessment of daily weights is one of the most useful noninvasive diagnostic tools. The daily weight is used to validate intake and output measurements. A 1-kg gain in body weight is equal to a 1000-mL fluid gain. Record the weight at the same time each day and with the same scale. Many critical care beds have built-in scales, which simplify the procedure. When the patient is weighed, ensure that the scale is properly calibrated and that the same number of bed linens and pillows are weighed with the patient each time. Recognize signs and symptoms of fluid volume overload, which can lead to pulmonary edema and severe respiratory distress (see Clinical Alert box).

CLINICAL ALERT

Fluid Volume Overload

Signs and symptoms of fluid volume overload include hypertension, edema, crackles, dyspnea, neck vein distension, weight gain, decreased urine output, decreased hematocrit, presence of an S_3 heart sound, and fatigue.

Infection is the most common and serious complication of AKI.[36] Nurses play a key role in preventing infections. Indwelling urinary catheters are not routinely inserted because they increase the risk of infection, and many patients remain oliguric for 8 to 14 days. Strict aseptic technique with all IV lines (central and peripheral), including temporary access devices used for dialysis, is also of extreme importance, both at the time of insertion and during daily maintenance.

Another key role of the nurse in preventing AKI is monitoring *trough* blood medication levels. Nurses are responsible for obtaining the trough blood levels at the appropriate times to ensure accurate results. Medication dosage adjustments must be made to prevent accumulation of the medication and toxic side effects. For example, aminoglycoside doses are based on medication levels and the patient's estimated creatinine clearance. A *trough blood level* is drawn just before the next dose is given and is an indicator of how well the body has cleared the medication.

CRITICAL JUDGMENT ACTIVITY

Which cues should be assessed in the care of older adult patients that increase their susceptibility to the development of acute kidney injury (AKI)?

MEDICAL MANAGEMENT OF ACUTE KIDNEY INJURY

Once AKI has developed, management is primarily supportive in nature.[14] The interventions should remain the same as those that were used to prevent its development. In addition, prevention of complications (e.g., hyperkalemia, metabolic acidosis, anemia) and fostering recovery of the kidney are paramount.[14] Management may include providing nutritional supplementation and initiating renal replacement therapy.[6] Medications may need to be discontinued or dosages adjusted. Specifically, analgesics, antivirals, antifungals, antimicrobials, diabetic agents, allopurinol, baclofen, colchicine, digoxin, lithium, low-molecular-weight heparin, and novel anticoagulants will need to be evaluated.[14] The use of a balanced crystalloid solution is recommended for patients who require fluid resuscitation, as opposed to a colloid or 0.9% normal saline.[14]

Prerenal Causes

AKI from prerenal conditions is usually reversible if renal perfusion is quickly restored; therefore early recognition and prompt treatment are essential. Prompt replacement of extracellular fluids and aggressive treatment of shock may help prevent AKI. Hypovolemia is treated in numerous ways, depending on the cause. Blood loss may necessitate blood transfusions, whereas patients with pancreatitis or peritonitis are usually treated with balanced crystalloid solution. Patients with cardiac instability usually require positive inotropic medications, antidysrhythmic medications, preload- or afterload-reducing medications, or a mechanical cardiac assist device. Hypovolemia from intense vasodilation may require vasoconstrictor medications, fluid replacement, and antibiotics (if the patient has sepsis) until the underlying problem has been resolved. Invasive or noninvasive hemodynamic monitoring may be considered in the management of fluid balance (see Chapter 9, Hemodynamic Monitoring).

Intrarenal Causes: Acute Tubular Necrosis

Common interventions for the patient with ATN include medication therapy, dietary management such as protein and electrolyte restrictions, management of fluid and electrolyte imbalances, and renal replacement therapies such as intermittent hemodialysis or continuous renal replacement therapy (CRRT). Considering the detrimental effect of AKI, the focus is on prevention. The most important preventive strategies are identification of patients at risk and elimination of potential contributing factors. Aggressive treatment must begin at the earliest sign of renal dysfunction.

Postrenal Causes

Postrenal obstruction should be suspected whenever a patient has an unexpected decrease in urine volume. Postrenal conditions are usually resolved with the insertion of an indwelling bladder catheter, either transurethral or suprapubic. Occasionally, a ureteral stent may be placed if the obstruction is caused by calculi or carcinoma.

In general, maintenance of cardiovascular function and adequate intravascular volume are the two key goals in the prevention of AKI. Box 16.6 summarizes important measures for preventing AKI.

Pharmacological Management Considerations

Fluid imbalances, retention of toxins, electrolyte disturbances, and metabolic acidosis are the physiological consequences of AKI. Management of AKI includes careful selection of medications to treat the physiological consequences of AKI and protect the kidney from additional injury. Medication therapy for the patient with AKI poses a challenge because most medications or their metabolites are eliminated from the body by the kidneys. Medication dose adjustments are often necessary to prevent toxic levels and adverse reactions. Assessment of renal function by creatinine clearance is often used to assist with medication dosing. The pharmacokinetic characteristics of the medication to be given, the route of elimination, and the extent of protein binding are also considered. Clinical pharmacists assist in determining optimal medication dosages for critically ill patients.

Many medications are removed by dialysis, and extra medication doses are often required to avoid suboptimal medication

BOX 16.6 Measures to Prevent Acute Kidney Injury

Avoid Nephrotoxins
- Use iso-osmolar radiocontrast media.
- Limit contrast volume to less than 100 mL.
- Use antibiotics cautiously with appropriate dose modification.
- Monitor medication levels (e.g., aminoglycosides).
- Stop certain medications (e.g., NSAIDs, ACE inhibitors, ARBs) before high-risk procedures.

Optimize Volume Status Before Surgery or Invasive Procedures
- Aim for urinary output greater than 40 mL/h.
- Keep mean arterial pressure greater than 70 mm Hg.
- Hydrate with 0.9% normal saline before and after procedures requiring radiocontrast media.
- Hold diuretics on the day before and the day of procedures.

Reduce Incidence of Nosocomial Infections
- Use indwelling urinary catheters judiciously.
- Remove indwelling urinary catheters when no longer needed.
- Use strict aseptic technique with all IV lines.

Implement Tight Glycemic Control in the Critically Ill

Aggressively Investigate and Treat Sepsis

ACE, Angiotensin-converting enzyme; *ARBs,* angiotensin receptor blockers; *NSAIDs,* nonsteroidal antiinflammatory drugs.

levels. Medications that are primarily water soluble, such as vitamins and phenobarbital, should be administered after dialysis. Medications that become bound to proteins or lipids or are metabolized by the liver are not removed by dialysis and can be administered at any time.

Diuretics. Diuretics are prescribed to increase urine output, thereby increasing the elimination of fluid and urinary solutes. The mechanism of action for most diuretics is to decrease the reabsorption of sodium in the renal tubules. Water remains with sodium in the tubules and is eliminated as urine. Other solutes, including potassium, chloride, calcium, and magnesium, are also influenced by sodium reabsorption rates. Urinary excretion of these electrolytes is typically increased with the administration of diuretics. Table 16.6 lists diuretic classes and mechanisms of action.

IV Fluid Replacement. Fluid volume replacement is indicated for the management of sepsis and other prerenal causes of AKI, usually with a balanced solution. Balanced solutions have an ion concentration like that of plasma, which is important because low-ion-balance solutions may affect acid-base balance as hydrogen and chloride ions shift. The ability to correct ion balance is impaired in AKI. Hyperchloremic acidosis can result because of chloride ion excess when 0.9% normal saline is used.

Dietary Management

Dietary management in patients with AKI is important. Energy expenditure in catabolic patients with AKI is much higher than normal. Dialysis also contributes to protein catabolism. The loss of amino acids and water-soluble vitamins in the dialysate solution used during dialysis constitutes another drain on the patient's nutritional stores. The overall goal of dietary management for AKI is provision of adequate energy, protein, and micronutrients such as multivitamins, folic acid, and iron supplements to maintain homeostasis in patients who may be extremely catabolic. If the patient is unable to ingest or tolerate an adequate oral nutritional intake, enteral feedings or total parenteral nutrition is prescribed. Nutritional support must supply the patient with sufficient nonprotein glucose calories, essential amino acids, fluids, electrolytes, and essential vitamins. Adequate nutrition not only prevents further catabolism, negative nitrogen balance, muscle wasting, and other uremic complications but also enhances the patient's tubular regenerating capacity, resistance to infection, and ability to combat other multisystem dysfunctions (see Chapter 7, Nutritional Therapy). The provider may also prescribe early renal replacement therapy to treat the increased fluid volume from enteral or total parenteral nutrition.

Management of Fluid, Electrolyte, and Acid-Base Imbalances

Fluid Imbalance. Volume overload is managed by dietary restriction of salt and water and administration of diuretics. In addition, dialysis or other renal replacement therapies may be indicated for fluid control.

Electrolyte Imbalance. Common electrolyte imbalances in AKI are listed in the Laboratory Alert box. Hyperkalemia is common in AKI, especially if the patient is hypercatabolic. Hyperkalemia occurs when potassium excretion is reduced because of the decrease in GFR. Sudden changes in the serum potassium level can cause dysrhythmias, which may be fatal. Fig. 16.6 shows the electrocardiographic changes commonly seen in hyperkalemia.

Three approaches are used to treat hyperkalemia: (1) reduce the body potassium content, (2) shift the potassium from outside the cell to inside the cell, and (3) antagonize the membrane effect of the hyperkalemia. Only dialysis and administration of cation exchange resins (sodium polystyrene sulfonate [Kayexalate]) reduce plasma potassium levels and total body potassium content in patients with renal dysfunction. In the past, sorbitol was combined with sodium polystyrene sulfonate powder for administration; however, because their concomitant use has been implicated in cases of colonic intestinal necrosis, this combination is not recommended.[37] Other treatments only "protect" the patient for a brief time until dialysis or cation exchange resins can be instituted. Table 16.7 summarizes medications used in the treatment of hyperkalemia.

Hyponatremia generally results from water overload. However, as nephrons are progressively damaged, the ability to conserve sodium is lost, and major salt-wasting states can develop, causing hyponatremia. Hyponatremia is treated with fluid restriction, specifically restriction of free water intake. Alterations in serum calcium and phosphorus levels occur frequently in AKI because of abnormalities in excretion, absorption, and metabolism of the electrolytes. Mild degrees of hypermagnesemia are common in AKI secondary to decreased renal excretion.

TABLE 16.6 Diuretic Class and Mechanism of Action

Diuretic Class	Mechanism of Action
Loop diuretics (furosemide, bumetanide)	Inhibit sodium, potassium, and chloride ion transport across the tubule membrane
Thiazide diuretics (hydrochlorothiazide, chlorthalidone)	Inhibit sodium and chloride transport across the tubule membrane
Carbonic anhydrase inhibitors (acetazolamide)	Inhibit hydrogen ion secretion and bicarbonate reabsorption, which reduces sodium reabsorption in the proximal tubules
Aldosterone antagonists (spironolactone)	Inhibit action of aldosterone in the tubules, decrease sodium reabsorption, and decrease potassium secretion in the collecting tubules
Sodium channel blockers (triamterene, amiloride)	Block entry of sodium ion into sodium channel, decrease sodium ion reabsorption, and decrease potassium secretion in the collecting tubules

! LABORATORY ALERT

Acute Kidney Injury

Laboratory Test	Normal Range	Critical Value[a]	Significance
Potassium (K^+)	3.5-5 mEq/L	>6.5 mEq/L	**Hyperkalemia:** potential for heart blocks, asystole, ventricular fibrillation; may cause muscle weakness, diarrhea, and abdominal cramps
Sodium (Na^+)	136-145 mEq/L	<120 mEq/L	**Hyponatremia**: potential for lethargy, confusion, coma, or seizures; may cause nausea, vomiting, and headaches
Total calcium (Ca^{++})	9.0-10.5 mg/dL	<6.0 mg/dL	**Hypocalcemia:** potential for seizures, muscle cramps, laryngospasm, stridor, tetany, heart blocks, and cardiac arrest; may see positive Chvostek's or Trousseau's sign
Magnesium (Mg^{++})	1.3-2.1 mEq/L	>3.0 mEq/L	**Hypermagnesemia:** potential for bradycardia and heart blocks, lethargy, coma, hypotension, hypoventilation, weak-to-absent deep tendon reflexes, nausea, and vomiting

[a]Critical values may vary by facility and laboratory.
Data from Pagana K, Pagana T. *Mosby's Diagnostic & Laboratory Test Reference*. 16th ed. St. Louis: Elsevier; 2023.

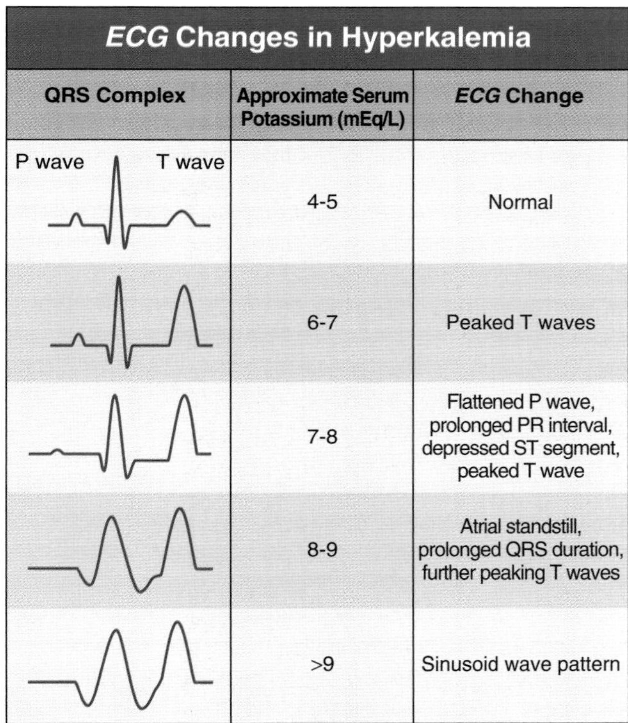

Fig. 16.6 Electrocardiographic *(ECG)* changes seen in hyperkalemia. (From Weiner D, Linas S, Wingo C. Disorders of potassium metabolism. In: Feehally J, Floege J, Tonelli M, Johnson R, eds. *Comprehensive Clinical Nephrology*. 6th ed. St. Louis, MO: Elsevier; 2019.)

CHECK YOUR UNDERSTANDING

5. Upon admission to the critical care unit, the patient's serum potassium is 8.1 mEq/L. Tall peaked T waves, prolonged QRS duration, and bradycardia are noted. Which *initial* pharmacological intervention is *most appropriate* for this situation?
   A. Regular insulin 10 units administered with 50 mL dextrose 50% IV
   B. Kayexalate enema
   C. Calcium chloride 5 to 10 mL of a 10% solution administered by IV injection
   D. Albuterol 10 to 20 mg administered by nebulizer over 20 minutes

Acid-Base Imbalance. Metabolic acidosis is the primary acid-base imbalance seen in AKI. Box 16.7 summarizes the etiology and signs and symptoms of metabolic acidosis in AKI. Treatment of metabolic acidosis depends on its severity. In mild metabolic acidosis, the lungs compensate by excreting carbon dioxide. Patients with a serum bicarbonate level of less than 15 mEq/L and a pH of less than 7.20 are usually treated with continuous infusion of sodium bicarbonate. The goal of treatment is to raise the pH to a value greater than 7.20. Rapid correction of the acidosis should be avoided, however, because tetany may occur due to hypocalcemia. The pH determines how much ionized calcium is present in the serum; the more acidic the serum, the more ionized calcium is present. If the metabolic acidosis is rapidly corrected, the serum ionized calcium level decreases as the calcium binds with albumin and other substances such as phosphate and sulfate. For this reason, IV calcium gluconate may be prescribed. Renal replacement therapies also may correct metabolic acidosis because they remove excess hydrogen ions, and bicarbonate is added to the dialysate and replacement solutions.

Renal Replacement Therapy

Renal replacement therapy (RRT) is the primary treatment for the patient with AKI. The incidence of RRT has increased because of the severity of illness and presence of either sepsis, decompensated heart failure, hepatic failure, cardiac surgery, or mechanical ventilation.[38] The decision to initiate renal replacement therapy is based on the fluid, electrolyte, acid-base, and metabolic status of each patient.[6] RRT options include intermittent hemodialysis, CRRT, prolonged intermittent renal replacement therapies (PIRRTs; a combination of the former two modalities), and peritoneal dialysis.[38]

Definition. *Dialysis* is defined as the separation of solutes by differential diffusion through a porous or semipermeable membrane that is placed between two solutions. The various dialysis methods are distinguished by the type of semipermeable membrane and the two solutions that are used.

TABLE 16.7 Pharmacology

Medications to Treat Hyperkalemia

Medication	Action/Use	Dosage/ Route	Side Effects	Nursing Implications
Sodium polystyrene sulfonate (Lokelma; Kayexalate)	↑ Fecal excretion of potassium by exchanging sodium ions for potassium ions	*Oral:* 15 g 1-4 times daily *Rectal:* 30-50 g via enema q1-2 h initially prn then q6h prn	Constipation Fecal impaction in the elderly Hypernatremia Hypokalemia Nausea and vomiting	Available as a powder or suspension. Mix powder with full glass of liquid and chill to increase palatability. Do not mix oral powder with orange juice. Do not mix with sorbitol.
Insulin and dextrose	Shifts potassium temporarily from the extracellular fluid (blood) into the intracellular fluid; dextrose helps prevent hypoglycemia	*IV:* Initial dose 5-10 units regular insulin and 50 mL of 50% dextrose IV push	Hyperglycemia Hypoglycemia Hypokalemia	If the serum glucose level is >250–300 mg/dL, the provider may order only the insulin.
Sodium bicarbonate	Shifts potassium temporarily from the extracellular fluid (blood) to the intracellular fluid	*IV:* 50-100 mEq/L push	Hypernatremia Hypokalemia Pulmonary edema	Do not mix with any other medications to prevent precipitation. May be used in patient with severe metabolic acidosis.
Albuterol	Adrenergic agonist ↑ plasma insulin concentration; shifts potassium to intracellular space	*Inhalation:* 10-20 mg over 15 min	Angina Hypertension Irritability Nervousness Palpitations Tachycardia	Note that the dose used is much higher than that used in treating pulmonary conditions. Use concentrated form (5 mg/mL) to minimize the volume to be inhaled.
Calcium gluconate	Emergent management of life-threatening hyperkalemia, stabilizes cardiac cell membrane	*IV:* 5-8 mL of 10% solution (500-800 mg) max 3 g IV, slow injection	Bradycardia Hypotension Necrosis if infiltrated Syncope	Has no effect on lowering serum potassium. Has an almost immediate effect on ECG appearance. Be sure IV is patent to prevent extravasation.
Calcium chloride	Emergent management of life-threatening hyperkalemia, stabilizes cardiac cell membrane	*IV:* 5-10 mL of 10% solution (500-1000 mg) slow injection	Bradycardia Hypotension Necrosis if infiltrated Syncope	Has no effect on lowering serum potassium. Has an almost immediate effect on ECG appearance. Be sure IV is patent; prevent extravasation.

ECG, Electrocardiogram; *PO,* by mouth; *prn,* as needed; *q,* every.

Data from Gahart B, Nazareno AR, Ortega M. *Gahart's 2019 Intravenous Medications: A Handbook for Nurses and Health Professionals.* St. Louis, MO: Elsevier; 2019; Skidmore-Roth L. *Mosby's 2023 Nursing Drug Reference.* 36th ed. St. Louis: Elsevier; 2023.

BOX 16.7 Metabolic Acidosis in Acute Kidney Injury

Etiology

- Inability of kidney to excrete hydrogen ions; decreased production of ammonia by the kidney (normally assists with hydrogen ion excretion).
- Retention of acid end products of metabolism, which use available buffers in the body; inability of kidney to synthesize bicarbonate.

Signs and Symptoms

- Low pH of arterial blood (pH <7.35)
- Low serum bicarbonate
- Increased rate and depth of respirations to excrete carbon dioxide from the lungs (compensatory mechanism); known as *Kussmaul respirations*
- Low partial pressure of carbon dioxide ($PaCO_2$)
- Lethargy and coma if severe

Indications for Renal Replacement Therapy. The most common reasons for initiating RRT in AKI are hyperkalemia, hyponatremia, hyperphosphatemia, volume overload, anuria, poisoning or intoxication, azotemia, metabolic acidosis (pH <7.20), severe oliguria, complications from uremia (e.g., encephalopathy, neuropathy, pericarditis), and progressive AKI.[5,14,38,39] Dialysis is usually started early during the renal dysfunction trajectory, before uremic complications occur.

The most optimal time to start RRT has not been determined. Weighing of the risks and benefits of early initiation or watchful waiting must take place. Early initiation is associated with timelier optimization of the conditions for which RRT may be indicated. Risks associated with RRT include complications with vascular access (e.g., infection, hemorrhage, clotting) and hypotension and bleeding from anticoagulation used to maintain patency of the circuit.[38,40]

Principles and Mechanisms. Dialysis therapy is based on two physical principles that operate simultaneously: diffusion and ultrafiltration. *Diffusion* (or clearance) is the movement of solutes, such as urea, from the patient's blood to the dialysate cleansing fluid, across a semipermeable membrane (the hemofilter). Substances such as bicarbonate may also cross in the opposite direction, from the dialysate through the semipermeable membrane into the patient's blood. Movement of solutes across the semipermeable membrane depends on the following:

- The number of solutes on each side of the semipermeable membrane; typically, the patient's blood has larger amounts of solutes such as urea, creatinine, and potassium
- The surface area of the semipermeable membrane (the size of the hemofilter)
- The permeability of the semipermeable membrane
- The size and charge of the solutes
- The rate of blood flowing through the hemofilter
- The rate of dialysate cleansing fluid flowing through the hemofilter

Ultrafiltration is the removal of plasma water and some low-molecular-weight particles by using a pressure or osmotic gradient. Ultrafiltration is primarily aimed at controlling fluid volume, whereas dialysis is aimed at decreasing waste products and treating fluid and electrolyte imbalances.[41]

Vascular Access. An essential component of all renal replacement therapies is adequate, easy access to the patient's bloodstream. Several types of vascular access (Figs. 16.7 and 16.8), including percutaneous venous catheters, arteriovenous fistulas, and arteriovenous grafts, are used for hemodialysis.

Temporary percutaneous catheters are commonly used in patients with AKI because they can be used immediately. The typical catheter has a double lumen and a wide bore (11.5 to 13.5 French) and is 15, 20, or 24 cm long. Three-lumen catheters are also available to provide access for infusions and central venous pressure measurement. The internal jugular vein is preferred for insertion of these catheters due to optimal blood flow with less risk of a pneumothorax. If not possible, catheter placement preference is the femoral vein.[16] The subclavian site is not recommended because of the risk of subclavian vein stenosis.[16] Routine replacement of hemodialysis catheters to prevent infection is not recommended, and the decision to remove or replace the catheter is based on clinical need and/or signs and symptoms of infection.[16]

An *arteriovenous fistula* is an internal, surgically created communication between an artery and a vein. The most frequently created fistula anastomoses the radial artery and the cephalic vein in a side-to-side or end-to-side manner. The anastomosis permits blood to bypass the capillaries and flow directly from the artery into the vein. The vein is forced to dilate to accommodate the increased pressure that accompanies the arterial blood. This method produces a vessel that is easy to cannulate but requires 4 to 6 weeks before it is mature enough to use.

Arteriovenous grafts are created with the use of several types of prosthetic materials. Most commonly, polytetrafluoroethylene (Teflon) grafts are placed under the skin and are surgically anastomosed between an artery (usually brachial) and a vein (usually antecubital). The graft site usually heals within 2 to 4 weeks.

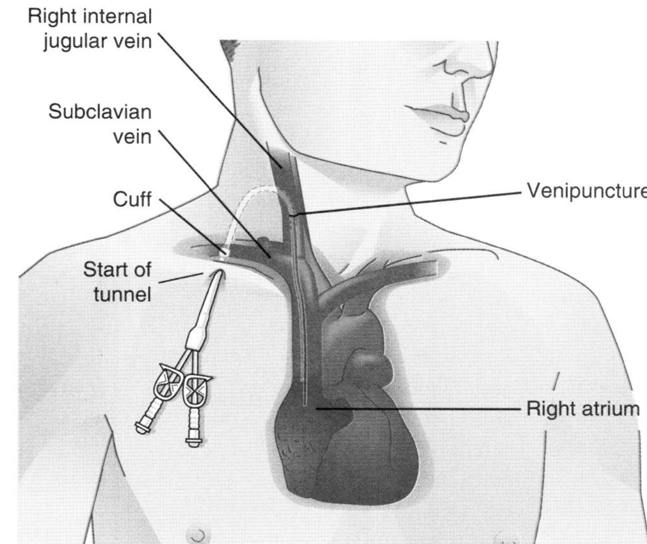

Fig. 16.7 Central venous catheter used for hemodialysis. (From Headley CM. Acute kidney injury and chronic kidney disease. In: Harding MM, Kwon J, Hagler D. *Lewis's Medical-Surgical Nursing: Assessment and Management of Clinical Problems*. 9th ed. St. Louis, MO: Mosby; 2023.)

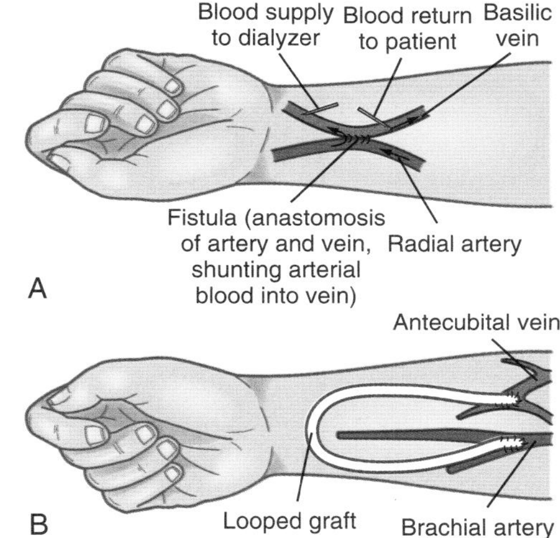

Fig. 16.8 Hemodialysis access devices. **A**, Arteriovenous fistula. **B**, Arteriovenous graft. (From Headley CM. Acute kidney injury and chronic kidney disease. In: Harding MM, Kwon J, Hagler D. *Lewis's Medical-Surgical Nursing: Assessment and Management of Clinical Problems*. 9th ed. St. Louis, MO: Mosby; 2023.)

Nursing care of arteriovenous fistula or graft. Protect the vascular access site. Auscultate an arteriovenous fistula or graft for a bruit and palpate for the presence of a thrill or buzz every 8 hours. Do not use the extremity that has a fistula or graft for drawing blood specimens, obtaining blood pressure measurements, or administering IV therapy or intramuscular injections. Such actions produce pressure changes within the altered vessels that could result in clotting or rupture. Alert other healthcare personnel of the presence of the fistula or graft by posting a large sign at the head of the patient's bed that indicates which arm should be used. Evaluate the presence and strength of the pulse distal to the fistula or graft at least every 8 hours. Inadequate collateral circulation past the fistula or graft may result in loss of this pulse. Notify the provider immediately if no bruit is auscultated, no thrill is palpated, or the distal pulse is absent.

Nursing care of percutaneous catheters. Strict aseptic technique must be applied to any percutaneous catheter placed for dialysis. Transparent, semipermeable polyurethane dressings are recommended because they allow continuous visualization for assessment of signs of infection. Replace transparent dressings on temporary percutaneous catheters every 7 days or per institution protocol and no more than once a week for percutaneous catheters unless the dressing is soiled or loose. Monitor the catheter site visually when changing the dressing or by palpation through an intact dressing. Tenderness at the insertion site, swelling, erythema, or drainage is reported to the provider. To prevent accidental dislodgement, minimize manipulation of the catheter. Do not use the catheter to administer fluids or medications or to sample blood unless a specific order is obtained. Three-lumen catheters permit infusions, medication administration, and blood sampling through the specified lumen not dedicated to RRT. Trained personnel may instill medication in the catheter to maintain patency and clamp the catheter when not in use.

Hemodialysis. Intermittent hemodialysis is the most frequently used RRT for treatment of AKI.[16] Hemodialysis consists of simply cleansing the patient's blood through a hemofilter using diffusion and ultrafiltration. Water and waste products of metabolism are easily removed. Hemodialysis is efficient and corrects biochemical disturbances quickly. Treatments are typically 3 to 4 hours long and are performed in the critical care unit at the patient's bedside. Because each hemodialysis treatment is only 3 to 4 hours long, no more than 2 to 3 liters of fluid can be removed in each session, even in patients with hemodynamic stability. The net balance is minimally negative because critically ill patients often receive the same amount of fluid throughout the 24-hour day.[42] Patients with AKI may be hemodynamically unstable and unable to tolerate intermittent hemodialysis.[42] In those instances, other methods of renal replacement therapy, such as peritoneal dialysis or CRRT, are considered.

Complications. Several complications are associated with hemodialysis. Hypotension is common and is usually the result of preexisting hypovolemia, excessive amounts of fluid removal, or excessively rapid fluid removal. Other factors that contribute to hypotension include left ventricular dysfunction from preexisting heart disease or medications, autonomic dysfunction resulting from medication or diabetes mellitus, and inappropriate vasodilation resulting from sepsis or antihypertensive medication therapy. Dialyzer membrane incompatibility may also cause hypotension.

Dysrhythmias may occur during dialysis. Causes of dysrhythmias include a rapid shift in the serum potassium level, clearance of antidysrhythmic medications, preexisting coronary artery disease, hypoxemia, or hypercalcemia from rapid influx of calcium from the dialysate solution.

Muscle cramps may occur during dialysis, but they occur more commonly in chronic renal failure. Cramping is thought to be caused by ischemia of the skeletal muscles resulting from aggressive fluid removal. The cramps typically involve the legs, feet, and hands and occur most often during the last half of the dialysis treatment.

A decrease in the arterial oxygen content of the blood can occur in patients undergoing hemodialysis. Usually, the decrease ranges from 5 to 35 mm Hg (mean, 15 mm Hg) and is not clinically significant except in the unstable critically ill patient. Several theories have been offered to explain the hypoxemia, including leukocyte interactions with the hemofilter and a decrease in carbon dioxide levels resulting from either an acetate dialysate solution or a loss of carbon dioxide across the semipermeable membrane.

Dialysis disequilibrium syndrome often occurs after the first or second dialysis treatment or in patients who have had sudden, large decreases in BUN and creatinine levels because of the hemodialysis. Because of the blood-brain barrier, dialysis does not deplete the concentrations of BUN, creatinine, and other uremic toxins in the brain as rapidly as it decreases those substances in the extracellular fluid. An osmotic concentration gradient established in the brain allows fluid to enter until the concentration levels equal those of the extracellular fluid. The extra fluid in the brain tissue creates a state of cerebral edema for the patient, which results in severe headaches, nausea and vomiting, muscle fasciculations, mental confusion, and occasionally seizures.[42] The incidence of dialysis disequilibrium syndrome may be decreased using shorter, more frequent dialysis treatments.

Infectious complications associated with hemodialysis include vascular access infections and hepatitis C. Vascular access infections are usually caused by a break in sterile technique, whereas hepatitis C is usually acquired through blood transfusions.

Hemolysis, air embolism, and hyperthermia are rare complications of hemodialysis. Hemolysis can occur when the patient's blood is exposed to incorrectly mixed dialysate solution. An air embolism can occur when air is introduced into the bloodstream through a break in the dialysis circuit. Hyperthermia may result if the temperature control devices on the dialysis machine malfunction. Complications of hemodialysis are summarized in Box 16.8.

BOX 16.8 Complications of Dialysis

- Hypotension
- Cramps
- Bleeding or clotting
- Dialyzer reaction
- Hemolysis
- Dysrhythmias
- Infections
- Hypoxemia
- Hyperthermia
- Hypothermia
- Pyrogen reactions
- Dialysis disequilibrium syndrome
- Vascular access dysfunction
- Technical errors (incorrect dialysate mixture, contaminated dialysate, air embolism)

Nursing care. The patient receiving hemodialysis requires specialized monitoring and interventions by the critical care nurse. Monitor vital signs before, during, and following each treatment. Monitor laboratory values and report abnormal results to the nephrologist and dialysis staff. Weigh the patient daily to monitor fluid status. On the day of dialysis, do not administer dialyzable (water-soluble) medications until after treatment. Consult the dialysis nurse or pharmacist to determine which medications to withhold or administer. Supplemental doses are administered as ordered after dialysis. Administration of antihypertensive medications is avoided for 4 to 6 hours before treatment. Doses of other medications that lower blood pressure (e.g., analgesics, sedatives) are reduced, if possible. Assess the percutaneous catheter, fistula, or graft frequently; report unusual findings such as loss of bruit, redness, or drainage at the site. After dialysis, assess the patient for signs of bleeding, hypovolemia, dialysis disequilibrium syndrome, or other adverse events.

CLINICAL EXEMPLAR

Person-Centered Care

During intermittent hemodialysis treatment, the patient shared with the nurse feeling more physically weak and worsened tingling in his feet since being hospitalized. The nurse knew that some patients with renal disease experience some degree of uremic polyneuropathy that could be exacerbated before experiencing the onset of critical illness. The nurse was aware that polyneuropathy can be very debilitating for individuals because it can cause a variety of symptoms affecting quality of life, including chronic pain, changes in sensation in the affected extremities, and alterations in muscle activity that may restrict mobility. The nurse gathered more information from the patient about the physical weakness, tingling sensation, pain, and leg cramps. The nurse also asked the patient about activity goals after hospital discharge. He said he enjoyed playing golf and long walks but also shared that it was harder for him to engage in activities the past few years because of leg discomfort. The nurse spoke with the provider, shared data she gathered from the patient, suggested a focused physical therapy consult to optimize mobility, and provided individualized education on safety concerns associated with the polyneuropathy.

Continuous Renal Replacement Therapy. CRRT is a pillar for managing critically ill patients with AKI. It is a continuous extracorporeal blood purification system managed by the bedside critical care nurse. It is like conventional intermittent hemodialysis in that a hemofilter is used to facilitate the processes of ultrafiltration and diffusion. It differs in that CRRT provides slow removal of solutes and water rather than the rapid removal of water and solutes that occurs with intermittent hemodialysis.[39]

Indications. The clinical indications for CRRT are like those for intermittent hemodialysis, including volume overload, hyperkalemia, acidosis, uremia, and hemodynamic stability. It is frequently selected for patients with AKI because of the ability to provide a gentle correction of uremia and fluid imbalances while minimizing hypotension.

Principles. The first CRRT systems were introduced in the 1970s. The extracorporeal circuit consisted of an arterial access catheter, hemofilter, and venous return catheter. The patient's blood pressure determined the flow rate through the circuit. Arteriovenous systems are no longer used because of therapy limitations related to patient-dependent blood flow and concern for complications related to arterial cannulation. Venovenous circuits are currently the standard for RRT. Improvements in dual-lumen venous catheters, mechanical blood pumps, and user-friendly RRT cassette circuits and monitors have increased the safety and efficiency of venovenous replacement therapies. In venovenous therapy, two venous accesses or a dual-lumen venous catheter is used. Blood is pulled from the access port of the dual-lumen dialysis catheter or from one of two single-lumen venous catheters by the negative pressure gradient created by a blood pump. The blood travels through the hemofilter and returns to the patient via the return port of the dual-lumen venous dialysis catheter or via a second venous catheter (Fig. 16.9).

Four types of continuous venovenous replacement therapies are used (Table 16.8):

1. Slow continuous ultrafiltration (SCUF)
2. Continuous venovenous hemofiltration (CVVH)
3. Continuous venovenous hemodialysis (CVVHD)
4. Continuous venovenous hemodiafiltration (CVVHDF)

Slow continuous ultrafiltration (SCUF), also known as *isolated ultrafiltration,* is used to remove plasma water in cases of volume overload. SCUF can remove 3 to 6 L of ultrafiltrate per day. Solute removal is minimal and therefore is not indicated for patients with conditions requiring removal of uremic toxins and correction of acidosis. A large-bore vascular access device is needed to help ensure sufficient blood flow.[43]

Continuous venovenous hemofiltration (CVVH) is used to remove fluids and solutes through the process of convection, which is the transfer of solutes across the semipermeable membranes of the hemofilter. As plasma moves across the membrane (ultrafiltration), it carries solute molecules. Increasing the volume of plasma water that crosses the hemofilter membranes increases the amount of solute removed. Replacement solution is added to replenish plasma water and electrolytes lost because of the high ultrafiltration rate. Replacement solutions typically are commercially prepared and contain electrolytes and a bicarbonate or lactate base. Calcium, magnesium, and phosphorus are not present in bicarbonate-based replacement solutions because they will form precipitates; these electrolytes will be administered separately. Replacement solutions can be administered before the hemofilter (predilution) or after the hemofilter (postdilution).

Continuous venovenous hemodialysis (CVVHD) is like CVVH in that ultrafiltration removes plasma water. It differs in that dialysate solution is added around the hemofilter membranes to facilitate solute removal by the process of diffusion. Because the dialysate solution is constantly refreshed around the hemofilter membranes, the solute clearance is greater with this therapy, and therefore it can be used to treat both volume overload and azotemia.[44]

Continuous venovenous hemodiafiltration (CVVHDF) combines ultrafiltration, convection, and diffusion to maximize fluid and solute removal. It is useful for the management of volume overload associated with requirements for high solute clearance.[44]

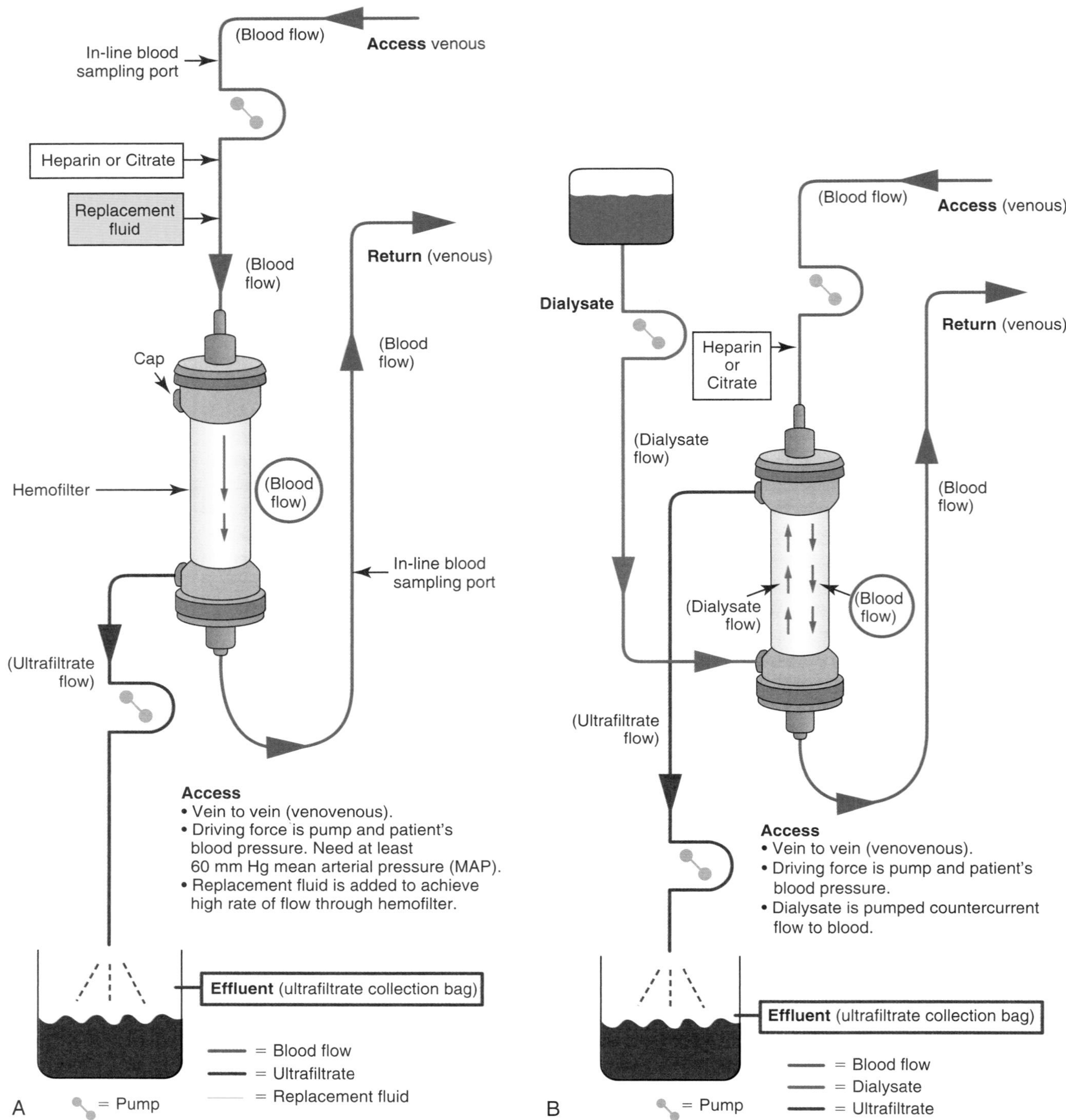

Fig. 16.9 A, Schematic diagram of continuous venovenous hemofiltration (CVVH). B, Schematic diagram of continuous venovenous hemodialysis (CVVHD). (From Urden L, Lough M, Stacy K, eds. *Critical Care Nursing: Diagnosis and Management*. 8th ed. St. Louis, MO: Mosby; 2018.)

Automated devices are marketed to facilitate delivery of the various CRRT therapies (Fig. 16.10).

Anticoagulation. The efficiency of the hemofilter can decline over time or fail suddenly because of clogging or clotting. Clogging results from the accumulation of protein and blood cells on the hemofilter membrane.[39] Filter clotting is the result of progressive loss of the hollow fibers within the hemofilter.[39] In most situations, CRRT requires some form of intervention to prevent clogging and clotting. During CRRT, the patient's blood comes in contact with the extracorporeal circuit, which causes activation of the coagulation cascade.[39] Heparin is used to inhibit coagulation and extend the life of the hemofilter.

TABLE 16.8 Continuous Renal Replacement Therapies

Modality	Name	Purpose	Vascular Access Required	Description
SCUF	Slow continuous ultrafiltration	Fluid removal	Dual-lumen venous catheter or two large venous catheters	Venous blood is circulated through a hemofilter and returned to the patient through a venous catheter; ultrafiltrate (fluid removed) is collected in a drainage bag as it exits the hemofilter.
CVVH	Continuous venovenous hemofiltration	Fluid and some uremic waste product removal	Dual-lumen venous catheter or two large venous catheters	Venous blood is circulated through a hemofilter and returned to the patient through a venous catheter; replacement fluid is used to increase flow through the hemofilter; ultrafiltrate (fluid removed) is collected in a drainage bag as it exits the hemofilter.
CVVHD	Continuous venovenous hemodialysis	Fluid and maximal uremic waste product removal	Dual-lumen venous catheter or two large venous catheters	Venous blood is circulated through a hemofilter (surrounded by a dialysate solution) and returned to the patient through a venous catheter; replacement solution may be used to improve convection; ultrafiltrate (fluid and waste products removed) is collected in a drainage bag as it exits the hemofilter.
CVVHDF	Continuous venovenous hemodiafiltration	Maximal fluid and uremic waste product removal	Dual-lumen venous catheter or two large venous catheters	Venous blood is circulated through a hemofilter (surrounded by a dialysate solution) and returned to the patient through a venous catheter; replacement solution is used to maintain fluid balance; ultrafiltration (fluid and waste products removed) is collected in a drainage bag as it exits the hemofilter.

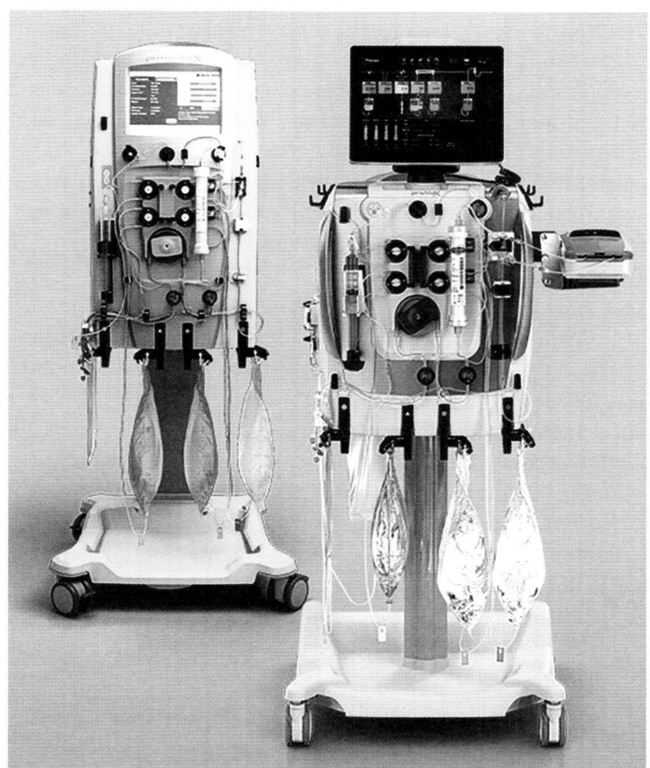

Fig. 16.10 Prismaflex and PrisMax continuous renal replacement therapy systems. (Courtesy Baxter, Deerfield, IL.)

However, heparin may be contraindicated if there is a risk of bleeding or heparin-induced thrombocytopenia.

An alternative to heparin during CRRT is citrate. Citrate chelates calcium in the serum and inhibits activation of the coagulation cascade.[38] Systemic anticoagulation is minimal because the liver quickly converts citrate to bicarbonate, increasing the risk of metabolic alkalosis. Citrate is infused into the circuit above the filter. Close monitoring of serum ionized calcium levels and calcium replacement through a separate venous line are required. Bicarbonate-based replacement solutions should not be used with citrate therapy.

Nursing care. The critical care nurse is responsible for monitoring the patient receiving CRRT. In some critical care units, the CRRT system is set up by the dialysis staff but maintained by critical care nurses after additional training. Monitor the patient's hemodynamic status hourly, including fluid intake and output. Monitor temperature because significant heat can be lost when blood is circulating through the extracorporeal circuit. Specialized devices are available to warm the dialysate or replacement fluid or to rewarm the blood returning to the patient.

Assess ultrafiltration volume hourly and administer replacement fluid per protocol. Assess the hemofilter every 2 to 4 hours for clotting (as evidenced by dark fibers or a rapid decrease in the amount of ultrafiltration without a change in the patient's hemodynamic status and changes in access pressures). If clotting is suspected, flush the system with 50 to 100 mL of 0.9% normal saline and observe for dark streaks or clots. If clots are present, the system may have to be changed. Monitor results of serum chemistries, clotting studies, and other tests. Assess the CRRT system frequently to ensure that the filter and lines are always visible, kinks are prevented, and the blood tubing is warm to the touch. Assess the ultrafiltrate for blood (pink-tinged to frank blood), which is indicative of membrane rupture. Use sterile technique during vascular access dressing changes.

Nutrition. Ensure the patient is receiving adequate nutrition. Patients' nutritional needs should be determined by the losses associated with AKI, in general, and CRRT losses specifically.[45]

Carbohydrates. Anticoagulation of the CRRT circuit with citrate is associated with approximately 300 kcal/day. When other forms of anticoagulation are used, the energy load ranges from 500 to 1200 kcal/day. These energy loads do not account for replacement fluids that were non–glucose containing; in this case, there would be a decreased number of calories gained. If glucose-free replacement fluids are used, there may be an associated glucose loss of up to 40 to 80 g/day.[45]

Proteins and amino acids. Increased protein catabolism is associated with critical illness and AKI. There is a redistribution of amino acids to tissues from lean body mass, which results in negative nitrogen balance and muscle wasting. There is also amino acid loss in CRRT ultrafiltrate. Nitrogen loss may be as high as 25 g/day. Currently, intake of 1.3 g/kg/day of protein is recommended for patients who are critically ill. It is further recommended that 10 to 15 additional grams of protein should be given to patients on CRRT to account for amino acid losses. It is unclear if the increase in protein intake affects patient outcomes.[45]

Lipids. Lipids should account for at least 30% to 35% of patient energy supply. This is essential to mitigate deficiency of essential fatty acids.[45]

Electrolytes and minerals. Because CRRT is associated with solute removal, monitoring of the patient's electrolyte status is essential. Observation of sodium, potassium, phosphorus, and magnesium levels for metabolic derangements on a regular basis is vital.[45]

Micronutrients. Due to the adsorption of vitamins and trace elements by the hemofilter, there is potential for deficiencies in vitamin C, folate, and thiamine. Loss of selenium and other micronutrients has also been suggested. Each of these micronutrients should be replaced, although there is no agreement on the amount of required supplementation.[45]

Complications of CRRT. Complications associated with CRRT are categorized as either catheter related, extracorporeal circuit related, or physiologic. Catheter-related complications include hemorrhage, infection, clotting, venous stenosis, pneumothorax, hemothorax, cardiac dysrhythmias, air embolism, visceral injury, and traumatic arteriovenous fistula. Complications related to the circuit include an allergic reaction to part of the circuit, clotting, hemolysis, and air embolism. Physiological complications include hypotension and electrolyte imbalances (i.e., low phosphorus, calcium, potassium, or magnesium). Medication dosing errors are also possible.[38,46]

Prolonged Intermittent Renal Replacement Therapies (PIRRTs). PIRRT is a form of dialysis that includes both convective (i.e., hemofiltration) and diffusive (i.e., hemodialysis) therapies for an extended period of time, often 6 to 18 hours, but is intermittent (i.e., a few times a week) as the patient becomes more hemodynamically stable.

CHECK YOUR UNDERSTANDING

6. Which lab result should the nurse anticipate as a complication of CRRT?
   A. Phosphorus 5.1 mg/dL
   B. Calcium 7.8 mg/dL
   C. Potassium 5.7 mEq/L
   D. Sodium 151 mEq/L

Peritoneal Dialysis. Peritoneal dialysis is the removal of solutes and fluid by diffusion through a patient's own semipermeable membrane (the peritoneal membrane) with a dialysate solution that has been instilled into the peritoneal cavity.[47] The peritoneal membrane surrounds the abdominal cavity and lines the organs inside the abdominal cavity. This RRT is not commonly used for the treatment of AKI because of its comparatively slow ability to alter biochemical imbalances. With peritoneal dialysis, a prescribed amount and type of dialysate fluid is infused into the abdominal cavity by gravity via a tunneled catheter. The fluid remains in the abdominal cavity for a predetermined amount of time (dwell time) and is then drained by gravity and discarded.[48]

Indications. Clinical indications for peritoneal dialysis include acute and chronic kidney injury, severe water intoxication, electrolyte disorders, and drug overdose. Advantages of peritoneal dialysis include easy and rapid assembly of the equipment, relatively inexpensive cost, minimal danger of acute electrolyte imbalances or hemorrhage, and easily individualized dialysate solutions. In addition, automated peritoneal dialysis systems are available. Disadvantages of peritoneal dialysis are that it requires at least 36 hours for a therapeutic effect to be achieved, biochemical disturbances are corrected slowly, access to the peritoneal cavity is sometimes difficult, and the risk of peritonitis is high. Contraindications to peritoneal dialysis are rare but include a patient not having a sufficiently clean environment, a lack of physical or cognitive ability or a care partner to perform the exchanges, and scarring of the peritoneal cavity.[47]

Complications. Although rare, many complications can result from peritoneal dialysis. These complications can be divided into two categories: infectious and noninfectious. Infectious complications include peritonitis and exit-site or tunnel infections.[47,49] Noninfectious complications are either catheter related (impaired flow, leak, or pain during dialysate instillation or drainage) or are due to intraabdominal pressure (back pain hernia from muscle strain from fluid dwelling in the abdomen) or metabolic derangements (hypokalemia or metabolic syndrome). Patients may develop hyperglycemia and hypertonicity with associated weight gain from the glucose contained in the dialysate. This is more likely to occur in patients with diabetes mellitus.[50]

Nursing care. Use aseptic technique when handling the peritoneal catheter and connections. Observe for peritonitis, the most common complication of peritoneal dialysis. Peritonitis is manifested by abdominal pain, cloudy peritoneal fluid, fever and chills, nausea and vomiting, ileus, and difficulty in draining fluid from the peritoneal cavity.[51,52]

Transplantation. Kidney transplantation is a therapeutic option for patients with end-stage kidney disease. Refer to the Transplant Considerations box for criteria and patient management after kidney transplantation.

TRANSPLANT CONSIDERATIONS

Kidney Transplantation

Criteria for Transplant Recipients

Usually the recipient is younger than age 80 years, has an estimated life expectancy of 2 years or more, and is expected to have an improved quality of life after transplantation. Patients with active substance use disorders or poor treatment compliance and who lack psychosocial support before and after transplant are not considered good transplant candidates. Most transplant centers require patients to be malignancy-free for 2 to 5 years prior to transplant, based on the type of cancer.

Patient Management

The kidney from a living donor functions almost immediately after transplantation; however, a cadaver kidney may have delayed function, and temporary hemodialysis may be needed. Careful monitoring of fluid and electrolyte balance is imperative, often every 4 to 6 hours in the immediate postoperative period.[1] Fluid balance may be determined by clinical assessment and hemodynamic monitoring. Chronic anemia is a consequence of end-stage renal disease (ESRD) and may limit tissue oxygen delivery; therefore, hemoglobin and hematocrit levels are monitored closely.

Maintenance immunosuppressive medications may consist of a calcineurin inhibitor (tacrolimus [Prograf] or cyclosporine [Neoral]) or mycophenolate mofetil (CellCept). These medications inhibit T-cell proliferation and differentiation, deplete lymphocytes, and inhibit macrophages. Early induction medications may include a lymphocyte-depleting agent such as basiliximab. Low-dose steroids may be used, although they are generally avoided, given the associated complications.[2] Potential kidney recipients at high immunological risk may receive plasmapheresis to decrease rejection risk with human leukocyte antigen (HLA) incompatibility.

Complications

Complications seen in the postoperative phase of care may be classified as *surgical* or *physiological*. Surgical-related complications include urine leak and arterial and venous bleeding caused by anastomotic failure. This may require reoperation for surgical repair or placement of a stent. Arterial or venous thrombosis and renal artery stenosis may also occur. Acute tubular necrosis is a physiological complication and may cause delayed graft function. Patients may need to restart dialysis until kidney function returns.

Complications associated with immunosuppressive therapy may include nephrotoxicity, hypertension, hyperlipidemia, bone loss, new-onset diabetes mellitus, and infection.[3] High-doses of immunosuppression therapy can increase susceptibility to infection; therefore, the patient and family must be knowledgeable of the signs and symptoms. Common signs of infection include low-grade fever, malaise, fatigue, nausea, and decreased urine output. One of the most common infections is cytomegalovirus (CMV), which presents as a fall in white blood cell count, fatigue, and fever.

A common cause of death after a kidney transplant is cardiovascular disease. Immunosuppression therapy, especially corticosteroids and calcineurin inhibitors, can contribute to the development of hypertension and diabetes mellitus, which play a role in the progression of atherosclerosis and lipid disorders.

Preventing Rejection

The evolution of immunosuppression therapy has lowered rejection rates after kidney transplant, but compliance with therapy is essential. *Acute rejection* rates have decreased to about 10% and typically occur within days to 3 months after transplantation and can either be T-cell mediated or antibody mediated. Acute rejection is diagnosed based on clinical presentation and biopsy findings. Symptoms of rejection include fever, edema, gross hematuria, pain, increased blood urea nitrogen and creatinine, weight gain, elevated blood pressure, and decreased urine output. Treatment strategies differ between T-cell mediated and antibody mediated but may include high-dose "pulse" methylprednisolone steroid therapy, thymoglobulin, and muromonab-CD3.[3] Chronic rejection occurs months to years after transplantation and is caused by chronic kidney allograft dysfunction. This is often secondary to fibrosis and intimal hyperplasia within vessels in the transplanted organ and is accompanied by hypertension and proteinuria. Risk factors include frequency of acute rejection episodes, transplant infectious disease, early ischemia reperfusion injury, and poor medication compliance.[4] During posttransplant follow-up, serum levels of immune-modulating agents, typically tacrolimus or cyclosporine, are closely monitored to allow drug titration and maintenance of therapeutic levels.

References

1. Baker RJ, Mark PB, Patel RL, et al. Renal association clinical practice guideline in postoperative care in the kidney transplant recipient. *BMC Nephrol.* 2017;18(1):174.
2. Woodle ES, Gill JS, Clark S, Stewart D, Alloway R, First R. Early corticosteroid cessation vs long-term corticosteroid therapy in kidney transplant recipients: long-term outcomes of a randomized clinical trial. *JAMA Surg.* 2021;156(4):307–314. https://doi.org/10.1001/jamasurg.2020.6929.
3. Cooper JE. Evaluation and treatment of acute rejection in kidney allografts. *Clin J Am Soc Nephrol.* 2020;15(3):430–438. https://doi.org/10.2215/CJN.11991019.
4. Lai X, Zheng X, Mathew JM, Gallon L, Leventhal JR, Zhang ZJ. Tackling chronic kidney transplant rejection: challenges and promises. *Front Immunol.* 2021;12:661643. https://doi.org/10.3389/fimmu.2021.661643.

Chelsea Sooy, BSN, RN, CCTC
Melissa A. Kelley, RN, CPTC

Acute and progressive decline in renal function is common in the critical care unit setting. It significantly contributes to patients' morbidity and mortality.[4] Meticulous nursing care and high levels of clinical judgment, clinical inquiry, and caring practices are essential for optimal patient outcomes.

CASE STUDY

Mr. B, age 32 years, was admitted to the critical care unit from the emergency department after successful cardiopulmonary resuscitation. Prior to admission, a family member placed an emergency call after Mr. B failed to report to work. Upon arrival, emergency responders found Mr. B unresponsive and in a contorted position on his back, with his lower legs flexed underneath his buttocks. A syringe and tourniquet were noted nearby. Agonal respirations were present, and Mr. B was intubated and manual bag ventilation begun. During transport to the emergency department, chest compressions were initiated for the onset of pulseless electrical activity. While in the emergency department, return of spontaneous circulation was achieved. Mechanical ventilation was initiated, and an indwelling temperature-sensing urinary catheter was placed. The preliminary toxicology screen report was positive for opiates and cocaine. The findings of the computed tomography (CT) scan of the head were consistent with anoxic injury.

Upon arrival to the critical care unit, a central line catheter was placed, and targeted temperature management was initiated with a programmable cooling/warming system. Infusions of vasoactive medications, norepinephrine, and balanced crystalloid infusions were required to achieve and maintain a mean arterial pressure of 65 mm Hg. An echocardiogram indicated global hypokinesis with a preliminary diagnosis of stress-induced

Continued

CASE STUDY—cont'd

cardiomyopathy. Life-threatening serum laboratory values were present, including potassium 8.5 mEq/L, lactate 11.8 mmol/L, and creatinine 4.71 mg/dL.

IV insulin and dextrose solution was administered for the emergent management of hyperkalemia. Urine output was less than 0.3 mL/kg/h, and a temporary dialysis catheter was placed for the initiation of continuous venovenous hemofiltration (CVVH).

Deep tissue injury was present on the buttocks and sacrum at the time of admission. Purple discoloration and edema were present on the thighs, extending to the lower legs. The feet were blue, with blistering evident. Posterior tibial and dorsalis pedis pulses were absent. Emergent compartment fasciotomies were performed 24 hours after admission. Seventy-two hours after admission, bilateral transfemoral amputations were performed.

After 2 weeks, Mr. B transitioned from CVVH to hemodialysis 3 days per week and was transferred to a rehabilitation center for brain injury recovery and mobility assistance after his double amputations.

Questions

1. How would you list and link risk factors that predisposed this patient to development of acute kidney injury (AKI)?
2. Argue the benefits of CVVH over other forms of dialysis in the care of Mr. B.
3. At the time of admission, Mr. B received IV insulin and dextrose solution for the management of life-threatening hyperkalemia. What are the risks and benefits of this intervention for treatment of hyperkalemia?
4. Identify possible causes and intervention priorities for the patient's elevated lactate level.

NURSING SELF-CARE

Preventing Nurse Burnout

1. Identification
    - Inability to cope with stressful work situations
    - Depersonalization
    - Reduction of personal fulfillment
    - Emotional exhaustion
2. Interventions
    - Development of teamwork and improvement courses
    - Yoga
    - Nursing supervision and implementation of individually planned care
    - Communication skill training
    - Intervention focused on the meaning of job satisfaction
    - Changes in the workplace
    - Cognitive coping strategies
    - Web-based stress management program
    - Strategies to manage stress, improving job satisfaction
    - Program to combat compassion fatigue
    - Improvement in work environment
    - Mental attention training
    - Reiki, healing touch, therapeutic massage, Jin Shin, Jyutsu
    - Resilience training program
    - Mindfulness-based course
    - Spiritual Pain Assessment Sheet
    - Meditation
    - Cognitive-behavioral interventions
    - Psychological Empowerment Program
    - Interventional workshop
    - Psychosocial intervention
    - Incentives to exercise, eat a healthy diet, reduce stress, and improve interpersonal relationships
    - Public management policies in nursing
    - Professional identity development program
    - Welfare program sessions

From de Oliveira SM, de Alcantara Sousa LV, do Socorro Vieira Gadelha M, Barbosa V. Prevention actions of burnout syndrome in nurses: an integrated literature review. *Clin Pract Epidemiol Ment Health.* 2019;15:64–73.

KEY POINTS

- Modifiable risk factors of AKI include anemia, hypertension, elevated cholesterol levels, low albumin levels, mechanical ventilation, administration of nephrotoxic drugs, rhabdomyolysis, and sepsis.
- It is important to obtain a thorough patient history. Kidney-related symptoms provide valuable clues to assist the clinician in completing a focused assessment.
- Patients with kidney disease may not have any presenting signs or symptoms, including pain, aside from obstruction of the urinary tract. They may present with an illness risk factor, such as sepsis, that is associated with the development of AKI.
- The etiology of AKI is defined as prerenal, intrarenal, and postrenal, and injury is often multifactorial, associated with hypoperfusion, direct nephron injury, and tubular obstruction.
- The most common reasons for initiating RRT in AKI are hyperkalemia, hyponatremia, hyperphosphatemia, volume overload, anuria, poisoning or intoxication, azotemia, metabolic acidosis (pH <7.20), severe oliguria, complications from uremia (e.g., encephalopathy, neuropathy, pericarditis), and progressive AKI. Dialysis is usually started early during the renal dysfunction trajectory, before uremic complications occur.
- Nursing care includes continuous assessment of possible complications associated with RRT, including vascular access loss, infection, electrolyte imbalances, dysrhythmias, inadequate nutrition, and hemodynamic changes.

REFERENCES

1. National Institute of Diabetes and Digestive and Kidney Diseases. Your kidneys and how they work. https://www.niddk.nih.gov/health-information/kidney-disease/kidneys-how-they-work#:~:text=Your%20kidneys%20remove%20wastes%20and,and%20potassium%E2%80%94in%20your%20blood. Updated July 2018. Accessed February 19, 2023.
2. Ellison D, Farrar FC. Kidney influence on fluid and electrolyte balance. *Nurs Clin N Am*. 2018;53:469–480.
3. Kaufman DP, Basit H, Knohl S. Physiology, glomerular filtration rate. https://www.ncbi.nlm.nih.gov/books/NBK500032/. Updated July 17, 2023. Accessed March 25, 2024.
4. Gehr TWB, Schoolwerth AC. Clinical assessment of renal function. In: Vincent J-L, Abraham E, Moore FA, Kochanek PM, Fink MP, eds. *Textbook of Critical Care*. 11th ed. Philadelphia, PA: Elsevier; 2017:712–717.
5. Elhassan EA, Schrier RW. Acute kidney injury. In: Vincent J-L, Abraham E, Moore FA, Kochanek PM, Fink MP, eds. *Textbook of Critical Care*. 11th ed. Philadelphia, PA: Elsevier; 2017:773–783.
6. Matuszkiewicz-Rowińska J, Małyszko J. Acute kidney injury, its definition, and treatment in adults: guidelines and reality. *Pol Arch Intern Med*. 2020;130(12):1074–1080. https://doi.org/10.20452/pamw.15373.
7. Ronco C, Billomo R, Kellum JA. Acute kidney injury. *Lancet*. 2019;394(10212):1949–1964.
8. Goyal A, Daneshpajouhnejad P, Hashmi MF, et al. Acute kidney injury. *StatPearls*. https://www.ncbi.nlm.nih.gov/books/NBK441896. Updated February 16, 2022. Accessed February 19, 2023.
9. van Dijk T, Rahaminov R, Chagnac A, et al. The effect of cause, timing, kidney function recovery, and recurrent events on the prognosis of acute kidney injury in kidney transplant recipients. *Clin Transplant*. 2022. https://doi.org/10.1111/ctr.13398.
10. Marahrens B, Amann K, Asmus K, et al. Renal replacement therapy-requiring acute kidney injury due to tubulointerstitial nephritis and uveitis syndrome: case report. *J Med Case Reports*. 2021;15:629.
11. Rachoin J-S, Weisberg LSS. Renal replacement therapy in the ICU. *Crit Care Med*. 2019;47(5):715–721.
12. Edelstein CL. Biomarkers of acute kidney injury. In: Vincent J-L, Abraham E, Moore FA, Kochanek PM, Fink MP, eds. *Textbook of Critical Care*. 11th ed. Philadelphia, PA: Elsevier; 2017:718–725.
13. Scott M, McCall G. Fifteen-minute consultation: how to identify and treat children with acute kidney injury. *Arch Dis Child Educ Pract Ed*. 2022. https://doi.org/10.1036/archdischild-2020-3198928.
14. Wiersema R, Koeze J, Eck R, et al. Clinical examination findings as predictors of acute kidney injury in critically ill patients. *Acta Anaesthesiol Scand*. 2022;64(1):69–74.
15. Mercado MG, Smith DK, Guard EL. Acute kidney injury: diagnosis and management. *Am Fam Physician*. 2019;100(11):687–694.
16. Marieb EN, Hoehn KN. *Human Anatomy & Physiology*. 11th ed. New York, NY: Pearson; 2019:974–1011.
17. Kidney Disease Improving Global Outcomes (KDIGO) Acute Injury Work Group. KDIGO clinical practice guideline for acute kidney injury. *Kidney Int*. 2012;2(1):1–138.
18. de Mendonca A, Vincent JL, Suter PM, et al. Acute renal failure in the ICU: risk factors and outcome evaluated by the SOFA score. *Intensive Care Med*. 2000;26(7):915–921.
19. Bayrakci N, Ozkam G, Sakaci M, et al. The incidence of acute kidney injury and its association with mortality in patients diagnosed with COVID-19 followed up in intensive care unit. *Ther Apher Dial*. 2022;26(5):889–896. https://doi.org/10.1111/1744-9987.13790.
20. Rasmussen S, Kandler K, Nielsen R, Jakobsen PC, Ranucci M, Ravn HB. Association between transfusion of blood products and acute kidney injury following cardiac surgery. *Acta Anaesthesio Scand*. 2020;64(10):1397–1404. https://doi.org/10.1111.aas.13664.
21. Asfar P, Radermacher P, Ostermann M. MAP of 65: target of the past? *Intensive Care Med*. 2018;44:1551–1552.
22. Rogers, JL. Alterations of renal and urinary tract function. In: Rogers, JL. *McCance & Huether's Pathophysiology: The Biologic Basis for Disease in Adults and Children*. 9th ed. St. Louis: Elsevier; 2024:1233-1270.
23. Mutnuri S. Acute tubular necrosis. https://emedicine.medscape.com/article/238064-overview. Updated March 15, 2021. Accessed August 29, 2022.
24. Basu A. Contrast-induced nephropathy. https://emedicine.medscape.com/article/246751-overview. Updated November 19, 2021. August 29, 2022.
25. Ramachandran P, Jayakumar D. Contrast-induced acute kidney injury. *Crit Care Med*. 2020;24(suppl 3):S122–S125.
26. Subramaniam RM, Suarez-Cuervo C, Wilson RF, et al. Effectiveness of prevention strategies for contrast-induced nephropathy: a system review and meta-analysis. *Ann Intern Med*. 2016;164(6):406–416.
27. De Guzman MM. Rhabdomyolysis. https://emedicine.medscape.com/article/1007814-overview. Updated August 30, 2020. Accessed April 19, 2022.
28. Gaut JP, Kiapis H. Acute kidney injury pathology and pathophysiology: a retrospective review. *Clin Kidney J*. 2021;14(2):526–536.
29. Yokota LG, Sampaio BM, Rocha EB, et al. Acute kidney injury in elderly patients: narrative review on incidence, risk factors, and mortality. *Int J Nephrol Renovasc Dis*. 2018;2018:217–224.
30. Gameiro J, Goncalves M, Pereira M, et al. Obesity, acute kidney injury and mortality in patients with sepsis: a cohort analysis. *Ren Fail*. 2018;40(1):120–126.
31. Barrett MP, Moore D, Smith FG, et al. The impact of body mass index on mortality in patients with acute kidney injury: a systematic review protocol. *Syst Rev*. 2018;173(2018). https://doi.org/10.1186/s13643-018-0825-3.
32. Erstad BL, Barletta JF. Drug dosing in the critically ill obese patient: a focus on medications for hemodynamic support and prophylaxis. *Crit Care*. 2021;25(1):77. https://ccforum.biomedcentral.com/articles/10.1186/s13054-021-03495-8.
33. Szczepanski J, Griffin A, Novotny S, et al. Acute kidney injury in pregnancies complicated with preeclampsia or HEELP syndrome. *Front Med*. 2020;7:22. https://doi.org/10.3389/fmed.2020.00022.
34. Joyce EL, Kane-Gill SL, Fuhrman DY, et al. Drug-associated acute kidney injury. *Pediatr Nephrol*. 2017;32(1):59–69.
35. Chalmers C. Applied anatomy and physiology and the renal disease process. In: Thomas N, ed. *Renal Nursing: Care and Management of People with Kidney Disease*. 5th ed. London, UK: Wiley Blackwell; 2019:21–58.
36. Rosinger AY, Pontzer H, Raichlen DA, et al. Age-related decline in urine concentration may not be universal: comparative study from the U.S. and two small-scale societies. *Am J Phys Anthropol*. 2019;168(4):705–716.
37. Workeneh BT. Acute kidney injury. https://emedicine.medscape.com/article/243492-overview. Updated December 24, 2020. Accessed April 20, 2022.
38. Skidmore-Roth L. *Mosby's 2023 Nursing Drug Reference*. 36th ed. St. Louis: Elsevier; 2023.

39. Tandukar S. Continuous renal replacement therapy. Who, when, why, and how. *Chest*. 2019;155(3):626–638.
40. Saunders, H. Continuous renal replacement therapy. *StatPearls*. https://www.ncbi.nlm.nih.gov/books/NBK556028/. Updated July 31, 2021. Accessed February 19, 2023.
41. Jeong R. Timing of renal-replacement therapy in intensive care unit-related acute kidney injury. *Curr Opin Crit Care*. 2021;27(6):573–581.
42. Hall J. Diuretics, kidney diseases. In: Hall J, ed. *Guyton and Hall Textbook of Medical Physiology*. 13th ed. Philadelphia, PA: Elsevier; 2022.
43. Bellomo R, Baldwin I, Ronco C, et al. ICU-based renal replacement therapy. *Crit Care Med*. 2021;49(3):406–418.
44. Cody N, McGarvey C, McAuley DF, et al. Feasibility of slow continuous ultrafiltration for treatment of fluid overload in critical illness: in vitro investigation of venous access options. [Thematic poster session.] *Am J Respir Crit Care Med*. 2021;203:A2863.
45. See EJ, Bellomo R. How I prescribe continuous renal replacement therapy. *Crit Care*. 2021;25. https://ccforum.biomedcentral.com/articles/10.1186/s13054-020-03448-7.
46. Sabatino A, Di Mario F, Fiaccadori E. Nutritional management of patients treated with continuous renal replacement therapy. In: Kopple J, Massry S, Kalantar-Zadeh K, et al., eds. *Nutritional Management of Renal Disease*. 4th ed. St. Louis, MO: Elsevier; 2021:863–876.
47. Ng Y-H, Ganta K, Davis H, et al. Vascular access site for renal replacement therapy in acute kidney injury: a post hoc analysis of the ATN study. *Front Med*. 2017;4:40. https://doi.org/10.3389/med.2017.00040.
48. Teitelbaum I. Peritoneal dialysis. *N Engl J Med*. 2021;385:1786–1795.
49. Roberts JR. Diagnosing peritoneal dialysis complications in the ED. *Emerg Med News*. 2022;44(2):12–13.
50. Salzer WL. Peritoneal dialysis-related peritonitis: challenges and solutions. *Int J Nephrol Renovasc Dis*. 2018;11:173–186.
51. Gibb J, Xu Z, Rohrscheib M, et al. Hyperglycemic crisis in an anuric peritoneal dialysis patient with profound and symptomatic hypertonicity. *Cureus*. 2018;10(5):e2566.
52. Daley BJ. Peritonitis and abdominal sepsis clinical presentation. https://emedicine.medscape.com/article/180234-clinical. Updated July 23, 2019. Accessed April 20, 2022.

17

Hematological and Immune Disorders

Leslie Smith, DNP, APRN-CNS, AOCNS, BMTCN
Susan Smith, DNP, APRN, ACNS-BC

INTRODUCTION

Hematological and immunological functions are necessary for gas exchange, tissue perfusion, nutrition, acid-base balance, protection against infection, and hemostasis. These complex, integrated responses are easily disrupted because most critically ill patients experience some abnormalities in hematological and immune function. This chapter provides a general overview of the pertinent anatomy and physiology of these organ systems and the typical alterations in red blood cells (RBCs), immune activity, and coagulation function encountered in the acute and critical care settings. Table 17.1 defines key terms used in this chapter. Guidelines are also presented for assessment and plans for care, including strategies needed by novice critical care nurses who care for patients at risk for or experiencing these disorders.

REVIEW OF ANATOMY AND PHYSIOLOGY

Blood was recognized as being essential to life in as early as the 1600s, but the specific composition and characteristics of blood were not defined until the 20th century. Blood has four major components: (1) a fluid component called *plasma,* (2) *circulating solutes* such as ions, (3) *serum proteins,* and (4) *cells.* Plasma makes up about 55% of blood volume and is the transportation medium for important serum proteins, such as albumin, globulin, fibrinogen, prothrombin, and plasminogen. The hematopoietic cells make up the remaining 45% of blood volume. Hematopoietic cells are classified into myeloid and the lymphoid cells or lineage. The myeloid and lymphoid lineages arise from the bone marrow.[1] Characteristics of blood and potential alterations that may occur in critically ill patients are shown in Table 17.2.

Hematopoiesis refers to the production of blood cells and plasma in the body. All cells of the blood arise from the progenitor or pluripotent hematopoietic stem cell. The cells in the blood consist of both the cells of the immune system as well as red blood cells and platelets. Hematopoiesis is described in detail below.

During the course of our lifetimes, we are exposed to millions of pathogens. Our bodies have built up defenses, in the form of the immune system, to prevent these pathogens from overwhelming us. The immune system is a complex network of cells, organs and biochemicals that work together to protect the body. Cells of the immune system consist of the white blood cells (WBCs), lymphocytes, and monocytes/macrophages. Organs of the immune system consist of lymph nodes, skin and mucus membranes, bone marrow, and specialized lymph tissues. Proteins, for example, complement and antibodies are the biochemicals of the immune system.

The first line of defense of the immune system is the skin and mucus membranes. If pathogens get through the skin or mucus membranes, our immune system is activated. Immunity can be classified as innate immunity, adaptive immunity, and passive immunity. These types of immunity will be described in the physiology review.

Hematopoiesis

Hematopoiesis is defined as the formation and maturation of blood cells. The pluripotent hematopoietic stem cell is the progenitor cell for all cells in the blood. In adults, the bone marrow is the primary site for hematopoiesis; secondary hematopoietic organs that participate in this process include the spleen, liver, thymus, lymphatic system, and lymphoid tissues. During gestation, the yolk sac and liver are the primary sites of hematopoiesis.[2] Negative feedback mechanisms within the body induce the bone marrow's pluripotent hematopoietic stem cells to differentiate into separate blood cell types (Fig. 17.1) including erythrocytes (RBCs), leukocytes (WBCs), monocytes/macrophages, thrombocytes (platelets), and lymphocytes.[3]

Some hematopoietic stem cells, designated as $CD34^+$ cells, also remain in the bone marrow stroma or hematopoietic stem cell compartment for self-renewal. This ensures there is a supply of hematopoietic stem cells ready for division and differentiation during a person's lifetime. Hematopoietic and immunological organs and key functions are summarized in Fig. 17.2.

Components and Characteristics of Blood

Erythrocytes. *Erythrocytes* (RBCs) are flexible, biconcave disks without nuclei whose primary function is to deliver an oxygen-carrying molecule called hemoglobin throughout the body. This physiological configuration permits RBCs to travel at high speeds and to navigate small blood vessels, exposing more surface area for gas exchange. In each cubic millimeter (mm^3) of blood, there are approximately 5 million RBCs.[1]

RBCs are generated from precursor *stem cells* under the influence of a growth factor called *erythropoietin.* Erythropoietin is secreted by the kidneys in response to a

TABLE 17.1 Hematology and Immunology Key Terms

Term	Definition
Active (adaptive) immunity	A term used when the body actively produces cells and mediators that result in destruction of the antigen.
Anemia	A reduction in the number of circulating red blood cells or hemoglobin that leads to inadequate oxygenation of tissues; subtypes are named by etiology (e.g., aplastic anemia means "without cells") or by cell appearance (e.g., macrocytic anemia has large cells).
Antibody	Immunoglobulin that is created by specific lymphocytes and designed to immunologically destroy a specific foreign antigen.
Anticoagulants	Factors inhibiting the clotting process.
Antigen	Any substance that is capable of stimulating an immune response in the host.
Autoimmunity	Situation in which the body abnormally sees self as nonself and an immune response is activated against those self tissues.
Bone marrow transplantation	Replacement of defective bone marrow with marrow that is functional; described in terms of the source of the transplant (e.g., autologous comes from self, allogeneic comes from another person).
CAR-T	T cells that are reengineered to produce chimeric antigen receptors (CARs) on their surface. The CARs target a specific receptor on the tumor cell to attack the cancer.
Cellular immunity	Production of cytokines in response to foreign antigen.
Coagulation pathway	A predetermined cascade of coagulation proteins that is stimulated by production of the platelet plug and occurs progressively, producing a fibrin clot; there are two pathways (intrinsic and extrinsic) triggered by different events that merge into a single sequence of events leading to a fibrin clot; clotting may be initiated by either or both pathways.
Coagulopathy	Disorder of normal clotting mechanisms; most often used to describe inappropriate bleeding but can also refer to clotting.
Cytokines	Cell-killer substances or mediators secreted by white blood cells; when secreted by a lymphocyte, they are called lymphokines, and secretions from monocytes are called monokines.
Dendritic cell	A phagocyte that presents antigens on its surface to other immune cells (lymphocytes, neutrophils, etc.) and initiates the adaptive immune response. Dendritic cells are present in tissues throughout the body, such as skin.
Disseminated intravascular coagulation (DIC)	Disorder of hemostasis characterized by exaggerated microvascular coagulation and intravascular depletion of clotting factors with subsequent bleeding; also called consumption coagulopathy.
Ecchymosis	Blue or purplish hemorrhagic spot on skin or mucous membrane; round or irregular, nonelevated.
Epistaxis	Bleeding from the nose.
Erythrocyte	Red blood cell.
Fibrinolysis	Breakdown of fibrin clots that naturally occurs 1-3 days after clot development.
Hemarthrosis	Blood in a joint cavity.
Hematemesis	Bloody emesis.
Hematochezia	Blood in stool; bright red.
Hematoma	Raised, hardened mass indicative of blood vessel rupture and clotting beneath the skin surface; if subcutaneous, it appears as a blue-purple or purple-black area; may occur in spaces such as the pleural or retroperitoneal area.
Hematopoiesis	Development of the early blood cells (erythrocytes, leukocytes, thrombocytes), encompassing their maturation in the bone marrow or lymphoreticular organs.
Hematuria	Blood in the urine.
Hemoglobinuria	Hemoglobin in the urine.
Hemoptysis	Coughing up blood from the airways or lungs.
Hemorrhage	Copious, active bleeding.
Hemostasis	A physiologic process involving hematologic and nonhematologic factors that lead to formation of a platelet or fibrin clot to control the loss of blood.
Human immunodeficiency virus (HIV)	A retrovirus that transcribes its RNA-containing genetic material into DNA of the host cell nucleus; this virus has a propensity for the immune cells, replacing the RNA of lymphocytes and macrophages and causing an immunodeficient state.
Humoral immunity	Production of antibodies in response to foreign proteins.
Immunocompromised	Quantitative or qualitative defects in white blood cells or immune physiology; may be congenital or acquired and may involve a single element or multiple processes; immune incompetence leads to lack of normal inflammatory, phagocytic, antibody, or cytokine responses.
Immunoglobulin	A specific type of antibody named by its molecular structure (e.g., immunoglobulin A).
Innate immunity	The first line of defense against harmful organisms that does not need to be learned by the immune system. Examples include neutrophils, monocytes/macrophages, cytokines, skin, tears, and gastric juice (this is an abbreviated list).
Leukocyte	General term for white blood cells; there are three major subtypes: granulocytes (neutrophils, basophils, eosinophils), lymphocytes, and monocytes.
Lymphoreticular system	Cells and organs containing immunologically active cells.
Macrophage (monocyte)	Differentiated monocyte that migrates to lymphoreticular tissues of the body.

TABLE 17.1 **Hematology and Immunology Key Terms—cont'd**

Term	Definition
Melena	Blood pigments in stool; dark or black.
Menorrhagia	Excessive bleeding during menstruation.
Neutropenia	Serum neutrophil count lower than normal; predisposes patients to infection.
Passive immunity	A situation in which antibodies against a specific disease are transferred from another person.
Petechiae	Small, red or purple, nonelevated dots indicative of capillary rupture; often located in areas of increased pressure (e.g., feet or back) or on the chest and trunk.
Primary immunodeficiency	Congenital disorders in which some part of the immune system fails to develop.
Procoagulants	Factors enhancing clotting mechanisms.
Purpura	Large, mottled bruises.
Reticulocytes	Slightly immature erythrocytes that are able to continue some essential functions of red blood cells.
Secondary or acquired immunodeficiency	Immune disorder resulting from factors outside the immune system and involving the loss of a previously functional immune defense.
Thrombocyte	Platelet.
Thrombocytopenia	Serum platelet count lower than normal; predisposes individuals to bleeding as a result of inadequate platelet plugs.
Thrombosis	Creation of clots; usually refers to excess clotting.
Tissue anergy	Absence of a "wheal" tissue response to antigens and evidence of altered antibody capabilities.
Tolerance	The body's ability to recognize self as self and therefore mount a rejection response against nonself but not self tissues.
Transfusion	IV infusion of blood or blood products.

TABLE 17.2 **Characteristics of Blood**

Characteristic	Normal	Alterations
Color	Arterial: bright red Venous: dark red or crimson	Hypochromic (light color) in anemia Lighter color in dilution
pH	Arterial: 7.35-7.45	<7.35: acidosis >7.45: alkalosis
Specific gravity	Plasma: 1.026 Red blood cells: 1.093	— —
Viscosity	3.5-4.5 times that of water	Loss of plasma volume or increased cell production increases viscosity. Abnormal immunoglobulin (e.g., in multiple myeloma) increases viscosity.
Volume	Plasma volume: 45 mL/kg Cell volume: 30 mL/kg Average male: about 5000 mL	Fat tissue contains little water, so total blood volume best correlates to lean body mass. Women have more fat, and therefore blood volume is usually lower than that in men. Plasma volume rises with progression of pregnancy. Volume increases with immobility and decreases with prolonged standing; this may be the result of changes in pressure in the glomerulus and glomerular filtration rate. Blood volume is highest in neonates and lowest in the older adult. Lack of nutrients causes decreased red blood cell and plasma formation. Increased environmental temperature increases blood volume.

perceived decrease in perfusion or tissue hypoxia. Maturation of RBCs takes 4 to 5 days, and their lifespan is about 120 days. *Reticulocytes* are immature RBCs that are released when there is a demand for RBCs that exceeds the number of available mature cells. Reticulocytes are active but less effective than mature cells and circulate about 24 hours before maturing. The spleen and liver are important for removal and clearance of senescent RBCs.[1]

The RBC contains *hemoglobin,* which binds with oxygen in the lungs and transports it to the tissues. The rate of erythrocyte production increases when oxygen transport to tissues is impaired, and it decreases when tissues are hypertransfused or exposed to high oxygen tension. The oxygen affinity for hemoglobin is modulated primarily by the concentration of 2,3-diphosphoglycerate (2,3-DPG) and depends on the blood pH and body temperature. Erythrocytes are also vital for maintenance of acid-base balance because they transport carbon dioxide away from the tissues.[4]

Platelets. *Platelets,* or *thrombocytes,* are the smallest of the formed elements of the blood. A normal platelet count ranges from 150,000 to 400,000 per mm^3 of blood. Platelets are created by hematopoietic stem cells in response to thrombopoietin, a hormone produced by the liver that stimulates megakaryocytes

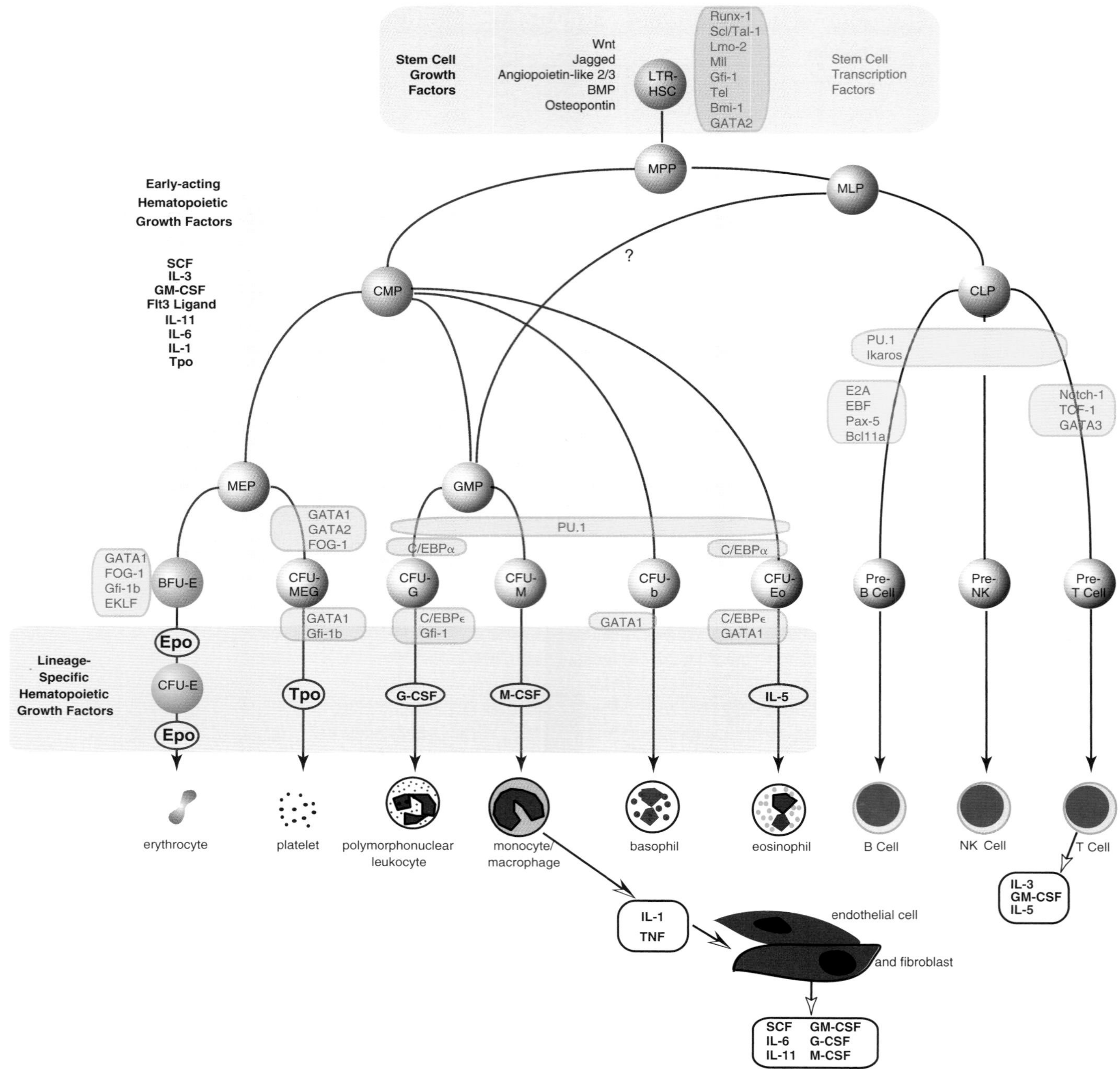

Fig. 17.1 This figure illustrates the hierarchical relationships of multipotent hematopoietic stem cells, progenitors, and mature cells of the myelopoietic, erythrocyte, and platelet lineages together with major growth factors, cytokines, and their actions. The involved growth factors and cytokines have overlapping actions during hematopoietic differentiation, as indicated, and, for most lineages, optimal development requires a combination of early-acting and late-acting factors (From Sieff CA, Zon LI. Anatomy and physiology of hemotopoiesis. In: Orkin S, Fisher D, Look AT, et al. eds. *Nathan and Oski's Hematology of Infancy and Childhood.* 8th ed. Philadelphia: Elsevier; 2015.)

to become platelets. Platelets have a lifespan of 8 to 12 days, but they may be used more rapidly if there are vascular injuries or clotting stimuli. Two-thirds of the platelets circulate in the blood. The spleen stores the remaining one-third and may become enlarged if excess or rapid platelet removal occurs. In patients who have had a splenectomy, 100% of the platelets remain in circulation.[1,5]

Platelets are the first responders in the clotting response, and they form a platelet plug that temporarily repairs an injured vessel. Platelets also release mediators that are necessary for completion of clotting. These mediators include histamine and serotonin, which contribute to vasospasm; adenosine diphosphate, which assists platelet adhesion and aggregation; and calcium and phospholipids, which are

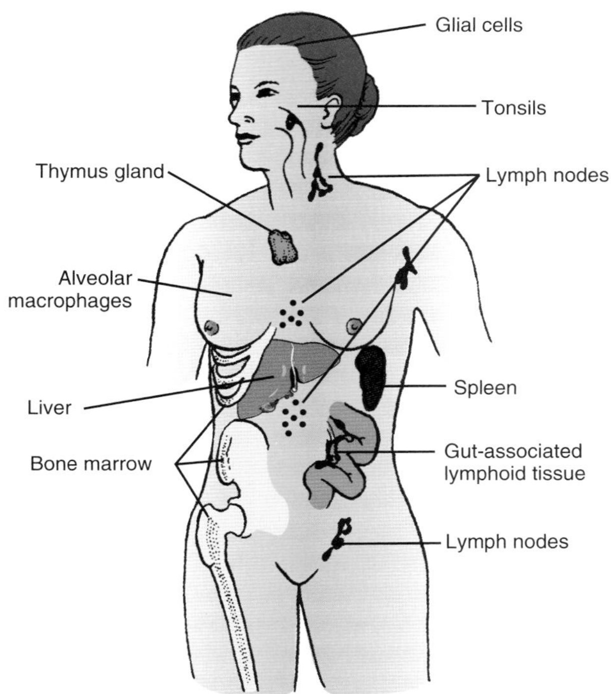

Organ	Key Functions
Bone marrow	Site of production for all hematopoietic cells.
Liver	The liver produces clotting factors, produces bile from RBC breakdown, and detoxifies many substances in the blood; its proper functioning is essential for normal hemostasis and metabolism. The liver filters and stores blood in addition to its many other metabolic functions.
Lymph nodes	Storage site for lymphocytes. Part of the continuous lymphatic system that filters foreign matter.
Spleen	The spleen is a highly vascular organ involved in the production of lymphocytes; the filtering and destruction of erythrocytes; the filtering and trapping of foreign matter, including bacteria and viruses; and the storage of blood. Although it is not necessary for survival, the spleen plays an important role in hemostasis and protection against infection.
Thymus gland	The thymus gland and lymph nodes are also part of the hematopoietic system; they are primarily involved in immunologic functions.
Tonsils, glial cells, alveolar macrophages, gut-associated lymphoid tissue	Lymphoid tissue responsive to antigens passing the initial barrier defenses, and possessing some inflammatory properties.

Fig. 17.2 Hematopoietic organs and their functions. *RBC,* Red blood cell. (Modified from Black JM, Hawks JH, eds. *Medical-Surgical Nursing: Clinical Management for Positive Outcomes*. 8th ed. Philadelphia: Saunders Elsevier; 2009.)

necessary for clotting.[5] During circulation, platelets also may adhere to roughened or sheared surfaces, such as blood vessel walls or indwelling catheters. Platelets also play a role in immunity through wound repair and resolution of the inflammatory process.[6]

Leukocytes. *Leukocytes* (WBCs) are part of the innate immune system. The average number of total WBCs ranges from 5000 to 10,000 per mm^3 in the adult. Cells vary in appearance, function, storage site, and lifespan. Specific characteristics of WBC development and life cycle are shown in Table 17.3.

Leukocytes are released into the bloodstream for transport to the tissues, where they perform specific functions.[7] WBCs play a key role in the defense against infectious organisms and foreign antigens. They produce and transport factors such as antibodies that are vital in maintaining immunity. Numbers of WBCs are increased in circumstances of inflammation, tissue injury, allergy, or invasion of pathogenic organisms. Their numbers are diminished in states of malnutrition, advancing age, and immune disease.[8]

WBCs are classified according to their structure (granulocytes or agranulocytes), their function (phagocytes or immunocytes), and their affinity for certain dyes. The *granulocytes* (or *polymorphonuclear leukocytes*) include neutrophils, eosinophils, and basophils, all of which function in phagocytosis.[7,9] When the reference to granulocytes is made, neutrophils is what is often meant. The *agranulocytes* consist of *monocytes and macrophages* (phagocytes) and *lymphocytes* (immunocytes).[7,9]

Neutrophils. Neutrophils are the most numerous of the granulocytes, constituting 54% to 62% of the WBC differential count.[9] Neutrophils are the "first responders" to sites of infection or inflammation. The *differential count* measures the percentage of each type of WBC present in the venous blood sample. These cells are divided into segmented neutrophils, in which filaments in the cell give the nuclei an appearance of having lobes, and band neutrophils, which are immature and have a thicker or U-shaped nucleus. Normally, band neutrophils constitute only about 3% to 5% of WBCs. The phrase *a shift to the left* refers to an increased number of "bands," or band neutrophils, compared with mature neutrophils on a complete blood count (CBC) report. The presence of bands generally indicates an acute bacterial infectious process that draws on the WBC reserves in the bone marrow and causes less mature forms to be released. Similarly, a *shift to the right* indicates an increased number of circulating mature cells and may be associated with liver disease, Down's syndrome, or megaloblastic or pernicious anemia.[9]

The survival time of neutrophils is short. Once released from the bone marrow, they circulate in the blood for less than 24 hours before migrating to the tissues, where they live for another few days. When serious infection is present, neutrophils may live only hours as they phagocytize infectious organisms.[9] Because of this short lifespan, medications that affect rapidly multiplying cells (e.g., chemotherapeutic agents) quickly decrease the neutrophil count and alter the patient's ability to fight infection.

Neutrophils exert their lethal effects against bacteria and foreign invaders through phagocytosis and the release of neutrophil elastase and cathepsin G, which are proteases that activate cytokines that kill organisms. Neutrophils are also responsible for ingesting cellular debris and dead tissue. Certain inherited immunodeficiency diseases, such as chronic granulomatosis disease (CGD), lack the enzyme nicotinamide adenine

TABLE 17.3 Overview of Leukocytes

Cell Type	Characteristics	Development and Migration	Lifespan
Granulocytes			
Neutrophils or segmented neutrophils and "bands"	Large granules and horseshoe-shaped nuclei that differentiate and become multilobed Bands are immature neutrophils that have an unsegmented nucleus	Mature in the bone marrow. Maturing granulocytes that are no longer dividing accumulate as a reserve in the bone marrow. Normally, about a 5-day supply is present in the bone marrow. In the adult, neutrophils make up 50%-80% of the total WBC count. A large number of bands in the WBC count can indicate infection. Granulocyte colony-stimulating factor (G-CSF) or granulocyte-macrophage stimulating factor (GM-CSF) are cytokines responsible for the differentiation of progenitor cells to neutrophils. There are 30–40 times more neutrophils present in the marrow than there are in circulation.	Average of 12 h in the circulation About 2-3 days in the tissues
Eosinophils	Have large, round granules that contain red-staining basic mucopolysaccharides and multilobed purple-blue nuclei	Eosinophils increase in reaction to a foreign protein such as parasitic infection or cancer. Eosinophils comprise 0%-2% of the WBC count.	Unknown
Basophils	Coarse blue granules conceal the segmented nucleus Granules contain histamine, heparin, and acid mucopolysaccharides	Basophils are 0%-1% of the total WBC. Basophils release histamine during an allergic reaction.	Unknown
Agranulocytes			
Lymphocytes	Small cells with a large, round, deep-staining, single-lobed nucleus and very little cytoplasm Cytoplasm is slightly basophilic and stains pale blue	T lymphocytes constantly circulate, following a path from the blood, to the lymphatic tissue, through the lymphatic channels, and back to the blood through the thoracic duct. B lymphocytes are largely noncirculating; they remain mainly in the lymphoid tissue and may differentiate into plasma cells.	Lifespan varies Small populations of memory lymphocytes survive for many years Most T lymphocytes of the peripheral lymphatic tissue recirculate about every 10 h Mature plasma cells have a survival time of 2-3 days
Monocytes/ Macrophages	Monocytes are large mononucleated cells with a kidney-shaped nucleus Monocytes form the mononuclear phagocytic system	Macrophages are named for their tissue of origin (alveolar macrophages, etc.). Macrophages are important for phagocytizing pathogens, cellular debris, and dead tissue. They are considered the clean-up crew of the immune system.	Monocytes live 1-3 days in bone marrow and 8-72 h in blood Monocytes become macrophages once in the tissue and can live up to 80 days
Natural killer (NK) cells	Natural killer cells are specialized lymphocytes that provide rapid responses to virus-infected cells or cancer cells, promoting rapid immune reaction	Arise from the lymphoid system.	Comprise 10% of circulating lymphocytes

WBC, White blood cell.

dinucleotide phosphate (NADPH) oxidase, which is produced by the granules of neutrophils and is responsible for killing infectious organisms. People with this condition have multiple infections over their lifetime from organisms, including unusual infections cause by aspergillus and enteric bacteria.

Eosinophils. Eosinophils are larger than neutrophils and make up 1% to 3% of the WBC count.[1,9] They are important in the defense against allergens and parasites and are thought to be involved in the detoxification of foreign proteins. Eosinophils are found largely in the tissues of the skin, lungs, and gastrointestinal tract. Eosinophils respond to chemotactic mechanisms that trigger them to participate in phagocytosis, but they also contain bactericidal substances and lysosomal enzymes that aid in the destruction of invading organisms.

Basophils. The basophil has large granules that contain heparin, serotonin, and histamine. They participate in the body's inflammatory and allergic responses by releasing these substances. Basophils, which constitute less than 1% of the WBC differential, play an important role in acute systemic allergic reactions and inflammatory responses.[9]

Monocytes. Monocytes are the largest of the leukocytes and constitute 1% to 10% of the WBC differential.[1,9] Once they migrate from the bloodstream into the tissues, monocytes mature into tissue macrophages, which are powerful phagocytes. Monocytes are the scavengers of the immune system. They phagocytose debris, dead tissue and cells and destroy cancer cells. In the lung, these tissue macrophages are alveolar macrophages; in the liver, Kupffer cells; and in connective tissue, histiocytes. Like eosinophils, macrophages contain lysosomal enzymes and bactericidal substances. When activated by antigens, macrophages secrete substances called monokines that act as chemical communicators between the cells involved in the immune response. Although monocytes may circulate for only 36 hours, they can survive for months or even years as tissue macrophages.[9] A rare genetic disorder called MonoMAC syndrome causes people to have a low monocyte count. This disorder puts them at risk for lifetime infections and leukemia.

Lymphocytes. Lymphocytes are derived from lymphocytic precursor cells and are made of the B and T lymphocytes, as well as the natural killer (NK) cells. In the adult, approximately 25% to 33% of the total WBCs are lymphocytes.[1,9] These cells are part of the adaptive immune system. Lymphocytes circulate in and out of tissues and may live for days or years, depending on the type. They contribute to the body's defense against microorganisms, but they are also essential for tumor immunity (surveillance for abnormal cells), delayed hypersensitivity reactions, autoimmune diseases, and foreign tissue rejection. Lymphocytes are responsible for specific immune responses and participate in two types of immunity: *humoral immunity,* which is mediated by B lymphocytes; and *cellular immunity,* which is mediated by T lymphocytes.

B and T lymphocytes originate in the bone marrow and are designated by markers on their surfaces. B lymphocytes mature in the lymph nodes, spleen, and other specialized lymphoid tissues such as the Peyer's patch in the intestines. B cells perform in antibody production or humoral immunity. The majority of T lymphocytes mature in the thymus. T cells assist B cells in humoral immunity and differentiate into different types: cytotoxic, helper, regulatory, and memory T cells. B lymphocytes are distinguished by CD19 and CD20 (CD, meaning cluster of differentiation), among others. T lymphocytes are designated by CD8 (cytotoxic T cells), CD4 (helper T cells), and multiple other immunosurface markers. NK cells are specialized lymphocytes that provide rapid responses to virus-infected cells or cancer cells, promoting rapid immune reaction. NK cells originate in the bone marrow, lymph nodes, spleen, tonsils, and thymus. NK cells are distinguished by the CD3 and CD56+ phenotype.

CHECK YOUR UNDERSTANDING

1. An 83-year-old patient is admitted to the critical care unit for severe pneumonia. The WBC is 26k µL. The patient also demonstrates a shift to the left on the CBC differential, which is indicative of an acute bacterial infection. Which of the following laboratory results would you expect to see?
   - A. Decreased number of basophils
   - B. Decreased number of eosinophils
   - C. Increased number of immature neutrophils (bands) compared to mature neutrophils
   - D. Increased number of mature neutrophils compared to immature neutrophils (bands)

Immune Anatomy

Immune activity involves an integrated, multilevel response against invading pathogens. It requires both WBCs of the hematopoietic system and the secondary hematopoietic organs, termed the *lymphoreticular system.* The lymphoreticular system consists of lymphoid tissue, lymphatic channels and nodes, and phagocytic cells that engulf and process foreign materials (Fig. 17.2).

The body's ability to resist and fight infection is called *immunity.* The human body is constantly exposed to normal and unusual microorganisms that are capable of causing disease. The healthy person's immune system recognizes potential pathogens and destroys them before tissue invasion occurs; however, the person with a dysfunctional immune system is at risk of overwhelming, life-threatening infection.

Immune Physiology

The immune response protects the body from disease by recognizing, processing, and destroying foreign invaders. It aids in the removal of damaged cells and defends the body against the proliferation of abnormal or malignant cells. The recognition of nonself molecules called *antigens* is the key triggering activity of the immune system. Microorganisms (e.g., bacteria, viruses, fungi, parasites), abnormal or mutated cells, transplanted cells, nonself protein molecules (e.g., vaccines), and nonhuman molecules (e.g., penicillin) can act as antigens. These antigens are detected by the body as foreign, or nonself, and are destroyed by immunological processes. The body's response to an antigen is determined by factors such as genetics, amount of antigen, and route of exposure. In autoimmunity, the body abnormally sees self as nonself, and an immune response is activated against those tissues. Autoimmunity can result from injury to tissues, infection, or malignancy, although in many cases, the cause is not known. An example of an autoimmune disease is systemic lupus erythematosus (SLE).[1,7]

An intact and healthy immune system consists of both natural (nonspecific) defenses and acquired (specific) defenses. *Innate immunity* refers to immunity that is present at birth. Monocytes/macrophages, neutrophils, and complement belong to the innate immune system. *Passive immunity* is that which is transferred from another person, as when maternal antibodies are transferred to the newborn through the placenta.[9] The nonspecific defenses are the first line of protection and include the processes of inflammation and phagocytosis. When nonspecific mechanisms fail to protect the body from invasion, the specific defenses of humoral and cellular immunity are put into action. *Adaptive immunity* is a term used when the body actively produces cells and mediators that result in destruction of the antigen.

Nonspecific Defenses. The body's nonspecific defenses consist of the physical and chemical barriers to invasion, the protective and repairing processes of inflammation and phagocytosis, and other substances that stimulate the body to fight back. The body's first line of defense against infection consists of physical and chemical barriers.

Epithelial surfaces. The epithelial surfaces are those that are exposed to the environment. Intact skin and mucous membranes provide a protective covering; they also secrete substances that have antimicrobial effects. For example, sweat glands produce a lysozyme, which is an antimicrobial enzyme; and sebaceous glands secrete sebum, which has antimicrobial and antifungal properties. The skin constantly exfoliates, a process that sloughs off bacterial and chemical hazards. These same epithelial surfaces are colonized by "normal" bacterial flora that protect the body from microorganisms by occupying space on the epithelium, preventing pathogen attachment.

Epithelial surfaces also have unique physical and chemical properties that protect them from pathogen invasion. For example, mucus and cilia work together to trap and remove harmful substances in the respiratory tract. The motility of the intestines maintains an even distribution of bacterial flora, thereby preventing overgrowth or invasion of pathogens, and promotes evacuation of harmful microbes. Chemical barriers to pathogenic entry include the unique pH of the skin and mucosa of the gastrointestinal and urinary tracts. This pH inhibits the growth of many microorganisms. Immunoglobulin (Ig)A (also called *secretory IgA*) and phagocytic cells are biological factors present in respiratory and gastrointestinal secretions. They are essential for destruction of particular pyogenic bacteria.[9,10]

Inflammation and phagocytosis. The second line of defense involves the processes of inflammation and phagocytosis. Inflammation is initiated by cellular injury, is necessary for tissue repair, and is harmful when uncontrolled. When cellular injury occurs, a process called *chemotaxis* generates both a mediator and a neutrophil response. Mediator substances (e.g., histamine, serotonin, kinins, lysosomal enzymes, prostaglandin, platelet-activating factor, clotting factors, and complement proteins) are released at the site of injury. These mediators cause vasodilation, increase blood flow, induce capillary permeability, and promote chemotaxis and phagocytosis by neutrophils. Inflammatory symptoms such as redness, heat, pain, and swelling are sequelae of these responses. *Complement* proteins enhance the antibody activity, phagocytosis, and inflammation.[9,10]

Neutrophils are attracted and migrate to areas of inflammation or bacterial invasion, where they ingest and kill invading microorganisms by phagocytosis. The inflammatory response is a rapid process initiated by granulocytes (i.e., neutrophils, basophils, and eosinophils) and macrophages. Granulocytes arrive within minutes after cellular injury. Once phagocytes have been attracted to an area by the release of mediators, a process called *opsonization* occurs, in which antibody and complement proteins attach to the target cell and enhance the phagocyte's ability to engulf the target cell. Once the bacteria have been engulfed, they are killed and digested within the cell by lysosomal enzymes. Exudate formation at the inflammatory site has three functions: dilute the toxins produced, deliver proteins and leukocytes to the site, and carry away toxins and debris.[9]

Infectious organisms that escape the local phagocytic responses may be engulfed and destroyed in a similar fashion by tissue macrophages within the lymphoreticular organs. The portal circulation of the spleen and liver filters most of the blood, removing infectious organisms before they infect tissues. In the lymphatic system, pathogenic substances are filtered by the lymph nodes and are phagocytized by tissue macrophages. Here, they may also stimulate immune responses by the lymphoid cells.

Other nonspecific defenses. Another nonspecific defensive activity is the release of cytokines and chemokines from WBCs, which are either proinflammatory, antiinflammatory, or both. These naturally occurring biological response modifiers, which include interleukins (ILs), tumor necrosis factor (TNF), colony-stimulating factors, monoclonal antibodies, and interferons (IFNs), mediate various interactions among immune system cells.[10] At least 30 human ILs exist. An example is IL-1, which is a proinflammatory cytokine. It is an endogenous pyrogen that increases body temperature in infection, thereby inhibiting the growth of temperature-sensitive pathogens. IL-1 also activates phagocytes and lymphocytes and acts as a growth factor for many cells. The IFNs have antitumor and antiviral activity and include 20 subtypes of IFN-alpha, two subtypes of IFN-beta, and IFN-gamma.

Through recombinant DNA technology, IFNs and other naturally occurring substances can be produced synthetically for the treatment of many disorders. IFNs, colony-stimulating factors, and monoclonal antibodies are some examples of biological therapies currently approved for the treatment of certain malignant disorders.[10]

CLINICAL JUDGMENT ACTIVITY

Identify disorders that may be associated with anemia in the critically ill patient. Determine assessment variables and nursing interventions in the management of the individual with symptomatic anemia.

Specific Defenses. *Specificity* refers to the finding that an immune response stimulates cells to develop immunity for a specific antigen. Two types of specific immune responses exist: humoral immunity and cell-mediated immunity. They are not mutually exclusive but act together to provide immunity.

Humoral immunity. Humoral immunity is mediated by B lymphocytes and involves the formation of antibodies (immunoglobulins) in response to specific antigens that bind to their receptor sites. Antigen binding activates the differentiation of B lymphocytes into plasma cells that produce specific antibodies in response to those antigens.[7] Five classes of immunoglobulins exist: IgG, IgM, IgA, IgD, and IgE. The clinical features and abnormalities associated with these immunoglobulins are described in Table 17.4.

TABLE 17.4 **Immunoglobulins**

Antibody	Description	Normal Value
IgG	Most abundant immunoglobulin Major influence with bacterial disease Crosses the placenta Coats microorganisms to enhance phagocytosis Activates complement	75% of total 500-1600 mg/dL
IgM	Primary immunoglobulin response to antigen, with levels increased by 7 days after exposure Present mostly in the intravascular space Causes antigenic agglutination and cell lysis via complement activation	10% of total 60-280 mg/dL
IgA	Found on mucosal surfaces of respiratory, GI, and GU systems, preventing antigen adherence Influential with bacteria and some viral organisms First antibody formed after exposure to antigen but rapidly diminishes as IgG increases Does not cross the placenta but passes to newborn through colostrum and breast milk Deficiency caused by congenital autosomal dominant or recessive disease or related to anticonvulsant use Deficiency (<5 mg/dL) manifests as chronic sinopulmonary infection	15% of total 90-450 mg/dL
IgD	Activates B lymphocytes to become plasma cells, which are the key immunoglobulin-producing cells	1% of total 0.5-3.0 mg/dL
IgE	Attaches to mast cells and basophils on epithelial surfaces and enhances release of histamine and other vasoactive mediators responsible for the "wheal and flare" reaction Important for allergic responses, inflammatory reactions, and parasitic infections	0.002% of total 0.01-0.04 mg/dL

GI, Gastrointestinal; *GU*, genitourinary.

Once antibodies have been synthesized and released, they bind to their specific antigen and form an antigen-antibody complex that activates phagocytosis and complement proteins. Antibodies cannot destroy pathogens by themselves, but they mark the antigen for other cells to kill the pathogen. This humoral response is regulated by the activity of T lymphocytes. Helper T cells promote B-lymphocyte activity and the production of antibodies, whereas suppressor T cells reduce the humoral response. Dendritic cells present the processed antigens to the lymphocytes, which act as a messenger between the innate and adaptive immune systems and stimulate the growth and differentiation of B and T lymphocytes.

The body generates both primary and secondary humoral responses. In the *primary response,* antigens that have evaded the nonspecific defenses are engulfed and processed by macrophages. In this first exposure, antibodies of the IgM subtype appear and predominate, and IgG appears later. During this primary response, the immunoglobulins develop an immunological memory for antigens. Then, when any subsequent exposure to the antigen occurs, a quicker, stronger, and longer-lasting IgG-mediated *secondary response* occurs. IgG antibodies predominate and may be detectable in the serum for decades.[7]

Adaptive or cell-mediated immunity. Adaptive immunity is mediated by T lymphocytes and is a more delayed reaction than the humoral response. Cell-mediated immunity occurs only when there is direct contact with sensitized lymphocytes. It is important in viral, fungal, and intracellular infections and is the mechanism involved in transplant rejection and recognition of neoplastic cells.

Cell-mediated immunity is initiated by macrophage recognition of nonself (foreign) materials. The macrophages trap, process, and present such materials to T lymphocytes, which then migrate to the site of the antigen, where they complete antigen destruction. Once contact is made with a specific antigen, the T lymphocytes differentiate into helper/inducer T cells, suppressor T cells, and cytotoxic killer cells. Although these T cells are microscopically identical, they can be distinguished by proteins present on the cell surface called CDs. Helper T cells (also known as CD4 cells because they carry a CD4 marker) enhance the humoral immune response by stimulating B cells to differentiate and produce antibodies.[7] Suppressor T cells reduce and suppress the humoral and cell-mediated responses. The ratio of helper/suppressor T cells is normally 2:1, and an alteration in this ratio may cause disease.[15] For example, a depressed ratio (a decrease of helper T cells in relation to suppressor T cells) is found in individuals with HIV, whereas a higher ratio (a decrease in suppressor T cells in relation to helper T cells) is a feature of an autoimmune disease.

Cytotoxic or killer T cells (CD8 marker) participate directly in the destruction of antigens by binding to and altering the intracellular environment, which ultimately destroys the cell. Killer T cells also release cytotoxic substances into the antigen cell that cause cell lysis. Killer T cells additionally provide the body with immunosurveillance capabilities that monitor for abnormal cells or tissue. This mechanism is responsible for the rejection of transplanted tissue and the destruction of single malignant cells.[11]

Another important component of the adaptive immune system is the major histocompatibility complex (MHC) or proteins. The MHCs are important for recognition of self versus nonself cells. There are two types of MHCs: MHC Class I and MHC Class II. MHC Class I transports viral peptides within an infected cell to the surface of the dendritic cell. As the dendritic cell passes through the thymus, immature T cells will differentiate into cytotoxic (CD8) T cells. The CD8 T cells in turn now recognize the virus and attack it. MHC Class II proteins work the same as the MHC Class I proteins but recognize antigens that are floating in the body's fluids that need to be destroyed.

LIFESPAN CONSIDERATIONS

Older Adults

- Immunosenescence refers to changes in the immune system associated with aging. Immunosenescence is associated with increased inflammation (known as inflammaging),[12] increased risk of infection, malignancy, and autoimmune disorders.
- Older adults have a decreased percentage of marrow space occupied by hematopoietic tissue, which may result in ineffective erythropoiesis, especially after blood loss.
- The number of T and B cells produced is decreased. The thymus starts to decline in middle age along with decreased function of T cells, which can delay hypersensitivity and increase risk of infection. Antibody production from the B cells declines, and the ability of the B and T cells to interact together to respond to infection and immunizations is limited.
- Autoimmune antibodies appear, increasing the risk of autoimmune disorders.
- Possible increased levels of IgA and IgG increase the risk of infection.
- Iron deficiency anemia may be observed in patients with occult gastrointestinal bleeding or underlying malignancy.
- Changes in bone marrow reserve, immune function, lean body mass, hepatic function, and renal function contribute to the challenges of caring for this rapidly expanding, vulnerable population.

Pregnant People

- Although pregnancy does not confer generalized immunosuppression, there is a dampening of the inflammatory response as well as a decrease in cytotoxic adaptive immunity.[13] This is to prevent maternal rejection of the fetus.
- Further, the trophoblast cells of the embryo protect the fetus from destruction by the maternal immune system.[14]
- The neutrophil count begins to increase in the second month of pregnancy and plateaus in the second or third trimester.
- The platelet count declines steadily as the pregnancy progresses but remains in the normal range.
- The major hematologic changes during pregnancy include expanded plasma volume, physiologic anemia, mild neutrophilia in some individuals, and a prothrombotic state that does not require intervention.
- Iron deficiency is common in pregnancy because of the increased demand for iron.
- Pregnancy loss before 20 weeks' gestation affects 15% to 20% of pregnant individuals in the United States.[13] Approximately 60% of miscarriages are attributed to genetic abnormalities of the embryo, but the rest are attributed to implant failure. It is unclear if there is an immunological reason behind the implant failures.
- Obstetrical complications (e.g., placenta previa, maintained fetus or placenta, abruptio placenta, gestational thrombocytopenia, preeclampsia/eclampsia, HELLP [hemolysis, elevated liver enzymes, and low platelet count] syndrome) may lead to disseminated intravascular coagulation (DIC), infection, coagulation issues, renal failure, and liver failure.

Hemostasis

Hemostasis is a physiological process involving platelets, blood proteins (clotting factors), and vasculature. This process involves the formation of blood clots to stop bleeding from injured vessels and natural anticoagulant and fibrinolytic systems to limit clot formation. Many substances that may activate the clotting system, including collagen, proteases, and bacterial endotoxins, are released during tissue destruction. The three physiological mechanisms that trigger clotting in the body are tissue injury, vessel injury, and the presence of a foreign body in the bloodstream. When one of these trigger factors is present, a series of physical events occurs that results in a fibrin clot.

Although the events of hemostasis are sequential, they require integration of components from the hematopoietic and coagulation systems. Within seconds after injury, platelets are attracted and adhere to the site of injury. The activated platelets then undergo changes in shape to expose receptors on their surfaces. RBCs increase the rate of platelet adherence by facilitating migration of platelets to the site and by liberating adenosine diphosphate (ADP), which enables platelets to stick to the exposed tissue (collagen). The exposed receptors on the activated platelet surfaces are capable of binding fibrinogen, an essential component underlying platelet aggregation. Serotonin and histamine are released by the adhered platelets and cause immediate constriction of the injured vessel to lessen bleeding. Vasoconstriction is followed by vasodilation, bringing the necessary cellular products of the inflammatory response to the site. With minor vessel injury, *primary hemostasis* is temporarily achieved with platelet plugs, usually within seconds. During *secondary hemostasis*, the platelet plug is solidified with fibrin, an end product of the coagulation pathway, and requires several minutes to reach completion[5,9] (Fig. 17.3).

Coagulation Pathway. In the classic theory, coagulation is viewed as occurring through two distinct pathways, *intrinsic* and *extrinsic*, that share a common "final" pathway, the formation of insoluble fibrin.[5,9] The in vitro model (Fig. 17.4A) illustrates the classic theory of coagulation.

Both pathways begin with an initiating event and involve a cascading sequence of clotting factor activation precipitated by a preceding reaction. The soluble clotting factors become insoluble fibrin. When blood is exposed to subendothelial collagen or is "injured," factor XII is activated, which initiates coagulation via the *intrinsic pathway*. In the *extrinsic pathway*, tissue injury precipitates release of a substance known as *tissue factor*, which activates factor VII. Factor VII is key in initiating blood coagulation, and the two pathways intersect at the activation of factor X.[5,9] Both coagulation pathways lead to a *final common pathway* of clot formation, retraction, and fibrinolysis.

In patients, coagulation occurs via the in vivo model (Fig. 17.4B). In patients, tissue factor is the major factor for initiating coagulation (Fig. 17.4B). The coagulation factors are plasma proteins that circulate as inactive enzymes, and most are synthesized in the liver. Vitamin K is necessary for synthesis of factors II, VII, IX, and X and proteins C and S (anticoagulation factors). For this reason, liver disease and vitamin K deficiency are commonly associated with impaired hemostasis.[5]

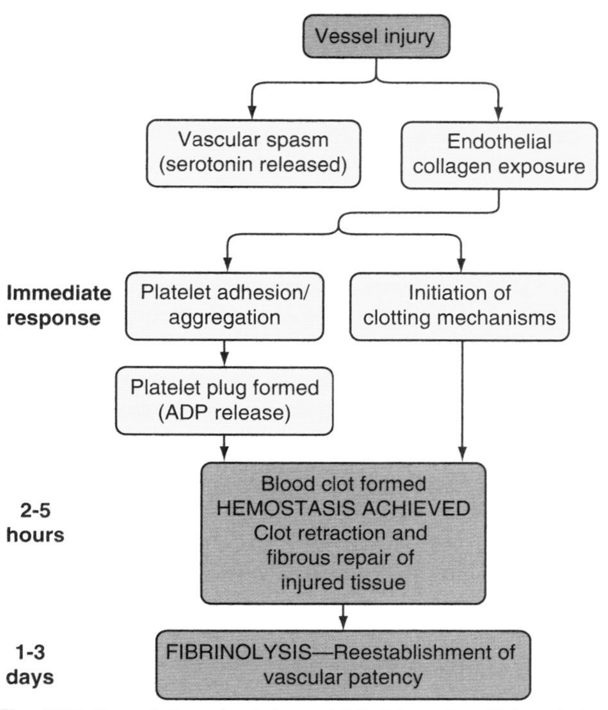

Fig. 17.3 Coagulation physiology. *ADP*, Adenosine diphosphate.

Coagulation Antagonists and Clot Lysis. Activation of the clotting factors, inhibition of these activated clotting factors, and production of circulating anticoagulant proteins maintain the balance of the coagulation processes. Normal vascular endothelium is smooth and intact, preventing the collagen exposure that initiates the intrinsic clotting pathway. Rapid blood flow dilutes and disperses clotting factors. Clotting factors that are not contained within a formed clot are filtered and removed from circulation by the liver. Several plasma proteins, including antiplasmin and antithrombin III, are present to localize clotting at the site of injury. When coagulation protein levels are deficient, clotting may become inappropriately widespread, such as in disseminated intravascular coagulation (DIC). The most potent anticoagulant forces are the fibrin threads, which absorb 85% to 90% of thrombin during clot formation and antithrombin III, which inactivates thrombin that is not contained within the clot. Heparin, which is produced in small quantities by basophils and tissue mast cells, acts as a potent anticoagulant. Heparin combines with antithrombin III to increase the effectiveness of the latter. This complex removes several of the activated coagulation factors from the blood.[5]

Once blood vessel integrity has been restored via hemostasis, blood flow must be reestablished. This goal is accomplished by the fibrinolytic system, which breaks down clots *(lysis)* and

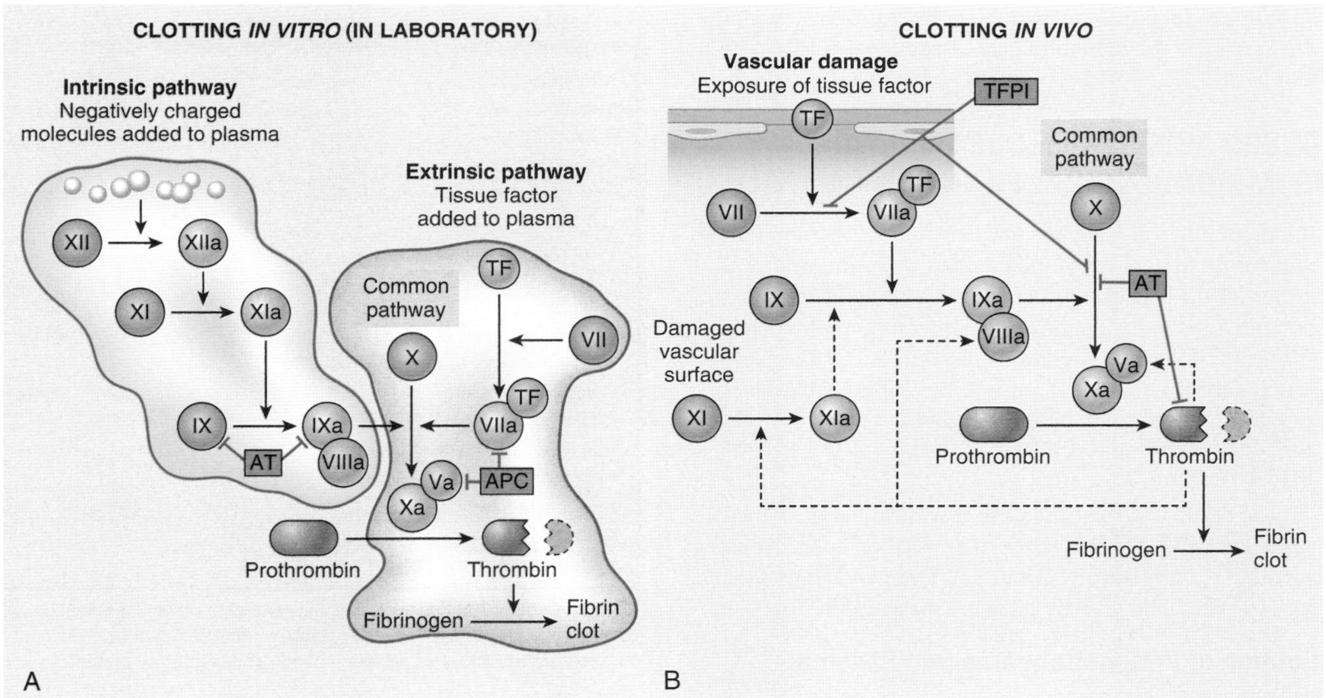

Fig. 17.4 Coagulation pathways. **A**, Classic theory of coagulation in vitro illustrating separate intrinsic and extrinsic pathways. **B**, Coagulation in vivo; clotting initiated by release of tissue factor *(TF)*. *APC*, Antigen-presenting cell; *AT*, antithrombin; *TFPI*, tissue factor pathway inhibitor. (From McCance KL. Structure and function of the hematological system. In: McCance KL, Huether SE, eds. *Pathophysiology: The Biologic Basis for Disease in Adults and Children*. 8th ed. St. Louis, MO: Mosby; 2019:890-925.)

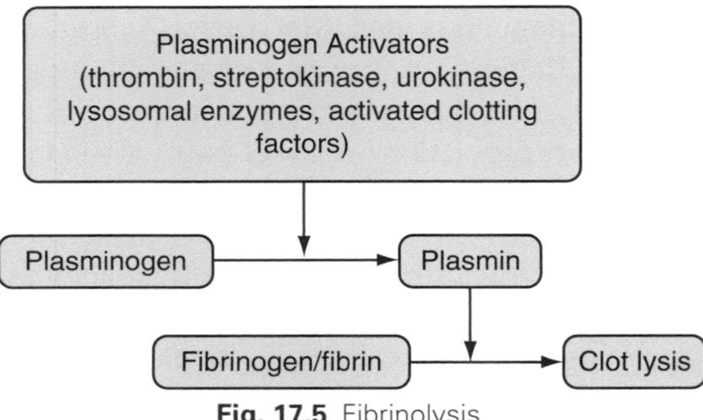

Fig. 17.5 Fibrinolysis.

removes them. *Fibrinolysis* occurs 1 to 3 days after clot formation and is mediated by plasmin, an enzyme that digests fibrinogen and fibrin (Fig. 17.5). The plasma protein plasminogen is the inactive form of plasmin. It is incorporated into the blood clot as the clot forms and cannot initiate clot lysis until it is activated. Substances capable of activating plasminogen include tissue plasminogen activator, thrombin, fibrin, factor XII, lysosomal enzymes, and urokinase.[5] Thrombin and plasmin are key for maintaining the balance between coagulation and lysis. Fibrinolysis is active within the microcirculation, where it maintains the patency of the capillary beds. Larger vessels contain less plasminogen activator, a characteristic that may predispose them to clot formation.

When plasmin digests fibrinogen, fragments known as *fibrin split products,* or *fibrin degradation products,* are produced and function as potent anticoagulants. In cases of excessive clotting and clot lysis, these molecules contribute to the coagulopathy. Fibrin split products are not normally present in the circulation but are seen in some hematological disorders and with thrombolytic therapy.

FOCUSED ASSESSMENT OF HEMATOLOGICAL AND IMMUNOLOGICAL FUNCTION

An understanding of both normal and disrupted hematological and immunological system activities is paramount to good assessment skills and use of therapeutic interventions. Nursing assessment involves evaluation of risk factors for hematological and immunological alterations, assessment of the patient's concerns, performance of a focused physical examination, and interpretation of pertinent laboratory tests.

Patient History

A complete health history includes an assessment of prior medical and surgical problems, allergies, use of medication or homeopathic remedies, and family history. Conditions that may indicate hematological or immunological disorders are presented in Box 17.1.

Evaluation of Patient Concerns and Physical Examination

Inspect the patient's general appearance. Ask the patient if they have had altered sleep/rest patterns, increased fatigue, acute illness, chronic disease, or inability to complete daily activities without fatigue. The most common manifestations of either hematological or immunological disease include altered oxygenation, bleeding or clotting abnormalities, infection, or inflammation. The most important assessment parameters for detection of anemia, bleeding, and infection are shown in Table 17.5. Transplantation may be indicated for a variety of hematological or immunological disorders (see Transplant Considerations box).

BOX 17.1 Conditions That May Indicate Hematologic or Immunological Problems[a]

Hematologic Disorders

- Alcohol use disorder
- Allergies
- Anemia of any kind
- Benzene exposure (gasoline, dry cleaning chemicals)
- Blood clots
- Delayed wound healing
- Excess bleeding
- Jaundice
- Liver disease
- Medications: allopurinol, antibiotics, anticoagulants, anticonvulsants, antidiabetics, antidysrhythmics, antiinflammatory agents, aspirin derivatives, chemotherapy, histamine blockers
- Neoplastic disease
- Pertinent surgical procedures: hepatic resection, partial or total gastric resection, splenectomy, tumor removal, valve replacement
- Pesticide exposure
- Poor nutrition
- Previous transfusion of blood or blood products
- Radiation: occupational, environmental
- Recurrent infection
- Renal disease
- Substance use disorder

Immunological Disorders

- Alcohol use disorder
- Allergies
- Anorexia or weight loss
- Bone tenderness or joint pain
- Delayed wound healing
- Diabetes mellitus
- Diarrhea
- Fever
- Liver disease
- Lymphadenopathy
- Medications: antibiotics, antiinflammatory agents, corticosteroids, chemotherapy, immunosuppressives
- Nausea and vomiting
- Neoplastic disease
- Night sweats
- Pertinent surgeries: hepatic resection, lung resection, small bowel resection, splenectomy, tumor removal
- Pesticide exposure
- Poor nutrition
- Previous transfusion of blood or blood products
- Radiation: occupational, environmental
- Recurrent infections
- Renal disease
- Substance use disorder

[a] This chart does not correlate specific risks with particular disease conditions because many overlap. History information should be supplemented with physical examination and laboratory test information.

TABLE 17.5 Physical Assessment for Hematological and Immune Disorders

Body System	Anemia	Bleeding	Infection[a]
Neurological	Difficulty concentrating Dizziness Fatigue Somnolence Vertigo	*Bleeding into brain (cerebrum, cerebellum):* alteration in level of consciousness, focal deficits such as unequal pupils or motor movement, headache Bleeding into potential spaces	*Encephalitis:* confusion, lethargy, difficulty arousing, headache, visual difficulty or photosensitivity, nausea, hypertension *Meningitis:* lethargy and somnolence, confusion, nuchal rigidity
Head and neck	Headache Tinnitus	*Bleeding into eye:* visual disturbances, frank hemorrhagic conjunctiva, bloody tears *Bleeding into nasopharyngeal area:* nasal stuffiness, epistaxis *Oral bleeding:* petechiae of buccal mucosa or gums, hemorrhagic oral lesions *Bleeding into subcutaneous tissue of head or neck:* enlarged, bruised areas, raccoon's eyes, bruising	*Conjunctivitis:* reddened conjunctiva, excess tearing of eye, puslike exudates from eye, blurred vision, swelling of eyelid, eye itching *Otitis media:* earache, difficulty hearing, itching inner ear, ear drainage *Sinusitis:* discolored nasal mucus, nasal congestion, face pain, eye pain, blurred vision *Oropharyngeal:* oral ulcerations or plaques, halitosis, reddened gums, abnormal papillae of the tongue, sore throat, difficulty swallowing *Lymphadenitis:* swollen neck lymph glands, tender lymph glands, a lump left when patient swallows
Pulmonary	Air hunger Anxiety Dyspnea Tachypnea	*Alveolar bleeding:* crackles on breath sound assessment, alveolar fluid on radiography, low oxygen saturation *Upper airway bleeding* (e.g., trachea, bronchi): hemoptysis *Pleural space bleeding:* decreased breath sounds, unequal chest excursion	*Bronchitis:* persistent cough, sputum production, gurgles in upper airways, wheezes in upper airways, hypoxemia and/or hypercapnia *Pneumonia:* chest discomfort pronounced with inspiration, persistent cough, sputum production, diminished breath sounds, crackles or gurgles, asymmetrical chest wall movement, labored breathing, nasal flaring with breathing, hypoxemia *Pleurisy:* chest discomfort pronounced with inspiration, sides of chest more painful, usually unilateral discomfort, splinting with deep breaths
Cardiovascular	Clubbing of digits Heart murmur Hypotension Nail beds pale Capillary refill slow Peripheral pulses weak and thready Tachycardia	*Pericardial bleeding:* dyspnea, chest discomfort, hypotension, narrow pulse pressure, muffled heart sounds, increased jugular venous distension *Vascular bleeding:* visible blood, hematoma, or bruising of subcutaneous tissue	*Myocarditis:* dysrhythmias, murmurs or gallops, elevated jugular venous pulsations, weak thready pulses, hypotension, point of maximal impulse shifted laterally *Pericarditis:* constant aching discomfort in the chest unrelieved by rest or nitrates; pericardial rub; muffled heart sounds
Gastrointestinal	Abdominal pain Constipation Splenic enlargement, tenderness	*Upper GI bleeding:* hematemesis, vomiting (coffee-ground appearance) *Lower GI bleeding:* melena *Hepatic or splenic rupture:* acute abdominal pain, abdominal distension, rapid-onset hypotension with hematocrit and hemoglobin *Hemorrhagic pancreatitis:* acute abdominal pain, abdominal distension, hypotension with hematocrit and hemoglobin	*Gastritis:* nausea, vomiting within 30 min after eating, heme-positive emesis, gastric pain that is initially improved by eating *Infectious diarrhea:* more than six loose stools per day, clay-colored or foul-smelling stools, abdominal cramping or distension *Cholelithiasis/pancreatitis:* epigastric pain, intolerance to high-fat meal, clay-colored stools, nausea and vomiting, hyperglycemia, hypocalcemia, ↓ albumin, ↑ lipase and amylase *Hepatitis:* jaundice, right upper quadrant discomfort, hepatomegaly, elevated transaminases and bilirubin, fatty food intolerances, nausea and vomiting, diarrhea
Genitourinary	—	*Bladder spasms with distended bladder* Hematuria	*Urethritis:* painful urination, difficulty urinating, genitourinary itching *Cystitis:* small frequent urination, feeling of bladder fullness *Nephritis:* flank discomfort, oliguria, protein in urine *Vaginitis:* itching or vaginal discharge
Musculoskeletal	Muscle fatigue Muscle weakness	Altered joint mobility Painful or swollen joints Warm, painful, swollen muscles	*Arthritis:* joint discomfort, swollen and warm joints *Myositis:* aching muscles, weakness
Dermatological	Cyanosis Jaundice (hemolytic anemia) Pallor Poor skin turgor Skin cool to touch	Bleeding from line insertion sites, puncture wounds, skin tears Ecchymosis Petechiae	*Superficial skin infection:* rashes, itching, raised and/or discolored skin lesions, open-draining skin lesions *Cellulitis:* redness, warmth and swelling of subcutaneous tissue area, radiating pain from area toward middle of body
Hematological/immunological	—	—	*Bacteremia:* positive blood culture

[a]Signs and symptoms presented in this chart are unique features of each process and do not include the common constitutional signs and symptoms seen with all infections, such as fever, chills, malaise, leukocytosis, positive tissue culture for microorganisms, or increased erythrocyte sedimentation rate.
GI, Gastrointestinal.

TRANSPLANT CONSIDERATIONS

Hematopoietic Stem Cell

Indications

Hematopoietic stem cell transplantation (HSCT) may be considered as treatment for a variety of hematological or immunological diseases in which the stem cells do not function properly. These include conditions of abnormal RBC production (e.g., sickle cell disease), hematological malignancies (e.g., leukemia, lymphoma, myeloma, myelodysplastic syndrome), lack of normal blood cell production (e.g., aplastic anemia), and immune system disorders (e.g., severe combined immunodeficiency syndrome). Transplantation of stem cells may help correct the underlying physiological problem. HSCT is classified by the source of the donor stem cells: bone marrow, peripheral blood stem cells, or umbilical cord blood.[1-4]

Categories

Allogeneic transplant: patient receives stem cells from a sibling, parent, or unrelated donor (not immunologically identical).

Reduced intensity or non-myeloablative transplant: lower doses of chemotherapy or radiation are administered prior to allogenic transplantation. This may also be called a minitransplant.

Autologous transplant: patient receives his or her own stem cells after treatment with chemotherapy or radiation.

Syngeneic transplant: patient receives stem cells from his or her identical twin (immunologically identical match).

Tandem transplant: type of autologous transplant in which high-dose chemotherapy and stem cell transplantation are performed in two sequential courses.

Tissue Typing

Proteins on the surface of leukocytes, called human leukocyte antigens (HLAs), are present on both donor and recipient cells—this is the basis of recognition of self versus nonself. HLA-matching between donor and recipient is essential for determining an appropriate donor and ensuring the new cells take root in the bone marrow and start making new cells, a process known as engraftment. Even with closely HLA matched cells, the donor cells can still recognize the patient's organs and tissues as foreign and destroy them in a process known as graft-versus-host disease (GVHD). In addition, the patient's immune system may recognize the donor stem cells as foreign and destroy them; this is known as graft rejection. The higher the number of matching HLAs, the greater the chance that the transplant will be successful. Following the transplant, engraftment occurs when stem cells repopulate the bone marrow and are able to reconstitute the immune system. This usually occurs 2 to 4 weeks after transplant. Patients have complete blood counts checked frequently. A steady increase in white blood cells and absolute neutrophil count indicates engraftment is occurring.[1,2]

Complications

Complications occur at any time during the HSCT continuum, from the pre-engraftment stage to day 30 after transplantation; early after engraftment, usually between days 30 and 100; and late after transplantation, more than 100 days after transplantation of donor stem cells. HSCT patients are susceptible to severe infections due to their profoundly immunocompromised state resulting from their disease process, bone marrow ablation in preparation for transplantation, and posttransplantation immunosuppressive therapy.

Complications include bacterial, fungal, protozoal, or viral infections; bleeding; sepsis; GVHD (acute or chronic); sinusoidal obstructive syndrome (previously called hepatic veno-occlusive disease); weight gain; painful hepatomegaly; jaundice; and respiratory complications. Short-term side effects include nausea, vomiting, fatigue, anorexia, mucositis, alopecia, and skin reactions. Potential long-term risks related to pretransplantation chemotherapy and radiation include infertility, cataracts, new cancers, and damage to major organs.

References

1. Balassa K, Danby R, Rocha V. Haematopoietic stem cell transplants: principles and indications. *Br J Hosp Med (Lond)*. 2019;80(1):33–39. https://doi.org/10.12968/hmed.2019.80.1.33.
2. Lee JY, Hong SH. Hematopoietic stem cells and their roles in tissue regeneration. *Int J Stem Cells*. 2020;13(1):1–12. https://doi.org/10.15283/ijsc19127.
3. Khaddour K, Hana CK, Mewawalla P. Hematopoietic Stem Cell Transplantation. In: *StatPearls*. Treasure Island, FL: StatPearls Publishing; 2023. [Internet] https://www.ncbi.nlm.nih.gov/books/NBK536951/#_NBK536951_pubdet_.
4. National Cancer Institute, National Institutes of Health, Stem Cell Transplants in Cancer Treatment. https://www.cancer.gov/about-cancer/treatment/types/stem-cell-transplant. Updated October 3, 2023, Accessed December 20, 2023.

Chelsea Sooy, BSN, RN, CCTC
Melissa A. Kelley, RN, CPTC

Diagnostic Tests

Hematological and immunological abnormalities are usually diagnosed using the patient's clinical profile in conjunction with a few key laboratory tests. The most invasive microscopic examinations of the bone marrow or lymph nodes (i.e., biopsy studies) are done only if laboratory tests are inconclusive or an abnormality in cellular maturation is suspected (i.e., aplastic anemia, leukemia, or lymphoma).

The first screening diagnostic tests performed are a CBC with differential and a coagulation profile. The CBC evaluates the cellular components of the blood.[1,3] The CBC reports the total RBC count and RBC indices, hematocrit, hemoglobin, WBC count and differential, platelet count, and cell morphologies. A summary of common hematological diagnostic laboratory tests, their normal values, and general implications of abnormal findings is shown in Table 17.6 (RBCs and WBCs) and Table 17.7 (coagulation).

SELECTED ERYTHROCYTE DISORDERS

Many pathological conditions affect the erythrocytes, ranging from mild anemias to life-threatening RBC lysis. A decrease in functional RBCs with a resulting oxygenation deficit is termed *anemia;* it is a common problem in critically ill patients. *Polycythemia,* a disorder in which the number of circulating RBCs is increased, is seen less often but can affect hypoxic patients (e.g., in chronic obstructive pulmonary disease). It leads to increased blood viscosity and thrombotic complications. Red blood cells also transport carbon dioxide and help distribute nitric oxide throughout the body, but transport of these gases is not dependent on the concentration of RBCs and is normal in patients with anemia.[15]

CHECK YOUR UNDERSTANDING

2. An older patient with a history of alcohol use disorder is admitted for urgent appendicitis and peritonitis. Based on initial lab results, which precaution(s) is a priority nursing intervention to be implemented? Admission labs: WBC 14.2/mm^3; RBC 3.2/mm^3; MCV 116; MCHC 27%; platelets 110/mm^3; B_{12} 188 pg/mL.
   A. Nutrition consult
   B. Fall precautions
   C. Bleeding precautions
   D. Contact isolation precautions

TABLE 17.6 Functions and Normal Values of Blood Cells

Test	Reason Evaluated	Normal Value	Alterations
Red Blood Cells (RBCs)			
Erythrocytes (RBCs)	Respiration Oxygen transport Acid-base balance	5 million/mm^3	↑ In polycythemia, dehydration ↓ In anemia, fluid overload, hemorrhage
Mean corpuscular volume (MCV)	Average size of each RBC; reflects maturity	80-100 femtoliter	↑ In nutrition deficiency ↓ In iron deficiency
Mean corpuscular hemoglobin (MCH)	Average amount of hemoglobin in each RBC	26-34 picograms	↓ In disorders of hemoglobin production
Mean corpuscular hemoglobin concentration (MCHC)	Average concentration of hemoglobin within a single RBC	31%-38%	↓ In cells with hemoglobin deficiency
Reticulocyte count	Immature RBCs released when suddenly in demand	1%-2% of total RBC count	↑ In recent blood loss or with chronic hemolysis
Serum folate	Amount of available vitamin for RBC development	95-500 mcg/mL	↓ In malnutrition or folic acid deficiency
Serum iron level	Iron stores within the body	40-160 mcg/dL	↓ With inadequate iron intake or inadequate absorption (e.g., gastric resection)
Total iron binding capacity (TIBC)	Reflection of liver function and nutrition	250-400 mcg/dL	↓ In chronic illness (e.g., infection, neoplasia, cirrhosis)
Ferritin level	Precursor to iron; reflects body's ability to create new iron stores	15-200 ng/mL	↓ Levels demonstrate inability to regenerate iron stores and hemoglobin
Transferrin level	Protein that binds to iron for removal or recirculation after RBCs are hemolyzed	200-400 mg/dL	↓ With excess hemolysis
Haptoglobin level	Protein that binds with heme for removal or recirculation after RBCs are hemolyzed	40-240 mg/dL	↓ With excess hemolysis
White Blood Cells (WBCs)			
Leukocytes (WBCs)	Inflammatory and immune responses Defend against infection, foreign tissue	4500-11,000/mm^3	↑ In inflammation, tissue necrosis, infection, hematological malignancy ↓ In bone marrow depression (e.g., radiation, immune disorders), chronic disease
Granular Leukocytes			
Neutrophils	Polymorphonuclear neutrophils Phagocytosis of invading organisms	50%-70% of WBCs	↑ In inflammation, infection, surgery, myocardial infarction ↓ In aplastic anemia, in hepatitis, with some pharmacological agents
Eosinophils	Defend against parasites; detoxification of foreign proteins Phagocytosis	1%-5% of WBCs	↑ In allergic attacks, autoimmune diseases, parasitic infections, dermatological conditions ↓ In stress reactions, severe infections
Basophils	Release heparin, serotonin, and histamine in allergic reactions; inflammatory response	0-1% of WBCs	↑ After splenectomy and with hemolytic anemia, radiation, hypothyroidism, leukemia, chronic hypersensitivity ↓ In stress reactions
Nongranular Leukocytes			
Monocytes	Mature into macrophages; phagocytosis of necrotic tissue, debris, foreign particles	1%-8% of WBCs	↑ In bacterial, parasitic, and some viral infections; chronic inflammation ↓ In stress reactions
Lymphocytes	Defend against microorganisms	20%-40% of WBCs	↑ In bacterial and viral infections, lymphocytic leukemia ↓ In immunoglobulin deficiency
B lymphocytes	Humoral immunity and production of antibodies	270-640/mm^3	↑ In bacterial and viral infections, lymphocytic leukemia ↓ In immunoglobulin deficiency, stress
T lymphocytes	Cell-mediated immunity	500-2400/mm^3	↓ With chemotherapy, immunodeficiencies, HIV, end-stage renal disease, immunosuppressive medications

Continued

TABLE 17.6 Functions and Normal Values of Blood Cells—cont'd

Test	Reason Evaluated	Normal Value	Alterations
Platelets			
Thrombocytes (platelets)	Blood clotting; hemostasis	150,000-400,000/mm^3	↑ In polycythemia vera, after splenectomy, with certain cancers ↓ In leukemia, bone marrow failure, DIC, hemorrhage, hypersplenism, radiation exposure, large foreign bodies in blood (e.g., aortic balloon pump), hypothermia, hyperthermia, severe infection

DIC, Disseminated intravascular coagulation; *RBCs*, red blood cells; *WBCs*, white blood cells.

TABLE 17.7 Common Coagulation Profile Studies

Test	Normal Value	Critical Value	Comments
Activated clotting time (ACT)	70-120 sec Therapeutic range for anticoagulation: 150-600 sec	Not specified	Used to monitor heparin therapy and detect clotting factor deficiencies
Activated partial thromboplastin time (aPTT)	30-40 sec	>70 sec	Used to monitor heparin therapy and detect clotting factor deficiencies ↑ With anticoagulation therapy, liver disease, vitamin K deficiency, DIC
Prothrombin time (PT) International normalized ratio (INR)	11-12.5 sec 0.8-1.1 INR Therapeutic range for anticoagulation: 1.5-2.0 times control value	PT >20 sec INR >5	Evaluates extrinsic pathway; used to monitor oral anticoagulant therapy ↑ With warfarin therapy, liver disease, vitamin K deficiency, obstructive jaundice
Fibrinogen level	200-400 mg/dL	<100 mg/dL associated with spontaneous bleeding	↓ In DIC and fibrinogen disorders ↑ In acute infection, in hepatitis, with oral contraceptive use
Fibrin degradation products (FDPs)	<10 mcg/mL	>40 mcg/mL	Evaluates hematologic disorders ↑ In DIC, fibrinolysis, thrombolytic therapy
Fibrin D-dimer	<0.4 mcg/mL	Not specified	Presence diagnostic for DIC
Platelet count	150,000-400,000/mm^3	<20,000/mm^3	Measures number of circulating platelets ↓ In thrombocytopenia
Platelet aggregation test	Varies; 3-5 min	Not specified	Measure of platelet function and aids in evaluation of bleeding disorders Prolonged in von Willebrand disease, acute leukemia, idiopathic thrombocytopenic purpura, liver cirrhosis, aspirin use
Calcium Ionized calcium	9-10.5 mg/dL 4.5-5.6 mg/dL	<6.0 mg/dL <2.2 mg/dL	↓ With massive transfusions of stored blood

DIC, Disseminated intravascular coagulation.
From Pagana KD, Pagana TJ, Pagana TN. *Mosby's Manual of Diagnostic and Laboratory Test.* 15th ed. St. Louis, MO: Elsevier; 2021.

Anemia

Pathophysiology. The term *anemia* refers to a reduction in the number of circulating RBCs or hemoglobin that leads to inadequate oxygenation of tissues. Although symptoms vary depending on the type, cause, and severity of the anemia, the basic clinical findings are the same. As oxygenation delivery is decreased, tissues become hypoxic and 2,3-DPG increases, causing hemoglobin to release oxygen. Blood flow is redistributed to areas where oxygenation is most vital, such as the brain, heart, and lungs. Anemia is described as mild, moderate, or severe based on symptoms, irrespective of actual RBC serum values. Patients are able to adjust and compensate to lower RBC levels when the condition is chronic or slow in onset. Severity of clinical symptoms is related to the degree of tissue hypoxia and the pathogenesis of the anemia.[15]

Anemia is classified by its origin or by the microscopic appearance of the RBCs. Hematologists typically use the microscopic classifications (e.g., microcytic, hypochromic), but critical care nurses plan care using the etiological classifications. Causes of anemia include (1) blood loss (acute or chronic), (2) impaired production, (3) increased RBC destruction, or (4) a combination of these.[15] Iron deficiency anemia is the most common type of anemia.

In adults, anemia usually results from chronic blood loss. Anemia can also result from chronic disease (anemia of inflammation), renal disease from erythropoietin deficiency, malignancy and congenital problems (Diamond-Blackfan anemia), folate and vitamin B_{12} deficiencies, and other rarer disorders. RBCs can also be destroyed, leading to anemia. Reasons for RBC destruction include hemoglobinopathies (e.g., sickle cell disease), RBC enzyme defects such as *glucose-6-phosphate dehydrogenase (G6PD)* mutations, and hemolysis due to autoimmune processes or mechanical causes (such as hemolytic uremic syndrome [HUS]).

Iron is essential for not only the synthesis of hemoglobin but also for erythropoiesis. Iron deficiency anemia is the most common cause of anemia in adults and usually results from chronic blood loss.

Haptoglobin is a protein that is made by the liver. Haptoglobin circulates in the plasma and binds to hemoglobin when RBCs die. This lab test is ordered if hemolysis is suspected. It is a sensitive indicator of hemolysis, as only minimal hemolysis is needed to deplete circulating haptoglobin.[16] The types of anemia are described in Table 17.8.

Assessment and Clinical Manifestations. Signs and symptoms of anemia begin gradually and initially include fatigue, weakness, and shortness of breath.[15] Signs and symptoms are related to three physiological effects of reduced RBCs: (1) decreased circulating volume caused by loss of RBC mass, (2) decreased oxygenation of tissues resulting from reduced hemoglobin binding sites, and (3) compensatory mechanisms implemented by the body in its attempt to improve tissue oxygenation. Decreased circulating volume is manifested by clinical findings reflective of low blood volume (e.g., tachycardia, hypotension, low urine output) and the effects of gravity on the lack of volume (e.g., orthostasis). Tissue hypoxia from inadequate oxygen delivery results in compensatory activities, including an increased depth and rate of respiration to increase oxygen availability, tachycardia to increase oxygen delivery, and the shunting of blood away from nonvital organs to perfuse the vital organs.[15] These compensatory mechanisms are a result of hypoxia-inducible factors (HIFs), which cause an upregulation of erythropoietin, angiogenesis, energy metabolism, and iron balance.[15]

Inadequate oxygenation of the tissues can ultimately lead to end-organ dysfunction. The disorders of anemia have their own classic clinical features, but the principal effect is the result of decreased oxygen-carrying capacity of the blood.[15] Laboratory findings across all anemias include a decreased RBC count and decreased hemoglobin and hematocrit values. Table 17.8 shows characteristics of the most common anemias, clinical presentation, diagnostic tests, nursing implications, and management.

Medical Intervention. Medical treatment is focused on identifying and treating the cause of the anemia. Supplemental oxygen and blood component therapy may be required to support the cardiopulmonary system. In anemia associated with blood loss, initial treatment is with IV administration of volume expanders (crystalloid or colloid) with or without transfusion of packed RBCs. Products that stimulate erythropoietin production may be ordered. For certain types of anemia, cause-specific interventions may be indicated. Splenectomy may be performed for hemolytic anemia, and bone marrow transplantation (BMT) may be preferred for refractory aplastic anemia. In sickle cell disease (SCD), oxygenation and correction of dehydration are important for the prevention and reversal of erythrocyte sickling.

Nursing Care. Nurses address problems common to the anemic patient. Problems vary and may include low cardiac output, decreased tissue perfusion, and altered gas exchange; risk for bleeding; fatigue and decreased exercise tolerance; pain; and skin alterations. The patient problems and interventions from the Collaborative Care Plan found in Chapter 1, Overview of Critical Care Nursing, apply and are tailored to the patient with anemia.

Nursing management of anemia is based on a continuous, thorough assessment and the prescribed medical treatment. Monitor vital signs, the electrocardiogram (ECG), hemodynamic parameters, heart and lung sounds, peripheral pulses to assess tissue perfusion, and gas exchange. In addition, assess mental status, urine output, and skin color and temperature. Be alert for tachycardia and orthostatic hypotension, indicators that the patient's cardiovascular system is not adequately compensating for the anemia. Provide comfort measures to prevent or treat pain and monitor closely for signs of infection. Institute fall precautions along with bleeding precautions if the patient is at risk for further blood loss.

Carefully monitor laboratory results, such as the CBC, particularly the hemoglobin and hematocrit levels. Other vital nursing interventions include promoting rest and oxygen conservation; administering blood components, medication therapy, and IV fluids; and monitoring the patient's responses to the therapy. The desired goal of treatment and nursing intervention is optimal tissue perfusion, oxygenation, and gas exchange.

CLINICAL JUDGMENT ACTIVITY

Describe nursing interventions and rationales for reducing the risk of hospital-acquired infections for the immunosuppressed patient.

WHITE BLOOD CELL AND IMMUNE DISORDERS

Many pathological conditions are classified as WBC or immune disorders. They may involve the WBCs themselves or other complementary immune processes. The immune system can fail to develop properly, lose its ability to react to invasion by pathogens, overreact to harmless antigens, or turn immune functions against self. Regardless of the cause, WBC and immune disorders or treatments suppress the mechanisms needed for inflammation and combating infection. Because the clinical features and complications are similar among a variety of disorders, this first section addresses general causes, signs and symptoms, and management of

TABLE 17.8 Anemias

Marrow Failure to Produce RBCs	Aplastic Anemia	Hemolytic Anemia	Sickle Cell Anemia (Hemolytic Subtype)	Vitamin B_{12} Deficiency	Folic Acid Deficiency	Iron Deficiency
Pathophysiology						
Disorder or bone marrow toxin damages the erythrocyte precursors, leading to ↓ RBC production	Disorder or bone marrow toxin damages hematopoietic stem cells and results in ↓ production of RBCs, WBCs, and platelets.	Stimulus causes extrasplenic destruction of the RBC, leading to hemolyzed RBC fragments in the circulating bloodstream; cell fragments ↑ blood viscosity and slow blood flow, leading to ischemia and/or infarction. Extrasplenic hemolysis also leads to ↑ levels of circulating bilirubin and unbound iron	Presence of abnormal Hgb causes RBCs to assume a sickle or crescent shape Sickling alters the blood viscosity, leading to microvascular occlusion; sickling crisis leads to hypoxia, thrombosis, and infarction in tissues and organs	Pernicious anemia is caused by decreased gastric production of HCl and intrinsic factor, which play a role in vitamin B_{12} absorption.	Malabsorption of dietary folic acid results from lack of intake or absorption	Body's iron stores are inadequate for RBC development; Hgb-deficient RBCs result
Etiology						
Disorders: Bone metastases *Medications:* Chemotherapy agents Antiretroviral agents *Toxic exposures:* Radiation to long bones	*Disorders:* Immune suppression Transplantation Pregnancy Vitamin B_{12} deficiency *Viral infection:* EBV, CMV *Medications:* Anticonvulsants Antidysrhythmics Antiinflammatory agents Chloramphenicol Quinines *Toxic exposures:* Benzene Arsenic Herbicides, insecticides Lacquers; paint thinners Radiation exposure Toluene (glue)	*Abnormal RBC membrane or Hgb:* Anemia of chronic disease Hereditary RBC shape disorders Paroxysmal nocturnal hemoglobinuria Porphyria Sickle cell disease G6PD deficiency Thalassemias *Immune reaction:* Autoimmune hemolytic syndrome BMT hemolytic transfusion reaction Autoimmune diseases *Physical damage to RBCs:* Blunt trauma Extracorporeal circulation Prosthetic heart valves Thermal injury *Unknown:* IgA deficiency Cocaine use Snake or spider bite	Hereditary hemolytic anemia caused by abnormal amount of hemoglobin S in relation to hemoglobin A.	Familial incidence related to autoimmune response with gastric mucosal atrophy. Higher incidence in autoimmune disorders: SLE, myxedema, Graves' disease. Common in Northern Europeans; rare in children and Black and Asian populations. Occurs postoperatively with gastric surgery.	Common in infants, adolescents, pregnant and lactating women, alcoholic patients, older adults, cancer, intestinal disease (jejunitis, small bowel resection), prolonged use of anticonvulsants or estrogens, excessive cooking of foods.	Present in 10%-30% of all American adults; primarily from dietary deficiency. Also in pregnant and lactating people, infants, adolescents. Malabsorption such as diarrhea, gastric resection, blood loss, or intravascular hemolysis.
Nursing Implications						
Monitor diet and medications that interfere with marrow production of cells[22]	*High risk of infection and bleeding:* implement bleeding precautions Administer transfusions cautiously; exposure to antigens may enhance rejection if BMT is required later.	Begin plasma reinfusion at a rate of 25 mL/h for 15 min, then 100 mL/h. Assess for hypersensitivity. Assess for fluid shifts into the interstitial spaces during infusion or within 6-12 h after infusion. Monitor for vomiting, pain at infusion site, diarrhea.	Incurable, although severity remains consistent throughout lifetime. Common cause of death is intracranial thrombosis or hemorrhage.	Lifetime treatment requires ongoing patient teaching. Heart failure prevention. Special oral hygiene. Monitor for persistent neurological deficits.	Foods high in folic acid: beef, liver, peanut butter, red beans, oatmeal, asparagus, broccoli	Monitor for allergic reactions to iron. Give oral supplements with straw to prevent staining teeth; causes skin irritation and iron deposits.

TABLE 17.8 Anemias—cont'd

Marrow Failure to Produce RBCs	Aplastic Anemia	Hemolytic Anemia	Sickle Cell Anemia (Hemolytic Subtype)	Vitamin B_{12} Deficiency	Folic Acid Deficiency	Iron Deficiency
Clinical Presentation						
↓ Production of cells in the earliest phase: bone marrow failure resulting in low RBC count Signs and symptoms are those common in profound anemia	Symptoms of infection, bleeding, and anemia occur simultaneously; earliest symptoms are usually the result of WBC dysfunction. Platelet production abnormalities lead to bleeding symptoms within 7-10 days, followed by symptoms of anemia.	Rapid hemolysis of RBCs leads to spleen uptake with enlarged and tender spleen; metabolism of RBCs often leads to excess bilirubin with jaundice, itching, and abdominal pain.	Hyperviscosity and poor perfusion (e.g., altered mentation, hypoxemia) sickled cells removed from circulation, causing enlarged and tender spleen; long-term sickling and thrombosis causes ↓ joint mobility, joint swelling and pain, gut dysfunction, cardiac failure, and risk for stroke, peripheral edema, and decreased urine output when in crisis.	Inhibited growth of all cells: anemia, leukopenia, thrombocytopenia. Demyelination of peripheral nerves to spinal cord. Triad: weakness, sore tongue, paresthesias.	Similar to vitamin B_{12} deficiency but without neurological symptoms. *Signs:* poor oxygenation, dizziness, irritability, dyspnea, pallor, headache, oral ulcers, tachycardia	Classic: "pica" (desire to eat nonfood items), ice or dirt cravings *Cardiovascular/ respiratory compromise:* hypoxia, fatigue, headache, cracks in mouth corners, smooth tongue, paresthesias, neuralgias
Diagnostic Tests						
CBC used as screening test Bone marrow aspiration and biopsy confirm maturation failure	CBC used as screening test: ↓reticulocyte, platelet, RBC, and WBC counts Bone marrow aspiration and biopsy reflect absence of precursor or stem cells	Reticulocytes usually ≥4% total RBC count ↑ Total bilirubin ↑ Direct bilirubin ↓ Transferrin ↓ Haptoglobin	Hgb electrophoresis abnormality. Stained blood smear reveals sickle cells.	Schilling test ↓ Hgb and RBC ↑ MCV ↓ MCHC ↓ WBC ↓ Platelets ↑ LDH	Macrocytosis Serum folate <4 mg/dL Abnormal platelet appearance ↑ Reticulocyte count	↓ Hct and Hgb ↓ Iron level with ↑ binding capacity ↓ Ferritin level ↓ RBC with hypochromia and microcytes ↓ MCHC
Management						
Erythropoietin per dosing guidelines (Procrit, Aranesp)	Eliminate cause Bone marrow stimulants Corticosteroids Immunosuppressive agents for autoimmune process Chelating (iron binding) agents Limit transfusions when possible to ↓ risk of rejection Allogeneic BMT	Staphylococcal protein A is capable of trapping IgG complexes that are thought to cause RBC autoantibodies. If autoantibodies are present, give immunosuppressive agents. Administer antiplatelet medications (e.g., salicylic acid).	Administer large volumes of IV fluids to dilute viscous blood. Oxygen therapy reduces sickling. Treat infections early. Manage extreme pain (result of ischemia); Gene transplants used experimentally.	Vitamin B_{12} 30 mcg IM or deep SC for 5-10 days then 100-200 mcg IM or deep SC every month.	Folic acid 0.25-1 mg/day PO	Ferrous sulfate 325 mg PO tid and ascorbic acid to aid absorption

BMT, Bone marrow transplantation; *CBC*, complete blood count; *CMV*, cytomegalovirus; *EBV*, Epstein-Barr virus; *G6PD*, glucose-6-phosphate dehydrogenase; *HCl*, hydrochloride; *Hct*, hematocrit; *Hgb*, hemoglobin; *IgA*, immunoglobulin A; *IgG*, immunoglobulin G; *IM*, intramuscular; *LDH*, lactate dehydrogenase; *MCHC*, mean corpuscular hemoglobin concentration; *MCV*, mean corpuscular volume; *PO*, orally; *RBCs*, red blood cells; *SC*, subcutaneously; *SLE*, systemic lupus erythematosus; *tid*, three times daily; *WBCs*, white blood cells.

immunological suppression. This is followed by in-depth discussions of specific WBC and immune disorders.

The Immunocompromised Patient

Pathophysiology. The *immunocompromised* patient is one who has defined quantitative or qualitative defects in WBCs or immune physiology. The defect may be congenital or acquired, and it may involve a single element or multiple processes. Regardless of the cause, the physiological outcome is immune incompetence—lack of normal inflammatory, phagocytic, antibody, or cytokine responses. Immunocompromise in the critically ill is caused by many factors. Immune incompetence is often asymptomatic until pathogenic organisms invade the body and create infection. Infection is the leading cause of death in immunocompromised patients.

Assessment and Clinical Manifestations. The risk for infection is the primary clinical problem for those with immune compromise. A detailed and comprehensive assessment containing the patient's history, physical examination findings, and laboratory studies is paramount for rapid detection of infection. In addition to existing immunodeficiency disease and life-threatening illness, immune defenses are altered by invasive procedures, inadequate nutrition, and the presence of opportunistic pathogens. Many of the medications and treatments administered in critical care depress the patient's immune system. Evaluate the patient's medical and social histories, current medications, and risk factors for infection (Table 17.9). Immunosuppressed patients do not respond to infection with typical signs and symptoms of inflammation (see Clinical Alert box).

! CLINICAL ALERT

Infection in Immunocompromised Patients

Immunocompromised patients do not have typical signs and symptoms of infection.

- Erythema, swelling, and exudate formation are usually not evident, as exudate (i.e., pus) is not able to form due to a lack of neutrophils.
- Symptoms of infection may be absent, masked, or present atypically.
- Fever, defined as a temperature greater than 100.4°F (38°C), is considered the cardinal and sometimes the only symptom of infection. However, some patients with infection do not have a fever.
- Patients are also more likely to describe pain at the site of infection, although physical inflammatory signs may be absent.
- Increased or worsening fatigue, malaise, and lethargy.

Reference

Haidar G, Singh N. Fever of unknown origin. *N Engl J Med. 2022;386(5):463–477.* https://doi.org/10.1056/NEJMra2111003.

TABLE 17.9 Risk Factors for Infection in the Immunocompromised Patient

Patient Characteristic	Physiological Mechanism of Risk of Infection
Host Characteristics	
Alcohol use disorder	↓ Neutrophil activity Hepatic/splenic congestion also slows phagocytic response
Substance use disorder	Chronic altered barrier defense leads to reduced WBCs and slowed phagocytic responses Constant viral exposure may also alter T-cell function
Aging	*Slowed phagocytosis:* bacterial infection, more rapid dissemination of infection *Slowed macrophage activity:* more fungal infection, more visceral infection *Atrophy of thymus:* ↑ risk of viral illness ↓ *Antigen-specific immunoglobulins:* diminished immune memory
Frequent hospitalizations	Frequent exposure to environmental organisms other than own normal flora Potential exposure to resistant organisms and other people's organisms through cross-contamination
Malnutrition	*Inadequate WBC count:* infection ↓ *Neutrophil activity:* bacterial infection, at risk of infection *Impaired phagocytic function:* bacterial infection *Impaired integumentary/mucosal barrier:* general infection risk ↓ *Macrophage mobilization:* risk of fungal or rapidly disseminating infection ↓ *Lymphocyte function:* ↑ risk of viral and opportunistic infection Thymus and lymph node atrophy with iron deficiency
Stress	Induces ↑ release of adrenal hormones (cortisol), which causes ↓ circulating eosinophils and lymphocytes
Immune Defects and Disorders	
Lymphopenia	↓ Antibody response to previously exposed antigens ↓ Recognition and destruction of viral and opportunistic organisms
Macrophage dysfunction or destruction	Altered response to fungi Inadequate antigen-antibody response Greater potential for visceral infection
Neutropenia	Inadequate neutrophils to combat pathogens (especially bacteria)
Splenectomy	Inability to recognize and remove encapsulated bacteria (e.g., streptococcus) Compromised reticuloendothelial system and ↓ antibodies lead to frequent and early bacteremia

TABLE 17.9 Risk Factors for Infection in the Immunocompromised Patient—cont'd

Patient Characteristic	Physiological Mechanism of Risk of Infection
Disease Processes	
Burns	Physiological stressor thought to ↓ phagocytic responses Altered barrier defenses allowing pathogen entry Protein loss through skin leads to malnutrition-related immunocompromise
Cancer	Structural disruption may lead to bone marrow or lymphatic abnormalities Certain cancers have specific immune defects (e.g., diminished phagocytic activity, T-cell defects) Radiation therapy destroys lymphocytes and causes shrinkage of lymphoid tissue Chemotherapy causes ↓ lymphocytes and alters proliferation and differentiation of stem cells
Cardiovascular disease	Inadequate tissue perfusion slows WBC response to tissue with pathogenic organism
Diabetes mellitus	↓ Numbers of neutrophils Hyperglycemia causes ↓ phagocytic activity and immunoglobin defects Vascular insufficiency leads to slowed phagocytic response to pathogens Neuropathy and glycosuria predispose to ↓ bladder emptying and urinary tract infections
Gastrointestinal disease	↓ Bowel motility allows normal flora to translocate across the gastrointestinal wall to the bloodstream
Hepatic disease	↓ Neutrophil count
Infectious diseases	↓ Phagocytic activity Hypermetabolism with infection accelerates phagocytic cell use and death Certain viral and opportunistic infections ↓ bone marrow production of WBCs
Pulmonary disease	Inadequate oxygenation suppresses neutrophil activity
Renal disease	↓ Neutrophil activity caused by uremic toxins ↓ Immunoglobulin activity
Traumatic injuries	Altered barrier defenses allowing pathogen entry Type of infection depends on source and severity of injury (e.g., soil or water contamination, skin flora)
Medications and Treatments	
Antibiotics	Normal flora destroyed, enhanced resistant organism growth, fungal superinfection
Immunosuppressive agents and corticosteroids	↓ Phagocytic activity Altered T-cell recognition of pathogens, especially viruses ↓ Interleukin-2 production leads to increased risk of malignancy ↓ IgG production Lack of immune memory to recall antibodies to previously encountered pathogens
Invasive devices	Altered barrier defenses allowing entry of pathogens, especially skin organisms
Surgical procedures/wounds	Normal flora may be translocated by surgical procedure Altered barrier defenses caused by surgical entry Stress of surgery and anesthetic agents reduces neutrophil activity
Transfusion of blood products	Risk of transfusion-transmitted infections undetected by donor screening: cytomegalovirus, hepatitis, HIV Exposure to foreign antigens in blood products causes T-lymphocytic immune suppression and increases risk of infection

IgG, Immunoglobulin G; *WBC*, white blood cell.

Laboratory results that reflect leukopenia, lymphopenia, low CD4 counts, and decreased Ig levels may demonstrate disorders of immune components.[1] A common test of the humoral (antibody) response to antigens is a skin test with intradermal injection of typical pathogens capable of initiating an antibody response. Absence of a "wheal" tissue response to the antigens (called *tissue anergy*) is evidence of altered antibody capabilities.

Patient Problem. The primary problem for the immunocompromised patient is decreased immunity with potential for systemic and local infection.

Medical Intervention. *Primary immunodeficiencies,* which are deficiencies in the immune response, are treated with specific replacement therapy or BMT. These treatments aim to reverse the cause of the immune dysfunction and prevent infectious complications. If the serum IgG level is less than 300 mg/dL, an infusion of Ig may be ordered to reverse the cause of the immune dysfunction. Gene replacement therapy is an emerging treatment for selected disorders.[17]

In *secondary immunodeficiencies,* the underlying causative condition is treated. For example, malnutrition is corrected, or doses of immunosuppressive medications are adjusted. Risk factors for infection are carefully assessed and avoided. For example, assess the need for invasive lines and use meticulous aseptic technique when managing lines. Patients who have HIV infection or are recovering from organ transplantation have defined CD4 or immune suppression levels that place them at risk for specific infections.[18] These patients often receive antimicrobial prophylaxis against infections with herpes simplex, *Candida albicans, Pneumocystis jirovecii, Mycobacterium avium-intracellulare, Mycobacterium tuberculosis,* and cytomegalovirus.

Nursing Intervention. Nursing interventions focus on protecting the patient from infection. Provide a protective environment to reduce the risk of infection. For patients that receive HSCT, high-efficiency particulate air (HEPA) filtration and laminar airflow in single-patient rooms are recommended to prevent infection with airborne microorganisms.

Hand washing is the best way to prevent infection. Nursing staff members play an important role in ensuring skin integrity and sterile technique when procedures are unavoidable. Other important hygiene measures include general bathing with antimicrobial soaps, oral care, perineal care, and advocating for early removal of invasive devices and lines.

General health promotion including adequate fluid, nutrition, and sleep is important in bolstering the patient's defenses against infection. Dietary restriction, such as prohibiting raw fruits and vegetables, is controversial and not standardized.[19] Nursing interventions are presented in the Plan of Care for the Immunocompromised Patient.

Neutropenia

Pathophysiology. Neutropenia is defined as an absolute neutrophil count of less than 1500 cells/mm^3 of blood. Neutropenia occurs as a result of inadequate production or excess destruction of neutrophils. Patients with low neutrophil counts are predisposed to infections because of the body's reduced phagocytic ability.[9] Neutropenia is classified based on the patient's predicted risk for infection: mild (1000 to 1500 cells/mm^3), moderate (500 to 1000 cells/mm^3), and severe (<500 cells/mm^3).[1]

Assessment and Clinical Manifestations. Obtain thorough medical and social histories to identify risk factors for neutropenia. Common causes include acute or overwhelming infections, radiation exposure, exposure to chemicals and medications, or other disease states (Box 17.2). No specific signs or symptoms indicate a low neutrophil count; therefore it is essential to evaluate the patient carefully for risk factors for neutropenia and clinical findings consistent with infection. Many patients describe fatigue or malaise that coincides with the drop in counts and precedes infectious signs and symptoms.

Examine every body system for physical findings of infection. Typical signs may not be evident. Pain such as sore throat or urethral discomfort may be indicative of an infected site. Areas of heavy bacterial colonization (e.g., oral mucosa, perineal area, venipuncture and catheter sites) have the highest risk of infection; however, the most common clinical infections are pneumonia and sepsis. Additional signs or symptoms of systemic infection include a rise in temperature from its normal set point, chills, and accompanying tachycardia.

BOX 17.2 Causes of Neutropenia

Malnutrition
- Calorie deficiency
- Deficiency of iron, protein, and/or vitamin B

Health States
- Addison disease
- Anaphylactic shock
- Brucellosis
- Chronic fever or illness
- Cirrhosis
- Diabetes mellitus
- Advanced age
- Hypothermia
- Infection (any severe bacterial or viral disease)
- Renal trauma

Medications and Substances
- Alcohol
- Alkylating agents, antineoplastic and immunosuppressive (e.g., cyclophosphamide)
- Allopurinol (Zyloprim)
- Anticonvulsants (e.g., phenytoin)
- Antidysrhythmics (e.g., procainamide, quinidine)
- Antimicrobials (e.g., aminoglycosides, chloramphenicol, sulfonamides, trimethoprim-sulfamethoxazole)
- Antiretroviral agents (e.g., zidovudine)
- Antitumor antibiotics (e.g., bleomycin, doxorubicin [Adriamycin])
- Arsenic
- Phenothiazines (e.g., prochlorperazine)

PLAN OF CARE

For the Immunocompromised Patient

Patient Problem

Decreased Immunity/Potential for Systemic and Local Infection. Risk factors include immunocompromise or immunosuppression, invasive procedures, and presence of opportunistic pathogens.

Desired Outcomes
- Absence of fever, redness, swelling, pain, and heat.
- WBC and differential, urinalysis, and cultures within normal limits.
- Chest radiographical study without infiltrates.
- Absence of adventitious breath sounds.

PLAN OF CARE—cont'd

Nursing Assessments/Interventions	Rationales
• Establish baseline assessment with documented history, physical examination, and laboratory study results.	• Establish trends to guide and monitor treatment.
• Follow universal precautions, including hand hygiene.	• Decrease risk of infection.
• Plan nurses' assignments to reduce the possibility of infection spread between patients.	• Decrease spread of infection.
• Be careful handling secretions and excretions that are known to be infected.	• Prevent cross-contamination.
• Monitor visitors for any recent history of communicable diseases.	• Prevent infection.
• Clean all multipurpose equipment (e.g., oximeter probes, noninvasive BP cuffs, bed scale slings, electronic thermometers) between uses.	• Prevent cross-contamination.
• Assess patient for signs and symptoms of infection.	• Guide early recognition and treatment.
• Monitor vital signs and temperature at least every 4 hours; report and investigate any elevation in temperature; rectal temperatures are not recommended.	• Assess for infection.
• Monitor laboratory results: WBC and differential, blood, urine, sputum, wound, and throat cultures.	• Assess for infection.
• Report abnormal results.	
• Note the presence of chills, tachycardia, oliguria, or altered mentation that may indicate sepsis; report subtle changes to provider.	• Assess for infection.
• Encourage incentive spirometry and change of position every 1-2 hours.	• Prevent atelectasis.
• Avoid breaks in the skin and mucous membranes: ○ Change position every 2 hours; avoid moisture contact with skin. ○ Provide skin lubricants and moisture barriers as indicated. ○ Provide meticulous oral and bathing hygiene.	• Maintain intact skin—the first line of defense.
• Use strict aseptic technique for dressing changes.	• Prevent infection.
• Avoid stopcocks in IV systems; use closed injection of site systems.	• Stopcocks can harbor bacteria and are an entry site for any infectious agent.
• Limit invasive devices and procedures whenever possible.	• Decrease risk for infection.
• Use private room; limit visitors; prohibit fresh and artificial flowers and plants.	• Fresh flowers and plants have a potential to introduce pathogenic organisms. Artificial flowers and plants collect dust.[20]
• Ensure that sleep needs are being met.	• Enhance resistance to infection and aid in healing.
• Control glucose levels.	• Hyperglycemia compromises phagocytic activity.
• Change oxygen setups with humidification (e.g., nasal cannula) every 24 hours.	• Prevent bacterial growth.
• Obtain cultures for first fever (38.0°C; temperature measured twice, 4 hours apart) and for new fever (38.3°C) after 72 hours on an antimicrobial regimen: ○ Blood cultures from two different peripheral sites, if possible. ○ Blood cultures from existing vascular access devices. ○ Urine culture. ○ Sputum culture, if obtainable. ○ Stool culture, if obtainable. ○ Culture of open lesions or wounds.	• Identify site(s) of infections and guide antimicrobial treatment.
• Administer antimicrobial therapy as ordered within 1 hour of the fever. • Measure antimicrobial peak and trough levels as ordered.	• Treat infection and assess effectiveness of antibiotics. Prompt administration of antibiotics within 1 hour in a neutropenic patient decreases mortality associated with sepsis.
• Be alert to superinfection with fungal flora anytime 7-10 days after initiation of antibiotics.	• Assess complications of antibiotic therapy; oral or topical nystatin may be indicated.

Patient Problem

Weight Loss. Risk factors include NPO status; anorexia, nausea, and vomiting; and painful oral mucosa.

Desired Outcomes

- Adequate caloric and protein intake.
- Ideal or stable body weight.
- Laboratory values remain within normal limits (total protein, serum albumin, electrolytes, hemoglobin, and hematocrit).

Continued

PLAN OF CARE—cont'd

Nursing Assessments/Interventions	Rationales
• Assess baseline nutritional status: ○ Height and weight ○ BMI ○ Laboratory values ○ Assess presence of weakness ○ Fatigue ○ Infection ○ Other signs of malnutrition	• Obtain baseline assessment. Consult with dietitian to screen patient using a validated malnutrition screening tool. Patients should be screened within 24 hours of admission per The Joint Commission.[21]
• Obtain dietary consultation to determine nutrients and intake required. • Administer enteral or parenteral nutritional therapy as ordered and observe response.	• Optimize nutritional therapy to reduce risks.
• Establish food preferences, encourage meals from home, and provide relaxed atmosphere during meals.	• Tailor nutritional support based on patient's preferences.
• Determine deterrents to adequate intake: ○ Fasting (NPO) status ○ Presence of anorexia, nausea, vomiting, stomatitis	• Assess risks for decreased nutrition.
• Monitor daily weight, laboratory values, protein and caloric intake, and I&O	• Monitor nutritional status.
• Encourage small, frequent, high-calorie, and high-protein meals.	• Promote adequate intake.
• Provide meticulous mouth care before and after meals.	• Maintain oral mucosa and facilitate oral intake.
• Administer antiemetics as needed, 30 min before meals.	• Encourage adequate intake.

BMI, Body mass index; *BP*, blood pressure; *I&O*, intake and output; *NPO*, nothing by mouth; *WBC*, white blood cell. Adapted from Snyder J, Sump C. *Swearingen's All-in-One Nursing Care Planning Resource*, 6th ed. Elsevier; 2024.

Absolute neutrophil count. The diagnostic test indicated when neutropenia is suspected is the WBC count with differential. Neutrophils are the "first responders" of the immune system; the absolute neutrophil count (ANC) result is valuable in determining whether the patient is neutropenic. The differential demonstrates the percentage of each type of WBC circulating in the bloodstream. Calculate the ANC by multiplying the total WBC count (without a decimal point) times the percentages (with decimal points) of polymorphonuclear leukocytes (polys; also called segs or neutrophils) and bands (immature neutrophils):

$$\text{WBC} \times (\text{segs} + \text{bands}) \times 100$$

Example:
Total WBC: 7000
Segs: 10% (0.1)
Bands: 10% (0.1)

$$7000 \times (0.1 + 0.1) = 1400$$

ANC is 1400—patient has mild neutropenia.

This gives a number that is translated into the categories of mild, moderate, or severe neutropenia.

Patient Problem. The specific problem related to all patients with neutropenia is potential for systemic and local infection.

Medical Intervention. Medical treatment of neutropenia is aimed at preventing and treating infection while reversing the cause of the neutropenia. Patients with anticipated neutropenia, such as those receiving antineoplastic or antiretroviral therapy, may be given bone marrow growth factors. Also known as *colony-stimulating factors* (CSFs), these agents enhance bone marrow regeneration of granulocyte colony-stimulating factor (G-CSF), macrophage colony-stimulating factor (M-CSF), or both cell lines (GM-CSF).[22]

Prophylactic antiinfective agents may be ordered to prevent infection, and potent broad-spectrum antimicrobial agents are ordered when there is evidence of infection. In sepsis accompanying neutropenia, granulocyte transfusions may be used to supplement the neutrophil count, though this therapy is not without risk.

Nursing Intervention. Nursing care of patients with neutropenia is the same as that for all immunocompromised patients (refer to the Plan of Care for the Critically Ill Patient with Potential for Decreased Immunity or Infection found in Chapter 1, Overview of Critical Care Nursing). Desired patient outcomes related to medical and nursing interventions include absence of infection, negative cultures, and an absolute neutrophil count of 1500 cells/mm^3 or higher.

Malignant White Blood Cell Disorders: Leukemia, Lymphoma, and Multiple Myeloma

Pathophysiology. Malignant diseases involving WBCs are termed leukemia, lymphoma, or plasma cell neoplasm (multiple myeloma). They are differentiated by the cell type affected and by the stage of cell development when malignancy occurs. Regardless of the specific neoplastic disorder, deficiency of functional WBCs is a common problem. The unique pathophysiological and clinical characteristics of these disorders are described in Table 17.10. Despite normal serum cell counts, WBC activity is always impaired, and infection is the most common complication in all these disorders.

TABLE 17.10 **Malignant White Blood Cell Disorders**

Leukemia	Lymphoma	Multiple Myeloma
Pathophysiology		
Cancer involving any of the WBCs during the early phase of maturation within the bone marrow.	Cancer affecting the lymphocytes after their bone marrow maturation, when they reside within the lymph node.	Cancer involving the mature and differentiated immunoglobulin-producing macrophage called a plasma cell; the malignancy is primarily manifested by excess abnormal immunoglobulin.
Classification		
Acute leukemia: excess proliferation of immature cells *Chronic leukemia:* excess proliferation of mature cells Leukemias are further classified according to whether they originate in the lymphocyte cell line or are nonlymphocytic.	Hodgkin's and non-Hodgkin's subtypes have more subclassifications denoting the maturity of the cell involved and the aggressiveness of the malignancy.	Disease is classified as limited or extensive depending on plasma viscosity, bone manifestations, presence of hypercalcemia, and renal involvement.
Risk Factors		
Chromosomal abnormalities Viral infection Radiation Herbicides and pesticides Benzene and toluene Immunosuppressive therapy	Chromosomal abnormalities Alkylating agents Viral infection Radiation Herbicides and pesticides Benzene and toluene Immunosuppressive therapy Alkylating agents Autoimmune disease	Advanced age Male sex African American descent Chronic hypersensitivity reactions Autoimmune diseases
Clinical Manifestations		
Fever Constitutional symptoms: fatigue, malaise, weakness, night sweats Easy bruising and bleeding from mucous membranes (e.g., gums) Bone pain	Enlarged (>2 cm), nontender lymph node(s) Usually immovable and irregularly shaped Masses in body cavities or other organs (e.g., peritoneal cavity, lungs)	Thrombotic events: deep vein thrombosis, pulmonary embolism, cerebral infarction Bone pain Renal failure
Acute Complications		
Leukostasis DIC Tumor lysis syndrome	Airway obstruction Superior vena cava syndrome Bowel obstruction Neoplastic tamponade Pleural effusion	Hyperviscosity Renal failure Hypercalcemia
Staging		
All patients are viewed as having systemic disease or late-stage disease.	Classified by number of lymph nodes involved, number of lymph node groups, whether involved nodes are only above the diaphragm or on both sides of the diaphragm, and how many extranodal sites are involved.	Disease is classified as limited when there are only elevated abnormal immunoglobin levels; it is described as extensive when there are bone lesions, hypercalcemia, or renal dysfunction.
Diagnostic Tests		
CBC shows either ↓ WBCs or large number of immature WBCs (blasts), ↓ RBCs, ↓ platelets Bone marrow aspiration and biopsy	Lymph node biopsy CT scans Chemistry: alkaline phosphatase	Bence Jones protein in urine Immunoglobulin electrophoresis Plasma viscosity
Medical Management		
Systemic chemotherapy BMT	Radiation therapy for single node or node group if above the diaphragm for control or remission Radiation used if palliation of tumor is the goal of therapy Systemic chemotherapy for multinode involvement, aggressive tumor subtypes Autologous BMT for patients with high risk of relapse Allogeneic BMT for patients with residual disease, especially involving bone marrow	Systemic chemotherapy provides an average of only 14-36 months of remission. BMT or "double" BMT may increase survival. Radiation therapy used to palliatively treat bone lesions.

Continued

TABLE 17.10 Malignant White Blood Cell Disorders—cont'd

Leukemia	Lymphoma	Multiple Myeloma
Nursing Care Issues		
Infection control practices Bleeding precautions	Infection control practices Edema management Monitoring for lymphoma masses compressing body organs	Infection control practices Safe mobility Thrombosis precautions Aspiration precautions if hypercalcemic

BMT, Bone marrow transplant; *CBC*, complete blood count; *CT*, computed tomography; *DIC*, disseminated intravascular coagulation; *RBCs*, red blood cells; *WBCs*, white blood cells.

Assessment and Clinical Manifestations. Malignant hematological diseases have common risk factors, such as genetic mutations (see Genetics box); viral infection (especially retroviral); exposure to radiation, carcinogens, benzene derivatives, or pesticides; and T-lymphocyte immune suppression (e.g., high-dose steroids, immunosuppressive medications after transplantation). Other risk factors that are unique to specific malignancies are included in Table 17.10.

Assessment findings common to all malignant WBC disorders involve alterations in the immunological response to injury or microbes. As in other disorders affecting WBC function, minimized inflammatory reactions and responses to pathogens are typical. Fever is particularly difficult to interpret; it may be a manifestation of the disease process or may accompany an infectious complication. General signs and symptoms such as fatigue, malaise, myalgia, activity intolerance, and night sweats are nonspecific indicators of immune disease. Each malignant WBC disorder is also associated with signs and symptoms representative of the cell line and location of the malignancy. For example, bone pain is common in multiple myeloma, whereas lymph node enlargement is more representative of lymphoma.[23] When symptoms overlap into more than one component of the immune system, it is often difficult to differentiate among these disorders.

Knowledge of oncological emergencies associated with these malignant diseases is also important. Oncological emergencies may be a consequence of the cancer itself or of a specific treatment plan (Table 17.10). These complications are likely to precipitate admission to the critical care unit and are associated with significant morbidity and mortality.[24]

Patient Problems. The patient problems associated with hematological malignancies vary. Common problems include an increased risk for infection, decreased tissue perfusion, and risk of bleeding.

Medical Intervention. Each major subtype of hematological malignancy is associated with slightly different presenting symptoms, prognostic variables, and treatment implications. The treatment plan is based on the stage of the definitive diagnosis established by histopathology.

Therapy commonly includes chemotherapy and biotherapy. Stem cell transplant and CAR-T (chimeric antigen receptor T cells) are used in selected cases. Surgery may be performed to establish a pathological diagnosis by excisional or incisional biopsy, but it has no other significant role in the management of hematological malignancies. Radiation may be used to treat lymphoma if the disease is limited to a single node or node group.

The complexity of treatment is illustrated in the following examples. Leukemia is considered a *systemic* disease at diagnosis. Treatment of acute leukemia requires a complex chemotherapy treatment plan called *induction* chemotherapy, and it is associated with a period of severe cytopenia that requires supportive care and transfusion therapy. The management of chronic myelogenous leukemia has been improved with the development of tyrosine kinase inhibitors (TKIs), oral agents that result in high remission rates.[25] Therapy for multiple myeloma involves careful staging and a choice of induction chemotherapy plans, leading to autologous stem cell transplantation for most patients. Radiation therapy is used palliatively to control the pain associated with bone lesions. Because of the rapid application of advances in molecular biology, there has been a dramatic improvement in remission and cure rates for most hematological malignancies.

Nursing Intervention. The care of patients with hematological malignancies is similar to that for all immunocompromised patients; however, specialized management of cancer therapies must be incorporated into the individual care plan. Oncology nursing references for chemotherapy administration guidelines, management of nausea and vomiting related to acute therapy, and oncological treatment modalities are available from the Oncology Nursing Society (ONS) at https://www.ons.org/.

? CLINICAL JUDGMENT ACTIVITY

Link therapeutic benefits and risks that are associated with interventions and medications that may adversely impact the hematological or immunological health of critically ill patients.

GENETICS

Factor V Leiden: An Inherited Clotting Disorder

Factor V Leiden is an *autosomal dominant* thrombophilic disorder inherited by 35% or more individuals in the United States.[1] Thrombophilia describes an increased tendency to form abnormal blood clots. Thrombophilia leads to venous thromboembolism (VTE) or deep vein thrombosis (DVT) and pulmonary embolism (PE).

The clotting cascade has proteins that start the clotting process and stop the cascade so that clots stop growing. Factor V is a clotting factor essential in converting prothrombin to thrombin in the clotting cascade. When Factor V Leiden disease occurs, there is a *gain-of-function*, i.e., increased thrombophilia and clotting.[1]

The genetic variation in Factor V Leiden is a *missense* variation or mutation. The missense mutation results in *F5* coding for a substitute amino acid during the *translation* of DNA to a protein. Although 12 mutations for Factor V have been identified, only eight are considered pathological.[2] Females with Factor V Leiden are more likely to experience miscarriage because of thrombophilia, particularly during the second or third trimester.[2]

Age, obesity, injury, smoking, surgery, pregnancy, and estrogen-based medications increase the risk of developing abnormal blood clots in people with Factor V Leiden thrombophilia. The interaction of a genetic variation with the environment and lifestyle is a *multifactorial* genetic condition. For those with *F5* mutations, the gene-environment-lifestyle interactions influence the onset, severity, and manifestations of thrombophilia.[3] There is a 30-fold increased risk for VTE among biological females who use hormonal contraceptives or hormone replacement therapy or are pregnant when they inherit Factor V Leiden variants.[2]

Factor V Leiden disease leads to thrombophilia by creating a variant protein (Factor V) resistant to activated protein C, an endogenous clotting cascade protein contributing to clot dissolution. Individuals with two copies of the *F5* variant gene have a *homozygous* inheritance pattern—these individuals experience a 10-fold increase in VTE during their lifespan. Compared to noncarriers, a *heterozygous* inheritance (i.e., a single copy of the variant gene) leads to a 3 to 5-fold increased risk of VTE throughout their lifespan.

Like most inherited diseases, assessing genetic risk starts with obtaining a personal and family history. If two or more first-degree relatives were diagnosed with unprovoked VTE in a three-generation family tree, consider this a significant indicator of *F5* genetic disease.[3] An unprovoked VTE (i.e., VTE *not* associated with cancer, immobility, surgery, or trauma) should lead to further serum analysis, such as clotting time analyses or thrombin generation-based assays. Factor V Leiden mutation occurs too infrequently to recommend routine genetic screening.[3]

Clotting time-based assays are generally used to screen for thrombophilia.[4] More sensitive and specific tests for thrombophilia are thrombin generation-based assays.[4] *Genotypic tests*, completed with serum analyses of clotting-related factors, are sometimes labeled a thrombotic screen.

A positive genetic test for Factor V Leiden has several clinical implications. Clinicians may offer long-term anticoagulation to reduce future thrombotic events, although there is limited evidence to support the exact duration of therapy.[3] Managing thrombophilia during pregnancy requires specialized knowledge and close monitoring. Some patients may never experience VTE despite inheriting a Factor V Leiden variant.[1]

Clinicians need to be aware of the legal and ethical implications of offering a genetic test.[5] In the United States, the *Genetic Information Nondiscrimination Act (GINA)* bans genetic discrimination related to health insurance eligibility and coverage, regulating employers.[6] The Affordable Care Act also prevents insurers from declining coverage based on preexisting genetic conditions among most employer-provided coverage.[6] The results of an individual genetic test shared with relatives can impact relationships and perception of health. Uncertainty around the risk versus manifestation of a condition can be confusing and fraught with misinterpretation by patients, their family members, and clinicians.

Direct-to-consumer genetic testing is widely available (e.g., 23andMe, Ancestry). However, the nuances around the interpretation of genetic results and meaningful support for decisions to seek treatment are not generally provided by commercial self-pay services. Nurses and advanced practice nurses need to use knowledge of genomic testing for various conditions to counsel patients and advocate for clear communication about genomic, personalized health care.[7]

References

1. Zhang Y, Zhang Z, Shu S, et al. The genetics of venous thromboembolism: a systematic review of thrombophilia families. *J Thromb Thrombolysis*. 2021;51(2):359–369. https://doi.org/10.1007/s11239-020-02203-7.
2. Kujovich JL, Factor V. Leiden Thrombophilia. In: Adam MP, Everman DB, Mirzza GM, Pagon RA, Wallace SE, eds. *Gene Reviews*. The University of Seattle; 1999. Updated 2022. https://www.ncbi.nlm.nih.gov/books/NBK1368/.
3. Morrow M, Lynch-Smith D. Factor V Leiden: development of VTE in surgery and trauma patients: a systematic review. *Dimens Crit Care Nurs*. 2022;41(4):190–199. https://doi.org/10.1097/DCC.0000000000000529.
4. Morimont L, Donis N, Bouvy C, Mullier F, Dogne JM, Douxfils J. Laboratory testing for the evaluation of phenotypic activated protein C resistance. *Semin Thromb Hemost*. 2022. https://doi.org/10.1055/s-0042-1757136.
5. Braverman G, Shapiro ZE, Bernstein JA. Ethical issues in contemporary clinical genetics. *Mayo Clin Proc Innov Qual Outcomes*. 2018;2(2):81–90. https://doi.org/10.1016/j.mayocpiqo.2018.03.005.
6. Joly Y, Dupras C, Pinkesz M, Tovino SA, Rothstein MA. Looking beyond GINA: policy approaches to address genetic discrimination. *Annu Rev Genomics Hum Genet*. 2020;21:491–507. https://doi.org/10.1146/annurev-genom-111119-011436.
7. Flowers E, Leutwyler H, Shim JK. Direct-to-consumer genomic testing: are nurses prepared? *Nursing*. 2020;50(8):48–52. https://doi.org/10.1097/01.NURSE.0000684200.71662.09.

Chris Winkelman, PhD, ACNP-BC, CCRN, CNE, FAANP, FCCM

Genetic terms: *missense, translation, heterozygous, homozygous, autosomal dominant, genotypic tests, multifactorial, gain-in-function variation, GINA*

SELECTED IMMUNOLOGICAL DISORDERS

Primary Immunodeficiency

In primary immunodeficiencies, the dysfunction exists in the immune system. Most primary immunodeficiencies are congenital disorders related to a single gene defect. There are over 200 known primary immunodeficiencies. The onset of symptoms may occur within the first 2 years of life or in the second or third decade of life. These defects of the immune system typically result in frequent or recurrent infections and sometimes predispose the affected individual to unusual or severe infections.[23] Primary immunodeficiencies also predispose the patient to the development of leukemia and lymphoma. Disorders are grouped by the specific immunological disruption.

Secondary Immunodeficiency

Secondary or acquired immunodeficiencies result from factors outside the immune system; they are not related to a genetic defect and involve loss of a previously functional immune defense system. Acquired immunodeficiency syndrome (AIDS) is the most notable secondary immunodeficiency disorder caused by an infection. Aging, dietary insufficiencies, malignancies, stressors (i.e., emotional, physical), immunosuppressive therapies, and certain diseases such as diabetes or sickle cell disease are additional conditions that may be associated with acquired immunodeficiencies. Risk factors for infections in immunocompromised patients are described in Table 17.9.

HIV and AIDS

Pathophysiology. HIV is a retrovirus that transcribes its RNA-containing genetic material into the DNA of the host cell nucleus by using an enzyme called reverse transcriptase.[25] HIV causes AIDS by depleting helper T cells, CD4 cells, and macrophages.[25,26] Seroconversion is manifested by the presence of HIV antibodies and usually occurs 2 to 4 weeks after the initial infection. Seroconversion is associated with flulike symptoms such as fever, sore throat, headache, malaise, and nausea that usually last 1 to 2 weeks. This is followed by a decrease in the HIV antibody titer as infected cells are sequestered in the lymph nodes. The earlier stages of HIV infection may last for as long as 10 years and may produce few or no symptoms, although viral particles are actively replacing normal cells. This phenomenon is evident through the decreasing CD4 cell count as the disease progresses.[26] As the CD4 cell count decreases, the patient becomes more susceptible to opportunistic infections, malignancies, and neurological disease. AIDS is the final stage of HIV infection and is defined as a CD4 count of below 200 cells/mm^3 and development of one or more opportunistic infections, regardless of their cell count. Fig. 17.6 shows the progression of disease and common clinical manifestations. It is estimated that 99% of untreated HIV-infected individuals will progress to AIDS.[25,26] People with untreated AIDS can live around 3 years. Treatment of HIV is with combined antiviral medication regimens that reduce viral replication, thus slowing the progression to AIDS. HIV is now considered a chronic disease for many individuals who are compliant with antiretroviral therapy, often dying of non-HIV related illnesses such as cancer, heart disease, or complications of diabetes.[27]

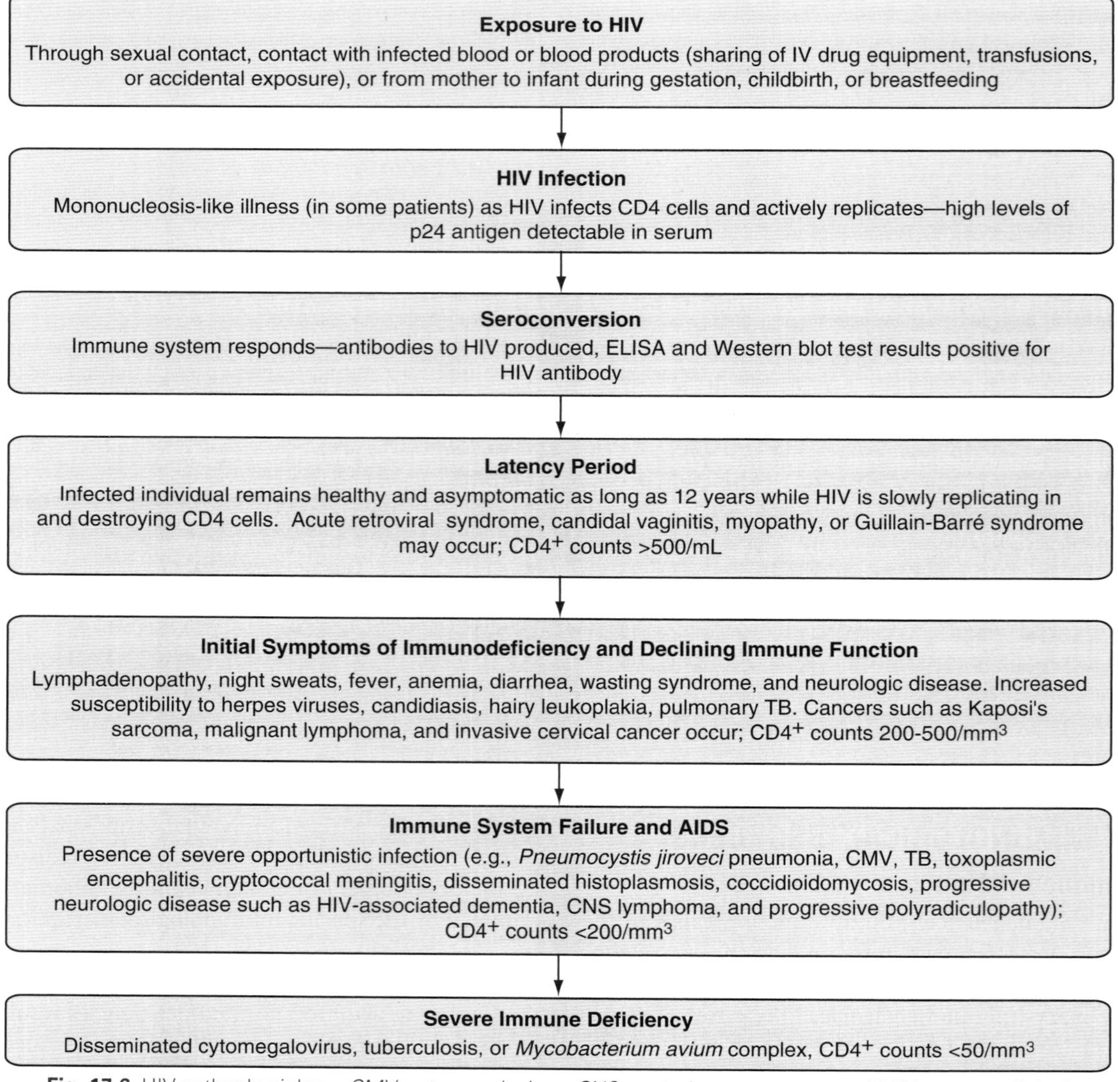

Fig. 17.6 HIV pathophysiology. *CMV,* cytomegalovirus; *CNS,* central nervous system; *ELISA,* enzyme-linked immunosorbent assay; *TB,* tuberculosis.

Prevalence of HIV in the United States continues to rise because of declining death rates from infection as a result of treatment with antiretrovirals.[25] Up to 15% of HIV-positive patients in the United States do not know they are HIV positive. Patients with HIV and AIDS are at risk of developing malignancies such as Kaposi's sarcoma, non-Hodgkin's lymphoma, and invasive cervical cancer.[27]

HIV is transmitted through exposure to infected body fluids, blood, or blood products. Common modes of transmission include rectal or vaginal intercourse with an infected person; IV drug use with contaminated equipment; transfusion with contaminated blood or blood products; and accidental exposure through needlesticks, breaks in the skin, and gestation or childbirth (transmission from mother to fetus). Risk of transmission is more likely when the infected person has advanced disease, although transmission of HIV can occur at any time or during any stage of infection. Since the 1980s, all blood products are screened for HIV, hepatitis virus, and human T-cell lymphotropic virus. HIV transmission to healthcare workers is rare.[25]

Assessment and clinical manifestations. The initial phase of HIV infection may be asymptomatic or may manifest as an acute seroconversion syndrome with symptoms similar to those of mononucleosis. This is followed by symptomatic disease as HIV progressively destroys immune cells.[27] Diagnosis of HIV infection is based on the presence of one of the core antigens of HIV or the presence of antibodies to HIV. Core antigens are tested through protein electrophoresis. HIV antibodies are detected by enzyme-linked immunosorbent assay (ELISA) and are confirmed by the Western blot test and polymerase chain reaction (PCR). Positive antibody test results are accurate for the presence of HIV infection, although a negative test result does not rule out HIV infection. Additional laboratory findings in HIV that has progressed to AIDS may include an abnormal helper-to-suppressor T-cell ratio (<1.0), leukopenia, and thrombocytopenia.

Patient problems. Nursing care of the patient with AIDS is complex and is tailored to the clinical manifestations of the disease. Patient problems commonly associated with AIDS may include decreased gas exchange, severely compromised immunity and potential for systemic infection, diarrhea, weight loss, delirium or decreased memory, acute and chronic pain, and fatigue.

Medical intervention. Medical treatment consists of primary control of HIV invasion of CD4 cells through antiretroviral therapy. Antiretroviral medications are categorized as nucleoside reverse transcriptase inhibitors, nonnucleoside reverse transcriptase inhibitors, and protease inhibitors. The specific agents used and the most appropriate strategies of combination therapy are a rapidly evolving field. Ensuring antiretroviral therapy is maintained during admission to the critical care unit is essential to maintain immune system support.[28]

Equally important to quality of life are prevention and management of opportunistic infections. Antimicrobials are administered to prevent high-risk opportunistic infections when predefined CD4 levels are reached. Additional treatment may include respiratory support, nutritional support, administration of blood products or IV fluids, administration of analgesics, and physical therapy.

Nursing intervention. Nursing care of persons living with HIV/AIDS (PLWHA) infection requires complex assessment and intervention skills. Evaluate the neurological status, mouth, respiratory status, abdominal symptoms, and peripheral sensation. As with all immunosuppressed patients, implement interventions to reduce infection risk. (see Plan of Care for the Immunocompromised Patient). These patients provide additional clinical challenges because of their multisystem clinical complications. Carefully monitor response to medications; persons with HIV have an increased risk of overlapping toxic effects as a result of polypharmacy from antiretrovirals and other medications.[28]

Desired patient outcomes of medical treatment and nursing interventions include reducing HIV viral load through medication adherence, absence of infection, adequate oxygenation, adequate nutrition and hydration, skin integrity, and absence of pain. Complications such as diarrhea and seizures are controlled. Reinforce the understanding the patient has of disease transmission regardless of viral load; the disease progression; and symptoms of opportunistic infections, treatments, and medications.

Nurse interactions with patients and family are important. Recognition of personal biases and avoidance of stigmatizing language or behaviors requires self-awareness. Delivery of care that is safe, respectful, and nonjudgmental helps to establish trust and promote more effective patient coping during acute and critical illness.[28]

CLINICAL EXEMPLAR

Diversity, Equity, and Inclusion

A female patient (she/her) recently emigrated from Eswatini, Africa, escaping violence and poverty. She is admitted with atypical pneumonia. In the course of the diagnostic workup she is diagnosed with HIV and AIDS. The patient was unaware of her HIV status. The nurse providing care to the patient understands the potential impact of this diagnosis for the patient, including her recent immigration status, lack of access to healthcare resources, language barriers, and sociocultural adjustments to the United States.

The nurse mobilizes resources within the hospital to activate social services, ethnically appropriate education, community resources, and follow-up care with a Ryan White HIV/AIDS center (https://ryanwhite.hrsa.gov/hiv-care/services). Interventions to support the patient postdischarge with her new diagnosis are incorporated into her plan of care to facilitate her ability to receive care and optimize the HIV/AIDS infection management once she recovers from the pneumonia and is discharged. Critical care nurses have a unique opportunity to provide safe, unbiased, and compassionate care to patients with HIV and AIDS who are often stigmatized as a result of their diagnosis.[28]

COVID-19

Severe acute respiratory syndrome coronavirus-2 (SARS-CoV-2) is the virus that causes coronavirus disease (COVID-19), is a highly infectious virus that spread quickly between people and has multiple presentations ranging from asymptomatic to severe illness.[29,30] The rapid transmission through several routes, however, mainly by respiratory droplets, created challenges in containing the spread of the virus. The World Health Organization (WHO) declared a global pandemic in March 2020.[31] Deaths attributed to the COVID-19 virus reached 6,808,544 worldwide as of April 2023, with 1,102,529 confirmed deaths in the United States.[31]

Coronaviruses

Coronaviruses (CoVs) are single-strand RNA viruses that were first discovered in the late 1960s and have been associated with illnesses of varying intensity.[30,32] These viruses are susceptible to mutation, leading to identification of more than 40 variations and more mutations evolving.[29,30,32] CoVs can infect humans, bats, pigs, cows, dogs, cats, pangolins, and birds.[30-32] Human-to-human transmission is most common via direct transmission, contact, and airborne particles.[30] Coughing, sneezing, and oral mucosa, and mucous membranes are common modes of viral spread.[32] SARS-CoV-2 belongs to the species of acute respiratory syndrome coronavirus (SARS-CoV). SARS-CoV was responsible for a severe outbreak in 2002, spreading to 30 countries, and the Middle Eastern respiratory syndrome coronavirus (MERS-CoV) emerged in 2012, presenting with similar acute respiratory tract infections and renal failure.[29,30,32] The emergence of SARS-CoV-2 was first identified in Wuhan, China in December 2019, leading the WHO to officially name the disease COVID-19.[30,31]

Pathophysiology. COVID-19 is an infectious disease caused by SARS-CoV-2, which attaches to the host cell at the angiotensin-converting enzyme 2 receptor. This interaction causes a release of numerous immune mediators, such as cytokines and chemokines, aimed at destroying the virus. There is a direct injury to the cell from the virus and unregulated host immune response, referred to as a cytokine storm. The unregulated immune response and release of proinflammatory cytokines triggers a complex cascade of physiologic events resulting in capillary leak, hypotension, hypoxia, DIC, bone marrow suppression with pancytopenia, and progressing to organ dysfunction (e.g., ARDS, renal, hepatic, and cardiac dysfunction, sepsis and shock).[29,30]

As an RNA virus, SARS-CoV-2 constantly evolves through random mutations; each new mutation can potentially increase or decrease infectiousness and virulence of the disease. These mutations can increase the virus' ability to evade our adaptive immunity from past infection or vaccination. Data on the emergence, transmission, and clinical relevance of each new variant evolves rapidly. This has an effect on how new variants might affect transmission rates, disease progression, vaccine development, and efficacy of treatments.[30]

Assessment and Clinical Manifestations. Patients with COVID-19 can experience clinical manifestations ranging from no symptoms to critical illness. The most common presentation is acute respiratory failure, sepsis, and progression to multiple organ failure. Patients at greatest risk of severe infection were older and had one or more chronic health condition (i.e., cardiac, renal, or pulmonary diseases, diabetes mellitus, immune disorders).[30,32] Patients with severe infections often present with significant coagulation abnormalities similar to DIC, although laboratory results vary. Most striking is an abnormally elevated D-dimer levels in almost 50% of patients.[29] Patients with a high D-dimer level have an increased need for mechanical ventilation and risk of death. Patients with severe disease often present with mild thrombocytopenia with platelet counts between 100 and 150 $\times$ 10^9/L and prolonged global coagulation tests.[30]

Nonspecific clinical manifestations included fever, cough, dyspnea, myalgias, nausea, vomiting, and diarrhea. Assessment of pulmonary function, specifically hypoxia and hypoxemia, is a key assessment parameter for defining severity of illness. Initial evaluation may include chest imaging, ECG, and laboratory testing including CBC with differential, metabolic profile, and liver and renal function tests. Inflammatory markers such as C-reactive protein (CRP), D-dimer and ferritin may also be measured. COVID-19 has been associated with a prothrombotic state with increased levels of fibrin, fibrin degradation products, and fibrinogen. Antithrombotic therapy may be needed.[30,32]

Patient Problems. As the disease progresses, the patient's clinical status can change. Patients who are ≥65 years of age, live in a nursing home or long-term care facility, are not vaccinated against COVID-19 or who have a poor response to COVID-19 vaccination, and those who have chronic conditions are at highest risk of more severe disease. Racial and ethnic minorities and other marginalized groups are also at higher risk of infection as a result of their inability to socially isolate and/or lack of access to health care.[29,30]

Patients with moderate illness have a saturation of peripheral oxygen (SpO_2) ≥94% on room air and evidence of lower respiratory disease on clinical exam. Patients with severe illness require supplemental oxygen to maintain adequate SpO_2. The respiratory rate may be over 30 breaths/minute, and lung infiltrates will be >50%. Patients who progress to critical illness may develop respiratory failure, septic shock, and/or multiple organ dysfunction syndrome (MODS).[29,30,33]

Patient problems and sequalae of COVID-19 infection vary greatly. Long COVID, or post-acute sequelae of COVID, presents with multiple diverse symptoms in approximately 10% of the population that had severe infection.[34,35] The syndrome is associated with all ages; however, the highest percentage of documented cases are individuals 36-50 years of age.[34,35] Patient symptoms associated with long COVID are different for each person. However, most common symptoms include fatigue, difficulty breathing and chronic cough, chest pain and fast-beating heart palpitations, difficulty concentrating, headaches, insomnia, abdominal discomfort, coagulopathies, microclots, joint or muscle pain, changes to menstrual cycles, and erectile dysfunction.[34,35] The management and long-term outcomes of long COVID are poorly understood, and the symptoms may last for years or be life long.[34,35]

Medical Intervention. Vaccination does not eliminate the risk of SARS-CoV-2 infection, but it does reduce the risk of morbidity and mortality.[31,33,34] Studies are ongoing to find treatments that may be helpful either pre-prophylaxis or post-prophylaxis exposure. Hospitalized patients who do not require supplemental oxygen can be treated with remdesivir.[31,33] Those who are hospitalized and requiring supplemental oxygen can receive remdesivir or dexamethasone with remdesivir. Baricitinib or tocilizumab may be added to this regimen. Patients should only receive broad-spectrum antibiotics in the case of proven or suspected bacterial infection.[30,31,33]

Patients with COVID-19 can develop hypoxic respiratory failure. Those who become critically ill require hemodynamic management, oxygenation, and possibly mechanical ventilation or extracorporeal membrane oxygenation (ECMO). Studies are ongoing to find other antiviral or immunomodulator medications to treat COVID-19. Dexamethasone with either baricitinib or tocilizumab can be added if the patient requires high-flow oxygen, noninvasive ventilation, mechanical ventilation, or ECMO.[29,30,33]

Nursing Intervention. Nursing care for the patient with COVID-19 is primarily supportive. Patients can be hospitalized for long periods of time. As the virus has mutated, risks associated with disease morbidity and mortality have changed. Nurses should take care to prevent the sequelae of critical illnesses such as hospital-acquired infection, VTE, and delirium. Patients who require prone positioning may be either nonventilated or mechanically ventilated and are at risk for pressure injury development (see Chapter 15, Acute Respiratory Failure). They should also be carefully assessed and managed for pain and anxiety, particularly if there is a need to use neuromuscular blocking agents. Effects of psychosocial aspects of critical illness must also be addressed for the patient and family.[29,35]

BLEEDING DISORDERS

Patients with abnormal hemostasis often require critical care treatment. A general approach to assessing and managing the bleeding patient is included, followed by a more thorough discussion of thrombocytopenia and DIC.

The Bleeding Patient

Pathophysiology. Bleeding disorders, also referred to as *coagulopathies,* are caused by abnormalities in one of the stages of clotting. Disorders may be inherited (e.g., hemophilia, von Willebrand disease) or acquired (e.g., vitamin K deficiency, DIC).[36,37] Coagulopathies induce bleeding manifestations, and many care principles are universal. This section addresses the universal care of patients with disorders of coagulation.

Assessment and Clinical Manifestations. A patient with abnormal bleeding requires careful collection of medical and social histories. Assess for medical disorders and medications known to interfere with platelets, coagulation proteins, or fibrinolysis. Disruptions in hemostasis commonly occur with renal disease, hepatic or gastrointestinal disorders, or malnutrition. Medications that may alter hemostasis include aminoglycosides, anticoagulants, antiplatelet agents, cephalosporins, histamine blockers, nitrates, sulfonamides, sympathomimetics, and vasodilators.

The physical examination is extremely important. Although many patients with bleeding disorders demonstrate active bleeding from body orifices, mucous membranes, and open lesions or IV line sites, equal numbers of patients have less obvious bleeding. The most susceptible sites for bleeding are existing openings in the epithelial surface. Mucous membranes have a low threshold for bleeding because the capillaries lie close to the membrane surface, and minor injury may damage and expose vessels. Substantial blood loss can occur in any coagulopathy, resulting in hypovolemic shock. A general overview of assessment findings that indicate bleeding is included in Table 17.5.

Diagnostic tests are performed to evaluate the cause of the bleeding disorder and the extent of blood loss. The CBC provides quantitative values for RBCs and platelets. When the disorder arises from coagulation protein or clot lysis abnormalities, screening coagulation tests for fibrinogen level, prothrombin time (PT), and activated partial thromboplastin time (aPTT) are ordered. Point-of-care tests for hemoglobin, hematocrit, and aPTT are important resources to obtain immediate feedback on the patient's status. In certain disease states, the results of additional specialized tests, such as bleeding time and level of fibrin degradation products, are monitored.

A thromboelastogram (TEG) is a newer noninvasive test that quantitatively measures the ability of the blood to form a clot. The test is done to identify hypercoagulable states, identify accelerated fibrinolysis, and assess the function of platelets and coagulation factors. Results may be used to guide treatment. Table 17.11 provides information about TEG.

Patient Problems. A patient with a hemostatic disorder can bleed in any body system. The major patient problems include potential for bleeding and hypovolemic shock, potential for skin and tissue breakdown, and acute pain.

Medical Intervention. Medical treatment for bleeding patients depends on the suspected cause. Component-specific replacement transfusions are preferred over whole blood because they provide more targeted treatment of the bleeding disorder. Transfusion thresholds are established based on laboratory values and patient-specific variables, particularly patient symptoms and clinical presentation. In general, the threshold for RBC transfusion is a hematocrit level of 28% to 31% and hemoglobin level 7 g/dL to 8 g/dL, based on the patient's cardiovascular tolerance (see Evidence-Based Practice box). If angina or orthostasis is present, a higher threshold may be maintained. The threshold for transfusing platelets is usually between 20,000 and 50,000/mm^3 of blood. Cryoprecipitate is usually infused if the fibrinogen level is lower than 100 mg/dL. Fresh frozen plasma is used to correct a prolonged PT and aPTT or a specific factor deficiency. A summary of blood product components, clinical indications, and nursing implications is included in Table 17.12.

When the cause of bleeding is unknown or multifactorial, nonspecific interventions aimed at stopping bleeding are used.

These include local and systemic procoagulant medications and therapies. Local therapies to stop bleeding are used when systemic anticoagulation is necessary for treatment of another health condition (e.g., myocardial infarction, ischemic stroke, pulmonary embolism). Local procoagulants act by direct tissue contact and initiation of a surface clot.

Systemic procoagulant medications may be used judiciously to enhance vasoconstriction (e.g., vasopressin), enhance clot formation (e.g., somatostatin), or prevent fibrinolysis (e.g., aminocaproic acid). Each agent has significant adverse effects that must be considered before implementation. All may enhance clot production and induce thrombotic vascular or neurological events. They may be contraindicated if the patient has simultaneous procoagulant risk factors.

Nursing Intervention. Patients with bleeding disorders often have multisystem manifestations. Administration of fluids and blood products is a priority nursing intervention that requires careful consideration of the patient's specific coagulation defect. If the patient's blood does not clot because of thrombocytopenia, administration of RBCs before platelets will result in RBC loss from disrupted vascular structures.

Additional nursing interventions specific to the patient with a coagulopathy include weighing dressings to assess blood loss, assessing fluids for occult blood, observing for oozing and bleeding from skin and mucous membranes, and leaving clots undisturbed. Precautions such as limiting invasive procedures (including indwelling urinary catheters and rectal temperature measurement) are also important.

CLINICAL JUDGMENT ACTIVITY

Identify and prioritize nursing and medical interventions for the bleeding patient.

PLAN OF CARE

For the Patient With a Bleeding Disorder

Patient Problem

Potential for bleeding/hemorrhage due to depletion of clotting factors or platelets.

Desired Outcomes

- Absence of bleeding.
- Stable vital signs.
- Oriented to person, place, and time; no changes in mental status.

Nursing Assessments/Interventions	Rationales
• Regularly assess LOC and monitor vital signs.	• Changes in mentation and vital signs can indicate hemorrhage.
• Prevent excess pressure when taking BP.	• Frequent BP readings can cause bleeding under the cuff.
• Assess for abdominal pain and distension.	• May indicate GI bleeding.
• Assess stool, urine, vomitus, and nasogastric drainage for occult blood.	• Bleeding initially may be undetectable.
• Regularly assess puncture sites.	• May detect external bleeding.
• Post "bleeding precautions" sign.	• Alert all caregivers to the potential for bleeding and to use caution when implementing care and treatments.
• Ensure no administration of rectal medications, IM injections, or flossing of teeth.	• Prevent disruption in skin and mucous membranes.
• Recognize signs and symptoms of subcutaneous bleeding (e.g., oozing, ecchymoses, hematomas).	• Assess for bleeding disorders.
• Administer blood products as ordered.	• Correct deficiencies.
• Administer procoagulants (e.g., somatostatin, estrogen) as ordered.	• Promote clotting and decrease bleeding.
• Administer topical hemostatic agents, if indicated.	• Decrease bleeding from skin lesions.

Patient Problem

Potential for skin and tissue breakdown due to altered circulation.

Desired Outcome

- Skin and tissue remain intact.

Nursing Assessments/Interventions	Rationales
• Regularly assess skin and mucous membranes for changes.	• Changes in color, sensation, and temperature may occur.
• Reposition patient every 2 hours; provide good skin and oral care.	• Promote circulation.
• Keep extremities warm.	• Prevent tissue hypoxia and improve circulation.
• Elevate any limb that is bleeding.	• Reduce blood flow to the area to prevent further blood loss.
• Use alternatives to tape for dressings.	• Tape can damage fragile skin.

BP, Blood pressure; *GI*, gastrointestinal; *IM*, intramuscular; *LOC*, level of consciousness.
Data from Snyder J, Sump C. *Swearingen's All-in-One Nursing Care Planning Resource*, 6th ed. Elsevier; 2024.

TABLE 17.11 Thromboelastogram (TEG) Parameters

Parameter	Clotting Phase Assessed	Normal Values	Implications
Reaction time (R)	Activation—time to activate the intrinsic pathway and initiate clot (amplitude 2 mm)	5-10 min	Dependent on clotting factors Prolonged R time may indicate need for FFP
Kinetics (K)	Amplification—time to form a clot with a certain level of strength (amplitude 20 mm)	1-3 min	Dependent on fibrinogen Prolonged time may indicate need for FFP or cryoprecipitate
Alpha angle (A)	Propagation—characterization of maximal speed of thrombus generation, fibrin deposition, and cross-linking	53-72 degrees	Dependent on fibrinogen Narrow angle may indicate need for cryoprecipitate and/or platelets
Maximum amplitude (MA)	Termination—maximal strength of the clot; measures amplitude of TEG curve	50-70 min	Dependent on platelets and interaction of fibrin with clotting factors GP IIb/IIa Low amplitude may indicate need for platelets
Lysis at 30 min (A30 or LY30)	Fibrinolytic—speed of fibrinolysis	0%-8%	Represents fibrinolysis Higher percentage may indicate need for tranexamic acid

FFP, Fresh frozen plasma; *TEG*, thromboelastogram.
Adapted from Shaydakov M, Sigmon DF, Blebea J. Thromboelastography (TEG). *Stat Pearls*. Treasure Island, FL: Stat Pearls Publishing; 2022. https://www.ncbi.nlm.nih.gov/books/NBK537061/#_NBK537061_pubdet_.

Thrombocytopenia

Pathophysiology. A quantitative deficiency of platelets is called *thrombocytopenia*. By definition, this is a platelet count of less than 150,000/mm^3.[36] A value of 50,000/mm^3 is considered critically low, and spontaneous bleeding may occur but often not until the platelet count falls below 20,000/mm^3. Fatal hemorrhage is a great risk when the count is lower than 10,000/mm^3, but some patients with immune thrombocytopenia can tolerate levels as low as 5000 mm^3.[36] The pathophysiology may be related to decreased production of platelets by the bone marrow, increased destruction of platelets, or sequestration of platelets (abnormal distribution).[23]

Assessment and Clinical Manifestations. Many critical care therapies and medications interfere with platelet production and cause thrombocytopenia. Thorough medical, social, and medication histories can help identify factors that can cause thrombocytopenia (Box 17.3). Heparin-induced thrombocytopenia (HIT) can occur and is described in Box 17.4.[23,36]

Clinically, the presenting symptoms of thrombocytopenia are petechiae, purpura, and ecchymosis, with oozing from mucous membranes. The patient may also have melena, hematuria, or epistaxis.

EVIDENCE-BASED PRACTICE

Red Blood Cell Transfusion

Problem

Transfusion of RBCs is not a benign procedure. It is associated with complications, including transfusion reactions and acute lung injury. Determining clinical indicators for transfusion, including thresholds, is important.

Clinical Question

What outcomes are associated with RBC transfusions? What clinical indicators and thresholds should be used to trigger transfusion orders?

Evidence

The systematic review by Carson and colleagues evaluated 48 trials involving 21,433 patients across clinical specialties. The hemoglobin concentration used to define restrictive transfusion (N=36) is a threshold between 7 g/dL and 8 g/dL, compared to the liberal transfusion threshold of 9 g/dL to 10 g/dL. Participants assigned to receive blood at lower blood counts were 41% less likely to receive a blood transfusion than those who were given blood at higher thresholds. The risk of dying within 30 days of the transfusion did not differ between groups.

The authors concluded that it was not harmful to the participants' health status to give blood at lower or higher blood counts. The amount of blood patients received and the risk of patients receiving blood transfusions unnecessarily would be substantially reduced if lower blood counts were used. Because transfusions can have harmful effects, the safety implications are appreciated, supporting more restrictive hemoglobin thresholds to guide blood transfusion decisions.

Implications for Nursing

The transfusion of RBCs can be avoided in most patients with hemoglobin levels above 7 to 8 g/dL. The safety of transfusion in certain clinical subgroups, including those with acute coronary syndrome, myocardial infarction, neurological injury, traumatic brain injury, acute neurological disorders, stroke, thrombocytopenia, cancer, hematological malignances, and bone marrow failure, is unknown. Blood is a limited resource, and the procedure itself comes with potential risk. Thus evaluating clinical presentation and symptoms for need may decrease the incidence of posttransfusion issues, including infection (e.g., pneumonia, wound infection, blood poisoning); heart attacks, strokes, and problems with blood clots. The patient's underlying comorbidities must be considered in decision making. Monitor serial hemoglobin levels and assess patients for signs and symptoms related to lower hemoglobin and hematocrit levels.

Level of Evidence

A—Systematic Review

Reference

Carson JL, Stanworth SJ, Dennis JA, et al. Transfusion thresholds for guiding allogeneic red blood cell transfusion. *Cochrane Database Syst Rev*. 2021. https://doi.org/10.1002/14651858.CD002042.pub5.

TABLE 17.12 Summary of Blood Products and Administration

Blood Component	Description	Actions	Indications	Administration	Complications
Whole blood	RBCs, plasma, and stable clotting factors	Restores oxygen-carrying capacity and intravascular volume	Symptomatic anemia with major circulating volume deficit Massive hemorrhage with shock	Donor and recipient must be ABO and Rh compatible Use microaggregate filter *Rate of infusion:* 2-4 units/h but more rapid in cases of shock	Hemolytic reaction Allergic reaction Hypothermia Electrolyte disturbances Citrate intoxication Infectious diseases
RBCs	RBCs centrifuged from whole blood	Restores oxygen-carrying capacity and intravascular volume	Symptomatic anemia when patient is at risk for fluid overload Acute hemorrhage	Donor and recipient must be ABO and Rh compatible Use microaggregate filter *Rate of infusion:* 2-4 units/h but more rapid in cases of shock	Infectious diseases Hemolytic reaction Allergic reaction Hypothermia Electrolyte disturbances Citrate intoxication
Leukocyte-poor cells or washed RBCs	RBCs from which leukocytes and plasma proteins have been reduced	Restores oxygen-carrying capacity and intravascular volume	Symptomatic anemia with patient history of repeated, febrile, nonhemolytic transfusion reactions Acute hemorrhage	Donor and recipient must be ABO and Rh compatible Use microaggregate filter *Rate of infusion:* 2-4 units/h but more rapid in cases of shock	Allergic reaction Hemolytic reaction Hypothermia Electrolyte disturbances Citrate intoxication Infectious diseases
Fresh frozen plasma	Plasma rich in clotting factors with platelets removed	Replaces clotting factors	Deficit of coagulation factors as in DIC, liver disease, and massive transfusions Major trauma with signs or symptoms of hemorrhage	Donor and recipient must be ABO compatible, but it is not necessary to be Rh compatible *Rate of infusion:* 10 mL/min	Allergic reaction Febrile reactions Circulatory overload Infectious diseases
Platelets	Removed from whole blood	Increases platelet count and improves hemostasis	Thrombocytopenia Platelet dysfunction (prophylactically for platelet counts 10,000-20,000/mm^3), evidence of bleeding with platelet count <50,000/mm^3	Do not use microaggregate filter; use component filter obtained from blood bank ABO testing is not necessary but is usually done Usually, 6 units are given at one time	Infectious diseases Allergic reactions Febrile reactions
Cryoprecipitate antihemophilic factor	Coagulation factor VIII with 250 mg of fibrinogen and 20%-30% of factor XIII	Replaces selected clotting factors	Hemophilia A, von Willebrand disease Hypofibrinogenemia Factor XIII deficiency Massive transfusions	Repeat doses may be necessary to attain desired serum level *Rate of infusion:* approximately 10 mL of diluted component per minute	Allergic reactions Infectious diseases

TABLE 17.12 Summary of Blood Products and Administration—cont'd

Blood Component	Description	Actions	Indications	Administration	Complications
Albumin	Prepared from plasma	Expands intravascular volume by increasing oncotic pressure	Hypovolemic shock Liver failure	Special administration set *Rate of infusion:* over 30-60 min	Circulatory overload Febrile reaction
Granulocytes	Prepared by centrifugation or filtration leucopheresis, which removes granulocytes from whole blood	Increases the leukocyte level	Decreased WBCs, usually from chemotherapy or radiation	Must be ABO and Rh compatible *Rate of infusion:* 1 unit over 2-4 h; closely observe for reaction	Rash Febrile reaction Hepatitis
Plasma proteins	Pooled from human plasma	Expands intravascular volume by increasing oncotic pressure	Hypovolemic shock	ABO compatibility not necessary *Rate of infusion:* over 30-60 min	Circulatory overload Febrile reaction

DIC, Disseminated intravascular coagulation; *RBCs,* red blood cells; *WBCs,* white blood cells.

BOX 17.3 Causes of Thrombocytopenia

Bone Marrow Suppression
- Aplastic anemia
- Burns
- Cancer chemotherapy
- Exposure to ionizing radiation
- Nutritional deficiency (vitamin B_{12}, folate)

Interference With Platelet Production (Other Than Nonspecific Marrow Suppression)
- Alcohol
- Histamine$_2$-blocking agents
- Histoplasmosis
- Hormones
- Thiazide diuretics

Platelet Destruction Outside the Bone Marrow
- Artificial heart valves
- Cardiac bypass machine
- Heat stroke
- Heparin
- Infections: severe or sepsis
- Intraaortic balloon pump
- Large-bore IV lines
- Splenic sequestration of platelets
- Sulfonamides
- Transfusions
- Trimethoprim-sulfamethoxazole

Immune Response Against Platelets
- Idiopathic thrombocytopenic purpura
- Mononucleosis
- Thrombotic thrombocytopenic purpura
- Vaccinations
- Viral illness

Interference With Platelet Function
- Cirrhosis
- Diabetes mellitus
- Hypothermia
- Malignant lymphomas
- Nonsteroidal antiinflammatory agents
- Omega 3 (fish oil)
- Sarcoidosis
- Scleroderma
- Systemic lupus erythematosus
- Thyrotoxicosis
- Uremia

Medications
- Aminoglycosides
- Dextran
- Diazepam
- Digitoxin
- Dopamine
- Epinephrine
- Loop diuretics
- Nonsteroidal antiinflammatory agents
- Omega 3 (fish oil)
- Phenothiazines
- Phenytoin
- Salicylate derivatives
- Tricyclic antidepressants
- Vitamin E

BOX 17.4 Heparin-Induced Thrombocytopenia

Definition

Heparin-induced thrombocytopenia (HIT) is defined as a decrease of 50% or more from the highest platelet count after heparin has been initiated to nadir of approximately 20×10^9/L. It usually occurs 5 to 10 days after the start of heparin therapy. However, delayed-onset HIT can develop after heparin has been discontinued, and spontaneous (autoimmune) HIT can develop in the absence of exposure to heparin; however, the timing may be unclear. Heparin binds to platelet factor 4 (PF4), forming an antigenic complex on the surface of the platelets. Some patients develop an antibody to this complex, which stimulates removal of platelets by splenic macrophages, and thrombocytopenia develops. The primary complication of HIT is not bleeding, but hypercoagulability and thrombosis.

Risks

The risk for HIT is 10-fold higher among those receiving unfractionated heparin as opposed to low-molecular-weight heparin (LMWH). HIT also occurs more frequently in patients who have had major surgery. The 4Ts score for estimating the pretest probability of HIT is calculated including the categories: thrombocytopenia (acute), timing of fall in platelet count or other sequelae, thrombosis or other sequelae, and other cause for thrombocytopenia. The pretest probability score of 6-8 is high; 4-5 is intermediate; and 0-3 is low.

Complications

Major complications are thromboembolic in nature. These include deep vein thrombosis, pulmonary embolism, myocardial infarction, thrombotic stroke, arterial occlusion in limbs, and disseminated intravascular coagulation (DIC).

Diagnosis

HIT usually develops 5 to 10 days after initiation of heparin therapy; however, rapid-onset HIT can occur within the first hours after heparin exposure. Clinical criteria include a 50% decrease from the highest level after heparin is started and a new thrombosis or anaphylactoid reaction after heparin bolus. PF4-heparin antibody tests are done if clinical criteria are present.

Treatment

HIT is treated by discontinuing all heparin products, including heparin flushes and heparin-coated infusion catheters. Treatment focuses on administration of medications that inhibit thrombin formation or cause direct thrombin inhibition: argatroban (Novastan), danaparoid (Orgaran), fondaparinux (Arixtra), or bivalirudin (Angiomax). Treatment with warfarin, LMWH, aminocaproic acid, or platelets is avoided because these agents may exacerbate the prothrombotic state.

From Greinacher A, Selleng S. Thrombocytopenia. In: Vincent JL, Abraham E, Moore FA, et al., eds. *Textbook of Critical Care*. 7th ed. Philadelphia: Elsevier; 2017:79-83.e1.

Patient Problems. Patients with thrombocytopenia have many of the same problems as listed under the care of the bleeding patient. An additional problem is altered body image due to petechiae and ecchymosis (see Clinical Alert box).

! CLINICAL ALERT

Bleeding Disorders

Inspect all body surfaces for overt bleeding, such as bruising or petechiae, bleeding gums, unexplained nose bleeds, or heavy menstrual bleeding. Internal bleeding is more difficult to recognize because it may occur even without a known injury, and symptoms are often subtle.

Medical Intervention. Medical treatment of thrombocytopenia includes infusions of platelets or growth factors, such as romiplostim, to stimulate the bone marrow to produce more platelets; however, growth factors can take days to increase the platelet count. Patients who require multiple platelet transfusions are evaluated for infusion of single-donor platelet products or HLA-matched platelets to prevent destruction of platelets by the recipient's immune system. For every unit of single-donor platelets, the platelet count is expected to increase by 5000 to 10,000/mm^3. Patients who receive many platelet transfusions can become refractory, or alloimmunized, to the different platelet antigens and may benefit from receiving platelets that are a match for their own HLA type. After multiple platelet transfusions, febrile and allergic transfusion reactions are common; they can be reduced by administration of acetaminophen and diphenhydramine before transfusion.

Some thrombocytopenia conditions are autoimmune induced and may respond to filtration of antibodies via plasmapheresis or immune suppression with corticosteroids. When the spleen is enlarged and tender and these other supportive therapies are unsuccessful, splenectomy can alleviate the autoimmune reaction.

Nursing Intervention. Nursing interventions for the patient with thrombocytopenia are similar to those listed for the bleeding patient. Recognize and limit factors that can deplete or shorten the lifespan of platelets. For example, high fever and high metabolic activity (e.g., seizures) prematurely destroy platelets. Desired patient outcomes include adequate tissue perfusion, skin integrity, prompt recognition and treatment of bleeding, and absence of pain.

CHECK YOUR UNDERSTANDING

3. When the patient's hematological and immunological systems are compromised, it is not uncommon to require transfusions of several different types of blood products. Which patient condition would warrant the administration of platelets as the first consideration?
   A. Anemia
   B. Thrombocytopenia
   C. Vitamin K deficiency
   D. Neutropenia

Disseminated Intravascular Coagulation

Pathophysiology. DIC is a serious disorder of hemostasis that is characterized by simultaneous clotting and bleeding. The syndrome is always caused by an underlying disease process and is not a disease itself. DIC can develop acutely or be a chronic condition. Acute DIC is life-threatening. Acute DIC develops rapidly and is the most serious form of acquired coagulopathy. Patients with chronic DIC may have more subtle clinical and laboratory findings. Sepsis is the most common cause of acute DIC, but malignancies and inflammatory state can also lead to DIC.[23,36,37]

In DIC, the coagulation cascade is abnormally activated, leading to coagulation and fibrinolysis. Blood is exposed to a procoagulant factor, which activates clotting. The procoagulant factor can come from different sources. Examples include blood vessel injury, such as in trauma, which can release procoagulant enzymes or phospholipids, "cancer procoagulant" with malignancy that activates factor X, or bacterial products that cause

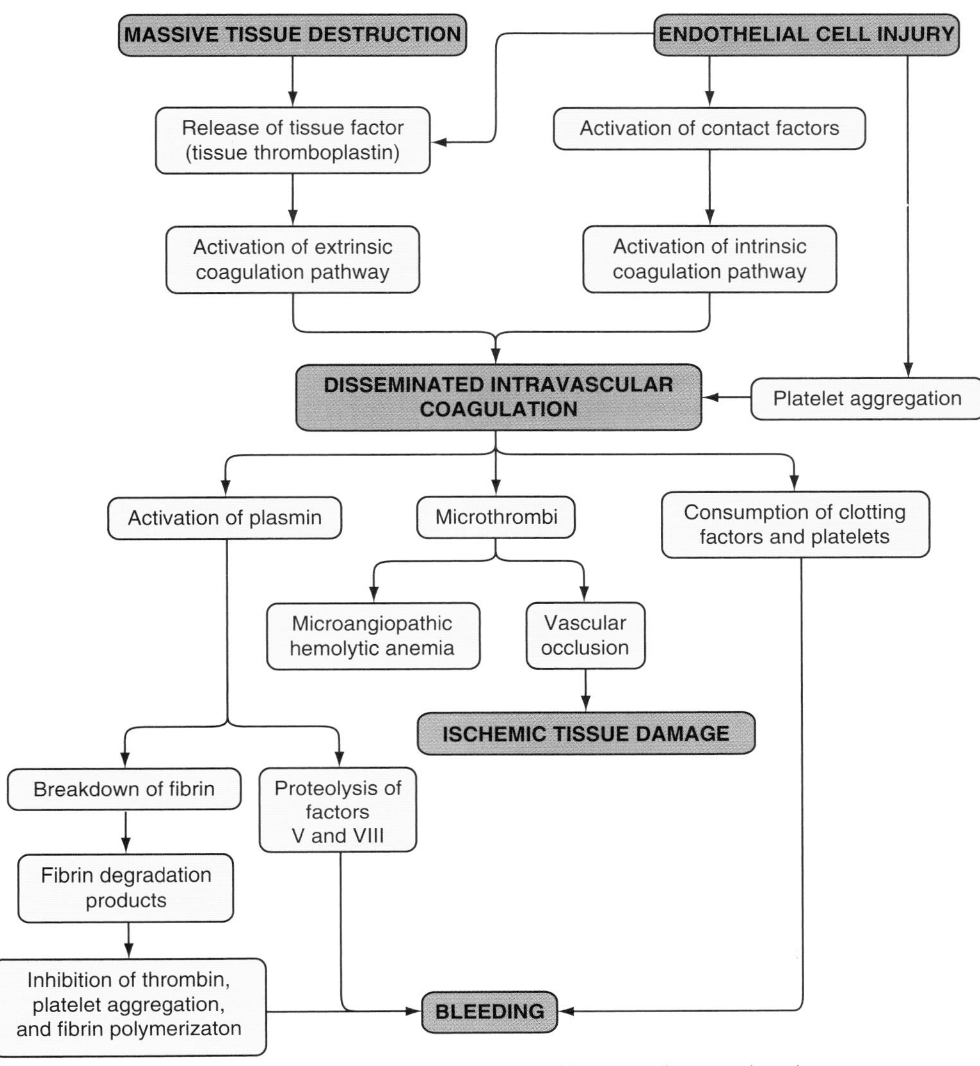

Fig. 17.7 Pathophysiology of disseminated intravascular coagulopathy.

inflammation and activate coagulation. The body responds to this clotting by activating fibrinolysis to break up the clots. End-organ damage occurs from the clotting or bleeding (Fig. 17.7). Clotting in the microvasculature of the patient with DIC causes organ ischemia and necrosis. The skin, lungs, and kidneys are most often damaged. Thrombophlebitis, pulmonary embolism, cerebrovascular accident, gastrointestinal bleeding, and renal failure may result from thrombosis. In addition, microvasculature thrombosis may result in cyanosis of the fingers and toes; purpura fulminans; or infarction and gangrene of the digits, the tip of the nose, or the penis.[23,37]

Assessment and Clinical Manifestations. DIC is always a secondary complication of excessive clotting stimuli and may be triggered by vessel injury caused by disease states, tissue injury, or a foreign body in the bloodstream. Sepsis, multisystem trauma, malignancy, and burns are the main risk factors for DIC.[23,38] Recognition of potential risk factors and conscientious monitoring of the high-risk patient can facilitate early intervention (see Table 17.13 for a summary of common risk factors for DIC).

Clinically, the patient with DIC first develops microvascular thrombosis. Thrombosis leads to organ ischemia and necrosis that may manifest as changes in mental status, angina, hypoxemia, oliguria, or nonspecific hepatitis. Cyanosis and infarction of the fingers, toes, and tip of the nose may occur if the DIC is severe. After a thrombotic phase of hours to a few days, depletion of clotting factors and clot lysis cause excessive bleeding. Early signs may include occult blood in the stool, emesis, and urine. Capillary fragility and depleted clotting factors often appear early as mucosal or subcutaneous tissue bleeding seen as gingival bleeding, petechiae, or ecchymosis. Overt bleeding ranges from mild oozing from venipuncture sites to massive hemorrhage from all body orifices. Occult bleeding into body cavities, such as the peritoneal and retroperitoneal spaces, is detected by changes in vital signs or other classic signs of blood loss.[37]

No singular lab test is diagnostic of DIC. Diagnosis of DIC is based on recognition of pertinent risk factors, clinical symptoms, and the results of laboratory studies. Lab tests that assist in the diagnosis of DIC are thrombocytopenia, PT, aPTT, decreased fibrinogen, and increased D-dimer level.[38] Altered laboratory values in DIC are described in the Laboratory Alert box.

TABLE 17.13 Causes of Disseminated Intravascular Coagulation

Cause	Examples
Infections	Bacterial (especially gram-negative), fungal, viral, mycobacterial, protozoan, rickettsia
Trauma	Burns, crush or multiple injuries, snakebite, severe head injury
Obstetric causes	Abruptio placentae, placenta previa, amniotic fluid embolism, retained dead fetus, missed abortion, eclampsia, hydatidiform mole, septic abortion
Hematologic/immunologic disorders	Transfusion reaction, transplant rejections, anaphylaxis, acute hemolysis, transfusion of mismatched blood products, autoimmune disorders, sickle cell crisis
Oncologic disorders	Carcinomas, leukemias, metastatic cancer
Miscellaneous	Extracorporeal circulation, pulmonary or fat embolism, anoxia, acidosis, hyperthermia or hypothermia, hypovolemic shock, ARDS, sustained hypotension, shock

ARDS, Acute respiratory distress syndrome.
From Marti-Carvajal AJ, Anand V, Ivan S. Treatment for disseminated intravascular coagulation in patients with acute and chronic leukemia. *Cochrane Database Syst Rev.* 2015;15(6):CD008562; Costello RA, Nehring SM. Disseminated Intravascular Coagulation. In: *StatPearls.* Treasure Island (FL): StatPearls Publishing; 2022.

! LABORATORY ALERT

Disseminated Intravascular Coagulation

Test	Normal Value[a]	Alteration
Platelet count	150,000-400,000/mm^3	Decreased
Prothrombin time (PT)	11-16 sec	Increased
Activated partial thromboplastin time (aPTT)	30-45 sec	Increased
Thrombin time (TT)	10-15 sec	Increased
Fibrinogen	150-400 mg/dL	Decreased
D-dimer assay	<100 mcg/L	Increased

[a]Critical values vary by facility and laboratory.

Patient Problems. DIC is likely to involve multiple systems that encompass both thrombotic and hemorrhagic manifestations. Patient problems may include potential for bleeding or hemorrhage, decreased peripheral tissue perfusion, fluid volume deficit, excessive clotting, impaired skin integrity, and acute pain.

Medical Intervention. Medical treatment of DIC is aimed at identifying and treating the underlying cause, stopping the abnormal coagulation, and controlling the bleeding. Correction of hypotension, hypoxemia, and acidosis is vital, as is treatment of infection if it is the triggering factor. If the cause is obstetrical, evacuation of the uterus for retained fetal tissue or other tissue must be performed. Blood volume expanders and crystalloid IV fluids, such as Lactated Ringer's solution or 0.9% normal saline, are given to counteract hypovolemia caused by blood loss, along with necessary blood products (see Chapter 12, Shock, Sepsis, and Multiple Organ Dysfunction Syndrome).

Blood component therapy is used to replace deficient platelets and clotting factors and to treat hemorrhage. Platelet infusions are usually necessary because of consumptive thrombocytopenia. Administration of platelets is the highest priority for transfusion because platelets provide the clotting factors needed to establish an initial platelet plug at any bleeding site. Fresh frozen plasma is administered for fibrinogen replacement. It contains all clotting factors and antithrombin III; however, factor VIII is often inactivated by the freezing process, necessitating administration of concentrated factor VIII in the form of cryoprecipitate. Transfusions of packed RBCs are given to replace cells lost through hemorrhage.

Heparin is a potent thrombin inhibitor and may be administered, in low doses, to block the clotting process that initiates DIC. Heparin is given to prevent further clotting and thrombosis that may lead to organ ischemia and necrosis. Although heparin's antithrombin activity prevents further clotting, it may increase the risk of bleeding and can cause further problems. Its use in patients with DIC is controversial.[39] Other pharmacological therapy in DIC includes the administration of synthetic antithrombin III, which also inhibits thrombin.[39] Antithrombin III concentrates may shorten the course of the disease and may increase the survival rate. Administration of aminocaproic acid (Amicar) inhibits fibrinolysis by interfering with plasmin activity. Fibrinolytics should be given only if other treatments have been unsuccessful and hemorrhage is life-threatening; there is no clear evidence of risk versus benefit with their use. Supportive care with transfusions remains the standard of care for DIC management.

Nursing Intervention. Nursing care of the patient with DIC is aimed at prevention and recognition of thrombotic and hemorrhagic events. Assessment for complications facilitates prompt and aggressive interventions. Psychosocial support for the patient and family is critical in these circumstances. It is important to inform the patient and family that DIC can take days to resolve once treatment of the underlying cause is started.

Pain relief and promotion of comfort are important nursing priorities. Assess the location, intensity, and quality of the patient's pain, along with the patient's response to discomfort. Optimize care to prevent vasoconstriction, which contributes to tissue ischemia and its associated discomfort. Relief of discomfort also reduces oxygen consumption, which is important for these patients with limited circulatory flow. Administer pain medication as ordered and before painful procedures. Positioning, with support and proper body alignment and frequent changes, also enhances the patient's level of comfort.

Monitor the results of coagulation laboratory studies for evidence of disease resolution. As fewer clots are created, the platelet count and fibrinogen level are among the first laboratory values to return to normal. The levels of fibrin degradation products and D-dimer fall, and antithrombin III levels rise, as fibrinolysis slows. Other coagulation tests are less sensitive and are not usually assessed.

CHECK YOUR UNDERSTANDING

4. Identify the medical condition that is least likely to predispose a patient to disseminated intravascular coagulation (DIC).
   A. Gram-negative bacterial infections
   B. Abruptio placentae
   C. Transfusion reaction
   D. Acute renal failure

CASE STUDY

Mr. F. is a 62-year-old male with acute myelogenous leukemia diagnosed 15 months ago. He received induction (high-dose) chemotherapy, which resulted in disease remission. He received additional chemotherapy over the next 4 months and underwent an allogeneic peripheral blood stem cell transplant (identical-matched donor; his sister). He was started on standard immunosuppressive medications to prevent graft-versus-host disease (GVHD). Forty-three days after his transplant, Mr. F. was diagnosed with steroid refractory GVHD with widespread skin sloughing, severe diarrhea, and nausea/vomiting, with no response to high-dose steroid treatment. He has been on high-dose steroids for several weeks and now presents to the critical care unit with pneumonia and sepsis, requiring intubation and pressors.

Questions

1. List risk factors for Mr. F that may have contributed to the development of GVHD.
2. Describe priority interventions in the of care for the patient experiencing chronic GVHD.
3. Identify key nursing interventions for this patient with steroid refractory GVHD.

KEY POINTS

- Nursing assessment of critically ill patients must include assessment for hematologic and immunologic derangements.
- Immunocompromised critically ill patients are at risk for serious infection and death from infectious disease processes.
- Coagulopathies can be inherited or acquired and can lead to substantial blood loss, causing critical illness.
- HIV is a chronic illness that, when untreated, can lead to AIDS and severe immune compromise.
- DIC is the most serious bleeding disorder. Sepsis is the most common cause of DIC.
- COVID-19 is a disease with propensity for causing critical illness.

REFERENCES

1. Turner K.C. Structure and Function of the Hematologic Systems. In: Rodgers, J eds. *McCance & Huether's Pathophysiology: The biologic Basis for Diseases in Adults and Children*. 9th ed. Elsevier. 2023:892–924.
2. Ghiaur G, Jones R. Hematopoiesis. In: Lazarus HM, Schmaier AH, eds. *Concise Guide to Hematology*. 2nd ed. Springer; 2019. Page numbers?
3. Wilson A, Trumpp A. Bone-marrow haematopoietic-stem-cell niches. *Nat Rev Immunol*. 2006;6(2):93–106. https://doi.org/10.1038/nri1779.
4. Hall JE, Hall ME. Transport of oxygen and carbon dioxide in blood and tissue fluids. In: Hall JE, ed. *Guyton and Hall Textbook of Medical Physiology*. 14th ed. Philadelphia, PA: Saunders; 2021:521–530.
5. Hall JE, Hall ME. Hemostasis and blood coagulation. In: Hall JE, ed. *Guyton and Hall Textbook of Medical Physiology*. 14th ed. Philadelphia, PA: Saunders; 2021:477–488.
6. McDonald B, Dunbar M. Platelets and intravascular immunity: guardians of the vascular space during bloodstream infections and sepsis. *Front Immunol*. 2019;10:2400. https://doi.org/10.3389/fimmu.2019.02400. PMID: 31681291; PMCID: PMC6797619.
7. Hall JE, Hall ME. Resistance of the body to infection: II. Immunity and the allergy innate immunity. In: Hall JE, ed. *Guyton and Hall Textbook of Medical Physiology*. 14th ed. Philadelphia, PA: Saunders; 2021:459–470.
8. Yeager JJ. Infection and inflammation. In: Meiner SE, Yeager JJ, eds. *Gerontologic Nursing*. 6th ed. St. Louis, MO: Elsevier; 2019:230–240.
9. Hall JE, Hall ME. Resistance of the body to infection: I. Leukocytes, granulocytes, the monocyte-macrophage system, and inflammation. In: Hall JE, ed. *Guyton and Hall Textbook of Medical Physiology*. 14th ed. Philadelphia, PA: Saunders; 2021:449–458.
10. Patton KT, Thibodeau GA. Innate immunity. In: Patton KT, Thibodeau GA, eds. *Anatomy and Physiology*. 11th ed. St. Louis, MO: Elsevier; 2022:746–758.
11. McGloughlin SA, Paterson DL. Infections in the immunocompromised patient. In: Vincent JL, Abraham E, Moore FA, et al., eds. *Textbook of Critical Care*. 7th ed. Philadelphia, PA: Elsevier; 2017:889–895.e1.
12. Franceschi C, Garagnani P, Parini P, Giuliani C, Santoro A. Inflammation: a new immune-metabolic viewpoint for age-related diseases. *Nat Rev Endocrinol*. 2018;14(10):576–590. https://doi.org/10.1038/s41574-018-0059-4.
13. Tsuda S, Nakashima A, Shima T, Saito S. New paradigm in the role of regulatory t cells during pregnancy. *Front Immunol*. 2019;10:573. https://doi.org/10.3389/fimmu.2019.00573.
14. Tong M, Abrahams VM. Immunology of the Placenta. *Obstet Gynecol Clin North Am*. 2020;47(1):49–63. https://doi.org/10.1016/j.ogc.2019.10.006. PMID: 32008671.
15. Hall JE, Hall ME. Red Blood Cells, Anemia, and Polycythemia. In: Hall Je, Hall ME, eds. *Guyton and Hall Textbook of Medical Physiology*. 14th ed. Philadelphia, PA: Saunders; 2021:439–447.
16. Barcellini W Fattizzo. BClinical applications of hemolytic markers in the differential diagnosis and management of hemolytic anemia. *Dis Markers*. 2015;2015:635670. 224 Sirisha Kundrapu and Jaime Noguez.
17. Segundo GRS, Condino-Neto A. Treatment of patients with immunodeficiency: Medication, gene therapy, and transplantation. *J Pediatr (Rio J)*. 2021;97 Suppl 1(Suppl 1):S17–S23. https://doi.org/10.1016/j.jped.2020.10.005.
18. Paris K, Wall LA. The Treatment of Primary Immune Deficiencies: Lessons Learned and Future Opportunities. [published online ahead of print, 2022 Jul 1]. *Clin Rev Allergy Immunol*. 2022:1–12. https://doi.org/10.1007/s12016-022-08950-0.
19. Snyder, J & Sump C. *Swearingen's All-in-One Nursing Care Planning Resource*. 6th ed. Elsevier, 2024

20. Braga CC, Taplitz RA, Flowers CR. Clinical implications of febrile neutropenia guidelines in the cancer patient population. *J Oncol Pract*. 2019;15(1):25–26. https://doi.org/10.1200/JOP.18.00718.
21. The Joint Commission. *When is it require to perform a nutritional, functional, and pain assessment or screen?*; 2022. Retrieved from https://www.jointcommission.org/standards/standard-faqs/critical-access-hospital/provision-of-care-treatment-and-services-pc/000001652/.
22. Theyab A, Algahtani M, Alsharif KF, et al. New insight into the mechanism of granulocyte colony-stimulating factor (G-CSF) that induces the mobilization of neutrophils. *Hematology*. 2021;26(1):628–636. https://doi.org/10.1080/16078454.2021.1965725.
23. McConnell, S, Brashers VL. Alterations in hematologic function. In: Rodgers, J ed. *McCance & Huether's Pathophysiology: The Biologic Bases for Disease in Adults and Children*. 9th ed. Elsevier. 2024:925-986.
24. Gould Rothberg BE, Quest TE, Yeung SJ, et al. Oncologic emergencies and urgencies: a comprehensive review. *CA Cancer J Clin*. 2022;72(6):570–593. https://doi.org/10.3322/caac.21727.
25. Centers for Disease Control and Prevention. *HIV Surveillance Report*. Vol. 29. http://www.cdc.gov/hiv/library/reports/hiv-surveillance.html. Published August 2022. Accessed April 24, 2023.
26. Gopalappa C, Farnham PG, Chen YH, Sansom SL. Progression and Transmission of HIV/AIDS (PATH 2.0). *Med Decis Making*. 2017;37(2):224–233. https://doi.org/10.1177/0272989X16668509.
27. Kwong JCE. HIV update: an epidemic transformed. *Am J Nurs*. 2019;119(9):30–39. https://doi.org/10.1097/01.NAJ.0000580156.27946.e4.
28. Graham L, Makic MBF. Nursing Considerations for Patients With Hiv in Critical Care Settings. *AACN Adv Crit Care*. 2020;31(3):308–317. https://doi.org/10.4037/aacnacc2020969.
29. Munro N, Scordo KA, Richmond MM. COVID-19: an immunopathologic assault. *AACN Adv Crit Care*. 2020;31(3):268–280. https://doi.org/10.4037/aacnacc2020802.
30. Rahman S, Montero MTV, Rowe K, Kirton R, Kunik Jr F. Epidemiology, pathogenesis, clinical presentations, diagnosis and treatment of COVID-19: a review of current evidence. *Expert Rev Clin Pharmacol*. 2021;14(5):601–621. https://doi.org/10.1080/17512433.2021.1902303.
31. Mahase ECOVID-19. WHO declares pandemic because of "alarming levels" of spread, severity and inaction. *BMJ*. 2020;368:M1036.
32. Sharma A, Ahmad Farouk I, Lal SK. COVID-19: a review on the novel coronavirus disease evolution, transmission, detection, control and prevention. *Viruses*. 2021;13(2):202. https://doi.org/10.3390/v13020202.
33. COVID-19 Treatment Guidelines Panel. Coronavirus Disease 2019 (COVID-19) Treatment Guidelines. National Institutes of Health. Available at https://www.covid19treatmentguidelines.nih.gov/. Accessed March 29, 2023.
34. Davis HE, McCorkell L, Vogel JM, Topol EJ. Long COVID: major findings, mechanisms and recommendations. *Nat Rev Microbiol*. 2023;21(3):133–146. https://doi.org/10.1038/s41579-022-00846-2.
35. Centers for Disease Control and Prevention. *Long COVID or Post COVID conditions*; 2022. Last updated December 16 https://www.cdc.gov/coronavirus/2019-ncov/long-term-effects/index.html.
36. Patton KT, Thibodeau GA. Blood. In: Patton KT, Thibodeau GA, eds. *Anatomy and Physiology*. 11th ed. St. Louis, MO: Elsevier; 2022:606–633.
37. Spring J, Munshi L. Hematology emergencies in critically ill adults: benign hematology. *Chest*. 2022;161(5):1285–1296. https://doi.org/10.1016/j.chest.2021.12.650.
38. Smith L. Disseminated intravascular coagulation. *Semin Oncol Nurs*. 2021;37(2):1–4. https://doi.org/10.1016/j.soncn.2021.151135.
39. Papageorgiou C, Jourdi G, Adjambri E, et al. Disseminated intravascular coagulation: an update on pathogenesis, diagnosis, and therapeutic strategies. *Clin Appl Thromb Hemost*. 2018;24(9_suppl):8S–28S. https://doi.org/10.1177/1076029618806424.

18

Gastrointestinal Alterations

Eleanor R. Fitzpatrick, DNP, RN, AGCNS-BC, ACNP-BC, CCRN

INTRODUCTION

Body cells require water, electrolytes, and nutrients (i.e., carbohydrates, fats, and proteins) to obtain the energy necessary to fuel body functions. The primary function of the alimentary tract (i.e., oropharyngeal cavity, esophagus, stomach, and small and large intestines) and accessory organs (i.e., pancreas, liver, and gallbladder) is to provide the body with a continual supply of nutrients. In addition, food must move through the system at a rate slow enough for digestive and absorptive functions to occur but also fast enough to meet the body's needs. Meeting these goals requires the appropriate and timely movement of nutrients through the gastrointestinal (GI) tract *(motility)*, the presence of specific enzymes to break down nutrients *(digestion)*, and the existence of transport mechanisms to move the nutrients into the bloodstream *(absorption)*. Each part is adapted for specific functions, including food passage, storage, digestion, and absorption.

This chapter provides a brief physiological review of each section of the GI system and of the general assessment of the GI system. This provides the foundation for the discussion of GI disorders commonly encountered in the critical care setting: acute upper GI bleeding, acute pancreatitis, and liver failure. Assessment, treatment, and nursing care for common GI disorders are discussed.

REVIEW OF ANATOMY AND PHYSIOLOGY

Gastrointestinal Tract

The anatomical structure of the GI system is shown in Fig. 18.1. It comprises the alimentary canal (beginning at the oropharynx and ending at the anus) and the accessory organs (i.e., pancreas, liver, and gallbladder) that empty their products into the canal at certain points. A review of the anatomy of the gut wall is provided as an introduction to this section because it is the foundation for the understanding of absorption of nutrients and GI protective mechanisms.

Gut Wall. The GI tract begins in the esophagus and extends to the rectum. It is composed of multiple tissue layers.

Mucosa. The innermost layer, the mucosa, is physiologically the most important. This layer is exposed to food substances and therefore plays a role in nutrient metabolism. The mucosa is also protective. The cells in this layer are connected by tight junctions that produce an effective barrier against large molecules and bacteria. They also protect the GI tract from bacterial colonization. The goblet cells in the mucosa secrete mucus, which provides lubrication for food substances and protects the mucosa from excoriation.

In the stomach, the special architecture of cells of the mucosa and the mucus that is secreted are known as the *gastric mucosal barrier*. This physiological barrier is impermeable to hydrochloric acid, which is normally secreted in the stomach, but it is permeable to other substances, such as salicylates, alcohol, steroids, and bile salts. Disruption of this barrier by these types of substances plays a role in ulcer development. In addition, these cells have a special feature—they regenerate rapidly. Because of this characteristic, disruptions in the mucosa can be quickly healed.

Submucosa. The second layer of the gut wall, the submucosa, is composed of connective tissue, blood vessels, and nerve fibers. The muscular layer follows this layer and is the major layer of the wall. The serosa is the outermost layer.

Beneath the mucosa, submucosa, and muscular layer are various nerve plexuses that are innervated by the autonomic nervous system. Disturbances in these neurons in a given segment of the GI tract cause a lack of motility.

Oropharyngeal Cavity

Mouth. Swallowing is a complex mechanism involving oral, pharyngeal, and esophageal stages. Food substances are ingested into the oral cavity primarily by the intrinsic desire for food, called *hunger*. Food in the mouth is initially subject to mechanical breakdown by the act of chewing *(mastication)*. Chewing of food is important for digestion of all foods, but particularly for digestion of fruits and raw vegetables, because they require the cellulose membranes around their nutrients to be broken down. The muscles used for chewing are innervated by the motor branch of the fifth cranial nerve.

Salivary glands. Saliva is the major secretion of the oropharynx. It is produced by three pairs of salivary glands: submaxillary, sublingual, and parotid. Saliva is rich in mucus, which lubricates food. Salivary amylase, a starch-digesting enzyme, is also secreted. Stimuli such as sight, smell, thoughts, and taste of

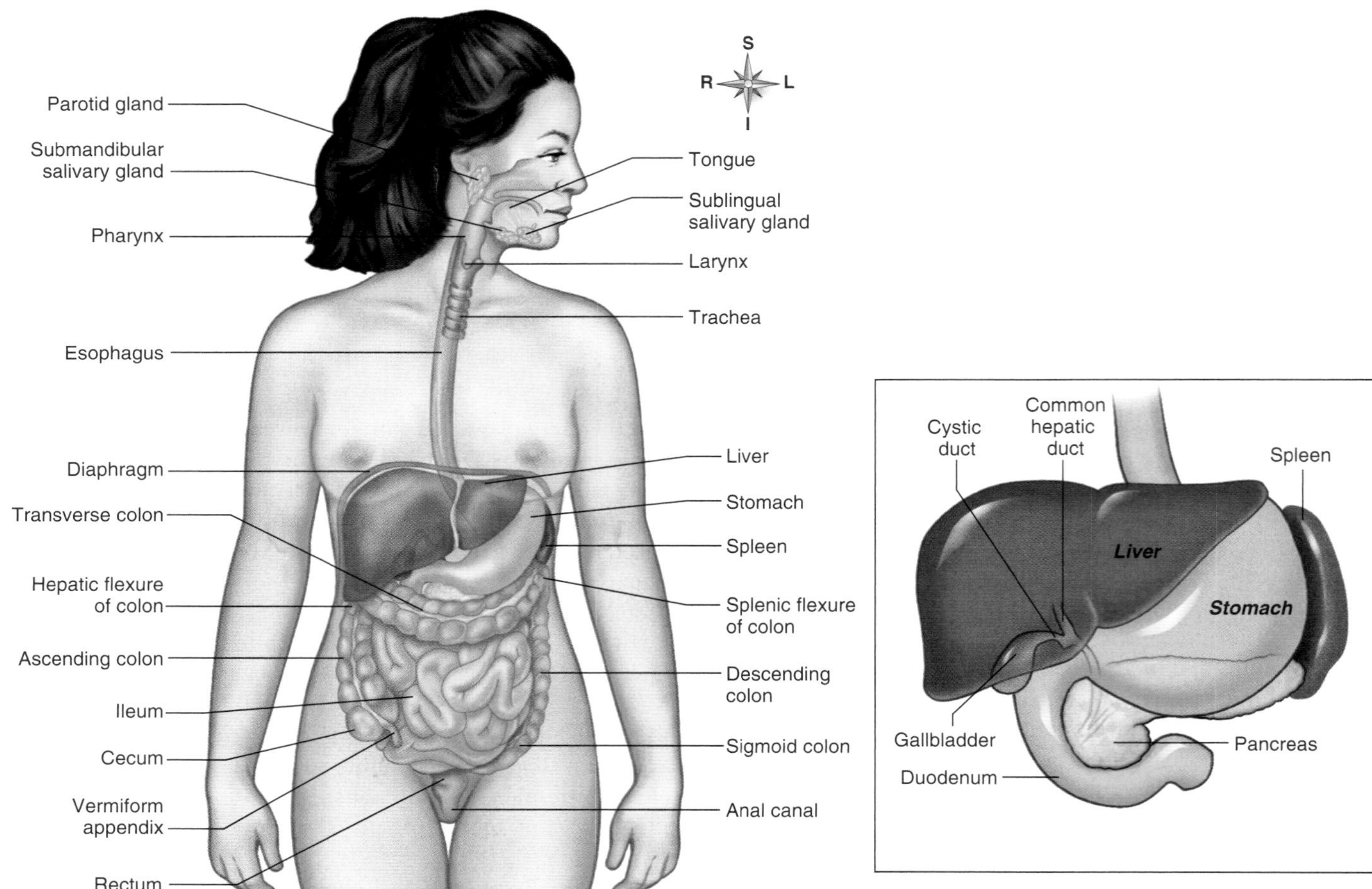

Fig. 18.1 The gastrointestinal system. (From Patton KT, Thibodeau GA. *Anthony's Textbook of Anatomy and Physiology*. 20th ed. St. Louis, MO: Mosby; 2013.)

food stimulate salivary gland secretion. Parasympathetic stimulation promotes a copious secretion of watery saliva. Conversely, sympathetic stimulation produces a scant output of thick saliva. The normal daily secretion of saliva is 1200 mL.

Pharynx. The role of the pharynx in swallowing is complex, as the pharynx serves several other functions, the most important of which is respiration. The pharynx participates in the function of swallowing for only a few seconds at a time to aid in the propulsion of food, which is triggered by the presence of fluid or food in the pharynx. Box 18.1 outlines the three broad stages of swallowing.

BOX 18.1 Stages of Swallowing

Oral: Voluntary
- Initiation of the swallowing process, usually stimulated by a bolus of food in the mouth near the pharynx

Pharyngeal: Involuntary
- Passage of food through the pharynx to the esophagus

Esophageal: Involuntary
- Promotes passage of food from the pharynx to the stomach

Esophagus. Once fluid or food enters the esophagus, it is propelled through the lumen by the process of *peristalsis,* which involves relaxation and contraction of esophageal muscles that are stimulated by the bolus of food. This process occurs repeatedly until the food reaches the lower esophageal sphincter, which is the last centimeter of the esophagus. This area is normally contracted, thus preventing reflux of gastric contents into the esophagus, a phenomenon that would damage the esophageal lining by exposure to gastric acid and enzymes. Waves of peristalsis cause this sphincter to relax and allow food to enter the stomach. Mucosal layers in the esophagus secrete mucus, which protects the lining from damage by gastric secretions or food and serves as a lubricant.[1]

Stomach. The stomach is located at the distal end of the esophagus. It is divided into four regions: the *cardia,* the *fundus,* the *body,* and the pylorus, sometimes referred to as the *antrum* (Fig. 18.2). The muscular walls form multiple folds that allow for greater expansion of the stomach. The motor functions of the stomach include storing food until it can be accommodated by the lower GI tract, mixing food with gastric secretions until it forms a semifluid mixture called *chyme,* and slowly emptying

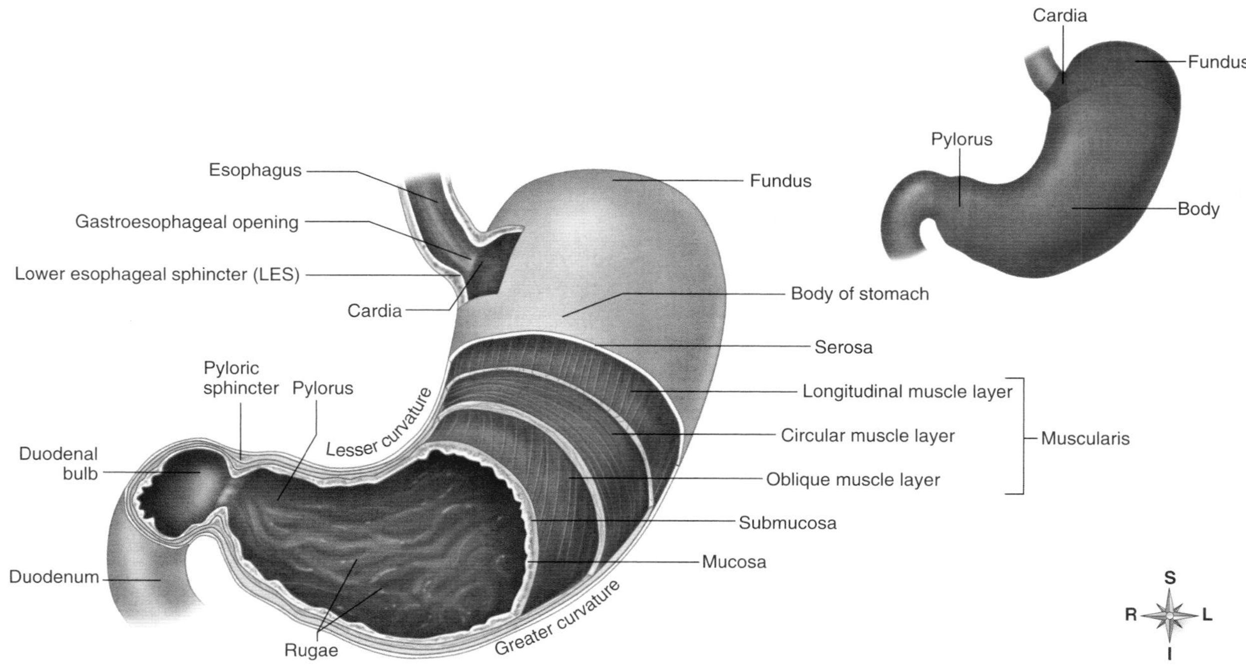

Fig. 18.2 The stomach. (From Patton KT, Thibodeau GA. *Anthony's Textbook of Anatomy and Physiology.* 21st ed. St. Louis, MO: Mosby; 2018.)

the chyme into the small intestine at a rate that allows for proper digestion and absorption. Motility is accomplished through peristalsis. The distal end of the stomach opens into the small intestine; this opening is surrounded by the pyloric sphincter, which prevents duodenal reflux.[1]

Gastric secretions are produced by mucus-secreting cells that line the inner surface of the stomach and by two types of tubular glands: oxyntic (gastric) glands and pyloric glands. Table 18.1 summarizes the major gastric secretions.[2]

An oxyntic gland is composed of three types of cells: mucous neck cells, parietal cells, and chief cells. *Mucous cells* secrete a viscid and alkaline mucus that coats the stomach mucosa, thereby providing protection and lubrication for food transport. *Parietal cells* secrete hydrochloric acid solution, which begins the digestion of food in the stomach. Hydrochloric acid is very acidic (pH 0.8). Stimulants of hydrochloric acid secretion include vagal stimulation, gastrin, and the chemical properties of chyme. Histamine, which stimulates the release of gastrin, also stimulates the secretion of hydrochloric acid. The acidic environment of the stomach promotes the conversion of pepsinogen, a proteolytic enzyme secreted by *chief cells,* to pepsin. Pepsin begins the initial breakdown of proteins. Pepsin is active only in a highly acidic environment (pH <5); therefore, hydrochloric acid secretion is essential for protein digestion.

An essential protein secreted only by the stomach's parietal cells is *intrinsic factor.* Intrinsic factor is necessary for the absorption of vitamin B_{12} in the ileum. Vitamin B_{12} is critical for the formation of red blood cells (RBCs), and a deficiency in this vitamin causes anemia.

TABLE 18.1 Gastric Secretions

Gland/Cells	Secretion
Cardiac gland	Mucus
Mucous neck cells	Mucus
Parietal cells	Water Hydrochloric acid Intrinsic factor
Chief cells	Pepsinogen Mucus
Pyloric gland	Mucus

The stomach also secretes fluid that is rich in sodium, potassium, and other electrolytes. Loss of these fluids via vomiting or gastric suction places the patient at risk for fluid and electrolyte imbalances and acid-base disturbances (Table 18.2).

Small Intestine. The segment spanning the first 10 to 12 inches of the small intestine is called the *duodenum.* This anatomical area is physiologically important because pancreatic juices and bile from the liver empty into this structure. The duodenum also contains an extensive network of mucus-secreting glands called *Brunner glands.* The function of this mucus is to protect the duodenal wall from digestion by gastric juice. Secretion of mucus by Brunner glands is inhibited by sympathetic stimulation, which leaves the duodenum unprotected from gastric juice. This inhibition is one of the reasons why this area of the GI tract is the site for more than 50% of peptic ulcers.

The segment spanning the next 7 to 8 feet of the small intestine is called the *jejunum,* and the remaining 10 to 12 feet comprise the *ileum.* The opening into the first part of the large intestine is protected by the *ileocecal valve,* which prevents reflux of colonic contents back into the ileum.

The movements of the small intestine include mixing contractions and propulsive contractions. The chyme in the small intestine takes 3 to 5 hours to move from the pylorus to the ileocecal valve, although this activity is greatly increased after meals. Digestion and absorption of foodstuffs occur primarily in the small intestine. The anatomical arrangement of villi and microvilli in the small intestine greatly increases the surface area in this part of the intestine and accounts for its substantial digestive and absorptive capabilities. Located on the entire surface of the small intestine are small pits called *crypts of Lieberkühn,* which produce intestinal secretions at a rate of 2000 mL/day. These secretions are neutral in pH and supply the watery vehicle necessary for absorption.[1]

In the small intestine, digestion of carbohydrates, fats, and proteins begins with degradation by pancreatic enzymes that are secreted into the duodenum. Pancreatic juice contains enzymes necessary for digesting all three of these major nutrients (Table 18.3). It also contains large quantities of bicarbonate ions, which play an important role in neutralizing the acidic chyme that is emptied from the stomach into the duodenum. Pancreatic juice is secreted primarily in response to the presence of chyme in the duodenum.

The small intestine also handles absorption of water, electrolytes, and vitamins. Up to 10 L of fluid enter the GI tract daily, but the fluid composition of stool is only about 200 mL. Sodium is actively reabsorbed in the small intestine. In the ileum, chloride is absorbed, and sodium bicarbonate is secreted. Potassium is absorbed and secreted in the GI tract. Vitamins, with the exception of B_{12}, and iron are absorbed in the upper part of the small bowel. Vitamin B_{12} is absorbed in the terminal ileum in the presence of intrinsic factor.

TABLE 18.2 Electrolyte and Acid-Base Disturbances Associated With the Gastrointestinal Tract

Fluid Loss	Imbalances
Gastric juice (e.g., vomiting, excessive suction)	Metabolic alkalosis Potassium deficit Sodium deficit Fluid volume deficit
Small intestine juice/large intestine juice (e.g., recent ileostomy, diarrhea)	Metabolic acidosis Potassium deficit Sodium deficit Fluid volume deficit
Bile or pancreatic fluid (e.g., biliary or pancreatic fistula	Metabolic acidosis Sodium deficit Fluid volume deficit

Large Intestine. The large intestine, or colon, is anatomically divided into the ascending colon, transverse colon, descending colon, and rectum (Fig. 18.3). The functions of the colon are absorption of the water and electrolytes from the chyme and storage of fecal material until it can be expelled. The proximal half of the colon performs primarily absorptive activities, whereas the distal half performs storage activities. The characteristic contractile activity in the colon is called *haustration;* it propels fecal material through the tract. A mass movement moves feces into the rectal vault, and then the urge to defecate is elicited. The mucosa of the large intestine is lined with crypts of Lieberkühn, but the cells contain very few enzymes. Rather, mucus is secreted, which protects the colon wall against excoriation and serves as a medium for holding fecal matter together.[1]

Accessory Organs

Pancreas. The pancreas is located in both upper quadrants of the abdomen, with the *head* in the upper right quadrant and the *tail* in the upper left quadrant. The head and tail are separated by a midsection called the *body of the pancreas* (Fig. 18.4). Because the pancreas lies retroperitoneally, it cannot be palpated; this characteristic also explains why diseases of the pancreas can cause pain that radiates to the back. In addition, a well-developed pancreatic capsule does not exist, and this may explain why inflammatory processes of the pancreas can freely spread and affect the surrounding organs (e.g., stomach and duodenum).

The pancreas has both *exocrine* functions (production of digestive enzymes) and *endocrine* functions (production of insulin and glucagon). The cells of the pancreas, called *acini,* secrete the major pancreatic enzymes that are essential for normal digestion (Table 18.3). Trypsinogen and chymotrypsinogen are secreted in an inactive form so that autodigestion of the gland does not occur. Bicarbonate is also secreted by the pancreas and plays an important role in enabling the pancreatic enzymes to break down foodstuffs. After breakdown by pancreatic enzymes, food is further digested by enzymes in the small intestine and is absorbed into the bloodstream. The presence of acid in the stomach stimulates the duodenum to produce the hormone secretin, which stimulates pancreatic secretions. Protein substances in the duodenum stimulate the production of cholecystokinin, which also stimulates the secretion of pancreatic enzymes.[1]

TABLE 18.3 Pancreatic Enzymes and Their Actions

Enzyme	Action
Carboxypeptidase[a]	Digests proteins
Cholesterol esterase	Digests fats
Chymotrypsin[a]	Digests proteins
Deoxyribonuclease	Digests proteins
Pancreatic amylase	Digests carbohydrates
Pancreatic lipase	Digests fats
Ribonuclease	Digests proteins
Trypsina	Digests proteins

[a]Activated only after it is secreted into the intestinal tract.

The endocrine functions of the pancreas are accomplished by groups of alpha and beta cells that compose the islets of Langerhans. *Beta cells* secrete insulin, and *alpha cells* secrete glucagon. Both are essential to carbohydrate metabolism. When beta cells are affected by disease, blood glucose levels can increase.[1]

The exocrine and endocrine functions of the pancreas are essential to digestion and carbohydrate metabolism, respectively. Pancreatic dysfunction can predispose the patient to malnutrition and accounts for many clinical problems.

The pancreatic response to low-flow states (i.e., decreased cardiac output) or hypotension is often ischemia of the pancreatic cells. This ischemia plays a role in the release of cardiotoxic factors (myocardial depressant factor), which decrease cardiac output. Pancreatic ischemia can also result in acute pancreatitis.

Liver. The liver is the largest internal organ of the body; it is located in the right upper abdominal quadrant. The basic functional unit of the liver is the liver lobule (Fig. 18.5). Hepatic cells are arranged in cords that radiate from the central vein into the periphery. Blood from portal arterioles and venules empties into channels called *sinusoids*. Lining the walls of the sinusoids are specialized phagocytic cells called *Kupffer cells*. These cells remove bacteria and other foreign material from the blood.[1]

The liver has a rich blood supply. It receives blood from both the hepatic artery and the portal vein, which drains structures of the GI tract. The blood supplied to the liver by these two vessels accounts for approximately 25% of the cardiac output.

The liver performs more than 400 functions. Hepatic functions can be classified into four major functions: metabolic, vascular, secretory, and storage. These actions are summarized in Box 18.2.

Metabolic functions.

Carbohydrate metabolism. The liver plays an important role in the maintenance of a normal blood glucose concentration. When the concentration of glucose increases to greater

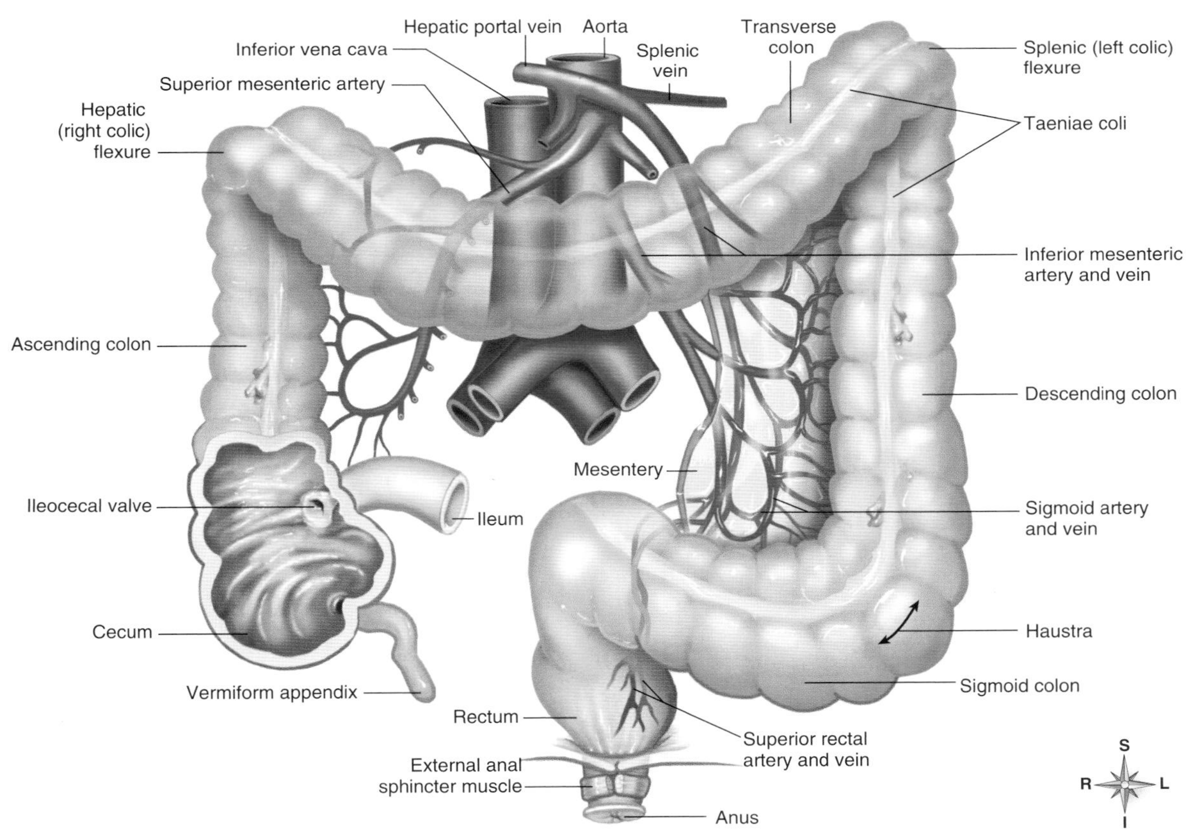

Fig. 18.3 The large intestine. (From Patton KT, Thibodeau GA. *Anthony's Textbook of Anatomy and Physiology*. 21st ed. St. Louis, MO: Mosby; 2018.)

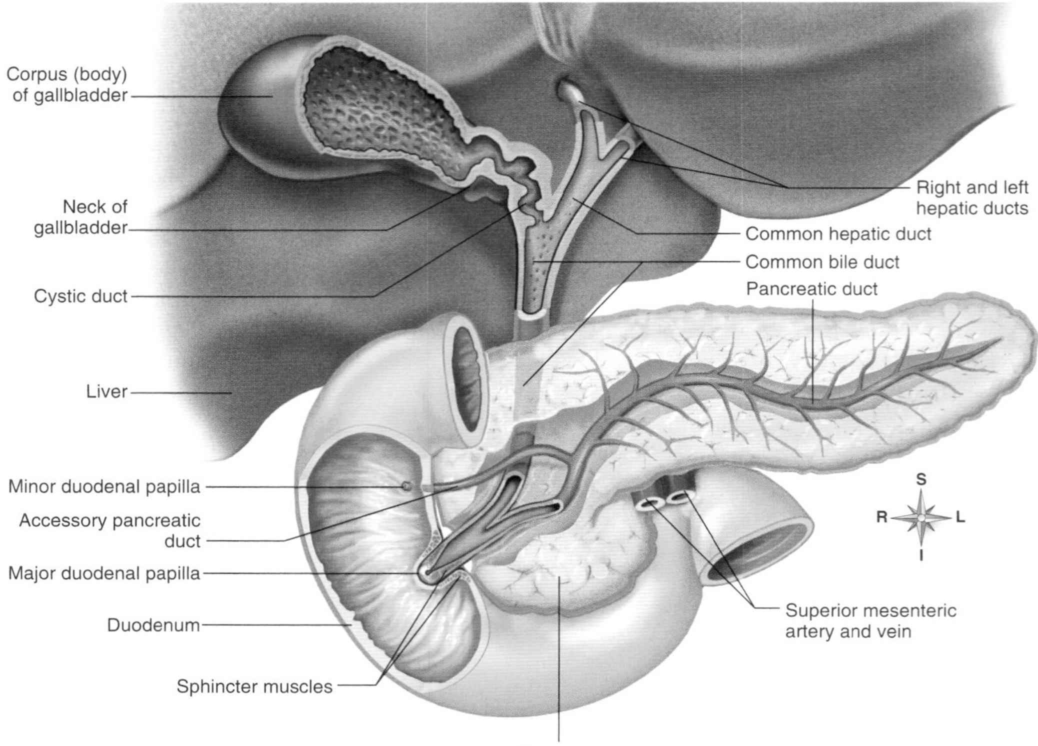

Fig. 18.4 The pancreas and gallbladder. (From Patton KT, Thibodeau GA. *Anthony's Textbook of Anatomy and Physiology*. 21st ed. St. Louis, MO: Mosby; 2018.)

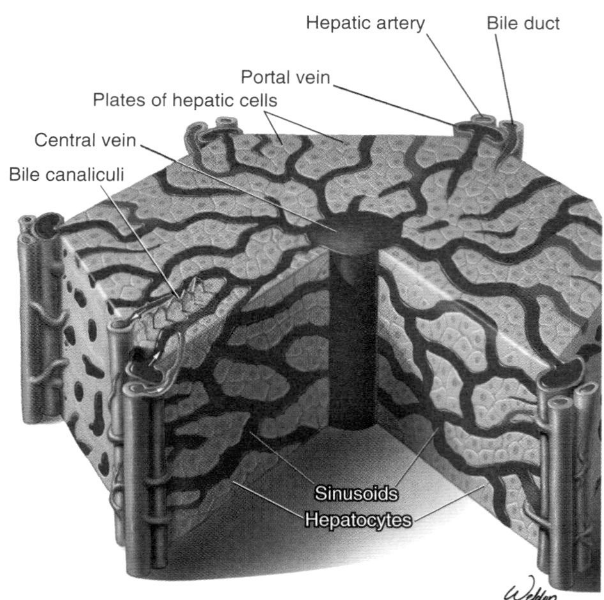

Fig. 18.5 The normal liver lobule.

BOX 18.2 Functions of the Liver

Metabolic Functions

- Carbohydrate, fat, and protein metabolism
- Synthesis of prothrombin (factor I), fibrinogen (factor II), and factors VII, IX, and X
- Removal of activated clotting factors
- Detoxification of medications, hormones, and other substances

Vascular Functions

- Blood storage
- Blood filtration

Secretory Functions

- Production of bile
- Secretion of bilirubin
- Conjugation of bilirubin

Storage Functions

- Blood
- Glucose
- Vitamins (A, B_{12}, D, E, K)
- Fat

than normal levels, it is stored as glycogen *(glycogenesis)*. When blood glucose levels decrease, glycogen stored in the liver is split to form glucose *(glycogenolysis)*. If blood glucose levels decrease to less than normal and glycogen stores are depleted, the liver can make glucose from proteins and fats *(gluconeogenesis)*.

Fat metabolism. Almost all cells in the body are capable of lipid metabolism; however, the liver metabolizes fats so rapidly that it is the primary site for these functions. The liver is also the primary site for the conversion of excess carbohydrates and proteins to triglycerides.

Protein metabolism. All nonessential amino acids are produced in the liver. Amino acids must be deaminated (cleared of ammonia) to be used for energy by cells or converted into carbohydrates or fats. Ammonia is released and removed from the blood by conversion to urea in the liver. The urea that is secreted by the liver into the bloodstream is then excreted by the kidneys.

With the exception of gamma globulins, the liver also produces all plasma proteins in the blood. The major types of plasma proteins are albumins, globulins, and fibrinogen. *Albumin* maintains blood oncotic pressure and prevents plasma loss from the capillaries. *Globulins* are essential for cellular enzymatic reactions. *Fibrinogen* helps to form blood clots.

Production and removal of blood clotting factors. The liver synthesizes fibrinogen (factor I), prothrombin (factor II), and factors VII, IX, and X. Vitamin K is essential for the synthesis of other clotting factors. The liver also removes active clotting factors from the circulation, which prevents clotting in the macrovasculature and microvasculature.

Detoxification. The liver detoxifies medications, hormones, and other toxic substances into inactive forms for excretion. This process is usually accomplished by conversion of the fat-soluble compounds to water-soluble compounds that are excreted via the bile or the urine.

Vascular functions.

Blood storage. Resistance to blood flow in the liver (hepatic vascular resistance) is normally low. Any increase in pressure to the veins of the liver causes blood to accumulate in the sinusoids, which can store up to 400 mL of blood. This blood volume serves as a compensatory mechanism in cases of hypovolemic shock; blood from the liver is shunted into the circulation to increase blood volume.

Blood filtration. Kupffer cells line the sinusoids. They cleanse the blood of bacteria and foreign material that have been absorbed through the GI tract. These cells are extremely phagocytic and normally prevent almost all bacteria from reaching the systemic circulation.

Secretory functions.

Bile production. The secretion of bile is a major function of the liver. Bile is composed of water, electrolytes, bile salts, phospholipids, cholesterol, and bilirubin. Approximately 500 to 1000 mL of bile is produced daily. Bile salts emulsify fats and foster their absorption. The bile salts are reabsorbed in the terminal portion of the ileum and are then transported back to the liver, where they can be used again. Bile travels to the gallbladder via the common bile duct, where it is stored and concentrated.

Bilirubin metabolism. Bilirubin, a physiologically inactive pigment, is a metabolic end product of the degradation of hemoglobin (Hgb). Bilirubin enters the circulation bound to albumin and is *unconjugated*. This portion of the bilirubin is reflected in the *indirect* serum bilirubin level. Accumulation of unconjugated bilirubin is toxic to cells. In the liver, bilirubin is *conjugated* with glucuronic acid. Conjugated bilirubin is soluble and is excreted in bile. Some conjugated bilirubin returns to the blood and is reflected in the *direct* serum bilirubin level.

Excess bilirubin accumulation in the blood results in *jaundice*. Jaundice has several categories, including hepatocellular, hemolytic, and obstructive. Viral hepatitis is the most common cause of *hepatocellular jaundice* (jaundice caused by hepatic cell damage). Cirrhosis and liver cancer also decrease the liver's ability to conjugate bilirubin. *Hemolytic jaundice* results from increased RBC destruction, such as that resulting from blood incompatibilities or sickle cell disease. *Obstructive jaundice* is usually caused by gallbladder disease (e.g., gallstones).[1,2]

Storage functions.

Storage, synthesis, and transport of vitamins and minerals. The liver plays a central role in the storage, synthesis, and transport of various vitamins and minerals. It functions as a storage depot principally for vitamins A, D, and B_{12}, accumulating, respectively, up to 3-, 10-, and 12-month supplies of these nutrients to prevent states of deficiency.

Gallbladder. The gallbladder is a saclike structure that lies beneath the right lobe of the liver (Figs. 18.1 and 18.4). Its primary function is the storage and concentration of bile. The gallbladder holds approximately 70 mL of bile. Bile salts are secreted into the duodenum when nutrients are ingested. The gallbladder is connected to the duodenum by the common bile duct. Bile flow is controlled by contraction of the gallbladder and relaxation of the sphincter of Oddi, which is located at the junction of the common bile duct and the duodenum. Contraction of the gallbladder is controlled by hormonal *(cholecystokinin)* and central nervous system signals and is initiated by the presence of food in the duodenum. Bile salts emulsify fats and assist in the absorption of fatty acids.[1]

Neural Innervation of the Gastrointestinal System

Functions of the GI system are influenced by neural and hormonal factors. The autonomic nervous system exerts multiple effects. Parasympathetic cholinergic fibers, or medications that mimic parasympathetic effects, stimulate GI secretion and motility. Sympathetic stimulation, or medications with adrenergic effects, tends to be inhibitory. Parasympathetic and sympathetic fibers also innervate the gallbladder and the pancreas. Other neural regulators of gastric secretions are stimulated by sight, smell, and thoughts of food and by the presence of food in the mouth. In this phase (cephalic), the brain centers reflexively cause parasympathetic stimulation of gastric secretions by chief and parietal cells.

Hormonal Control of the Gastrointestinal System

The GI tract is considered to be the largest endocrine organ in the body. Hormones that influence GI function include those produced by specialized cells in the GI tract and those produced by other endocrine organs (i.e., pancreas and gallbladder). GI hormones modulate motility, secretion, absorption, and maturation of GI tissues. Table 18.4 summarizes the common GI hormones and their actions.

Blood Supply of the Gastrointestinal System

The blood supply to organs within the abdomen is referred to as the *splanchnic circulation*. The GI system receives the largest percentage of the cardiac output. Approximately one-third of the cardiac output supplies these tissues. The superior and inferior mesenteric and celiac arteries supply the stomach, small and large intestines, pancreas, and gallbladder. The liver has a dual blood supply and receives part of its supply from the hepatic artery. Circulation to the GI system is unique in that venous blood draining the system empties into the portal vein, which perfuses the liver. The portal vein supplies 70% to 75% of liver blood flow.

CHECK YOUR UNDERSTANDING

1. The nurse is preparing to receive a patient status post motor vehicle collision with a significant liver laceration. The patient is currently hemodynamically stable. Given the physiology of the liver, what assessments and interventions should the nurse expect to initiate?
   A. Serial hemoglobin and hematocrit
   B. Frequent vital sign monitoring
   C. Serial abdominal exams
   D. All of the above

A large percentage of cardiac output perfuses the GI tract; therefore, the GI tract is a major source of blood flow during times of increased need, such as during exercise or as a compensatory mechanism in hemorrhage. Conversely, prolonged occlusion or hypoperfusion of a major artery supplying the GI tract can lead to mucosal ischemia and eventually necrosis. Necrosis of intestinal villi can destroy the GI tract's barrier to harmful toxins and bacteria. These bacteria can then enter the blood supply and cause septic shock.

Lifespan Considerations

Older Adults. Changes related to the aging process include decreased salivation, or xerostomia (dry mouth syndrome), which may change the patient's taste perception; delayed esophageal and bowel emptying; increased bowel emptying, which may lead to anxiety about incontinence; decreased thirst sensation, which may lead to a reduction of fluid intake; decreased gastric secretions; and altered drug metabolism. The most common GI disorders in older patients are functional bowel disorders such as chronic constipation, irritable bowel syndrome, peptic ulcer disease (PUD), and neoplasms. Upper abdominal discomfort in an older patient may be associated with coronary artery disease.[3–5]

Older populations are at risk for malnutrition or undernutrition and for vitamin and mineral deficiencies resulting from a reduction of olfactory, gustatory, and visual food perception that can lead to a decrease in appetite.[5] Malnutrition is one of the most relevant conditions that negatively influence the health of older people. Malnourished patients have an increased hospital length of stay and are more susceptible to infections. Oral nutritional support is important to correct malnutrition and for patients at risk for malnutrition. Oral nutritional supplements (ONS) may be used as an adjunct in a patient's nutritional management.[5] ONS are defined as the supplementary oral intake of dietary food for special medical purposes in addition to normal foods. ONS are usually liquids, but they are also available in other forms such as powders, dessert-style servings, or bars. Use of ONS has been shown to decrease hospital complications and readmission, increase protein intake, and improve weight in the older adult.[5] Additional considerations are outlined in the Lifespan Considerations box.[3–5]

TABLE 18.4 Actions of Gastrointestinal Hormones

Action	Gastrin	Cholecystokinin	Secretin	Gastric Inhibitory Peptide
Acid secretion	Stimulates	Stimulates	Inhibits	Inhibits
Gastric motility	Stimulates	Stimulates	Inhibits	—
Gastric emptying	Inhibits	Inhibits	Inhibits	Inhibits
Intestinal motility	Stimulates	Stimulates	Inhibits	—
Mucosal growth	Stimulates	Stimulates	Inhibits	—
Pancreatic HCO_3^- secretion	Stimulates	Stimulates	Stimulates	No effect
Pancreatic enzyme secretion	Stimulates	Stimulates	Stimulates	No effect
Pancreatic growth	Stimulates	Stimulates	Stimulates	—
Bile HCO_3^- secretion	Stimulates	Stimulates	Stimulates	No effect
Gallbladder contraction	Stimulates	Stimulates	Stimulates	—

—, Not yet tested; HCO_3^-, bicarbonate.

GENETICS

Cytochrome P450 Enzymes and the Patient's Response to Medications

Pharmacogenomics focuses on the expressed genome and techniques to study drug responses (e.g., proteomics, metabolomics, and gene expression). It includes genetic technology that guides medication development and testing. *Pharmacogenetics* is more specific, referring to the individual variability for genetic inheritance. However, the two terms are often used interchangeably, and the abbreviation "PGx" describes the selection of drugs or doses based on an individual's genetic profile. The most common genetic variations influencing patient response to medications affect metabolism.

The cytochrome *P450 (CYP450)* genes are the source of production for 70% to 80% of enzymes involved in the metabolism of medications.[1] *Cytochrome,* meaning "colored cell," refers to the red heme molecule in CYP450 enzymes. The P450 portion of the name is derived from the wavelength of light absorbed in mass spectrography (i.e., at 450 nanometers).[1] The name of each *CYP450* gene begins with CYP, followed by a number associated with a specific group within the *CYP* genes. Next, a letter represents the gene's subgroup, and a number is assigned to the gene within the subgroup. To illustrate, the gene in group 2, subgroup D, gene 6, is labeled *CYP2D6.*

CYP450 enzymes also break down toxins produced by normal cell functions, detoxify ingested procarcinogens such as nitrates, and alter harmful substances such as hydrocarbons from cigarette smoke. The CYP450 enzymes synthesize fatty acids, cholesterol, prostaglandins, and hormones. The CYP450 enzymes are abundant in the liver and also found in the intestines, lungs, and other tissues.

Polymorphism is a genetic variation. Not all polymorphisms result in pathology. Most polymorphisms are *single nucleotide polymorphisms* (SNP). *SNPs* occur in base-pair substitutions with a frequency of 1% or greater in the population. The base pair substitutions can occur anywhere in the DNA, with over 600,000 occurring in protein-coding regions. Most polymorphisms in CYP450 are SNPs.

Polymorphisms of CYP450 enzymes are numerous. Many polymorphisms affect the function of enzymes. Individuals may inherit low-, normal-, or high-functioning enzymes and be genotyped as poor (slow), intermediate or extensive (normal), and ultra-rapid metabolizers. These categories are *phenotypes*, or observable characteristics of an individual resulting from the interaction of one's *genotype* with the environment. The CYP450 enzyme variants are present in 1% to 15% of the US population.[1]

When an individual is a slow metabolizer, a drug has reduced inactivation due to the reduced volume or function of one or more CYP450 enzymes. For medications that are prodrugs like codeine and clopidogrel, slow-metabolizing CYP450 enzymes cannot convert the prodrug into an active form; therapeutic blood levels are not achieved. When an individual is genotyped as ultra-rapid, the increased breakdown of the drug leads to rapid medication clearance and ineffective treatment. Toxic effects may manifest early or with greater severity due to either poor or ultra-rapid metabolism. Inheriting two *alleles*—two copies of a gene—for an ultra-rapid or slow metabolizing polymorphism can magnify altered degradation and risk for toxicity or adverse drug-related outcomes.

Foods, body temperature, pH, medications, and environmental factors also affect the activity of CYP450 enzymes. For example, grapefruit reduces the function of CYP450 enzymes in the gastrointestinal tract, resulting in greater serum levels of some oral medications when taken following a meal with this citrus fruit. Genotyping is only one factor to consider, but it is a factor that is increasingly determined by both patients using commercial testing and astute clinicians.

The CYP2D6 enzymes metabolize many beta-blockers, antidysrhythmics, antiplatelets, antipsychotics, and selective serotonin reuptake inhibitors.[1] Reduced function of *CYP2D6* is linked to increased incidence of bradycardia from some beta-blockers and dysrhythmias from lengthening the QTc interval with antipsychotics.[2,3] *CYP2D6* function may explain the ineffective treatment of bipolar disease.[2]

The CYP2D6 enzymes have specific clinical implications for codeine administration. Patients with inherited low CYP2D6 enzymatic activity cannot convert codeine to its active form; therefore, codeine provides no pain relief, and adjusting the dose does not change this response. Conversely, individuals who inherit a genotype that results in ultra-rapid metabolism experience a quick conversion of codeine into morphine, causing unanticipated respiratory depression and sedation.

Genetic variations other than CYP450 metabolizing enzymes contribute to inter- and intra-individual variations in drug response. Other metabolizing enzymes (i.e., phase 2 enzymes in the liver), transporters, and receptor/post-receptor mechanism polymorphism cause gene-drug response variations. These variations and effects can be important to prescribing and monitoring drug response decisions. The US Federal Drug Administration (FDA) has a list of 70-plus drugs that have recommendations for genetic testing.[3]

Precision medicine is an approach to care that uses variability in genes, environment, and lifestyle to diagnose and treat individuals. In addition to the FDA, the Clinical Pharmacogenetics Implementation Consortium lists indications for genetic testing for nearly 450 drugs.[4] Clinical genotyping can limit trial-and-error dosing and avoid adverse effects from a dose that is too high or too low based on the individual's metabolic genetic profile. Genotyping results are not affected by an underlying disease or co-administration of other medications and do not change over time.

Use of pharmacogenetic testing to personalize treatment is increasing. Multiple researchers are investigating tools to assess the impact of genetic variants and patient characteristics on drug effectiveness.[5] However, clinicians, including nurses, often do not have the knowledge and skills to interpret these tools or genetic tests.[6,7] Individuals have access to commercial pharmacogenetic tests. The clinical implications of a commercial test are not always clear to patients who may decide to stop a medication based on testing. Genomic literacy is essential to providing the benefits of genetic testing and precision medicine.

Genetic terms: *pharmacogenomics, pharmacogenetics, polymorphism, allele, single nucleotide polymorphism (SNP), phenotype, genotype, precision medicine.*

References

1. Correia MA. Drug biotransformation. In: Katzung BG, Vanderah TW, eds. *Basic and Clinical Pharmacology.* 15th edition. New York, NY: McGraw-Hill LANGE; 2022:1–20. online pages.
2. Dong AN, Tan BH, Pan Y, Ong CE. Cytochrome P450 genotype-guided drug therapies: an update on current states. *Clin Exp Pharmacol Physiol.* 2018;45(10):991–1001. https://doi.org/10.1111/1440-1681.12978.
3. Federal Drug Administration. *Table of Pharmacogenetic Associations.* https://www.fda.gov/medical-devices/precision-medicine/table-pharmacogenetic-associations#section1. Updated October 26, 2022. Accessed December 27, 2023.
4. Clinical Pharmacogentics Implementation Consortium (CPIC). *Genes-Drugs.* https://cpicpgx.org/genes-drugs/. Updated Jun 21, 2022. Accessed December 27, 2023.
5. Thomas CD, Franchi F, Keeley EC, et al. Impact of the ABCD-GENE score on clopidogrel clinical effectiveness after PCI: a multi-site, real-world investigation. *Clin Pharmacol Ther.* 2022;112(1):146–155. https://doi.org/10.1002/cpt.2612.
6. Flowers E, Leutwyler H, Shim JK. Direct-to-consumer genomic testing: are nurses prepared? *Nursing.* 2020;50(8):48–52. https://doi.org/10.1097/01.NURSE.0000684200.71662.09.
7. Haga SB, Kim E, Myers RA, Ginsburg GS. Primary care physicians' knowledge, attitudes, and experience with personal genetic testing. *J Pers Med.* 2019;9(2). https://doi.org/10.3390/jpm9020029.

Chris Winkelman, PhD, ACNP-BC, CCRN, CNE, FAANP, FCCM

Pregnancy. GI discomforts that frequently occur during pregnancy include nausea and vomiting, gastroesophageal reflux disease (GERD), hemorrhoids, and pelvic floor disorders, including constipation and fecal incontinence.[6,7] Nausea and vomiting during pregnancy may be caused by gastric motility disturbances and pregnancy-associated alterations as a result of differing reactions to taste and smell and involvement of behavioral and psychological factors. GERD, which is the abnormal reflux of gastric contents into the esophagus, is experienced by 30% to 80% of pregnant people, and about one-third of pregnant people complain of hemorrhoids.[7,8] GERD symptoms are similar to those of heartburn. In pregnant people, contributing factors include obesity, increased intra-abdominal pressure, and a decrease in lower esophageal sphincter pressure.[7,8] Constipation is a common symptom experienced by pregnant people in the first trimester, and it affects up to 25% of pregnant people for up to 3 months after delivery.[7,8] Hyperemesis gravidarum, which is defined as persistent nausea and vomiting after 6 to 8 weeks of gestation, occurs in less than 1% of pregnant people. Severe nausea and vomiting from hyperemesis gravidarum can lead to dehydration, postural hypotension, tachycardia, electrolyte imbalances, ketosis, muscle wasting, and weight loss.[6,9,10]

Pica, the compulsive consumption of nonfood items, can also occur during pregnancy. The etiology of pica is not well understood. It has been suggested that mineral deficiencies (e.g., iron, zinc) may be a contributing factor. The most common cravings are for dirt *(geophagia)*, ice *(pagophagia)*, and laundry or corn starch *(amylophagia)*. Cravings for cigarette ashes, burnt matches, stones, coffee grounds, paint chips, clay, baking soda, lead-based paint, and sand have also been reported.[11]

Other, less common pregnancy GI disorders reported in the literature include obstetric cholestasis, acute fatty liver, diarrhea, inflammatory bowel diseases such as Crohn's disease and ulcerative colitis, irritable bowel syndrome, appendicitis, gallbladder disease, pancreatitis, cirrhosis, and hepatitis.[6,12,13] The Lifespan Considerations box highlights these changes and related nursing implications.[6–14]

LIFESPAN CONSIDERATIONS

Older Adults

- Provide oral care to keep mucous membranes moist in periods of decreased salivation.
- Older adults may experience delayed esophageal emptying. Symptoms include complaints of bloating or regurgitation when drinking a large amount of fluid with meals.
- Dysphagia increases the risk for aspiration, especially during meals. Elevate the patient's head of bed during mealtime or feedings.
- Assess for problems during feeding such as tremors, dementia, and functional impairments.
- Because of decreased senses of taste, sight, and smell, providing adequate nutrition to those receiving oral feedings is challenging. Obtain dietary consultation to assist with meal planning and administer oral nutritional supplements as ordered.
- Decreased gastric acid secretion may result in anemia, which can lead to hypoxemia. Assess the patient's complete blood count, arterial blood gases, and pulse oximetry values, as appropriate.
- Older adults are at higher risk for complications of gallbladder disease, such as pancreatitis, because of an increased incidence of gallstones. Assess for signs and symptoms of cholecystitis.
- Blood flow to the liver decreases by almost half by age 85, which may lead to an impaired medication metabolism. Assess the patient for medication toxicity and consult with the clinical pharmacist to identify the need for adjusting medication dosages.
- Some medications (i.e., nifedipine and verapamil) cause rectosigmoid dysmotility and severe constipation. Assess the need for medication and provide interventions to prevent or treat constipation.
- The older adult may also experience diarrhea from increased bowel emptying. Use of laxatives and nonsteroidal antiinflammatory drugs (NSAIDs) can cause bowel disturbances. Assess bowel function and medication side effects.

Pregnant People

- Pregnancy can cause decreased gastric motility, resulting in nausea and vomiting. Assess the patient for signs and symptoms of dehydration and complications. Administer recommended first-line therapy for nausea as prescribed (e.g., doxylamine succinate and vitamin B_6).
- Pregnancy increases levels of female sex hormones, which in turn can decrease lower esophageal sphincter pressure resulting in heartburn, regurgitation, and/or gastroesophageal reflux disease (GERD). Assess nutritional status, diet, and physical activity. Instruct the patient to avoid lying in a supine position after meals, consider nonpharmacological remedies that are safe in pregnancy (e.g., ginger root), administer first-line medications of antacids and sucralfate, and consider alginate preparations if antacids do not provide relief.
- Constipation may occur because of decreased colonic motility and increased pressure on the rectosigmoid colon. Assess the patient's fluid and fiber intakes and administer laxatives and bulking agents, as prescribed. Do not discontinue oral iron.
- Weight gain and increased pelvic pressure can cause engorgement of rectal veins, inflammation of the anal mucosa, varicose veins of the anus and rectum, and hemorrhoids. Prevent constipation and obtain nutritional consultation for dietary changes to increase fluids and fiber. Administer supplemental fiber as prescribed. Apply warm soaks, witch hazel pads, and topical creams such as hydrocortisone-pramoxine to provide pain relief.
- Diarrhea or frequent stools may also occur during pregnancy, particularly at term when labor is near. However, diarrhea can also be a symptom of a more serious disease. Monitor stool frequency and other symptoms accompanied with diarrhea such as fever or severe abdominal pain lasting for more than 48 hours, as these can be signs of an illness caused by infective agents such as bacteria, viruses, and protozoa. Assess the onset of the diarrhea, stool frequency, the patient's recent travel history, recent antibiotic use, employment history, food and water intake, and contact with ill family members. Anticipate obtaining stool cultures. Instruct the patient on hand washing and avoidance of contaminated foods. Other nonpharmacological treatments include oral hydration with salt- or sugar-containing fluids and consuming bland foods or a BRAT diet (bananas, rice, applesauce, and toast). Instruct the patient to avoid milk and high-fat foods. Loperamide (Imodium) can be used in pregnancy in the absence of bloody diarrhea. Antibiotics may be indicated for infectious diarrhea.
- Pica, or compulsion to consume nonfood items, may occur in pregnancy. Treatment of pica is tailored to the patient and the nonfood item consumed.
- Assess the patient for anemia. Obtain laboratory tests to determine the underlying cause.
- Pregnant people are more vulnerable to hepatitis E virus (HEV). In HEV, there is no apparent increase in mortality rate and no reports of fetal transmission.
- In pregnant people who are positive for hepatitis B surface antigen with viral DNA present in the serum, the risk of transmission to the neonate is high during delivery. Routine screening for hepatitis B virus (HBV) infection is warranted to minimize the transmission risk. Pregnant patients, in their third trimester of pregnancy, may be treated with lamivudine (Epivir) to decrease HBV transmission.
- Anal sphincter weakness may occur during and after pregnancy, and fecal incontinence has been reported as early as 12 weeks' gestation. Treatment includes dietary modification and fiber supplementation. Loperamide (Imodium) may be given as a pharmacological intervention. Pelvic floor muscle training or physical therapy may alleviate symptoms of fecal incontinence. Surgical intervention is typically reserved for when other options have failed.

GENERAL ASSESSMENT OF THE GASTROINTESTINAL SYSTEM

A comprehensive assessment of the abdomen includes a history, inspection, auscultation, percussion, and palpation. Use the four-quadrant method (right upper, right lower, left upper, and left lower) to map the abdomen for descriptive purposes by drawing imaginary lines crossing at the umbilicus. Use these landmarks to describe symptoms, such as pain.

History

Unless an emergency situation requires immediate intervention, begin assessment of the GI system by obtaining a history. Question the patient about past problems with indigestion, difficulty swallowing *(dysphagia)*, pain on swallowing, nausea and vomiting, heartburn, belching, abdominal distension or bloating, diarrhea, constipation, and bleeding. Note that problems such as anorexia, fatigue, and headache may relate to specific GI ailments. Explore symptoms in terms of when they became apparent, any precipitating factors, what treatment was sought, factors that relieved or made the symptoms worse, and whether the symptom is current. Obtain a weight history that includes usual and ideal body weight along with a history of fluctuations, acute weight loss, and interventions or treatments for weight loss.

Pain assessment is challenging. Pain receptors in the abdomen are less likely to be localized and are mediated by common sensory structures projected to the skin. Therefore, it is often difficult to distinguish the pain of a peptic ulcer or cholecystitis from that of a myocardial infarction. Abdominal pain is often caused by engorged mucosa, pressure in the mucosa, distension, or spasm. Visceral pain is likely to cause pallor, perspiration, bradycardia, nausea and vomiting, weakness, and hypotension. Increasing intensity of pain, especially after surgery or other intervention, is always significant and usually signifies complicating factors such as inflammation, gastric distension, hemorrhage into tissue or the peritoneal space, or peritonitis. Obtain a description of the location and the type of pain in the patient's own words.

Obtain a history of any GI surgical procedures, including the specific types and dates. Also, record a list of current medications because many medications have GI side effects.

Inspection

Inspect the abdomen, focusing on the following characteristics: skin color and texture, symmetry and contour of the abdomen, masses and pulsations, and peristalsis and movement. Record findings.

Skin Color and Texture. Observe for pigmentation of skin (jaundice), lesions, discolorations, old or new scars, and vascular and hair patterns. Assess general nutrition and hydration status.

Symmetry and Contour of Abdomen. Note the size and shape of the abdomen and the presence of visible protrusions and adipose distribution. Always investigate abdominal distension, particularly in the presence of pain, because it usually indicates trapped air or fluid within the abdominal cavity.

Masses and Pulsations. Look for any obvious abdominal masses, which are best observed on deep inspiration. Pulsations, if they are seen, usually originate from the aorta.[27]

Peristalsis and Movement. Motility of the stomach may be reflected in movement of the abdomen in lean patients, and this is a normal sign. However, strong contractions are abnormal and indicate the presence of disease.

Auscultation

Auscultation of bowel sounds is a noninvasive and simple method to assess GI motility and function, and it is valuable in the examination of patients with acute abdominal pain.[15] Bowel sounds are high-pitched, gurgling sounds caused by air and fluid as they move through the GI tract. Typically, bowel sounds are auscultated before palpation. However, research has found that the order of auscultation, whether before or after palpation, does not affect bowel sound frequency. Given these findings, if no bowel sounds are audible on the initial assessment, auscultation can be done after palpation.[15,16] Position the patient for proper auscultation. A supine position with the patient's arms at the sides or folded at the chest is usually recommended. Place a pillow under the patient's knees to relax the abdominal wall.

Bowel sounds are best heard with the diaphragm of the stethoscope and are systematically assessed in all four quadrants of the abdomen. Assess the frequency and character of the sounds. The frequency of bowel sounds has been estimated at 5 to 35 per minute, and the sounds are usually irregular. The amount of time required for bowel sounds to be auscultated ranges from 30 seconds to 7 minutes. Therefore, assess for bowel sounds for at least 5 minutes before determining that bowel sounds are absent.[15] Box 18.3 reviews common causes of increased, decreased, and absent bowel sounds as they relate to acute illness.[15] Diagnosis should not be based solely on auscultation, but from a complete assessment and diagnostic evaluation.

Thorough auscultation can reveal additional findings beyond just bowel sounds. Vascular sounds such as bruits may be heard; they indicate dilated, tortuous, or constricted vessels. Venous

BOX 18.3 Causes of Changes in the Frequency of Bowel Sounds

Causes of Decreased or Absent Bowel Sounds

- Gangrene
- Intestinal ischemia
- Late bowel obstruction
- Paralytic ileus
- Peritonitis
- Reflux ileus
- Surgical manipulation of bowel

Causes of Increased Bowel Sounds

- Bleeding esophageal varices
- Bleeding ulcers or electrolyte disturbances
- Diarrhea
- Early pyloric or intestinal obstruction
- Subsiding ileus

hums are normally heard from the inferior vena cava. A hum in the periumbilical region in a patient with cirrhosis indicates obstructed portal circulation. Peritoneal friction rubs may be heard and may indicate infection, abscess, or tumor.[15]

Percussion

Percussion provides information about the structure of abdominal organs and tissues and is aimed at detecting fluid, gaseous distension, and masses. Because of the presence of gas within the GI tract, percussed tympany predominates. Solid masses are dull on percussion. Impaired tympany or a dullness in sound quality may be related to an abnormality. For example, a solid mass in the abdomen changes the percussion note. Percussion that produces a dull note in the midline of the lower abdomen in a male patient most likely represents a distended urinary bladder. Organ borders of the liver, spleen, and stomach may also be ascertained with the use of percussion.

Palpation

Palpation is the use of touch to determine the characteristics of an area of the body, including skin elevation or depression, warmth, tenderness, pulses, and crepitus. Palpation is also used to evaluate the major organs with respect to shape, size, position, mobility, consistency, and tension. Perform palpation last because it often elicits pain or muscle spasm. Deep abdominal tenderness and rebound tenderness must be differentiated. Rebound tenderness occurs when pain is elicited after deep palpation when the examiner's hand is quickly released. Rigidity or guarding of the abdomen is also noted. Masses in the liver, spleen, kidneys, gallbladder, or descending colon can be palpated. A pulsatile mass palpated in the abdomen might be an abdominal aneurysm, and an acutely tender mass that descends with inspiration in the right upper quadrant might be an inflamed gallbladder.

CHECK YOUR UNDERSTANDING

2. An older adult patient presents to a hospital's emergency department with a chief complaint of constipation for 1 week. The patient has a medical history of hypertension, diabetes, and hyperlipidemia. The patient has been taking calcium supplements for a year. What should the nurse perform first?
   A. Ask the provider to discontinue the patient's calcium supplements.
   B. Instruct the patient and family member to increase the patient's fluid intake.
   C. Assess the patient for abdominal pain and usual diet.
   D. Administer a stool softener, as ordered.

ACUTE GASTROINTESTINAL BLEEDING

Pathophysiology

Many causes of acute GI bleeding necessitate admission of a patient to the critical care unit. Box 18.4 reviews the most common causes of this emergency condition.

BOX 18.4 Causes of Gastrointestinal Bleeding

Causes of Upper Gastrointestinal Bleeding
- Duodenal ulcer
- Esophageal or gastric varices
- Gastric ulcer
- Mallory-Weiss tear

Causes of Lower Gastrointestinal Bleeding
- Cancer
- Diverticulosis
- Hemorrhoids
- Inflammatory disease
- Polyps
- Vascular ectasias

Peptic Ulcer Disease. PUD is characterized by a break in the mucosa that extends through the entire mucosa and into the muscle layers, damaging blood vessels and causing hemorrhage or perforation into the GI wall (Fig. 18.6).[17,18] Duodenal and gastric ulcers are the most common types of PUD and the most common causes of upper GI bleeding. The ulcer in PUD is a crater surrounded by acutely or chronically inflamed cells. Over time, the inflamed tissue is replaced by necrotic tissue, then by granulation tissue, and finally by scar tissue.[19,20]

The secretion of acid is important in the pathogenesis of ulcer disease. Acetylcholine (a neurotransmitter), gastrin (a hormone), and secretin (a hormone) stimulate the chief cells, which stimulate acid secretion. Parietal cell mass is observed 1.5 to 2 times more often in people with PUD than in those without the disease, increasing the potential for greater hydrochloric acid secretion. Complications of PUD include bleeding, perforation, gastric outlet obstruction, and gastric cancer.[19,20] Risk factors for the development of PUD are presented in Box 18.5. Contributing factors in ulcer formation are shown in Box 18.6. Infection with *Helicobacter pylori* bacteria is a major cause of duodenal ulcers.[19,20] Chronic use of nonsteroidal antiinflammatory drugs (NSAIDs) is also a contributing cause of PUD in patients with *H. pylori* infection. Treatment choices include standard triple therapy, sequential therapy, quadruple therapy, and levofloxacin-based triple therapy (see Pharmacological Therapy).[18,21] Selected studies of GI function are reviewed in Table 18.5. Characteristics of gastric and duodenal ulcers are presented in Table 18.6.

Stress Ulcer. Stress-related mucosal bleeding, or stress ulcer, is an acute form of peptic ulcer that often accompanies severe illness, systemic trauma, or neurological injury.[21] Ischemia is the primary etiology associated with stress ulcer formation. Ischemic ulcers develop within hours after an event such as hemorrhage, multisystem trauma, severe burns, heart failure, or sepsis.[21] The shock, anoxia, and sympathetic responses decrease mucosal blood flow, leading to ischemia. Patients at high risk for stress ulcer development include those receiving positive-pressure ventilation for more than 48 hours; on extracorporeal life support; with coagulopathies; who have a history of GI bleeding or ulceration in the past year; with traumatic brain or spinal cord injuries; or with thermal injuries over 35% or more of their total body surface area.[22]

Stress ulcers that develop as a result of burn injury are often called *Curling ulcers*. Stress ulcers associated with severe head trauma or brain surgery are called *Cushing ulcers*. The decreased

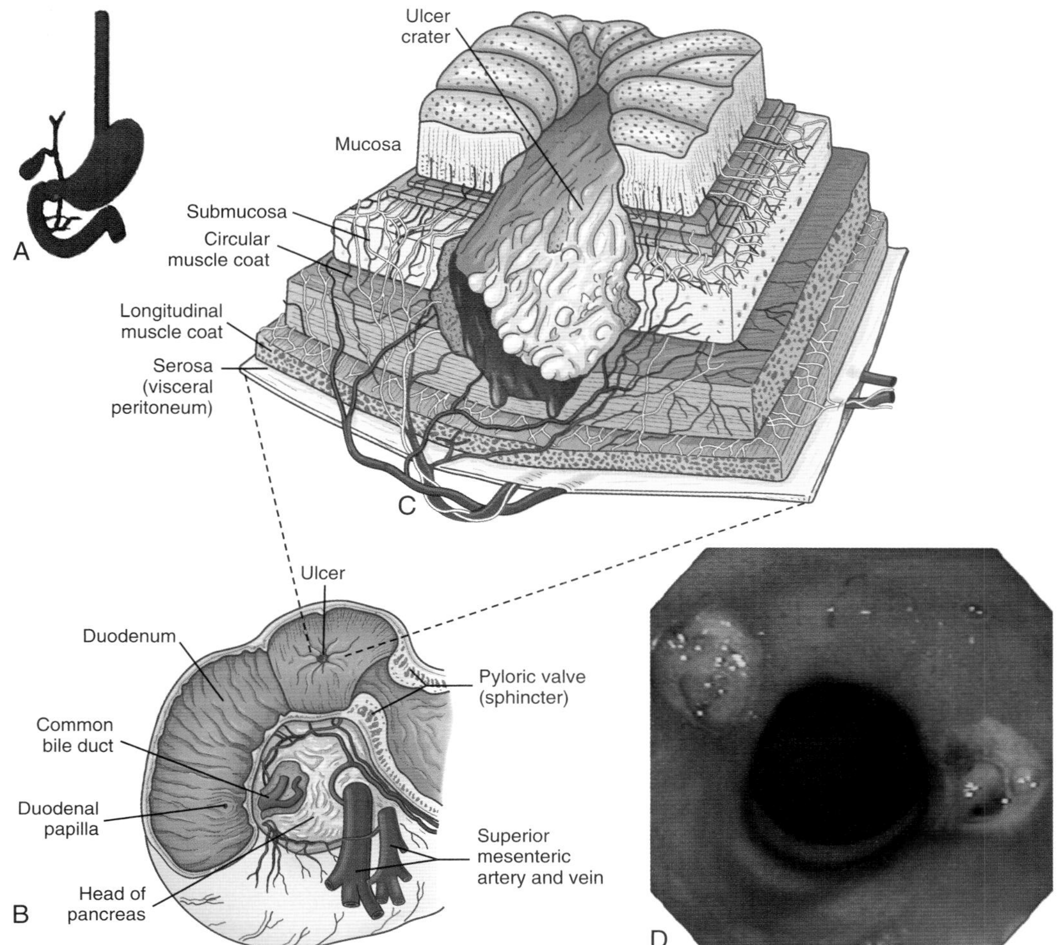

Fig. 18.6 Duodenal ulcer. **A**, Location of the ulcer in the gastrointestinal tract, location noted via the *red dot*. **B**, Placement of the ulcer from outside the gastrointestinal lumen. **C**, Deep ulceration in the duodenal wall extending as a crater through the entire mucosa and into the muscle layers. **D**, Bilateral duodenal ulcers in a person using nonsteroidal antiinflammatory drugs. (**A**, **B**, **C**, from Rogers J. *McCance and Huether's Pathophysiology: The Biologic Basis for Disease in Adults and Children*. 9th ed. St. Louis, MO: Elsevier; 2024. **B**, Courtesy David Bjorkman, MD, University of Utah School of Medicine, Department of Gastroenterology, Salt Lake City, UT.)

BOX 18.5 Risk Factors for Peptic Ulcer Disease

- Alcohol consumption
- *Helicobacter pylori* infection: elevates levels of gastrin and pepsinogen and releases toxins and enzymes that promote inflammation and ulceration
- Nonsteroidal antiinflammatory drugs (NSAIDs): inhibit prostaglandins
- Smoking: stimulates acid secretion

BOX 18.6 Contributing Factors to Ulcer Formation

- Increased number of parietal cells in the gastric mucosa
- Gastrin levels that remain higher for longer after eating
- Gastrin levels that continue to stimulate secretion of acid and pepsin
- Failure of feedback mechanism
- Rapid gastric emptying that overwhelms buffering capacity
- Association of *Helicobacter pylori* with mucosal epithelial cell necrosis
- Decreased mucosal bicarbonate secretion

mucosal blood flow and hypersecretion of acid caused by overstimulation of the vagal nuclei are associated with Cushing ulcers.[19,20]

Administration of histamine receptor (H2 receptor) antagonists and proton pump inhibitors (PPIs) may be used for stress ulcer prophylaxis (SUP) in critically ill patients (see Evidence-Based Practice box). Critically ill patients at risk for the development of stress-related mucosal bleeding may benefit from the administration of either a PPI or an H2 receptor antagonist, both of which have been found to decrease the rate of GI bleeding. However, PPIs may be superior to H2 receptor antagonists at reducing the risk of GI bleeding.[23]

SUP measures are, at the time of this writing, recommended by the Institute for Healthcare Improvement as part of a "bundle" of best practices for care of the critically ill adult, specifically

TABLE 18.5 Selected Studies of Gastrointestinal Function

Test	Normal Findings	Clinical Significance
Stool studies	*Fat:* 2–6 g/24 h	Steatorrhea can result from intestinal malabsorption or pancreatic insufficiency
	Occult blood (guaiac test): none	Positive test is associated with either active or a recent history of bleeding
Gastric acid stimulation	11–20 mEq/h after stimulation	Increased with duodenal ulcers Decreased with gastric atrophy or gastric carcinoma
Glucose breath test or D-xylose	Negative for hydrogen and CO_2	May indicate intestinal bacterial overgrowth
Urea breath test	Negative for isotopically labeled CO_2	Presence of *Helicobacter pylori* infection

CO_2, Carbon dioxide.
Modified from Turner KC. Structure and function of the digestive system. In: Rogers J, ed. *McCance and Huether's Pathophysiology: The Biologic Basis for Disease in Adults and Children.* 9th ed. St. Louis, MO: Elsevier; 2024:1285a-1317.

TABLE 18.6 Characteristics of Gastric and Duodenal Ulcers

Characteristic	Gastric Ulcer	Duodenal Ulcer
Incidence		
Age at onset	50–70 years	20–50 years
Family history	Usually negative	Positive
Gender prevalence	Equal in females and males	Equal in females and males
Stress factors	Increased	Average
Ulcerogenic medications	Normal use	Increased use
Cancer risk	Increased	Not increased
Pathophysiology		
Abnormal mucus	May be present	May be present
Parietal cell mass	Normal or decreased	Increased
Acid production	Normal or decreased	Increased
Serum gastrin	Increased	Normal
Serum pepsinogen	Normal	Increased
Associated gastritis	More common	Usually not present
Helicobacter pylori	May be present (60%–80%)	Often present (95%–100%)
Clinical Manifestations		
Pain	Upper abdomen	Upper abdomen
	Intermittent	Intermittent
	Pain-antacid-relief pattern	Pain–antacid or food-relief pattern
	Food-pain pattern	Nocturnal pain common
Clinical course	Chronic ulcer without pattern of remission and exacerbation	Pattern of remissions and exacerbations for years

From Spain SR. Alterations of digestive function. In: Rogers J, ed. *McCance and Huether's Pathophysiology: The Biologic Basis for Disease in Adults and Children.* 9th ed. St. Louis, MO: Elsevier; 2024:1318-1374.

SUP for prevention of ventilator-associated pneumonia or ventilator-associated events. SUP is an important intervention for mechanically ventilated patients because of their increased risk of developing stress ulcers in the mucosa of the upper GI tract. The development of stress ulcers may result in the need for blood transfusion or corrective interventions, all of which may increase ventilator days, critical care length of stay, and the risk of infection.[21–23]

EVIDENCE-BASED PRACTICE

Preventing Upper Gastrointestinal Bleeding in Critically Ill Patients

Problem

There is evidence to support that upper gastrointestinal (GI) bleeding from stress ulcers contribute to increased morbidity and mortality in critically ill patients. However, the incidence of stress-induced GI bleeding in critical care units has decreased, and not all critically ill patients may need prophylactic treatment. In addition, stress ulcer prophylaxis may be associated with negative effects, such as or pneumonia and virulent forms of *Clostridium difficile* (see Clinical Alert box).

Clinical Questions

In critically ill patients, what is the relative impact of proton pump inhibitors (PPIs), H2 receptor antagonists, sucralfate, or no GI bleeding (GIB) prophylaxis (or stress ulcer prophylaxis) on outcomes important to patients?

Evidence

Medline, PubMed, Embase, Cochrane Central Register of Controlled Trials, trial registers, and literature outside of traditional publishing sources were searched up to March 2019. A total of 72 randomized controlled trials of 12,660 patients were included. PPIs and H2 receptor antagonists probably reduce the risk of clinically significant GIB in high-risk and highest-risk patients when compared to placebo or no prophylaxis. The reduction in bleeding may be unimportant in patients with low risk. Both PPIs and H2 receptor antagonists may increase the risk for pneumonia. Though the quality of evidence is variable, the results provided no support for any effect on hospital or critical care length of stay, duration of mechanical ventilation, mortality, or *C. difficile* infection.

Implications for Nursing

Critically ill patients with more risk factors for the development of stress ulcers may benefit from prophylaxis with PPIs and H2 receptor antagonists to prevent upper GIB. The risk of pneumonia may be increased with the addition of these medications; therefore, nurses should adhere to ventilator-associated pneumonia prevention bundles to reduce the patient's risk of infection. Once the patient's risk decreases (e.g., extubation, resolution of coagulopathies), stress ulcer prophylaxis should be discontinued given the increased risk of harm without improvement in patient outcomes.

Level of Evidence

A—Systematic review and meta-analysis

Reference

Wang Y, Ye Z, Ge L, et al. Efficacy and safety of gastrointestinal bleeding prophylaxis in critically ill patients: systematic review and network meta-analysis. *BMJ.* 2020;368:l6744. https://doi.org/10.1136/bmj.l6744.

CLINICAL ALERT

Clostridium difficile Infection

- *Clostridium difficile*, a gram-positive, spore-forming anaerobic bacillus, is a common cause of antibiotic-associated diarrhea and can result in *C. difficile* infection (CDI).
- *C. difficile* produces two exotoxins, toxin A and toxin B. The organism colonizes the mucosal lining of the colon, especially in immunocompromised patients. It also attacks the normal gastrointestinal microbes (gut flora) that have been altered as a result of antibiotics or other causes.
- Toxins cause mucosal injury and inflammation, resulting in pseudomembranous colitis. This occurs when *C. difficile* toxins cause cell death and erosion of areas of the intestinal mucosal lining, leaving a shallow ulcer on the surface. Mucus and inflammatory cells flow out from the ulcer, producing the watery diarrhea.
- Some patients progress to severe disease with toxicity and shock, requiring admission to a critical care unit and/or surgical therapy with colectomy. Some patients succumb to severe disease with the development of toxic megacolon or septic shock.

Risk Factors

- Antibiotic exposure (most commonly to fluoroquinolones)
- Institutionalization
- Advanced age
- Preexisting severe illness

Diagnosis

- Detection of enterotoxins (toxins A and B) in stool specimens.
- Nucleic acid amplification testing (NAAT), a polymerase chain reaction (PCR) test, is an accurate test to identify the gene that controls toxins A and B and to diagnose CDI in symptomatic patients. If NAAT is negative, no further testing is indicated. If NAAT is positive, a *C. difficile* toxin antigen enzyme immunoassay (EIA) is performed to identify *C. difficile* toxins A and B. The EIA has a good positive predictive value for CDI but may also detect colonization. A negative *C. difficile* toxin antigen EIA has a low negative predictive value.
- Endoscopic (colonoscopy) determination of pseudomembranous colitis.

Treatment Based on Clinical Judgment

- Discontinue offending antibiotics, if possible.
- First-line treatment is oral fidaxomicin; however, vancomycin is an acceptable alternative based on available resources.
- Oral metronidazole is an alternative for nonsevere CDI.
- Other interventions include withdrawing antibiotic therapy, repleting volume and electrolyte losses, avoiding antiperistaltic agents, and strict adherence to infection control practices.
- Some cases are refractory to treatment and may recur. Recurrent disease may be treated with additional antibiotics and/or fecal microbiota transplant.

Prevention

- Nurses have an important role in the prevention of transmission of this disease.
- The main routes of *C. difficile* transmission include: the hands of clinical staff, an inadequately cleaned room formerly occupied by a CDI patient, and contaminated medical equipment.

Reference

Johnson S, Lavergne V, Skinner AM, et al. Clinical Practice Guideline by the Infectious Diseases Society of America (IDSA) and Society for Healthcare Epidemiology of America (SHEA): 2021 Focused Update Guidelines on Management of Clostridioides difficile Infection in Adults. *Clin Infect Dis.* 2021;73(5):e1029-e1044. https://doi.org/10.1093/cid/ciab549.

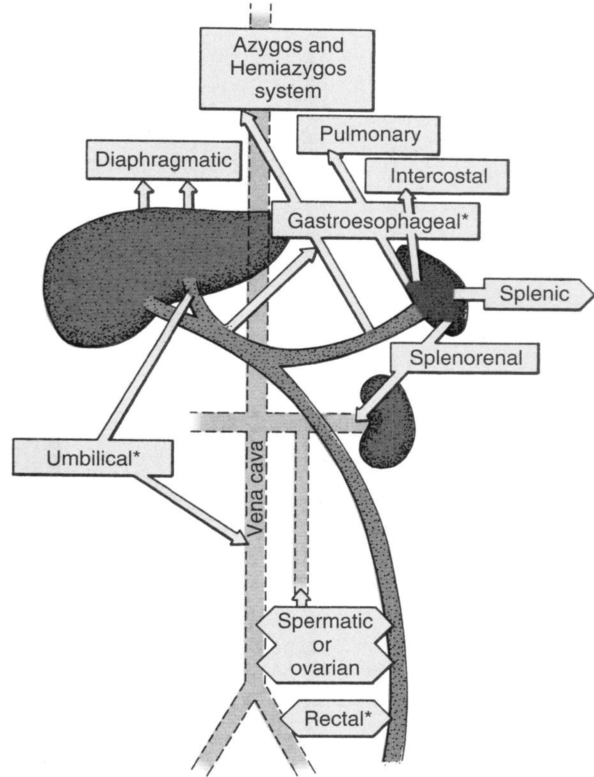

Fig. 18.7 The liver and collateral circulation. *Indicates most common sites.

Mallory-Weiss Tear. A Mallory-Weiss tear is an arterial hemorrhage resulting from an acute longitudinal tear in the gastroesophageal mucosa. Mallory-Weiss tears account for 10% to 15% of upper GI bleeding episodes. They are associated with long-term use of NSAIDs or aspirin and with excessive alcohol consumption. The upper GI bleeding usually occurs after episodes of forceful retching. Bleeding usually resolves spontaneously; however, lacerations of the esophagogastric junction may cause massive GI bleeding, requiring surgical repair.

Esophageal Varices. In chronic liver failure, liver cell structure and function are impaired, resulting in increased portal venous pressure, called *portal hypertension* (see discussion of Hepatic Failure). As a result, part of the venous blood in the splanchnic system is diverted from the liver to the systemic circulation by the development of connections to neighboring low-pressure veins. This phenomenon is called *collateral circulation.* The most common sites for the development of these collateral channels are the submucosa of the esophagus and rectum, the anterior abdominal wall, and the parietal peritoneum. Fig. 18.7 shows a liver with collateral circulation. The normal portal venous pressure is 2 to 6 mm Hg. As these veins experience increases in pressure, they become distended with blood, the vessels enlarge, and varices develop when the pressure exceeds 10 mm Hg. The varices tend to bleed when the portal venous pressures reach 12 mm Hg. The most common sites for development of these varices are the esophagus and the upper portion of the stomach.[24,25]

Assessment

Clinical Presentation. Patients manifest blood loss from the GI tract in several ways. Vomiting or drainage from a nasogastric tube that yields blood or coffee groundlike material is associated with upper GI bleeding. However, blood or coffee groundlike contents may not be present if bleeding has ceased or if the bleeding arises beyond a closed pylorus. Upper GI bleeding commonly manifests with *hematemesis,* which is bloody vomitus that is either bright red, indicating fresh blood, or has the appearance of coffee grounds, resulting from older blood that has been in the stomach long enough for the gastric juices to act on it. Blood from an upper GI bleed may also pass via the colon as melena. *Melena* is shiny, black, foul-smelling stool that results from the degradation of blood by stomach acids or intestinal bacteria. Bright red or maroon blood *(hematochezia)* is usually a sign of a lower GI source of bleeding, but it may be observed with massive upper GI bleeding (>1000 mL). Often, GI blood loss is occult (not visible) and is detected only by testing the stool with a chemical reagent *(guaiac)* (Table 18.5). Stool and nasogastric drainage can test positive with guaiac for up to 10 days after a bleeding episode.

Upper GI bleeding may also be accompanied by mild epigastric pain or abdominal distress. Pain arises from the acid bathing the ulcerated crater.

Finally, patients with acute upper GI bleeding may manifest clinical signs and symptoms of blood loss. Rapidly assess for hemodynamic stability associated with bleeding and collaborate with the multiprofessional team to determine whether the bleeding is acute or chronic in etiology. Patients with acute upper GI bleeding commonly have signs or symptoms of hypovolemic shock. Fig. 18.8 describes the pathophysiology of acute upper GI bleeding.

Nursing Assessment. Initial evaluation of the patient with upper GI bleeding involves rapid assessment of the severity of blood loss, hemodynamic stability, and the necessity for fluid resuscitation. Monitor signs of hypovolemic shock (see Chapter 12, Shock, Sepsis, and Multiple Organ Dysfunction Syndrome). Changes in blood pressure and heart rate depend on the amount of blood loss, the suddenness of the blood loss, and the degree of cardiac and vascular compensation. Monitor vital signs at least every 15 minutes. As blood loss exceeds 1000 mL, the shock syndrome progresses, causing decreased blood flow to the skin, lungs, liver, and kidneys. Hypotension is an advanced sign of shock.

Hypertension is a common comorbid condition in those at risk of GI bleeding. Conditions such as chronic hypertension or cardiovascular disease often mask signs of shock and make resuscitative attempts difficult. In the chronically hypertensive patient, normal values for predicting perfusion do not apply; therefore, assess other parameters, such as level of consciousness and urinary output. Decreasing blood pressure is often associated with increasing blood loss.

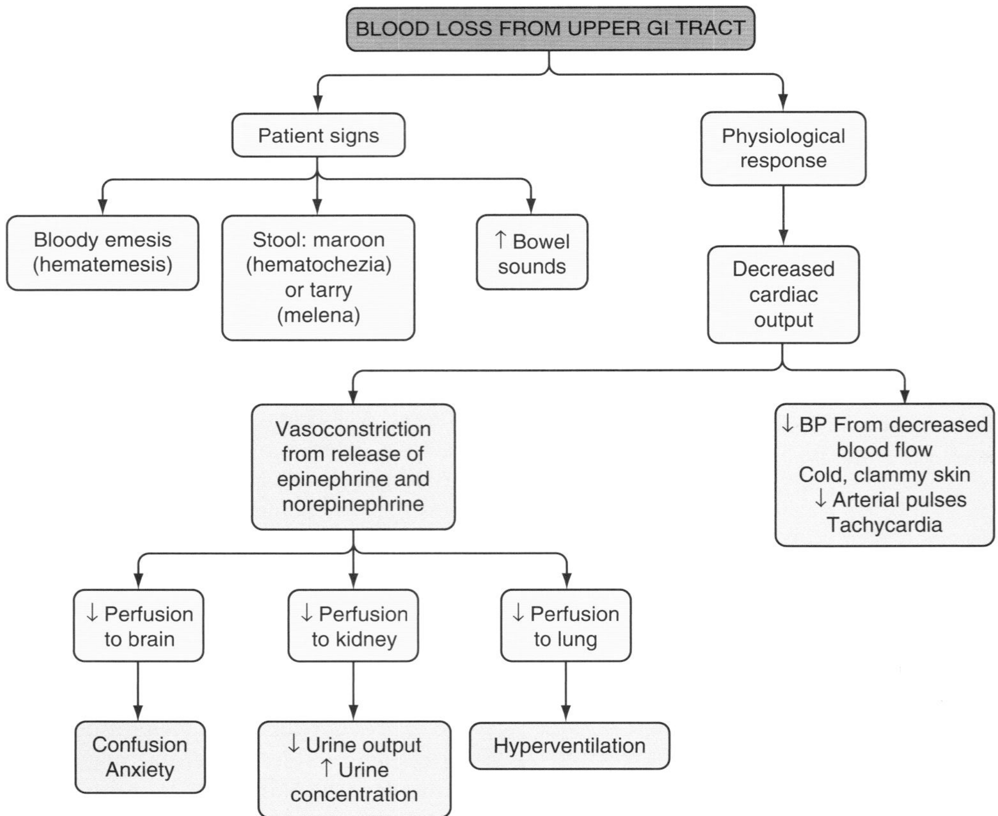

Fig. 18.8 Pathophysiology flow diagram of acute upper gastrointestinal *(GI)* bleeding. *BP,* Blood pressure.

Hemodynamic monitoring (see Chapter 9, Hemodynamic Monitoring) may be initiated to evaluate the patient's hemodynamic response to blood loss and resuscitative measures. An electrocardiogram (ECG) may show ST-segment depression or flattening of the T waves, both of which indicate decreased coronary blood flow resulting in ischemia.

Abdominal assessment may reveal a soft or distended abdomen. Bowel sounds most often are hyperactive as a result of the sensitivity of the bowel to blood.

In addition to the physical examination, obtain a history to identify whether there have been previous episodes of bleeding or surgery for bleeding; a family history of bleeding; or a current illness or disease that may lead to bleeding, such as a coagulopathy, cancer, or liver disease. Also assess for drug or alcohol use disorders and other risk factors.

Medical Assessment

Laboratory studies. The common laboratory studies ordered for a patient with acute upper GI bleeding are listed in Box 18.7. Although a complete blood count is always ordered, the hematocrit (Hct) value does not change substantially during the first few hours after an acute bleeding episode. During this time, do not underestimate the severity of the bleeding. Only when extravascular fluid enters the vascular space to restore volume does the Hct value decrease.

BOX 18.7 Abnormal Laboratory Values of Upper Gastrointestinal Bleeding

Arterial Blood Gases
Metabolic acidosis
Respiratory alkalosis

Coagulation Profile
Prothrombin time, partial thromboplastin time: Usually ↑

Complete Blood Count
Hematocrit: Normal, then ↓
Hemoglobin: Normal, then ↓
Platelet count: Initially ↑, then ↓
White blood cell count: ↑

Gastric Aspirate for pH and Guaiac
Guaiac positive
Possibly acidotic pH

Liver Function Tests
Serum enzyme levels: ↓

Serum Chemistry Panel
Ammonia: Possibly ↑
Blood urea nitrogen, creatinine: ↑
Calcium: Normal or ↓
Glucose: Hyperglycemia common
Lactate: ↑
Potassium: ↓, then ↑
Sodium: ↓

This effect is further complicated by fluids and blood products administered during the resuscitation period. Platelet and white blood cell (WBC) counts may be increased, reflecting the body's attempt to restore homeostasis. An electrolyte profile is also indicated. Decreases in levels of potassium and sodium are common as a result of the accompanying vomiting. Later, serum sodium levels may increase as a result of the loss of vascular volume. The glucose level is often increased (related to the stress response). Increases in the levels of blood urea nitrogen (BUN) and creatinine reflect decreased perfusion to the liver and kidneys. Liver function tests, clotting profiles, and serum ammonia levels are ordered to rule out preexisting liver disease. An arterial blood gas analysis is ordered to evaluate the patient's acid-base and oxygenation status. Respiratory alkalosis is common with GI bleeding because of patient anxiety and the effects of the sympathetic nervous system. As shock progresses, the patient may develop metabolic acidosis as a result of anaerobic metabolism. Hypoxemia may also be present as a result of decreased circulating Hgb levels.

Esophagogastroduodenoscopy and other diagnostic tests. Esophagogastroduodenoscopy (EGD) is the procedure of choice for the diagnosis and treatment of active upper GI bleeding and for the prevention of rebleeding. This procedure allows for direct mucosal inspection with the use of a flexible, fiberoptic scope. The procedure can be done at the bedside, which is an advantage when caring for a critically ill patient. Endoscopic evaluation of the source of the bleeding is not usually undertaken until the patient is hemodynamically stable. Small bowel endoscopy is a safe option for identifying bleeding, and video capsule endoscopy provides diagnostic accuracy in hemodynamically stable patients. When diagnostic testing is unable to identify elusive bleeding, patients may undergo interventional radiological examination to locate active bleeding.[18] Barium studies may be performed for some patients to determine the presence of peptic ulcers, the site(s) of bleeding, and the presence of tumors and inflammatory processes.[18–21]

Patient Problems

The problem most commonly observed in patients with acute GI bleeding is the potential for hypovolemic shock resulting from blood loss (see Chapter 12, Shock, Sepsis, and Multiple Organ Dysfunction Syndrome).

Nursing and Medical Considerations

The management of acute GI bleeding initially consists of treatment to restore hemodynamic stability, followed by diagnosis of the cause of bleeding and initiation of specific and supportive therapies (Box 18.8). The nurse's role during the initial management of acute GI bleeding includes assessment, carrying out prescribed medical therapy, monitoring the patient's physiological and psychosocial responses to the interventions, monitoring for complications of the disease process or treatment

BOX 18.8 Management of Upper Gastrointestinal Bleeding

Hemodynamic Stabilization	Definitive and Supportive Therapies

• Colloids
• Isotonic crystalloids
• Blood or blood products
	• Pharmacological therapies
	  o H2 receptor antagonists
	  o Proton pump inhibitors
	• Endoscopic therapies
	  o Sclerotherapy
	  o Heater probe
	  o Laser
	  o Endoclips
	  o Band ligation
	• Surgical therapies

regimen, and providing supportive care. In addition, the nurse supports the patient and family and explains the diagnostic tests and medical therapies.

Hemodynamic Stabilization. For patients who are hemodynamically unstable, establish immediate venous access using a large-bore IV catheter and begin volume resuscitation (see Chapter 12, Shock, Sepsis, and Multiple Organ Dysfunction Syndrome). For the restoration of vascular volume, infuse blood products and fluids as rapidly as the patient's cardiovascular status allows and until vital signs return to baseline.

Patients who continue to bleed or who have an excessively low Hct value (<25%) and clinical symptoms of blood loss may be resuscitated with blood and blood products. The decision to use blood products is based on laboratory data and clinical examination. Blood is transfused to improve oxygenation (by increasing the number of RBCs) or to improve coagulation (by replacing platelets and plasma). If the patient is hemodynamically unstable and hemorrhaging, implementation of a massive transfusion protocol (MTP) may be warranted (see Chapter 12, Shock, Sepsis, and Multiple Organ Dysfunction Syndrome, and Chapter 20, Trauma and Surgical Management). The Hct value may not initially reflect actual blood volume during the first 24 to 72 hours after a hemorrhage and until vascular volume is restored. A reasonable goal for blood transfusions is a Hgb value greater than 7 g/dL or Hct of 30%, but these goals are individually determined based on clinical assessments.[26,27] One unit of packed RBCs usually increases the Hgb value by 1 g/dL and the Hct value by approximately 3%, but this effect is influenced by the patient's intravascular volume status and whether the patient is actively bleeding. Carefully monitor the patient for complications of blood transfusion therapy: hypocalcemia, hyperkalemia, infection, increased ammonia levels, hypothermia, and anaphylactic reactions.

Gastric Lavage. The use of gastric lavage is somewhat controversial, and its use has not demonstrated benefit in clinical outcomes; therefore, it is not routinely used before upper endoscopy. Though infrequently used, gastric lavage before endoscopy for acute upper GI bleeding is safe and may provide better visualization of the gastric fundus. Insert a large-bore nasogastric tube and connect it to suction. If lavage is ordered, instill 200 to 300 mL of room-temperature 0.9% normal saline via the nasogastric tube and gently remove the gastric contents by intermittent suction or gravity until the secretions are clear. After lavage, the nasogastric tube may be removed or left in place. Nasogastric tubes left in place can increase hydrochloric acid secretion in the stomach and cause increased bleeding. Carefully document the nature of the nasogastric secretions or vomitus, such as color, amount, and pH.[28,29]

Pharmacological Therapy. The best treatment of acute GI bleed is prevention and is accomplished through appropriate use of SUP with H2 receptor antagonists and PPIs. Pharmaclogical treatment of acute GI bleed often includes the use of a PPI. Once diagnostics are completed, the pharmacological interventions are tailored to the etiology of the acute GI bleed and may include PPI mucosal barrier enhancers, and antibiotics. Table 18.7 describes the treatments commonly used to decrease gastric acid secretion or reduce the effects of acid on the gastric mucosa.

Antibiotics. *H. pylori* infection is often associated with PUD. Triple-agent therapy with a PPI and two antibiotics for 14 days is the recommended treatment for eradication of *H. pylori.* The first-line treatment for *H. pylori* infection consists of triple therapy with a PPI (e.g., esomeprazole, omeprazole, pantoprazole) plus the antibiotics amoxicillin and clarithromycin.[17] In case first-line therapy fails, quadruple therapy has proven effective.[17] This second-line therapy consists of a PPI or H2 receptor antagonist, bismuth, metronidazole, and a tetracycline. Alternatively, a 10-day course of levofloxacin may be administered as a second-line therapy for *H. pylori* infections after the initial treatment regimen. European guidelines recommend sequential therapy, which includes 5 days of amoxicillin therapy with a PPI followed by 5 days of clarithromycin, metronidazole, and a PPI.[30]

Endoscopic Therapy. Endoscopic intervention is the treatment of choice for upper GI bleeding, and several endoscopic therapies have been developed. EGD is performed only after the patient is stabilized hemodynamically but within 24 hours after manifestation of the GI bleeding.[31–32] The advantage of endoscopic therapies is that they can be applied during the diagnostic procedure. *Sclerotherapy* involves injecting the bleeding ulcer with a necrotizing agent. The agents most commonly used are morrhuate sodium, ethanolamine, and tetradecyl sulfate. These agents work by traumatizing the endothelium, causing necrosis and eventually sclerosis of the bleeding vessel. Thermal methods of endoscopic therapy include use of the heater probe, laser photocoagulation, and electrocoagulation to tamponade the vessel. Endoclipping—band dilators and hemoclips—may

TABLE 18.7 **PHARMACOLOGY**

Treatments to Decrease Gastric Acid Secretion and/or Reduce Acid Effects on Gastric Mucosa

Medication	Action/Use	Dose/Route	Side Effects	Nursing Implications
Histamine (H2 receptor) Antagonists				
Cimetidine	Inhibits H2-receptors of gastric parietal cells to inhibit gastric acid secretion	*Oral:* 300 mg q6h Renal dose adjusments required (variable in the literature)	Most H2-receptor antagonists do not have any side effects. Some have the following side effects: Diarrhea Headache Dizziness Rash Tiredness	Monitor for presence of vomiting of blood, blood in stools, unintentional weight loss, difficulty swallowing, persistent abdominal pain.
Famotidine	Same	*Oral/Intravenous:* 20 mg bid PO or IV	Same	Same
Nizatidine	Same	*Oral:* CrCl 20–50 150 mg daily CrCl <20 150 mg q48h	Same	Same
Proton Pump Inhibitors				
Esomeprazole (Nexium)	Inhibit gastric acid secretion by specific inhibition of the hydrogen-potassium–adenosine triphosphatase enzyme system	*Intravenous:* 20–40 mg daily IV, up to 10 days	Abdominal pain Constipation Diarrhea Flatulence Headaches Nausea Vomiting	Monitor for presence of blood in vomit or stool, unintentional weight loss, difficulty swallowing, abdominal pain, or persistent vomiting.
Lansoprazole (Prevacid)	Same	*Oral:* 30 mg daily PO	Same	Same
Omeprazole (Prilosec)	Same	*Oral:* 20–40 mg daily PO	Same	Same
Pantoprazole (Protonix)	Same	*Oral/intravenous:* 40 mg daily PO or IV ***For treatment of GI Bleed:*** *Intravenous:* 80 mg IVP x1 followed by 40 mg IVP q12h or 8 mg/hr x 48-72 hrs followed by 40 mg IVP q12h	Same	Same
Mucosal Barrier Enhancers				
Sucralfate	Reduce the effects of acid secretion; promote healing	*Oral:* 1 g qid, 1 h AC and qHS/PO	Constipation Dizziness Lightheadedness Severe allergic reactions	Assess for presence of dizziness. May have sensitivity to the aluminum in it

AC, before meals; *bid*, twice a day; *GI*, gastrointestinal; *H2*, histamine; *IVP*, intravenous push; *PO*, by mouth; *q*, every; *qHS*, every hour of sleep.
From Skidmore-Roth L. *Mosby's 2023 Nursing Drug Reference*. 36th ed. St. Louis, MO: Elsevier; 2023; Cimetidine injection: Package insert. Drugs.com. https://www.drugs.com/pro/cimetidine-injection.html. Updated March 27, 2023. Accessed December 27, 2023.

be used to provide hemostasis and to decrease the incidence of rebleeding.

During EGD, assist with procedures and monitor for untoward effects. Maintain the airway and observe the patient's breathing during endoscopy. Assist in positioning the patient in a left lateral reverse Trendelenburg position to help prevent respiratory complications. Other common complications of sclerotherapy include fever and oozing from the bleeding site.

Surgical Therapy. Surgery may be considered for patients who have massive GI bleeding. The patient is usually admitted to a critical care unit for initial management and stabilization in preparation for emergency surgery. The most common reason for emergency surgery is massive rebleeding that occurs within 8 hours of admission. Patients may also become surgical candidates if they continue to bleed despite aggressive medical intervention. Criteria for delayed surgery vary, but it is usually

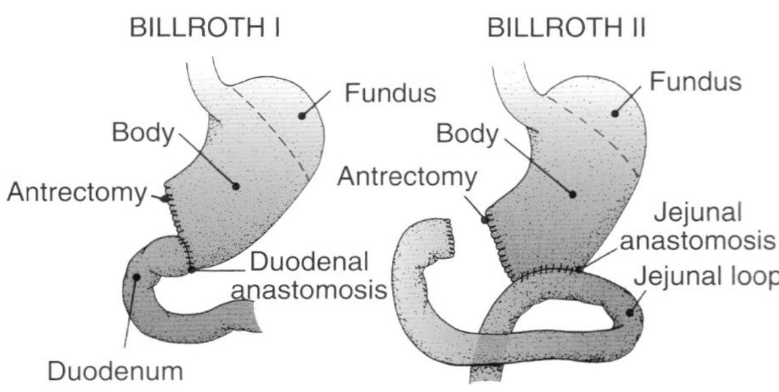

Fig. 18.9 Billroth I and II procedures.

considered in those who require more than 8 units of blood within a 24-hour period.

Surgical therapies for PUD include gastric resection (antrectomy, gastrectomy, gastroenterostomy, vagotomy) and combined operations to restore GI continuity (Billroth I, Billroth II) or to prevent complications of the surgery (vagotomy and pyloroplasty). An *antrectomy* may be performed for duodenal ulcers to decrease the acidity of the duodenum by removing the antrum, which secretes gastric acid. A *vagotomy* decreases acid secretion in the stomach by dividing the vagus nerve along the esophagus. A *pyloroplasty* may be performed in conjunction with a vagotomy to prevent stomach atony, a common complication of the vagotomy procedure. A *Billroth I* procedure involves vagotomy, antrectomy, and anastomosis of the stomach to the duodenum. A *Billroth II* procedure involves vagotomy, resection of the antrum, and anastomosis of the stomach to the jejunum (Fig. 18.9). A perforation can be treated by simple closure with the use of a patch to cover the gastric mucosal hole (omental patch) or by excision of the ulcer and suturing of the surrounding tissue.

Impaired emptying of solids or liquids from the stomach into the small intestine (gastric outlet obstruction) may also necessitate surgical intervention. The major symptoms of obstruction are vomiting and continued pain localized in the epigastrium.

Postoperative nursing care is focused on preventing and monitoring potential complications. Fluid and electrolyte imbalances are common from loss of fluids during the surgical procedure, surgical drains, and a nasogastric tube that may be left in place to decompress the stomach. In addition, the GI system may not function normally after surgery, with resulting nausea, vomiting, ileus, or diarrhea. Providing adequate nutrition is important to promote wound healing, and a dietitian consult is highly recommended. In cases of prolonged ileus after surgery, total parenteral nutrition may be considered. Monitor for signs and symptoms of wound infection: erythema, swelling, tenderness, drainage, fever, and increased WBC count. A systemic infection may result from peritonitis if perforation has allowed stomach or intestinal contents to spill into the peritoneum. Postoperative rupture of the anastomosis may also lead to this complication.

Pain is an important postoperative nursing concern. Abdominal incisions are associated with postoperative discomfort because of their anatomical location. Implement incentive spirometry and other pulmonary hygiene measures to reduce the risk of postoperative lung infections. Pulmonary infections are common because incisional pain impairs the ability to cough and breathe deeply. A program supporting early mobility can also improve respiratory function in critically ill patients.[33] Early and progressive mobility of postoperative patients may improve functional outcomes and decrease length of stay.[33,34]

Several problems are associated with the postoperative care of patients with upper GI bleeding. These problems include potential infection; acute pain; potential for fluid, electrolyte, and acid-base imbalances; potential for impaired nutrition; potential for decreased multisystem tissue perfusion; and decreased gas exchange (refer to the Collaborative Care Plan found in Chapter 1, Overview of Critical Care Nursing).

Recognition of Potential Complications. Perforation of the gastric mucosa is the major GI complication of PUD (see Clinical Alert box). The most common signs of perforation are an abrupt onset of abdominal pain followed rapidly by signs of peritonitis. Emergent surgery is indicated for treatment. Fluid and electrolyte resuscitation and treatment of any immediate complication are the priorities. These patients almost always have nasogastric tubes placed for gastric decompression. Broad-spectrum antibiotics are also usually prescribed before surgery. H2 receptor antagonists and PPIs may or may not be indicated, depending on the cause of the upper GI bleeding. Mortality rates for patients with perforation range from 10% to 40%, depending on the age and condition of the patient at the time of surgery.

Treatment of Variceal Bleeding

Bleeding esophageal or gastric varices are usually a medical emergency because they cause massive upper GI blood loss. The patient typically develops hemodynamic instability and signs and symptoms of shock. Often, the cause of the bleeding is unknown unless the patient has a history of cirrhosis or has previously bled from varices. Initial treatment of esophageal and gastric varices is the same. Top priorities include hemodynamic stabilization and establishment of a patent airway. Gastric lavage may be used to clear the stomach and to document the amount of blood loss. Diagnosis of the cause of the bleeding through endoscopy is a priority before definitive treatment for the varices can be started.[35,36]

Somatostatin or Octreotide. Somatostatin or octreotide (a long-acting somatostatin) may be ordered to slow or stop bleeding. These medications decrease splanchnic blood flow, reduce portal pressure, and have minimal adverse effects. Octreotide is given to stabilize patients before definitive treatment is performed.[37,38] Octreotide is recommended for patients with

! CLINICAL ALERT

Acute Gastric Perforation

- Abdominal tenderness
- Abrupt onset of severe abdominal pain
- Boardlike abdomen
- Leukocytosis
- Presence of free air on radiography
- Bowel sounds are usually absent

variceal upper GI bleeding, and it can be used as adjunctive therapy for nonvariceal upper GI bleeding.[18,19,21] Octreotide is given as an IV loading dose followed by an infusion for 2 to 5 days. Postprandial hyperglycemia may occur in nondiabetic patients receiving octreotide.[39] Monitor for both hypoglycemia and hyperglycemia.[18,19,21]

Vasopressin. Vasopressin (Pitressin) is a synthetic antidiuretic hormone (Box 18.9). Vasopressin lowers portal pressure by vasoconstriction of the splanchnic arteriolar bed. Ultimately, it decreases pressure and flow in liver collateral circulation channels to decrease bleeding and may be used as an adjunct to therapy in acute bleeding episodes.[40,41] However, vasopressin does not improve survival rates from active variceal bleeding and is rarely used because of its adverse effects.[36,42] Vasopressin may be considered if octreotide cannot be used.

Endoscopic Procedures. *Sclerotherapy* is another option for the treatment of bleeding varices. After the varices are identified, the sclerosing agent is injected into the varix and the surrounding tissue. Usually, several applications of the sclerosing agent are needed several days apart to decompress the bleeding varix.

Endoscopic band ligation is another treatment for varices.[35,42] Under endoscopy, a rubber band is placed over the varix. This treatment results in thrombosis, sloughing, and fibrosis of the varix.

Transjugular Intrahepatic Portosystemic Shunting. *Transjugular intrahepatic portosystemic shunting (TIPS)* is a nonsurgical treatment for recurrent variceal bleeding after sclerotherapy. TIPS has been used primarily to treat the major consequences of portal hypertension, such as bleeding and ascites, or as a bridge to liver transplantation in cirrhotic patients.[42,43] Placement of the shunt is performed with the use of fluoroscopy. A stainless steel stent is placed between the hepatic and portal veins to create a portosystemic shunt in the liver and decrease portal pressure.[42,43] A lower portal pressure decreases pressure within the varix, thereby decreasing the risk of acute hemorrhage.

Approximately 10% to 20% of patients do not stop bleeding after endoscopic treatment combined with somatostatin infusion, and others rebleed within the first couple of days after cessation of the initial bleed. After a second unsuccessful endoscopic attempt, the TIPS procedure is used as a treatment option. Although TIPS is also commonly used for other indications, such as Budd-Chiari syndrome, acute variceal bleeding, and hepatic hydrothorax, the best available evidence supports use of TIPS in secondary prevention of variceal bleeding and in refractory ascites.[42,43] Early preemptive TIPS can be the first choice for high-risk patients such as those with uncontrolled variceal bleeding, severe portal hypertension, a Child-Pugh score of B with active bleeding, or a Child-Pugh score of C up to 13 points.[42,43] The Child-Pugh score estimates mortality in liver disease, typically cirrhosis, with scores B and C indicating significant functional compromise and decompensated disease, respectively.

BOX 18.9 Vasopressin (Pitressin) Therapy

Mechanism of Action

Vasoconstrictor: constricts the splanchnic vascular bed, contracts intestinal smooth muscle, and lowers portal vein pressure

Dose

Given by IV, although it may be given intraarterially. IV infusion is started at 0.2–0.4 unit/min and increased by 0.2 unit/min each hour until hemorrhage is controlled, to a maximum dose of 0.8 unit/min. The infusion should not be continued for longer than 24 h at the highest effective dose. Wean slowly.

Side Effects

- *Gastrointestinal:* cramping, nausea, vomiting, diarrhea
- *Cardiovascular:* dizziness, diaphoresis, hypertension, cardiac dysrhythmias, exacerbation of heart failure
- *Neurological:* tremors, headache, vertigo, decreased level of consciousness
- *Integumentary:* pallor, localized gangrene

Nursing Considerations

- Monitor for angina and dysrhythmias.
- Infuse through a central line.
- Assess serum sodium.
- Assess neurological status.

From Collins, Shelly R. Elsevier's 2023 Intravenous Medications. 39th ed. St. Louis, MO: Elsevier; 2022.

Esophagogastric Tamponade. If bleeding continues despite therapy, esophagogastric balloon tamponade therapy may provide short-term, temporary control. Inflation of the balloon ports applies pressure to the vessels supplying the varices to decrease blood flow, thereby stopping the bleeding. Three types of tubes are used for tamponade: Sengstaken-Blakemore, Minnesota, and Linton tubes. The adult *Sengstaken-Blakemore tube* has three lumina: one for gastric aspiration (similar to that in a nasogastric tube), one for inflation of the esophageal balloon, and one for inflation of the gastric balloon (Fig. 18.10). The *Minnesota tube* has an additional lumen that allows for aspiration of esophageal secretions. The Minnesota tube is commonly used because it

CLINICAL EXEMPLAR

Quality and Safety

The nurse manager was very concerned about the increasing rates of *Clostridium difficile* infection (CDI) on the unit. The nurse manager and nurse educator spent a great deal of time educating the clinical nurses and technicians on the unit in the prevention of this healthcare-acquired infection (HAI). However, the rates continued to increase. The nurse manager realized data on CDI risk factors and transmission specific to the unit were needed.

The nurse manager and educator collaborated with the Infection Prevention and Informatics departments to develop a hand hygiene audit tool. The tool would be used by two volunteers monitoring hand washing on the unit. If any personnel did not comply with the hand washing policies and procedures, they were respectfully educated by the observers in real-time. Audits identified that the hand washing compliance rate was low and needed improvement. During this time, the leaders also observed that stool specimens were being ordered and sent on patients without appropriate indications for testing.

The nurse manager and educator developed a CDI bundle and a unit-based decision tree for *C. difficile* testing. The CDI bundle (i.e., a group of best practices for the care of hospitalized patients) included contact isolation precautions, hand washing on entering and exiting the room, an isolation cart outside of the room, and disinfecting equipment removed from a patient's room. The nursing leadership believed that this bundle was in line with the culture of safety and quality on the unit. The decision tree included avoiding stool specimens if a patient was on laxatives; stopping laxatives and watching for resolution of diarrhea; placing the patient on contact isolation precautions without testing and re-evaluating in 24 hours; and discontinuing unnecessary IV antibiotics or changing to the oral route. The manager and educator developed reference cards, which were printed and laminated for the multiprofessional team's reference.

Over the next few months, hand washing compliance rates improved as more observers provided real-time hand hygiene feedback. A reduction in CDI rates were also observed with improved hand hygiene practices and implementation of the CDI bundle and decision tree. As the nurses developed their knowledge and confidence of the CDI bundle and decision tree, they were able to educate many providers on appropriate ordering of *C. difficile* stool specimens. They also became more cognizant of the antibiotics that their patients were receiving and discussed their necessity during multiprofessional rounds. Given the successes on the unit, the hand washing audit tool, CDI bundle, and decision tree were spread to all of the other inpatient units.

allows for suction of secretions above and below the balloon. The *Linton tube* has a gastric balloon only, with lumens for gastric and esophageal suction; it is reserved for those with bleeding gastric varices.

Regardless of type, the balloon tip is inserted into the stomach, and the gastric balloon is inflated and clamped. The tube is then withdrawn slowly until resistance is met so that pressure is exerted at the gastroesophageal junction. Correct positioning and traction are maintained by the use of an external traction source or a nasal cuff around the tube at the mouth or nose. External traction can be attached to a helmet or to the foot of the bed with over-bed traction and weights. Proper amounts of traction are essential because too little traction lets the balloon fall away from the gastric wall, resulting in insufficient pressure on the bleeding vessels, whereas too much traction causes discomfort, gastric ulceration, or vomiting. If bleeding does not stop with inflation of the gastric balloon, the esophageal balloon is inflated and clamped (Sengstaken-Blakemore or Minnesota tube). Normal inflation pressure of the esophageal balloon is 20 to 45 mm Hg.

Monitor balloon lumen pressures and the patency of the system. The gastric balloon port placement below the gastroesophageal junction must be confirmed by radiographic images. Defer to the provider's orders, but typically, deflate the balloon every 8 to 12 hours to decompress the esophagus and gastric mucosa. During this procedure, assess the status of the bleeding and be prepared for hemostasis. Deflate the esophageal balloon before deflating the gastric balloon; otherwise, the entire tube will displace upward and occlude the airway.

Spontaneous rupture of the gastric balloon, upward migration of the tube, and occlusion of the airway are possible complications that need to be assessed. Esophageal rupture may occur and is characterized by the abrupt onset of severe pain.

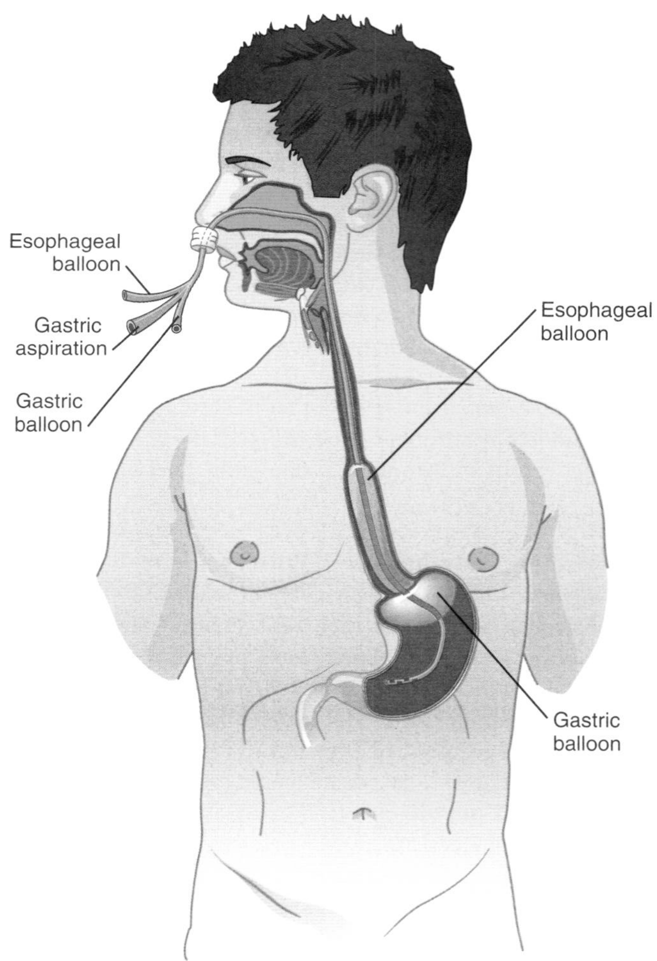

Fig. 18.10 Sengstaken-Blakemore tube. (From Good VS, Kirkwood PL, eds. *AACN Advanced Critical Care Nursing.* 2nd ed. Philadelphia, PA: Saunders; 2017.)

In the event of either of these two life-threatening emergencies, all three lumina are cut and the entire tube is removed. For this reason, ensure that scissors are at the patient's bedside at all times. Endotracheal intubation is strongly recommended to protect the airway if the patient requires balloon tamponade treatment.

Other complications of esophagogastric tamponade include ulcerations of the esophageal or gastric mucosa. In addition, lesions can develop around the mouth and nose as a result of the traction devices. Clean and lubricate the areas around the traction devices to prevent skin breakdown. Suction the nasopharynx frequently because the tube insertion results in an increase in secretions, and the patient's swallowing reflex is decreased. Irrigate the nasogastric tube at least every 2 hours to ensure patency and to keep the stomach empty. This measure helps prevent aspiration and prevents accumulation of blood in the stomach, which is especially important in the patient with liver failure. Ammonia is a byproduct of the protein in blood breaking down and cannot be detoxified by the patient with liver failure.[44,45]

Surgical Interventions. Permanent decompression of portal hypertension is achieved only through surgical creation of a *portocaval shunt* that diverts blood around the blocked portal system. In these operations, a connection is made between the portal vein and the inferior vena cava that diverts blood flow into the vena cava to decrease portal pressure. Several variations of this procedure exist, including the end-to-side shunt and the side-to-side shunt (Fig. 18.11). Other surgical techniques for reduction of portal pressure include splenorenal and mesocaval shunting.

Surgical shunts decrease rebleeding but do not improve survival. The procedure is associated with a higher risk of encephalopathy and makes liver transplantation, if needed, more difficult. Therefore, surgical shunts are rarely performed.[41] A temporary increase in ascites occurs after all of these procedures, and careful assessments and interventions are required during the care of these patients (see discussion of Hepatic Failure).

ACUTE PANCREATITIS

Acute pancreatitis is an acute inflammatory disease of the pancreas. The intensity of the disease ranges from mild, in which the patient has abdominal pain and elevated blood amylase and lipase levels, to extremely severe, which results in multiple organ failure. In 85% to 90% of patients, the disease is self-limited (mild acute pancreatitis), and patients recover rapidly. However, the disease can run a fulminant course and is associated with high mortality rates. Severe acute pancreatitis develops in 25% of patients with acute pancreatitis. Management of severe pancreatitis requires intensive nursing and medical care.

Pathophysiology

Acute pancreatitis is an inflammation of the pancreas with the potential for necrosis of pancreatic cells resulting from premature activation of pancreatic enzymes. It is one of the most common pancreatic diseases. Each year, about 300,000 patients are hospitalized in the United States because of pancreatitis.[46] Normally, pancreatic juices are secreted into the duodenum, where they are activated. These enzymes are essential for the metabolism of carbohydrates, fats, and proteins. The most common theory regarding the development of pancreatitis is that an injury or disruption of pancreatic acinar cells allows leakage of pancreatic enzymes into pancreatic tissue. The leaked enzymes (trypsin, chymotrypsin, and elastase) become activated in the tissue and start the process of *autodigestion*. The activated enzymes break down tissue and cell membranes, causing edema, vascular damage, hemorrhage, necrosis, and fibrosis.[46,47] These now toxic enzymes and inflammatory mediators are released into the bloodstream and cause injury to vessels and organ systems, such as the hepatic and renal systems. Acute pancreatitis starts as a localized pancreatic inflammation and is usually accompanied by a compensatory antiinflammatory response syndrome (CARS). Excessive CARS makes the patient susceptible to infection.[46] Box 18.10 reviews the major systemic complications of acute fulminating pancreatitis.

Acute pancreatitis has numerous causes (Box 18.11), but the most common are alcohol ingestion and biliary disease. Many medications can initiate acute pancreatitis as a result of ingestion of toxic doses or a medication reaction. Pancreatitis may

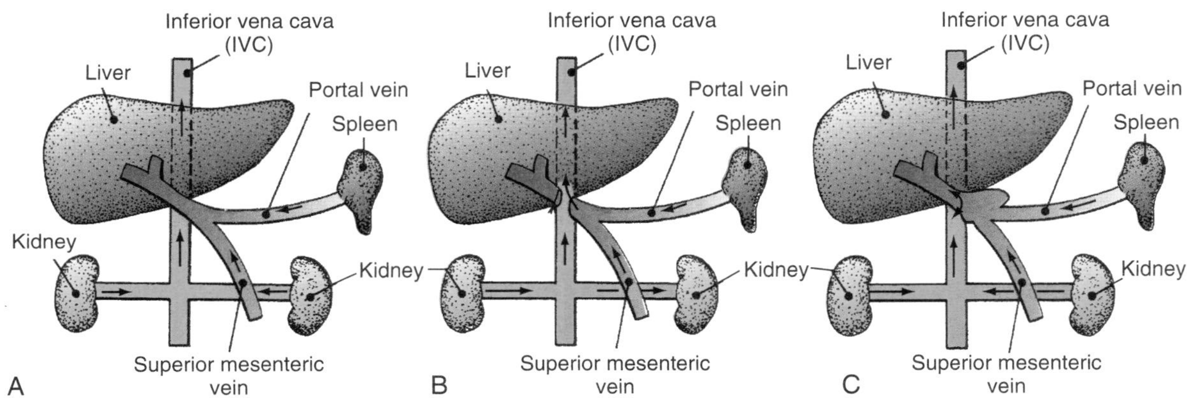

Fig. 18.11 Types of portocaval shunt. **A,** Normal portal circulation. **B,** End-to-side shunt. **C,** Side-to-side shunt.

also develop after blunt or penetrating abdominal trauma and after endoscopic exploration of the biliary tree.

Most patients with mild acute pancreatitis are treated with IV hydration and analgesia. Severe acute pancreatitis is treated with intensive hemodynamic and pulmonary management, nutritional support, infection control, and pharmacological agents.[46,47]

Metabolic complications of acute pancreatitis include hypocalcemia and hyperlipidemia, which are related to the areas of fat necrosis. Hypocalcemia is a major complication and usually indicates a more serious manifestation of acute pancreatitis. Various hormone imbalances, particularly parathyroid hormone imbalance, also occur in pancreatitis.[46,48]

Assessment

History and Physical Examination. A diagnosis of acute pancreatitis is based on clinical examination and the results of laboratory and radiological tests (Box 18.12). Nurses conduct initial and ongoing assessments, monitor and report physical and laboratory data, and coordinate the multiprofessional plan of care.

Patients who have organ failure at admission or within 72 hours of disease onset have a complicated clinical course with persistence of multisystem dysfunction. Multiple organ dysfunction syndrome (MODS) triggers additional mechanisms that lead to the translocation of bacteria and subsequent sepsis. Early and persistent organ failure in patients with acute pancreatitis is an indicator of a prolonged hospital stay and an increased risk of mortality.[46,49,50]

Most patients with acute pancreatitis develop severe abdominal pain. It is most often epigastric or midabdominal pain that radiates to the back. The pain is caused by edema, chemical irritation and inflammation of the peritoneum, and irritation or obstruction of the biliary tract.[46,48,51]

Nausea and vomiting are also common symptoms and are caused by hypermotility or paralytic ileus secondary to the pancreatitis or peritonitis. Abdominal distension accompanies the bowel symptoms, along with accumulation of fluid in the peritoneal cavity.[46,48] This fluid contains enzymes and kinins that increase vascular permeability and dilate the blood vessels. Hypotension and shock occur from the intravascular volume

BOX 18.10 Systemic Complications of Acute Pancreatitis

Cardiovascular
- Cardiac dysrhythmias
- Hypovolemic shock
- Myocardial depression

Gastrointestinal
- Gastrointestinal bleeding
- Pancreatic abscess
- Pancreatic pseudocyst

Hematological
- Coagulation abnormalities
- Disseminated intravascular coagulation

Metabolic
- Hyperglycemia
- Hyperlipidemia
- Hypocalcemia
- Metabolic acidosis

Pulmonary
- Acute respiratory distress syndrome
- Atelectasis
- Pneumonia
- Pleural effusion
- Hypoxemia

Renal
- Acute renal failure
- Azotemia
- Oliguria

BOX 18.11 Causes of Acute Pancreatitis

- Alcohol consumption
- Biliary disease
  - Common bile duct obstruction
  - ERCP procedure
  - Gallstones
- Heredity
- Hypercalcemia
- Hypertriglyceridemia
- Idiopathic
- Infections
- Medications
  - Azathioprine
  - Corticosteroids
  - Estrogen
  - Furosemide
  - Octreotide
  - Pentamidine
  - Sulfonamides
  - Thiazide diuretics
- Traumatic injury of the pancreas
- Tumors of pancreatic ductal system or metastatic tumors

ERCP, Endoscopic retrograde cholangiopancreatography.

BOX 18.12 Abnormal Laboratory Values of Pancreatitis

Albumin: ↓ or ↑
Alkaline phosphatase: ↑ with biliary disease
Bilirubin, AST, LDH: ↑
Calcium: ↓
Glucose: ↑ with islet cell damage
Hematocrit: ↑ with dehydration; ↓ with hemorrhagic pancreatitis
Potassium: ↓
Serum and urine amylase: ↑
Serum isoamylase: ↑
Serum lipase: ↑
White blood cell count: ↑

AST, Aspartate transaminase; *LDH*, lactate dehydrogenase.

depletion, leading to myocardial insufficiency. Fever and leukocytosis are also symptoms of the inflammatory process.

Patients with more severe pancreatic disease may have ascites, jaundice, or palpable abdominal masses. Two rare signs that may be present in any disease associated with retroperitoneal hemorrhage are a bluish discoloration of the flanks *(Grey Turner's sign)* or around the umbilical area *(Cullen's sign)*, indicative of blood in these areas.[46,48,51] Bleeding due to pancreatitis may arise from the erosion of local blood vessels by pancreatic enzymes. Because of the potential increase in abdominal size, measure and record the abdominal girth at least every 4 hours to detect internal bleeding (see Clinical Alert box).

! CLINICAL ALERT

Signs and Symptoms of Acute Pancreatitis

- Abdominal guarding, distension
- Cullen's sign
- Dehydration
- Fever
- Grey Turner's sign
- Nausea and vomiting
- Pain

Diagnostic Tests. Acute pancreatitis is diagnosed based on clinical findings, the presence of associated disorders, and laboratory testing. Pain associated with acute pancreatitis is similar to that associated with PUD, gallbladder disease, intestinal obstruction, or acute myocardial infarction. These similarities exist because pain receptors in the abdomen are poorly differentiated as they exit the skin surface. Because the clinical history, presenting signs and symptoms, and physical findings mimic those of many other GI and cardiovascular disorders, endoscopic and transabdominal ultrasound studies and computed tomography (CT) scans are performed to determine the extent of involvement and the presence of complications.

Serum lipase and amylase tests are the most specific indicators of acute pancreatitis because these enzymes are released as the pancreatic cells and ducts are destroyed. An elevated serum amylase level is a characteristic diagnostic feature. Amylase levels usually rise within 12 hours of symptom onset and return to normal within 3 to 5 days. Isoamylase P value is more specific to the diagnosis of acute pancreatitis, as the pancreas is the only organ to produce this isoenzyme; therefore, when it is elevated, this is because of pancreatic disease. Some laboratories are equipped to measure this isoenzyme, which is sensitive and specific to the diagnosis of acute pancreatitis, even later in the course of the disease. Isoamylase P values remain elevated in 80% of patients with pancreatitis 1 week after onset.[52] Serum lipase levels increase within 4 to 8 hours of clinical symptom onset and then decrease within 8 to 14 days. Serum trypsin levels are very specific for pancreatitis but may not be readily available. Urine trypsinogen-2 and urine amylase levels are also elevated. The C-reactive protein level increases within 48 hours and is a marker of severity. The ratio of amylase clearance to creatinine clearance by the kidney can be diagnostic. Other conditions associated with increased serum amylase levels are listed in Box 18.13.[46,48,51]

Other common laboratory abnormalities associated with acute pancreatitis include an elevated WBC count resulting from the inflammatory process and an elevated serum glucose level resulting from beta cell damage and pancreatic necrosis. Hypokalemia may be present because of associated vomiting. Hyperkalemia may be a systemic complication in the presence of acute renal failure. Hypocalcemia is common with severe disease and usually indicates pancreatic fat necrosis. Serum albumin and protein levels may decrease as a result of the movement of fluid into the extracellular space. Intravascular fluid losses may result in an increase in albumin levels. Increases in serum bilirubin, lactate dehydrogenase, and aspartate transaminase levels and prothrombin time are common in the presence of concurrent liver disease. Serum triglyceride levels may increase dramatically and be a causative factor in development of the acute inflammatory process. Arterial blood gas analysis often shows hypoxemia and retained carbon dioxide levels, which indicate respiratory failure.[53,54]

CT modalities and magnetic resonance imaging (MRI) are also used to confirm the diagnosis. Contrast-enhanced CT reliably detects pancreatic necrosis located in the parenchyma. It is considered the gold standard for diagnosing pancreatic necrosis and for grading acute pancreatitis.[53,54] The Balthazar CT severity index is a scoring system that ranges from 0 to 10 and is obtained by adding points attributed to the extent of the inflammatory process to the volume of pancreatic necrosis. A higher index is associated with increased severity of disease. MRI can better detect necrosis in the peripancreatic collections. However, an acutely ill patient might not tolerate this procedure.[46,53–55] Endoscopic retrograde cholangiopancreatography (ERCP) combines radiography with endoscopy and may assist in diagnosis.

BOX 18.13 Conditions Associated With Increased Serum Amylase Levels

- Acute pancreatitis
- Biliary tract disease
- Burns
- Cerebral trauma
- Chronic alcohol use disorder
- Diabetic ketoacidosis
- Gynecological disorders
- Intra-abdominal disease (e.g., perforation, obstruction, aortic disease, peritonitis, appendicitis)
- Pneumonia
- Pregnancy
- Prostatic disease
- Renal insufficiency
- Salivary gland disease
- Shock
- Tumors

Predicting the Severity of Acute Pancreatitis. Patients with acute pancreatitis can develop mild or fulminant disease. The prognosis of pancreatitis is based on classification criteria. One prognostic scoring system was developed by Ranson[56] (Box 18.14). This system considers the number of signs present within the first 48 hours after admission; these directly relate to the patient's morbidity and mortality. In Ranson's research, patients with fewer than three signs had a 1% mortality rate; those with three or four signs had a 15% mortality rate; those with five or six signs had a 40% mortality rate; and those with seven or more signs had a 100% mortality rate.

The Atlanta Classification is accepted worldwide as the first clinically reliable classification system. This system defines severe acute pancreatitis as the presence of three or more Ranson criteria or a score of 8 or higher on the Acute Physiology and Chronic Health Evaluation (APACHE II). The APACHE III prognostic system is similar to that of APACHE II, with the addition of several variables (e.g., diagnosis and prior treatment location). High APACHE III and five or more Ranson criteria can predict multiple complications or death in critically ill patients.[46,49,53,57]

There are several other scoring systems that have been used to determine the severity of acute pancreatitis. These include the Glasgow Coma Scale, the bedside index of severity in acute pancreatitis (BISAP), and the modified CT severity index. There are several other novel scoring systems under development to evaluate the severity and outcomes of acute pancreatitis. Another scale used to predict mortality is the Sequential Organ Failure Assessment (SOFA).[57–59]

Patient Problems

Actual or potential patient problems associated with acute pancreatitis or with systemic complications of the disease process are found in the Collaborative Care Plan found in Chapter 1, Overview of Critical Care Nursing. These problems include acute pain; decreased multisystem tissue perfusion; potential for infection; potential for fluid, electrolyte, and acid-base imbalances; and potential for impaired nutrition. Tailor these problems and nursing interventions to the patient's presentation (i.e., to address hemodynamic instability and pain).

BOX 18.14 Ranson Criteria for Predicting Severity of Acute Pancreatitis[a]

At Admission or on Diagnosis

- Age >55 years (>70 years)
- Leukocyte count >16,000/mm^3 (>18,000/mm^3)
- Serum AST level >250 IU/L
- Serum glucose level >200 mg/dL (>220 mg/dL)
- Serum LDH level >350 IU/L (>400 IU/L)

During Initial 48 Hours

- Base deficit >4 mEq/L (>5 mEq/L)
- Decrease in hematocrit >10%
- Estimated fluid sequestration >6 L (>4 L)
- Increase in blood urea nitrogen level >5 mg/dL (>2 mg/dL)
- Partial pressure of arterial oxygen <60 mm Hg
- Serum calcium level <8 mg/dL

[a]Criteria values for nonalcoholic acute pancreatitis (shown in parentheses) differ from those in alcohol-related disease.
AST, Aspartate transaminase; *LDH,* lactate dehydrogenase.
Modified from Ranson JC. Risk factors in acute pancreatitis. *Hosp Pract (Off Ed).* 1985;20(4):69-73.

Nursing and Medical Interventions

Nursing and medical priorities for the management of acute pancreatitis include several interventions. Managing respiratory dysfunction is a high priority. Replace fluids and electrolytes to maintain or replenish vascular volume and electrolyte balance. Administer analgesics for pain control. Supportive therapies are aimed to provide early oral or enteral nutrition.

Fluid Replacement. In patients with severe acute pancreatitis, fluid collects in the retroperitoneal space and peritoneal cavity. Patients sequester up to one-third of their plasma volume. Initially, most patients develop some degree of dehydration and, in severe cases, hypovolemic shock. Hypovolemia and shock are major causes of death early in the disease process. Fluid replacement is a high priority in the treatment of acute pancreatitis.

Fluid replacement helps maintain perfusion to the pancreas and kidneys, reducing the potential for complications. The IV solutions ordered for fluid resuscitation are usually colloids or crystalloids, typically Lactated Ringer's solution; however, fresh frozen plasma and albumin also may be administered. Aggressive IV fluid administration with crystalloids at 5 to 10 mL/kg/h is often required to maintain hemodynamic stability. Vigorous IV fluid replacement at 20 mL/kg/h for 8 to 12 hours is indicated if the patient manifests symptoms of hypotension and tachycardia.[46,55]

Evaluating the effectiveness of fluid replacement includes accurate monitoring of intake and output. A decrease in urine output is an early and sensitive measure of hypovolemia and hypoperfusion. Monitor vital signs and skin temperature. Although patient responses vary, reasonable goals are to maintain a mean arterial pressure of more than 60 to 70 mm Hg and a heart rate of less than 100 beats/min.[60] Warm extremities indicate adequate peripheral circulation.

Patients with severe manifestations of the disease may require invasive, minimally invasive, or noninvasive hemodynamic monitoring to evaluate fluid status and response to treatment. Pulmonary artery pressure monitoring is a sensitive measure of volume status and left ventricular filling pressure. The less invasive methods for hemodynamic monitoring identify stroke volume and stroke volume variation and can determine if patients are volume responsive or if other interventions such as vasopressors may be indicated (see Chapter 9, Hemodynamic Monitoring). Echocardiograms via bedside point of care ultrasound (POCUS) provide important information about volume requirements through assessment and measurement of the inferior vena cava.

Patients with severe disease who do not respond to fluid therapy alone may need vasopressors to support blood pressure. Patients with acute hemorrhagic pancreatitis may also need packed RBCs in addition to fluid therapy to restore intravascular volume.

New Modalities. Surgical decompression of *abdominal compartment syndrome* (ACS, also referred to as intraabdominal hypertension) may be used to relieve retroperitoneal edema, fluid collections in the abdomen, ascites, ileus, and overly aggressive use of fluid therapy in patients with severe acute pancreatitis. ACS is defined as intraabdominal pressure higher than

20 mm Hg with new-onset organ failure. ACS is seen early in about 30% of patients with severe acute pancreatitis and is associated with multiple organ dysfunction.[61]

Pentoxifylline has been shown to decrease inflammation, bacterial translocation, and infections. It is a methylxanthine derivative that improves blood flow by increasing erythrocyte and leukocyte flexibility; it also stimulates production of cytokines. Clinical trials for off-label use in pancreatitis are underway at the time of this writing, and some have shown improved patient outcomes.[62]

Electrolyte Replacement. Hypocalcemia (serum calcium level <8.5 mg/dL) is a common electrolyte imbalance. It is associated with a high mortality rate. Calcium is essential for many physiological functions: catalyzing impulses for nerves and muscles, maintaining the integrity of cell membranes and vessels, clotting blood, strengthening bones and teeth, and increasing contractility in the heart. A sign of hypocalcemia on the ECG is lengthening of the QT interval. Severe hypocalcemia (serum calcium level <6 mg/dL) may cause tetany, seizures, and respiratory distress. A positive Chvostek sign, or facial muscle twitching in response to tapping the cheek, Trousseau sign, or carpopedal spasm of the hand and wrist after insufflation of a blood pressure cuff may also be observed. Place patients with severe hypocalcemia on seizure precaution status and ensure respiratory support equipment is readily available (e.g., oral airway, suction). Monitor calcium levels, administer replacement as ordered, and monitor the patient's response to calcium replacement. Monitor serum albumin levels because true serum calcium levels can be evaluated only in comparison with serum albumin levels. Also monitor for calcium toxicity, indicated by lethargy, nausea, shortening of the QT interval, and decreased excitability of nerves and muscles. Hypomagnesemia may also be present in patients with hypocalcemia, and magnesium replacement may be required.

Potassium is another electrolyte that may need to be replaced early in the treatment regimen. Hypokalemia is associated with cardiac dysrhythmias, muscle weakness, hypotension, decreased bowel sounds, ileus, and irritability. Potassium is replaced via an infusion pump according to the unit protocol.

Hyperglycemia is not a common complication of acute pancreatitis, because most of the pancreatic gland must be necrosed before the insulin-secreting islet cells are affected. More commonly, hyperglycemia is a result of the body's stress response to acute illness.

Nutritional Support. Nasogastric suction for decompression and "nothing by mouth" status have been the classic treatments for patients with acute pancreatitis to suppress pancreatic exocrine secretion by preventing the release of secretin from the duodenum. Because secretin, which stimulates pancreatic secretion production, is stimulated when acid is in the duodenum, gastric suction has been a primary treatment. Nasogastric suctioning may also reduce nausea, vomiting, and abdominal pain. A nasogastric tube is essential in patients with ileus, severe gastric distension, and a decreased level of consciousness to prevent complications resulting from pulmonary aspiration.

However, trends in nutritional management are changing. Early nutritional support may be ordered to prevent atrophy of gut lymphoid tissue, prevent bacterial overgrowth in the intestine, and increase intestinal permeability. Immediate oral feeding in patients with mild acute pancreatitis is safe and may accelerate recovery.[46,48,50,55] The enteral route is still preferred for providing nutrition in patients with severe acute pancreatitis (see Chapter 7, Nutritional Therapy).[46,48,51,55]

CHECK YOUR UNDERSTANDING

3. A patient is admitted with chronic nonsteroidal antiinflammatory drug (NSAID) use and a recently diagnosed duodenal ulcer. The patient states that, 3 days ago, they had a positive urea breath test. Based on the patient's history, what treatment would you expect to initiate or continue?
   A. Esomeprazole, amoxicillin, and clarithromycin
   B. Famotidine, bismuth, metronidazole, and a tetracycline
   C. Famotidine and sucralfate
   D. Esomeprazole and levofloxacin

Comfort Management. Pain control is a nursing priority in patients with acute pancreatitis, not only because the disorder produces extreme patient discomfort, but also because pain increases the patient's metabolism and thus increases pancreatic secretions. The pain of pancreatitis is caused by edema and distension of the pancreatic capsule, obstruction of the biliary system, and peritoneal inflammation from pancreatic enzymes. Pain is often severe and unrelenting and is related to the degree of pancreatic inflammation.

Perform a baseline pain assessment early after the patient's admission. Include information about the onset, intensity, duration, and location (local or diffuse) of the pain. Analgesic administration is a nursing priority. Adequate pain control generally requires the use of IV opiates, often in the form of a patient-controlled analgesia (PCA) pump. If a PCA pump is not ordered, administer pain medications as needed. NSAIDs are also part the mainstay of pain management based on randomized controlled trial evidence. NSAIDs are effective in management of pain associated with acute pancreatitis and limit the need for rescue analgesia use. The adverse effects of opioid use and the potential for misuse has led to an increased use of NSAIDs for pancreatitis-associated pain. NSAIDs should be avoided in patients with acute kidney injury.[63] Traditionally, opiate analgesics (e.g., morphine) were thought to cause spasm of the sphincter of Oddi and to exacerbate pain; however, opioid analgesia is now commonly used based upon evidence of its effectiveness. Depending on the patient's hemodynamic status, position the patient to relieve some of the discomfort. Epidural analgesia may also be used to treat the pain of acute pancreatitis.[63,64]

CLINICAL JUDGMENT ACTIVITY

A 50-year-old patient is admitted with hematemesis and reports having dark stools for the past 12 hours. Which of the following admission data is the best indicator of the amount of blood lost?

Blood pressure	95/60 mm Hg (supine)
Heart rate	125 beats/min
Respiratory rate	28 breaths/min
Hematocrit	27%
Hemoglobin	14 g/dL

Pharmacological Intervention. Various pharmacological therapies have been researched in the treatment of acute pancreatitis. Medications given to rest the pancreas have been studied—specifically, anticholinergics, glucagon, somatostatin, cimetidine, and calcitonin—but these have not been shown to be effective. Prevention of stress ulcers is achieved through the use of H2 receptor antagonists and PPIs.

Prophylactic antibiotics to prevent infection in patients with acute pancreatitis is not recommended by experts or professional organizations. Treatment with antibiotics is recommended only for patients with infected pancreatic necrosis (confirmed by fine needle aspiration or clinically suspected), infection-related shock, or systemic inflammatory response syndrome (SIRS). If infected pancreatic necrosis is identified, antibiotic therapy should be effective against pancreatic and GI organisms. Appropriate treatment with antibiotics may prevent the need for surgical intervention in some patients.[46,48,55]

Treatment of Systemic Complications. Multisystemic complications of acute pancreatitis are related to the ability of the pancreas to produce many vasoactive substances that affect organs throughout the body. These complications are summarized in Box 18.10.

Pulmonary complications are common in patients with both mild and severe manifestations of the disease. Arterial hypoxemia, atelectasis, pleural effusions, acute respiratory distress syndrome (ARDS), and pneumonia have been identified in many patients with acute pancreatitis. Accumulation of fluid in the peritoneum causes restricted movement of the diaphragm. Arterial oxygen saturation via pulse oximetry is continuously monitored, and arterial blood gases are assessed as needed. Treatment of hypoxemia includes supplemental oxygen and vigorous pulmonary hygiene, such as deep breathing, coughing, and frequent position changes. Some patients may need intubation to ensure adequate ventilation; others can be maintained with noninvasive ventilation modes. Pulmonary emboli have also been documented as a complication of acute pancreatitis. Careful fluid administration is necessary to prevent fluid overload and pulmonary congestion. Patients with severe disease may develop acute respiratory failure.

Close monitoring and management of other systemic complications of acute pancreatitis, such as coagulation abnormalities and hemorrhage, cardiovascular failure and dysrhythmias, and acute renal failure, are also important. Coagulation defects in acute pancreatitis are similar to disseminated intravascular coagulation (DIC) and are associated with a high mortality rate. The cardiac depression associated with acute pancreatitis may vary. The presence of hypovolemic shock is a grave presentation; astute cardiovascular monitoring and volume replacement are required to reverse this serious complication. Impaired renal function has been documented in many patients.

Local GI complications of acute pancreatitis include pancreatic pseudocyst and abdominal abscess. Suspect a pseudocyst in any patient who has persistent abdominal pain with nausea and vomiting, a prolonged fever, and an elevated serum amylase level. CT can be helpful in diagnosing the location and size of the pseudocyst. Early recognition and treatment of a pancreatic pseudocyst are important because this condition is associated with a high mortality rate. Signs and symptoms of an abdominal abscess include an increased WBC count, fever, abdominal pain, and vomiting. CT provides a definitive diagnosis.

Surgical Therapy. Pancreatic resection for acute necrotizing pancreatitis may be performed to prevent systemic complications of the disease process. In this procedure, dead or infected pancreatic tissue is surgically removed while most of the gland is preserved.[46,47,55] Many surgical treatment modalities, including laparoscopic techniques, are available. The indication for surgical intervention is clinical deterioration of the patient despite conventional treatments or the presence of peritonitis. In addition, minimally invasive techniques are also used prior to surgery in what is known as the "step-up approach." This is now the first-line intervention for infected pancreatic necrosis and may obviate the need for open surgical procedures. Percutaneous drains and video-assisted retroperitoneoscopic debridement (VARD) are used as well as endoscopic placement of stents or necrosectomy to remove necrotic, infected tissue.[49,65]

Surgery may also be indicated for pseudocysts; however, surgery is usually delayed because some pseudocysts resolve spontaneously. Surgical or interventional treatment of a pseudocyst can be performed through internal or external drainage or needle aspiration. Acute surgical intervention may be required if the pseudocyst becomes infected or perforated. Surgery may also be performed when gallstones are the cause of the acute pancreatitis. A cholecystectomy is usually performed.

CLINICAL JUDGMENT ACTIVITY

The nurse is caring for a patient who is admitted with acute abdominal pain and vomiting. His admission vital signs and laboratory values include the following:

Blood pressure	94/72 mm Hg
Heart rate	114 beats/min
Respiratory rate	32 breaths/min
Potassium	3.0 mEq/L
Calcium	7.0 mg/dL
Arterial oxygen saturation	88%
Serum amylase	280 IU/L
Serum lipase	320 IU/L

1. What is the suspected medical diagnosis, and what findings support this diagnosis?
2. What are the priority nursing interventions?

HEPATIC FAILURE

Chronic liver disease, or cirrhosis, is the 12th leading cause of death in the United States, accounting for at least one million deaths annually.[45,66,67] End-stage liver disease is characterized as deterioration from a compensated to an uncompensated state. Critically ill patients with end-stage liver disease have a mortality rate of 50% to 100%.[67] Hepatic failure also results from chronic liver disease, in which healthy liver tissue is replaced by fibrotic tissue. This form of liver failure is called *cirrhosis.* Finally, liver cells can be replaced by fatty cells or tissue; this is known as *nonalcoholic fatty liver disease.*[69,70]

Pathophysiology

Normal liver architecture is pictured in Fig. 18.5. The basic functional unit of the liver is called the *lobule*. The liver lobule is uniquely made in that it has its own blood supply, which allows the liver cells *(hepatocytes)* to be exposed continuously to blood. Hepatic failure results when the liver is unable to perform its many functions (Box 18.2). Liver failure results from necrosis or a decrease in the blood supply to liver cells. This problem is most often caused by hepatitis or inflammation of the liver.

Hepatitis. *Hepatitis* is an acute inflammation of the hepatocytes. This inflammation is accompanied by edema. As the inflammation progresses, blood supply to the hepatocytes is interrupted, causing necrosis and breakdown of healthy cells. Blood may back up in the portal system, causing *portal hypertension*.

Liver cells have the capacity to regenerate. Over time, liver cells that become damaged are removed by the body's immune system and replaced with healthy liver cells. Therefore, most patients with hepatitis recover and regain normal liver function.

Hepatitis is most often caused by a virus. Several hepatitis viruses have been identified, and they are termed hepatitis A, B, C, D, E, and G. Researchers continue to study other viruses that may be associated with acute hepatitis. Modes of transmission are summarized in Box 18.15. Characteristics of hepatitis in terms of type, route of transmission, severity, and prophylaxis are presented in Table 18.8.

Assessment. Patients with hepatitis are often asymptomatic. In many patients, prodromal symptoms of anorexia, nausea, vomiting, abdominal pain or distension, and fatigue may be present. Symptoms then progress to a low-grade fever, an enlarged and tender liver, and jaundice (see Clinical Alert box).[1]

BOX 18.15 Modes of Transmission for Hepatitis

- Invasive medical procedures using contaminated equipment
- Direct contact with contaminated fluids or objects (e.g., birth, sexual contact)
- Percutaneously through mucous membranes
- Transfusion of contaminated blood and blood products

From Hepatitis. World Health Organization. https://www.who.int/news-room/questions-and-answers/item/hepatitis. Accessed December 27, 2023.

! CLINICAL ALERT

Signs and Symptoms of Fulminant Hepatic Failure (Acute Liver Failure)

- Chills
- Convulsions
- Decreased level of consciousness, coma
- Hyperexcitability
- Insomnia
- Irritability
- Jaundice
- Lethargy
- Nausea and vomiting
- Sudden onset of high fever

Assessment of risk factors often assists in the diagnosis of hepatitis. Laboratory tests show elevated liver function enzymes. The diagnosis is confirmed by identifying antibodies specific to each type of hepatitis. Recovery from acute hepatitis varies from a few weeks to a few months, depending on the severity of illness. Hepatitis B, C, D, and G may progress to chronic forms.[70]

Patient problems. Many patient problems are associated with viral hepatitis. These include fatigue; potential for bleeding; potential for infection; potential for impaired nutrition; nausea; and potential for skin abrasions.

Nursing and medical interventions. No definitive treatment for acute inflammation of the liver exists. Goals for medical and nursing care include providing rest and assisting the patient in obtaining optimal nutrition. Most patients are cared for at home unless the disease becomes prolonged or fulminant failure develops. Medications to help the patient rest or to decrease agitation must be closely monitored because most of these medications require clearance by the liver, which is impaired during the acute phase.

Maintenance of the nutritional status of the patient is a nursing priority. Loss of appetite, nausea, and vomiting may persist for weeks. Administer antiemetics to reduce symptoms. Collaborate

TABLE 18.8 Characteristics of Hepatitis

Type	Route of Transmission	Severity	Prophylaxis
Hepatitis A	Fecal-oral, parenteral, sexual	Mild	Hygiene, immune serum globulin, HAV vaccine, Twinrix[a]
Hepatitis B	Parenteral, sexual	Severe, may be prolonged or chronic	Hygiene, HBV vaccine, Twinrix[a]
Hepatitis C	Parenteral	Mild to severe	Hygiene, screening blood, interferon-alpha
Hepatitis D	Parenteral, fecal-oral, sexual	Severe	Hygiene, HBV vaccine
Hepatitis E	Fecal-oral	Severe in pregnant people	Hygiene, safe water
Hepatitis G	Parenteral, sexual	Unknown	Unknown

[a]A bivalent vaccine containing the antigenic components, a sterile suspension of inactivated hepatitis A virus combined with purified surface antigen of the hepatitis B virus.
HAV, Hepatitis A virus; *HBV*, hepatitis B virus.
Modified from Turner KC. Structure and function of the digestive system. In: Rogers J, ed. *McCance and Huether's Pathophysiology: The Biologic Basis for Disease in Adults and Children.* 9th ed. St. Louis, MO: Elsevier; 2024:1285a–1317.

with a dietitian to develop a nutritional plan. Offer small, frequent, palatable meals and supplements. Regularly assess intake and output, daily weight, serum albumin level, and nitrogen balance as ongoing nutritional evaluation. Instruct patients to avoid drinking alcohol or taking over-the-counter medications that can cause liver damage. Box 18.16 lists common hepatotoxic medications.

Liver transplantation is the standard of care for patients with progressive, irreversible acute or chronic liver disease when there are no other medical or surgical options. Some of the leading indications for liver transplantation are alcohol-related liver disease, nonalcoholic steatohepatitis, liver carcinoma, and hepatitis C (see the Transplantation Considerations box).[69,71] The antiviral medications now available to treat hepatitis C have decreased the need for liver transplants performed for this disease. These medications are prescribed according to the identified genotype of the virus.

TRANSPLANT CONSIDERATIONS

Liver

Criteria for Transplant Recipients

Indications for liver transplantation include refractory, irreversible liver disease that can be either acute or chronic. The recipient must be able to survive the operation and recovery with significant survival and quality of life benefits.

Contraindications for liver transplantation include active extrahepatic malignancy, severe cardiopulmonary disease, uncontrolled sepsis, active alcohol or illicit substance use disorder, uncontrolled or untreated human immunodeficiency virus (HIV), persistent noncompliance or lack of social support, and technical or anatomic barriers to liver transplantation.[1] Waiting list placement is determined primarily by the Model for End-Stage Liver Disease (MELD) score. The MELD score is calculated using serum creatinine, serum bilirubin, and international normalized ratio to predict survival. The higher the MELD score, the higher the patient is ranked on the list.

Patient Management

Immediate postoperative management is focused on maintaining blood pressure and optimizing end-organ perfusion. Signs the new liver is functioning, include resolution of metabolic acidosis and coagulopathy, a decrease in bleeding, and hemodynamic stability.[2] Immunosuppressive medications consist of triple therapy—a calcineurin inhibitor (tacrolimus [Prograf] or cyclosporine [Neoral]), a corticosteroid (prednisone), and mycophenolate mofetil (CellCept) or azathioprine (Imuran). These medications inhibit T-cell proliferation and differentiation, deplete lymphocytes, and inhibit macrophages. If used, induction immunosuppression therapy with basiliximab (monoclonal antibody) or high-dose steroids may begin in the operating room before implantation of the donor liver. This is in an effort to delay using calcineurin inhibitors to protect renal function. Posttransplant, immune modulation agents, such as tacrolimus or cyclosporine, are titrated based on serum levels.

Complications

Postoperative complications include bleeding, renal failure, infection, pleural effusions, fluid and electrolyte imbalances, biliary leaks, and biliary obstruction or stricture at anastomosis sites.[3] Vascular complications such as portal vein thrombosis and arterial thrombosis may also occur, which can lead to primary liver nonfunction and urgent relisting for liver transplantation. Biliary stones (cast syndrome) and recurrent cholangitis are other possible complications. Bacterial and fungal infections occur most frequently in the first few months; viral infections, especially cytomegalovirus (CMV), are more prevalent in the months after transplantation.[4] Complications associated with immunosuppressive therapy affect all body systems and include nephrotoxicity, hypertension, hyperlipidemia, bone loss, new-onset diabetes mellitus, and increased risk of infection and malignancy.[4]

Preventing Rejection

Compliance with immunosuppressive therapy is essential. *Acute rejection* occurs days to 3 months after transplantation and involves the activation and proliferation of T cells with destruction of liver tissue. Acute rejection accounts for approximately 40% of all rejection episodes. *Chronic rejection* occurs months to years after transplantation and may lead to the need for retransplantation.[3]

Rejection may be suspected if aspartate aminotransferase (AST), alanine aminotransferase (ALT), or bilirubin increase. A biopsy is performed to confirm diagnosis. Symptoms of rejection include abdominal discomfort, fatigue, fever, jaundice, ascites, dark urine, and loss of appetite. Most rejection is reversible if diagnosed and treated early; therefore, compliance with scheduled laboratory testing is important. Management of acute rejection includes increasing the dosages of current immunosuppressive medications. Patient and family education on the optimal use of immunosuppressive medications and strict compliance with dosing schedules is another strategy to mitigate rejection risks.

References

1. Mahmud N. Selection for liver transplantation: indications and evaluation. *Curr Hepatol Rep*. 2020;19(3):203–212. https://doi.org/10.1007/s11901-020-00527-9.
2. Keegan MT, Kramer DJ. Perioperative care of the liver transplant patient. *Crit Care Clin*. 2016;32(3):453–473. https://doi.org/10.1016/j.ccc.2016.02.005.
3. Choudhary NS, Saigal S, Bansal RK, Saraf N, Gautam D, Soin AS. Acute and chronic rejection after liver transplantation: what a clinician needs to know. *J Clin Exp Hepatol*. 2017;7(4):358–366. https://doi.org/10.1016/j.jceh.2017.10.003.
4. Di Maira T, Little EC, Berenguer M. Immunosuppression in liver transplant. *Best Pract Res Clin Gastroenterol*. 2020:46–47:101681. https://doi.org/10.1016/j.bpg.2020.101681.

Chelsea Sooy, BSN, RN, CCTC
Melissa A. Kelley, RN, CPTC

Hepatitis can lead to acute hepatic failure. The clinical manifestations of this disorder are discussed herein. Special precautions must be taken to prevent spread of the virus when caring for the patient with hepatitis. These include *universal precautions* while handling items contaminated with the patient's body secretions, including patient care items such as thermometers, dishes, and eating utensils.

Cirrhosis. Cirrhosis causes severe alterations in the structure and function of liver cells. It is characterized by inflammation and liver cell necrosis that may be focal or diffuse. Fat deposits may also be present. The enlarged liver cells cause compression of the liver lobule and lead to increased resistance to blood flow and portal hypertension. Necrosis is followed by regeneration of liver tissue but not in a normal fashion. Fibrous tissue is laid down over time, which distorts the normal architecture of the liver lobule. These fibrotic changes are usually irreversible and result in chronic liver dysfunction. Table 18.9 characterizes the types of cirrhosis.

Nonalcoholic Fatty Liver. The term *fatty liver* refers to an accumulation of excessive fats in the liver; it is morphologically distinguishable from cirrhosis. Alcohol use disorder is the most common cause of fatty liver. However, other disorders unrelated to alcohol use can result in the development of what is termed nonalcoholic fatty liver disease (NAFLD). The causes of this entity include obesity, diabetes, hepatic resection, starvation, and total parenteral nutrition. Damage caused by the fat deposits may result in liver dysfunction, failure, and death.[69,72]

BOX 18.16 Common Hepatotoxic Medications

Analgesics
- Acetaminophen (Tylenol)
- Salicylates (aspirin)

Anesthetics
- Halothane (Fluothane)

Anticonvulsants
- Phenytoin (Dilantin)
- Phenobarbital

Antidepressants
- Monoamine oxidase inhibitors

Antimicrobial Agents
- Isoniazid
- Nitrofurantoin (Macrodantin)
- Rifampin
- Silver sulfadiazine (Silvadene)
- Tetracycline

Antipsychotic Medications
- Haloperidol (Haldol)

Cardiovascular Medications
- Quinidine sulfate

Hormonal Agents
- Antithyroid medications
- Oral contraceptives
- Oral hypoglycemics (tolbutamide)

Sedatives
- Chlordiazepoxide (Librium)
- Diazepam (Valium)

Others
- Cimetidine (Tagamet)

Assessment of Hepatic Failure

Presenting Clinical Signs. Initial clinical signs of hepatic failure are vague and include weakness, fatigue, loss of appetite, weight loss, abdominal discomfort, nausea and vomiting, and change in bowel habits. As destruction in the liver progresses, the systemic effects of the disease become apparent. Impaired liver function results in loss of the normal vascular, secretory, and metabolic functions of the liver (Box 18.2). The functional sequelae of liver disease are divided into three categories: (1) portal hypertension, (2) impaired liver metabolic processes, and (3) impaired bile formation and flow. These derangements and their clinical manifestations are summarized in Box 18.17.

Portal hypertension. Portal hypertension causes two main clinical problems for the patient: hyperdynamic circulation and development of esophageal or gastric varices. Liver cell destruction causes shunting of blood and increased cardiac output. Vasodilation is also present, which causes decreased perfusion to all body organs, even though the cardiac output is very high. This phenomenon is known as *high-output failure* or *hyperdynamic circulation*. Clinical signs and symptoms are those of heart failure and include jugular vein distension, pulmonary crackles, and decreased perfusion to all organs. Initially, the patient may have hypertension, flushed skin, and bounding pulses. When a patient experiences low blood pressure, dysrhythmias are common. Increased portal venous pressure causes the formation of varices that shunt blood to decrease pressure. These varices can cause massive upper GI bleeding.[73] Splenomegaly is also associated with portal hypertension.

Impaired metabolic processes. The liver is the most complex organ because it carries out many metabolic processes. Liver failure causes altered metabolism of carbohydrates, fats, and proteins; decreased synthesis of blood clotting factors; decreased removal of activated clotting components; decreased metabolism of vitamins and iron; decreased storage functions; and decreased detoxification functions.

Altered carbohydrate metabolism may result in unstable blood glucose levels. The serum glucose level may increase to more than 200 mg/dL. This condition is termed *cirrhotic diabetes*. Altered carbohydrate metabolism may also result in malnutrition and a decreased stress response. Hypoglycemia may also be seen secondary to depletion of hepatic glycogen stores and decreased gluconeogenesis.[68,74]

Altered fat metabolism may result in a fatty liver. Fat is used by all cells for energy. Altered metabolism may cause fatigue and decreased activity tolerance in many patients. Alterations

TABLE 18.9 Characteristics of Cirrhosis Types

Type	Cause	Consequences	Sequelae
Alcoholic (Laennec's)	Chronic alcohol use disorder	Fatty liver Fibrotic tissue replaces liver cells	Acetaldehyde, a toxic metabolite of alcohol ingestion, causes liver cell damage and death
Biliary	Long-term obstruction of bile ducts	Decrease in bile flow	Degeneration and fibrosis of the ducts
Cardiac	Severe long-term right-sided heart failure	Decreased oxygenation of liver cells	Cellular death
Postnecrotic	Exposure to hepatotoxins or chemicals, infection, or metabolic disorder	Massive death of liver cells	Development of liver cancer

in skin integrity are common in chronic liver disease and are related to this metabolic dysfunction. Bile salts are not adequately produced, which leads to an inability of the small intestine to metabolize fats. Malnutrition often results.

BOX 18.17 Clinical Signs and Symptoms of Liver Disease

Cardiac
- Activity intolerance
- Dysrhythmias
- Edema
- Hyperdynamic circulation
- Portal hypertension

Dermatological
- Jaundice
- Pruritus
- Spider angiomas

Electrolytes
- Hypernatremia
- Hypokalemia
- Hyponatremia (dilutional)

Endocrine
- Increased aldosterone
- Increased antidiuretic hormone

Fluid Alterations
- Ascites
- Decreased volume in vascular space
- Water retention

Gastrointestinal
- Abdominal discomfort
- Decreased appetite
- Diarrhea
- Malnutrition
- Nausea and vomiting
- Varices or gastrointestinal bleeding

Hematological
- Anemia
- Disseminated intravascular coagulation
- Impaired coagulation

Immune System
- Increased susceptibility to infection

Neurological
- Hepatic encephalopathy

Pulmonary
- Dyspnea
- Hepatopulmonary syndrome
- Hyperventilation
- Hypoxemia
- Ineffective breathing patterns

Renal
- Hepatorenal syndrome

Protein metabolism, albumin synthesis, and serum albumin levels are decreased. Albumin is necessary for colloid oncotic pressure to hold fluid in the intravascular space and for nutrition. Low albumin levels are also associated with the development of ascites, a complication of hepatic failure. Globulin is another protein that is essential for the transport of substances in the blood. Fibrinogen is an essential protein that is necessary for normal clotting. A low plasma fibrinogen level, coupled with decreased synthesis of many blood clotting factors, predisposes the patient to bleeding. Clinical signs and symptoms range from bruising and nasal and gingival bleeding to frank hemorrhage. DIC may also develop.

Kupffer cells in the liver play an important role in fighting infections throughout the body. Loss of this function predisposes the patient to severe infections, particularly sepsis caused by gram-negative bacteria.

The liver also removes activated clotting factors from the general circulation to prevent widespread clotting in the system. Loss of this function predisposes the patient to clot formation and complications such as pulmonary embolus.

Decreased metabolism and storage of vitamins A, B_{12}, and D; iron; glucose; and fat predispose the patient to many nutritional deficiencies. The liver loses the function of detoxifying medications, ammonia, and hormones. Loss of ammonia conversion to urea in the liver is responsible for many of the altered thought processes seen in liver failure because ammonia is allowed to enter the central nervous system directly. These alterations range from minor sensory perceptual changes, such as tremors, slurred speech, and impaired decision-making, to dramatic confusion or profound coma.

Hormonal imbalances are common in liver disease. The most important physiological imbalance is the activation of aldosterone and antidiuretic hormone, which contribute to the fluid and electrolyte disturbances commonly found in liver disease. Sodium and water retention and portal hypertension lead to third-spacing of fluid from the intravascular space into the peritoneal cavity *(ascites).* The resultant decrease in plasma volume causes activation of compensatory mechanisms in the body to release antidiuretic hormone and aldosterone, causing further water and sodium retention. The *renin-angiotensin system* is also activated, which causes systemic vasoconstriction. The kidneys are most severely affected, and urine output decreases because of impaired perfusion. Sexual dysfunction is common in patients with liver disease, and this can lead to self-concept alterations. Dermatological lesions that occur in some patients with liver failure, called *spider angiomas,* are related to an endocrine imbalance. These vascular lesions may be venous or arterial and represent the progression of liver disease.

Impaired bile formation and flow. The liver's inability to metabolize bile is reflected clinically in an increased serum bilirubin level and a staining of tissue by bilirubin (i.e., jaundice). Jaundice is generally present in patients with a serum bilirubin level higher than 3 mg/dL.

Patient Problems

Refer to the Plan of Care for the Patient With Liver Failure for a detailed description of patient problems, specific nursing interventions, and selected rationales. Other interventions are discussed in the Collaborative Care Plan found in Chapter 1, Overview of Critical Care Nursing.

PLAN OF CARE

For the Patient With Liver Failure

Patient Problem

Potential for Delirium. Risk factors include cerebral accumulation of ammonia, medications that require liver metabolism, GI bleeding, and decreased perfusion states.

Desired Outcomes

- Orientation to person, place, and time.
- Free of injury.

Nursing Assessments/Interventions	Rationales
• Monitor ammonia levels and conduct ongoing neurological assessments.	• Assess trends in neurological status and response to treatment.
• Determine patient's baseline personality and memory by asking the patient's family and friends.	
• Observe for asterixis and report to the provider.	• May be present in advanced disease states.
• Administer lactulose as indicated and monitor results.	• Reduce ammonia levels and improve neurological status.
• Reduce the risk of stress ulcer–related bleeding through stress ulcer prophylaxis administration.	• Prevent bleeding, which may lead to hepatic encephalopathy.
• Use sedatives and analgesics judiciously.	• Drug metabolism is impaired in hepatic failure.
• Prevent and treat infection, dehydration, and electrolyte or acid-base disturbances.	• Assess for altered mental status associated with elevated ammonia level. • Shifting electrolytes may further alter the patient's mental status.
• Reorient the patient and provide safety support during periods of impaired mentation.	• Provide orientation and reduce risk for injury.

Patient Problem

Potential for Bleeding/Hemorrhage. Risk factors include portal hypertension and altered coagulation factors.

Desired Outcomes

- Orientation to person, place, and time.
- Bruising absent.
- Hemoglobin and hematocrit within normal limits for the patient.
- Absent of signs of hypovolemic shock:
  - Systolic blood pressure >90 mm Hg
  - Heart rate <100 beats/min

Nursing Assessments/Interventions	Rationales
• Assess vital signs every 1 to 2 hours or more frequently if vital signs are abnormal.	• Assess for bleeding and need for prompt treatment; esophageal varices, portal hypertension, peptic ulcers, or Mallory-Weiss tears are common in hepatic failure and can lead to significant bleeding. • Patients with varices treated with banding or sclerotherapy may require more frequent monitoring given the risk of perforation and subsequent hemorrhage.
• Immediately notify the provider of signs and symptoms of bleeding (i.e., bruising, weakness, pallor, hematemesis, altered vital signs, agitation, mental status changes).	• Assess for hemorrhage and initiate interventions.
• Reduce the risk of stress ulcer–related bleeding through stress ulcer prophylaxis administration.	• Reduce risk for peptic ulcers. • Reduce the impact of hemodynamic and inflammatory changes, which may damage the gastric mucosa.

Patient Problem

Fluid Overload. Risk factors include portal hypertension and compromised regulatory mechanisms.

Desired Outcomes

- Normal lung sounds (i.e., absence of crackles, rales).
- Respiratory rate <20 breaths/min.
- Edema decreasing or absent.
- Abdominal girth decreasing.

Continued

PLAN OF CARE—cont'd

For the Patient With Liver Failure

Nursing Assessments/Interventions	Rationales
• Monitor and document weight and I&O.	• Output should equal or exceed intake. • Weight loss, especially when using diuretics, should not exceed 0.5 kg/day to prevent electrolyte imbalance.
• Monitor electrolytes, especially Na^+ and K^+; report critical values to the provider.	• Hyponatremia associated with water retention occurs in the late stages of hepatic failure. • Hypokalemia is common in chronic alcoholic liver disease.
• Assess for and report dyspnea and bibasilar crackles.	• Indicate pulmonary edema.
• Provide frequent mouth care to minimize thirst.	• Reduce thirst without compounding fluid volume excess.
• Apply compression stockings or sequential compression devices.	• Reduce peripheral edema.
• Monitor skin integrity.	• Edema increases risk for device-related pressure injuries.

GI, gastrointestinal; *I&O*, intake and output; *K^+*, potassium; *Na^+*, sodium.
Adapted from Swearingen PL, Wright JD. *Swearingen's All-in-One Nursing Care Planning Resource*. 5th ed. St. Louis, MO: Elsevier; 2019.

Nursing and Medical Interventions

Nursing and medical management for the patient with liver failure is aimed at supportive therapies and early recognition and treatment of complications associated with the disease process. Management of acute liver failure challenges the best skills of the multiprofessional team.

Diagnostic Tests. Altered laboratory results in patients with liver disease (Box 18.18) are a direct result of the destruction of hepatic cells (liver enzymes) or of impaired liver metabolic processes.

Parenchymal tests such as liver biopsy can be performed to study the liver cell architecture directly. The liver is characteristically small and has a marked decrease in functioning hepatic cell structures. This characteristic allows for a definitive diagnosis of the cause of the hepatic failure. An ultrasound study may detect impaired bile flow.

Supportive Therapy. Hemodynamic instability and decreased perfusion to core organs are the end result of portal hypertension and hyperdynamic circulation. Invasive monitoring may be used in the critically ill patient, but it must be weighed in terms of the potential for infection in a patient with an impaired immune response. Administration of vasoactive medications and fluids may be ordered to support blood pressure and kidney perfusion, and close monitoring by the nurse is needed. Portal hypertension also predisposes the patient to esophageal and gastric varices, which have the potential to bleed.

The patient with liver failure is at risk for bleeding complications because of decreased synthesis of clotting factors. Protect patients who have a prolonged prothrombin time, partial thromboplastin time, and decreased platelet count from injury by padding the side rails and assisting with all activities. Keep venipuncture and other needlesticks to a minimum. Blood products may be ordered in severe cases. PPIs and H2 receptor antagonists are ordered to prevent gastritis and bleeding from stress ulcers.

Administration of all medications metabolized by the liver must be restricted. The administration of such medications could cause acute liver failure in a patient with chronic disease.[74]

BOX 18.18 Abnormal Laboratory Values of Liver Failure

Albumin: ↓
Ammonia: ↑
Bile pigments
  Total bilirubin: ↑
  Direct or conjugated: ↑
  Cholesterol: ↑
Coagulation tests
  Prothrombin time: Prolonged
  Partial thromboplastin time: Prolonged
Enzymes
  APT: ↑
  AST: ↑
  ALT: ↑
  GGT: ↑
Urine
  Bilirubin: ↑
  Urobilinogen: ↑

ALT, Alanine transaminase; *APT*, alkaline phosphatase; *AST*, aspartate transaminase; *GGT*, gamma-glutamyl transpeptidase.

Support for the Failing Liver. Advances have been made in the development of artificial support of liver function, spurred on by the shortage of donor organs and the high incidence of mortality related to acute or chronic liver failure.[68,74,75] Bioartificial liver devices (BLDs) were developed to partially replace the synthetic and regulatory function of the liver besides detoxifying the patient's plasma. BLDs may serve as a bridge to liver transplantation or support liver function long enough to allow regeneration of normal liver function.[67,71,74,76]

Another type of support is the Molecular Adsorbents Recirculating System (MARS), an extracorporeal albumin dialysis technique that uses an albumin-impregnated membrane to remove both protein-bound and water-soluble toxins from the blood (Fig. 18.12).[75,76] Cytokines are believed to play an important role in acute-on-chronic liver failure. Cytokines can be cleared from plasma by MARS and by another system, known as fractionated plasma separation, adsorption, and dialysis (i.e., Prometheus). However, at the time of this writing, neither of these treatments are able to change serum cytokine levels.

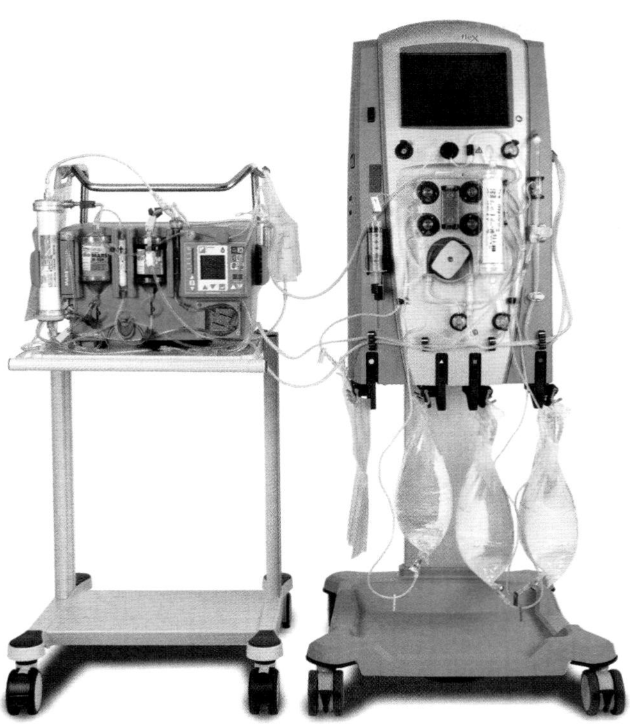

Fig. 18.12 Molecular adsorbent recirculating system (MARS). (From Baxter. All rights reserved. https://usrenalacute.baxter.com/therapies/mars.)

CHECK YOUR UNDERSTANDING

4. A nurse is assessing a patient who presents with an altered mental status. The assessment reveals pulmonary crackles and jugular venous distention. The patient's current blood pressure is 94/62 mm Hg, with dysrhythmias observed on monitor. The patient was admitted 3 months prior for an upper GI bleed. Which of the following appropriately identifies the patient's disease process?
   A. Type 1 diabetes
   B. Pancreatitis
   C. Peptic ulcer disease
   D. Liver disease

CLINICAL JUDGMENT ACTIVITY

A 45-year-old business executive is admitted to the telemetry unit. The patient tells the nurse that they travel a lot for business and recently returned from a trip to Mexico. During the initial assessment, the patient tells the nurse that they are not married and relates that they frequently have unprotected sex with multiple partners. History includes persistent abdominal pain, nausea with occasional vomiting, fatigue, and decreased appetite. Initial vital signs and laboratory results include the following:

Heart rate	70 beats/min
Urine	Clear and dark yellow
Aspartate transaminase (AST)	20 IU/L
Alanine transaminase (ALT)	70 IU/L
Serum albumin	3.2 mg/dL
Total serum bilirubin	1.5 mg/dL

1. What is the most likely diagnosis?
2. What precautions should the nurse take while caring for this patient?

Treatment of Complications

Ascites. Impaired handling of salt and water by the kidneys and other abnormalities in fluid homeostasis predispose the patient to an accumulation of fluid in the peritoneum, known as *ascites.* Ascites is problematic because, as more fluid is retained, it pushes up on the diaphragm, thereby impairing breathing. Regularly assess respiratory rate, breath sounds, and pulse oximetry values. Monitor and record abdominal girth at the level of the umbilicus to assess for increased fluid accumulation. Position the patient in a semi-Fowler's position to promote diaphragm movement. Encourage frequent deep-breathing and coughing exercises and changes in position to facilitate full or optimal breathing. Some patients may require intubation and mechanical ventilation until medical management of the ascites is accomplished. Ascites may also result in *abdominal compartment syndrome.*[51,73] Box 18.19 lists the physiological effects that can occur with this complication.

Ascites is medically managed through a low-sodium diet, fluid restriction, and diuretic therapy. Diuretics must be administered cautiously; however, if the intravascular volume is depleted too quickly, acute renal failure may be induced. Closely monitor the serum creatinine level, the BUN level, and urine output for early detection of renal impairment. Also monitor electrolyte levels, particularly serum potassium and sodium levels, when diuretics are administered.

Paracentesis, in which ascitic fluid is withdrawn through percutaneous needle aspiration, is another medical therapy for ascites. Closely monitor vital signs during this procedure, especially as fluid is withdrawn. Major complications include sudden loss of intravascular pressure (decreased blood pressure) and tachycardia. To prevent these complications, 1 to 2 L of fluid is usually withdrawn at one time. However, large volume paracentesis (LVP) with up to 6 L of fluid withdrawn is performed in cases of end-stage liver disease with rapid re-accumulation of ascites.[45,51,69] Very close monitoring of patients undergoing LVP is required to avoid hemodynamic compromise and to intervene quickly should this occur. Document the amount, color, and character of peritoneal fluid obtained. Often, a specimen of the fluid is sent to the laboratory for analysis. Measure the patient's abdominal girth before and after the procedure. Albumin administration is recommended to increase colloid osmotic pressure and to decrease loss of fluid into the peritoneal cavity.[77]

Peritoneovenous shunting is a surgical procedure used to relieve ascites resistant to other therapies. The provider may insert a *LeVeen shunt* by placing the distal end of a tube in the peritoneum and tunneling the other end under the skin into the jugular vein or superior vena cava. A valve that opens and closes according to pressure gradients allows ascitic fluid to flow into the superior vena cava. The patient's breathing normally triggers the valve. During inspiration, pressure increases in the peritoneum and decreases in the vena cava, thereby allowing fluid to flow from the peritoneum into the general circulation. Major complications of this therapy include hemodilution, shunt clotting, wound infection, leakage of ascitic fluid from the incision, and bleeding problems.

A variation of this procedure is the *Denver shunt,* which involves placement of a pump in addition to the peritoneal catheter (Fig. 18.13).[51] The Denver shunt is used to treat both cirrhotic and pleural ascites. Fluid is allowed to flow through

BOX 18.19 Physiological Effects of Abdominal Compartment Syndrome

Cardiovascular
- Decreased venous return
- Increased systemic vascular resistance and intrathoracic pressure
- Reduction in cardiac output

Gastrointestinal
- Impaired lymphatic, venous, and arterial flow
- Poor healing of anastomoses

Hepatic and Renal
- Decreased blood flow to liver and kidneys
- Functional impairment of both organs

Neurological
- If an increased intracranial pressure is present (i.e., head trauma), the intra-abdominal hypertension can exacerbate pressures in the head

Respiratory
- Atelectasis
- Impaired ventilation
- Pneumonia
- Respiratory failure

the pump from the peritoneum into the general circulation at a uniform rate to increase blood volume and renal blood flow; retain nutrients and improve nutritional status; increase diuresis; improve mobility and respiration; and relieve massive, refractory ascites. The popularity and use of the Denver shunt has been limited because of associated adverse events, including shunt occlusion, peritoneal infection, ascitic leak, bleeding, DIC, pneumothorax, and pneumoperitoneum.[68]

Portal Systemic Encephalopathy. *Portal systemic encephalopathy,* commonly known as *hepatic encephalopathy,* is a functional derangement of the central nervous system that causes altered levels of consciousness and cerebral manifestations ranging from confusion to coma. Impaired motor ability is often present as well. *Asterixis,* a flapping tremor of the hand, is an early sign of hepatic encephalopathy that can be assessed by the nurse.

The exact cause of hepatic encephalopathy is unknown, but abnormal ammonia metabolism is hypothesized to be the primary cause. Increased serum ammonia levels interfere with normal cerebral metabolism. In acute liver failure, signs and symptoms of this disorder may appear rapidly; in chronic liver failure, they often occur over time. Many conditions precipitate the development of hepatic encephalopathy, including fluid and electrolyte and acid-base disturbances, increased protein intake, portosystemic shunts, blood transfusions, GI bleeding, and many medications such as diuretics, analgesics, narcotics, and sedatives. Progression of hepatic encephalopathy can be divided into stages (Box 18.20).

Management of hepatic encephalopathy involves addressing precipitating factors such as infection, GI bleeding, and electrolyte and acid-base imbalances. Measures for decreasing ammonia production are necessary. Lactulose, neomycin, and metronidazole are medications ordered to reduce bacterial breakdown of protein in the bowel.[68]

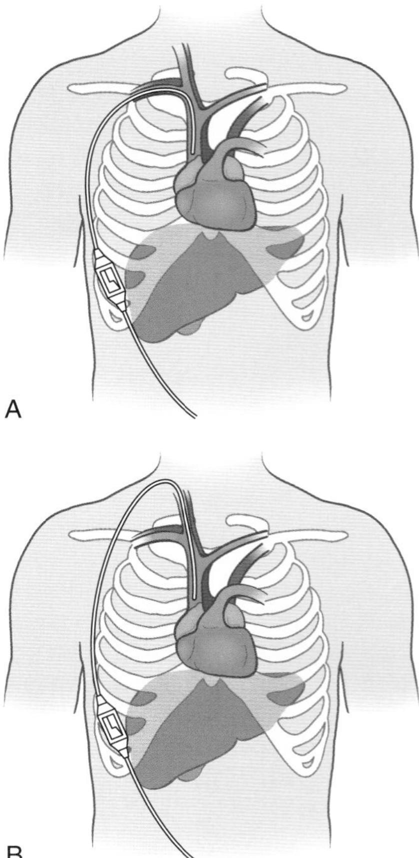

Fig. 18.13 The Denver shunt. Percutaneous placement of the venous and peritoneal catheters of a Denver ascites shunt. The venous catheter may be placed into the subclavian vein (**A**) or the internal jugular vein (**B**).

BOX 18.20 Stages of Portal Systemic Encephalopathy

Stage 1
- Impaired decision-making
- Slurred speech
- Tremors

Stage 2
- Asterixis
- Drowsiness
- Loss of sphincter control

Stage 3
- Dramatic confusion
- Somnolence

Stage 4
- Gastrointestinal alterations
- Profound coma
- Unresponsiveness to pain

Lactulose is the first-line treatment for hepatic encephalopathy. Lactulose creates an acidic environment in the bowel that causes the ammonia to leave the bloodstream and enter the colon. Ammonia becomes trapped in the bowel. Lactulose also has a laxative effect that allows for elimination of the ammonia. Lactulose is given orally or via a rectal enema.

Neomycin and metronidazole are second-line treatments for hepatic encephalopathy. Neomycin is a broad-spectrum antibiotic that destroys the normal bacteria found in the bowel, thereby decreasing protein breakdown and ammonia production. This medication is toxic to the kidneys and cannot be given to patients with renal failure. Daily renal function studies are monitored when neomycin is administered. Metronidazole does not cause diarrhea, and it is not nephrotoxic. Metronidazole may cause epigastric discomfort, which may in turn result in poor compliance with long-term treatment.

Restriction of medications that are toxic to the liver is another important treatment. Collaborate with the clinical pharmacist to review all medications that are metabolized by the liver.

In the past, treatment was aimed at reducing protein intake given the metabolism of protein to ammonia. This theory has been dispelled, and patients should not limit the protein in their diet. Protein is necessary to meet the metabolic needs of patients with liver disease with encephalopathy. Protein intake should be at least 1.2–1.5 g/kg/day. Up to 2 g/kg/day is recommended if the patient is already malnourished.[68,78]

Nursing measures for protecting the patient with an altered mental status from harm are a priority. Patients with hepatic encephalopathy may need to be sedated to prevent them from doing harm to themselves or to others. Sedatives and analgesics metabolized by the liver must be used judiciously to avoid oversedation.

Hepatorenal syndrome. Acute renal failure that occurs with liver failure is called *hepatorenal syndrome.* The pathophysiology of this disorder is not well understood, but it is associated with end-stage cirrhosis and ascites, decreased albumin levels, and portal hypertension. Decreased urine output and an increased serum creatinine level usually occur acutely. The prognosis for the patient with hepatorenal syndrome is generally poor because therapies to improve renal function are usually ineffective.[68,79] The goals of general medical therapies are to improve liver function while supporting renal function. Fluid administration and diuretic therapy are used to improve urine output. Medications that are toxic to the kidney are discontinued. Occasionally, hemodialysis is used to support renal function if there is a chance for an improvement in liver function. Kidney function may improve if liver transplantation is performed as a treatment option for the hepatic failure. Because of the poor prognosis in patients who are not candidates for a liver transplantation, it is appropriate for the critical care nurse to begin to address end-of-life decisions with the patient and family (see Chapter 4, Palliative and End-of-Life Care).[6,30,56,68,79,80] This is done with consideration of the individual nurse's comfort level, as well as the organizational policy and family dynamics.[80]

Hepatopulmonary Syndrome. *Hepatopulmonary syndrome* (HPS) is a pulmonary complication that is observed in patients with chronic liver disease, portal hypertension, or both. HPS occurs because of intrapulmonary vascular dilation that may induce severe hypoxemia. HPS is defined as a triad of liver disease, increased alveolar-arterial oxygen gradient, and intrapulmonary vascular dilations. Patients with HPS experience hypoxia as a result of ventilation-perfusion mismatch, pulmonary capillary vasodilation, and limitations of oxygen diffusion. Pulse oximetry and arterial blood gas measurements are useful screening tools for HPS. Current medical and surgical therapies for HPS include oxygen and TIPS; liver transplantation is the definitive treatment to improve symptoms and survival.[81] The current 1- and 5-year survival rates for patients who received liver transplantation are 86% to 90% and 72% to 80%, respectively.[71]

Patient Outcomes

Outcomes for the patient with liver failure are included in the Plan of Care for the Patient With Liver Failure and the Collaborative Plan of Care for the Critically Ill Patient found in Chapter 1, Overview of Critical Care Nursing).

CASE STUDY

The critical care nurse receives report from the emergency department of a 47-year-old patient with a week-long history of severe abdominal pain that worsens with food intake. The pain is associated with nausea and vomiting. The patient is oriented to person and place; however, the patient is disoriented to day and time and is described as "lethargic." A nasogastric tube and urinary catheter were placed and IV access was established in the emergency department.

Vital signs include the following: heart rate, 110 beats/min; respirations, 30 breaths/min; blood pressure, 104/56 mm Hg; and temperature, 38°C.

Laboratory values include the following: white blood cell count, 19,000/mm^3; hematocrit, 38%; sodium, 148 mEq/L; potassium, 4.0 mEq/L; chloride, 114 mEq/L; blood urea nitrogen, 25 mg/dL; creatinine, 1.0 mg/dL; glucose, 180 mg/dL; amylase, 500 IU/L; and lipase, 600 IU/L.

Questions

1. What further data should the critical care nurse request from the nurse in the emergency department?
2. What interventions and treatments would the nurse expect to initiate upon admission to the critical care unit?
3. Aggressive IV fluid administration with crystalloids at 5 to 10 mL/kg/h was initiated in the emergency department to maintain hemodynamic stability. How could the nurse determine if the intervention was effective?
4. What further assessment data would be valuable for long-term management of this patient?

KEY POINTS

- The GI system comprises the alimentary canal and the accessory organs (i.e., pancreas, liver, and gallbladder) that empty their products into the canal at certain points.
- Functions of the GI system are influenced by neural and hormonal factors.
- The splanchnic circulation supplies blood to organs within the abdomen and accounts for approximately one-third of the cardiac output. The liver is unique in that it is partially perfused by the portal vein.
- Etiologies of acute GI bleeding commonly observed in critical care include peptic ulcer disease, stress-related mucosal bleeding, Mallory-Weiss tears, and esophageal varices. Acute GI bleeding may constitute a medical emergency, as the patient can rapidly develop hemodynamic instability and shock.
- The initial treatment of acute GI bleeding is similar regardless of cause and includes stabilizing the patient and initiating the prescribed medical treatment. Definitive treatment can begin once the etiology of the bleeding is identified via endoscopy.
- Critically ill patients receiving positive-pressure ventilation for more than 48 hours; on extracorporeal life support; with coagulopathies; who have a history of GI bleeding or ulceration in the past year; with traumatic brain or spinal cord injuries; or with thermal injuries over 35% or more of their total body surface area may benefit from SUP with either a PPI or H2 receptor antagonist to reduce the risk of GI bleeding.
- Serum lipase and amylase are released as the pancreatic cells and ducts are destroyed; therefore, these tests are the most specific indicators of acute pancreatitis.
- Once acute pancreatitis is diagnosed, priorities include managing respiratory dysfunction, replacing fluids and electrolytes, administering analgesics for pain control, and providing early oral or enteral nutrition with the goal of avoiding progression to multiple organ dysfunction.
- Viral hepatitis is a common cause of liver failure. Though the initial signs and symptoms of liver failure are vague, as the disease progresses the systemic effects become apparent with the development of portal hypertension, impaired liver metabolic processes, and impaired bile formation and flow.
- The treatment of liver failure is mostly supportive; however, the artificial support of liver function with bioartificial liver devices or the Molecular Adsorbents Recirculating System may be used as a bridge to medical recovery or transplantation.
- Complications of liver failure include ascites, encephalopathy, and HPS. Ascites can be medically managed via diet and diuretics, with paracentesis, or a combination of these therapies. Lactulose is the first-line treatment for hepatic encephalopathy. The definitive treatment for HPS is liver transplant.

REFERENCES

1. Turner KC. Structure and function of the digestive system. In: Rogers J, ed. *McCance and Huether's Pathophysiology: The Biologic Basis for Disease in Adults and Children*. 9th ed. St. Louis, MO: Elsevier; 2024:1285a–1317.
2. Patton KT, Bell F, Thompson T, Williamson P. Chapter 63: principles of gastrointestinal function – motility, nervous control, and blood circulation. In: Patton KT, Bell F, Thompson T, Williamson P, eds. *Anatomy and Physiology*. 11th ed. St. Louis, MO: Elsevier; 2022.
3. Deb B, Prichard DO, Bharucha AE. Constipation and fecal incontinence in the elderly. *Curr Gastroenterol Rep*. 2020;22(11):54.
4. Kang SJ, Cho YS, Lee TH, et al. Medical management of constipation in elderly patients: systematic review. *J Neurogastroenterol Motility*. 2021;27(4):495–512.
5. Volkert D, Beck AM, Cederholm T, et al. ESPEN practical guideline: clinical nutrition and hydration in geriatrics. *Clin Nutrit*. 2022;41(4):958–989.
6. Eke AC. An update on the physiologic changes during pregnancy and their impact on drug pharmacokinetics and pharmacogenomics. *J Basic Clin Physiol Pharmacol*. 2021. https://doi.org/10.1515/jbcpp-2021-0312, 10.1515/jbcpp-2021-0312.
7. Graves CR, Hill WC, Owens MY, et al. Gastrointestinal diseases complicating pregnancy. In: Reece EA, Leguizamon GF, Macones GA, et al., eds. *Clinical Obstetrics: The Fetus and Mother*. 4th ed. Philadelphia, PA: Wolters Kluwer; 2022:598–624.
8. Morgan JA, Morgan KH, Lewis DF. Gastrointestinal diseases. In: Evans AT, ed. *& DeFranco, E. Manual of Obstetrics*. 9th ed. Philadelphia: Wolters Kluwer Health; 2021:269–285.
9. Lowe SA, Steinweg KE. Review article: management of hyperemesis gravidarum and nausea and vomiting in pregnancy. *Emerg Med Australasia*. 2022;34(1):9–15.
10. Mares R, Morrow A, Shumway H, et al. Assessment of management approaches for hyperemesis gravidarum and nausea and vomiting of pregnancy: a retrospective questionnaire analysis. *BMC Pregnancy Childbirth*. 2022;22(1):609.
11. Schnitzler E. The neurology and psychopathology of pica. *Curr Neurol Neurosci Rep*. 2022;22(8):531–536. https://doi.org/10.1007/s11910-022-01218-2.
12. Terrault NA, Williamson C. Pregnancy-associated liver diseases. *Gastroenterol*. 2022;163(1):97–117. e1.
13. Verma D, Saab AM, Saab S. A systematic approach to pregnancy-specific liver disorders. *Gastroenterol Hepatol*. 2021;17(7):322–329.
14. De Seymour JV, Beck KL, Conlon CA. Nutrition in pregnancy. *Obstet, Gyn & Reproduct Med*. 2022. https:// doi.org/10.1016/j.ogrm.2022.08.007.
15. DiLeo TL, Henn MC. Perfecting the gastrointestinal physical exam: findings and their utility and examination pearls. *Emerg Med Clin N Am*. 2021;39(4):689–702.
16. Çalış AS, Kaya E, Mehmetaj L, et al. Abdominal palpation and percussion maneuvers do not affect bowel sounds. *Turk J Surg*. 2019;35(4):309–313. https://doi.org/10.5578/turkjsurg.4291.
17. Costable NJ, Greenwald DA. Upper gastrointestinal bleeding. *Clin Geri Med*. 2021;37(1):155–172.
18. Laine L, Barkun A, Saltzman J, et al. ACG clinical guideline: upper gastrointestinal and ulcer bleeding. *Am J of Gastroenterol*. 2021;116:899–917.

19. Barkun A, Almadi M, Kuipers K, et al. Management of nonvariceal upper gastrointestinal bleeding: guideline recommendations from the international consensus group. *Annals of Int Med.* 2019;171(11):805–826.
20. Orbis-Canamares P, Arbeloa A. New trends and advances in non-variceal gastrointestinal bleeding-series II. *J Clin Med.* 2021;10:3045.
21. Awadalla M, Desimone M, Wassef W. Updates on management of nonvariceal upper gastrointestinal bleeding. *Curr Opin Gastroenterol.* 2019;35:517–523.
22. Saeed M, Bass S, Chaisson NF. Which ICU patients need stress ulcer prophylaxis? *Cleve Clin J Med.* 2022;89(7):363–367. https://doi.org/10.3949/ccjm.89a.21085.
23. Al-Dorzi HM, Arabi YM. Prevention of gastrointestinal bleeding in critically ill patients. *Curr Opin Crit Care.* 2021;27(2):177–182.
24. Douglas QZ. Variceal bleeds in patients with cirrhosis. *Crit Care Nurs Clin North Am.* 2022;34(3):303–309.
25. Rodge GA, Goenka U, Goenka MK. Management of refractory variceal bleed in cirrhosis. *J Clin Exp Hepatol.* 2022;12(2):595–602.
26. Stolow E, Moreau C, Sayana H, et al. Management of non-variceal upper GI bleeding in the geriatric population: an update. *Curr Gastroenterol Rep.* 2021;23(4):5.
27. Villanueva C, Colomo A, Bosch A, et al. Transfusion strategies for acute upper gastrointestinal bleeding. *N Engl J Med.* 2013;368(1):11–21. https://doi.org/10.1056/NEJMoa1211801. [published correction appears in N Engl J Med. 2013 Jun 13;368(24):2341].
28. Wilkins T, Wheeler B, Carpenter M. Upper gastrointestinal bleeding in adults: evaluation and management. *Am Fam Physician.* 2020;101(5):294–300.
29. Patel V, Nicastro A. Upper gastrointestinal bleeding. *Clin Colon Rectal Surg.* 2020;33(1):42–44.
30. Malfertheiner P, Megraud F, O'Morain CA, et al. Management of Helicobacter pylori infection-the Maastricht V/Florence consensus report. *Gut.* 2017;66:6–30.
31. Mullady DK, Wang AY, Waschke KA. AGA clinical practice update on endoscopic therapies for non-variceal upper gastrointestinal bleeding: expert review. *Gastroenterol.* 2020;159(3):1120–1128.
32. Kate V, Sureshkumar S, Gurushankari B, Kalayarasan R. Acute upper non-variceal and lower gastrointestinal bleeding. *J Gastrointest Surg.* 2022;26(4):932–949. https://doi.org/10.1007/s11605-022-05258-4.
33. Schujmann DS, Teixeira Gomes T, Lunardi AC, et al. Impact of a progressive mobility program on the functional status, respiratory, and muscular systems of ICU patients: a randomized and controlled trial. *Crit Care Med.* 2020;48(4):491–497. https://doi.org/10.1097/CCM.0000000000004181.
34. Zang K, Chen B, Wang M, et al. The effect of early mobilization in critically ill patients: a meta-analysis. *Nurs Crit Care.* 2020;25(6):360–367. https://doi.org/10.1111/nicc.12455.
35. Edelson JC, Basso JE, Rockey DC. Updated strategies in the management of acute variceal hemorrhage. *Curr Opin Gastoenterol.* 2021;37(3):167–172.
36. Edelson JC, Mitchell NE, Rockey DC. Endohepatology - current status. *Curr Opin Gastoenterol.* 2022;38(3):216–220.
37. Baiges A, Hernández-Gea V. Management of liver decompensation in advanced chronic liver disease: ascites, hyponatremia, and gastroesophageal variceal bleeding. *Clin Drug Investig.* 2022;42(Suppl 1):25–31. https://doi.org/10.1007/s40261-022-01147-5.
38. Douglas QZ. Variceal bleeds in patients with cirrhosis. *Crit Care Nurs Clin North Am.* 2022;34(3):303–309. https://doi.org/10.1016/j.cnc.2022.04.006.
39. Collins SR. *Elsevier's 2023 Intravenous Medications.* 39th ed. St. Louis, MO: Elsevier, Inc; 2023.
40. Maydeo A, Patil G. How to approach a patient with gastric varices. *Gastroenterology.* 2022;162(3):689–695. https://doi.org/10.1053/j.gastro.2021.12.277.
41. Radu P, Prunoiu VM, Strâmbu V, et al. The portosystemic shunt for the control of variceal bleeding in cirrhotic patients: past and present. *Can J Gastroenterol Hepatol.* 2022;2022:1382556. https://doi.org/10.1155/2022/1382556.
42. Rodge GA, Goenka U, Goenka MK. Management of refractory variceal bleed in cirrhosis. *J Clin Exp Hepatol.* 2022;12(2):595–602.
43. Bettinger D, Thimme R, Schultheis M. Implantation of transjugular intrahepatic portosystemic shunt (TIPS): indication and patient selection. *Curr Opin Gastoenterol.* 2022;38(3):221–229.
44. Aller de la Fuente R. Nutrition and chronic liver disease. *Clin Drug Investig.* 2022;42:55–61.
45. Tapper EB, Ufere NN, Huang DQ, et al. Review article: current and emerging therapies for the management of cirrhosis and its complications. *Aliment Pharmacol Ther.* 2022;55(9):1099–1115.
46. Mederos MA, Reber HA, Girgis MD. Acute pancreatitis: a review. *JAMA.* 2021;325(4):382–390.
47. Leonard-Murali S, Lezotte J, Kalu R, et al. Necrotizing pancreatitis: a review for the acute care surgeon. *Am J Surg.* 2020;221(2021):927–934.
48. Gliem N, Ammer-Herrmenau C, Ellenrieder V, et al. Management of severe acute pancreatitis: an update. *Digestion.* 2021;102(4):503–507. 2021.
49. MacGoey P, Dickson EJ, Puxty K. Management of the patient with acute pancreatitis. *BJA Educ.* 2019;19(8):240–245. 2019.
50. Zheng Z, Ding YX, Qu YX, et al. A narrative review of the mechanism of acute pancreatitis and recent advances in its clinical management. *Am J Transl Res.* 2021;13(3):833–852.
51. Will V, Rodrigues SG, Berzigotti A. Current treatment options of refractory ascites in liver cirrhosis–A systematic review and meta-analysis. *Digest Liver Dis.* 2022;54(8):1007–1014.
52. Ashraf H, Colombo JP, Marcucci V, Rhoton J, Olowoyo O. A clinical overview of acute and chronic pancreatitis: the medical and surgical management. *Cureus.* 2021;13(11):e19764. https://doi.org/10.7759/cureus.19764.
53. Lee PJ, Papachristou GI. Management of severe acute pancreatitis. *Curr Treat Options Gastroenterol.* 2020;18:670–681.
54. Sinonquel P, Laleman W, Wilmer A. Advances in acute pancreatitis. *Curr Opin Crit Care.* 2021;27(2):193–200.
55. Boxhoorn L, Voermans RP, Bouwense SA, et al. Acute pancreatitis. *Lancet.* 2020;396:726–734.
56. Ranson JC. Risk factors in acute pancreatitis. *Hosp Pract.* 1985;20(4):69–73.
57. Vivian E, Cler L, Conwell D, et al. Acute pancreatitis task force on quality: development of quality indicators for acute pancreatitis management. *Am J Gastroenterol.* 2019;114(8):1322–1342.
58. Ketwaroo G, Sealock RJ, Freedman S, et al. Quality of care indicators in patients with acute pancreatitis. *Digestive Dis Sci.* 2019;64(9):2514–2526.
59. Crockett SD, Wani S, Gardner TB, et al. American Gastroenterological Association Institute guideline on initial management of acute pancreatitis. *Gastroenterol.* 2018;154(4):1096–1101. 2018.
60. Sarkar S, Singh S, Rout A. Mean arterial pressure goal in critically ill patients: a meta-analysis of randomized controlled trials. *J Clin Med Res.* 2022;14(5):196–201. https://doi.org/10.14740/jocmr4702.

61. Siebert M, Le Fouler A, Sitbon N, Cohen J, Abba J, Poupardin E. Management of abdominal compartment syndrome in acute pancreatitis. *J Visc Surg*. 2021;158(5):411–419. https://doi.org/10.1016/j.jviscsurg.2021.01.001.
62. Vege SS, Atwal T, et al. Pentoxifylline treatment in severe acute pancreatitis: a pilot, double-blind, placebo-controlled, randomized trial. *Gastroenterol*. 2015;149(2):318–320.e3. 2015.
63. Cai W, Liu F, Wen Y, et al. Pain management in acute pancreatitis: a systematic review and meta-analysis of randomised controlled trials. *Front Med (Lausanne)*. 2021;8:782151. https://doi.org/10.3389/fmed.2021.782151.
64. Pandanaboyana S, Huang W, Windsor JA, et al. Update on pain management in acute pancreatitis. *Curr Opin Gastoenterol*. 2022;38(5):487–494.
65. Heckler M, Hackert T, Hu K, Halloran CM, Büchler MW, Neoptolemos JP. Severe acute pancreatitis: surgical indications and treatment. *Langenbecks Arch Surg*. 2021;406(3):521–535. https://doi.org/10.1007/s00423-020-01944-6.
66. Rowe IA. Lessons from epidemiology: the burden of liver disease. *Dig Dis*. 2017;35(4):304–309.
67. Scaglione S, Kliethermes S, Cao G, et al. The epidemiology of cirrhosis in the United States: population-based study. *J Clin Gastroenterol*. 2015;49(8):690–696.
68. Kaplan A, Rosenblatt R. Symptom management in patients with cirrhosis: a practical guide. *Curr Treatment Options Gastroenterol*. 2022;20:144–159. 2022.
69. Muthiah MD, Cheng Han N, Sanyal AJ. A clinical overview of non-alcoholic fatty liver disease: a guide to diagnosis, the clinical features, and complications-what the non-specialist needs to know. *Diabetes Obes Metab*. 2022;24(Suppl 2):3–14. https://doi.org/10.1111/dom.14521.
70. Centers for Disease Control and Prevention. What is Viral Hepatitis? https://www.cdc.gov/hepatitis/abc/index.htm. Updated March 9, 2023. Accessed May 2, 2023.
71. Kassel CA, Wilke TJ, Fremming BA, et al. Clinical updates in liver transplantation. *J Cardiothor Vasc Anes*. 2022;00(2022):1–9.
72. Sheka AC, Adeyi O, Thompson J, et al. Nonalcoholic steatohepatitis: a review. *JAMA*. 2020;323(12):1175–1183.
73. Kulkarni AV, Rabiee A, Mohanty A. Management of portal hypertension. *J Clin Exp Hepatol*. 2022;12(4):1184–1199.
74. Vasques F, Cavazza A, Bernal W. Acute liver failure. *Curr Opin Crit Care*. 2022;28(2):198–207.
75. Saliba F, Bañares R, Larsen FS. Artificial liver support in patients with liver failure: a modified DELPHI consensus of international experts. *Int Care Med*. 2022;48:1352–1367.
76. Johnson G, Dave S, Teeter W. Molecular adsorbent recirculating system therapy for acute liver failure: institutional indications. *Crit Care Med*. 2022;50(1):4.
77. Yoshiji H, Nagoshi S, Akahane T, et al. Evidence-based clinical practice guidelines for Liver Cirrhosis 2020. *J Gastroenterol*. 2021;56(7):593–619. https://doi.org/10.1007/s00535-021-01788-x.
78. Aller de la Fuente R. Nutrition and chronic liver disease. *Clin Drug Investig*. 2022;42:55–61.
79. Bera C, Wong F. Management of hepatorenal syndrome in liver cirrhosis: a recent update. *Therapeutic Adv in Gastroenterol*. 2022;15. https://doi.org/10.1177/17562848221102679.
80. Rogal SS, Hansen L, Patel A. AASLD practice guidance: palliative care and symptom-based management in decompensated cirrhosis. *Hepatol*. 2022;76(3):819–853.
81. Raevens S, Boret M, Fallon MB. Hepatopulmonary syndrome. *JHEP Reports*. 2022;4(9):100527.

19

Endocrine Alterations

Amanda Brown, MSN-Ed, RN

INTRODUCTION

The endocrine system is composed of multiple glands throughout the body that form a communication network linking all body systems. The endocrine glands synthesize and release hormones to control and regulate metabolic processes such as energy production, fluid and electrolyte balance, and response to stress. This system is closely linked to and integrated with the nervous system. This chapter describes both the endocrine response to critical illness and the crises that occur because of imbalances in hormones from the pancreas, adrenal glands, thyroid gland, and posterior pituitary gland.

Older adult patients with endocrine disorders present diagnostic and treatment challenges. Responses to endocrine dysfunction are blunted, and many of the compensatory mechanisms are lost with advanced age.[1,2] Lifespan Considerations boxes are integrated throughout the chapter to highlight information specific to older adults and pregnant people.

HORMONAL REGULATION

Hormone release occurs in response to a change in the cellular environment or as part of the process of maintaining regulated levels of certain hormones or substances in the body. One or more of the following mechanisms regulate the release of hormones: (1) chemical factors (i.e., blood glucose levels) (2) endocrine factors (one endocrine gland controls another endocrine gland), and (3) neural control.[2]

Hypothalamus and Pituitary Glands

In particular, the hypothalamus and the pituitary gland play major roles in hormonal regulation. The hypothalamus manufactures and secretes several releasing or inhibiting hormones that are conveyed to the pituitary. The pituitary gland responds to these hormones by increasing or decreasing hormone secretion, thus regulating circulating hormone levels. This system is designed as a feedback control mechanism. Positive feedback stimulates the release of a hormone when serum hormone levels are low. Negative feedback inhibits the release of hormones when serum hormone levels are high. Examples of how these feedback systems work to control circulating levels of cortisol are provided in Fig. 19.1 Similar feedback systems control the secretion and inhibition of other hormones outside hypothalamic-pituitary control.

Stress of Critical Illness

Diseases involving the hypothalamus, the pituitary gland, and the primary endocrine organs (i.e., pancreas, adrenal glands, and thyroid gland) interfere with normal feedback mechanisms and the secretion of hormones. Crisis states occur when these diseases are untreated or undertreated or when the patient is physiologically or psychologically stressed.

The stress of critical illness provokes a significant response by the endocrine system. Excess glucose in the blood occurs because of the release of *counterregulatory hormones* that promote hepatic gluconeogenesis and decreased peripheral use of glucose, with resulting relative hypoinsulinemia. Adrenal insufficiency can occur due to insult or damage to the gland itself (primary); dysfunction of the hypothalamus, pituitary, or both (secondary); or whenever cortisol levels are inadequate for the demand (relative). Thyroid hormone balance is disrupted by changes in peripheral metabolism that cause a decrease in triiodothyronine (T_3) levels. Pituitary and hypothalamus dysfunction as a result of brain tumor, trauma, or surgery can cause significant fluid and electrolyte imbalances that complicate critical illness.

HYPERGLYCEMIA IN THE CRITICALLY ILL PATIENT

Critically ill patients are at high risk for hyperglycemia from many different stressors, including disease states, illness-related hormonal responses to stress, and the critical care environment. Box 19.1 reviews risk factors associated with the development of increased blood glucose levels.

Although stress-induced hyperglycemia is a normal physiological response due to the *fight-or-flight* mode, glucose elevation is associated with poor outcomes in hospitalized patients with and without a formal diagnosis of diabetes mellitus (DM). Hyperglycemia in acutely ill patients has been linked to increased morbidity and mortality, increased length of stay, impaired immune function, cerebral ischemia, osmotic diuresis, poor wound healing, increased thrombosis, vasoconstriction with resulting hypertension, decreased respiratory muscle function, neuronal damage, and impaired gastric motility.[3] Therapy aimed at establishing euglycemic levels contributes to improved patient outcomes.

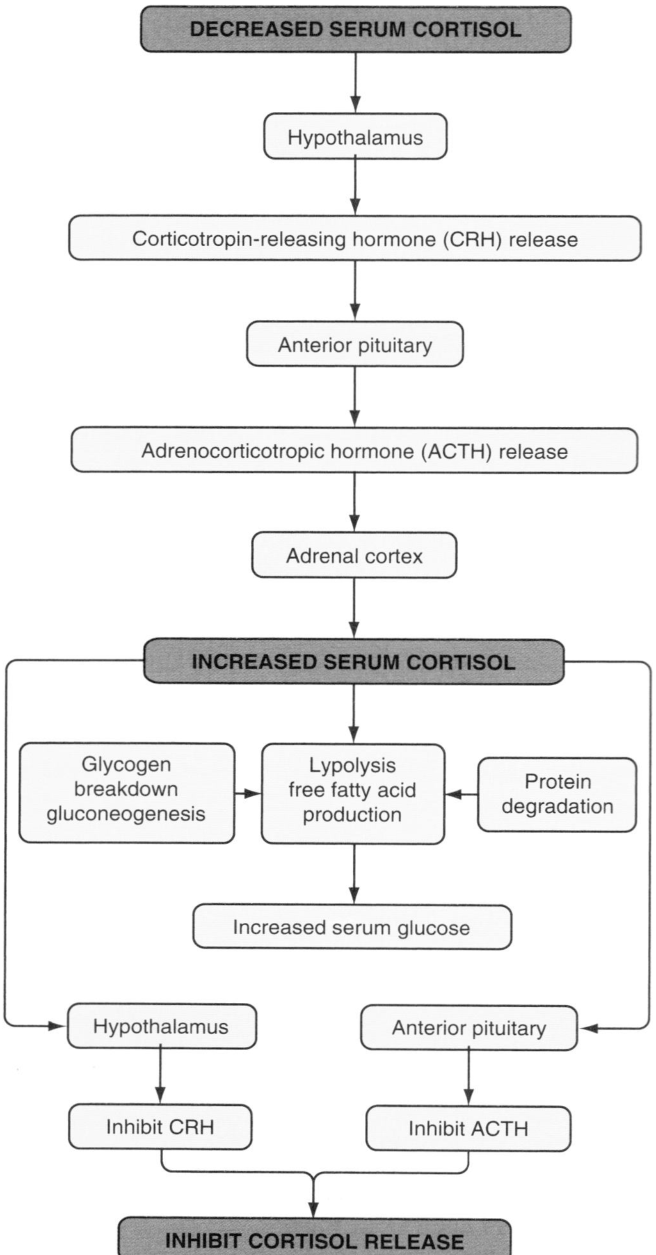

Fig. 19.1 Feedback system for cortisol regulation.

Achieving Optimal Glycemic Control

Critically ill patients with diabetes are most effectively managed with insulin therapy regardless of their usual home self-management regimen.[3] Fig. 19.2 and Table 19.1 provide a review of the insulin action profiles of various insulin products and common insulin regimens. Achieving glycemic control in the hospital can be challenging; however, effective glycemic control in hospitalized patients improves patient outcomes and can shorten hospital length of stay and reduce hospital costs. In recent decades, debate surrounding the effectiveness of tight versus moderate glycemic control has occurred. A 2001 landmark study published by Van den Berghe and colleagues showed that intensive insulin control of hyperglycemia in a critically ill surgical population decreased mortality and morbidity.[1,4] The findings of this study led many hospitals to institute tight glycemic control protocols in critically ill patients as a standard of care. Subsequent studies conducted in broader populations have demonstrated higher rates of mortality in nonsurgical populations and significantly higher rates of severe hypoglycemia in patients who were on intensively controlled glycemic protocols, raising questions about the degree of glycemic control that should be maintained in critically ill individuals.[1]

BOX 19.1 Risk Factors for the Development of Hyperglycemia in the Critically Ill Patient

- Preexisting diabetes mellitus, diagnosed or undiagnosed
- Comorbidities such as obesity, pancreatitis, cirrhosis, hypokalemia
- Stress response release of cortisol, growth hormone, catecholamines (e.g., epinephrine and norepinephrine), glucagon, glucocorticoids, cytokines (e.g., interleukin-1, interleukin-6, and tumor necrosis factor)
- Advanced age
- Lack of muscular activity
- Relative insulin deficiency or insulin resistance
- Administration of exogenous catecholamines, glucocorticoids
- Administration of dextrose solutions, nutritional support
- Medication therapy such as thiazides, beta-blockers, highly active antiretroviral therapy (HAART), phenytoin, tacrolimus, cyclosporine

In response, the American Diabetes Association and the American Association of Clinical Endocrinologists issued a joint statement on inpatient glycemic control. Current guidelines recommend an initial target glucose level of no greater than 180 mg/dL; targets of 140 to 180 mg/dL are appropriate for most critically ill patients once insulin therapy has been initiated.[1,3] Glycemic targets at the lower end of this range may be most beneficial. Glycemic targets of 110 to 140 mg/dL may be appropriate for select critically ill patients if the target can be achieved without significant hypoglycemia.[1] Glycemic targets of 110 mg/dL or less are no longer recommended for critically ill individuals.[1,5] The effectiveness of inpatient treatment may be improved if it is based on pre-admission glycemia; however, current practice does not usually take this into account when determining glycemic targets.[1,3] It is recommended that a hemoglobin A1c (HbA1C) should be measured for all patients admitted to the hospital with DM or hyperglycemia if it has not been measured in the last 3 months.[1,3]

Glycemic Protocols

Continuous intravenous (IV) delivery of short-acting insulin guided by an evidence-based protocol is the preferred method to achieve glycemic targets and optimize patient safety.[1,5] These protocols include frequent glucose monitoring every 30 minutes to 2 hours and insulin dosage adjustments based on patient-specific glucose targets to ensure the appropriate insulin dosage and minimize the incidence of hypoglycemia. Standardized computer-based insulin protocols can improve the quality of glucose control and minimize variability in treatment.[3] The key elements for glycemic control protocols are described in Box 19.2.

Most glucose monitoring in the hospital occurs through point-of-care glucose meters and capillary blood taken from fingersticks. In the critical care setting, it is important to note that point-of-care meters are not as accurate as serum glucose measurements. Capillary blood glucose readings may be affected by perfusion, edema, anemia, or medications used in the hospital.[1,3] Capillary glucose results that do not correlate with the patient's clinical status should be confirmed through a serum glucose measurement. Currently, continuous blood glucose monitoring devices are not approved for monitoring glucose in acute and critically ill patients. However, current research is exploring the efficacy of continuous blood glucose monitoring devices for management and treatment during critical illness.

CLINICAL EXEMPLAR

Quality and Safety

A group of nurses from the critical care unit and an endocrinology advanced practice nurse practitioner noticed that the organization's quality scores for patients with severe hyperglycemia (glucose >300 mg/dL) were above the national aggregate for comparable-size units. The nurses were cognizant that hyperglycemia is associated with increased mortality and morbidity, longer hospital stays, and associated costs. They understood that extreme physiological stress, changes in nutrition, steroid use, and variability in practice patterns all contribute to critical care unit hyperglycemia.

Identified gaps for reducing hyperglycemia in the unit included a need for more user-friendly insulin infusion titration guides, medical resident resistance to ordering the insulin infusion protocol, lack of education about severe hyperglycemia for the nurses and rotating residents, and a lack of guidance for titration of insulin during steroid use. A 1-year comprehensive audit of hyperglycemia was instituted to screen for hyperglycemia events. Results indicated that while the overall number of hyperglycemia events was low (n = 50), a potential communication gap existed, as 46% of nurses did not notify a provider when two consecutive hyperglycemic events occurred as directed by the insulin infusion protocol.

The nurses decided to focus on improving glucose management by implementing several interventions to mitigate severe hyperglycemia. The interventions implemented by the nurses included the following :

- Education of medical and nursing staff on nurse-driven diabetes protocols, insulin infusion, and steroid guidance.
- Set expectations for nurses to notify the provider if there are two consecutive blood glucose levels greater than 300 mg/dL in a 12-hour period.
- Staff to report severe hyperglycemia episodes at safety huddles.
- Identify nurse champions to use a generated report to audit hyperglycemic episodes. Data included provider contact, actions taken, documentation, and causes, with individual nurse follow-up as needed.
- Monthly review of hyperglycemia audits at staff meetings.
- Posting of monthly hyperglycemia data in a secure location for feedback, with an area for staff comments and suggestions for ongoing improvement ideas.

Results indicated that 2 years prior to the intervention, process control chart data for the unit's hyperglycemia management practice were well above the national aggregate. After interventions, the hyperglycemia rates were closer to or below the national average. Moreover, the continued vigilance has helped sustain this important nurse-led quality and safety initiative.

References

Neelon L, Basawil K, Whitney L et al. Critical care nurse–led quality improvement hyperglycemia reduction initiative. *J Nurs Care Qual.* 2019;34(2):91-93. https://doi.org/10.1097/NCQ.0000000000000380.

Rovida S, Bruni A, Pelaia C et al. Nurse led protocols for control of glycaemia in critically ill patients: a systematic review. *Intensive Crit Care Nurs.* 2022;71:103247. https://doi.org/10.1016/j.iccn.2022.103247.

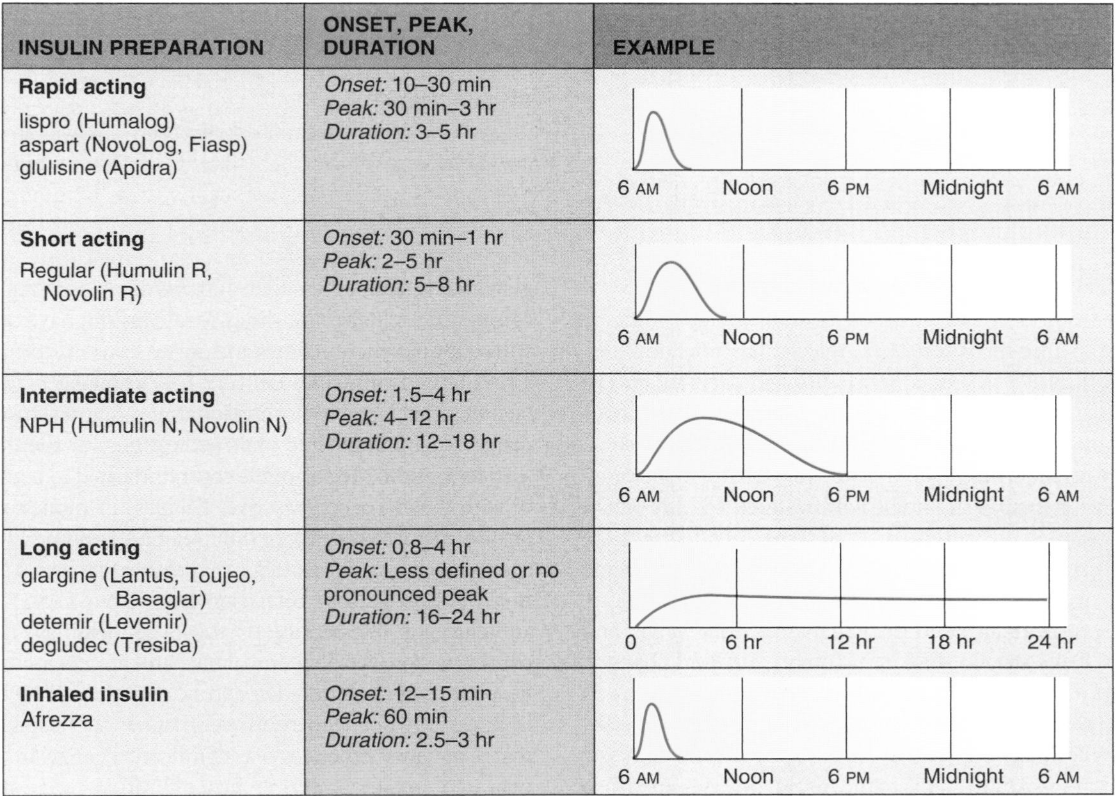

INSULIN PREPARATION	ONSET, PEAK, DURATION	EXAMPLE
Rapid acting lispro (Humalog) aspart (NovoLog, Fiasp) glulisine (Apidra)	*Onset:* 10–30 min *Peak:* 30 min–3 hr *Duration:* 3–5 hr	6 AM Noon 6 PM Midnight 6 AM
Short acting Regular (Humulin R, Novolin R)	*Onset:* 30 min–1 hr *Peak:* 2–5 hr *Duration:* 5–8 hr	6 AM Noon 6 PM Midnight 6 AM
Intermediate acting NPH (Humulin N, Novolin N)	*Onset:* 1.5–4 hr *Peak:* 4–12 hr *Duration:* 12–18 hr	6 AM Noon 6 PM Midnight 6 AM
Long acting glargine (Lantus, Toujeo, Basaglar) detemir (Levemir) degludec (Tresiba)	*Onset:* 0.8–4 hr *Peak:* Less defined or no pronounced peak *Duration:* 16–24 hr	0 6 hr 12 hr 18 hr 24 hr
Inhaled insulin Afrezza	*Onset:* 12–15 min *Peak:* 60 min *Duration:* 2.5–3 hr	6 AM Noon 6 PM Midnight 6 AM

Fig. 19.2 Commercially available insulin preparations showing onset, peak, and duration of action. From Dickinson J. Diabetes mellitus. In: Harding M, Kwong J, Roberts D et al., eds. *Lewis's Medical-Surgical Nursing: Assessment and Management of Clinical Problems.* 12th ed. St. Louis, MO: Elsevier; 2023.

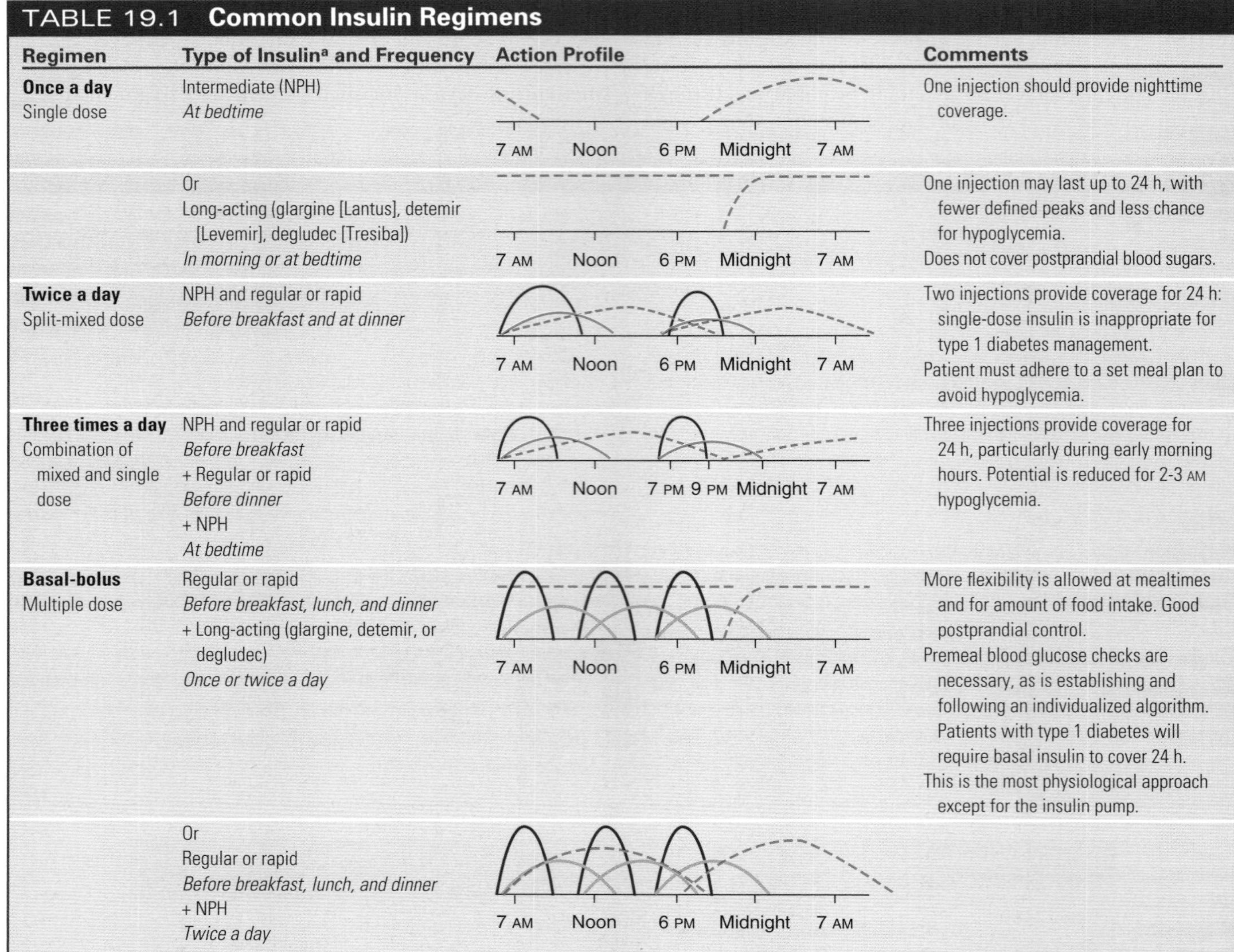

TABLE 19.1 **Common Insulin Regimens**

Regimen	Type of Insulin[a] and Frequency	Action Profile	Comments
Once a day Single dose	Intermediate (NPH) *At bedtime*	7 AM Noon 6 PM Midnight 7 AM	One injection should provide nighttime coverage.
	Or Long-acting (glargine [Lantus], detemir [Levemir], degludec [Tresiba]) *In morning or at bedtime*	7 AM Noon 6 PM Midnight 7 AM	One injection may last up to 24 h, with fewer defined peaks and less chance for hypoglycemia. Does not cover postprandial blood sugars.
Twice a day Split-mixed dose	NPH and regular or rapid *Before breakfast and at dinner*	7 AM Noon 6 PM Midnight 7 AM	Two injections provide coverage for 24 h: single-dose insulin is inappropriate for type 1 diabetes management. Patient must adhere to a set meal plan to avoid hypoglycemia.
Three times a day Combination of mixed and single dose	NPH and regular or rapid *Before breakfast* + Regular or rapid *Before dinner* + NPH *At bedtime*	7 AM Noon 7 PM 9 PM Midnight 7 AM	Three injections provide coverage for 24 h, particularly during early morning hours. Potential is reduced for 2-3 AM hypoglycemia.
Basal-bolus Multiple dose	Regular or rapid *Before breakfast, lunch, and dinner* + Long-acting (glargine, detemir, or degludec) *Once or twice a day*	7 AM Noon 6 PM Midnight 7 AM	More flexibility is allowed at mealtimes and for amount of food intake. Good postprandial control. Premeal blood glucose checks are necessary, as is establishing and following an individualized algorithm. Patients with type 1 diabetes will require basal insulin to cover 24 h. This is the most physiological approach except for the insulin pump.
	Or Regular or rapid *Before breakfast, lunch, and dinner* + NPH *Twice a day*	7 AM Noon 6 PM Midnight 7 AM	

[a]Insulin types include rapid acting (lispro, aspart, glulisine), short acting (regular), intermediate acting (NPH), and long acting (glargine, detemir).
Images from Dickinson J. Diabetes mellitus. In: Harding M, Kwong J, Roberts D et al., eds. *Lewis's Medical-Surgical Nursing: Assessment and Management of Clinical Problems.* 12th ed. St Louis, MO: Elsevier; 2023:1292.

Insulin Transition Protocols

The transition from IV to subcutaneous insulin therapy must be carefully timed to limit the risk for hyperglycemia. Transition protocols have been shown to reduce morbidity and decrease cost of care.[1] Most patients may be transitioned from IV to subcutaneous insulin when they are eating regular meals or when their clinical condition warrants transfer to a lower-intensity level of care.[1] Subcutaneous basal insulin should be administered 2 hours before the insulin infusion is discontinued.[6] It is recommended that the subcutaneous insulin regimen for a non–critically ill patient include basal, nutritional, and correction insulin components.[1] Protocols are additionally individualized to the patient based on weight and renal function. Daily insulin dose adjustments, IV fluid changes, and retiming of point-of-care glucose monitoring may be required for significant glucose elevations and to account for significant changes in dietary intake imposed by "nothing by mouth" status or nausea and vomiting. Adjustments to the insulin dose regimen also may be required if the patient is receiving enteral feedings, parenteral nutrition, or high-dose glucocorticoids or if the patient's blood glucose level falls to less than 100 mg/dL. Insulin regimens that are composed exclusively of sliding-scale insulin have been associated with poor patient outcomes and are no longer recommended as the only method of insulin delivery for hospitalized patients.[1] Many facilities that use basal-nutritional-correctional insulin protocols discontinue antidiabetic oral medications for the duration of the hospitalization. Metformin is contraindicated in acute renal failure or with the use of contrast dye. Thiazolidinediones, such as pioglitazone, increase the risk of fluid retention and heart failure. Other agents, such as sulfonylureas, may increase the risk for hypoglycemia. Sodium-glucose cotransporter protein 2 (SGLT2) inhibitors and glucagon-like peptide 1 (GLP-1) agonists have the potential to contribute to electrolyte imbalance and are not well studied in the hospitalized population. Dipeptidyl peptidase 4 (DPP-4) inhibitors likewise have not been extensively studied for hospital use. Because many patients experience a significant change in their diabetes treatment regimen during hospitalization, accurate medication reconciliation and effective discharge education are critical for all hospitalized patients who are being treated for diabetes.

BOX 19.2 Key Components of a Glucose Management Protocol

- Obtain frequent plasma blood glucose measurements, taking into consideration awareness of previous blood glucose levels, insulin dose adjustments, and individual patient parameters.
- Verify point-of-care blood glucose value with laboratory analysis, especially with changes in patient condition (e.g., sepsis, vasoactive agents, acetaminophen administration).
- Review concentration of insulin infusion, with the intention of avoiding hypoglycemia.
- Initial IV insulin bolus dose if appropriate, accounting for characteristics of individual patients and goal glucose range.
- Institute proactive measures for titration to increase or decrease insulin infusion based on glucose levels incorporated into nurse-directed protocols.
- Initiate interventions for:
  - Hypoglycemia, should it occur
  - Interruption of feeding, either parenteral or enteral
  - Transport of the patient from the critical care unit for diagnostic testing
  - Discontinuation of the IV insulin infusion
  - Transfer of the patient from the critical care unit

Data from Compton F, Ahlborn R, Weidehoff T. Nurse-directed blood glucose management in a medical intensive care unit. *Crit Care Nurse.* 2017;37(3):30-41. Rovida S, Bruni A, Pelaia C et al. Nurse led protocols for control of glycaemia in critically ill patients: a systematic review. *Intensive Crit Care Nurs.* 2022;71:103247. https://doi.org/10.1016/j.iccn.2022.103247.

CHECK YOUR UNDERSTANDING

1. The critical care nurse has just completed the second blood glucose bedside assessment. The results of both blood glucose values are as follows: 315 mg/dL at 0900 and 350 mg/dL at 1300. Determine the priority nursing actions given the findings.
   A. Assess the patient for signs of dehydration.
   B. Report the hyperglycemia findings at the change-of-shift safety huddle.
   C. Notify the provider, as two consecutive blood glucose measurements >300 mg/dL require intervention.
   D. Determine who oversees the monthly review of hyperglycemia audits at the next staff meeting to report the event.

PANCREATIC ENDOCRINE EMERGENCIES

The pancreas has a complex role in digestion and metabolism. The exocrine function of the pancreas facilitates conversion of food to fuel for the body's cells through the release of enzymes that aid digestion. The endocrine function of the pancreas regulates blood sugar.

Review of Physiology

DM is a metabolic disease of glucose imbalance resulting from alterations in insulin secretion, insulin action, or both.[7] The two most common types of DM are type 1 and type 2. Type 1 DM is primarily caused by the destruction of pancreatic islet beta cells, which results in an *absolute insulin deficiency* and a tendency to develop ketoacidosis. In most cases, type 1 DM is an autoimmune disorder. A subset of patients, primarily of African American or Asian ancestry, may experience a genetic but nonimmunological form of type 1 diabetes.[7]

Type 2 is the most common form of diabetes. It results from the combination of insulin resistance and insulin secretory defects, which causes a *relative insulin deficiency*.[7] A combination of cardiovascular risk factors, including hypertension, atherogenic dyslipidemia, and hyperglycemia, makes up the *cardiometabolic risk syndrome* and significantly increases the risk of developing type 2 DM. The other causes of DM include insulin resistance during pregnancy (gestational diabetes mellitus, or GDM), medications such as corticosteroids, thiazide diuretics, some HIV medications and atypical antipsychotic agents, genetic disorders such as cystic fibrosis, pancreatic damage, viruses, and disorders of the pituitary and adrenal glands.[7] In addition, polycystic ovary syndrome is strongly associated with the development of obesity and insulin resistance and places a female at significant risk for the development of GDM and type 2 DM later in life.[7]

Genetics. Genetic factors have a strong role in the development of type 1 DM (see Genetics box). For example, rates of type 1 DM are particularly high in people from Scandinavia. Genetic alterations may play a role in the development of type 2 DM and related conditions, such as obesity and the cardiometabolic risk syndrome. The incidence of type 2 DM in the United States is higher among Hispanics or Latinos, African Americans, Native Americans, Alaska Natives, Asian Americans, and Pacific Islanders.[7]

Hyperglycemic Crises

Pathogenesis. Diabetic ketoacidosis (DKA) and hyperosmolar hyperglycemic state (HHS) are endocrine emergencies. The underlying mechanisms in DKA and HHS are reduced circulating insulin as a result of decreased insulin secretion (DKA) or ineffective action of insulin (HHS) coupled with a concomitant elevation of counterregulatory hormones (Fig. 19.3). Together, this hormonal mix leads to increased hepatic and renal glucose production and decreased use of glucose in the peripheral tissues compounded by osmotic diuresis caused by glycosuria that leads to dehydration and electrolyte abnormalities.[8] Historically, DKA was described as the crisis state in individuals with type 1 DM, whereas HHS was thought to occur only in individuals with type 2 DM. However, both DKA and HHS may occur in individuals with either type of DM.

Etiology of diabetic ketoacidosis. Numerous factors precipitate DKA (Box 19.3). In many patients, DKA is the initial indication of previously undiagnosed type 1 DM and is more commonly seen in individuals with type 1 DM than type 2 DM. In the critically ill, the presence of coexisting autoimmune disorders of the thyroid and adrenal glands must be considered, especially in unstable patients with type 1 DM.[9] In addition, the multiple endocrine changes that accompany pregnancy alter insulin needs, which escalate rapidly in the second and third trimesters.[10] Pregnant people with type 1 DM are at increased risk for DKA.[10] Signs and symptoms of DKA characteristically develop over a short period, and patients seek medical help early because of the associated symptoms.

The incidence of recurrent DKA is higher in females and peaks in the early teenage years. The risk of recurrent DKA is

GENETICS

Type 2 Diabetes: Complex Genetics

Type 2 diabetes mellitus (T2DM) does not display a pattern of single-gene inheritance. Nonetheless, T2DM is highly associated with inheritance. Offspring of two parents with T2DM have a significant risk for a similar diagnosis—as much as a sixfold increase over the general population.[1]

T2DM is an example of a *multifactorial* (complex) *polygenic* disease. *Complex disease* or multifactorial conditions suggest that pathology results from the interaction among genes, environment, and lifestyle. *Polygenic* means that more than one gene is implicated in the development of the disease. More than 150 DNA variations are associated with the risk of developing T2DM, and these polymorphisms are beginning to be clustered to provide additional diagnostic and treatment information.[1] Most polymorphisms associated with T2DM act by changing the amount, timing, and location of *gene expression*. Gene expression is the process by which a gene produces a product, including *transcription* and *translation*.

Genome-wide association studies (GWASs) have contributed to our understanding of the heterogeneity of T2DM. A genome-wide association study is an approach that involves rapidly scanning markers across the complete sets of genomes across many people to find genetic variations associated with a particular disease.[2] The use of GWAS builds information about genetic variations that contribute to multifactorial diseases such as diabetes, asthma, cancer, and mental illness.

Many genetic polymorphisms related to T2DM are linked to insulin secretion and resistance. Some contributing genetic polymorphisms are found in the genome's *intron* (noncoding) regions. Others are found in the *exon* or protein-coding regions. Both regions can be affected by environmental and lifestyle factors. There is evidence that lifestyle changes can decrease the occurrence of T2DM despite a genetic predisposition for T2DM. For example, 14 weeks of physical training in prediabetic, postmenopausal women altered the expression of many genes associated with hyperglycemia.[3]

Epigenetics helps explain the linkages between genetic risk and environment-lifestyle in the onset and progression of T2DM. Epigenetics examines changes in gene function that are inheritable but do not involve a change in DNA sequence. Most gene function changes result from DNA methylation or histone modifications. For example, changes to DNA methylation are associated with the onset and severity of retinopathy, an all-to-common complication of T2DM.[4]

Gene function—epigenetics—related to T2DM is altered by diet, smoking, and alcohol intake. Diet can alter DNA methylation, histone modifications, messenger RNA (mRNA), and microRNA (miRNA) expression. These epigenetic changes influence the onset and progression of T2DM, including complications such as nephropathy, vascular disease, and neuropathy.[5,6] Epigenetics holds promise for strategies to delay the onset of T2DM and reduce its associated complications' severity. It may be that subtypes of T2DM are more amenable to environment-lifestyle changes. The ultimate goal of examining epigenetics is to build phenotypic-associated interventions that target patient-centered outcomes.

Metabolomics, the large-scale study of small molecules—metabolites—within a cell, tissue, and organ, is also being used to guide treatment for T2DM. Metabolomics uses technology developed during genomic studies to build knowledge around global biological systems like glucose regulation and use in humans. For example, the function of the adipose tissue is influenced by complex interactions between genetics, epigenetics, and the environment.[7] The presence and type of adipose tissue are implicated in the cause and severity of T2DM. Understanding how to influence adipose tissue crosstalk with other body systems may create new treatment approaches for T2DM.

Multifactorial, polygenic disorders are common. The use of GWASs is building information about genetic variations that contribute to multifactorial diseases such as diabetes, asthma, cancer, and mental illness. Proteomics, metabolomics, and epigenetic studies are genomic-derived laboratory techniques. They are refining our understanding of gene and environment-lifestyle interactions. Ultimately these approaches will contribute to individual, precise diagnostics and interventions.

Genetic terms: *multifactorial conditions, complex disease, polygenetic disorders, gene expression, translation, transcription, intron, exon, genome-wide association studies (GWASs), deoxyribonucleic acid (DNA), micro- and messenger ribonucleic acid (miRNA and mRNA), epigenetics, metabolomics.*

References

1. Udler MS. Type 2 diabetes: multiple genes, multiple diseases. *Curr Diab Rep.* 2019;19(8):55-62. https://doi.org/10.1007/s11892-019-1169-7.
2. National Institutes of Health. *Genome wide association studies fact sheet.* National Human Genome Research Institute. Last updated August 17, 2020. https://www.genome.gov/about-genomics/fact-sheets/Genome-Wide-Association-Studies-Fact-Sheet. Accessed January 18, 2024.
3. Yumi Noronha N, da Silva Rodrigues G, Harumi Yonehara Noma I et al. 14-weeks combined exercise epigenetically modulated 118 genes of menopausal women with prediabetes. *Front Endocrinol (Lausanne).* 2022;13:895489. https://doi.org/10.3389/fendo.2022.895489.
4. Barnstable CJ. Epigenetics and degenerative retinal diseases: prospects for new therapeutic approaches. *Asia Pac J Ophthalmol (Phila).* 2022;11(4):328-334. https://doi.org/10.1097/APO.0000000000000520.
5. Kushwaha K, Garg SS, Gupta J. Targeting epigenetic regulators for treating diabetic nephropathy. *Biochimie.* 2022;202:146-158. https://doi.org/10.1016/j.biochi.2022.08.001.
6. Zhou JY, Park S. Regular exercise, alcohol consumption, and smoking interact with the polygenetic risk scores involved in insulin sensitivity and secretion for the risk of concurrent hyperglycemia, hypertension, and dyslipidemia. *Nutrition.* 2021;91-92:111422. https://doi.org/10.1016/j.nut.2021.111422.
7. Wang L, Qiu Y, Gu H et al. Regulation of adipose thermogenesis and its critical role in glucose and lipid metabolism. *Int J Biol Sci.* 2022;18(13):4950-4962. https://doi.org/10.7150/ijbs.75488.

Chris Winkelman, PhD, ACNP-BC, CCRN, CNE, FAANP, FCCM

also higher in patients with DM diagnosed at an early age and in those of lower socioeconomic status. The causes of recurrent DKA are unclear but include physiological, psychosomatic, and psychosocial factors. Psychological problems complicated by eating disorders in younger patients with type 1 DM may contribute to 20% of recurrent DKA.[8]

Euglycemic DKA can be difficult to recognize because the patient's blood glucose is less than 250 mg/dL; however, signs of metabolic acidosis and ketones in the blood and/or urine are present.[11] The patient may complain of nausea, vomiting, general malaise, lethargy, fatigue, loss of appetite, and abdominal pain but may not have polyuria or mental status changes.[9] Though the risk of DKA in patients being treated with SGLT2 inhibitors is small, this class of medications increases DKA risk two- to fourfold in type 2 DM and up to 5% in type 1 DM.[8] Euglycemic DKA is mostly associated with conditions with low glycogen reserves and/or increased rates of glucosuria, such as pregnancy, liver disorders, alcohol intoxication, glycogen storage diseases, and poor oral intake or starvation states.[8,12]

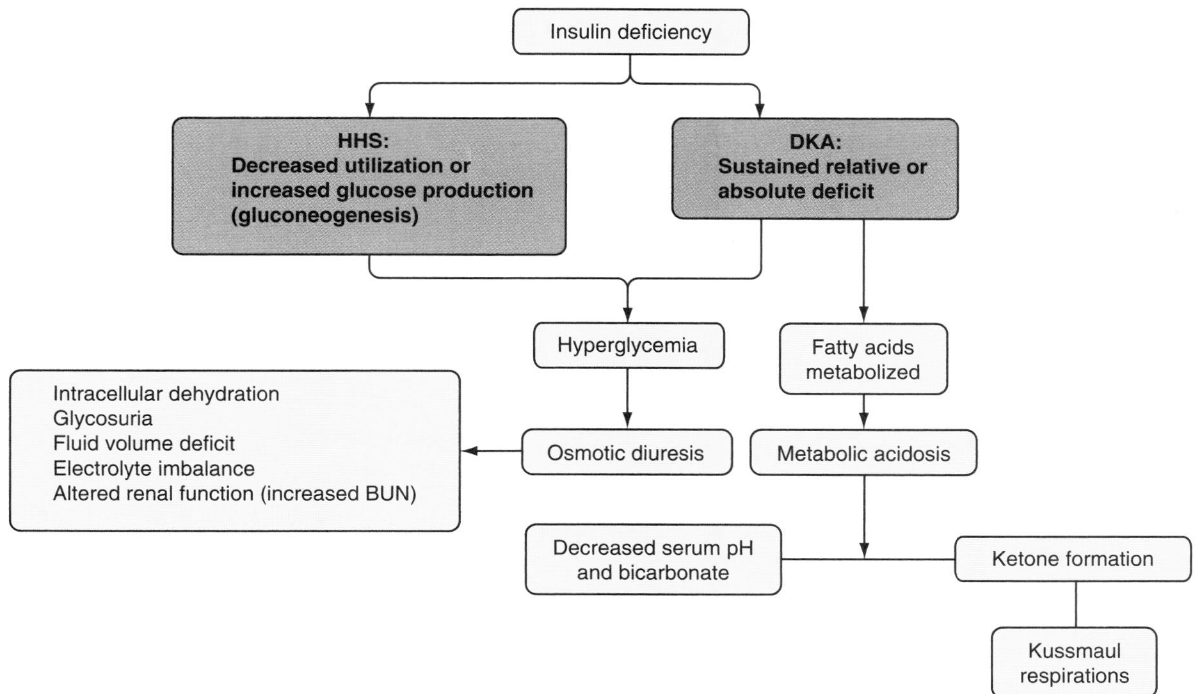

Fig. 19.3 Pathophysiology of diabetic ketoacidosis *(DKA)* and hyperosmolar hyperglycemic state *(HHS)*. *BUN,* Blood urea nitrogen.

BOX 19.3 Factors Leading to Diabetic Ketoacidosis and Hyperosmolar Hyperglycemic State

Common Factors
- *Infections:* pneumonia, urinary tract infection, sepsis, or abscess
- Omission of diabetic therapy or inadequate treatment
- New-onset diabetes mellitus
- *Preexisting illness:* cardiac, renal diseases
- *Major or acute illness:* myocardial infarction, cerebral vascular accident, pancreatitis, trauma, surgery, renal disease
- *Other endocrine disorders:* hyperthyroidism, Cushing disease, pheochromocytoma
- Stress
- High-calorie parenteral or enteral nutrition

DKA-Specific Factors
- Malfunction of insulin pump
- Insulin pump infusion set site problems (infection, disconnection, catheter kinking or migration)
- Increased insulin needs secondary to insulin-resistant states (pregnancy, puberty, before menstruation)

HHS-Specific Factors
- Decreased thirst mechanism
- Difficulty accessing fluids (e.g., nursing home resident)

Medications
- Steroids (especially glucocorticoids)
- Beta-blockers
- Thiazide diuretics
- Calcium channel blockers
- Phenytoin
- Epinephrine
- Psychotropic agents, including tricyclic antidepressants
- Sympathomimetics
- Analgesics
- Cimetidine
- Calcium channel blockers
- Immunosuppressants
- Diazoxide
- Chemotherapeutic agents
- SGLT2 inhibitors
- "Illicit drugs" such as cocaine, Ecstasy

DKA, diabetic ketoacidosis; *HHS,* hyperosmolar hyperglycemic state; *SGLT2,* sodium-glucose cotransporter protein 2.

Etiology of hyperosmolar hyperglycemic state. HHS is usually precipitated by a physiological stressor (i.e., infection, critical illness) that results in insulin resistance and increased serum glucose. It is more commonly seen in patients who have type 2 DM or no prior history of DM and may be the initial presentation of type 2 DM in younger adults.[13] However, most patients who develop this condition are older adults with decreased compensatory mechanisms to maintain homeostasis in hyperosmolar states. High-calorie parenteral and enteral feedings that exceed the patient's ability to metabolize glucose can induce HHS. Several medications are associated with the development of the disorder. The major etiological factors of HHS are included in Box 19.3.

Pathophysiology of Diabetic Ketoacidosis. Several significant intracellular and extracellular shifts occur in DKA and HHS (Fig. 19.4). In both disorders, high extracellular glucose levels produce an osmotic gradient between the intracellular and extracellular spaces, causing fluid to translocate out of the cells.[8] This process is called *osmotic diuresis.* When serum glucose levels exceed the renal threshold (approximately 200 mg/dL), glucose is lost through the kidneys *(glycosuria).* As glycosuria and osmotic diuresis progress, urinary losses of water, sodium, potassium, magnesium, calcium, and phosphorus occur. This cycle of osmotic diuresis causes increases in serum osmolality, further compensatory fluid shifts from the intracellular to the intravascular space, and worsening dehydration.

Typically, body water losses in DKA total 6 L.[8] The evolving hyperosmolarity further impairs insulin secretion and promotes a state of insulin resistance known as *glucose toxicity.*[9] The glomerular filtration rate in the kidney decreases in response to the severe fluid volume deficits, resulting in decreased glucose excretion (causing increased serum glucose levels) and hemoconcentration. The altered neurological status frequently seen in these patients is partially the result of cellular dehydration and the hyperosmolar state.

The absolute or relative insulin deficiency that precipitates DKA leads to decreased glucose uptake, increased fat mobilization with release of fatty acids, accelerated gluconeogenesis (synthesis of glucose from noncarbohydrates), glycogenolysis (breakdown of glycogen to glucose), and ketogenesis (formation of ketone bodies).[9] Without insulin, the liberated glucose cannot be used, further increasing serum blood glucose and urine glucose concentrations and worsening osmotic diuresis. As nitrogen accumulates in peripheral tissues, blood urea nitrogen (BUN) rises. Serum electrolytes, particularly potassium, may be falsely elevated in relation to the actual intracellular level. Breakdown of protein stores stimulates the shift of intracellular potassium into the extracellular serum (hyperkalemia). This additional circulating potassium may also be lost as a result of osmotic diuresis (hypokalemia). Total body potassium deficits are common and must be considered in the overall management of DKA. Because of the fluid volume and potassium shifts, serum potassium values must be interpreted with caution in patients with DKA.[6]

The fat cells are broken down into free fatty acids that are released into the blood and transported to the liver, where they are oxidized into ketone bodies (β-hydroxybutyrate, acetoacetate, and acetone). Accumulation of the ketone bodies results in ketoacidosis. Inadequate buffering of the excess ketone acids by circulating bicarbonate results in metabolic acidosis as the ratio of carbonic acid to bicarbonate ions increases.

Euglycemic DKA may occur in patients who are taking SGLT2 inhibitors. In these patients, ketones are elevated from a relative insulin deficiency brought on by SGLT2 inhibitor–induced glucosuria and reduced carbohydrate intake.[6,12] The respiratory system attempts to compensate for excess carbonic acid by "blowing off" carbon dioxide (CO_2), a weak acid. Kussmaul respirations, characterized by an increased rate and depth of breathing, and an acetone ("fruity") breath odor are classic clinical signs of DKA associated with this compensatory process.

In addition, patients with DKA may have an accumulation of lactic acid (lactic acidosis). The resulting dehydration may cause decreased perfusion to core organs, with consequent hypoxemia and worsening of the lactic acidosis. Excess lactic acid results in an increased *anion gap* (increased body acids). Sodium, potassium, chloride, and bicarbonate are responsible for maintaining a normal anion gap (<16 mEq/L). Ketone accumulation causes an increase in the anion gap greater than 16 mEq/L. To calculate the anion gap, see Box 19.4.

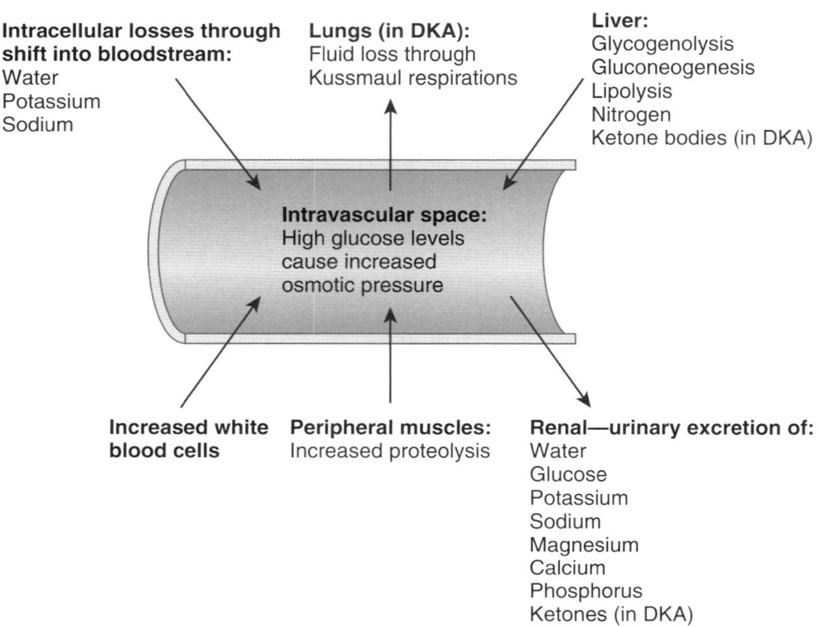

Fig. 19.4 Intracellular and extracellular shifts in hyperglycemic crises. *DKA,* Diabetic ketoacidosis.

BOX 19.4 Calculation of the Anion Gap

The anion gap is calculated as the difference between the measured concentrations of sodium (Na^+) and potassium (K^+), the major anions, and those of chloride (Cl^-) and bicarbonate (HCO_3^-), the major cations:

$$\left(Na^+ + K^+\right) - \left(Cl^- + HCO_3^-\right)$$

The normal serum anion gap is 8 to 16 mEq/L. An elevated value indicates the accumulation of acids, such as is present in diabetic ketoacidosis.

In summary, cells without glucose starve and begin to use existing stores of fat and protein to provide energy for body processes (gluconeogenesis). Fats are metabolized faster than they can be stored, resulting in an accumulation of ketone acids, a byproduct of fat metabolism in the liver. Ketone acids accumulate in the bloodstream, where hydrogen ions dissociate from the ketones. The more acidotic the patient becomes, the less able the body is to metabolize these ketones. The net result in DKA is an additional increase in serum glucose, nitrogen levels, plasma osmolality, and metabolic acidosis.

CHECK YOUR UNDERSTANDING

2. A 67-year-old patient on an SGLT2 inhibitor agent for heart failure complains of increasing fatigue, shortness of breath, and loss of appetite. What additional data should the nurse obtain before contacting the provider?
   A. Weight, urine output last hour, blood pressure, and respiratory rate
   B. Presence of ketones in urine, blood pressure, heart rate, and respiratory rate
   C. Blood glucose, presence of ketones in urine, blood pressure, heart rate, and respiratory rate
   D. Oxygen saturation, respiratory rate, weight, and nutrition history

Pathophysiology of Hyperosmotic Hyperglycemic State. The pathophysiology of HHS is similar to that of DKA. However, in HHS, there are significantly lower levels of free fatty acids, resulting in a lack of ketosis but even higher levels of hyperglycemia, hyperosmolality, and severe dehydration (see Fig. 19.3).[13]

Ketoacidosis is usually not seen in patients with HHS because insulin levels in these patients are sufficient to prevent lipolysis and subsequent ketone formation.[9,13] Insulin resistance leads to difficulty in glucose utilization and an increase in counterregulatory hormones like glucagon, growth hormone, and cortisol, further worsening the inability of peripheral tissues to use insulin for metabolism. This leads to a continued increase in serum glucose levels. Persistence or worsening of the stressor precipitating HHS may allow the hyperglycemia to progress to a state of extreme insulin deficiency. The hyperglycemic state causes an osmotic movement of water out of the cells, leading to an expansion of the extracellular fluid volume and intracellular dehydration. The osmotic diuresis and resultant intracellular and extracellular dehydration in HHS are typically more severe than those found in DKA because HHS usually develops insidiously over a period of weeks to months. Alterations in neurological status are common because of cellular dehydration. The typical total body water deficit is greater in HHS, approximately 9 L.[8] By the time these patients seek medical attention, they are profoundly dehydrated and hyperosmolar.[14] HHS most commonly occurs in older adults with comorbid problems, such as renal insufficiency, heart failure, myocardial ischemia, and chronic lung disease.[9] These factors may limit the ability of providers to aggressively treat the condition, particularly regarding fluid resuscitation.[15] The mortality rate of HHS is 10 times higher than that of DKA in older adults.[13]

Assessment

Clinical presentation. The presenting symptoms of DKA and HHS are similar (Table 19.2). The severity of presenting symptoms is due to the degree of dehydration and electrolyte imbalances. The osmotic diuresis occurring from hyperglycemia results in signs of increased thirst (polydipsia), increased urine output (polyuria), and dehydration. Increased hunger (polyphagia) may be an early sign. Signs of intravascular dehydration are common as the physiological processes continue.[6]

Hyperglycemia and ketosis both contribute to delayed gastric emptying. Nausea and vomiting can occur and further worsen total body dehydration. Patients also report symptoms of weakness and anorexia. Abdominal pain and tenderness are common presenting symptoms, particularly in DKA, and are associated with dehydration and underlying pathophysiology, such as pyelonephritis, duodenal ulcer, appendicitis, and metabolic acidosis. Pain associated with DKA usually disappears with treatment of the dehydration. Significant weight loss occurs because of the fluid losses and an inability to metabolize glucose.

Altered states of consciousness range from restlessness, confusion, and agitation to somnolence and coma. Visual disturbances, especially blurred vision, are common in hyperglycemia. Generally, altered levels of consciousness are more pronounced in patients with HHS. This is due to the severity of hyperglycemia, serum hyperosmolality, and electrolyte disturbances. Seizures and focal neurological signs may also be present and often lead to misdiagnosis in patients with HHS.

In DKA, ketonuria and metabolic acidosis are seen. Kussmaul respirations and an acetone breath odor are additional clinical signs of ketosis. Later in the disease process, the respiratory status of the patient may be influenced by the neurological status, precipitating impaired breathing patterns and reduced gas exchange. Various degrees of changes in consciousness also occur due to the acidotic state. The flushed face associated with DKA is the result of superficial vasodilation. See the Lifespan Considerations box for additional information related to older adults and pregnant people.

Laboratory evaluation. Numerous diagnostic studies are used to evaluate for the presence of DKA and HHS, to rule out other diseases, and to detect complications (see Laboratory Alert box). In addition, cultures and tests are performed to determine any precipitating factors, such as infection or myocardial

TABLE 19.2 Manifestations of Diabetic Ketoacidosis and Hyperosmolar Hyperglycemic State

	Diabetic Ketoacidosis	Hyperosmolar Hyperglycemic State
Pathophysiology	Relative or absolute insulin deficiency resulting in cellular dehydration and volume depletion, acidosis, and protein catabolism	Insulin deficiency resulting in dehydration and hyperosmolality
Health history	History of type 1 diabetes mellitus (DM) or use of insulin Signs and symptoms of hyperglycemia before admission Can also occur in type 2 DM in severe stress	History of type 2 DM signs and symptoms of hyperglycemia before admission Occurs most frequently in older adults with preexisting renal and cardiovascular disease
Onset	Develops quickly	Develops insidiously
Clinical presentation	Flushed, dry skin Dry mucous membranes ↓ Skin turgor Tachycardia Hypotension Kussmaul respirations Acetone breath Altered level of consciousness Visual disturbances Polydipsia Nausea and vomiting Anorexia Abdominal pain	Flushed, dry skin Dry mucous membranes ↓ Skin turgor (may not be present in older adult) Tachycardia Hypotension Shallow respirations Altered level of consciousness (generally more profound and may include absent deep tendon reflexes, paresis, and positive Babinski sign)
Diagnostics	↑ Plasma glucose (average: 675 mg/dL) pH <7.30 ↓ Bicarbonate Ketosis Azotemia Electrolytes vary with state of hydration; often hyperkalemic Plasma hyperosmolality (average: 330 mOsm/kg)	↑ Plasma glucose (usually >1000 mg/dL) pH >7.30 Bicarbonate >15 mEq/L Absence of significant ketosis Azotemia Electrolytes vary with state of hydration; often hypernatremic Plasma hyperosmolality (average: 350 mOsm/kg) Hypotonic urine

infarction. Failing to identify underlying illnesses that may have precipitated the hyperglycemic crisis increases the risk of poor patient outcomes.

In DKA, an initial arterial blood gas analysis reflects metabolic acidosis (low pH and low bicarbonate level). The bicarbonate is initially low as circulating bicarbonate buffers the excess circulating hydrogen ions. The arterial partial pressure of carbon dioxide ($PaCO_2$) may be low, reflecting the respiratory system's compensatory mechanism, hyperventilation. Acidosis is subsequently monitored by venous pH, which correlates well with arterial pH but is easier to obtain and process. In DKA, the serum glucose is usually in the range of 250 mg/dL to 500 mg/dL.[6] The severity of DKA is determined by the pH, bicarbonate level, ketone values, and the patient's mental status.[8]

In HHS, the laboratory results are similar to those in DKA but with four major differences: (1) the serum glucose concentration in HHS is usually significantly more elevated than in DKA and may exceed 1000 mg/dL, (2) plasma osmolality is higher in HHS than in DKA and is associated with the degree of dehydration, (3) acidosis is not present or is very mild in HHS compared with DKA, and (4) ketosis is usually absent or very mild in HHS compared with DKA because of the availability of basal insulin.[8,13] Serum electrolyte concentrations may be low, normal, or elevated and are not reliable indicators of total body stores of electrolytes or water.

Nursing and Medical Interventions. Primary interventions in the treatment of DKA and HHS include respiratory support, fluid replacement, administration of insulin to correct hyperglycemia, replacement of electrolytes, correction of acidosis in DKA, prevention of complications, and patient teaching and support (see Evidence-Based Practice box).

Respiratory support. Assessment of the airway, breathing, and circulation is always the first priority in managing life-threatening disorders. Support airway and breathing as needed through the use of oral airways and oxygen therapy. In more severe cases, the patient may be intubated and require ventilatory support. Prevent aspiration by elevating the head of the bed. Collaborate with the provider to determine the need for nasogastric tube suction in a patient with impaired mentation who is actively vomiting.

Fluid replacement. Fluid replacement reduces insulin resistance by increasing intravascular volume *and* improving renal perfusion, which halts the actions of counterregulatory hormones.[6] Dehydration may progress to hypovolemic shock by the time of admission. Immediate IV access and rehydration must be initiated. In DKA, the typical water deficit approximates 100 mL/kg, and it may be as high as 200 mL/kg in HHS.[8] Monitor for signs and symptoms of hypovolemic shock, and assess vital signs and neurological status at least every hour initially. Changes in mentation may indicate a change in fluid status. In unstable patients,

LIFESPAN CONSIDERATIONS

Diabetes

Older Adults

- With aging, pancreatic endocrine function declines. Fasting glucose levels trend upward with age, and glucose tolerance decreases.[2] These changes are caused by a combination of decreased insulin production and increased insulin resistance, independent of any other coexisting disease states.
- Fifty percent of adults aged 65 years and older have elevated blood glucose levels and are at increased risk for diabetes (prediabetes).[15]
- The incidence of diabetes mellitus (DM) increases with age, and 30% of adults older than 65 years of age have diabetes, primarily type 2 DM.[7]
- Older adults are more prone to develop hyperosmolar hyperglycemic state.
- Older adults have a decreased sense of thirst; therefore this sign may not be observed during hyperglycemic crises.
- The risk for lack of awareness of hypoglycemia is higher in older adults.
- Older adults with diabetes are more likely to have comorbid conditions, such as cardiac or renal disease, and to take medications that make them more reactive to electrolyte imbalances.[15]
- Older adults are more likely to be affected by geriatric syndromes such as cognitive dysfunction, polypharmacy, depression, and pain.[15]
- Older adults with diabetes often respond more slowly to treatments.

Pregnant People

- Gestational diabetes mellitus (GDM) is glucose intolerance that develops or is first recognized during pregnancy.[10] Many females with GDM have previously undiagnosed type or type 2 DM.[9]
- Unless females have an increased risk, screen for GDM between the 24th and 28th weeks of pregnancy.[10] Individuals who develop GDM have a significant risk for type 2 diabetes and long-term metabolic and cardiovascular concerns later in life.[9]
- Screen pregnant people with risk factors for type 2 DM (e.g., polycystic ovarian syndrome, significant obesity) at the first prenatal appointment.
- GDM is managed with blood glucose monitoring, medical nutrition therapy, and exercise. Oral agents (e.g., metformin, glyburide) and insulin therapy are added to the GDM treatment regimen if initial glucose-lowering interventions fail.[10] The risks for the neonate include macrosomia, birth trauma, neonatal hypoglycemia, and hyperbilirubinemia.[10,16]
- Individuals with pregestational type 1 or type 2 DM require intensive monitoring before, during, and after a pregnancy. Blood levels of glycated hemoglobin (HbA1c) greater than 7% at the time of conception increase the risk for early pregnancy loss and major fetal malformations, including anencephaly and congenital heart defects.[10]
- People with a history of pregestational DM should seek preconception counseling, which includes interventions to optimize blood glucose, evaluate and treat chronic diabetes-related complications such as nephropathy and retinopathy, and assess for the risk of non–diabetes-related fetal and maternal risks.[10]
- Uncontrolled DM during pregnancy increases the risk for preeclampsia, intrauterine fetal demise, neonatal hyperbilirubinemia, and neonatal hypoglycemia.[16]
- All neonates of females who experienced DM during the pregnancy require intensive assessment for hypoglycemia after delivery.
- Blood glucose targets of less than 95 mg/dL fasting, less than 140 mg/dL 1 hour after meals, and less than 120 mg/dL 2 hours after meals are desired in pregnant people with DM.[10]
- Because many antihyperglycemic agents are contraindicated in pregnancy, prepregnancy DM medication regimens may require adjustment to limit fetal risks and achieve target glycemic levels. Intensive insulin therapy is indicated for management in most individuals with pregestational diabetes.
- The first trimester in pregnant people with pregestational type 1 DM is characterized by an increased risk of maternal hypoglycemia.[10]
- The influence of increasing levels of counterregulatory hormones such as growth hormone, cortisol, and glucagon causes the person to become more insulin resistant during the second and third trimesters of pregnancy.[10] Insulin demands may double in the later stages of pregnancy, necessitating frequent insulin dose adjustments. These increasing insulin demands increase the risk for development of diabetic ketoacidosis (DKA).
- Pregnant people with pregestational DM are often given insulin infusions during labor and immediately after delivery. Individuals with type 1 DM are at an exceptionally high risk for hypoglycemia in the days and weeks after delivery because of the rapid reductions in circulating counterregulatory hormones.[10]

monitor and record hemodynamic parameters at least every 15 minutes. Hemodynamic monitoring may be instituted to evaluate fluid requirements, monitor the patient's response to treatment, and watch for signs of hypervolemia from overaggressive replacement (Chapter 9, Hemodynamic Monitoring). This is particularly true for patients with HHS, who tend to be older and to have concurrent cardiovascular and renal disease. Measure intake and output hourly, and record weight daily. Evaluate the effectiveness of fluid replacement by assessing hemodynamic status, intake and output, laboratory measures, cardiopulmonary status, and the patient's general physical condition, particularly mental status.

Accepted guidelines for fluid replacement recommend 0.9% normal saline (0.9% NS) as the fluid of choice for fluid resuscitation. However, recent studies have shown that balanced isotonic solutions (i.e., Lactated Ringer's or Plasma-Lyte A) are effective alternatives for fluid resuscitation and may have shorter time to DKA resolution than 0.9% NS.[13,17] Fluid replacement usually starts with an initial bolus of 1 L. This is followed by an infusion of 10 to 15 mL/kg during the first hour if the patient is not in shock.[8,13] A rate of 20 mL/kg/h may be required if the patient shows clinical signs of shock. If the serum sodium level is elevated or normal, the IV fluid is changed to hypotonic saline (0.45% NS) and is infused at a slower rate to replace intracellular fluid deficits.[13] When the plasma glucose level approaches 250 mg/dL in DKA and 300 mg/dL in HHS, 5% to 10% dextrose is added to fluids to prevent hypoglycemia and assist in the resolution of ketosis.[6,13] The goal is to replace half of the estimated fluid deficit over the first 8 hours. The second half of the fluid deficit should be replaced during the next 16 hours of therapy so that the volume is restored in most patients within the first 24 hours of treatment.[8] Significant improvements in hyperglycemia may be seen with fluid resuscitation before initiation of insulin therapy. Hyperglycemia resolves more quickly than ketosis. IV fluids and insulin are continued until the acidosis is corrected.[6]

The goal of fluid resuscitation is normovolemia. Prevent hypervolemia, especially in patients with ischemic heart disease, heart failure, acute kidney injury, or chronic kidney

LABORATORY ALERT

Pancreatic Endocrine Disorders

Serum Laboratory Test	Critical Value[a]	Significance
Glucose	≥200 mg/dL (2 h postprandial or random)	Combined with symptoms, establishes diagnosis of diabetes mellitus
	≥126 mg/dL (fasting)	
	>250 mg/dL	Suggestive of DKA
	>600 mg/dL	Suggestive of HHS
	<70 mg/dL	Hypoglycemia
	<50 mg/dL	Critical hypoglycemia
Potassium	>6.1 mEq/L	Potential for heart blocks, bradydysrhythmias, sinus arrest, ventricular fibrillation, or asystole
	<3.0 mEq/L	Potential for ventricular dysrhythmias; muscle weakness, including respiratory arrest; will further decrease with insulin administration
Sodium	>160 mEq/L	May be a result of stress and profound dehydration
	<120 mEq/L	Usually associated with disorders other than diabetes
BUN	>100 mg/dL	Values >20 mg/dL may be observed due to protein breakdown and hemoconcentration
Bicarbonate	<10 mEq/L	Decreased in DKA due to immediate compensation for acidosis
pH	<7.3	Decreased in DKA due to accumulation of nonvolatile acids
Osmolality	>320 mOsm/kg H_2O	Elevated in DKA relative to dehydration; higher in HHS
Phosphorus	<1.0 mg/dL	May result in impaired respiratory and cardiac functions; values <2.5 mg/dL are often observed and will further decrease with insulin administration
Magnesium	<0.5 mEq/L	Depleted by osmotic diuresis; may coincide with decreased potassium and calcium levels; may result in dysrhythmias
β-Hydroxybutyrate	>3.0 mg/dL	Reflects blood ketosis in DKA
Anion gap	>16 mEq/L	Reflects blood ketosis in DKA

[a]Critical values vary by facility and laboratory.

BUN, Blood urea nitrogen; *DKA,* diabetic ketoacidosis; *HHS,* hyperosmolar hyperglycemic state.

From Pagana K, Pagana T, Pagana T. *Mosby's Diagnostic and Laboratory Test Reference.* 15th ed. St. Louis, MO: Elsevier; 2021.

EVIDENCE-BASED PRACTICE

Tight Glycemic Control

Problem

Tight glycemic control in critically ill patients has been debated. Issues and outcomes of achieving glycemic control need to be identified.

Clinical Question

What are the outcomes and issues associated with tight glycemic control in critically ill patients?

Evidence

Current systematic reviews and meta-analyses have critically evaluated the effect of tight glycemic control on mortality and hypoglycemic outcomes. Yamada and colleagues analyzed data from 36 randomized clinical trials and compared outcomes of various levels of glycemic control: tight (80 to <110 mg/dL), moderate (110 to <140 mg/dL), mild (140 to <180 mg/dL), and very mild (180 to 220 mg/dL). They found no reduction in mortality with tight glycemic control in critically ill patients. Severe hypoglycemia with tight control in comparison with mild or very mild control was noted.

Yao and colleagues conducted a systematic review and meta-analysis that included 57 randomized controlled trial studies and 21,840 patients in the analysis. Patients admitted to critical care managed by insulin protocols to maintain serum glucose at 140 to 180 mg/dL were found to have statistically reduced all-cause mortality, reduced infection rate, lower occurrence of acquired sepsis, and shorter length of stay.

Conclusion

Because tight glycemic control is associated with a greater risk of severe hypoglycemia, a target range of 140 to 180 mg/dL is recommended. Many IV insulin protocols used in critical care units and basal-nutrition-correction insulin protocols used in medical-surgical units have adopted these glycemic targets.

Implications for Nursing

Current evidence on inpatient glycemic management supports continuous IV insulin infusion protocols over traditional sliding-scale regimens. The use of insulin protocols improves glycemic control and reduces treatment-related complications, specifically hypoglycemia. Understanding how to use the insulin protocol to reach target glucose range improves patient outcomes.

Level of Evidence

A—Systematic review and meta-analysis

References

Yamada T, Shojima N, Noma H et al. Glycemic control, mortality, and hypoglycemia in critically ill patients: a systematic review and network meta-analysis of randomized controlled trials. *Intensive Care Med.* 2017;43(1):1-15.

Yao RQ, Ren C, Wu GS, Zhu YB, Xia ZF, Yao YM. Is intensive glucose control bad for critically ill patients? A systematic review and meta-analysis. *Int J Biol Sci.* 2020;16(9):1658-1675. http://doi.org/10.7150/ijbs.43447.

disease. Signs and symptoms of fluid overload are reviewed in Box 19.5. Rapid fluid administration may contribute to cerebral edema and osmotic demyelination syndrome (ODS). A rapid decrease in the plasma glucose level, combined with rapid fluid administration and concurrent insulin therapy (see next section), may lead to movement of water into brain cells, resulting in brain edema, which can be fatal. Assessment of neurological status during the initial phases of fluid replacement and glucose lowering is imperative.

Insulin therapy. Insulin dosing in HHS differs from dosing in DKA. Patients with HHS may not need insulin initially because serum glucose levels may improve with fluid resuscitation.[13] Before starting insulin therapy, fluid replacement therapy must be underway, and the serum potassium level must be greater than 3.3 mEq/L.[8] During the insulin infusion, monitor serum glucose levels hourly using a consistent monitoring method. It is important that serum glucose levels not be lowered too rapidly. A steady decrease of 50 to 70 mg/dL/h is recommended to prevent cerebral edema, which could result in seizures and coma.[8,13] Any patient who exhibits an abrupt change in level of consciousness after initiation of insulin therapy requires frequent blood glucose monitoring and institution of protective steps to prevent harm (e.g., seizure precautions). Treatment of acute cerebral edema usually involves administration of an osmotic diuretic (e.g., 20% mannitol solution). The goal is to restore normal glucose uptake by cells while preventing complications of excess insulin administration, such as hypoglycemia, hypokalemia, and hypophosphatemia. Hyperglycemic crises are commonly treated with IV insulin infusions because absorption is more predictable.

For DKA, an initial IV bolus of 0.1 unit/kg of regular insulin is administered, followed by a continuous infusion of 0.1 unit/kg/h. If the patient has severe acidosis or high baseline insulin requirements, an infusion of 0.2 to 0.3 units/kg/h may be required.[6] Maintain the initial insulin infusion rate until the pH exceeds 7.3 and bicarbonate concentration is greater than 18 mEq/L, at which time the insulin infusion may be decreased to 0.05 unit/kg/h with a target glucose value of 150 to 200 mg/dL until acidosis is completely resolved.[8,18] Patients with DKA may be transitioned to subcutaneous insulin when the blood glucose is 200 mg/dL or less when at least two of the following criteria are met: (1) venous pH is greater than 7.30, (2) serum bicarbonate level is greater than 18 mEq/L, and (3) calculated anion gap is 12 mEq/L or less.[8] Patients with mild to moderate DKA may be treated with hourly subcutaneous injections of rapid-acting insulin using a titration scale.

For patients with HHS, an insulin infusion at a rate of 0.05 to 0.1 units/kg/h with no bolus is recommended.[8,13] In patients with HHS, insulin infusion rates may be decreased to 0.2 to 0.5 unit/kg/h when the glucose values reach 300 mg/dL.[8] Target glucose values of 200 to 300 mg/dL should be maintained until the patient's mental status improves, at which time the patient may be transitioned to subcutaneous insulin therapy. For both DKA and HHS, subcutaneous insulin therapy should be initiated 1 to 2 hours before the IV insulin infusion is discontinued to avoid recurrence of hyperglycemia, acidosis, and ketogenesis.[13,18]

Electrolyte management. Potassium, phosphate, chloride, and magnesium replacement may be required, especially during insulin administration. Osmotic diuresis in DKA and HHS results in total body potassium depletion ranging from 400 to 600 mEq. The potassium deficit may be greater in HHS. Insulin therapy promotes translocation of potassium into the intracellular space, resulting in a further decrease in serum potassium levels.

The need for potassium therapy is based on serum laboratory results. In the absence of renal disease, insulin replacement and monitoring begin after (1) the first liter of IV fluid has been administered, (2) the serum potassium level is greater than 3.3 mEq/L, and (3) the patient is producing urine. At that point, 20 to 30 mEq/L/h of potassium may be added to each liter of fluid and augmented by additional doses of intermittent potassium infusions.[8] Maintain serum potassium levels between 4 and 5 mEq/L during the course of therapy. In the event that a patient is admitted with hypokalemia, insulin therapy should be withheld until potassium values exceed 3.3 mEq/L.[6,8] Maintain the integrity of the IV site to prevent extravasation. Monitor cardiac rhythm and respiratory status during potassium administration.

Hypophosphatemia occurs due to transcellular shifts and osmotic diuresis, but serum phosphate levels may remain normal. Insulin therapy may cause further reduction in phosphate levels. Phosphate replacement is not routine because there is a lack of supporting data of efficacy of replenishment during DKA and the risk for hypocalcemia.[6,18] Replacement may occur at a rate of 20 to 30 mEq/L added to replacement fluids when there is associated respiratory or cardiac dysfunction.[6,8] Phosphate replacement is used with extreme caution in patients with renal failure because these patients are unable to excrete phosphate and typically have underlying hyperphosphatemia.

Treatment of acidosis. Acidosis is a hallmark feature of DKA. However, many studies have shown that treatment with sodium bicarbonate is often not beneficial and may pose increased risks of hypoglycemia, cerebral edema, cellular hypoxemia secondary to decreased uptake of oxygen by body tissues, worsening hypokalemia, and development of central nervous system acidosis.[8] Therefore sodium bicarbonate is not routinely used to treat acidosis unless the serum pH is less than 7.0. Bicarbonate replacement is used only to bring the pH up to 7.1 but not to normal levels.[6] Serum blood gas analysis is done frequently to assess for changes in pH, bicarbonate, anion gap, $PaCO_2$, and oxygenation status. Once fluid and electrolyte imbalances are corrected and insulin is administered, the kidneys begin to conserve bicarbonate to restore acid-base homeostasis, and ketone formation ceases.

Patient and family education. A primary intervention to prevent DKA is patient education. Incorporate essential content into patient education: (1) manage blood glucose levels with

BOX 19.5 Signs and Symptoms of Fluid Overload

- Tachypnea
- Neck vein distension
- Tachycardia
- Crackles
- Increased pulmonary artery occlusion or right atrial pressures
- Declining level of consciousness

diet, exercise, and medication; (2) monitor HbA1C levels three or four times per year to assess long-term control of blood glucose levels, changing insulin needs, and psychosocial or behavioral factors that may affect control[7]; (3) maintain a regular schedule for eating, exercise, rest, sleep, and relaxation; (4) adjust the usual diabetic control regimen for illness (known as "sick day management"); and (5) identify strategies to prevent complications. If the patient has an episode of DKA while on insulin pump therapy, reeducate the patient about pump features, insulin pump safety, management of pump failure, and troubleshooting abnormal glucose levels. Instruct patients to avoid exercise and excessive activities when blood glucose levels exceed 240 mg/dL and urine ketones are present.

Patient Outcomes. Outcomes for a patient with DKA or HHS are included with specific aspects due to hyperglycemia management in the Plan of Care for the Patient with Hyperglycemic Crisis (see also the Collaborative Plan of Care for the Critically Ill Patient in Chapter 1, Overview of Critical Care Nursing).

Hypoglycemia

Hypoglycemia can be life-threatening and requires rapid assessment and treatment. Evaluating and treating the cause of the hypoglycemia is equally important in the care of acute and critically ill individuals.

CLINICAL JUDGMENT ACTIVITY

Insulin therapy is a critical intervention in the treatment of diabetic ketoacidosis (DKA) and hyperosmolar hyperglycemic state (HHS). Explain which crucial parameters must be monitored and the associated goals of each parameter to ensure optimal patient outcomes.

Pathophysiology. A hypoglycemic episode is defined as a decrease in the plasma glucose level to less than 70 mg/dL, with a critical hypoglycemic glucose level of less than 50 mg/dL. Hypoglycemic events may sometimes be referred to as *insulin shock or insulin reaction*. Glucose production falls behind glucose use, resulting in decreased blood glucose levels. Because the brain is an obligate user of glucose, the first clinical sign of hypoglycemia is a change in mental status. A hypoglycemic event activates the sympathetic nervous system, causing a rise in counterregulatory hormones, including glucagon, epinephrine, cortisol, and growth hormone. Those at highest risk for hypoglycemia are patients taking insulin; children and pregnant people with type 1 DM; patients with autonomic diabetic neuropathy; older adults with type 1 or type 2 DM; and patients with type 2 DM who are taking SGLT2 inhibitors, GLP-1 receptor agonists, sulfonylureas, thiazolidinediones, and exogenous insulin.[9,15]

PLAN OF CARE

For the Patient With Hyperglycemic Crisis

Patient Problem

Dehydration. Risk factors include osmotic diuresis, ketosis, increased lipolysis, and vomiting.

Desired Outcomes

- Normal serum glucose levels.
- Hemodynamic stability: normal sinus rhythm, blood pressure, heart rate, right atrial pressure, and pulmonary artery occlusion pressure within normal limits.
- Urine output greater than 0.5 mL/kg/h.
- Balanced intake and output.
- Stable weight.
- Warm, dry extremities.
- Normal skin turgor.
- Moist mucous membranes.
- Serum osmolality and serum electrolyte levels (sodium, potassium, calcium, phosphorus) within normal limits.
- pH within normal limits.

Nursing Assessments/Interventions	Rationales

• Assess fluid status:
  ○ Vital signs every hour until stable.
  ○ I&O measurements every 1-2 h.
  ○ Skin turgor, mucous membranes, thirst.
  ○ Consider insensible fluid losses.
  ○ Daily weight.
	• Provides clinical indications of hypovolemia and provides data for restoring cellular function.

• Initiate fluid replacement therapy:
  ○ Monitor for signs and symptoms of fluid overload.
  ○ Monitor effects of volume repletion.
	• Corrects volume deficit and prevents or treats hypovolemic shock; neurological status should improve as electrolytes normalize.

• Monitor neurological status closely.	• Mental status changes may indicate cerebral edema if glycemic correction is too rapid.

• Administer IV insulin infusion per hospital protocol:
  ○ Titrate therapy hourly based on glucose levels.
  ○ Provide a steady decrease in serum glucose levels; a decrease of 50-70 mg/dL/h is desired.
	• Prevent cerebral edema and potentially dangerous electrolyte abnormalities.

Continued

PLAN OF CARE—cont'd

Nursing Assessments/Interventions	Rationales
• Monitor glucose every hour via consistent method (serum or fingerstick capillary) during insulin infusion.	• Assess response to therapy and allow for immediate correction of glycemic abnormalities.
• Monitor for signs and symptoms of hypoglycemia.	• Hypoglycemia may occur if insulin dose exceeds patient's needs.
• Add dextrose to maintenance IV solutions once serum glucose level reaches 250 mg/dL in DKA or 300 mg/dL in HHS.	• Prevent relative hypoglycemia and a decrease in plasma osmolality that could result in cerebral edema.
• Monitor serum electrolyte levels (sodium, potassium, calcium, phosphorus); administer supplements according to protocols.	• Prevent complications of electrolyte imbalance; osmotic diuresis may result in increased excretion of potassium and hyponatremia.
• Assess causes of continuing electrolyte depletion (i.e., diuresis, vomiting, NG suction).	• Insulin therapy causes potassium and phosphate to shift to the intracellular space.
• Monitor pH.	• pH is the best indicator of acidosis and response to treatment. • Acidosis corrects more slowly than hyperglycemia. • Correction of hyperglycemia without correction of ketosis may result in recurrence of DKA.
• Administer bicarbonate only in severe acidosis (pH <7.0).	• Routine administration of bicarbonate has been associated with hypokalemia, hypoglycemia, cellular ischemia, cerebral edema, and CNS cellular acidosis.

Patient Problem

Need for Health Teaching (Patient and Family). Risk factors include the complexity of the disease process and treatment plan, as well as the health literacy of the learner.

Desired Outcomes

- Patient/family can describe the pathophysiology and causes of DKA and/or HHS; preventive interventions due to diet, exercise regimen, and medications; signs and symptoms of hypoglycemia and hyperglycemia; signs and symptoms of infections that require medical follow-up; sick day management; and emergency hypoglycemia management.
- Patient/family can identify the patient's individual glucose targets.
- Patient/family can demonstrate self-monitoring of blood glucose levels and administration of oral hypoglycemic medications and/or insulin therapy according to glucose values.

Nursing Assessments/Interventions	Rationales
• Assess patient/family's current diabetes self-management practices, ability to learn information, and psychomotor and sensory skills.	• Allow for individualization of patient's plan of care to match physical, psychosocial, and educational needs.
• Identify psychosocial factors that may preclude effective self-management.	• Address factors in patient education to promote self-management.
• Implement a teaching program that includes information on pathophysiology and causes of DKA or HHS; diet and exercise restrictions; individualized target glucose values; signs and symptoms of hypoglycemia and hyperglycemia, including interventions; and signs and symptoms of infection and illness, including interventions.	• Prevention of acute diabetes complications primarily rests with the patient and/or family who are capable and able to follow the self-management plan and act early on significant physiological changes.
• Demonstrate methods for blood glucose monitoring.	• Regular glucose monitoring is essential for patient self-management.
• If the patient takes insulin, demonstrate administration. • Review insulin pump use and abilities if used for treatment. • For each skill, have the patient demonstrate abilities with repeat demonstration.	• Ensure that patient/family has the ability to perform the skills involved in at-home monitoring, insulin delivery, and problem solving due to abnormal glucose findings before discharge.
• Review administration of hypoglycemic medications and/or insulin, including dosage, frequency, action, duration, side effects, and situations in which medication may need to be adjusted.	• Patients/family require a thorough knowledge of insulin therapy to optimize treatment. • Failure to adjust hypoglycemic medications to match changing glycemic demands may result in acute hyperglycemia or hypoglycemia.
• Consult with clinical dietitian regarding disease-specific nutrition and diet needs.	• Assists in identifying the appropriate diet based on the patient's condition and caloric needs.
• Encourage patient to wear a form of identification for diabetes.	• Assists in prompt recognition and treatment of complications should they occur.
• Provide written materials for all content taught; provide means for the patient to get questions answered after discharge and schedule follow-up diabetes self-management education after discharge.	• Effective diabetes self-management education is a collaboration between the patient, family, and the multiprofessional team. • Improve glycemic control and self-management outcomes.

CNS, Central nervous system; *DKA,* diabetic ketoacidosis; *HHS,* hyperosmolar hyperglycemic state; *I&O,* intake and output; *NG,* nasogastric.
Adapted from Snyder J, Sump C. *Swearingen's All-in-One Nursing Care Planning Resource.* 6th ed. St. Louis: Elsevier; 2024.

Hypoglycemia unawareness, also known as *hypoglycemia-associated autonomic failure,* describes a diabetes-related condition in which a patient does not recognize the onset of hypoglycemic signs and symptoms.[5] In this complication, the impairment of the autonomic nervous systems results in a blunted response to critically low glucose levels (see Clinical Alert box). Patients with hypoglycemia unawareness may remain asymptomatic while experiencing extremely low blood glucose levels. Patients who have other forms of autonomic neuropathy, such as orthostasis, gastroparesis, erectile dysfunction, and cardiac autonomic neuropathy, are also at higher risk for this condition. Those at highest risk of hypoglycemia unawareness include older adults because of their impeded stress responses and patients with diminished mental function resulting from dementia, concurrent illness, or other factors. Patients taking beta-blockers are at risk for decreased awareness of signs of hypoglycemia because of the medication's effect on the sympathetic nervous system. The pathophysiological mechanisms associated with acute hypoglycemia and the associated central nervous system and sympathetic symptoms are reviewed in Fig. 19.5.

! CLINICAL ALERT

Hypoglycemia Unawareness

Some patients have hypoglycemia unawareness, in which the individual may be asymptomatic despite extremely low blood glucose levels. Older adult patients and those taking beta-blockers are at especially high risk of hypoglycemic unawareness.

Etiology. Many hypoglycemic episodes in the hospital are preventable. The increased incidence of hypoglycemia in critically ill patients is associated with reduction in or discontinuation of nutrition without adjustment of insulin therapy (e.g., interruption of parenteral or enteral feedings during diagnostic examinations); decreased caloric intake due to missed or delayed meal; nausea and vomiting; anorexia; heart failure; kidney disease; liver disease; sepsis; and the use of or change in dosage of inotropic medications, vasopressor support, and glucocorticoid therapy.[1] Closely monitor patients receiving insulin therapy for hypoglycemia. Insulin requirements may be lower because of weight loss, renal insufficiency, increase in insulin dose, new prescription or adjustment in nondiabetic medications that affect blood glucose, and rotation of insulin injection sites from a hypertrophied area to one with unimpaired absorption. In addition, patients who use oral agents that promote production and release of endogenous insulin, such as long-acting sulfonylureas, are at risk for hypoglycemia. Amylin and agents that mimic or act on incretin hormones (e.g., exenatide and gliptins) also increase the risk for a hypoglycemic episode when they are combined with insulin or secretagogues. As a patient recovers from a stress event (e.g., infection illness, corticosteroid therapy, postpartum), the need for exogenous insulin decreases, and failure to adjust the insulin dose can precipitate hypoglycemia. Other major causes of hypoglycemia are reviewed in Box 19.6.

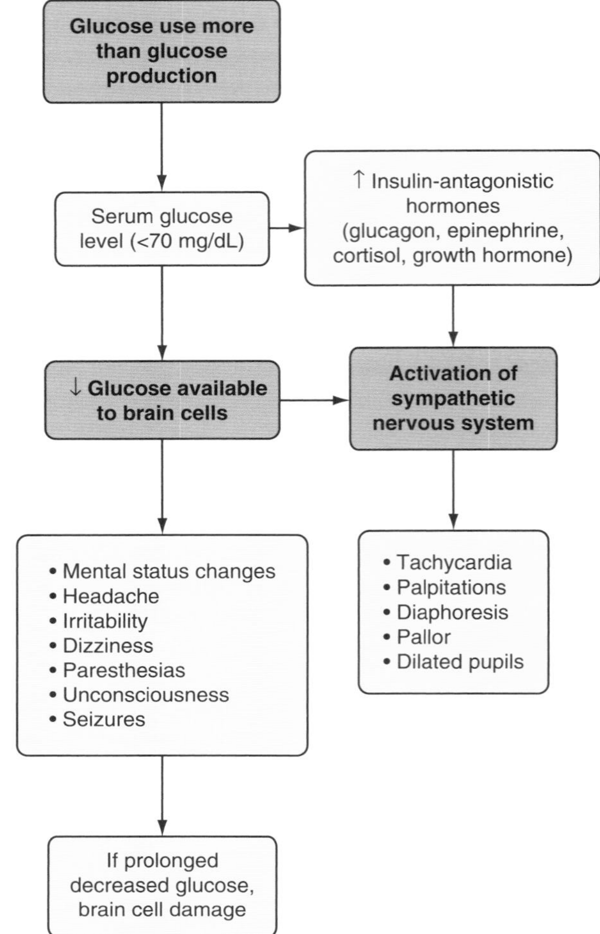

Fig. 19.5 Pathophysiology of hypoglycemia.

Both severe hypoglycemia and hypoglycemia unawareness place a patient at risk for injury secondary to falls and seizures. Patients with renal impairment or liver dysfunction are at particular risk for a severe hypoglycemic episode. Delayed degradation or excretion of hypoglycemic medications potentiates or prolongs the action of many diabetes medications. The resulting increase in circulating levels of active drug, including insulin, results in erratic glucose control. Close glucose monitoring and patient and family education on prevention, recognition, and treatment of hypoglycemia are critical to promote safety in these very high-risk patients.

Assessment

Clinical presentation. Common signs and symptoms of hypoglycemia are summarized in Table 19.3. Symptoms of hypoglycemia are categorized as (1) mild symptoms from autonomic nervous system stimulation that are characteristic of a rapid decrease in serum glucose levels and (2) moderate symptoms reflective of an inadequate supply of glucose to neural tissues that are associated with a slower, more prolonged decline in serum glucose levels. With a rapid decrease in serum glucose levels, there is activation of the sympathetic nervous system mediated by epinephrine release from the adrenal medulla. This compensatory fight-or-flight mechanism results in symptoms

BOX 19.6 Causes of Hypoglycemia

Excess Insulin or Oral Hypoglycemics
- Dose of insulin or oral hypoglycemics too high
- Islet cell tumors (insulinomas)
- Liver insufficiency or failure (impaired metabolism of insulin)
- Acute kidney injury (impaired inactivation of insulin)
- Autoimmune phenomenon
- Medications that potentiate action of antidiabetic medications (e.g., propranolol, oxytetracycline, antibiotics)
- Sulfonylureas in older adult patients
- Amylin and incretin mimetic diabetes agents

Decreased Oral, Enteral, or Parenteral Intake
Underproduction of Glucose
- Heavy alcohol consumption
- Medications: aspirin, disopyramide (Norpace), haloperidol (Haldol)
- Decreased production by liver
- Hormonal imbalances

Too-Rapid Use of Glucose
- Gastrointestinal surgery
- Extrapancreatic tumor
- Increased or strenuous exercise

TABLE 19.3 Signs and Symptoms of Hypoglycemia

DECREASE IN BLOOD SUGAR	
Rapid: Activation of Sympathetic Nervous System	**Prolonged: Inadequate Glucose Supply to Neural Tissues**
Nervousness	Headache
Apprehension	Restlessness
Tachycardia	Difficulty speaking
Palpitations	Difficulty thinking
Pallor	Visual disturbances
Diaphoresis	Paresthesia
Dilated pupils	Difficulty walking
Tremors	Altered consciousness
Fatigue	Coma
General weakness	Convulsions
Headache	Change in personality
Hunger	Psychiatric reactions
	Maniacal behavior
	Catatonia
	Acute paranoia

such as tachycardia; palpitations; tremors; cool, clammy skin; diaphoresis; hunger; pallor; and dilated pupils. The patient may also report feelings of apprehension, nervousness, headache, tremulousness, and general weakness.

Slower and more prolonged declines in serum glucose levels result in symptoms associated with inadequate glucose supply to neural tissues *(neuroglycopenia)*. These include restlessness, difficulty in thinking and speaking, visual disturbances, and paresthesias. The patient may have profound changes in level of consciousness, seizures, or both. Personality changes and psychiatric manifestations have been reported. Prolonged hypoglycemia may lead to irreversible brain damage and coma.[18]

Laboratory evaluation. In most patients, the confirming laboratory test for hypoglycemia is a serum or capillary blood glucose level lower than 70 mg/dL. Adults with a history of hypoglycemia unawareness, those who are cognitively impaired, and older adults at high risk for falls may have higher target glucose ranges and an individualized protocol for management of lower glucose values.[5] Assess the glucose level in all high-risk patients before initiating treatment. Obtain a history of baseline values before treatment because patients who have experienced elevated glucose levels for some time may complain of hypoglycemia-like symptoms when their glucose levels are corrected to a normal range. In patients with a known history of DM, obtain a thorough history of past experiences of hypoglycemia, including patient-specific associated signs and symptoms. Identify the glucose level at which symptoms appear, which varies from patient to patient. In addition, evaluate renal function in patients with long-standing diabetes who have a new history of recurrent hypoglycemia. Decreased renal function may result in impaired clearance of insulin and erratic glucose control in patients who are taking short-acting insulins, long-acting insulins, or oral insulin secretagogues (i.e., glipizide).

Patient Problems. The following problems may apply to a patient with a hypoglycemic episode:
- Potential for hypoglycemia due to excess circulating insulin in relation to available plasma glucose
- Changes in mental status due to decreased glucose delivery to the brain and nervous tissue
- Risk for seizures and falls due to altered neuronal function
- Need for health teaching due to hypoglycemia: prevention, recognition, and treatment of hypoglycemia

Nursing and Medical Interventions. Hypoglycemia management protocols should be implemented in the hospital to help provide a plan for preventing and treating hypoglycemia.[1] Protocols should provide direction on hypoglycemic glucose levels, frequency of monitoring glucose levels, treatment for hypoglycemic episodes, and recheck time frames.[1] After serum or capillary glucose levels have been confirmed, provide carbohydrates. The patient's neurological status and ability to swallow without aspiration determine the route to be used. Box 19.7 details a protocol for treatment of mild, moderate, and severe hypoglycemia. Box 19.8 lists common food substances that contain at least 15 g of carbohydrate. Reassess glucose levels 15 minutes after treatment. Repeat the treatment if the blood glucose level is less than 70 mg/dL.

In the event of hypoglycemia, temporarily withhold rapid-acting and short-acting insulins. If the patient has an insulin pump, suspend the pump for moderate or severe hypoglycemia, but do not remove the infusion catheter. Do not withhold longer-acting basal insulins in patients receiving subcutaneous insulin therapy who are experiencing hypoglycemia because this will increase the risk for hyperglycemia in all patients and for DKA in patients with type 1 DM.

CHECK YOUR UNDERSTANDING

3. Following an assessment of the blood glucose via fingerstick, a value of 54 mg/dL was obtained on the critical care patient. Determine the priority intervention using the 15/15 rule for glucose management.
   A. 1 glucose tablet and monitor blood glucose again in 15 minutes
   B. ¼ cup (2 ounces or 60 milliliters) of fruit juice and repeat again in 15 minutes
   C. 4 ounces skim or low-fat milk, then repeat fingerstick in 15 minutes to determine next intervention
   D. 1 tablespoon (15 grams) of sugar and repeat fingerstick in 15 minutes to determine effectiveness of intervention

BOX 19.7 Treatment of Hypoglycemia

Mild Hypoglycemia

- Patient is completely alert. Symptoms may include pallor, diaphoresis, tachycardia, palpitations, hunger, or shakiness. Blood glucose is less than 70 mg/dL. Patient is able to drink.
- *Treatment:* 15 g of carbohydrate by mouth

Moderate Hypoglycemia

- Patient is conscious, cooperative, and able to swallow safely. Symptoms may include difficulty concentrating, confusion, slurred speech, or extreme fatigue. Blood glucose is usually less than 50 mg/dL. Patient is able to drink.
- *Treatment:* 20 to 30 g of carbohydrate by mouth

Severe Hypoglycemia

- Patient is uncooperative or unconscious. Blood glucose is usually less than 50 mg/dL or patient is unable to drink.
- *Treatment with IV access:* 12.5 g of 50% dextrose in water solution ($D_{50}W$)
- *Treatment without IV access:* 1 mg of glucagon subcutaneously or intramuscularly and turn patient on the side or observe to avoid potential aspiration from nausea and vomiting side effect

BOX 19.8 15/15 Rule for Hypoglycemia Management

To treat low blood glucose, the 15/15 rule is usually applied. Eat 15 grams (g) of carbohydrates and then recheck your blood glucose 15 minutes later.

15 grams (g) of Carbohydrate Examples

- 3 to 4 glucose tablets[a]
- ½ to 1 tube of glucose gel[a]
- 4 ounces (1/2 cup) of fruit juice
- 1 Tbsp. corn syrup
- 8 ounces of milk—skim or low fat
- 1 Tbsp. of jam, preserves, jelly, honey, or sugar

If blood glucose is still low, repeat these steps.

[a]Ask your pharmacist or healthcare team about how much 15 grams is. From Centers for Disease Control and Prevention. *How to treat low blood sugar (Hypoglycemia).* https://www.cdc.gov/diabetes/basics/low-blood-sugar-treatment.html#print. Updated December 20, 2022. Accessed January 2024.

Perform neurological assessments to detect any changes in cerebral function due to hypoglycemia. Document baseline neurological status, including mental status, cranial nerve function, sensory and motor function, and deep tendon reflexes. Assess for seizure activity that may occur due to altered neuronal cellular metabolism during the hypoglycemic phase. If seizures are observed, describe the seizure event and associated symptoms. Institute seizure precautions, including padded side rails, oxygen, oral airway, bedside suction, and removal of potentially harmful objects from the environment. Neurological status is the best clinical indicator of effective treatment for hypoglycemia.

Patient and Family Education. Provide instruction to the patient and family members on the causes, symptoms, treatment, and prevention of hypoglycemia. Explain hypoglycemia associated with critical illness. Explore their understanding of the relationships of carbohydrate intake, actions of insulin or oral hypoglycemic agents, and activity changes and hypoglycemia risk.

Patients at risk for severe hypoglycemia may be considered for continuous glucose monitoring units and should be prescribed a glucagon emergency kit, with family and significant regular contacts instructed in its use. Encourage the patient to wear emergency medical identification and to perform a blood glucose test before driving. If the patient is at risk for nocturnal hypoglycemia, encourage storage of glucose gel at the bedside. Pregnant people with diabetes are at very high risk for hypoglycemia after delivery as the levels of insulin-resistant hormones drop quickly. Lactating individuals also may be at particular risk and may be encouraged to drink milk while nursing. In addition, instruct patients on the relationship between alcohol ingestion and hypoglycemia. Instruct patients to notify their diabetes care provider if two or more events of hypoglycemia are experienced within 1 week because the medication regimen may require adjustment.

CLINICAL JUDGMENT ACTIVITY

Identify the hazards of hypoglycemia and strategies to prevent hypoglycemic events.

ACUTE AND RELATIVE ADRENAL INSUFFICIENCY

Etiology

Hypofunction of the adrenal gland results from either primary or secondary mechanisms that suppress secretion of cortisol, aldosterone, and androgens. Primary mechanisms, such as Addison's disease, are those that cause destruction of the adrenal gland itself. At least 90% of the adrenal cortex must be destroyed before clinical signs and symptoms appear.[9] Primary disorders result in deficiencies of both glucocorticoids and mineralocorticoids.

Primary adrenal insufficiency has a variety of causes, including idiopathic autoimmune destruction of the gland; infection and sepsis; human immunodeficiency virus (HIV); tuberculosis; hemorrhagic destruction; and granulomatous infiltration from neoplasms, amyloidosis, sarcoidosis, or hemochromatosis.[9]

Idiopathic autoimmune destruction of the adrenal gland is the most common cause of adrenal insufficiency, accounting for 50% to 70% of cases.[9] Autoimmune adrenal destruction may have a genetic component that leads to atrophy of the gland. Genetic adrenal disease may affect just the adrenal gland, or it may be part of a constellation of autoimmune problems, such as autoimmune polyglandular disorder.[19] Young female individuals with spontaneous premature ovarian failure are at increased risk of developing the autoimmune form of adrenal insufficiency.[19]

Secondary mechanisms that can produce adrenal insufficiency are those that decrease adrenocorticotropic hormone (ACTH) secretion; this results in deficiency of glucocorticoids alone because mineralocorticoids are not primarily dependent on ACTH secretion. Mechanisms that can produce secondary adrenal insufficiency include abrupt withdrawal of corticosteroids, pituitary and hypothalamic disorders, and sepsis.[14] A more detailed listing of possible causes of primary and secondary adrenal insufficiency is given in Box 19.9.

The most common cause of acute adrenal insufficiency is abrupt withdrawal from corticosteroid therapy. Long-term corticosteroid use suppresses the normal *corticotropin-releasing hormone–ACTH–adrenal feedback systems* (see Fig. 19.1) and results in adrenal suppression. While it is difficult to accurately predict the degree of adrenal suppression caused by exogenous glucocorticoid therapy, longer-acting agents (e.g., dexamethasone) are more likely to produce suppression than shorter-acting corticosteroids (e.g., hydrocortisone). Once corticosteroid use has been tapered off, it may take several months for patients to resume normal secretion of endogenous corticosteroids. Therefore, knowledge of corticosteroid use is important in the care of critically ill patients because the resulting adrenal suppression may prevent a normal stress response and may put these patients at risk of an adrenal crisis.

Other medications may also contribute to adrenal suppression. For example, administration of etomidate to facilitate endotracheal intubation is associated with significant but temporary adrenal dysfunction and increased mortality.[19]

Infection and sepsis are among the most common causes of adrenal insufficiency in the critical care setting.[9] The proinflammatory state commonly seen in critical illness is thought to produce adrenal insufficiency by suppressing the hypothalamic-pituitary-adrenal axis. Glucocorticoid resistance and suppression of feedback mechanisms are postulated to contribute to low cortisol levels commonly seen in critical illness. Sepsis and septic shock can also cause thrombotic necrosis of the adrenal gland.[19]

BOX 19.9 Causes of Adrenal Insufficiency

Primary

- *Autoimmune disease:* idiopathic and polyglandular
- *Granulomatous disease:* tuberculosis, sarcoidosis, histoplasmosis, blastomycosis
- Cancer
- *Hemorrhagic destruction:* anticoagulation, trauma, sepsis
- *Infectious:* meningococcal, staphylococcal, pneumococcal, fungal (i.e., candidiasis), cytomegalovirus
- AIDS
- *Medications:* ketoconazole, aminoglutethimide, trimethoprim, etomidate, 5-fluorouracil (suppress adrenals); phenytoin, barbiturates, rifampin (increase steroid degradation)
- Irradiation
- Adrenalectomy
- Developmental or genetic abnormality

Secondary

- Abrupt withdrawal of corticosteroids
- Pathology affecting the pituitary, such as tumors, hemorrhage, irradiation, metastatic cancer, lymphoma, leukemia, sarcoidosis
- *Systemic inflammatory states:* sepsis, vasculitis, sickle cell disease
- Postpartum pituitary hemorrhage (Sheehan syndrome)
- Trauma, especially head trauma, or surgery
- Hypothalamic disorders

The concept of *relative adrenal insufficiency* has been debated for several years. The hypermetabolic state of critical illness may increase cortisol levels by as much as tenfold over baseline.[19] Patients with an inadequate physiological response to the demands of this hypermetabolic state have an increased mortality rate. The degree of response, how to best measure the response, and optimum treatment continue to be investigated.[19]

Review of Physiology

The manifestations of adrenal insufficiency result from a lack of adrenocortical secretion of glucocorticoids (primarily cortisol), mineralocorticoids (primarily aldosterone), or both. The deficiency of glucocorticoids is especially significant because their influence on the defense mechanisms of the body and its response to stress makes them essential for life.

Cortisol. Normally, cortisol is released in response to ACTH stimulation from the anterior pituitary gland (see Fig. 19.1). ACTH is stimulated by corticotropin-releasing hormone from the hypothalamus, which is influenced by circulating cortisol levels, circadian rhythms, and stress. Circadian rhythms affect ACTH and cortisol levels, creating peak levels of cortisol in the morning and the lowest levels around midnight. This normal diurnal rhythm can be overridden by stress. Release of cortisol increases the blood glucose concentration by promoting

BOX 19.10 Physiological Effects of Glucocorticoids (Cortisol)

- *Protein metabolism:* promotes gluconeogenesis, stimulates protein breakdown, and inhibits protein synthesis
- *Fat metabolism:* lipolysis and free fatty acid production; promotes fat deposits in face and cervical area
- *Opposes action of insulin:* glucose transport and use in cells
- *Inhibits inflammatory response:*
  - Suppresses mediator release (kinins, histamine, interleukins, prostaglandins, leukotrienes, serotonin)
  - Stabilizes cell membrane and inhibits capillary dilation
  - Formation of edema
  - Inhibits leukocyte migration and phagocytic activity
- *Immunosuppression:*
  - Proliferation of T lymphocytes and killer cell activity
  - Complement production and immunoglobulins
- Increases circulating erythrocytes
- *Gastrointestinal effects:* appetite; increases rate of acid and pepsin secretion in stomach
  - Increases uric acid excretion
  - Decreases serum calcium
  - Sensitizes arterioles to effects of catecholamines; increasing blood pressure
  - Increases renal glomerular filtration rate and excretion of water

glycogen breakdown and gluconeogenesis in the liver, increases lipolysis and free fatty acid production, increases protein degradation, and inhibits the inflammatory and immune responses. Cortisol also increases sensitivity to catecholamines, producing vasoconstriction, hypertension, and tachycardia (Box 19.10).

Aldosterone. A primary mineralocorticoid synthesized in the adrenal cortex that regulates the body's electrolyte and water balance in the renal tubules is aldosterone. Secretion of aldosterone is regulated primarily by the renin-angiotensin-aldosterone system. Renin is stored in the cells of the juxtaglomerular apparatus in the kidneys and is released in response to low plasma sodium levels, increased plasma potassium levels, decreased extracellular fluid volume, decreased blood pressure, and decreased sympathetic nerve activity.[20] Renin stimulates conversion of angiotensinogen to angiotensin I, which is then converted to angiotensin II in the lungs by angiotensin-converting enzyme. Angiotensin II causes vasoconstriction, which causes elevated systemic blood pressure and stimulates aldosterone secretion. Aldosterone acts in the kidneys on the ascending loop of Henle, the distal convoluted tubule, and the collecting ducts to increase sodium ion reabsorption and increase potassium and hydrogen ion excretion. Because reabsorption of sodium creates an osmotic gradient across the renal tubular membrane, antidiuretic hormone (ADH) is activated, causing water to be reabsorbed with sodium. The physiology of aldosterone release is summarized in Fig. 19.6.

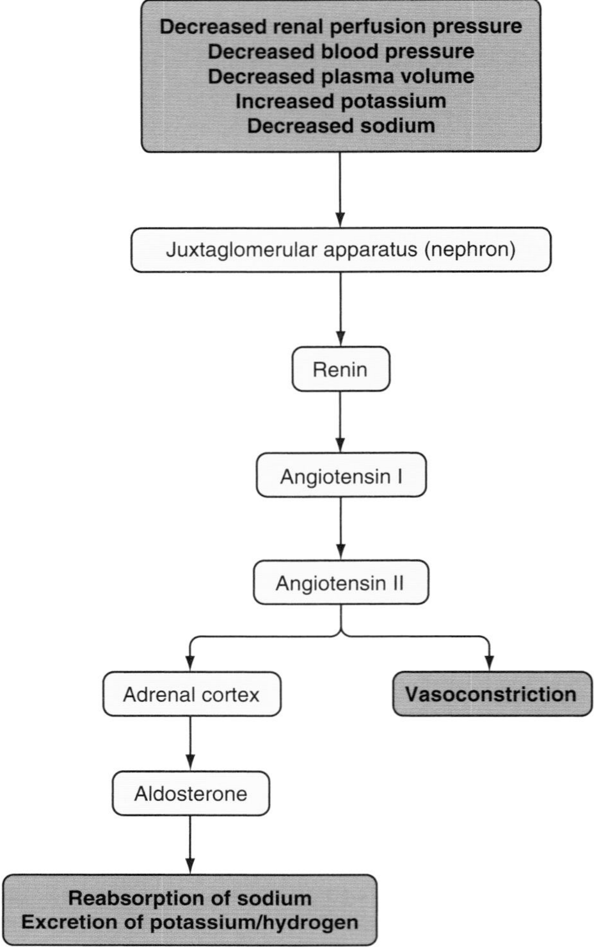

Fig. 19.6 Physiology of aldosterone release.

Pathophysiology of Adrenal Crisis

Adrenal crisis is a life-threatening absence of cortisol (glucocorticoid) and aldosterone (mineralocorticoid). A deficiency of cortisol results in decreased production of glucose, decreased metabolism of protein and fat, decreased appetite, decreased intestinal motility and digestion, decreased vascular tone, and diminished effects of catecholamines. If a patient with deficient cortisol is stressed, this deficiency can produce profound shock as a result of significant decreases in vascular tone caused by the diminished effects of catecholamines.[19]

Deficiency of aldosterone results in decreased retention of sodium and water, decreased circulating volume, and increased potassium and hydrogen ion reabsorption. These effects are seen in patients with underlying primary adrenal insufficiency but not in those with secondary adrenal insufficiency because aldosterone secretion is not primarily dependent on ACTH. A summary of the pathophysiological effects of adrenal insufficiency can be found in Fig. 19.7.

Assessment

Clinical Presentation. Adrenal crisis is a medical emergency that requires astute and rapid assessment. Box 19.11 identifies risk factors for adrenal crisis. Features of adrenal crisis are nonspecific and often attributed to other medical disorders. Signs and symptoms vary (see Fig. 19.6). Adrenal insufficiency may go undiagnosed until a crisis occurs and patients experience symptoms such as acute illness with fever, vomiting,

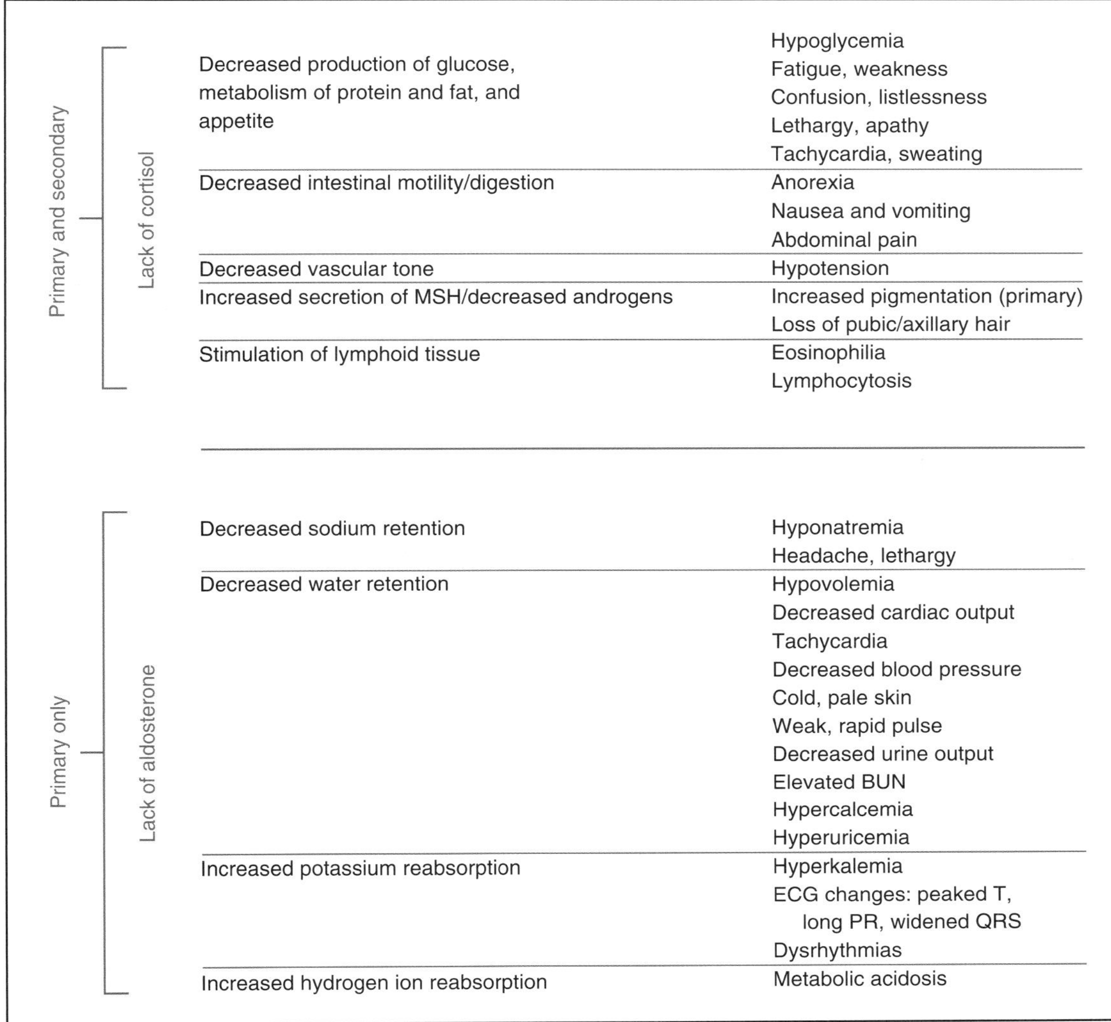

Fig. 19.7 Pathophysiological effects of adrenal insufficiency. *BUN,* Blood urea nitrogen; *ECG,* electrocardiogram; *MSH,* melanocyte-stimulating hormone.

BOX 19.11 Assessment of Risk Factors for Adrenal Crisis

Assess patients carefully for risk factors, predisposing factors, and physical findings associated with chronic adrenal insufficiency. Risk factors include the following:

- *Medication history:* steroids within the past year, phenytoin, barbiturates, rifampin
- *Illness history:* infection, cancer, autoimmune disease, diseases treated with steroids, irradiation of the head or abdomen, HIV-positive status
- *Family history:* autoimmune disease, Addison disease
- *Nutrition:* weight loss, decreased appetite
- *Miscellaneous:* fatigue, dizziness, weakness, darkening of skin, low blood glucose that does not respond to therapy, salt craving

hypotension, shock, decreased serum sodium level, increased serum potassium level, or hypoglycemia[18] (see Laboratory Alert box). Specific system disturbances are widespread. See the Lifespan Considerations box for additional information related to older adults and pregnant people.

LIFESPAN CONSIDERATIONS

Adrenal Disorders

Older Adults

- Use and clearance of cortisol decrease with age, resulting in increased serum cortisol levels. Cortisol secretion then decreases because feedback systems are intact, leading to lower cortisol levels in the older adult.
- The absolute level of cortisol needed to maintain homeostasis in an older adult is unknown.
- Poor nutrition and decreased stores of albumin (one of cortisol's binding proteins) may compound the decline in cortisol availability and response. This predisposes the older adult to dehydration, electrolyte imbalance, acid-base imbalance, and infection due to disorders of the adrenal cortex.[21]

Pregnant People

- Both corticotropin (adrenocorticotropic hormone, or ACTH) and cortisol levels are elevated in pregnancy and thus can exacerbate Cushing's syndrome during pregnancy.
- Acute adrenal crisis may be precipitated by the stress of labor and delivery.[22]
- Untreated adrenal insufficiency increases the risk of intrauterine growth restriction, suboptimal birth weight, and preterm delivery.[22]

! LABORATORY ALERT

Adrenal Disorders

Serum Laboratory Test	Critical Value[a]	Significance
Glucose	<70 mg/dL	Hypoglycemia
	<50 mg/dL	Severe hypoglycemia
Cortisol	<10 mcg/dL considered insufficiency	In severely ill or stressed patient, indicates insufficiency
Potassium	>6.1 mEq/L	Potential for heart blocks, bradydysrhythmias, sinus arrest, ventricular fibrillation, asystole
	<3.0 mEq/L	Potential for ventricular dysrhythmias
Sodium	>160 mEq/L	May be a result of stress and dehydration
	<120 mEq/L	From lack of aldosterone
BUN	>100 mg/dL	Values >20 mg/dL may be observed due to protein breakdown and hemoconcentration
pH	<7.25	Decreased from accumulation of acids and dehydration

[a]Critical values vary by facility and laboratory.
BUN, Blood urea nitrogen.
From Pagana K, Pagana T, Pagana T. *Mosby's Diagnostic and Laboratory Test Reference.* 16th ed. St. Louis, MO: Elsevier; 2023.

Cardiovascular system. Cardiovascular signs and symptoms in adrenal crisis are due to hypovolemia (decreased water reabsorption), decreased vascular tone (decreased effectiveness of catecholamines), and hyperkalemia. The most common presentation of adrenal crisis in critically ill patients is hypotension refractory to fluids and requiring vasopressors. The patient may also have symptoms of decreased cardiac output; weak, rapid pulse; dysrhythmias; and cold, pale skin. Changes in the electrocardiogram may result if there is significant hyperkalemia. Hypovolemia and vascular dilation may be severe enough in crisis to cause hemodynamic collapse and shock.

Neurological system. Neurological manifestations in adrenal crisis are due to decreases in glucose levels, protein metabolism, volume and perfusion, and sodium concentrations. Patients may complain of headache, fatigue that worsens as the day progresses, and severe weakness.[9] They may also exhibit mental confusion, listlessness, lethargy, apathy, psychoses, and emotional lability.

Gastrointestinal system. The gastrointestinal signs and symptoms in adrenal crisis are due to decreased digestive enzymes, intestinal motility, and digestion. Anorexia, nausea, vomiting, diarrhea, and vague abdominal pain are present in most patients.[9]

Genitourinary system. Diminished circulation to the kidneys from reduced circulating volume and hypotension decreases renal perfusion and glomerular filtration rate. Urine output may decline, and acute kidney injury may occur.

Laboratory Evaluation. Laboratory findings in a patient with acute adrenal crisis include hypoglycemia, hyponatremia, hyperkalemia, eosinophilia, increased BUN level, and metabolic acidosis (see Laboratory Alert box). Hypercalcemia or hyperuricemia is possible as a result of volume depletion.

The diagnosis of adrenal crisis is made by evaluating random total plasma cortisol levels.[19] The normal pattern of diurnal variation in cortisol levels is lost in the critically ill, making the timing of the test unimportant. In crisis, plasma cortisol levels are lower than 10 mcg/dL. Differentiation between primary and secondary adrenal insufficiency is accomplished by evaluating serum ACTH levels, which are elevated in primary insufficiency and normal or decreased in secondary insufficiency. Laboratory blood draws are usually collected during the morning hours.

A "normal" cortisol level in a critically ill patient may actually be abnormal and indicate an inadequate response.[19] A random total cortisol value lower than 10 mcg/dL can be life-threatening and warrants further evaluation. Cortisol levels are difficult to interpret in the context of critical illness, but guidelines recommend beginning corticosteroid replacement as soon as insufficiency is suspected.[19]

The technique for performing a cosyntropin (synthetic ACTH) stimulation is outlined in Box 19.12. The test determines baseline levels and response to stimulation. A standard dose of 250 mcg cosyntropin is given, and the expected response is an increase in cortisol level of 7 to 9 mcg/dL from the baseline. A patient whose cortisol level does not increase by this amount is deemed a nonresponder and has an increased risk of mortality.[19]

CHECK YOUR UNDERSTANDING

4. A provider orders a cosyntropin test to assess adrenal status. Examine the following statements and determine which is true regarding the test.
   A. Salivary cortisol levels provide an accurate assessment of the patient's response.
   B. Dexamethasone administration does not affect cortisol values, and it can be administered in emergency situations.
   C. Either 1 mcg (low dose) or 100 mcg (regular dose) of cosyntropin can be administered to assess the patient's response.
   D. Following cosyntropin administration, reassess cortisol level in 15 minutes.

BOX 19.12 Cosyntropin Stimulation Test

Standard Method
- Obtain baseline serum cortisol measurement less than 30 minutes before cosyntropin administration.
- Administer cosyntropin, 250 mcg up to 750 mcg IV over a 2-minute period.
- Measure the serum cortisol level 30 and 60 minutes after cosyntropin administration.
- In emergency situations, may treat with hydrocortisone.

Test Response
- *Expected response:* cortisol greater than 20 mcg/dL, or increase from baseline of greater than 9 mcg/dL
- *Primary aldosterone insufficiency:* cortisol level does not change from baseline and/or the change is less than 7 mcg/dL
- *Relative aldosterone insufficiency:* a change from baseline of less than 9 mcg/dL regardless of baseline level

Patient Problems. The following problems may apply to a patient with adrenal crisis based on assessment data:
- Hypovolemia due to deficiency of aldosterone hormone (mineralocorticoid) and decreased sodium and water retention
- Decreased peripheral tissue perfusion due to cortisol deficiency, resulting in decreased vascular tone and decreased effectiveness of catecholamines
- Nutrition deficit due to cortisol deficiency and resultant decreased metabolism of protein and fats, decreased appetite, and decreased intestinal motility and digestion
- Need for health teaching due to adrenal disorder: proper long-term corticosteroid management
- Low tolerance to activity due to use of endogenous protein for energy needs and loss of skeletal muscle mass as evidenced by early fatigue, weakness, and exertional dyspnea

Nursing and Medical Interventions. Many of the interventions for these patient problems are addressed in the Collaborative Plan of Care for the Critically Ill Patient (see Chapter 1, Overview of Critical Care Nursing). Adrenal crisis requires immediate recognition and intervention if the patient is to survive. Primary objectives in the treatment of adrenal crisis include identifying and treating the precipitating cause, replacing fluid and electrolytes, replacing hormones, and educating the patient and family. See the Evidence-Based Practice box for recommendations developed by a task force of critical care experts.

Fluid and electrolyte replacement. Fluid losses should be replaced with an infusion of 5% dextrose in 0.9% NS until signs and symptoms of hypovolemia stabilize. This not only reverses the volume deficit but also provides glucose to minimize hypoglycemia. The patient may need as much as 5 L of fluid in the first 12 to 24 hours to maintain adequate blood pressure and urine output and to replace the fluid deficit.

Hyperkalemia frequently responds to volume expansion and glucocorticoid replacement and may require no further treatment. In fact, the patient may become hypokalemic during therapy and may require potassium replacement. Acidosis also usually corrects itself with volume expansion and glucocorticoid replacement.

Hormone replacement. Initially, glucocorticoid replacement is a priority to address necessary hormone replacement. If adrenal insufficiency has not been previously diagnosed and the patient's condition is unstable, hydrocortisone sodium succinate (Solu-Cortef) is the medication of choice because it has both glucocorticoid and mineralocorticoid

EVIDENCE-BASED PRACTICE

Guidelines for Diagnosis and Management of Critical Illness–Related Corticosteroid Insufficiency in Critically Ill Patients

Corticosteroid insufficiency is common in critical illness. A multiprofessional task force representing critical care experts convened to develop evidence-based guidelines for managing critical illness–related corticosteroid insufficiency (CIRCI) in the critically ill. Recommendations were developed using a systematic approach based on rating of the evidence and were classified as strong or conditional. At least 80% of the task force members had to agree on a recommendation. The task force could not agree on a single test to reliably diagnose CIRCI; therefore, consider a change in cortisol of less than 9 mcg/dL after a 250-mg cosyntropin test or a random plasma cortisol of less than 10 mcg/dL to make the diagnosis. Recommendations are as follows:
- Avoid using methods other than plasma cortisol (e.g., salivary) for diagnosis and treatment (conditional, low-quality evidence).
- Recommend the 250-mcg adrenocorticotropic hormone (ACTH) test over the 1-mcg ACTH test for diagnosis of CIRCI (conditional, low-quality evidence).
- Administer hydrocortisone less than 400 mg/day IV for 3 or more days in those with septic shock unresponsive to vasopressors (conditional, low-quality evidence).
- Do not administer corticosteroids in patients with sepsis without shock (conditional, moderate-quality evidence).
- Administer methylprednisolone 1 mg/kg/day IV in those with early moderate to severe acute respiratory distress syndrome (conditional, moderate-quality evidence).
- Avoid corticosteroids for major trauma patients (conditional, low-quality evidence).

Level of Evidence

D—Peer-reviewed professional organizational standards

Reference

Annane D, Pastores SM, Rochwerg B et al. Guidelines for the diagnosis and management of critical illness–related corticosteroid insufficiency (CIRCI) in critically ill patients (part I): Society of Critical Care Medicine (SCCM) and European Society of Intensive Care Medicine (ESICM). *Intensive Care Med.* 2017;43:1751-1763. https://doi.org/10.1007/s00134-017-4919-5.

activities. A bolus dose of 100 mg IV is given, followed by continuous infusion of 10 mg/h, or 50 mg every 4 hours, or 75 to 100 mg every 6 hours, resulting in a total dose of 240 to 300 mg in 24 hours. After 24 to 48 hours, doses are tapered slowly to a desired maintenance dose.[19] Cortisone acetate may be given intramuscularly if the IV route is not available. The patient can be switched to oral replacement once oral intake is resumed. At lower doses (<100 mg/day of hydrocortisone), a patient with primary adrenal insufficiency may also require mineralocorticoid replacement. Fludrocortisone, 100 to 200 mcg PO daily, is added. A nutritional consideration, if the patient is experiencing excessive sweating or diarrhea, is to increase sodium intake to 15 mEq/day. Table 19.4 describes the medications used in the treatment of acute adrenal crisis.

Patient and Family Education. In a patient with known adrenal insufficiency and in those receiving corticosteroid therapy, adrenal crisis is preventable. Education of patients, family, and significant others is the key to prevention.

CLINICAL JUDGMENT ACTIVITY

Explain which patient population the nurse would expect to administer a cosyntropin stimulation test. Justify the priority nursing interventions for educating the patient and family about the diagnostic procedure. Determine which factors may affect the interpretation of the test results.

THYROID GLAND IN CRITICAL CARE

Review of Physiology

Thyroid hormones play a role in regulating the function of all body systems. Box 19.13 lists the physiological effects of thyroid hormones. The thyroid hormones thyroxine (T_4) and triiodothyronine (T_3) are secreted by the thyroid gland under the influence of the anterior pituitary gland via secretion of thyroid-stimulating hormone (TSH; also called *thyrotropin*), which in turn is influenced by thyroid-releasing hormone (TRH; also called *thyrotropin-releasing hormone*) from the hypothalamus. Thyroid hormones are highly bound to globulin, T_4-binding prealbumin, and albumin. Only the unbound (or free) fraction of the circulating hormone is biologically active. Regulation of these hormones occurs via positive and negative feedback mechanisms (Fig. 19.8).[23]

T_4 accounts for more than 90% of circulating thyroid hormones,[2,12] but half of all thyroid activity comes from T_3. T_3 is five times more potent, acts more quickly, and enters cells more easily than T_4.[23] T_3 is derived from conversion of T_4 in nonthyroidal tissue. Certain conditions and medications can block the conversion of T_4 to T_3, creating a potential thyroid imbalance. Possible causes for blocked conversion are listed in Box 19.14.

Effects of Aging

With aging, thyroid function declines. Hypothyroidism occurs in older adults, frequently with an insidious onset. The decrease in energy level; the feeling of being cold; the dry, flaky skin; and other signs are often mistakenly assumed to be part of aging but may be signs of decreased thyroid function.[9,23] Thyroid function

TABLE 19.4 PHARMACOLOGY

Medications Used to Treat Adrenal Crisis

Medication	Action/Uses	Dose/Route	Side Effects	Nursing Implications
Hydrocortisone (Solu-Cortef)	Mixed glucocorticoid and mineralocorticoid Antiinflammatory and immunosuppressive effects Salt-retaining (mineralocorticoid) effects in high doses	Individualized in adrenal crisis	Cushing's syndrome Electrolyte disorders Euphoria and other psychic symptoms Fluid retention Hyperglycemia Hypertension Infection Nausea and vomiting Peptic ulcers	Monitor serum glucose and electrolyte levels Watch for signs of fluid overload Observe for signs of infection (may be masked) Maintain adequate nutrition to avoid catabolic effects
Fludrocortisone (Florinef)	Pure mineralocorticoid Causes sodium and water retention and increases excretion of hydrogen, potassium, and water	*PO:* 100-200 mcg/day	Edema Headaches HF Hypertension Increased blood volume Weakness of extremities	Assess for signs of fluid overload Monitor serum sodium and potassium levels Use only in conjunction with glucocorticoids Restrict sodium intake if the patient has edema or fluid overload Not used to treat acute crisis; added as glucocorticoid dose is decreased

GI, Gastrointestinal; *h,* hour; *HF,* heart failure; *IM,* intramuscular; *PO,* orally; *q,* every.
Data from Gahart BL, Nazareno AR, Ortega MQ. *Gahart's 2023 Intravenous Medications.* 39th ed. St. Louis, MO: Elsevier; 2023; Skidmore-Roth L. *Mosby's 2023 Nursing Drug Reference.* 36th ed. St. Louis, MO: Elsevier; 2023.

BOX 19.13 Physiological Effects of Thyroid Hormones

Major Effects
- Metabolic activities of all tissues
- Rate of nutrient use and oxygen consumption for adenosine triphosphate (ATP) production
- Rate of growth
- Activities of other endocrine glands

Other Effects
- Regulate protein synthesis and catabolism
- Regulate body heat production and dissipation
- Gluconeogenesis and use of glucose
- Maintain appetite and gastrointestinal motility
- Maintain calcium metabolism
- Stimulate cholesterol synthesis
- Maintain cardiac rate, contractility, and output
- Affect respiratory rate, oxygen use, and carbon dioxide formation
- Affect red blood cell production
- Affect central nervous system affect and attention
- Produce muscle tone and vigor and provide normal skin constituents

should be assessed in any older adult patient through diagnostic laboratory testing. See the Lifespan Considerations box for additional information related to older adults and pregnant people.

Thyroid Function in the Critically Ill

During critical illness, stress-related changes occur in thyroid hormone balance. Initially, there is a decrease in plasma T_3 levels, known as *low-T_3 syndrome* or *euthyroid sick syndrome*.[23] These changes are thought to result from alterations in the peripheral metabolism of thyroid hormones, which may be an adaptation to severe illness in which the body attempts to reduce energy expenditure.[23] Alterations in thyroid hormone concentrations will improve as the acute illness resolves. However, this process may be prolonged, and full recovery to normal range may take weeks or months.[23]

In the chronically critically ill, additional thyroid hormone changes occur. Both T_3 and T_4 levels are reduced, as is TSH

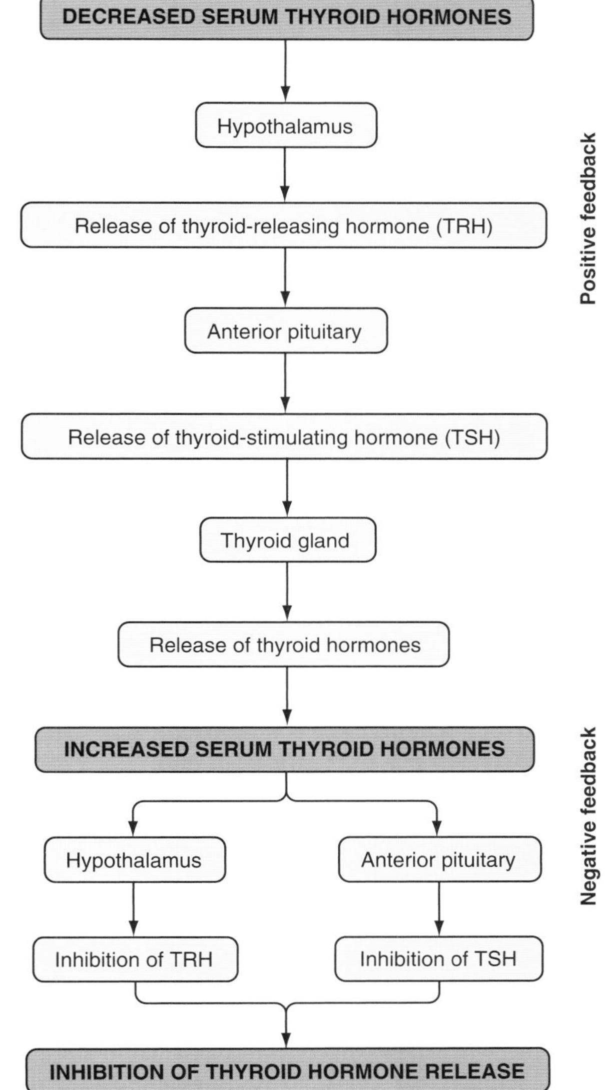

Fig. 19.8 Feedback systems for thyroid hormone regulation.

LIFESPAN CONSIDERATIONS

Thyroid Disorders

Older Adults
- Thyroid hormone levels decrease with age because of glandular atrophy, fibrosis, and inflammation.[2,21]
- Approximately 5% of older adults are affected by hypothyroidism.
- Detection of thyroid disease by assessment of signs or symptoms is more challenging in older adults. On clinical presentation, hypothyroidism can easily be confused with dementia.
- Lower amounts of thyroid medication are needed as replacement, and adjustments of dosage must be slower to prevent potentially dangerous side effects.
- Older adults are less likely to tolerate urgent treatment with liothyronine sodium.
- Older adults may not exhibit the typical signs of thyrotoxicosis. Anorexia, atrial fibrillation, apathy, and weight loss may already be present or misinterpreted.
- Goiter, hyperactive reflexes, sweating, heat intolerance, tremor, nervousness, and polydipsia are less commonly present in older adults.
- Symptoms of thyroid storm may manifest as hypomania, increasing angina, or worsening heart failure.

Pregnant People
- Thyroid hormones are increased during pregnancy as a result of increased synthesis of thyroxine-binding globulin.[9] Free levels are unchanged.

BOX 19.14 Factors That Block Conversion of Thyroxine to Triiodothyronine

- *Severe illness:* chronic renal failure, cancer, chronic liver disease
- Trauma
- Malnutrition, fasting
- *Medications:* glucocorticoids, propranolol, propylthiouracil, amiodarone
- Radiopaque contrast media
- Acidosis

secretion. The changes in chronic critical illness are not well understood but are thought to also include central neuroendocrine dysfunction.[23] Low T_3 state is a predictor of all-cause and cardiac mortalities in critically ill decompensated heart failure, and T_4 levels may serve as a poor prognostic indicator for patient recovery.[23]

THYROID CRISES

Thyroid disorders that have been previously diagnosed and adequately treated do not generally result in crisis states. However, if patients with thyroid disorders, especially undiagnosed thyroid disorders, are stressed either physiologically or psychologically, the results can be life-threatening. Hyperthyroidism must be explored as a causative factor in a patient with new-onset, otherwise unexplained rapid heart rates.

Etiology

Hyperthyroidism, or thyrotoxicosis, results from causes that increase thyroid hormone levels. The most frequent form of hyperthyroidism is *toxic diffuse goiter,* also known as *Graves' disease.*[9] It occurs most frequently in young (third or fourth decade), previously healthy females. A family history of hyperthyroidism is often present. Graves' disease is an autoimmune disease. Affected patients have abnormal thyroid-stimulating immunoglobulins that cause thyroid inflammation, diffuse enlargement, and hyperplasia of the gland.

Toxic multinodular goiter is the second most common cause of hyperthyroidism.[9] It also occurs more commonly in females, but the patients are typically older (fourth to seventh decades). Crises in patients with toxic multinodular goiter are commonly associated with heart failure or severe muscle weakness. Hyperthyroidism also occurs secondary to exposure to radiation, interferon-alpha therapy for viral hepatitis, and other events.[23] Administration of amiodarone, a heavily iodinated compound, can result in either hyperthyroidism or hypothyroidism.[23] Other possible causes of hyperthyroidism are listed in Box 19.15.

Hypothyroidism occurs due to deficient production of thyroid hormone by the thyroid gland. Hypothyroidism is the most common thyroid function disorder.[9] Common causes of hypothyroidism are autoimmune thyroiditis (Hashimoto's disease), iatrogenic loss of thyroid tissue after surgical or radioactive treatment for hyperthyroidism, head and neck radiation therapy, medications, and iodine deficiency.[9] Approximately 5% of adults have hypothyroidism due to a pituitary (secondary) or hypothalamic (tertiary) disorder. These and other less common causes of hypothyroidism are listed in Box 19.16.

BOX 19.15 Causes of Hyperthyroidism

Most Common
- Toxic diffuse goiter (Graves' disease)
- Toxic multinodular goiter
- Toxic uninodular goiter

Other Causes
- Triiodothyronine
- Exogenous iodine in a patient with preexisting thyroid disease: exposure to iodine load from radiographic contrast dyes, medications (amiodarone)
- Thyroiditis (transient)
- Postpartum thyroiditis
- *Medications:*
  - Nonsteroidal antiinflammatory medications
  - Salicylates
  - Tricyclic antidepressants
  - Thiazide diuretics
  - Insulin

Rare Causes
- Toxic thyroid adenoma—more common in the older adult
- Metastatic thyroid cancer
- Malignancies with circulating thyroid stimulators
- Pituitary tumors producing thyroid-stimulating hormone
- Acromegaly

Associations With Other Disorders[a]
- Pernicious anemia
- Idiopathic Addison disease
- Myasthenia gravis
- Sarcoidosis
- Albright syndrome

[a]The presence of these disorders in a patient with thyroid crisis increases the likelihood that the patient has underlying hyperthyroidism.

Thyrotoxic Crisis (Thyroid Storm)

Pathophysiology. *Thyroid storm* occurs in untreated or inadequately treated patients with hyperthyroidism; it is rare in patients with normal thyroid gland function.[9] The crisis is often precipitated by stress due to an underlying illness, general anesthesia, surgery, or infection. It can also be associated with stroke, DKA, and trauma. Uncontrolled hyperthyroidism produces a hyperdynamic, hypermetabolic state that results in disruption of many major body functions; without treatment, death may occur within 48 hours. The specific mechanism that produces thyroid storm is unknown but includes high levels of circulating thyroid hormones, an enhanced cellular response to those hormones, and hyperactivity of the sympathetic nervous system.[23] Thyroid hormones normally increase the synthesis of enzymes that stimulate cellular mitochondria and energy production. When excess thyroid hormones are present, the increased activity of these enzymes produces excessive thermal energy and fever. It is believed that the rapidity with which hormone levels rise may be more important than the absolute levels.

Assessment

Clinical presentation. The excess thyroid hormone activity of hyperthyroidism affects the body in many ways. Box 19.17 lists

BOX 19.16 Causes of Hypothyroidism

Primary Thyroid Disease

- Autoimmune (Hashimoto's thyroiditis)
- Radioactive iodine treatment of Graves' disease
- Thyroidectomy
- Congenital enzymatic defect in thyroid hormone biosynthesis
- Inhibition of thyroid hormone synthesis or release
- *Medications:*
    - Antithyroid medications
    - Iodides
    - Amiodarone
    - Lithium carbonate
    - Oral hypoglycemic agents
    - Dopamine
- Idiopathic thyroid atrophy

Secondary (Pituitary) or Tertiary (Hypothalamus) Disease

- Tumors
- Infiltrative disease (sarcoidosis)
- Hypophysectomy
- Pituitary irradiation
- Head injury
- Stroke
- Pituitary infarction

BOX 19.17 Progressive Signs of Hyperthyroidism

- *Cardiovascular:* Increased heart rate and palpitations. Hyperthyroidism may manifest as sinus tachycardia in a sleeping patient or as atrial fibrillation with a rapid ventricular response.
- *Neurological:* Increased irritability, hyperactivity, decreased attention span, and nervousness. In an older adult patient, these signs may be masked, and depression or apathy may be present.
- *Temperature intolerance:* Increased cold tolerance; heat intolerance; fever; excessive sweating; and warm, moist skin. Older patients may naturally lose their ability to shiver and may be less comfortable in the cold.
- *Respiratory:* Increased respiratory rate, weakened thoracic muscles, and decreased vital capacity are evident.
- *Gastrointestinal:* Increased appetite, decreased absorption (especially of vitamins), weight loss, and increased stools. Diarrhea is not common. Older adult patients may be constipated.
- *Musculoskeletal:* Fine tremors of tongue or eyelids, peripheral tremors with activity, and muscle wasting are noted.
- *Integumentary:* Thin, fine, and fragile hair; soft, friable nails; and petechiae. Young women generally have the more classic findings. Young men may notice an increase in acne and sweating. An older adult patient with dry, atrophic skin may not have significant skin changes.
- *Hematopoietic:* Normochromic, normocytic anemia and leukocytosis may occur.
- *Ophthalmic:* Pathological features result from edema and inflammation. Physical findings may include upper lid retraction, lid lag, extraocular muscle palsies, and sight loss. Exophthalmos is found almost exclusively in Graves' disease.

progressive signs associated with hyperthyroidism. Common findings in patients with thyroid storm, their significance, and the actions nurses can take to address each of these findings are listed in Table 19.5.

Thyroid storm has an abrupt onset. The most prominent clinical features of thyroid storm are severe fever, marked tachycardia (especially atrial tachydysrhythmias), heart failure, nausea, vomiting and diarrhea with subsequent fluid volume depletion, tremors, delirium, stupor, and coma.[9,23] The patient's ability to survive thyroid storm is determined by the severity of the hyperthyroid state and the patient's general health. The severity of the hyperthyroid state is not necessarily indicated by the serum levels of thyroid hormones but rather by tissue and organ responsiveness to the hormones.[23]

CHECK YOUR UNDERSTANDING

5. Determine which assessment parameter is consistent with thyroid storm.
    A. Heart rate >120 beats/minute at rest
    B. Oral temperature of 98.7°F (37°C)
    C. Alert and oriented to name, date, place, event
    D. Deep rapid respirations

Thermoregulation disturbances. Temperature regulation is lost. The patient's body temperature may be as high as 41.1°C (106°F). The increase in heat production and metabolic end products also causes the blood vessels of the skin to dilate. This enhances oxygen and nutrient delivery to the peripheral tissues and accounts for the patient's warm, moist skin.

Neurological disturbances. Thyroid hormones normally maintain alertness and attention. Excess thyroid hormones cause hypermetabolism and hyperactivity of the nervous system, resulting in agitation, delirium, psychosis, tremulousness, seizures, and coma.

Cardiovascular disturbances. Thyroid hormones play a role in maintaining cardiac rate, force of contraction, and cardiac output. The increase in metabolism and the stimulation of catecholamines produced by thyroid hormones cause a hyperdynamic heart. Contractility, heart rate, and cardiac output increase as peripheral vascular resistance decreases. These effects are magnified by the body's increased demand for oxygen and nutrients. In thyroid storm, the increased demands on the heart produce high-output heart failure and cardiovascular collapse if the crisis is not recognized and treated. Vascular collapse and shock due to cardiac decompensation and dehydration are indicators of poor prognosis.[23]

Patients experience palpitations, tachycardia (out of proportion to the fever), and a widened pulse pressure. Atrial fibrillation is common. A prominent third heart sound may be heard, as well as a systolic murmur over the pulmonic area, the aortic area, or both. Occasionally, a pericardial rub may be heard. In the absence of atrial fibrillation, frequent premature atrial contractions or atrial flutter may be present. In an older adult patient with underlying heart disease, worsening of angina or severe heart failure may herald thyroid storm.

Pulmonary disturbances. Thyroid hormones affect respiratory rate and depth, oxygen use, and CO_2 formation. Tissues need more oxygen due to hypermetabolism. This increased need for oxygen stimulates the respiratory drive and increases the respiratory rate. However, increased protein catabolism reduces protein in respiratory muscles (diaphragm

TABLE 19.5 **Thyroid Crises**

Clinical Concerns	Significance	Nursing Actions
Thyroid Storm		
Alterations in level of consciousness	Symptoms can be confused with other disorders (e.g., paranoia, psychosis, depression), especially in the older adult	Provide a safe environment. Assess for orientation, agitation, inattention. Control environmental influences. Implement seizure precautions.
↑ Cardiac workload due to hypermetabolic state; ↓ cardiac output	Can lead to heart failure and cardiovascular collapse	Assess for chest pain, palpitations. Monitor for cardiac dysrhythmias (e.g., atrial fibrillation or flutter) and tachycardia. Monitor blood pressure for widening pulse pressure. Auscultate for the development of an S_3 heart sound. Monitor hemodynamic status: SvO_2, SI, PAOP, RAP. Assess urine output. Evaluate response to therapy.
↑ Oxygen demand due to hypermetabolic state; ineffective breathing pattern	↑ Respiratory rate and drive can lead to fatigue and hypoventilation	Provide supplemental oxygen or mechanical ventilation as needed. Monitor respiratory rate and effort. Monitor oxygen saturation via pulse oximeter. Minimize activity.
Loss of ability to regulate with temperature	Inability to respond to fever exacerbates hypermetabolic demands	Monitor temperature and treat with acetaminophen and/or a cooling blanket as needed.
Myxedema Coma		
↓ Cardiac function	Hypotension and potential for pericardial effusion	Perform ECG monitoring (look for voltage in the QRS complexes, indicating effusion). Auscultate for diminished heart sounds. Monitor blood pressure for signs of hypotension.
Muscle weakness, hypoventilation, pleural effusion; ineffective breathing	Potential for respiratory acidosis and hypoxemia	Auscultate the lungs frequently. Monitor respiratory effort (rate and depth) and pattern. Maintain I&O (probable need for fluid restriction). Monitor ABGs/pulse oximetry and CBC (for anemia). Position for optimum respiratory effort.
Alteration in level of consciousness	Ranges from difficulty concentrating to coma Seizures can occur	Assess and maintain patient safety.
Loss of ability to regulate temperature	Inability to respond to cold	Monitor temperature. Control room temperature, provide rewarming measures.

ABGs, Arterial blood gases; *CBC,* complete blood count; *ECG,* electrocardiographic; *I&O,* intake and output; *PAOP,* pulmonary artery occlusion pressure; *RAP,* right atrial pressure; *SI,* stroke index; *SvO_2,* mixed venous oxygen consumption.

and intercostals). As a result, even with an increased respiratory rate, muscle weakness may prevent the patient from meeting the oxygen demand and may cause hypoventilation, CO_2 retention, and respiratory failure.

Gastrointestinal disturbances. Excess thyroid hormones increase metabolism and accelerate protein and fat degradation. Thyroid hormones also increase gastrointestinal motility, which may result in abdominal pain, nausea, and jaundice. Vomiting and diarrhea can occur, contributing to volume depletion during thyrotoxic crises.

Musculoskeletal disturbances. Muscle weakness and fatigue result from increased protein catabolism. Skeletal muscle changes are manifested as tremors. Thoracic muscles are weak, causing dyspnea. In thyrotoxic crises, patients are placed on bed rest to reduce metabolic demand.

Laboratory evaluation. The diagnosis of thyroid storm is made clinically. Thyroid hormone levels are elevated, but they are usually no higher than those normally found in uncomplicated hyperthyroidism. In any event, thyroid storm is a medical emergency, and the patient must be treated before these results are available. See the Laboratory Alert box for laboratory abnormalities that may occur in thyroid storm.

Patient Problems. The following problems may apply to a patient with thyroid storm based on assessment data:

- Hyperthermia due to loss of temperature regulation, increased metabolism, and increased heat production
- Risk for low cardiac output due to increased metabolic demands on the heart, extreme tachycardia, dysrhythmias, and heart failure
- Changes in breathing patterns and decreased gas exchange due to muscle weakness and decreased vital capacity resulting in hypoventilation and CO_2 retention and increased oxygen needs from hypermetabolism
- Inadequate nutrition due to increased requirement, increased peristalsis, and decreased absorption

! LABORATORY ALERT

Thyroid Disorders

Laboratory Test	Critical Value[a]	Significance
Thyroid Storm		
T_3, free (triiodothyronine)	>0.52 ng/dL	Hyperthyroidism
T_3, resin uptake	>35% of total	
T_4 (thyroxine)	>12 mcg/dL	
TSH	<0.01 milliunits/L	
Glucose	≥ 200 mg/dL (2 h postprandial or random); >140 mg/dL (fasting)	↑ Insulin degradation
Sodium	>150 mEq/L	May be a result of stress, dehydration, and/or hypermetabolic state
BUN	>20 mg/dL	↑ Due to protein breakdown and hemoconcentration
CBC	↓ RBCs ↑ WBCs	Normocytic, normochromic anemia
Calcium	>10.2 mg/dL	Excess bone resorption
Myxedema Coma		
T_3, free	<0.2 mg/dL	Hypothyroidism
T_3, resin uptake	<25% of total	
T_4	<5 mcg/dL	
TSH	>25 milliunits/L	
Sodium	<130 mEq/L	Dilutional from increased total body water
Glucose	<50 mg/dL	Hypoglycemia due to hypermetabolic state
CBC	↓ RBCs	Anemia due to vitamin B_{12} deficiency, inadequate folate or iron absorption
Platelets	<150,000 cells/mm^3	Risk for bleeding
pH	<7.35	Respiratory acidosis from hypoventilation

[a]Critical values vary by facility and laboratory.

From Pagana K, Pagana T, Pagana T. *Mosby's Diagnostic and Laboratory Test Reference*. 16th ed. St. Louis, MO: Elsevier; 2023.

BUN, Blood urea nitrogen; *CBC*, complete blood count; *RBCs*, red blood cells; *TSH*, thyroid-stimulating hormone (thyrotropin); *WBCs*, white blood cells.

- Decreased mobility and inability to tolerate activity due to muscle weakness, tremors, anemia, fatigue, and extreme energy expenditure
- Need for health teaching due to thyroid disorder: disease process, therapeutic regimen, and prevention of complications

Nursing and Medical Interventions. Refer to the Collaborative Plan of Care for the Critically Ill Patient (Chapter 1, Overview of Critical Care Nursing) for nursing interventions due to these patient problems. Thyroid storm requires immediate intervention if the patient is to survive. The primary objectives in the treatment of thyroid storm are antagonizing the peripheral effects of thyroid hormone, inhibiting thyroid hormone biosynthesis, blocking thyroid hormone release, providing supportive care, identifying and treating the precipitating cause, and providing patient and family education. Box 19.18 details the treatment of thyroid storm.

Antagonism of peripheral effects of thyroid hormones. Because it can take days or longer for treatment to affect circulating thyroid hormones, immediate action is necessary to minimize the systemic effects of thyroid storm. The mortality rate of thyroid storm has been significantly reduced since the introduction of beta-blockers to inhibit the effects of thyroid hormones. The medication used most frequently is propranolol (Inderal). Other beta-blockers, such as esmolol hydrochloride (Brevibloc) or atenolol (Tenormin), may also be used. Results are typically seen within minutes after IV administration and within 1 hour after oral treatment. IV effects last 3 to 4 hours. In addition, high-dose glucocorticoids are administered to block the conversion of T_4 to T_3, thereby decreasing the effects of thyroid hormone on peripheral tissues.

Inhibition of thyroid hormone biosynthesis. One of two thioamide medications may be administered to inhibit thyroid hormone biosynthesis: propylthiouracil and methimazole (Tapazole). Neither of these medications is available in IV form, but they may be given via a nasogastric or rectal tube if necessary.[23] In high doses, propylthiouracil inhibits conversion of T_4 to T_3 in peripheral tissues and results in a more rapid reduction of circulating thyroid hormone levels.[23] Methimazole may be used because of its longer half-life and higher potency.

The disadvantage of both propylthiouracil and methimazole is that they lack immediate effect. They do not block the release of thyroid hormones already stored in the thyroid gland, and weeks to months may be required to lower thyroid hormone levels to normal.

Blockage of thyroid hormone release. Iodide agents inhibit the release of thyroid hormones from the thyroid gland, inhibit thyroid hormone production, and decrease the vascularity and

BOX 19.18 Treatment of Thyroid Storm[a]

Antagonize Peripheral Effects of Thyroid Hormone

- Propranolol (Inderal): 1 to 3 mg IV, given 1 mg at a time IV bolus. After 2 minutes of no change, may be repeated once.
- Hydrocortisone: 100 mg IV q8h; or dexamethasone: 0.75 to 9 mg PO per day in divided doses q6-12h.

Inhibit Hormone Biosynthesis

- Propylthiouracil (PTU): PO loading dose of 200 to 400 mg q4h for 24h until thyrotoxicosis controlled, or
- Methimazole (Tapazole): up to 60 mg PO loading dose, divided into 3 doses q8h, then 5 to 15 mg PO daily.

Block Thyroid Hormone Release

Give 1 to 2 Hours After Propylthiouracil or Methimazole Loading Dose

- Saturated solution of potassium iodide (SSKI): 5 drops q6h PO, mixed in 240 mL of water, juice, milk, or broth.
- Alternatively, potassium iodide tablets: 250 mg PO tid.

Supportive Therapy

- Pharmacotherapy for heart failure or tachydysrhythmia.
- Correct fluid and electrolyte imbalances.
- Treat hyperthermia (avoid aspirin).
- High-calorie, high-protein diet.

Identify and Treat Precipitating Cause

Patient and Family Education

[a]Doses are approximate and may vary based on the individual situation.
PO, Orally; *tid,* three times daily.

size of the thyroid gland. Serum T_4 levels decrease approximately 30% to 50% with any of these medications, with stabilization in 3 to 6 days.

Saturated solution of potassium iodide (SSKI) or Lugol's solution may be given orally or sublingually. These medications must be administered 1 to 2 hours after antithyroid medications (propylthiouracil or methimazole) to prevent the iodide from being used to synthesize more T_4, which will worsen the hyperthyroidism.[23] Lithium carbonate inhibits the release of thyroid hormones but is more toxic, so it is used only in patients with an iodide allergy. Lithium carbonate is given orally or by nasogastric or rectal tube, and the dose is adjusted to maintain therapeutic serum levels. Glucocorticoids may be added to block conversion of T_4 to T_3 and may also minimize adrenal insufficiency that can accompany the crisis.[23]

Supportive care. Symptoms are aggressively treated. To manage fever, administer acetaminophen and consider applying cooling blankets or ice packs. Manage cardiac complications with prescribed pharmacotherapy. Administer oxygen to support the respiratory effort. Obtain orders for fluid replacements and monitor hemodynamic status. Provide nutritional support. Lastly, identify and treat or remove precipitating factors.

Patient and Family Education. Education of patients, families, and significant others is crucial in identifying and preventing episodes of thyroid storm. Teaching varies depending on the long-term therapy chosen for each patient (e.g., medications versus radioactive iodine or surgery).

Myxedema Coma

Pathophysiology. *Myxedema coma* is the most extreme form of hypothyroidism and is life-threatening.[9] Hypothyroidism disrupts the normal physiology of most body systems, occurs insidiously over months or years, and produces a hypodynamic, hypometabolic state. Myxedema coma in the absence of an associated stress or illness is uncommon, and infection is the most frequent stressor. The addition of stress to someone with hypothyroidism accelerates the metabolism and clearance of whatever thyroid hormone is present in the body. The patient experiences increased hormone use but decreased hormone production, which precipitates a crisis state. Myxedema coma should be suspected in patients with known hypothyroidism, patients with a surgical scar on the lower neck, and those patients who are unusually sensitive to medications or opioid agents.[23] Common findings in patients with myxedema coma are presented in Table 19.5, along with common findings of thyroid storm.

Etiology. Myxedema coma is the end stage of improperly treated, neglected, or undiagnosed hypothyroidism.[23] It is a life-threatening emergency with a mortality rate as high as 40% despite appropriate therapy.[23] Much of this mortality can be attributed to underlying illnesses. Most patients who develop myxedema coma are older adult females; it is rarely seen in young persons. It occurs more frequently in winter, related to the increased stress of exposure to cold in a person who is unable to maintain body heat. Known precipitating factors include hypothermia, infection, stroke, trauma, and critical illness. Medications that may precipitate myxedema coma include those that affect the central nervous system, such as opioids, anesthetics, barbiturates, sedatives, tranquilizers, lithium, and amiodarone.[23]

Assessment

Clinical presentation. The key features in myxedema coma are (1) altered mental status with varying degrees of change in level of consciousness and confusion, (2) dysfunctional thermoregulation leading to hypothermia, (3) cardiovascular depression, and (4) a precipitating factor.[18,23] Many of these patients may have had vague signs and symptoms of hypothyroidism for several years (Box 19.19). Alterations in renal perfusion leads to decrease water excretion and dilutional hypernatremia. Fluid collects in soft tissues, such as the face, and in joints and muscles. It can also produce pericardial effusion. The clinical picture of myxedema coma varies with the rate of onset and severity. Diagnosis is based on the clinical signs and symptoms, a high index of suspicion, and a careful history and physical examination.

Thermoregulation disturbances. Patients with hypothyroidism are unable to maintain body heat because of the decreased metabolic rate and decreased production of thermal

BOX 19.19 Progressive Signs of Hypothyroidism

- *Earliest signs:* Fatigue, weakness, muscle cramps, intolerance to cold, and weight gain.
- *Cardiovascular:* Bradycardia and hypotension.
- *Neurological:* Difficulty concentrating, slowed mentation, depression, lethargy, slow and deliberate speech, coarse and raspy voice, hearing loss, and vertigo.
- *Respiratory:* Dyspnea on exertion.
- *Gastrointestinal:* Decreased appetite, decreased peristalsis, anorexia, decreased bowel sounds, constipation, and paralytic ileus. However, the decreased metabolic rate also leads to weight gain.
- *Musculoskeletal:* Fluid in joints and muscles results in stiffness and muscle cramps.
- *Integumentary:* Dry, flaky, cool, coarse skin; dry, coarse hair; and brittle nails. The face is puffy and pallid; the tongue may be enlarged. The dorsa of the hands and feet are edematous. There may be a yellow tint to the skin from depressed hepatic conversion of carotene to vitamin A. Ecchymoses may develop from increased capillary fragility and decreased platelets.
- *Hematological:* Pernicious anemia and jaundice. Splenomegaly occurs in about 50% of patients. About 10% of patients have a decrease in neutrophils.
- *Ophthalmic:* Generalized mucinous edema in the eyelids and periorbital tissue.
- *Metabolic:* Elevated creatine phosphokinase, aspartate aminotransferase, lactate dehydrogenase, cholesterol, and triglyceride levels. Elevated cholesterol and triglyceride levels predispose persons with hypothyroidism to the development of atherosclerosis.

energy. Because of this, patients may present in crisis after being stressed by exposure to cold. Hypothermia is present in 80% of patients with myxedema coma, and temperatures can be as low as 26.7°C (80°F). Patients with temperatures lower than 32°C (88.6°F) have a grave prognosis. If a patient with myxedema coma has a temperature greater than 37°C (98.6°F), underlying infection should be suspected.

Neurological disturbances. The low metabolic rate and resulting decreased mentation produce both psychological and physiological changes. The patient in hypothyroid crisis may present with somnolence, delirium, seizures, or coma. Personality changes such as paranoia and delusions may be evident.

Cardiovascular disturbances. Cardiac function is depressed, resulting in decreases in heart rate, blood pressure, contractility, stroke volume, and cardiac output. The patient may develop a pericardial effusion or cardiac tamponade, making heart tones distant. The electrocardiogram has decreased voltage because of the pericardial effusion.

Pulmonary disturbances. The respiratory system responsiveness is depressed, producing hypoventilation, respiratory muscle weakness, and CO_2 retention. CO_2 narcosis may contribute to decreased mentation. As part of the picture of generalized mucinous edema and fluid retention, these patients may also develop pleural effusions or upper airway edema, further restricting their breathing.

Skeletal muscle disturbances. Slowed motor conduction produces decreased tendon reflexes and sluggish, awkward movements. Additionally, patients may experience muscle aching and joint stiffness.[9]

Laboratory Evaluation. Serum T_4 and T_3 levels and resin T_3 uptake are low in patients with myxedema coma. In primary hypothyroidism, TSH levels are high. If hypothyroidism is the result of disease of the pituitary gland or hypothalamus (i.e., secondary or tertiary hypothyroidism), TSH levels are inappropriately normal or low. As in patients with thyroid storm, if myxedema coma is suspected, treatment should not be delayed while awaiting these results to confirm the diagnosis.

Serum sodium levels may be low due to impaired water excretion due to inappropriate ADH secretion and cortisol deficiency, which frequently accompany hypothyroidism. The patient should be monitored for signs and symptoms of hyponatremia, such as weakness, muscle twitching, seizures, and coma.

Hypoglycemia is common and may be due to pituitary or hypophyseal disorders and/or adrenal insufficiency. Adrenal insufficiency may result in serum cortisol levels that are inappropriately low for stress. Laboratory manifestations of myxedema coma are summarized in Laboratory Alert: Thyroid Disorders.

Patient Problems. The following problems apply to a patient in myxedema coma based on assessment data:

- Low cardiac output due to decreased contractility, decreased heart rate, decreased stroke volume, pericardial effusion, and dysrhythmias
- Decreased gas exchange due to hypoventilation, muscle weakness, decreased respiratory rate, ascites, and pleural effusions
- Hypothermia due to inability of body to retain heat
- Excess fluid volume due to impaired water excretion
- Risk for injury due to altered mental status
- Activity intolerance due to muscle weakness
- Inadequate nutrition due to decreased appetite, decreased carbohydrate metabolism, and hypoglycemia
- Need for health teaching due to myxedema coma: disease process, therapeutic regimen, and prevention of complications

Nursing and Medical Interventions. Myxedema coma requires immediate intervention if the patient is to survive. The primary objectives in the treatment of myxedema coma are identifying and treating the precipitating cause, providing thyroid replacement, restoring fluid and electrolyte balance, providing supportive care, and providing patient and family education. Box 19.20 details the treatment of myxedema coma. It is important to achieve physiological levels of thyroid hormones without incurring the adverse effects of excess thyroid hormones. Also refer to the Collaborative Plan of Care for the Critically Ill Patient (see Chapter 1, Overview of Critical Care Nursing).

Thyroid replacement. The best method of thyroid replacement is controversial. Either levothyroxine sodium (Synthroid; T_4) or liothyronine sodium (Cytomel; T_3) can be used. Levothyroxine ultimately provides the patient with both T_4 and, through

BOX 19.20 Treatment of Myxedema Coma[a]

- Identification and treatment of underlying disorder.
- *Thyroid replacement:* levothyroxine initial, 300 to 500 mcg IV for one-dose maintenance, 50 to 100 mcg IV daily until patient can tolerate oral therapy; or liothyronine 25 to 50 mcg IV, with subsequent doses separated by at least 4 hours and not more than 12 hours; individualized dosing determined by monitoring of clinical condition and response.
- Restoration of fluid and electrolyte balance
  - Cautious administration of vasopressors.
  - *Hyponatremia:* fluid restriction.
  - *Hypoglycemia:* IV dextrose.
- Supportive care
  - Passive warming with blankets (do not actively warm).
  - Ventilatory assistance.
  - Avoid analgesic and sedative medications.
  - Adrenal hormone replacement until coexisting adrenal insufficiency is excluded: hydrocortisone, 100-mg IV bolus, then 100-mg IV infusion over the following day. Change to oral dosing when patient is stable.
  - Radiographic or ultrasound study of the chest to assess pleural effusion.
  - Echocardiogram to assess cardiac function and/or pericardial effusion.
- Patient and family education.

[a] Doses are approximate and may vary based on the individual situation.

peripheral conversion, T_3 replacement, whereas liothyronine sodium provides only T_3.

Levothyroxine sodium is commonly used for treatment. It has a smoother onset and a longer duration of effect. The preferred route is IV because absorption of oral or intramuscular levothyroxine is variable. The initial dose may be decreased if the patient has underlying factors such as angina, dysrhythmias, or other heart disease.

Liothyronine sodium has more pronounced metabolic effects, a more rapid onset (6 hours), and a shorter half-life (1 day) than levothyroxine. Because of liothyronine's potency, its administration may be complicated by angina, myocardial infarction, and cardiac irritability. For this reason, it is usually avoided in older adults.

The effects of levothyroxine are not as rapid as those of liothyronine, but its cardiac toxicity is lower. Serum levels of T_4 reach normal in 1 to 2 days. Levels of TSH begin to fall within 24 hours and return to normal within 10 to 14 days.

Fluid and electrolyte replacement. Thyroid replacement usually corrects hypotension or shock, but cautious volume expansion with saline also helps. Vasopressors are used with extreme caution because patients in myxedema coma are unable to respond to vasopressors until they have adequate levels of thyroid hormones available. Simultaneous administration of vasopressors and thyroid hormones is associated with myocardial irritability.

Hyponatremia usually responds to thyroid replacement and water restriction; the patient can resume water intake once thyroid hormones are replaced. If hyponatremia is severe (<120 mEq/L) or the patient is having seizures, hypertonic saline with or without a loop diuretic may be administered,[18] but only until symptoms disappear or the sodium level is at least 120 mEq/L.

If a patient has hypoglycemia, adrenal insufficiency, or both, glucose is added to IV fluids. Glucocorticoid administration is recommended for all patients if hypoadrenalism coexists with hypothyroidism. Hydrocortisone is the medication of choice for replacement. The adrenal abnormality may last for several weeks after thyroid replacement is begun, so this support is continued during that period.

Supportive care. Aggressively manage symptoms. Keep the room warm, and use passive rewarming methods (e.g., warming blankets) to treat and prevent hypothermia. Avoid medications that depress respiration, such as opioids. Assess and treat cardiac function. Monitor respiratory status and anticipate the need for mechanical ventilation.

Patient and Family Education. The education of patients, family, and significant others is critical in identifying and preventing episodes of myxedema coma.

SODIUM DISORDERS IN CRITICAL ILLNESS

Sodium disorders are common in critically ill patients and may occur as part of the pathophysiology of other endocrine disorders such as DKA, HHS, adrenal disorders, thyroid disorders, or pituitary disorders. Details of the sodium imbalances associated with specific endocrine crises, as well as the pathophysiology leading to the imbalance, can be found in the tables, boxes, and figures throughout this chapter.

Etiology

Hypernatremia, serum sodium >145 mEq/L, most commonly occurs due to excess loss of free water leading to increased serum osmolality and increased serum sodium. Loop diuretics, inability of the kidneys to concentrate urine, vomiting, diarrhea, and excessive sweating may lead to hypernatremia. Rarely, hypernatremia may occur due to hypervolemia as a result of infusion of hypertonic saline solutions, heart failure, or oversecretion of ACTH or aldosterone.[20] In this instance, the increase in total body sodium exceeds the increase in total body water. Older adult patients and patients with impaired mental status are at increased risk for developing hypernatremia.[24]

Hyponatremia, serum sodium <135 mEq/L, is the most common electrolyte disorder in hospitalized individuals, occurring in 30% of critical care cases, and is associated with increased morbidity and mortality.[25] Hyponatremia develops when sodium loss exceeds water loss or when total body water increase exceeds sodium increase. It may also occur due to osmotic fluid shifts from the intracellular to the extracellular environment that cause dilutional serum sodium. Associated causes of hyponatremia are fluid restoration therapy, adrenal insufficiency, prolonged vomiting, diuretics, syndrome of inappropriate antidiuretic hormone (SIADH; see Pituitary Gland: Antidiuretic Hormone Disorders in this chapter), hypothyroidism, glucocorticoid deficiency, or pneumonia.[20] Patients admitted for acute brain injuries (i.e., stroke, trauma, subarachnoid hemorrhage) are at increased risk for hyponatremia.

Assessment

Clinical Presentation. Patients with hypernatremia will have signs of hypovolemia, such as oliguria, weight loss, orthostatic hypotension, decreased jugular venous pressure, dry mucous membranes, and tachycardia. Patients also present with neurological alterations, including altered level of consciousness, confusion, or delirium.

Individuals experiencing mild hyponatremia may be asymptomatic, or they may experience nausea and vomiting. As hyponatremia worsens, neurological symptoms such as headache, lethargy, confusion, seizures, and coma may occur. In hypovolemic hyponatremia, loss of sodium accompanied by extracellular fluid losses leads to hypotension, tachycardia, and decreased urine output. Conversely, in hypervolemic hyponatremia, patients may experience edema, ascites, and jugular venous distention.

Nursing and Medical Management. Identification of the underlying cause of the sodium imbalance is important. Understanding the exact mechanism by which the sodium imbalance occurred helps to guide treatment and rate of correction. Management of sodium imbalances is determined by (1) severity of imbalance as determined by serum sodium; (2) central nervous system (CNS) symptoms associated with the imbalance, such as delirium, seizures, or coma; and (3) acuity of the sodium imbalance (onset <48 vs. >48 h).[24,26]

Hypernatremia. Treatment of hypernatremia in the critical care setting includes fluid replacement with hypotonic fluids (5% dextrose alternating with 0.45% NS). The rate of replacement is adjusted to avoid too-rapid correction of serum sodium. The recommended rate of correction for serum sodium is 0.5 mEq/L/h or 12 mEq/L/day.[26]

Hyponatremia. Treatment of hyponatremia includes slowly increasing serum sodium—no more than 12 mEq within the first 24 hours.[7] Too-rapid correction of hyponatremia can lead to cerebral edema and central pontine myelinolysis or ODS, a severe neurological syndrome that can lead to permanent brain damage or death.[26] Fluid restrictions are implemented for dilutional hypernatremia. Fluid replacement and tonicity of fluids depend on the etiology of the hyponatremia, severity, and associated symptoms.[26] Fluid and electrolyte replacement guidelines specific to the underlying endocrine etiology can be found in the treatment sections throughout this chapter.

PITUITARY GLAND: ANTIDIURETIC HORMONE DISORDERS

Review of Physiology

The primary function of ADH is regulation of water balance and serum osmolality. ADH (also known as *arginine vasopressin,* or AVP) is produced in the supraoptic and paraventricular nuclei of the hypothalamus. These nuclei are positioned near the thirst center and osmoreceptors in the hypothalamus (Fig. 19.9). Once produced, ADH is stored in neurons in the posterior pituitary until stimulation of the nuclei causes release of ADH from the posterior pituitary. Nuclei are stimulated in several ways (Fig. 19.10). Primary triggers for ADH release are increased serum osmolality, decreased blood volume (by >10%), and decreased blood pressure (5% to 10% drop). Other factors

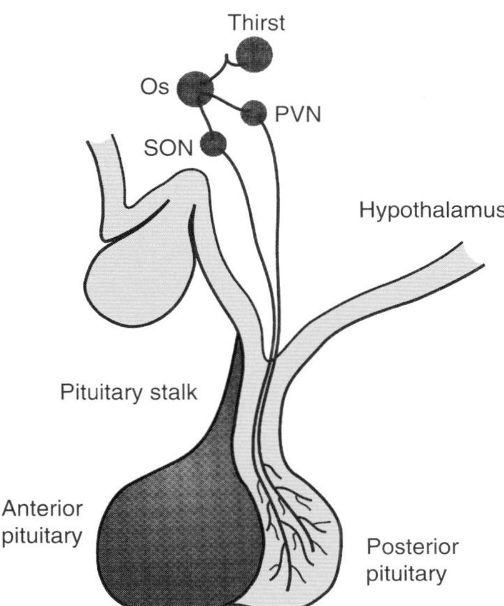

Fig. 19.9 The hypothalamic–posterior pituitary system. *Os,* Osmoreceptor; *PVN,* paraventricular nuclei; *SON,* supraoptic nuclei.

that stimulate ADH release are elevated serum sodium levels, trauma, hypoxia, pain, stress, and anxiety. Certain medications, such as analgesics, barbiturates, anesthetics, and chemotherapeutic agents, also stimulate ADH release (see Fig. 19.10).

Once released, ADH acts on the renal distal tubules and collecting ducts to cause water reabsorption. In high concentrations, ADH also acts on smooth muscles of the arterioles to produce vasoconstriction.

Two common disturbances of ADH are *diabetes insipidus* (DI) and SIADH. A less common ADH disorder is cerebral salt wasting (CSW), which is similar to SIADH but with important differences. Differentiating CSW from SIADH is crucial because of opposing management strategies. Table 19.6 compares the electrolyte and fluid findings associated with DI, SIADH, and CSW.[9]

Diabetes Insipidus

Etiology. Various disorders produce neurogenic DI (Box 19.21), but the primary cause is traumatic injury to the posterior pituitary or hypothalamus as a result of head injury or surgery.[27] Transient DI may be caused by trauma to the pituitary, manipulation of the pituitary stalk during surgery, or cerebral edema. Permanent DI occurs when more than 80% to 85% of hypothalamic nuclei or the proximal pituitary stalk is destroyed.

Nephrogenic DI may occur in genetically predisposed persons. It also may be acquired as a result of chronic renal disease, medications, or other conditions that produce permanent kidney damage or inhibit the generation of cyclic adenosine monophosphate in the tubules.[9]

Pathophysiology. DI results from an ADH deficiency *(neurogenic* or *central DI),* from ADH insensitivity *(nephrogenic DI),* or from excessive water intake *(secondary DI).*[9] Regardless of the cause, the effect is impaired renal conservation of water, resulting in polyuria (>3 L in 24 hours). As long as the thirst center remains intact and the person is able to respond to this thirst, fluid volume can be maintained. If the patient is unable

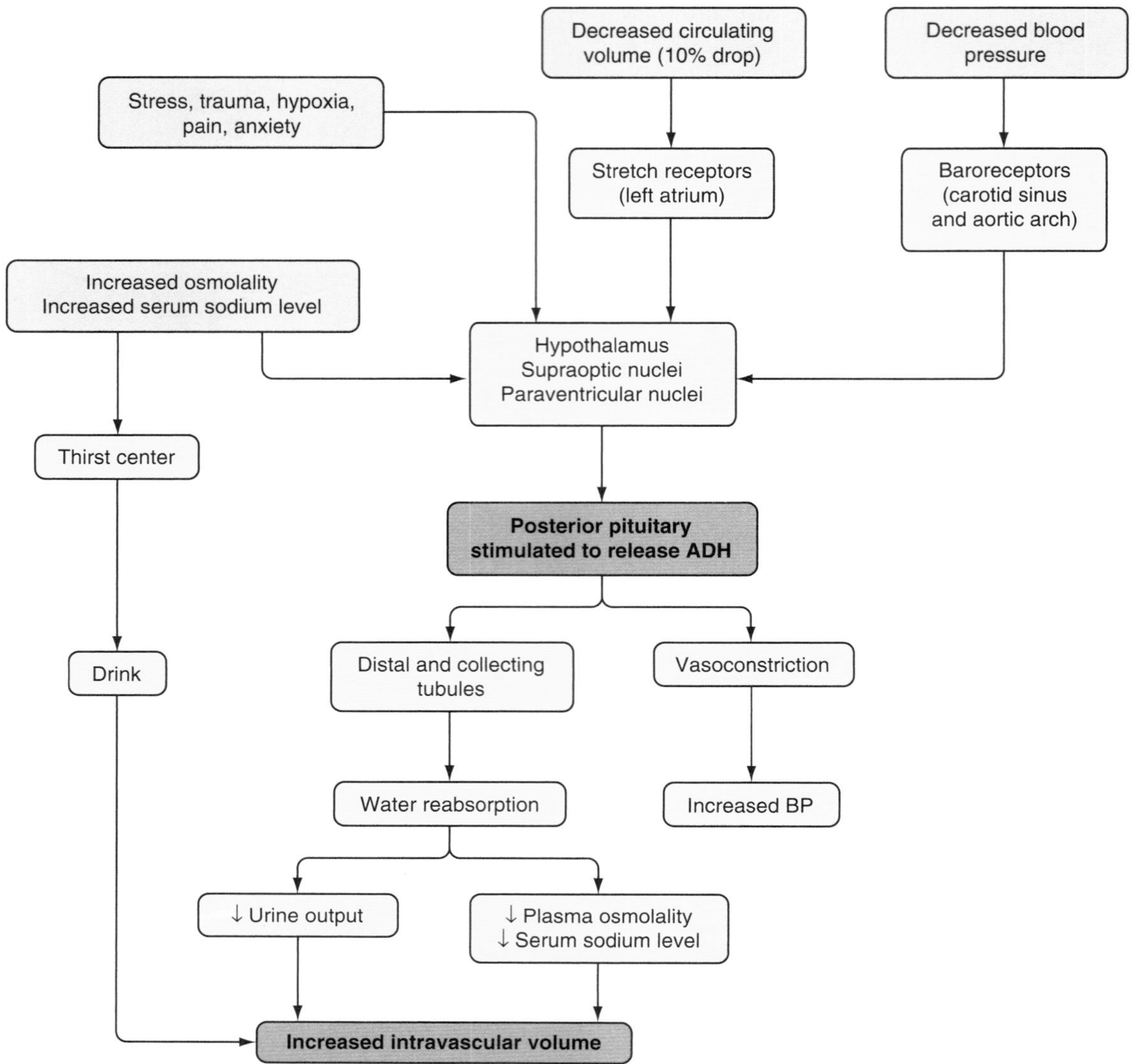

Fig. 19.10 Physiology of antidiuretic hormone *(ADH)* release. *BP,* Blood pressure.

TABLE 19.6 Electrolyte and Fluid Findings in Antidiuretic Hormone Disorders

Finding	Diabetes Insipidus	SIADH	Cerebral Salt Wasting
Plasma volume	Decreased	Increased	Decreased
Serum sodium	Increased	Decreased	Decreased
Serum osmolality	Increased	Decreased	Normal or increased
Urine sodium	Normal	Increased	Increased
Urine osmolality	Decreased	Increased	Normal or increased

SIADH, Syndrome of inappropriate antidiuretic hormone secretion.

to respond, severe dehydration results if fluid losses are not replaced.

Neurogenic DI occurs because of disruption of the neural pathways or structures involved in ADH production, synthesis, or release. Absent or diminished release of ADH from the posterior pituitary leads to free water loss and causes serum osmolality and serum sodium to rise. The posterior pituitary is unable to respond by increasing ADH levels; therefore, the kidneys are not stimulated to reabsorb water, and excessive water loss results.

In nephrogenic DI, the kidney collecting ducts and distal tubules are unresponsive to ADH; although adequate levels of ADH may be synthesized and released, the kidneys are unable to conserve water in response to ADH. In patients with secondary DI, compulsive high-volume water consumption causes polyuria.

Assessment

Clinical presentation. Neurogenic DI usually occurs suddenly with an abrupt onset of polyuria, as much as 5 to 15 L in 24 hours.[9,27] The onset of nephrogenic DI is more gradual.[9] In both types, the urine is pale and dilute. The thirst mechanism is activated in conscious patients, and polydipsia occurs. If the patient is unable to replace the water lost by responding to thirst, signs of hypovolemia, such as hypotension, decreased skin turgor, dry mucous membranes, tachycardia, weight loss, and low right atrial and pulmonary artery occlusion pressures,

BOX 19.21 Causes of Diabetes Insipidus

Antidiuretic Hormone Deficiency (Neurogenic)
- *Idiopathic:* familial, congenital, autoimmune, genetic
- Intracranial surgery, especially in region of pituitary
- *Tumors:* craniopharyngioma, pituitary tumors, metastases to hypothalamus
- *Infections:* meningitis, encephalitis, syphilis, mycoses, toxoplasmosis
- *Granulomatous disease:* tuberculosis, sarcoidosis, histiocytosis
- Severe head trauma, anoxic encephalopathy, or any disorder that causes increased intracranial pressure

Antidiuretic Hormone Insensitivity (Nephrogenic)
- Hereditary or idiopathic
- *Renal disease:* pyelonephritis, amyloidosis, polycystic kidney disease, obstructive uropathy, transplantation
- *Multisystem disorders affecting kidneys:* multiple myeloma, sickle cell disease, cystic fibrosis
- *Metabolic disturbances:* chronic hypokalemia or hypercalcemia
- *Medications:* ethanol, phenytoin, lithium carbonate, amphotericin, methoxyflurane

Secondary Diabetes Insipidus
- Idiopathic
- Psychogenic polydipsia
- *Hypothalamic disease:* sarcoidosis
- Excessive IV fluid administration
- *Medication-induced disease:* anticholinergics, tricyclic antidepressants

develop. Neurological signs and symptoms are seen with hypovolemia and hypernatremia.

Laboratory Evaluation. The classic signs of DI are an inappropriately low urine osmolality, decreased urine specific gravity, and a high serum osmolality. Corresponding to the low urine osmolality is a decreased urine specific gravity. Serum osmolality is greater than 295 mOsm/kg, and the serum sodium level is greater than 145 mEq/L. The presence of hypokalemia or hypercalcemia suggests nephrogenic DI. Other values, such as BUN, may be elevated as a result of hemoconcentration. Further testing to differentiate neurogenic and nephrogenic DI includes water deprivation studies. However, these tests are inappropriate in the critically ill population (see Laboratory Alert box).

Patient Problems. The following problems may apply to a patient with DI:
- Decreased fluid volume due to deficient ADH, insensitivity of renal cells to ADH, polyuria, and inability to respond to thirst
- Changes in mental status due to decreased cerebral perfusion, cerebral dehydration, and hypernatremia

Nursing and Medical Interventions. The primary goals of treatment are to identify and correct the underlying cause and restore normal fluid volume, osmolality, and electrolyte balance. Identifying the underlying cause is a necessary part of determining appropriate treatment, particularly medication therapy. Also refer to the Collaborative Plan of Care for the Critically Ill Patient (Chapter 1, Overview of Critical Care Nursing).

! LABORATORY ALERT

Pituitary Disorders

Laboratory Test	Critical Value[a]	Explanation
Diabetes Insipidus		
Sodium (serum)	>145 mEq/L	Free water loss due to absent or diminished release of ADH or lack of response by the kidneys results in hemoconcentration of sodium.
Osmolality (serum)	>295 mOsm/kg	Free water loss due to absent or diminished release of ADH or lack of response by the kidneys increases serum osmolality; normal in secondary DI.
Osmolality (urine)	<100 mOsm/kg	Free water loss into urine decreases urine osmolality.
Sodium (urine)	40-200 mEq/L	Urine sodium is not affected.
Urine specific gravity	<1.010	Free water loss decreases specific gravity
Syndrome of Inappropriate Antidiuretic Hormone Secretion		
Sodium (serum)	<135 mEq/L	Free water retention due to oversecretion of ADH dilutes sodium.
Osmolality (serum)	<280 mOsm/kg	Free water retention due to oversecretion of ADH decreases osmolality.
Osmolality (urine)	>100 mOsm/kg	Lack of water excretion increases urine osmolality.
Sodium (urine)	>200 mEq/L	Sodium is excreted in an attempt to excrete excess water.
Urine specific gravity	>1.020	Free water retention due to oversecretion of ADH increases specific gravity.
Cerebral Salt Wasting		
Sodium (serum)	<135 mEq/L	Kidneys are unable to conserve sodium.
Osmolality (serum)	<295 mOsm/kg	Hypovolemia decreases serum osmolality.
Osmolality (urine)	>100 mOsm/kg	Lack of water excretion increases urine osmolality.
Sodium (urine)	>200 mEq/L	Sodium wasting through renal tubules occurs.
Urine specific gravity	>1.020	Lack of water excretion increases urine specific gravity.

[a]Critical values vary by facility and laboratory.
ADH, Antidiuretic hormone; *DI,* diabetes insipidus.
From Pagana K, Pagana T, Pagana T. *Mosby's Diagnostic and Laboratory Test Reference*. 16th ed. St. Louis, MO: Elsevier; 2023.

Volume replacement. Monitoring for hypovolemia is a priority. Vital signs and urine output must be recorded at least every hour. This is particularly important in older adult patients, who are likely to have concurrent cardiovascular and renal disease. Additionally, accurate intake and output and daily weights are essential.

Patients who are alert and able to respond to thirst usually drink enough water to avoid symptomatic hypovolemia. However, critically ill patients who develop DI and older adult patients with cognitive impairments are frequently unable to recognize or respond to thirst, so fluid replacement is essential.

If the patient has symptoms of hypovolemia, the volume lost must be replaced. In addition, fluid is replaced every hour to keep up with current urine losses.[27] Correction of hypernatremia and replacement of free water are achieved by administration of hypotonic solutions of dextrose in water. If the patient has circulatory failure, 0.9% NS may be administered until hemodynamic stability and vascular volume are restored.[24] Plasma sodium should be monitored every 4 hours until sodium levels are stabilized.[27] Hemodynamic monitoring may be instituted to evaluate fluid requirements and monitor the patient's response to treatment.

Monitor the patient's neurological status frequently; alterations may indicate a change in fluid status, electrolyte status (e.g., sodium), or both. Avoid fluid overload from overly aggressive fluid replacement, particularly after hormone replacement therapy has been instituted.

Hormone replacement. Because of the decreased secretion of ADH, neurogenic DI is controlled primarily by administration of exogenous ADH preparations. These medications replace ADH and enable the kidneys to conserve water. They can be administered intravenously, intramuscularly, subcutaneously, intranasally, or orally. Injectable forms are typically more potent than the intranasal or oral forms. Absorption is more reliable through the IV route.

The drug most used for management is desmopressin (DDAVP), a synthetic analog of vasopressin.[27] Unlike aqueous vasopressin and lysine vasopressin, desmopressin has reduced vasoconstrictor effects and has a longer antidiuretic action (12 to 24 hours). Side effects are usually mild and include headache, nausea, and mild abdominal cramps; however, overmedication can produce water overload. Monitor the patient for signs of dyspnea, hypertension, weight gain, hyponatremia, headache, or drowsiness.

Nephrogenic diabetes insipidus. Nephrogenic DI is treated with sodium restriction, which decreases the glomerular filtration rate and enhances fluid reabsorption. Administration of thiazide diuretics may increase tubular sensitivity to ADH.

Patient and Family Education. Patients who have a permanent ADH deficit require education on the following: (1) pathogenesis of DI; (2) dose, side effects, and rationale for prescribed medications; (3) parameters for notifying the provider; (4) importance of adherence to medication regimen; (5) importance of recording daily weight measurements to identify weight gain; (6) importance of wearing an identification bracelet; and (7) importance of drinking according to thirst and avoiding excessive drinking.

Syndrome of Inappropriate Antidiuretic Hormone Secretion

Etiology. Central nervous system disorders such as head injury, infection, hemorrhage, surgery, and stroke stimulate the hypothalamus or pituitary, producing excess secretion of ADH. A common cause of SIADH is ectopic production of ADH by malignant disease, especially small cell carcinoma of the duodenum, stomach, pancreas, and lung.[9] The malignant cells synthesize, store, and release ADH and thus place control of ADH outside the normal pituitary-hypothalamus feedback loops. Other types of malignancies known to produce SIADH include Hodgkin's lymphoma, sarcoma, and squamous cell carcinoma of the tongue.

Nonmalignant pulmonary conditions such as tuberculosis, pneumonia, lung abscess, and chronic obstructive pulmonary disease can also produce SIADH. As with malignant cells, it is believed that benign pulmonary tissue is capable of synthesizing and releasing ADH in certain disease states.

Many medications are associated with the development of SIADH (Box 19.22). The mechanisms involved include increasing or potentiating the action of ADH, acting on the renal distal tubule to decrease free water excretion, or causing central release of ADH.[9]

Pathophysiology. SIADH occurs when the body secretes excessive ADH due to plasma osmolality. This occurs when there is a failure in the negative feedback mechanism that regulates the release and inhibition of ADH. The results are an inability to secrete dilute urine, fluid retention, and dilutional hyponatremia.[9] The primary treatment of SIADH is to restrict or withhold fluids.

Assessment

Clinical presentation. The clinical manifestations are primarily the result of water retention, hyponatremia, and hypoosmolality of the serum. The severity of the signs and symptoms is due to the rate of onset and the severity of the hyponatremia. See the Lifespan Considerations box for additional information related to older adults.

LIFESPAN CONSIDERATIONS

Pituitary Disorders

Older Adults

- An increase in secretion of antidiuretic hormone (ADH) occurs with aging and increases the risk for dilutional hyponatremia.
- Older adults are at greater risk for the syndrome of inappropriate antidiuretic hormone secretion (SIADH) from any cause.
- Older adult patients often fail to recognize and respond to thirst and therefore are at increased risk for dehydration.[26]

Central nervous system. Manifestations such as weakness, lethargy, mental confusion, difficulty concentrating, restlessness, headache, seizures, and coma may occur in response to hyponatremia and hypoosmolality. Hypoosmolality disrupts the

BOX 19.22 Causes of Syndrome of Inappropriate Antidiuretic Hormone

Ectopic Antidiuretic Hormone Production
- Small cell carcinoma of lung
- Cancer of prostate, pancreas, or duodenum
- Hodgkin's disease
- Sarcoma, squamous cell carcinoma of the tongue, thymoma
- *Nonmalignant pulmonary disease:* viral pneumonia, tuberculosis, chronic obstructive pulmonary disease, lung abscess

Central Nervous System Disorders
- Head trauma
- *Infections:* meningitis, encephalitis, brain abscess
- Intracranial surgery, cerebral aneurysm, brain tumor, cerebral atrophy, stroke
- Guillain-Barré syndrome, lupus erythematosus

Medications
- Angiotensin-converting enzyme inhibitors
- Amiodarone
- *Analgesics and narcotics:* morphine, fentanyl, acetaminophen
- *Antineoplastics:* vincristine, cyclophosphamide, vinblastine, cisplatin
- Barbiturates
- Carbamazepine (Tegretol) and oxcarbazepine (Trileptal)
- Ciprofloxacin
- General anesthetics
- Haloperidol (Haldol)
- Mizoribine
- Nicotine
- Nonsteroidal antiinflammatory medications
- Pentamidine
- *Serotonergic agents:* 3,4-methylenedioxymethamphetamine (MDMA; Ecstasy), selective serotonin reuptake inhibitors
- Thiazide diuretics
- Tricyclic antidepressants

Positive-Pressure Ventilation

intracellular-extracellular osmotic gradient and causes a shift of water into brain cells, leading to cerebral edema and increased intracranial pressure. A decrease in the serum sodium level to lower than 120 mEq/L in 48 hours or less is usually associated with serious neurological symptoms and a mortality rate as high as 50%. If hyponatremia develops more slowly, the body may be able to protect against cerebral edema; however, serum sodium <110 to 115 mEq/L can cause confusion, lethargy, and seizures.[9]

Cardiovascular system. Water retention produces edema, increased blood pressure, and elevated central venous and pulmonary artery occlusion pressures.

Pulmonary system. Fluid overload in the pulmonary system produces increased respiratory rate; dyspnea; adventitious lung sounds; and frothy, pink sputum.

Gastrointestinal system. Congestion of the gastrointestinal tract and decreased motility occur because of hyponatremia. This is manifested by nausea and vomiting, anorexia, muscle cramps, and decreased bowel sounds.

Laboratory Evaluation. The hallmark of SIADH is hyponatremia and hypoosmolality in the presence of concentrated urine. A low serum osmolarity should trigger inhibition of ADH secretion, resulting in loss of water through the kidneys and dilute urine (see Laboratory Alert: Pituitary Disorders).

High urinary sodium levels (>20 mEq/L) help differentiate SIADH from other causes of hypoosmolality, hyponatremia, and volume overload (e.g., heart failure). In SIADH, renal perfusion (a major stimulus for sodium reabsorption) is usually adequate, so sodium is not conserved, resulting in urinary sodium excretion. In a disorder such as heart failure, renal perfusion is low because of decreased cardiac output triggering reabsorption of sodium.

Hemodilution may decrease other laboratory values such as BUN, creatinine, and albumin. SIADH should be suspected in a patient with evidence of hemodilution and urine that is hypertonic relative to plasma.

Patient Problems. The primary problem for the patient with SIADH is fluid overload due to water retention from excess ADH.

Nursing and Medical Interventions. The goals of therapy are to treat the underlying cause, eliminate excess water, and increase serum osmolality. In many instances, treatment of the underlying disorder (e.g., discontinuation of a responsible medication) is all that is needed to return the patient's condition to normal. Also refer to the Collaborative Plan of Care for the Critically Ill Patient (Chapter 1, Overview of Critical Care Nursing).

Fluid balance. In mild to moderate cases (serum sodium level, 125 to 135 mEq/L), fluid intake is restricted to 800 to 1000 mL/day, with liberal dietary salt and protein intake.[9,25] Evaluate the patient's response by monitoring serum sodium levels, serum osmolality, and weight loss for a gradual return to baseline.

In severe, symptomatic cases (coma, seizures, serum sodium level <110 mEq/L), small amounts of hypertonic (1.5% to 3%) saline may be administered, following rigorous guidelines and with careful monitoring (Box 19.23). Strict adherence to rates of administration of hypertonic solutions and measurement of serial serum sodium levels are essential to prevent cerebral edema and central pontine myelinolysis. The risk of heart failure is also significant. A diuretic such as furosemide may be given during hypertonic saline administration to promote diuresis and free water clearance. Treatments for chronic or resistant SIADH are listed in Box 19.24.

Nursing. Prevention of SIADH may not be possible, but early detection and treatment may prevent more serious sequelae from occurring. Be aware of the populations at risk and monitor at-risk patients for clinical signs of alterations.

Closely monitor fluid and electrolyte balance. Weigh the patient daily. Record intake and output hourly and measure the urine specific gravity. Monitor for fluid overload by assessing for tachycardia, increased blood pressure, increased hemodynamic pressures, full bounding pulses, and distended neck veins. Monitor respiratory function for signs of tachypnea, labored respirations, shortness of breath, or fine crackles. Regularly

BOX 19.23 Nursing Considerations for Administration of 3% Sodium Chloride

- Central venous catheter preferred with higher concentrations and infusion rate.
- Administer via pump only.
- Rate should not exceed 50 mL/h.
- Monitor serum sodium levels every 4 hours; hold infusion if serum sodium level exceeds 155 mEq/L.
- Wean solution rather than stopping abruptly.
- Monitor level of responsiveness for evidence of decline (could indicate cerebral edema or worsening hyponatremia).
- Monitor lung sounds for crackles indicating pulmonary edema.
- Monitor intake and output every hour.

BOX 19.24 Treatments for Chronic or Resistant Syndrome of Inappropriate Antidiuretic Hormone Secretion[a]

- Water restriction of 800 to 1000 mL/day.
- Administration of loop diuretics in conjunction with increased salt and potassium intake is the safest method for treating chronic hyponatremia. The diuretic prevents urine concentration, and the increased salt and potassium intake increases water output by increasing delivery of solutes to the kidney.

[a]Doses are approximate and may vary based on the individual situation.
ADH, Antidiuretic hormone; *PO,* orally.

monitor potassium and magnesium levels for the need to replace diuresis-induced losses.

Adherence to fluid restriction is critical but difficult for patients. Ensure that the patient and family understand the importance of the restriction and that they are included in planning types and timing of fluids. Encourage patients to choose fluids high in sodium content, such as milk, tomato juice, and beef or chicken broth. To relieve some of the discomfort caused by fluid restriction, provide frequent mouth care, oral rinses without swallowing, chilled beverages, and hard candy.

Assess the patient's neurological status to monitor the effects of treatment and identify complications. Observe the patient for subtle changes that may indicate water intoxication, such as fatigue, weakness, headache, or changes in level of consciousness. Institute seizure precautions if the patient's sodium level decreases to less than 120 mEq/L.

Patient and Family Education. Some patients with SIADH may need long-term treatment, ongoing monitoring, or both. These patients and their families require instruction on the following: (1) early signs and symptoms to report to the healthcare provider—weight gain, lethargy, weakness, nausea, and mental status changes; (2) the significance of adherence to fluid restriction; (3) dose, side effects, and rationale for prescribed medications; and (4) the importance of daily weights.

Cerebral Salt Wasting

Etiology. Patients with any type of serious brain insult may develop CSW. Brain trauma, subarachnoid hemorrhage, ischemic stroke, spontaneous intracranial hemorrhage, and meningitis are associated with development of CSW.[25] CSW occurs in up to 40% of traumatic brain injury cases and is associated with increased morbidity and mortality.[25]

Pathophysiology. The exact pathophysiology of CSW is unknown. A defect in renal sodium transport has been suggested, and *renal salt wasting* has been proposed as a more accurate term for this condition.[7] Natriuretic peptides, which are commonly released in severe brain injury, and impaired aldosterone have been implicated as factors in defective renal sodium transport. However, research has produced conflicting data, and diagnosis of salt wasting in the absence of cerebral injuries is rare.[25]

Assessment

Clinical presentation. The findings associated with CSW are due to hypovolemia and hyponatremia. Signs of hypovolemia include decreased skin turgor, dry mucous membranes, tachycardia, weight loss, and hypotension. Signs of hyponatremia include weakness, lethargy, mental confusion, difficulty concentrating, restlessness, headache, seizures, and coma. Neurological signs and symptoms are seen with both hypovolemia and hyponatremia.

Laboratory Evaluation. An increased serum osmolality, decreased serum sodium, and increased urine sodium characterize CSW. Hemoconcentration may increase other laboratory values, such as BUN, creatinine, and albumin (see Laboratory Alert: Pituitary Disorders).

Patient Problems. The primary problem that may apply to a patient with CSW is low fluid volume and risk for dehydration due to lack of renal sodium retention and diuresis.

Nursing and Medical Interventions. The primary goal of treatment is to simultaneously restore both sodium and fluid volume. Replacing fluids without sodium may worsen the hyponatremia, resulting in life-threatening consequences. Both isotonic saline and hypertonic (1.5% to 3%) saline are used. Hypertonic saline is given in the presence of cerebral edema so that sodium levels increase at a rate of no more than 12 mEq/L in 24 hours, and 0.9% NS is administered to replace volume at a rate that matches urine output.[25] Once symptoms have resolved, hypertonic saline can be stopped. Serum sodium levels should be monitored every 4 to 6 hours to watch for recurrent drops in sodium.[25] Oral or IV fludrocortisone, 100 to 200 mcg daily, may be given to increase sodium retention in the renal tubules.[25] Refer to the Collaborative Plan of Care for the Critically Ill Patient (Chapter 1, Overview of Critical Care Nursing).

CLINICAL JUDGMENT ACTIVITY

Compare the laboratory of diabetes insipidus (DI), syndrome of inappropriate antidiuretic hormone secretion (SIADH), and cerebral salt wasting (CSW) and explain how they help differentiate these crises in patients with neurological injury.

CASE STUDY

A 68-year-old male is admitted to the critical care unit from the emergency department with respiratory failure and hypotension. His history is significant for type 2 diabetes mellitus, steroid-dependent chronic obstructive pulmonary disease, peripheral vascular disease, cigarette smoking, and alcohol use disorder. His medications at home include glipizide, prednisone, and a metered-dose inhaler with albuterol and ipratropium (Combivent). In the emergency department he received a single dose of ceftriaxone and etomidate for intubation.

On examination, he is intubated, on pressure-controlled ventilation, and receiving 0.9% normal saline at 200 mL/h and dopamine at 8 mcg/kg/min. His blood pressure is 86/50 mm Hg; heart rate, 126 beats/min; oxygen saturation, 88%; and temperature, 39.6°C. His cardiac rhythm shows sinus tachycardia and nonspecific ST-T wave changes. Arterial blood gas values are as follows: pH, 7.21; PaO_2, 83 mm Hg; $PaCO_2$, 50 mm Hg; and bicarbonate, 12 mEq/L. Other laboratory values are as follows: serum glucose, 308 mg/dL; serum creatinine, 2.1 mg/dL; and white blood cell count, 19,000/mm^3.

Questions

1. Identify which disease state you suspect this patient is experiencing and explain why.
2. Based on this patient's risk factors, determine which potential endocrine complications you anticipate.
3. What further laboratory studies would you want? Explain what results you anticipate.
4. What treatment goals and strategies do you anticipate implementing?
5. In providing patient and family education and support, explain which issues need to be addressed immediately and which can be delayed.

KEY POINTS

- Alterations in endocrine function may be due to hyposecretion or hypersecretion of hormones, alterations in transport of hormones, or alterations in receptor function.
- The most effective way to manage hyperglycemia is administration of insulin with a target glucose of 140 to 180 mg/dL.
- Many episodes of hypoglycemia are preventable. Accurate and consistent glucose assessment is key in preventing hypoglycemia.
- DKA and HHS occur due to relative or absolute insulin deficiency and increased amounts of counterregulatory hormones.
- In DKA, ketosis is present; in HHS, there is a lack of ketosis due to the presence of some insulin, which prevents lipolysis.
- Adrenal crisis occurs due to absence of cortisol (glucocorticoid) and aldosterone (mineralocorticoid) and may develop due to undiagnosed disease, abrupt withdrawal of glucocorticoid therapy, or stress associated with infection or critical illness.
- Thyrotoxicosis (thyroid storm) is a severe form of hyperthyroidism, and myxedema coma is a severe form of hypothyroidism. Both crises usually occur in undiagnosed or undertreated thyroid disorders in times of stress and illness and are life-threatening medical emergencies.
- SIADH is characterized by abnormally high ADH secretion; DI is characterized by abnormally low ADH secretion. CSW is similar to SI ADH, but it is important to differentiate between the two because treatment strategies differ.
- Sodium disorders, especially hyponatremia, are common in critically ill patients experiencing endocrine crises.
- Replacement of fluids and electrolytes should be controlled to prevent adverse neurological effects such as cerebral edema and osmotic demyelination syndrome.
- Frequent assessment and monitoring of neurologic, cardiac, respiratory, vascular, and electrolyte status are key nursing responsibilities for patients with endocrine disorders.

REFERENCES

1. American Diabetes Association. Diabetes care in the hospital: standards of medical care in diabetes. *Diab Care*. 2022;45(Suppl 1):S244–S253.
2. Turner KD, Brashers V. Mechanisms of hormonal regulation. In: Rogers J, McCance K, Huether S, eds. *Pathophysiology: The Biologic Basis for Disease in Adults and Children*. 9th ed. St. Louis, MO: Elsevier; 2023:662–648.
3. Alhatemi G, Aldiwani H, Alhatemi R, et al. Glycemic control in the critically ill: less is more. *Cleve Clin J Med*. 2022;89(4):191–199.
4. Van den Berghe G, Wouters P, Weekers F, et al. Intensive insulin therapy in critically ill patients. *N Engl J Med*. 2001;345(19):1359–1367.
5. American Diabetes Association. Glycemic targets: standards of medical care in diabetes. *Diab Care*. 2022;45(Suppl 1):S83–S96.
6. Long B, Willis G, Lentz S, et al. Diagnosis and management of the critically ill adult patient with hyperglycemic hyperosmolar state. *J Emerg Med*. 2021;61(4):365–375.
7. American Diabetes Association. Classification and diagnosis of diabetes: standards of medical care in diabetes. *Diab Care*. 2022;45(Suppl 1):S17–S38.
8. Gosmanov AR, Gosmanova EO, Kitabchi AE. Hyperglycemic crises: diabetic ketoacidosis (DKA) and hyperglycemic hyperosmolar state (HHS). In: Feingold KR, Anawalt B, Boyce A, et al., eds. *Endotext*. South Dartmouth, MA: MDText.com, Inc.; 2018. [Internet]. https://www.ncbi.nlm.nih.gov/books/NBK279052/.
9. Allen JA. Alterations of hormonal regulation. In: Rodgers J, ed. *McCance & Huether's Pathophysiology: The Biologic Basis for Disease in Adults and Children*. 9th ed. St. Louis, MO: Elsevier; 2023:688–718.
10. American Diabetes Association. Management of diabetes in pregnancy: standards of medical care in diabetes. *Diabetes Care*. 2022;45(Suppl 1):S232–S243.
11. Nasa P, Chaudhary S, Shrivastava PK, Singh A. Euglycemic diabetic ketoacidosis: a missed diagnosis. *World J Diabetes*. 2021;12(5):514–523. https://doi.org/10.4239/wjd.v23.i5.514.

12. Diaz-Ramos A, Eilber W, Marquez D. Euglycemic diabetic ketoacidosis associated with sodium-glucose cotransporter-2 inhibitor use: a case report and review of the literature. *Int J Emer Med*. 2019;12:27.
13. Long B, Willis G, Lentz S, et al. Evaluation and management of the critically ill adult with diabetic ketoacidosis. *J Emerg Med*. 2020;59(3):371–383.
14. Jacobi J. Management of endocrine emergencies in the ICU. *J Pharm Pract*. 2019;32(3):314–326.
15. American Diabetes Association. Older adults: standards of medical care in diabetes. *Diab Care*. 2022;45(Suppl 1):S195–S207.
16. Gojnic M, et al. Maternal and fetal outcomes among pregnant women with diabetes. *Int J Environ Res Public Health*. 2022;19:3684.
17. Self WH, Evans CS, Jenkins CA, et al. Clinical effects of balanced crystalloids vs saline in adults with diabetic ketoacidosis: a subgroup analysis of cluster randomized clinical trials. *JAMA Netw Open*. 2020;3(11):e2024596.
18. Cruz-Flores S. Neurological complications of endocrine emergencies. *Current Neurol Neurosci Rep*. 2021;21:21.
19. Gerlach H. Adrenal insufficiency. In: Vincent JL, Abraham E, Moore FA, et al., eds. *Textbook of Critical Care*. 7th ed. Philadelphia, PA: Elsevier; 2017:1024–1033.e2.
20. Felver L. The cellular environment. In: Rogers J, McCance K, Huether S, eds. *Pathophysiology: The Biologic Basis for Disease in Adults and Children*. 9th ed. St. Louis, MO: Elsevier; 2023:106–129.
21. Winton MB. Endocrine function. In: Meiner SE, Yeager JJ, eds. *Gerontologic Nursing*. 6th ed. St. Louis, MO: Elsevier; 2019:521–571.
22. Lee J, Torpy D. Adrenal insufficiency in pregnancy: physiology, diagnosis, management, and areas for future research. *Endocr Metab Disord*. 2023;24(1):57–69. https://doi.org/10.1007/s11154-022-09745-6.
23. Leung AM, Farwell AP. Thyroid disorders. In: Vincent JL, Abraham E, Moore FA, et al., eds. *Textbook of Critical Care*. 7th ed. Philadelphia, PA: Elsevier; 2017:1034-1-42.e2.
24. Brennan M, Mulkerrin L, O'Keefe ST, O'Shea PM. Approach to the management of hypernatremia in older hospitalized patients. *J Nutr Health Aging*. 2021;25(10):1161–1166.
25. Baba M, Alsbrook D, Williamson S, et al. Approach to the management of sodium disorders in the neuro critical care unit. *Curr Treat Options Neurol*. 2022;24:327–346.
26. Kheetan M, Ogu I, Shapiro JI, Khitan ZJ. Acute and chronic hyponatremia. *Front Med (Lausanne)*. 2021;8:693738. https://doi.org/10.3389/fmed.2021.
27. Brimioulle S. Diabetes insipidus. In: Vincent JL, Abraham E, Moor FA, et al., eds. *Textbook of Critical Care*. 7th ed. Philadelphia, PA: Elsevier; 2017:1043–1045.e1.

20

Trauma and Surgical Management

Linda Staubli, MSN, RN, CCRN, ACCNS-AG

INTRODUCTION

Trauma is defined as an injury or wound to a living tissue caused by external force.[1] In addition to the physical injury, trauma can also be a disordered psychic or behavioral state resulting from severe mental or emotional stress or physical injury.[1] Traumatic injury typically includes unintentional injuries and violence-related injuries and affects everyone, regardless of age, race, or economic status. Unintentional and violence-related injuries, including suicide, homicide, overdoses, motor vehicle crashes, and falls, were among the top 10 causes of death for all age groups in the United States.[2] Unintentional and violence-related injuries are costly and considered preventable. Therefore, an overarching goal in trauma care is prevention. However, when traumatic injuries occur, the priority is early and aggressive intervention to save life and limb. This chapter provides a review of trauma systems, the trauma team concept, the systematic and standardized approach to trauma care, and phases of trauma care. Because the nature of traumatic events usually requires surgical interventions, the postsurgical management of the trauma patient is discussed. Special populations, common traumatic injuries, and mass casualty incident response are also described.

TRAUMA IN THE UNITED STATES

Trauma Demographics

Trauma is frequently referred to as a disease of the young because unintentional injury is the leading cause of death in persons ages 1 to 44 years in the United States.[3] Motor vehicle collisions (MVCs) are a leading cause of injury death in the United States across all age groups, with more than 100 people dying every day.[4] In 2021 in the United States, more than 41,000 people died in MVCs, more than 2.1 million emergency department (ED) visits were due to injuries from MVCs, and deaths from crashes resulted in over $430 billion in total costs.[4] Fortunately, MVC injuries are preventable, and proven strategies can improve the safety of drivers on the road.

Another peak in trauma-related injuries occurs between the ages of 25 and 64 years, in which poisoning from prescription or illegal drugs is the leading cause of unintentional deaths; MVCs are the next-highest cause in this age group.[3] Nearly 106,699 drug overdose deaths occurred in the United States in 2021, and the age-adjusted rate of drug overdose deaths was more than 32.4 per 100,000 individuals.[5] In persons aged 65 and older, unintentional falls, followed by MVCs, are the leading cause of injury deaths.[3]

Trauma is a major healthcare and economic concern because of the loss of life, the societal burden in terms of lost productivity and increased disability of injured persons, and the consumption of healthcare resources. Economic factors associated with traumatic injury include both direct and indirect costs. Direct costs are related to the actual expense of treatment and rehabilitative care. Indirect costs are associated with lost work, physical and psychological disability (temporary and permanent), and lost productivity. Unintentional and violence-related injuries were among the top 10 causes of death in the United States for all age groups and caused nearly 27 million nonfatal emergency department visits.[2] The estimated economic cost of injuries in the United States was $4.2 trillion, including costs of medical care, work loss, and quality of life loss.[2]

Injury is a potentially preventable public health problem of enormous magnitude, whether measured by years of productive life lost, prolonged or permanent disability, or financial cost. Advocates of organized trauma systems identify prevention as an essential component of a structured approach to trauma care. Once a trauma injury happens, an organized and structured approach to trauma care is critical to improved outcomes with decreased patient morbidity and mortality.[6–10] Nurses play an essential role in the care of the patient after traumatic injury, from prevention to resuscitation through rehabilitation.

SYSTEMS APPROACH TO TRAUMA CARE

Trauma System

Trauma systems are effective in reducing the morbidity and mortality of severely injured individuals by providing care to all injured patients in an organized, coordinated manner across geographical areas and the continuum of care.[8–10] Optimal trauma care requires a systematic approach that is coordinated along the entire continuum of injury care, including intentional and unintentional injury prevention, prehospital advanced life-support interventions, rapid transport, acute hospital care with evidence-based trauma protocols and resources to care for injured patients, rehabilitation, and reassimilation of the injured individual into the community (Fig. 20.1).[9,10] This model of a

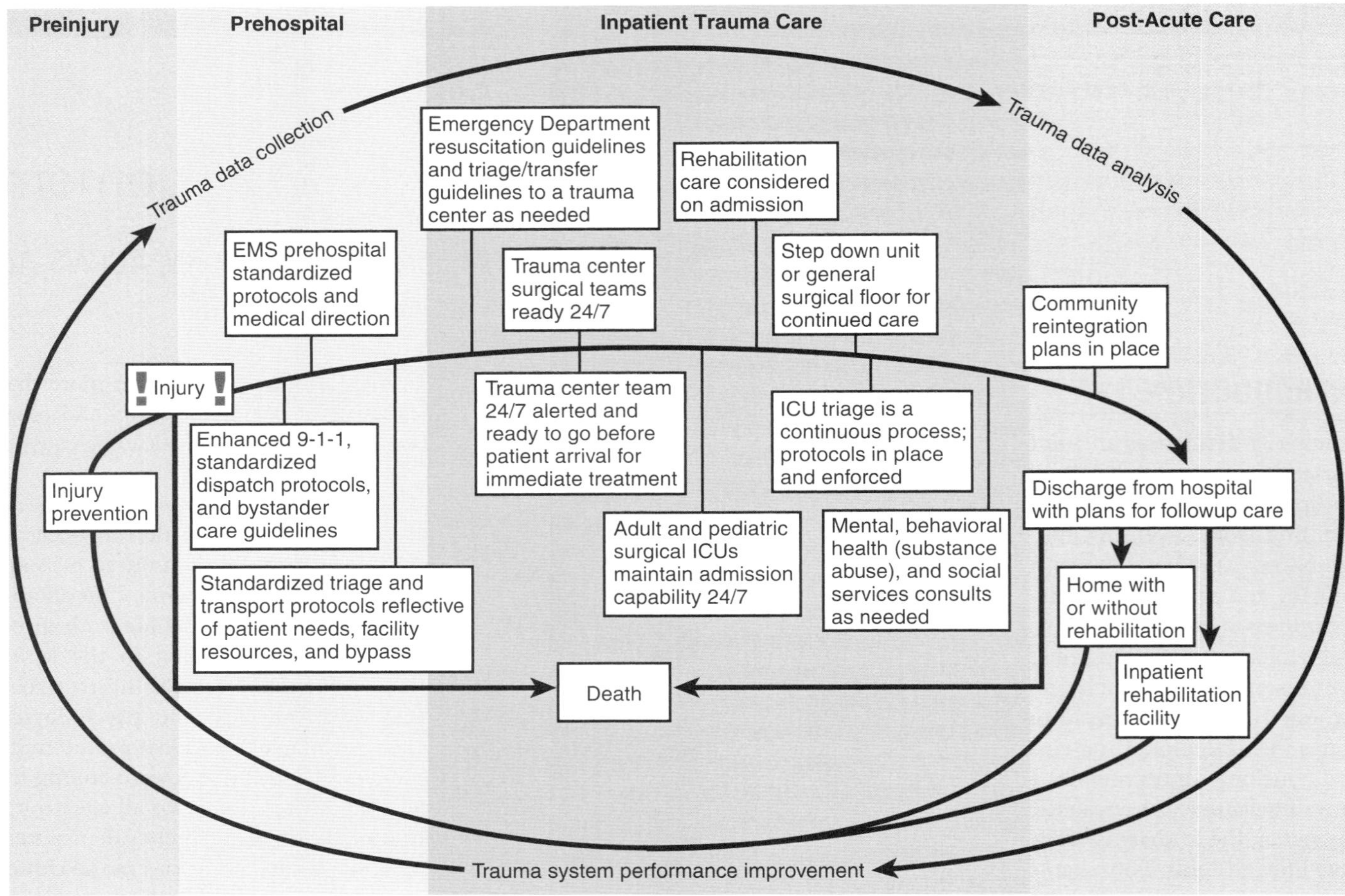

Fig. 20.1 A preplanned trauma care continuum. *EMS,* Emergency medical services; *ICU,* intensive care unit. (From U.S. Department of Health and Human Services [HHS], Health Resources and Services Administration. *Model Trauma System Planning and Evaluation.* Rockville, MD: HHS; 2006. https://www.facs.org/media/p0nfw0n0/hrsa-mtspe.pdf.)

trauma system expands care from a single center to multiple facilities. Specifically, a network of regional and state trauma systems allows for the best possible care to be delivered for the type and severity of traumatic injury by matching the patient's medical needs to the level of trauma hospital with the necessary resources. The goal of a trauma system is to facilitate and coordinate a multiprofessional response that matches the needs of injured patients to the capabilities of the trauma center.[9,10] A trauma system includes a combination of levels of designated trauma centers with other acute care facilities. Levels of trauma centers distinguish a difference in resources and expertise available within the specific hospital.[11]

Levels of Trauma Care

Formal categorization of trauma care facilities, based on resources and capabilities to meet the needs of an injured patient, is essential to provide optimal care. The American College of Surgeons (ACS) has established the process for categorizing hospitals based on minimum standards at each level. The ACS trauma system identifies three levels of trauma care: Levels I, II, and III (Table 20.1).[11] The organization conducts reviews of hospitals seeking trauma designation and provides consultations with hospitals, communities, and states regarding trauma centers. Hospitals of all designations collaborate to develop transfer agreements and treatment protocols that maximize patient survival. A current list of hospitals with verified trauma centers is published on the ACS website (http://www.facs.org/trauma/verified.html).

Trauma Continuum

Death caused by traumatic injury is historically described as having a trimodal distribution, implying that death due to injury occurs in one of three peaks. The first peak, labeled as *immediate death,* occurs within seconds to minutes from the time of injury. These patients are declared dead at the scene or shortly after arrival in an ED. Death is caused by severe injuries, such as apnea from severe brain or high spinal cord injury or massive hemorrhage.[6] Only trauma prevention will decrease deaths that occur in the first peak.

The second peak is labeled *early death.* It occurs within minutes to several hours after injury. Death results from severe injuries such as hemopneumothorax, ruptured spleen, liver laceration, pelvic fracture, or other multiple injuries associated with significant blood loss. The first hour of emergent care, called the "golden hour," focuses on rapid assessment, resuscitation, and treatment of life-threatening injuries.[6]

TABLE 20.1 American College of Surgeons Classification of Trauma Center Level

Level I	• Provides comprehensive trauma care • Serves as a regional resource center to provide leadership in education, outreach, and systems planning • Admits at least 1200 trauma patients annually or has at least 240 admissions with an Injury Severity Score (ISS) >15 • Provides 24-hour in-house availability of an attending surgeon, who will be in the emergency department on patient arrival or within 15 min for the highest level of activation • Conducts trauma research
Level II	• Provides comprehensive trauma care as a supplement to a Level I center • Meets the same attending surgeon expectations for care as a Level I center
Level III	• Provides immediate emergency care and stabilization of a patient before transfer to a higher level of care • Provides definitive care to patients with mild to moderate injuries • Serves a community that does not have immediate access to a Level I or II center

Modified from American College of Surgeons, Committee on Trauma. *Resources for Optimal Care of the Injured Patient*. Chicago, IL: American College of Surgeons, Committee on Trauma; 2022.

The third peak, *late death*, occurs several days to weeks after the initial injury. It is most often the result of sepsis, acute respiratory distress syndrome (ARDS), increased intracranial pressure (ICP), and multiple organ dysfunction syndrome (MODS).[6]

Since the seminal publication of a trimodal distribution of trauma deaths, the development of trauma systems has altered the distribution of deaths to a bimodal or unimodal pattern with an overall reduction in trauma mortality.[6,12] Specifically, there has been a continuous decrease in the incidence of late deaths.[12] This shifting distribution of death supports the central concept of trauma systems: matching patients' severity of injury to the available resources for optimal care at a designated trauma center to decrease the incidence of death after admission. Special resources, including early surgical management of injuries, are needed to decrease the morbidity and mortality of severely injured patients. Therefore the most critically injured patients should be cared for in higher-level trauma centers with the appropriate resources and expertise to maximize patient outcomes.

Injury Prevention

Traumatic injury prevention is an important aspect of trauma system effectiveness. In partnership with community organizations, trauma centers must have an organized approach to injury prevention that is prioritized based on local injury patterns.[13] Level I trauma centers must have a prevention coordinator, whereas lower-level trauma centers have someone with prevention efforts detailed in their job description.[13] Level I and Level II trauma centers must implement programs that address one of the major causes of injury in the community.[13]

Injury prevention occurs at three levels. *Primary prevention* involves interventions to prevent the event (e.g., driving safety classes, speed limits, campaigns against drinking and driving, fall prevention interventions, domestic violence prevention campaigns, drug awareness campaigns). *Secondary prevention* entails strategies to minimize the impact of the traumatic event (e.g., seat-belt use, airbags, advances in automobile construction, car seats, helmets, antibullying hotlines). *Tertiary prevention* refers to interventions to maximize patient outcomes after a traumatic event through emergency response systems, medical care, and rehabilitation.

Historically, traumatic events were considered accidents or events that resulted from human error, fate, or bad luck. Today, it is understood that injuries and violence are not random events. An individual's knowledge, risk-taking behaviors, beliefs, and decisions to engage in certain activities influence the outcomes of actions. The word *accident* conveys a message of randomness in which an individual cannot prevent the event. Because most traumatic events are considered preventable, this word has been removed from the discussion of traumatic injuries such as those sustained in MVCs. Changing the language—*motor vehicle collision* instead of *motor vehicle accident*—conveys the message that efforts can be implemented to prevent MVCs and that additional behaviors, such as wearing a seat belt, may minimize their impact.

Nurses are role models for trauma prevention within their families and communities and through political involvement. Simple efforts include writing letters to local and national policy makers to encourage changes in laws and enforcement of public policies favoring injury prevention, such as helmet and seat-belt laws, driving under the influence of drugs or alcohol laws, limiting access to firearms laws, and support programs to end domestic violence and bullying. Involvement in injury and violence prevention programs includes supporting community and national coalition networks for prevention, such as Mothers Against Drunk Driving and antibullying campaigns.[14] Nurses, as members of the frontline team, are poised to lead injury prevention by identifying patients at risk, educating patients and families, collaborating with injury-prevention specialists, and referring to community resources where available.[15]

Trauma Team Concept

The term *trauma team*, similar to a code team, refers to healthcare professionals who respond immediately to and participate in the initial resuscitation and stabilization of the trauma patient. Box 20.1 lists the composition of a typical trauma team. Trauma care begins in the field when the emergency medical services (EMS) team responds to an event. Trauma systems work with EMS teams to create protocols that maximize treatment in the field. Once a patient has been stabilized in the field, the EMS team communicates with the hospital en route, and the hospital trauma team is activated. Essential to the team approach is ensuring that each team member is preassigned and understands the specific responsibilities inherent in a particular team role. The trauma surgeon is ultimately responsible for the activities of the trauma team and acts as the team leader in

BOX 20.1 Multiprofessional Trauma Team

- Emergency medical services (EMS) response team
- Trauma surgeon (team leader)
- Emergency provider
- Anesthesiologist
- Trauma nurse team leader (coordinates and directs nursing care)
- Trauma resuscitation nurse (hangs IV fluids, blood, and medications; assists providers)
- Trauma scribe (records all interventions on the trauma flowsheet)
- Pharmacist
- Respiratory therapist
- Laboratory phlebotomist
- Radiology technician
- Social worker or pastoral services provider
- Hospital security officer
- Specialists (neurosurgeon, orthopedic surgeon, urological surgeon)

establishing rapid assessment, resuscitation, stabilization, and intervention priorities. Other team members, such as ED providers, consultants (e.g., orthopedic surgeons, neurosurgeons, otolaryngologists, thoracic surgeons, ophthalmologists, plastic surgeons), nurses, pharmacists, respiratory therapists, social workers, chaplains, and interventional radiologists, all have specific responsibilities. Each member of the trauma team is vital to meeting the needs of a patient with multiple traumatic injuries.

MECHANISM OF INJURY

Injury and death result from both unintentional events and deliberate actions such as violent aggression or suicide. The term *mechanism of injury* refers to how a traumatic event occurred, the injuring agent, and information about the type and amount of energy exchanged during the event. Knowledge of the mechanism of injury assists the trauma team in early identification and management of injuries that may not be apparent on initial assessment.[6,16] Understanding the mechanism of traumatic injury provides insight into the transfer of energy to the body, guiding the assessment and interventions to minimize the chance of missing injuries that are more subtle (e.g., organ contusions). Questions regarding mechanisms of injury are directed to the patient (if applicable), prehospital care providers, law enforcement personnel, or bystanders in an attempt to reenact the scene of the trauma (Box 20.2).

The transfer of energy with the human body causes traumatic injury. Energy may be kinetic (e.g., collisions, falls, blast injuries, penetrating injuries), thermal, electrical, chemical, or radiant. *Kinetic energy* is defined as mass multiplied by velocity squared. Therefore, the greater the mass and/or velocity (speed), the more significant the displacement of kinetic energy to body structures, resulting in more severe injury. The effects of the energy released and the resultant injuries depend on the force of impact, the duration of impact, the body tissue involved, the injuring agent, and the presence of associated risk factors. Understanding the mechanism of injury and resultant transfer of energy helps the trauma team anticipate injury patterns and interventions.[6,16] Injury patterns resulting from energy exchange are further described as blunt, penetrating, and blast injuries.

BOX 20.2 Sample Questions to Ask to Determine Mechanism of Injury and Potential Complications

- Was the patient wearing a seat belt?
- Was the airbag deployed?
- What was the speed of the vehicle on impact?
- Where was the patient located in the car? Driver? Passenger? Front seat or back seat?
- Was the patient wearing a helmet (e.g., for a bicycle, motorcycle, or snow sporting collision)?
- What type of weapon was used (e.g., length of knife, type and caliber of gun)?
- How far did the patient fall (or how far was the patient thrown by the impact)?
- How long was the patient in the field before emergency medical services (EMS) arrived?
- Was there a death in the vehicle or at the event?

Blunt Trauma

Blunt trauma is a common mechanism of injury. Blunt trauma can appear less obvious than other injury patterns, with minimal or no outward signs of injury.[16] It often results from MVCs, motorcycle collisions, assaults with blunt objects, falls, sports-related activities, and pedestrians struck by a motor vehicle. Blunt trauma may be caused by accelerating, decelerating, shearing, crushing, and compressing forces. Vehicular injury often results from a mechanism of acceleration-deceleration forces. The vehicle and the body accelerate and travel at an identified speed. In normal circumstances, the vehicle and body slow to a motionless state concurrently. However, when a vehicle stops abruptly, the body continues to travel forward until it comes in contact with a stationary object, such as the dashboard, windshield, or steering column. Injury occurs in the presence of rapid deceleration, when the movement ceases and contents within the body continue to travel within an enclosed space or compartment. An example of this occurs when a passenger's head strikes the windshield after the automobile collides with a cement barrier. The brain tissue strikes the cranium and is thrown back against the opposite side of the cranial vault, with a resulting coup-contrecoup injury. Fig. 20.2 shows potential sites of injury to an unrestrained passenger and driver as a result of blunt trauma.

CLINICAL JUDGMENT ACTIVITY

A patient presents to the trauma center after a motor vehicle collision en route to an antique automobile event. The patient was restrained by his seat belt; however, he was driving an antique car that did not have airbags. He was awake at the scene, but his level of consciousness quickly declined during transport by emergency medical services (EMS). Initial assessment revealed a 6-cm scalp laceration, a right closed femur fracture, four broken ribs, and possible cardiac and pulmonary contusions. Describe additional prehospital information that the nurse should elicit in anticipating care for this patient. Considering the mechanism and patterns of the injuries, determine and describe the immediate nursing management priorities for this patient.

Body tissues and structures respond to kinetic energy in different ways. Low-density porous tissues and structures, such as the lungs, tolerate energy transference and often experience little damage because of their elasticity. Conversely, organs such as the heart, spleen, and liver are less resilient because of their high-density tissue and decreased ability to release energy without resultant tissue damage.[17,18] These types of organs often present with lacerations, contusions, or rupture. The severity of injury resulting from a blunt force is contingent on the duration of energy exposure, the body organ involved, and the underlying structures. Blunt trauma requires expert clinical judgment and knowledge of the mechanism of injury to assess and diagnose actual and potential injuries because organ injury from blunt trauma may not be immediately visible.

Penetrating Trauma

Penetrating trauma results from foreign objects (e.g., knives, bullets, debris) entering through the skin barrier. Penetrating injuries are often more easily diagnosed and treated than blunt-force injuries because of the obvious signs of injury. Stab wounds and firearm-related injuries are common causes of penetrating injuries. Stab wounds are low-velocity injuries; the velocity is equal only to the speed with which the object was thrust into the body. The direct path of injury occurs when the impaled object contacts underlying vessels and tissues. Important considerations in a stabbing are the length and width of the impaling object and the presence of vital organs in the area of the stab wound.

Ballistic trauma is categorized as either low- or high-velocity injuries. Low-velocity weapons are shotguns and pistols. High-velocity weapons are assault weapons and rifles. The velocity; type of bullet, including caliber and material (missile); and trajectory in the body influence the transfer of energy that creates tissue injury.[19] As the missile penetrates the tissues, vessels are stretched and compressed, creating a cavity of tissue damage (referred to as a *cavitation*). Depending on the range, the distance from the weapon to the point of bodily impact, and the velocity of the missile, the cavitation may be as great as 30 times the diameter of the bullet.[19] As bullets travel through the body, damage to surrounding tissues and organs may occur. Knowledge of the type of bullet (e.g., size, round versus hollow point, shotgun pellet) influences the assessment as to the type of internal tissue damage that may have occurred. For example, air-filled organs such as the lungs and stomach tolerate high-velocity cavitation better than solid organs such as the liver, which have a greater propensity to shear or tear.[16] Assessment of the penetrating injuries from a gunshot involves examination of the entrance wound and, if applicable, the exit wounds. Penetrating injuries are monitored closely for subsequent complications, including organ damage, hemorrhage, and infection.

Blast Injuries

Blast injuries are forms of blunt and penetrating trauma. Energy exchanged from the blast causes tissue and organ damage. Blast injuries may occur as a result of construction site explosions, fireworks, and terrorist attacks. Penetrating injury may occur as a result of debris entering the body. The U.S. Department of Defense classifies blast injuries into five levels: primary, secondary, tertiary, quaternary, or quinary.[16,20]

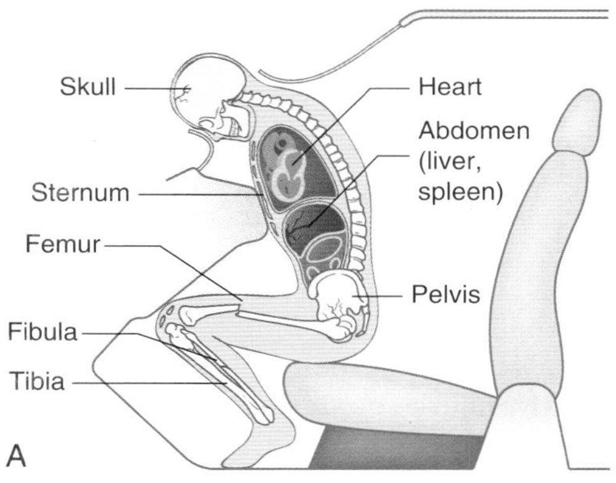

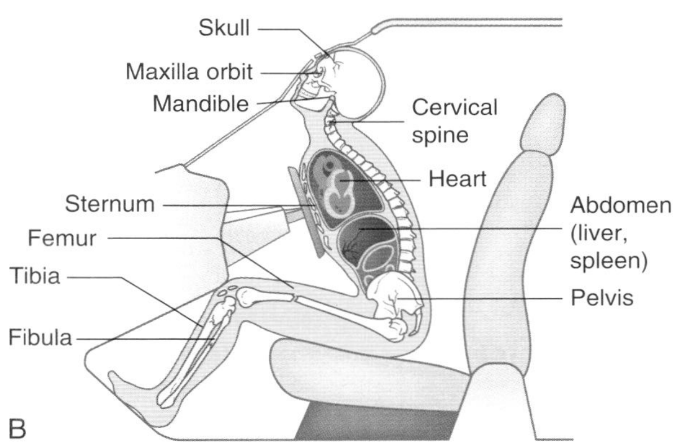

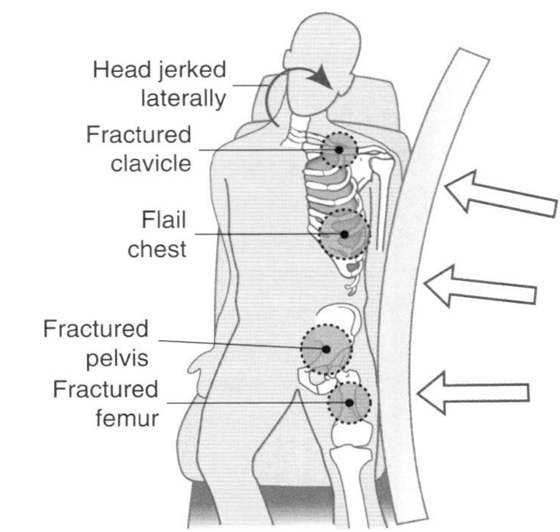

Fig. 20.2 Potential sites of blunt trauma injury to an unrestrained passenger and driver in a motor vehicle crash. A, Unrestrained passenger in front seat. B, Unrestrained driver. C, Lateral impact collision. (From Herm RL. Biomechanics and mechanism of injury. In: Cohen SS, ed. *Trauma Nursing Secrets*. Philadelphia, PA: Hanley & Belfus; 2003.)

The *primary* explosive blast generates shock waves that change air pressure, and tissue damage results from the pressure waves passing through the body. Initially after an explosion, there is a rapid increase in positive pressure for a short period, followed by a longer period of negative pressure. The increase in positive pressure injures gas-containing organs. The tympanic membrane ruptures, and the stomach, bowel, lungs, and brain may show evidence of contusion, acute edema, or rupture. Intraocular hemorrhage and intestinal rupture may occur from the first shock wave after an explosion. *Secondary* injuries occur from projectiles from the explosion, resulting in penetrating injuries and lacerations. *Tertiary* blast injuries result as the body is thrown or propelled by the force of the explosion, resulting in blunt tissue trauma, including closed head injuries, fractures, and visceral organ injury. *Quaternary* blast injuries occur as a result of chemical or thermal effects or exacerbations of existing conditions such as asthma attacks, panic attacks, or pregnancy complications. *Quinary* blast injuries are associated with hazardous materials, such as radiation from dirty bombs or environmental contamination.[16,20]

DISASTER AND MASS CASUALTY MANAGEMENT

A disaster is a sudden event in which local EMS, hospitals, and community resources are overwhelmed by the demands placed on them. Disasters can be caused by fire, weather (e.g., earthquake, hurricane, flood, tornado), explosions, terrorist activity, radiation or chemical spills, epidemic outbreaks, and human error (e.g., plane crash, mass-transit or multicar crash). An analysis of the National Emergency Medical Services Information system reported that just fewer than 10,000 mass casualty incidents (MCIs) occur annually in the United States.[21] Each disaster is unique, placing tremendous strain on local hospitals or communities to minimize mortality, injury, and destruction of property. Some MCIs are limited to individual hospitals, such as an MVC with multiple victims arriving simultaneously at a critical access hospital that overwhelms the hospital's resources.

Disasters also vary in terms of resource demand, depending on whether any warning was available before the event. For example, with impending weather disasters (e.g., hurricane), medical personnel can prepare a tentative plan for response, but some disasters (e.g., tornado, plane crash, industrial explosion) do not allow for preparation. Mass shootings are the most common and most closely tracked mass casualty event. In the United States, a mass shooting, in which four or more people are injured in a single event, occurs more than once a day on average.[22] The number and lethality of mass shooting incidents have been increasing. While current data is lacking a reported 50% increase in incidents, injuries, and deaths occurred between 2019 and 2021 alone.[22]

Hospital and Community Preparedness

Disaster planning and management response have long been considered a primary responsibility of trauma systems in conjunction with community municipalities. Emergency management is centered around four phases: mitigating the likelihood or limiting the impact of an event, emergency preparedness plans to improve the capability and capacity to manage an emergency, responding safely and effectively when the incident occurs, and recovering from the event.[16,23]

Hospital preparedness strategies improve a hospital and community's capability to respond to an emergency. Preparedness includes planning, training, and exercising for events that cannot be mitigated.[23] Hospitals have well-developed disaster plans (e.g., for weather-related emergencies, bombings, MCIs) that outline specific healthcare provider responses during an event. These plans describe the roles and responsibilities of all healthcare providers, including administrators and security personnel. All personnel are required to be familiar with the disaster response policy. Hospitals maintain active disaster phone call lists. When a disaster occurs, a coordinated effort within each hospital activates this phone list or texting system to contact all the people on the list. Individuals are informed when and where to respond to help with the disaster management. Both human resources and medical supplies are assessed.

Effective Responses Systems and Triage

Effective disaster response includes coordinated communications, triage, and surge capacity. The disaster response is aimed at reducing mortality and morbidity by doing the greatest amount of good for the greatest number of patients.[23,24] Several principles of disaster management and care for individuals injured in an MCI exist. For effective communication, an incident command system (ICS) provides the framework for a coordinated response from all agencies. The ICS exists at the local, state, and national levels, as well as a hospital incident command system (HICS).[24] Field triage is vital in determining how patients are transported to local hospitals and trauma centers. ICS and communication stations are established at the event site whenever possible and maintain contact with the hospital to facilitate efficient transport of patients. Effective, consistent, and accurate communication of the activities at the disaster site and effective management of the severity and volume of incoming victims at the hospitals are critical to successful disaster and MCI management.

Triage occurs at several points during a patient's course through the system: Primary triage occurs in the field by emergency medical services personnel to identify and prioritize the injured before emergency transport.[24,25] Secondary triage is performed immediately upon arrival to the hospital, by an emergency provider or trauma surgeon. Victims are triaged based on the severity of their injuries. Many mass casualty triage classification schemes exist. Traditional mass casualty triage systems involve *Sort, Assess, Lifesaving Intervention, Treatment/Transport (SALT)* and *Simple Triage and Rapid Treatment (START)* triage methodologies and commonly assign each victim to green (minor), yellow (delayed), red (immediate), or black (expectant) categories.[24,25] Black signifies that the patient is unlikely to survive given the severity of injuries, and palliative care and pain relief should be provided. Red (immediate) indicates emergent, life-threatening injuries requiring immediate medical attention. Yellow (delayed) means serious and potentially life-threatening injuries, but status is not expected to deteriorate significantly in the immediate future. Green indicates nonurgent injuries that the patient can likely self-treat.[24] The colored designations can be changed at any time due to clinical status. Patients receive treatment based on the assessment of their chance for survival matched to the resources available for medical intervention. Maximal treatment is provided to the victims; however, supplies are judiciously used to avoid running out of essential items. Matching resources to the trauma patient's needs is necessary to reduce morbidity and mortality.

NURSING SELF-CARE BOX

Recovering After a Trauma Disaster

The recovery phase includes restoration and resumption of normal operations, an after-action analysis for improvement, and staff recovery.[23] Disasters cause significant psychological stress both during the event and after the situation has been stabilized. The psychological well-being of the healthcare provider is acknowledged after a disaster event, and support should be easily accessible and highly encouraged.[23] Timely staff debriefing and employee assistance programs (EAPs) are recommended in the postdisaster phase. Current standards include debriefing after an event to identify opportunities and address the psychological stress on the individual and the team. Debriefing frequently occurs as a group discussion session involving all healthcare team members who participated in the disaster response; however, individual and ongoing psychological interventions may be necessary.

Evidence also suggests that healthcare professionals who engage in stress reduction, mindfulness techniques (e.g., meditation, self-awareness skills, reflective writing), and self-care activities such as regular exercise are more resilient when faced with difficult work situations such as trauma emergency response situations.[26]

EMERGENCY CARE PHASE: TRIAGE

Prehospital Care and Transport

The prehospital medical team provides initial on-scene assessment, management, and transport to the closest facility whose capabilities match the needs of the patient.[27] The ultimate goal of any EMS system is to get the patient to the right level of hospital care in the shortest span of time to optimize patient outcomes without duplicating services based on the maxim "right patient, right place, right time."[27]

Once EMS personnel arrive at the scene of an incident, they direct the situation and prepare the patient for transport. The time from injury to definitive care is a determinant of survival, particularly for those with major internal hemorrhage.[6,28] Treatment of life-threatening injuries is provided at the scene, with careful attention given to the airway with cervical spine immobilization, breathing, and circulation (ABC). Interventions include establishing an airway, providing ventilation, applying pressure to control hemorrhage, immobilizing the complete spine, and stabilizing fractures. Additional life-saving prehospital interventions may include maintaining spinal precautions, placing occlusive dressings on open chest wounds, and performing needle thoracotomy to relieve tension pneumothorax.[29]

Large-caliber IV or intraosseous (IO) access and administration of blood products or low-volume crystalloid solution (e.g., Lactated Ringer's solution) is initiated to restore lost volume and regain tissue perfusion.[30] Large-volume resuscitation is avoided because aggressive overresuscitation can precipitate complications such as inflammatory organ injury (e.g., ARDS, MODS), abdominal compartment syndrome, and worsening coagulopathy.[28,30,31] Fluid resuscitation is guided by vital signs and assessment of end-organ perfusion (i.e., goal-directed resuscitation). In trauma patients without a traumatic brain injury, permissive hypotension, where fluid is given to increase systolic blood pressure (SBP) without achieving normotension, is associated with decreased blood loss, decreased acidemia, decreased hemodilution, decreased thrombocytopenia, and decreased coagulopathy.[30] Fluid resuscitation that raises the blood pressure to normotensive or higher may disrupt tenuous early clots. Until the cause of hemorrhage is addressed in hemorrhagic shock, fluid resuscitation may be initiated to treat hypotension, with an SBP goal of 80 to 90 mm Hg.[30] If prehospital transport time is short (10 to 15 minutes), delayed resuscitation may be desired.[30] In patients with a traumatic brain injury (TBI), mortality is increased with low cerebral perfusion pressures. Therefore, permissive hypotension is contraindicated in TBI, and small aliquots of fluid (100 to 200 mL) are administered to maintain SBP >90 mm Hg or mean arterial pressure (MAP) >80 mm Hg.[30]

Ground or air transport is appropriate to move the patient from the scene of the injury to the trauma center. Considerations in the choice of transport include travel time, terrain, availability of air and ground units, capabilities of transport personnel, and weather conditions. Once the decision is made to transport a patient to a trauma center, the trauma team is notified. In most trauma centers, the initial resuscitation and stabilization of the trauma patient occurs in a designated resuscitation area, usually within the ED. Optimally, the trauma team responds before the patient's arrival and begins preparations based on the report of the patient's injuries and clinical status. Trauma patients in unstable conditions may be admitted directly to the operating room for resuscitation and immediate surgical intervention.

Trauma Triage

Triage of an injured patient to the appropriate trauma center based on assessment and established protocols is an essential component of a successful trauma system. *Triage* means sorting the patients to determine which patients need specialized care for actual or potential injuries. Triage decisions are often made by EMS personnel based on knowledge of the mechanisms of injury and rapid assessment of the patient's clinical status. Medical direction of this process occurs through voice communication and medical review of triage decisions.

Trauma is classified as minor or major, depending on the severity of injury. *Minor trauma* refers to a single-system injury that does not pose a threat to life or limb and can be appropriately treated in a basic emergency center. *Major trauma* refers to serious multiple-system injuries that require immediate intervention to prevent disability, loss of limb, or death. In some regions, an injury scoring system is used to objectively measure and convey the severity of injury an individual has sustained. Several scoring systems are used for this purpose.[32] The *Abbreviated Injury Scale* (AIS) divides the body into six regions and applies a severity score from 1 to 6 for each injury. The scores from the three most severely injured body regions are squared and added together to arrive at the *Injury Severity Score* (ISS). The risk for mortality increases with a higher ISS. An AIS score of 1 indicates minor injury, and a score of 6 indicates an unsurvivable injury (see https://www.aci.health.nsw.gov.au/get-involved/institute-of-trauma-and-injury-management/Data/injury-scoring/injury_severity_score).

Another scoring system that is used to objectively evaluate a patient's severity of neurological injury is the Glasgow Coma Scale (GCS). The lower the GCS score, based on three assessment parameters, the more severe the neurological injury, suggesting the need for emergent transport to a trauma center (see Chapter 14, Nervous System Alterations).

The development of and adherence to established triage criteria are essential for maintaining an effective system of optimal care for the trauma patient. Triage decisions are based on abnormal findings in the patient's physiological functions, the mechanism of injury, the severity of injury, the anatomical area of injury, or evidence of risk factors such as age and preexisting disease.[29] Prehospital personnel may elect to transport the patient to a trauma center in the absence of accepted triage criteria. This decision is most often based on visualization of the trauma incident and the patient's clinical condition.

Hospital Triage

Information obtained during the prehospital phase provides data to ensure a coordinated, life-saving approach in the management of trauma patients. Most traumatic events are considered "scoop and run" situations with short transport times to the closest appropriate trauma center; other patients may arrive at the hospital by private car. Triage continues after the patient arrives at the hospital to identify those patients who need immediate treatment as well as to match available resources with treatment needs based on injury mechanism and severity. Procedures exist within hospitals to activate the trauma team, including the operating room team for emergent surgical interventions.

EDs in trauma centers designate resuscitation rooms in a central location to facilitate a rapid initial assessment, stabilization, and determination of the immediate medical needs of the patient. The resuscitation room must always be in a state of readiness for the next trauma patient. Equipment needed for management of the airway with cervical spine immobilization, breathing, circulatory support, and hemorrhage control must be immediately available and easily accessible.

Preparation

The risk of coming in contact with body fluids in severely injured patients is high. The ACS recommends face mask, eye protection, water-impervious gown, and gloves as minimum precautions and protection for all healthcare providers when coming in contact with body fluids.[6]

EMERGENCY CARE PHASE: RESUSCITATION

Initial Patient Assessment

Patient survival after a serious traumatic event depends on a rapid and systematic assessment in conjunction with immediate resuscitative interventions. Priorities of care are based on the patient's clinical presentation, physical assessment, history of the traumatic event (mechanism of injury), and knowledge of any preexisting disease. Critical components of care that take immediate precedence include management of airway patency, ventilation, hemorrhage control, and stabilization of fractures. A systematic approach, using primary and secondary surveys, is implemented so that life-threatening emergencies are evaluated and addressed as a priority.

Primary and Secondary Surveys

The assessment begins with a primary survey and resuscitation adjuncts. The *primary survey* is the most crucial assessment tool in trauma care. This rapid, 1- to 2-minute evaluation is designed to identify life-threatening injuries accurately, establish priorities, and provide simultaneous therapeutic interventions. An **ABCDEFG** mnemonic is used to guide the *primary survey*: Across-the-room assessment for uncontrolled hemorrhage and **A**irway with cervical spine immobilization, **B**reathing and ventilation, **C**irculation with hemorrhage control, **D**isability or assessment of neurological status, **E**xposure with environmental considerations, **F**ull set of vital signs and **F**amily presence, and **G**ive comfort and **G**et resuscitation adjuncts.[6,16] **LMNOP** is the mnemonic used to outline the resuscitative adjuncts (i.e., **L**aboratory studies, **M**onitor cardiac rhythm, **N**asogastric/orogastric tube insertion, **O**xygen and ventilation assessment, and **P**ain management and psychosocial support). Life-threatening conditions are identified, and management is instituted simultaneously (Table 20.2).

The *secondary survey*, **HI,** is initiated after all actual or potential life-threatening injuries have been addressed and resuscitative efforts have been initiated. It is a methodical approach to obtain event **H**istory and a **H**ead-to-toe assessment of the patient. **I**nspect posterior is next. Assess each region of the body to minimize the potential for missing an injury or failing to grasp the significance of an injury. Assessment techniques of inspection, auscultation, and palpation are used to identify all injuries (Table 20.3).[16]

Information about actual and potential injuries are noted and used to establish diagnostic and treatment priorities. Radiological and ultrasound studies are completed according to a standardized trauma protocol or an assessment of suspected injuries. The sequence of diagnostic procedures is influenced by the patient's level of consciousness and hemodynamic stability, the mechanism of injury, and the identified injuries. As data are obtained, the team leader determines the need for consultation with specialty providers such as neurosurgeons or orthopedic surgeons. Supportive interventions such as management of pain

TABLE 20.2 Primary Survey: ABCDEFG

Assessment	Observations Indicating Impairment	Simultaneous Management
A = Airway • Open and patent • Maintain cervical spine immobilization • Patency of artificial airway (if present)	Shallow, noisy breathing (gurgling, snoring, stridor) Hoarse voice or inability to speak Decreased level of consciousness (GCS score ≤8) Trauma to face, mouth, or neck Evidence of inhalation injury Debris or foreign matter in mouth or pharynx	Suction the airway. Use jaw-thrust maneuver to open the airway while maintaining cervical spine stabilization. Consider airway adjuncts (nasal or oral airway) or a definitive airway (endotracheal intubation).
B = Breathing • Presence and effectiveness	Asymmetrical chest movement Absent, decreased, or unequal breath sounds Nasal flaring or accessory muscle use Pallor or cyanosis Dyspnea Open chest wounds Blunt chest injury Respiratory rate <8-10 or >20 breaths/min Tracheal shift	Administer oxygen at 10-15 L/min via non-rebreather device. Use a bag-mask device connected to oxygen at 15 L/min if preparing for a definitive airway (endotracheal intubation). See Table 20.4.
C = Circulation • Presence of major pulses • Presence of external hemorrhage • Skin color, temperature and moisture • Unstable pelvis	Weak, thready pulse HR >120 beats/min Pallor Systolic BP <90 mm Hg MAP <65 mm Hg Muffled heart sounds Obvious external hemorrhage Decreased level of consciousness	Apply direct pressure to site of bleeding. Consider a pelvic binder for an unstable pelvic fracture. Insert two large-caliber peripheral IV catheters. Initiate blood administration using a rapid infuser or other warming device and maintaining 1:1:1 ratio (packed RBCs: plasma: platelets).
D = Disability • Gross neurological status • Pupil size, equality, and reactivity to light • Spontaneous movements or moves to command	GCS score ≤13 Agitation Lack of spontaneous movement Posturing Lack of sensation in extremities	Consider need for CT. Consider alcohol level and/or toxicology screening. Consider ABG for evaluation of hypoxia and glucose level for assessment of hypoglycemia.
E = Expose patient with environmental control	Presence of soft tissue injury, crepitus, deformities, edema	Preserve clothing in paper bag for use as evidence. Maintain body temperature by covering the patient with warm blankets, using warmed IV fluids, and increasing the room ambient temperature.
F = Full set of vital signs and family presence		Obtain full set of vital signs (BP, HR, respiratory rate, temperature). Obtain oxygen saturation via pulse oximetry. Identify family; provide updates; facilitate family presence in accordance with patient and family wishes.
G = Get resuscitation adjuncts (LMNOP) • L—Laboratory studies (lactic acid, ABG, type and crossmatch)	Lactic acid levels >2 mmol/L reflect poor tissue perfusion Base deficit < −3 may indicate poor perfusion and tissue hypoxia	Obtain blood and specimens for type and crossmatch and other laboratory studies.
• M—Monitor cardiac rhythm	Dysrhythmias may indicate blunt cardiac trauma or electrolyte abnormalities PEA may indicate cardiac tamponade, tension pneumothorax, or significant hypovolemia	Connect patient to cardiac monitor.
• N—Nasogastric or orogastric tube consideration		Insert nasogastric or orogastric tube if indicated.
• O—Oxygen and ventilation assessment		Connect patient to pulse oximeter and $ETCO_2$ monitoring.
• P—Pain assessment and management and psychosocial support		Provide pharmacological and nonpharmacological pain management. Provide appropriate spiritual and psychosocial support.

ABG, Arterial blood gas; *BP*, blood pressure; *CT*, computed tomography; *$ETCO_2$*, end-tidal carbon dioxide; *GCS*, Glasgow Coma Scale; *HR*, heart rate; *MAP*, mean arterial pressure; *PEA*, pulseless electrical activity; *RBC*, red blood cell.
Modified from Emergency Nurses Association. *Trauma Nurse Core Course Provider Manual*. 8th ed. Jones and Bartlett; 2020.

TABLE 20.3 Secondary Survey: HI

Survey Activities	Actions	Inspection	Palpation	Auscultation
H = History 1. History of event: MIST • M—Mechanism of injury • I—Injuries sustained • S—Signs and symptoms in the field • T—Treatment in the field 2. Patient history: SAMPLE • S—Symptoms • A—Allergies • M—Medications • P—Past medical history • L—Last oral intake • E—Events and environmental factors **Head-to-toe Assessment**	Perform head-to-toe assessment Obtain information on allergies, current medications, past illnesses, pregnancies, last meal	*Head/face:* Inspect for wounds, ecchymosis, deformities, drainage, unusual drainage from ears or nose *Neck:* Inspect for wounds, ecchymosis, deformities, distended neck veins *Chest:* Inspect for breathing rate and depth, wounds, deformities, ecchymosis, use of accessory muscles, paradoxical movement *Abdomen:* Inspect for wounds, distension, ecchymosis, scars *Pelvis/perineum:* Inspect for wounds, deformities, ecchymosis, priapism, blood at the urinary meatus or in the perineal area *Extremities:* Inspect for ecchymosis, movement, wounds, deformities	*Head/face:* Palpate for tenderness, crepitus, deformities *Neck:* Palpate for tenderness, crepitus, deformities, tracheal position *Chest:* Palpate for tenderness, crepitus, subcutaneous emphysema, deformities *Abdomen:* Palpate all four quadrants for tenderness, rigidity, guarding, masses, femoral pulses *Pelvis/perineum:* Palpate the pelvis and rectal tone *Extremities:* Palpate for pulses, skin temperature, sensation, tenderness, deformities, crepitus	*Chest:* Auscultate breath and heart sounds *Abdomen:* Auscultate bowel sounds; observe for passing flatulence
I = Inspect Posterior Surfaces	Maintain cervical spine stabilization Logroll patient using three hospital personnel if spine clearance could not be completed with imaging prior	Inspect posterior surfaces for wounds, deformities, and ecchymosis	Palpate posterior surfaces for deformities and pain Assist provider with the rectal examination, if not previously completed	

Modified from Emergency Nurses Association. *Trauma Nurse Core Course Provider Manual*. 8th ed. Sudbury, MA: Jones and Bartlett; 2020.

and agitation, splinting of extremities, wound care, and administration of tetanus prophylaxis and antibiotics are completed. The primary and secondary surveys are repeated frequently to identify changes in the patient's status, indicating the need for additional intervention.[6] As initial life-threatening injuries are managed, other equally life-threatening problems and less severe injuries may become apparent, which can significantly affect the patient's prognosis.[6,16]

From the time of initial injury until the patient is stabilized in the ED or operating room, the trauma team resuscitates the patient. *Resuscitation* in trauma refers to reestablishing an effective circulatory volume and a stable hemodynamic status in the patient and is a central component of the primary and secondary surveys. The ABCDEFG of emergency care continues, and life-threatening injuries (e.g., pneumothorax, cardiac tamponade) are treated emergently. Each of these interventions is discussed in detail in the following sections.

CHECK YOUR UNDERSTANDING

1. The primary survey is to determine:
   A. All potential injuries and treatment
   B. Sequence for completing a head-to-toe examination
   C. Greatest life-threatening emergencies needing treatment
   D. The need for additional consultation teams and resources

Establish Airway Patency and Restrict Cervical Spine Motion

Every trauma patient has the potential for an ineffective airway, whether it occurs at the time of injury or develops during resuscitation. A patient may lose airway patency for many reasons, including obstruction, structural impairments, and an inability to protect the airway associated with a change in level of consciousness. The tongue, because of posterior displacement, is the most common cause of airway obstruction. Other causes of obstruction include foreign debris (i.e., blood or vomitus) and anatomical obstructions due to maxillofacial fractures. Direct injuries to the throat or neck can structurally impair the airway. Patients with an altered sensorium or high spinal cord injury may not be able to protect their airway.

Maintaining the patient's airway with simultaneous cervical spine protection is an important initial intervention.[6,16] Suspect a cervical spine injury in any patient with multisystem trauma until radiographic studies or clinical evaluation by an experienced provider determines otherwise. Until a cervical spinal injury has been cleared, manually stabilize the cervical spine by holding the head and neck in alignment or restrict cervical spine motion with a cervical collar when establishing the patient's airway. If a patient is unable to open his or her mouth, does not follow commands, or is unresponsive, use a jaw-thrust maneuver to open and assess the airway. Clear the airway of any foreign material such as blood, vomitus, bone fragments, or teeth by gentle suction with a tonsillar-tip catheter. Nasopharyngeal and oropharyngeal airways are the simplest artificial airway adjuncts used in patients with spontaneous respirations and adequate ventilatory effort. Both devices help prevent posterior displacement of the tongue. Do not insert an oropharyngeal airway in a conscious patient because it may induce gagging, vomiting, and aspiration; if an artificial airway is needed, a nasopharyngeal airway is better tolerated (see Chapter 10, Ventilatory Assistance).

A definitive airway may be required for a patient who presents with apnea, a low GCS score, severe maxillofacial fractures, or an inability to protect the airway.[16] Examples of definitive airways include endotracheal intubation and tracheostomy. Endotracheal intubation is the definitive nonsurgical airway management technique. Oral intubation is often preferred, but nasotracheal intubation is acceptable depending on circumstances and injury. Nasotracheal intubation is contraindicated if there are signs of facial, frontal sinus, basilar skull, or cribriform plate fractures.[6,16] Evidence of nasal fracture, raccoon eyes (bilateral ecchymosis in the periorbital region), Battle's sign (mastoid ecchymosis), and possible cerebrospinal fluid (CSF) leaks (rhinorrhea or otorrhea) are all signs of these injuries.[16] During intubation, precautions to restrict cervical spine movement are followed. Refer to Chapter 10, Ventilatory Assistance for intubation procedures. Rapid-sequence intubation (sequential administration of a sedative or anesthetic and a neuromuscular blocking agent) may be used to facilitate the procedure.

In rare circumstances, it may be difficult to intubate the patient. If endotracheal intubation is not feasible or has failed, an alternative airway device, such as a laryngeal mask airway (LMA), may be used until a definitive airway can be placed.[16] These devices are positioned above the glottis to facilitate immediate ventilation and oxygenation. An emergent cricothyroidotomy, a surgical intervention, is considered a last resort in establishing an airway.[16] Conditions that may require cricothyroidotomy include maxillofacial trauma, laryngeal fractures, severe oropharyngeal hemorrhage, or an inability to place an endotracheal tube through the vocal cords.[6,16]

Maintain Effective Breathing

Assess the patient frequently for sensorium, spontaneous breathing, respiratory rate and effort, heart rate and rhythm, breath sounds, symmetrical rise and fall of the chest, contusions or abrasions, skin color, tracheal position, and jugular venous distension. When spontaneous breathing is present but ineffective, consider the presence of a life-threatening condition if any of the following are present: altered mental status; central cyanosis; asymmetrical expansion of the chest wall; use of accessory muscles, abdominal muscles, or both; paradoxical movement of the chest wall during inspiration and expiration; diminished or absent breath sounds; tracheal shift from midline position; decreasing oxygen saturation via pulse oximetry; or distended jugular veins. Ineffective breathing patterns may be the result of certain traumatic injuries. These injuries and specific interventions are listed in Table 20.4 and discussed throughout this chapter. Breathing is supported by administering oxygen at 10 to 15 L/minute via a non-rebreather mask. If ventilation is ineffective, a bag-mask device is connected to an oxygen source at 10 to 15 L/min, and breaths are administered at a rate of 10 to 12 breaths per minute.[6,16] Interventions to restore normal breathing patterns are directed toward the specific injury or underlying cause of respiratory distress, with the goal of improving ventilation and oxygenation. Provide supplemental oxygen with ventilatory assistance (if applicable), position for effective ventilation, and evaluate interventions. Arterial blood gas analysis and diagnostic studies, including chest radiography and computed tomography (CT) imaging, may be completed to assist in determining the effectiveness of specific interventions.

Impaired oxygenation follows airway obstruction as a crucial problem after traumatic injury. Impaired gas exchange

TABLE 20.4 Specific Interventions for Ineffective Breathing Patterns

Etiology	Interventions
Decreased level of consciousness	Position the patient's head at midline with the head of the bed elevated Anticipate a computed tomography scan Implement interventions to prevent aspiration Prepare for intubation and mechanical ventilation
Spinal cord injury	Avoid hyperextension or rotation of the patient's neck Observe ventilatory effort and use of accessory muscles Maintain complete spinal immobilization Prepare for application of cervical traction tongs or a halo device Monitor motor and sensory function Monitor for signs of distributive (neurogenic) shock
Pneumothorax	Provide supplemental oxygen Prepare for chest tube insertion on affected side if patient is hemodynamically unstable
Tension pneumothorax	Prepare for decompression by needle thoracotomy with a 14-gauge needle in the second intercostal space at the midclavicular line on affected side Prepare for chest tube insertion on affected side
Open chest wound	Seal the wound with an occlusive dressing and tape on three sides Prepare for chest tube insertion on affected side
Massive hemothorax	Establish two 14- or 16-gauge peripheral IV catheters for blood administration Obtain blood for type and crossmatch Prepare for chest tube insertion on affected side Administer blood or blood products as ordered Anticipate and prepare for transfer to the operating room
Pulmonary contusion	Administer oxygen to avoid hypoxemia Prepare for possible endotracheal intubation and mechanical ventilation
Flail chest	Prepare for possible endotracheal intubation and mechanical ventilation Administer analgesics as ordered

can result from ineffective ventilation, an inability to exchange gases at the alveoli, or both. Possible causes include a decrease in inspired air, retained secretions, lung collapse or compression, atelectasis, or accumulation of blood in the thoracic cavity. Assess any patient who presents with multiple systemic injuries, hemorrhagic shock, chest trauma, and/or central nervous system trauma for impaired gas exchange. These conditions have the potential to affect the patient's intravascular volume status and oxygen-carrying capacity, interfere with the mechanics of ventilation, or interrupt the autonomic control of respirations. The nurse must be prepared to assist with endotracheal intubation and subsequent mechanical ventilation, needle thoracostomy, chest tube insertion, and restoration of circulating blood volume at any time during the resuscitation phase of care. Because conditions that compromise breathing may not manifest during the first assessment of airway or breathing, ongoing airway assessment is a nursing priority.

Maintain Circulation

The most common cause of impaired cardiac output and circulation after traumatic injury is hypovolemic shock from acute blood loss. Causes may be external (hemorrhage) or internal (hemothorax, hemoperitoneum, solid-organ injury, long bone or massive pelvic fractures). Initial management of actively bleeding patients includes hemorrhage control by applying pressure or a tourniquet to control bleeding, replacing circulatory volume with blood products, and surgery focused on hemorrhage control (damage-control surgery) rather than definitive surgical management.[33] In the face of hypovolemic shock from hemorrhage, early, rapid surgical intervention is life-saving and limb-saving.[6,33]

> **! CLINICAL ALERT**
>
> Uncontrolled hemorrhage is a major cause of death after injury. Early intervention is critical, and early application of direct pressure or tourniquet on the actively bleeding limb will minimize the likelihood of mortality from hemorrhage.[34] A national awareness campaign and call to action, ***Stop the Bleed***, encourages bystanders to become trained in how to control bleeding before emergency medical services arrive. This program includes training in direct pressure and tourniquet use.
>
> See https://www.stopthebleed.org/.

The management of hypovolemic shock focuses on finding and eliminating the cause of the bleeding and concomitant support of the patient's circulatory system with IV fluids and blood products (see Chapter 12, Shock, Sepsis, and Multiple Organ Dysfunction Syndrome). It is often difficult to assess blood loss, especially with internal hemorrhage from blunt trauma. Furthermore, when blood volume decreases, the sympathetic nervous system compensatory mechanisms in the body respond through tachycardia, narrowing pulse pressure, tachypnea, vasoconstriction, and decreased urine output. Signs and symptoms of hypovolemic shock may not be obvious until the patient is in a later stage of hypovolemic shock.[6,33] It is estimated that signs of hypotension may not be clinically obvious until a patient has lost more than 30% to 40% of blood volume.[6] Continually assess the patient for subtle changes in vital signs and end-organ function. Initiate hemorrhage control and fluid resuscitation when early signs and symptoms of blood loss are apparent or suspected rather than waiting for overt signs associated with a decreasing blood pressure.[6,33]

Perform Diagnostic Testing

Diagnostic testing is completed early in the resuscitative phase to determine injuries and potential sources of bleeding. Potential injuries to the chest, pelvis, and abdomen and suspected extremity fractures are assessed. Diagnostic studies include CT, radiography, *focused assessment with sonography for trauma (FAST)*, and *extended FAST (E-FAST)*. FAST is an ultrasound assessment that provides a rapid, noninvasive means of diagnosing accumulation of blood or free fluid in the peritoneal cavity or pericardial sac.[6,35–37] E-FAST simply extends the ultrasound examination to evaluate possible injuries in the chest, looking for hemothorax and pneumothorax. In the context of traumatic injury, free fluid identified on the FAST examination is usually due to hemorrhage. If free fluid or hemorrhage is found, a CT scan may be obtained and/or surgical interventions initiated immediately.[6,36,37] An echocardiogram, a 12-lead electrocardiogram (ECG), and continuous ECG with ST-segment monitoring may also be ordered to evaluate cardiac function, especially if the patient is showing signs of diminished cardiac output, if thoracic injury is present, or if the patient has a history of cardiovascular disease.

Pelvic fractures can be a hidden cause of hemorrhage because the retroperitoneum can be a site for significant blood loss. In the patient with blunt-force trauma and an unidentifiable cause of hypotension, radiographic evaluation and a pelvic examination are critical to identify an unstable pelvic fracture as a source of injury and bleeding. Apply a pelvic binder or sheet to stabilize the injury and minimize further bleeding.[6,16]

> **CHECK YOUR UNDERSTANDING**
>
> 2. A construction worker is admitted after falling approximately 15 feet from scaffolding. The nurse anticipates which priority intervention to evaluate sources of potential bleeding?
>   A. FAST or E-FAST
>   B. Complete metabolic laboratory test panel
>   C. Chest radiograph
>   D. Urinalysis

Perform Fluid Resuscitation

Venous access and infusion of volume are required for optimal fluid resuscitation in the trauma patient with hypovolemic shock. As a general rule, venous access is achieved rapidly with the largest-bore catheter possible to initiate early fluid resuscitation. Immediate management of severely injured trauma patients focuses on replacing lost intravascular volume and treating coagulopathy.[6] The provision of IV fluids and blood products is contingent on obtaining adequate vascular access to the patient's venous system. Insert at least two large-caliber peripheral IV catheters.[6,16] The preferred sites are the forearm or antecubital veins. If peripheral access cannot be obtained

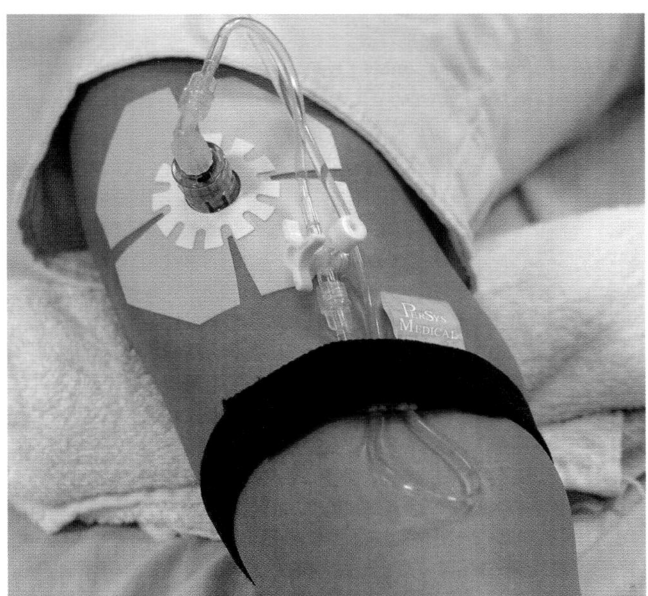

Fig. 20.3 Tibial insertion of an intraosseous (IO) device that is taped in place with IV extension attached to the needle for instillation of fluids and medications. (Courtesy Waismed, Ltd., Houston, TX.)

quickly, IO needles may be used for temporary access through bone in the sternum, leg (tibia), or arm (humerus) if the patient's injuries do not interfere with the procedure (Fig. 20.3).[6,16,33,38] IO access should not be performed in an extremity with a known or suspected fracture.[6] The IO access may be placed in the field by EMS personnel or in the ED. Resuscitation fluids, medications, and blood products can be administered through an IO device.[6,33,38] Potential complications with IO access include pain on instillation of fluids, extravasation of fluids, and compartment syndrome. A central venous catheter (single lumen or multiple lumen) may be necessary because of peripheral vasoconstriction and venous collapse. It may be beneficial as a resuscitation monitoring tool and for rapid administration of large volumes of fluid.

Appropriate initiation, timing, and choice of fluid used for resuscitation are pivotal in affecting patient outcomes. Continual assessment of fluid volume status is critical throughout resuscitation. Fluid resuscitation follows the principles of *damage-control resuscitation* involving two strategies: hypotensive and hemostatic resuscitation. Large volumes of crystalloid fluid resuscitation are associated with increased bleeding and mortality as a result of hemodilution and decreased clotting factors.[6,16] Current recommendations include smaller volumes of crystalloid solutions and the use of boluses to follow the principle of permissive hypotension and goal-directed therapy.[6,16] In trauma patients without a TBI, permissive hypotension aims to give fluid to increase SBP without achieving normotension. Until the cause of hemorrhage is addressed in hemorrhagic shock, fluid resuscitation may be initiated to treat hypotension for an SBP goal of 80 to 90 mm Hg.[30] Goal-directed therapy aims to optimize tissue and cellular oxygenation by preventing further losses through hemodilutional coagulopathy.[6,16] Because large volumes of crystalloid, especially 0.9% normal saline, are associated with poor patient outcomes by worsening acidosis and coagulopathy, current practice focuses on plasma and blood products as the primary resuscitation fluids.[6,16,28,39] Patients with massive hemorrhage lose clotting factors as well as red blood cells and plasma. To effectively stop bleeding, packed red blood cells (PRBCs), fresh frozen plasma (FFP), and platelets must be replaced. Coagulation factors are present in FFP and platelets, and to minimize coagulopathies, it is critical that PRBCs, FFP, and platelets are all administered as part of resuscitation. To support this practice, massive transfusion protocols have been developed with the intention of getting all blood components to the patient in a timely manner using a ratio-based transfusion of one part PRBCs to one part thawed plasma to one part platelets (1:1:1 ratio).[6,16,28,40] Some facilities have shown similar results using whole-blood transfusions.[41,42] This practice has been adopted from military settings where component therapy was less easily available. Type-specific blood may be administered, but in the event of life-threatening blood loss, unmatched type-specific or type O (universal donor) blood may be prescribed. Crossmatched type-specific blood should be instituted as soon as it is available. Massive transfusion often requires more than 5 units or more of blood products within a 3-hour period.[43]

Once laboratory data are available, resuscitation should be based on the laboratory findings and clinical evidence of ongoing bleeding.[40] A thromboelastography (TEG) or rotational thromboelastometry (ROTEM) test evaluates whole-blood coagulation, including platelet function, clot strength, and fibrinolysis, and assists the clinician in identifying whether a patient has normal hemostasis or a coagulopathy. If available, TEG or ROTEM may be used to monitor coagulation and guide blood product administration during massive transfusion.[16]

TEG results are displayed in a unique tracing as well as discrete values. If a coagulopathy is identified, the TEG results are used to identify the specific product used for treatment, including FFP, cryoprecipitate, or an antifibrinolytic or thrombolytic medication. TEG supports individualized resuscitation of trauma patients by tailoring massive transfusion to the dynamic biology of individual hemostasis.[39] Trials have demonstrated that TEG-directed resuscitation improves survival after injury and promotes appropriate use of hemostatic blood products.[39]

Monitor the patient's response to the initial fluid administration by assessing urine output (goal: 0.5 mL/kg/h in the adult), level of consciousness, heart rate, blood pressure, pulse pressure, and laboratory indices (e.g., serum lactate level, base deficit). Monitor the hemoglobin level, hematocrit value, plasma fibrinogen level, platelet count, prothrombin time (PT), and partial thromboplastin time (PTT). Also monitor for hypothermia, electrolyte imbalances, and dilutional coagulopathies. Other adjuncts, such as calcium chloride replacement and antifibrinolytic agents, such as tranexamic acid (TXA), should be considered.[16,40]

EVIDENCE-BASED PRACTICE

Effects of Tranexamic Acid on Death, Disability, Vascular Occlusive Events, and Other Morbidities In Patients with Acute Traumatic Brain Injury (Crash-3): A Randomized, Placebo-Controlled Trial

Problem

Intracranial bleeding is a common complication of traumatic brain injury (TBI) and increases the risk of death and disability. Although bleeding can start from the moment of impact, it often continues for several hours after injury. Previous research showed that in patients with trauma, early administration of tranexamic acid (TXA) reduces bleeding deaths by a third.[44,45] Since the CRASH-2 trial results, TXA has been included in guidelines for the care of patients with trauma, although patients with isolated TBI were specifically excluded. However, increased fibrinolysis is often seen in patients with TBI and predicts intracranial hemorrhage expansion. Therefore, early administration of TXA in patients with TBI might reduce intracranial hemorrhage expansion.

Clinical Question

Does timely TXA treatment reduce deaths from intracranial bleeding after TBI?

Evidence

In total, 7637 patients were included in the analysis, which excluded patients with a Glasgow Coma Scale (GCS) score of 3 or bilateral unreactive pupils at baseline. In this group, the risk of head injury–related death was 12.5% in the TXA group versus 14% in the placebo group (485 vs. 525 events: risk ratio [RR], 0.89; 95% confidence interval [CI], 0.80 to 1.00). The risk of early death, within 24 hours of injury, was reduced with TXA (112 [2.9%] TXA group vs. 147 [3.9%] placebo group; RR, 0.74; 95% CI, 0.58 to 0.94). Early treatment was more effective than later treatment in patients with mild and moderate head injury ($p = .005$), but time to treatment had no obvious effect in patients with severe head injury ($p = .73$). The risk of vascular occlusive events was similar in the TXA and placebo groups (RR, 0.98; 95% CI, 0.74 to 1.28). The risk of seizures was also similar between groups (1.09; 95% CI, 0.90 to 1.33).

Implications for Nursing

Before this study, TXA administration had been safely used to reduce intraoperative bleeding, and a previous large randomized controlled trial showed reduced mortality in trauma patients. The results of this study support early administration to patients with a mild to moderate TBI. Understanding the role of coagulopathy in the trauma triad of death is important for all trauma patients. Anticipating management of these elements is critical to improving mortality.

Level of Evidence

B—Multisite randomized controlled trial

References

CRASH-3 Collaborators. Effects of tranexamic acid on death, disability, vascular occlusive events and other morbidities in patients with acute traumatic brain injury (CRASH-3): a randomized, placebo-controlled trial. *Lancet.* 2019;394:1713-1723.

Brenner A, Belli A, Chaudhri R et al. Understanding the neuroprotective effect of tranexamic acid: an exploratory analysis of the CRASH-3 randomized trial. *Crit Care.* 2020;24:560. https://doi.org/10.1186/s13054-020-03243-4.

Banked blood products have high levels of citrate, which may induce transient hypocalcemia. Decreased serum calcium levels may lead to ineffective coagulation because calcium is a necessary cofactor in the coagulation cascade. Further inhibition of the clotting cascade is observed when platelet dysfunction develops secondary to hypothermia or metabolic acidosis. To address hypothermia risk, a fluid warmer or rapid infuser device should be used to administer warmed fluids and blood products during resuscitation. Antifibrinolytic agents, such as TXA, inhibit the activation of plasminogen, which is a substance responsible for dissolving clots. Management focuses on improving perfusion to the body tissues, increasing the patient's body temperature, and stabilizing coagulopathies. TEG and/or ROTEM can be helpful in determining the clotting deficiency and appropriate blood components to correct the deficiency.[6,16]

! LABORATORY ALERT

Laboratory Test	Normal Range	Critical Value[a]	Significance
Lactic acid (lactate)	0.6-2.2 mmol/L or 5-20 mg/dL (venous) 0.3-0.8 mmol/L or 4-7 mg/dL (arterial)	>2 mmol/L	• Lactate is a byproduct of anaerobic metabolism that results from inadequate tissue perfusion. • It is a marker for cellular hypoxia in hypovolemic/hemorrhagic shock. • Elevated lactate levels indicate widespread tissue hypoperfusion and are an independent predictor of more severe injury and poor outcomes in trauma patients.
Base deficit/excess	–2 to +2 mEq/L	–3 mEq/L +3 mEq/L	• Base deficit/excess represents the number of buffering anions in the blood. • A negative value (base deficit) indicates metabolic acidosis (e.g., lactic acidosis). It may indicate poor perfusion and tissue hypoxia. • A positive value (base excess) indicates metabolic alkalosis or a compensatory response to respiratory acidosis.
Ionized calcium	1.05-1.3 mmol/L	<0.55 mmol/L	• Hypocalcemia is a concern with massive transfusion because citrate is added as a preservative to banked blood to prevent coagulation. However, citrate binds with calcium, making it inactive and worsening coagulopathy.

[a]Critical values vary by facility and laboratory.

From Pagana K, Pagana T, Pagana T. *Mosby's Manual of Diagnostic and Laboratory Tests.* 16th ed. St. Louis, MO: Elsevier; 2023.

Assess for Neurological Disabilities

Assess for neurological disabilities by evaluating the patient's level of consciousness, pupillary size and reaction, and spontaneous and reflexive spinal movements. The GCS is the standard method for evaluating level of consciousness in the injured patient (see Chapter 14, Nervous System Alterations).[16] Accurate GCS assessment is limited in patients receiving sedating and analgesic agents and those who are intubated or unable to respond to the verbal component of the exam.[16] Consider possible neurological injuries based on the history of the injury (e.g., ejection from motor vehicle, fall, diving accident). Perform a complete sensory and motor neurological examination to identify the presence and level of spinal cord injury.

Use of recreational drugs and/or alcohol by the patient can mask neurological responsiveness, resulting in misleading findings. Hypotension, hypoventilation, and hypoglycemia can also alter the neurological examination. Hypotension decreases cerebral perfusion; therefore, consider the patient's response to interventions and the degree of tissue ischemia during the neurological examination. If an effective neurological examination cannot be conducted, management is based on knowledge of the traumatic event and the current neurological response. Management priorities focus on the premise that changes in level of consciousness are the result of the traumatic injury until proven otherwise. The key to neurological assessments is trending the results to detect improvement or deterioration and notifying the provider for prompt intervention (see Chapter 14, Nervous System Alterations).

Exposure and Environmental Considerations

Standard practice in trauma management is to remove all clothing and expose the patient to allow for full-body visualization and identification of all injuries. However, exposure decreases body temperature, and preventing hypothermia by maintaining body temperature is a critical nursing priority. Hypothermia, generally defined as a core body temperature of less than 35°C (95°F), is caused by a combination of accelerated heat loss and decreased heat production and is associated with increased hospital mortality.[47] Patients, and especially older persons, are more susceptible to hypothermia after severe injury, excessive blood loss, alcohol use, and massive fluid resuscitation. Body temperature continues to fall after clothing removal, contact with wet linens, and surgical exposure of body cavities during the initial assessment. Prolonged exposure to hypothermia is associated with the development of myocardial dysfunction, coagulopathies, reduced perfusion, dysrhythmias (bradycardia and atrial or ventricular fibrillation), and decreased metabolic rate.

The combination of hypothermia, coagulopathy, and acidosis is commonly referred to as trauma's *lethal triad of death*.[6,16,47] Even mild hypothermia in a trauma patient can result in devastating physiological consequences that affect the coagulation system, ultimately resulting in worsening hemorrhage and adverse patient outcomes. Minimize the negative effects of hypothermia by covering the patient with warm blankets, administering warmed IV fluids, warming the room, covering the patient's head, and using convection air blankets. Suggested techniques for rewarming are listed in Table 20.5.

TABLE 20.5 Rewarming Strategies

Type	Interventions
Passive external	Removal of wet clothing Warm room Decreased airflow over patient Blankets Head coverings
Active external	Radiant lights Fluid-filled warming blankets Convection air blankets
Active internal	Warmed gases to respiratory tract Warmed IV fluids, including blood Body cavity irrigation (peritoneal, mediastinal, pleural, gastric) Continuous arteriovenous rewarming Cardiopulmonary bypass

CHECK YOUR UNDERSTANDING

3. The "trauma triad of death" includes which conditions? (Select all that apply.)
   A. Hypothermia
   B. Acidosis
   C. Hypotension
   D. Tachycardia
   E. Coagulopathy

Full Set of Vitals and Family Presence

A full set of vital signs, including heart rate and rhythm, blood pressure, respiratory rate, pulse oximetry, and temperature, is monitored and trended to assess the effectiveness of resuscitation. Facilitate family presence during this part of the primary assessment and as soon as a trauma team member is able to act as a liaison to the family.[16] While some providers may have concerns about family presence during resuscitation and invasive procedures, family presence has been shown to be beneficial to the families, the team, and patients.[48–50]

Get Resuscitation Adjuncts and Give Comfort

Specific adjuncts are crucial to continue to assess and manage elements in the primary assessment (**LMNOP**): **L**aboratory studies, **M**onitoring, **N**asogastric or orogastric tube consideration, **O**xygenation and ventilation, and **P**ain and psychosocial management.[16] Laboratory studies, including lactate and base deficit, reflect the effectiveness of cellular perfusion, the adequacy of ventilation, and the success of fluid resuscitation (circulation). As a result of hypovolemia and hypoxemia, metabolic acidosis occurs secondary to a shift from aerobic to anaerobic metabolism and the production of lactic acid. Increases in lactate level and base deficit are accompanied by a decrease in tissue perfusion, with increased morbidity and mortality.[16,46] Monitor cardiac rhythm and rate: dysrhythmias may indicate blunt cardiac trauma. Insertion of a nasogastric or orogastric tube provides a route to decompress the stomach, preventing emesis and aspiration, and allows optimal inflation of the lungs. Pulse oximetry detects changes in oxygenation that may not be clinically observed. However, pulse oximetry relies on adequate peripheral perfusion. Capnography, or end-tidal carbon dioxide ($ETCO_2$) monitoring, provides immediate information about the patient's ventilation and perfusion status. Appropriate pain management and psychosocial support for the patient and family are important aspects of trauma care.[16]

Secondary Survey

The secondary survey begins after resuscitative efforts have been initiated and vital functions have been stabilized during the primary survey.[16] The secondary survey includes obtaining the **H**istory of the patient and the event, a **H**ead-to-toe assessment, and **I**nspection of the posterior surfaces. The patient's history begins with the prehospital report to understand the mechanism of injury to anticipate certain injuries. The **MIST** pneumonic can be used as a guide for the prehospital report: **M**echanism of injury, **I**njuries sustained, **S**igns and symptoms in the field, and **T**reatment prior to hospital arrival. The **SAMPLE** pneumonic is used to obtain important aspects of the patient and event history: **S**ymptoms associated with the injury, **A**llergies and tetanus status, **M**edications currently used, **P**ast medical and surgical history, **L**ast oral intake, and **E**vents and **E**nvironmental factors related to the injury. If the patient's family is present, ask about the patient's health history.

If the patient is responsive, eliciting symptoms is helpful to identify areas of pain and otherwise unrecognized injuries. For example, the trauma team might have identified a significant burn during the primary survey, and the patient might complain of pain in a nonburned area. This can identify the need for additional assessment and radiological imaging to rule out a fracture that might not have been recognized. When obtaining information regarding current medication use, identify medications that affect initial management, including anticoagulants and beta-blockers. Coagulopathy contributes to worsening hemorrhage and worse outcomes and may be reversed with other pharmaceutical agents or blood products in the resuscitation phase of trauma care. Warfarin may be emergently reversed using four-factor prothrombin complex concentrate to reduce bleeding prior to surgery or other interventions.[51] While obtaining the patient's history, consider medical or comorbid factors that will influence the necessary care of the patient or place the injured patient at greater risk for complications. For example, risk for death from injury increases in older age, children require specialized pediatric care, and pregnant patients of any gestational age warrant an early obstetric consult.[16]

Event and environmental considerations are related to the location and circumstances of the traumatic event. Environmental considerations are important in farming accidents, impalement with machinery or contaminated industrial equipment, exposure to contaminated water, or wound contamination with soil and road dirt. Initial attempts to cleanse the wound are not priorities in the emergency care phase of trauma management; however, once the patient is stabilized, the wounds are cleansed and debrided, and appropriate antibiotics are initiated.

During the head-to-toe assessment and inspection of posterior surfaces, identify all injuries using a systematic evaluation moving from the patient's head to the lower extremities and posterior surface.[16] Inspection, auscultation, palpation, and percussion are used. Assess the posterior surface after a patient has been cleared of spinal injuries, pelvic fractures, or other injuries that may be exacerbated by movement.[16] Logrolling a patient can cause secondary injuries from excess movement in the traumatically injured patient, including spinal cord injury of an unstable spine and hemorrhage from pelvic fractures.[16,52] The motion during logroll makes it very difficult to maintain spinal alignment. Alternative patient-handling methods that produce less movement, such as the six-plus lift-and-slide or roller boards, are available for transferring patients.[52] Incorporating these methods may require additional assistance from other departments. However, if a patient must still be turned using logroll prior to imaging, maintain cervical spine mobilization using additional team members to assist with logrolling the patient. Support the extremities and maintain vertebral column alignment of the torso, hips, and lower extremities. If possible, avoid turning the patient on an injured extremity. While inspecting for lacerations, abrasions, puncture wounds, deformity, and tenderness along the vertebral column, a provider also assesses rectal tone to assess for neurological disabilities.

Obtain information regarding the event to rule out nonaccidental trauma in pediatrics, older adult abuse, and intimate partner violence. Each state has regulations regarding reporting such events.

CHECK YOUR UNDERSTANDING

4. Assessment of the trauma patient's laboratory results suggests resuscitation efforts are ineffective. Which laboratory value should be reported to the provider for urgent intervention?
   A. Potassium (K^+) of 6.1 mEq/L
   B. Calcium (Ca^{++}) of 8.0 mg/dL
   C. Hematocrit (Hct) of 28.2%
   D. Lactate of 5 mmol/L

ASSESSMENT AND MANAGEMENT OF SPECIFIC INJURIES

This section discusses common traumatic injuries, which may be diagnosed and managed in the emergency care phase or in the subsequent critical care phase. Rapid assessment, resuscitation, and damage-control surgery to minimize bleeding in the emergency care phase, coupled with definitive surgical interventions in the critical care phase, have decreased mortality.[6,53] Damage-control surgery is intended to stop the bleeding, restore normothermia, and treat coagulopathies.[54] Definitive injury repair is completed later during planned operations after the patient has been resuscitated and stabilized.[16] However, not all injuries require surgical intervention. Ongoing assessment, management of specific organ injuries, and an awareness of the patient's response to the stress of the injury are vital during the resuscitative and critical care phase of trauma care.

Head Injuries

TBI is an injury that affects how the brain functions and is caused by a bump or jolt to the head or by a penetrating injury to the head.[55] It is a major cause of death and disability in the United States. Although TBIs affect people of all ages, some groups are at greater risk based on health disparities and also mechanism of injury resulting in the TBI. Falls are the leading cause of TBI, accounting for almost 50% of all TBI-related hospitalizations in the United States.[55] TBIs are associated with falls in adults ages 65 years and older, and people aged 75 years and older had the highest numbers and rates of TBI-related hospitalizations and deaths.[55] Among all age groups, firearm-related suicide is the most common cause of TBI-related deaths in the United States.[55] MVCs and assaults are other common causes of TBIs.

Patients who sustain TBIs may develop postconcussive syndrome days to months after the head injury. Assessment findings include persistent headache, memory and judgment impairment, dizziness and nausea, and attention deficits. If the symptoms persist, these patients may require ongoing evaluation, treatment, and extended rehabilitation before they are able to return to their previous level of activities.[16]

Head injury from blunt trauma typically occurs in the presence of acceleration, deceleration, or rotational forces. Injury may be focal or diffuse. Focal injuries include cerebral contusion, intracerebral hematoma, epidural hematomas, and subdural hematomas.[16] Following a blunt head injury, systemic changes (hypotension, hypoxia, anemia, hyperthermia) or intracranial changes (edema, intracranial hypertension, seizures) may result in alterations in the nervous system tissue. Early interventions and management for a patient with acute head trauma include the following: ensure adequate blood pressure to meet cerebral perfusion of at least 60 to 70 mm Hg; maximize ventilation and oxygenation through effective airway management; maintain the head in a midline position to enhance cerebral blood flow; elevate the head of bed to 30 degrees if not otherwise contraindicated, plan for CT imaging; prepare for insertion of an ICP monitoring device; conduct frequent neurological assessments (see Chapter 14, Nervous System Alterations).[16,56]

Lacerations to the scalp often result in significant bleeding. These wounds are cleansed, debrided, and sutured. Fractures of the skull may be linear, basilar, closed depressed, open depressed, or comminuted. Underlying brain injury may occur with skull fractures. Basilar skull fractures are located at the base of the cranium and potentially involve the five bones that form the skull base. The diagnosis is based on the presence of cerebrospinal fluid in the nose (rhinorrhea), in the ears (otorrhea), or both; ecchymosis over the mastoid area (Battle's sign); or hemotympanum (blood in the middle ear). Raccoon eyes or periorbital ecchymoses are present after a basilar skull fracture (see Chapter 14, Nervous System Alterations).

Spinal Cord Injury

Spinal cord injury (SCI) is a major neurological disability that is assessed early in the emergent phase of traumatic injury (see Chapter 14, Nervous System Alterations). Mechanisms of injury that may result in SCI include hyperflexion, hyperextension, axial loading, rotation, and penetrating trauma. Secondary injury can occur from progressive cell damage to the spinal cord, causing an inflammatory response.[6,16] The initial treatment of a patient with suspected SCI includes the ABCs of resuscitation, spine immobilization, and prevention of further injury through surgical stabilization of the spine. A complete sensory and motor neurological examination is performed during the disability assessment of the primary survey, and radiographic studies of the cervical spine are considered. A spinal CT scan may be performed to rule out occult injury. It is important to determine the approximate level of the SCI because higher cervical spine injuries may result in loss of phrenic nerve innervations, compromising the patient's ability to breathe spontaneously.

SCI causes a loss of sympathetic output, resulting in distributive shock with hypotension and bradycardia. Blood pressure may respond to IV fluids, but vasopressor medications are often required to compensate for the loss of sympathetic innervation and resultant vasodilation. The patient with an SCI presents complex challenges for the trauma team as they attempt to minimize loss of function associated with the injury. Proactive, aggressive, and comprehensive care is necessary to help the patient achieve optimal functional outcomes.

Thoracic Injuries

The thoracic region contains vital organs such as the heart, great vessels, and lungs. It is considered a critical region because injuries to the thoracic organs and structures can quickly become life-threatening. FAST and E-FAST are typically the first-line diagnostic tools used in the emergent evaluation of a patient presenting with thoracic injury, providing essential information for the immediate management of the trauma pat ient.[6,16,35–37]

Blunt Cardiac Injury, Cardiac Contusion, and Cardiac Tamponade. Blunt cardiac injury encompasses a wide range of clinical manifestations, from asymptomatic cardiac contusion to cardiac tamponade and cardiac rupture. Blunt cardiac trauma is most often a consequence of an MVC, a fall, blast injuries, or any mechanism of injury involving decelerating forces with direct thoracic or chest impact.[6,16]

Blunt trauma to the chest is the most frequent cause of cardiac contusion.[17] The force of the traumatic event bruises the heart muscle and can compromise effective heart functioning and cause dysrhythmias.[6,17] In the event of significant anterior chest trauma, obtain a 12-lead ECG and serum levels of cardiac isoenzymes and troponin to rule out ischemia or infarction. If conduction abnormalities are identified, ongoing monitoring for symptomatic cardiac dysrhythmias via continuous monitoring of the ECG is indicated for 24 hours.[6] With severe cardiac contusion injuries, inotropic medications are occasionally needed to support myocardial function.

Cardiac tamponade is a life-threatening condition caused by rapid accumulation of fluid (usually blood) in the pericardial sac. Cardiac tamponade may be caused by penetrating or blunt trauma to the chest.[6,16] It should also be suspected in any patient with chest and multisystem injuries who presents in shock and does not respond to aggressive fluid resuscitation. As the intrapericardial pressure increases, cardiac output is impaired because of decreased venous return. The development of pulsus paradoxus may occur, with a decrease in SBP during spontaneous inspiration. Blood, if unable to flow into the right side of the heart, causes increased right atrial pressure and distended neck veins. Classic signs of cardiac tamponade are hypotension, muffled or distant heart sounds, and elevated venous pressure (Beck's triad). Beck's triad may not be present until late in the development of tamponade. ECG changes may include multiple premature ventricular contractions (PVCs), atrial fibrillation, bundle branch block and ST-segment changes, or indications of a myocardial infarction.[6] FAST exam can facilitate early diagnosis of cardiac tamponade that may be treated by pericardiocentesis (needle aspiration of the pericardial sac) followed by a thoracotomy.[6,16,17] Pericardiocentesis is performed by the provider; a needle is used to aspirate blood from the pericardial sac. Removal of as little as 15 to 20 mL of blood may dramatically improve blood pressure. Anticipate and obtain equipment for an emergency thoracotomy in the event of cardiac arrest during the pericardiocentesis.

Aortic Disruption. Aortic disruption is produced by blunt trauma to the chest and frequently results in death at the scene of the traumatic event. Rapid deceleration forces produced by a head-on MVC, ejection, or fall can cause shearing forces and dissection of the aorta. The proximal descending aorta is at greatest risk, with injuries ranging from complete transection to hematomas. Although this injury has a high mortality, early diagnosis can prevent tearing of the innermost layer, exsanguination, and death.

Specific signs of traumatic aortic disruption are frequently absent but may include greater muscle strength in upper extremities compared to lower extremities or paraplegia.[6,16] Chest radiography and/or CT may demonstrate a widened mediastinum, tracheal deviation to the right, depressed left mainstem bronchus, first and second rib fractures, and left hemothorax.[6,16] The diagnosis is confirmed by angiography if available. Definitive, emergent surgical resection and repair are necessary with this injury.

Pneumothorax, Tension Pneumothorax, and Open Pneumothorax. Pneumothorax occurs when air escapes from the injured lung into the pleural space, altering the negative intrapleural pressure and resulting in a partial or complete collapse of the lung. The patient presents with respiratory distress, tachypnea, tachycardia, diminished or absent breath sounds on the injured side, and chest pain.[16] Pneumothorax may be confirmed by chest radiography or E-FAST.[36,57] Treatment is determined by the size of the pneumothorax as well as patient symptoms. If a patient is stable with a small pneumothorax, treatment focuses on providing supplemental oxygen. However, in patients who are unstable or likely to deteriorate, chest tube placement to evacuate the pleural air and reexpand the lung is necessary.[57,58]

Tension pneumothorax is a rapidly fatal emergency that is easily resolved with early recognition and intervention. It occurs when an injury to the chest allows air to enter the pleural cavity without a route for escape. With each inspiration, additional air accumulates in the pleural space, increasing intrathoracic pressure and leading to lung collapse. The increased pressure causes compression of the heart and great vessels toward the unaffected side, as evidenced by mediastinal shift and distended neck veins. The resulting decreased cardiac output and alterations in gas exchange are manifested by agitation, severe respiratory distress, absence of breath sounds on the affected side, hypotension, distended neck veins, and tracheal deviation away from the side of injury (Fig. 20.4). As intrathoracic pressure rises, venous return is compromised, and hypotension occurs. Cyanosis is a late manifestation of this life-threatening clinical

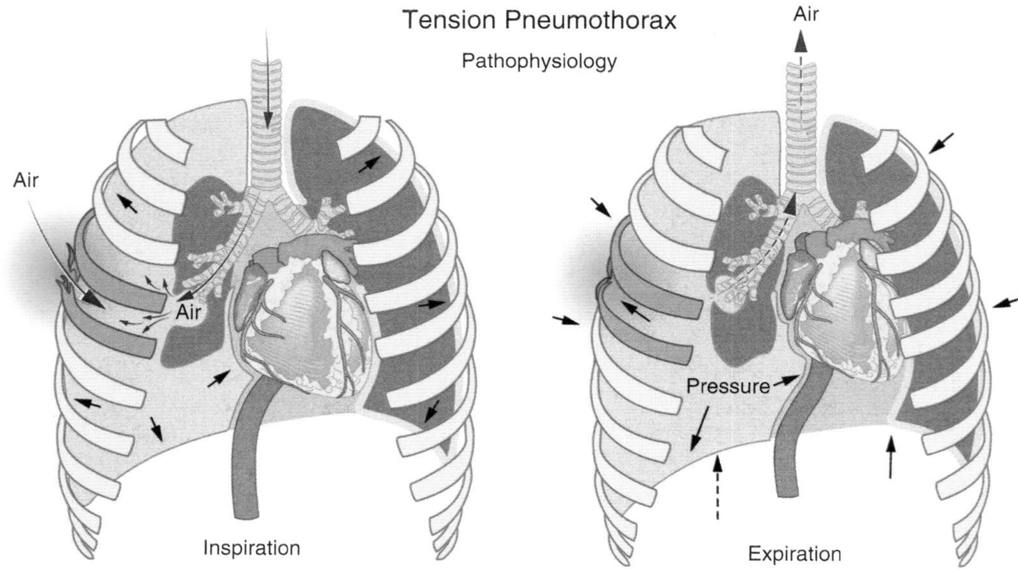

Fig. 20.4 Tension pneumothorax. Following a chest injury, air enters the pleural cavity on inspiration and, without a route to escape, pressure increases, compressing the heart and great vessels to the unaffected side (mediastinal shift). (Reprinted with permission, Cleveland Clinic Center for Medical Art & Photography ©2015-2019. All rights reserved.)

situation. The diagnosis of tension pneumothorax is based on the patient's clinical presentation. Never delay treatment to confirm the diagnosis by radiography.[6,16] Immediate decompression of the intrathoracic pressure is accomplished by needle thoracentesis followed by definitive treatment with a chest tube.[6,16,57,58]

Open pneumothorax is associated with penetrating chest trauma that allows air to enter the pleural space. In addition to the signs and symptoms of a pneumothorax, subcutaneous emphysema may also be present. Management of the open chest wound is accomplished with a nonporous dressing taped securely on three sides.[6,16] The fourth side is left open to allow for exhalation of air from within the pleural cavity. If the dressing becomes completely occlusive on all sides, air becomes trapped in the intrapleural space, and a tension pneumothorax may occur.

Hemothorax. Hemothorax is a collection of blood in the pleural space; it results from injuries to the heart, the great vessels, or the pulmonary parenchyma. Bleeding can be moderate (from intercostal vessels) or massive (from the aorta or subclavian or pulmonary vessels). Decreased breath sounds, hypotension, and respiratory distress may be seen.[6,16] Placement of a chest tube facilitates removal of blood from the pleural space, with resolution of ventilation and gas exchange abnormalities. Nursing interventions include managing the chest tube, closely observing the amount of blood drained from the pleural space, and monitoring the patient's hemodynamic response.

Pulmonary Contusion. Pulmonary contusion occurs as a result of rapid deceleration (as experienced in MVCs and falls), blunt impact, or blast forces to the chest. A contusion develops when capillary blood leaks into the lung parenchyma, resulting in inflammation and edema. The contusion may be localized or diffuse. The degree of respiratory distress is related to the size of the contusion, severity of injury at the alveolar-capillary membrane, and subsequent development of atelectasis.[16] Pulmonary contusions are often seen with other thoracic injuries. This injury is often difficult to detect because the initial chest radiographic study may be normal and is frequently only seen on CT scan with other injuries.[59] The clinical presentation includes worsening dyspnea, ineffective cough, hypoxia, chest wall abrasions, and chest pain.[16,59] Interventions focus on maintaining adequate oxygenation with supplemental oxygen, maintenance of fluid balance, and possibly mechanical ventilation. Administer fluids cautiously to avoid further lung edema.[16,59] Provide adequate pain relief with IV analgesics to optimize lung expansion and respiratory effort and to prevent complications, including atelectasis, pneumonia, and ARDS.

Rib Fractures and Flail Chest. Rib fractures are one of the most frequent diagnoses in trauma patients and the most common chest injury.[16,60] Rib fractures may lead to significant respiratory dysfunction and may indicate a serious injury to organs and structures below and near the rib cage. A high-impact force is needed to fracture the clavicle and first rib, with the risk of associated injuries of the head, neck, spinal cord, and great vessels.[6] Sternal injuries are usually not isolated due to the force required to fracture the sternum, and a severely displaced sternal fracture warrants concern for and anticipation of serious cardiac injury as well.[16] Assess for hemodynamic instability, which may indicate the presence of major vessel injury such as aortic disruption or injury to the subclavian artery. Injury to the liver, spleen, or kidney may accompany fractures of the lower ribs. The diagnosis of rib fractures is frequently made after a chest radiographic study. However, there are situations in which rib fractures are not visualized on chest radiographs and the diagnosis is made through clinical assessment.

The management of rib fractures depends on the number of ribs fractured, the degree of underlying injury, and the age of the patient. Assess the patient's ventilation and oxygenation and provide effective pain management. Provide education on coughing and deep-breathing exercises, the benefits of early ambulation, and pain management.[6,60] Effective pain management enables the patient to maximally participate in pulmonary exercises and improves outcomes in patients with rib fractures.

A flail chest is frequently defined as fractures of three or more adjacent ribs in two or more places, creating a free-floating segment of the rib cage. The flail segment results in paradoxical chest movement; the chest contracts inward with inhalation and expands outward with exhalation. Normal respiratory mechanics depend on a rigid chest wall to generate negative intrathoracic pressure for effective ventilation. The uncoordinated chest movement in flail chest; pain; and underlying injuries, including contusion or hemothorax, can impair effective ventilation.[16,60] The clinical presentation includes paradoxical chest movement, increased work of breathing, tachypnea, and eventually signs and symptoms of hypoxemia. Management frequently involves endotracheal intubation and mechanical ventilation with adequate pain control, which may include epidural analgesia or a regional block.[6,60] Internal surgical fixation of rib fractures may be used in some patients.[60] Position the patient to enhance ventilation and oxygenation, and provide frequent pulmonary care to prevent pneumonia.

CLINICAL JUDGMENT ACTIVITY

Determine which laboratory analysis to anticipate for a patient who experiences thoracic trauma and explain why. Describe why cardiac monitoring and/or a 12-lead electrocardiogram (ECG) is prescribed.

Abdominal Injuries

Abdominal injuries are often difficult to diagnose. A normal initial examination does not necessarily rule out intra-abdominal injury. The classic sign of abdominal injury is pain. However, pain cannot be used as an assessment tool if the patient has an altered sensorium, drug intoxication, or SCI with impaired sensation. Injuries to the intra-abdominal organs can cause significant bleeding and uncontrolled hemorrhage. The peritoneum can accommodate a significant blood volume, and abdominal distension might not be apparent until several liters of blood are in the peritoneal cavity.[61] Because hemodynamic instability from intraabdominal injuries arises from major hemorrhage, immediate management is focused on resuscitation with early use of blood products until definitive hemostasis can be achieved, usually through surgical intervention. In unstable patients with traumatic injury below the diaphragm and who are unresponsive, or transient responders to resuscitation, resuscitative endovascular balloon occlusion of the aorta (REBOA) may be considered.[61,62] A specially trained provider inserts a REBOA catheter through the femoral artery and inflates a balloon on the catheter in the distal thoracic aorta or the distal abdominal aorta to achieve aortic occlusion. This temporizing measure increases SBP and allows patient transport to an operating room for damage-control surgery.[61,62] Document the procedure as well as balloon inflation and/or deflation time.

The liver is the most commonly injured abdominal organ by blunt or penetrating trauma.[6,16] The patient may present with a history of right lower thoracic trauma, fractured lower right ribs, right upper quadrant ecchymosis, right upper quadrant tenderness, and hypotension. The diagnosis is confirmed with the use of FAST and/or abdominal CT. The degree of liver injury is graded on a scale of I to VI, with I representing a nonexpanding subcapsular hematoma and VI signifying hepatic avulsion. Angiographic embolization or surgical management is indicated for patients with high-grade liver injuries and signs of hemodynamic instability, in which there is expansion of the hemorrhage, a large laceration, or complete avulsion of the liver from its vascular supply.[16,63] Hemodynamically stable patients with a liver injury are managed nonoperatively with frequent monitoring (regular abdominal assessment and serial hemoglobin and hematocrit measurements).[6,16,62]

Splenic injury occurs most often as a result of blunt trauma to the abdomen, penetrating trauma to the left upper quadrant of the abdomen, or fracture of the anterior left lower ribs. The patient may present with left upper quadrant tenderness, peritoneal irritation, ecchymosis on the left flank *(Grey Turner's sign)*, and hypotension or signs of hypovolemic shock. An encapsulated hemorrhage of the spleen produces no immediate signs of bleeding. The diagnosis is confirmed by using the same tests as for liver injuries. Management of splenic injury is similar to that of liver injuries. Close monitoring of the patient is vital. Assess the patient's hemodynamic status and assess the abdomen for guarding, rebound tenderness, rigidity, or distension. Nonoperative management is the goal for hemodynamically stable patients, or angiography and embolization may be performed if the patient is hemodynamically stable with a moderate to severe laceration.[64] Operative intervention is performed in patients with hemodynamic instability and is often necessary after severe splenic injuries. A ruptured spleen is a life-threatening event that requires immediate surgical intervention. In pediatric patients, every effort is made to preserve splenic tissue because of its role in immune function. All patients who have undergone splenectomy are susceptible to infections, and administration of the pneumococcal, *Haemophilus influenzae* type b (Hib), meningococcal, and other vaccines is strongly recommended.[64]

Injuries to the stomach, small bowel, and large bowel are most frequently the consequence of penetrating trauma from gunshot wounds. Blast injuries can also cause injury to these hollow organs. Gastric and bowel injury is suspected based on the mechanism of injury, and surgical intervention is usually required. Postoperative complications include infection and difficulty maintaining nutrition.

Blunt trauma to the abdomen may also injure the kidneys; however, usually only one kidney is affected. The patient may present with costovertebral tenderness, microscopic or gross hematuria, bruising or ecchymosis over the 11th and 12th ribs, hemorrhage, and/or shock.[16] Diagnostic studies include FAST, CT, angiography, IV pyelography, and cystoscopy. For hemodynamically stable patients with minor injuries, management focuses on hydration and monitoring of kidney function, which includes adequacy of urine output; urinalysis; hematuria; blood urea nitrogen, creatinine, and electrolyte levels; and a complete blood count. Management of major and critical kidney injuries focuses on surgical intervention, including control of bleeding, repair of the injury, or nephrectomy. Postsurgical complications include refractory hypertension, hemorrhage, fistula formation, and infection.

Blunt trauma causing disruption of the pelvic structure is a challenging clinical problem because of the large vascular supply, nervous system pathways, location of urological structures, and articulation of the hip joint within the pelvic ring. Treatment of pelvic injuries often requires the expertise of many specialties (e.g., orthopedics, general surgery, neurosurgery, urology). Pelvic injuries occur most frequently in high-deceleration MVCs, pedestrian-vehicle impacts, and falls. The mortality rate from pelvic injuries is estimated at 5% to 30% and up to 50% in patients with open pelvic fractures.[6] Mortality is primarily related to hemorrhage and hemodynamic instability. Primary interventions focus on pelvic stabilization and aggressive fluid resuscitation to ensure adequate tissue perfusion. Initially, pelvic stabilization can be accomplished by tying a large sheet or pelvic binder around the patient's hips at the level of the greater trochanter to control the bleeding.[6,9,61,62] Early definitive treatment is accomplished through surgical repair in the operating room, although interventional radiology procedures that use embolization or coil techniques may also be used to stop the bleeding. Surgical repair may be required for internal or external fixation of complex pelvic fractures.

Musculoskeletal Injuries

Musculoskeletal injuries are rarely a priority in the emergent management after trauma unless there is an immediate threat to life or limb. Some musculoskeletal injuries result in significant hemodynamic instability (e.g., pelvic fractures, traumatic amputations). The injuries may be blunt or penetrating, and they may involve bone, soft tissue, muscle, nerves, and/or blood vessels. Injuries are classified as fractures, fracture-dislocations, amputations, and soft tissue trauma (crushing injuries to the soft tissue, nerves, vessels, or tendons). Knowing the mechanism of injury is important in evaluating musculoskeletal injuries because kinetic energy can be distributed from the bony impact to other areas of the body. For example, when a patient falls from a height, ankle fractures are likely, but energy displaced from the impact may also cause lumbar spine and pelvic fractures.

During the secondary survey, assess for limb swelling, ecchymosis, and deformity. A break in the skin integrity may indicate underlying fractures or dislocations without an otherwise obvious deformity. Assessment of neurovascular status is a critical component of assessing circulation in the injured extremity. The neurovascular assessment of the extremity is often described by the Six P's: pain, pallor, pulses, paresthesia, pressure, and paralysis. Loss of pulses is considered a late sign of diminished perfusion.[65,66] The presence of increased pain, pallor, and paresthesia supersedes loss of pulses and should be reported immediately to the trauma team.

Fractures involve a disruption of bony continuity. Radiographs are taken to diagnose fractures. Common types of fractures are shown in Fig. 20.5. If the skin is open at the fracture site, it is called an *open fracture;* if the skin is intact, it is called a *closed fracture.* Fractures are further classified into grades based on the degree of damage to the bone, soft tissues, vascular tissues, and nerves. Early treatment of a fracture involves immobilization with splints or application of traction. If the patient presents with an open fracture, antibiotics are administered within 1 hour of presentation, and the patient is taken to the operating room for irrigation and debridement within 24 hours.[67]

Traumatic amputation may be a partial or full amputation. The priority is to establish and maintain hemodynamic stability with hemorrhage control. Elevate the extremity and apply direct pressure over the artery above the bleeding site. Apply a tourniquet if direct pressure does not control bleeding until damage-control surgery can be completed.[34] These wounds usually require debridement and surgical closure.

Traumatic soft tissue injuries are categorized as contusions, abrasions, lacerations, puncture wounds, crush injuries, or avulsion injuries. Injury to the skin and soft tissues predisposes the individual to secondary complications, including localized and systemic infection. Assessment of soft tissue injury is part of the head-to-toe assessment in the secondary survey unless the loss of tissue (e.g., amputation) causes hemodynamic compromise. Contusions do not cause a break in the skin, but localized edema, ecchymosis, and pain occur. Abrasions ("road rash") occur when the skin experiences friction. Abrasions can be superficial, or they can cause deep tissue injury. Traumatic abrasions are frequently contaminated with debris implanted into the skin, resulting in traumatic tattooing. It can take hours to days to effectively remove the debris from the wound. Lacerations are usually caused by sharp objects, and they are treated with cleansing and suturing. Puncture wounds carry a heightened risk of infection.[68] Animal bites are notorious causes of puncture wounds. Suture or surgical closure of puncture wounds or other wounds with a high risk of infection may be delayed until the treatment for infection with irrigation and antibiotics has been completed.[68] Avulsion injuries result in stretching and tearing of the soft tissue and may tear nerves and vessels at levels different from the actual site of bone and tissue trauma. A crush injury may produce local soft tissue trauma or extensive damage distant from the site of injury. Crush injuries of the pelvis and/or both lower extremities or a prolonged entrapment can be limb- or life-threatening because prolonged compression produces ischemia and anoxia of the affected muscle tissue.[6] Third-spacing of fluid, localized edema, and increased compartment pressures cause secondary ischemia. Without aggressive intervention, these injuries can result in irreversible complications.

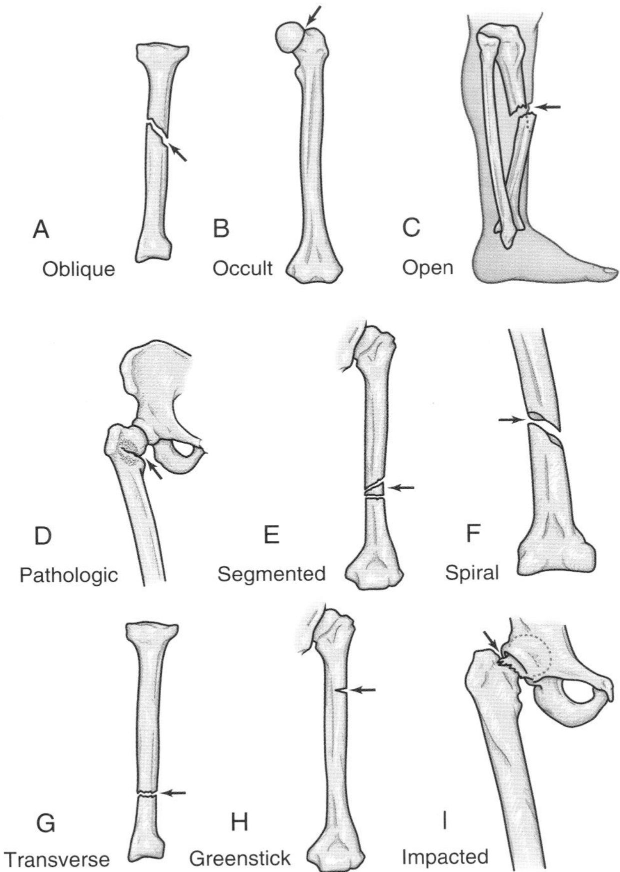

Fig. 20.5 Common types of fractures. **A**, Oblique: fracture at oblique angle across both cortices. Cause: direct or indirect energy, with angulation and some compression. **B**, Occult: fracture that is hidden or not readily discernible. Cause: minor force or energy. **C**, Open: skin broken over fracture; possible soft tissue trauma. Cause: moderate to severe energy that is continuous and exceeds tissue tolerances. **D**, Pathologic: transverse, oblique, or spiral fracture of bone weakened by tumor pressure or presence. Cause: minor energy or force, which may be direct or indirect. **E**, Segmented: fracture with two or more pieces or segments. Cause: direct or indirect moderate to severe force. **F**, Spiral: fracture that curves around cortices and may become displaced by twist. Cause: direct or indirect twisting energy or force with distal part held or unable to move. **G**, Transverse: horizontal break through bone. Cause: direct or indirect energy toward bone. **H**, Greenstick: break in only one cortex of bone. Cause: minor direct or indirect energy. **I**, Impacted: fracture with one end wedged into opposite end of inside fractured fragment. Cause: compressive axial energy or force directly to distal fragment. (From Smallheer A, Reeves GC. The musculoskeletal system. In: Rogers JL, Huether S, McCance K, eds., *Pathophysiology: The Biologic Basis for Disease in Adults and Children.* 9th ed. St. Louis, MO: Elsevier; 2023.)

All traumatic wounds are considered contaminated.[68] Wounds are cleansed and debrided to reduce the risk of infection. Ongoing assessment of the wound includes evaluating the healing and investigating any local or systemic signs and symptoms of infection (e.g., increased wound pain, swelling, fever, elevated white blood cell count, increased wound drainage). Tetanus toxoid administration and antibiotic therapy are also considered.

Complications. Complications of musculoskeletal injury include the systemic effects that may occur after a crush injury, such as compartment syndrome, rhabdomyolysis, hyperkalemia, venous thromboembolism (VTE), and fat embolism.

Compartment syndrome. Compartment syndrome occurs when the tissue pressure within a fascia-enclosed muscle compartment, such as an extremity, experiences increased pressure. The cause of increased pressure can be from internal or external sources. Internal sources include edema and hemorrhage; external forces include splints, immobilizers, and dressings. The closed muscle compartment of an extremity contains neurovascular bundles that are tightly covered by fascia. If the pressure is not relieved, compression of nerves, blood vessels, and muscles occurs, with resulting ischemia and necrosis of muscle and nerve tissue. The degree of damage depends on the amount of pressure and length of time during which perfusion is compromised. Unrecognized compartment syndrome can be limb-threatening. Muscle necrosis resulting in permanent loss of function and amputation can occur within 4 to 6 hours of ischemia.[6,16] Thorough and repeated nursing assessment for compartment syndrome is critical to quickly detect this complication and to save muscle.

The Six P's (pain, pressure, pallor, pulses, paresthesia, and paralysis) guide the assessment. Pain is a hallmark sign of compartment syndrome. Patients with developing compartment syndrome complain of increasing throbbing pain disproportionate to the injury, and narcotic administration does not relieve the pain. The pain is localized to the involved compartment and increases with passive muscle stretching. The area affected is firm. Paresthesia distal to the compartment, pallor, pulselessness, and paralysis are late signs and must be reported immediately to prevent loss of the extremity because muscle damage may already be irreversible.[65,66] In addition, elevate the affected limb to heart level to promote venous outflow and prevent further swelling. Compartmental pressure monitoring may be performed for definitive diagnosis. Treatment of compartment syndrome is immediate surgical fasciotomy in which the fascial compartment is opened to relieve the pressure.

Rhabdomyolysis. Rhabdomyolysis is a syndrome characterized by muscle damage and cellular destruction that results in release of intramuscular components, including myoglobin, a muscle protein, into the circulation. Causes of rhabdomyolysis include crush injuries, compartment syndrome, burns, and injuries from being struck by lightning. The classic signs of rhabdomyolysis include muscle pain, weakness, and dark-colored urine. Myoglobinuria (the excretion of myoglobin through the urine) is a marker of rhabdomyolysis and causes the urine to be a dark tea color. The myoglobin becomes trapped in the renal tubule, causing acute tubular necrosis, electrolyte and acid-base imbalances, and eventually acute kidney injury. Treatment of rhabdomyolysis is focused on aggressive fluid resuscitation to flush the myoglobin from the renal tubules and prevent acute kidney injury. Acute kidney injury is the most common systemic complication of rhabdomyolysis and is associated with a poor outcome (see Chapter 16, Acute Kidney Injury). Treatment includes targeting the underlying etiology and titration of IV fluids to achieve a urine output of 100 to 300 mL/h until the myoglobinuria is resolved.[69]

Hyperkalemia. Hyperkalemia may occur as a result of cellular damage. Potassium predominantly exists intracellularly; thus cellular destruction results in the release of large amounts of potassium into circulation, resulting in hyperkalemia. This places the patient at risk for life-threatening dysrhythmias. Calcium gluconate may be administered for cardiac protection until a more definitive treatment of the elevated potassium is implemented.[16] Tissue hypoperfusion and acidotic states may exacerbate hyperkalemia.

Venous thromboembolism. VTE is a significant complication of traumatic injury and accounts for significant morbidity and mortality in the injured patient.[70] The risk of VTE in trauma patients depends on the severity of injury, the type of injury (e.g., musculoskeletal injuries), the presence of shock, recent surgeries, vascular injury, and immobility. Trauma is a known risk factor for VTE secondary to decreased venous flow; diminished fibrinolysis; immobilization; and depletion of anticoagulants, such as antithrombim, in the acute phase.[70] Most trauma patients are hypercoagulable on admission, increasing the risk and prevalence of VTE.[71]

Thrombus formation is enhanced in the presence of Virchow's triad: vessel damage, venous stasis, and hypercoagulability. VTE usually results from a deep vein thrombosis (DVT) in the lower extremities, although it can form in the upper extremities as well. If the thrombus dislodges, it becomes an embolus and travels through the body's vasculature until it lodges in either the pulmonary artery or one of its smaller branches (pulmonary embolism). Once the embolus becomes lodged, blood flow is obstructed distally, and the tissues distal to the obstruction become hypoxic. Pulmonary vessels constrict in response to the hypoxia, resulting in ventilation-perfusion mismatches and hypoxemia. Prevention of VTE is essential. Unless contraindicated, pharmacological prophylaxis should be prescribed.[70] Encourage ambulation, evaluate the patient's overall hydration, and ensure that intermittent pneumatic compression or sequential compression devices are used properly.

Fat embolism syndrome. Fat embolism syndrome is a potential complication that accompanies traumatic injury to the long bones and pelvis that results in multiple skeletal fractures. Long bone injury may release fat globules into torn vessels and the systemic circulation. The fat particles act as emboli, traveling through the great vessels and pulmonary system, obstructing flow and causing hypoxia. Most instances of fat embolism are asymptomatic, but symptomatic patients demonstrate a classic triad of clinical signs 24 to 72 hours after injury: altered mental status; respiratory distress, including dyspnea, increased respiratory rate and effort, and hypoxemia (partial pressure of arterial oxygen [PaO_2] ≤60 mm Hg); and a petechial rash.[16,72] Other, nonspecific signs include tachycardia, hypotension, right heart strain, and fever.[72]

Prevention of fat embolism is the best treatment. Stabilization of extremity fractures to minimize both bone movement and the release of fatty products from the bone marrow must be accomplished as early as possible.[72] Treatment of fat embolism syndrome is primarily supportive and directed toward preservation of pulmonary function and maintenance of cardiovascular stability. Administration of supplemental oxygen and intubation with mechanical ventilation and positive end-expiratory pressure may be required to restore or maintain pulmonary function. Monitoring of the patient's cardiovascular stability is continued throughout the critical care phase, with particular attention to ECG and hemodynamic changes.

CHECK YOUR UNDERSTANDING

5. Assessment of the trauma patient suggests possible compartment syndrome. Which symptom should be reported to the provider for urgent evaluation and intervention to address possible compartment syndrome?
   A. Swelling of the broken extremity
   B. Increasing pain not relieved by pain medication
   C. Red discoloration of urine
   D. Dyspnea

CRITICAL CARE PHASE

The critical care phase for the patient with multisystem traumatic injuries requires the skills and collaboration of a variety of healthcare professionals. The patient experiences additional physiological stressors from the traumatic injury and subsequent surgeries, as well as disruption of the social or family unit. The nurse is central to the critical care phase, continually assessing the patient's progress, anticipating and evaluating for possible complications, encouraging family-centered care, and acting as the patient's advocate. Interventions that were initiated in the emergency care phase to treat and manage the traumatic injuries continue into the critical care phase.

Damage-Control Surgery

Patients with multiple injuries from traumatic events are at greatest risk of death from hemorrhage. Emergent surgical management is the gold standard for stopping hemorrhage and stabilizing life-threatening injuries. Extensive or complex surgeries during the resuscitation phase may affect patient outcomes due to the lethal triad of coagulopathy, hypothermia, and acidosis.[6,16] Thus, definitive surgery is deferred until resuscitation is complete and the patient is hemodynamically stable.[53]

Damage-control surgery emphasizes rapid surgical control of active hemorrhage while minimizing extensive or lengthy interventions for definitive treatment of traumatic injuries.[53] Damage-control surgery is described in five phases. The initial phase involves identifying the patient based on injury characteristics and presenting pathophysiology. The second phase involves an abbreviated surgery focused on bleeding control in conjunction with phase three, which is sequential assessment and reassessment of vital signs and urine output during the operative course. Frequently, drains are placed during damage-control surgery; thus monitoring the amount and type of drainage (e.g., bloody to serosanguinous) is important. Patients are returned to the critical care unit (phase four) for aggressive rewarming, ongoing resuscitation, and attainment of hemodynamic stability. Definitive surgical repair is completed during phase five, although this may occur in several operations.[53] Damage-control surgery is a life-saving measure to control hemorrhage while minimizing the risks associated with coagulopathy, hypothermia, and acidosis that are perpetuated during hemorrhage and extensive surgery.

Postoperative Management

Most critically ill trauma patients are admitted directly to the critical care unit after surgery. Preparation for admission of the patient provides a smooth transition in care from the operative phase to the critical care phase. In preparation for the patient, the nurse is responsible for several actions, including increasing the room temperature to manage or prevent anticipated hypothermia; obtaining IV infusion pumps; contacting the respiratory therapist for a ventilator; checking necessary monitoring equipment and room supplies (e.g., suction supplies, oxygen) to ensure that they are available once the patient is admitted; locating emergency supplies near the patient's room; and zeroing the bed scale to obtain an admission weight of the patient. The nurse frequently receives a report from the ED nurse before the patient goes to surgery; however, a thorough report from the anesthesiologist as part of handoff communication is essential for continuity of care. Elements of the handoff communication include a review of systems, past medical history, description of the injury, description of the intraoperative procedures, the patient's tolerance of the procedures, vital signs during the surgery and current vital signs, total intake (i.e., crystalloids, colloids, and blood products) and output (i.e., urine output, chest tube output, and estimated blood loss), laboratory values, medications administered (i.e., sedation, analgesia, neuromuscular blockade reversal agents, antibiotics, and vasoactive medications), IV access, location of chest tubes and other drains, and any complications that may have occurred during the intraoperative procedure.[73,74] The use of a standard checklist is recommended to ensure a safe and effective handoff from the operating room to the critical care unit.[73,74]

The initial assessment and management of the patient on admission to the critical care unit follow the same systematic primary and secondary survey approach. First, complete a rapid assessment of airway, breathing, circulation, disability, and exposure. Connect the patient to the bedside monitor and ventilator, and complete an assessment of vital signs, cardiac rhythm, pulse oximetry reading, level of consciousness, and pupil reactivity. Because hypothermia and the associated coagulopathy and acidosis abnormalities remain a concern postoperatively, keep the patient covered while assessing the body for surgical incisions, dressings, other injuries, and location and function of drainage devices (e.g., chest tubes, surgical drains). Complete a secondary survey with a head-to-toe assessment and inspection of the posterior surface of the patient by turning the patient. While turning the patient, remove soiled linens and place clean linens to help identify new bleeding. Reassess IV access and evaluate the patency of IV catheters, which may have become dislodged during transport. Trace all IV infusions from the IV fluid to the infusion pump and to the patient's IV access catheter. Calculate medication dosages and rates as part of the initial assessment. Empty all drainage devices and record the volume of output. If a chest tube is in place, mark (date/time) the amount of existing drainage on the external collection system.

Postoperative management of critically ill patients involves a systematic and thorough assessment and monitoring of respiratory and cardiovascular function, neuromuscular abilities, mental status, temperature, pain, drainage and bleeding, urine output, and resuscitation efforts. Patients may have an endotracheal tube in place when they are transferred to the critical care unit. Patients who do not require mechanical ventilation are extubated within minutes to hours after admission, depending on their ability to protect the airway after reversal of anesthesia and neuromuscular blocking agents. Other critically ill patients are maintained on mechanical ventilation until they are stable, their injuries are definitively repaired, and/or pulmonary pathological processes have resolved. Monitoring oxygenation and ventilation status is part of ongoing critical care management. Modifications in the ventilatory modes, adjuncts, and fraction of inspired oxygen (FiO_2) are made based on assessment.

After ensuring the stability of the patient's airway and the adequacy of ventilation, focus on hemodynamic assessment. This includes monitoring the heart rate, cardiac rhythm, blood pressure, respiratory rate, pulse oximetry, temperature, drainage (e.g., chest tubes, nasogastric tubes, wound or incisional drains), urinary output, IV fluids, and vasoactive medications. The common practice for monitoring these parameters is every 15 minutes for 1 hour, then hourly thereafter. More frequent monitoring is indicated if the patient is hemodynamically unstable. Additional hemodynamic values are obtained if the patient has a pulmonary artery catheter or an ICP monitor.

Assess the patient's mental status to ensure that a neurological event did not occur intraoperatively. Handoff communication from the anesthesia provider includes the most recent administration times and dosages of analgesic, amnesic, or sedative medications. This provides information on the estimated time of patient wakefulness. Check the patient's pupils for reactivity. Once the patient is awake, assess for alertness and orientation to person, place, and time, as well as the ability to follow commands. If the patient does not awaken, determine the cause of the unresponsive state. The team must determine whether the anesthetic agents, sedation, or analgesic medications are contributing factors. If it is determined that medications are not the contributing cause of the neurological impairment, the patient may require additional diagnostic testing, such as a CT scan of the head. Any alterations in the patient's clinical assessment must be analyzed by the multiprofessional team to determine whether intervention is necessary.

Measure the patient's temperature on admission and monitor at regular intervals. In the event of hypothermia, implement passive and active strategies to rewarm the patient to a normothermic state (see Table 20.5). Prevent shivering because it increases the metabolic rate and results in increased oxygen demands and the potential for hemodynamic instability. During the rewarming process, vasodilation and electrolyte shifts can occur; therefore, monitor the patient for decreases in blood pressure and dysrhythmias.

Obtain admission laboratory studies. The studies most frequently obtained postoperatively include a complete blood count, a complete metabolic panel, coagulation studies, an arterial lactate level, and an arterial blood gas analysis with base deficit. Finally, weigh the patient. The admission weight is important for ongoing assessment of the patient's fluid status and medication administration throughout the critical care unit admission. Once the assessment and initial interventions are completed, contact the family to coordinate updates and family presence.

Perform a complete physical assessment on all postoperative patients. Assess all body systems, including the neurological, cardiovascular, pulmonary, gastrointestinal, renal, hematological, immune, musculoskeletal, and integumentary systems. Continuous collection of assessment data guides therapies aimed at correcting identified problems or injuries and preventing or minimizing postinjury complications. Older adult patients are at increased risk of complications after traumatic injury because of age-related changes.

CLINICAL JUDGMENT ACTIVITY

Describe the nursing assessment and intervention priorities during the first postoperative hour once a patient is admitted to the critical care unit. Articulate strategies to incorporate patient and family-centered care during the immediate postoperative phase of nursing care. Identify mechanisms to improve communication and establish trust with the patient, family, and healthcare team.

Assess patients to determine their level of pain and the presence of nausea.[75] Multiple pain scales are available to assess the degree of pain (see Chapter 6, Comfort and Sedation). Postoperative orders include analgesic medication to be administered orally or intravenously (as needed or as a continuous infusion). If the patient's pain level cannot be assessed postoperatively because of the patient's lack of wakefulness or secondary to a neurological event, evaluate the pain by assessing other parameters, including increased heart rate and blood pressure, restlessness, facial grimacing, decreasing oxygen levels, and ventilator dyssynchrony. After administration of analgesia, reassess the patient's pain level.

Evaluate resuscitative efforts postoperatively to determine the effectiveness of fluid management. Establish baseline hemodynamic status, laboratory values (e.g., basic chemistry panel, arterial blood gases, arterial lactate level), and intake and output to determine the patient's fluid volume status and the degree of successful resuscitation. Hemoglobin levels, hematocrit values, and coagulation studies provide valuable information on whether the patient is bleeding or has a high probability of bleeding due to unavailable or ineffective clotting factors. The presence of abnormal values indicates the need for more aggressive resuscitation or blood component therapy.

LIFESPAN CONSIDERATIONS

Older Adults

- Falls are the most frequent cause of injury for the elderly population and the leading cause of injury-related deaths in individuals older than 65 years of age.[3] Falls result in fractures of the hips, arms, hands, legs, feet, pelvis, ribs, and vertebrae.
- Older adults can experience significant injury despite a seemingly trivial mechanism. Under-triage of older adults is associated with a twofold increase in the risk of mortality, so a lower threshold for trauma team activation is recommended for older adults.[76]
- Three factors contribute to a higher morbidity and mortality in this population: comorbidities, medications, and age-related physiological changes.[76,77]
- Physiological changes associated with aging and reduced physiological reserves predispose older adults to serious injury, prolonged recovery, and increased mortality. Older adults with poor functional status and multiple comorbidities such as disseminated cancer, chronic renal failure, and heart failure (HF) have worse outcomes after trauma.[78,79]
- Individuals with chronic hypertension may appear to have a normal blood pressure when, in fact, they are hypotensive. An older adult who is taking beta-blockers and a calcium channel blocker may have a blunted hemodynamic response to trauma.[76,79] Therefore slight changes in heart rate or blood pressure may signify unrecognized injury.
- Knowledge of current medications, specifically anticoagulants, steroids, cardiac medications (e.g., beta-blockers, calcium channel blockers), and nonsteroidal antiinflammatory drugs (NSAIDs), is important because they may increase the risk of injury and the risk of complications.
- The Beers Medication List is updated by the American Geriatric Society and provides information on medications and potential adverse reactions in the older adult.[77]

Pregnant People

- Trauma is a leading cause of nonobstetric mortality during pregnancy. Domestic violence and motor vehicle collisions (MVCs) account for a significant portion of trauma-related injuries during pregnancy.[80]
- Risk factors for additional injuries associated with the pregnant state include Rh exposure, placental abruption, uterine rupture, preterm labor, and fetal compromise.
- Advanced stages of pregnancy press up on the diaphragm, reducing functional residual capacity and challenging pulmonary mechanics (e.g., ventilation effort). Pregnant patients also have a marked increase in basal oxygen consumption; therefore continuously monitor oxygenation and ventilation. Administer supplemental oxygen by a nasal cannula, mask, or mechanical ventilation (if indicated).[16]
- The pregnant patient experiences significant changes in fluid volume status, which may make it harder to detect blood loss. The pregnant trauma patient may lose up to 40% of circulating volume before there is an appreciable drop in blood pressure.[6,16]
- Compression of the vena cava by the uterus can cause a significant reduction in cardiac output. The gravid uterus is moved off the inferior vena cava to increase venous return and cardiac output in the acutely injured pregnant people.[6,16,80] This can be achieved by manual displacement of the uterus or left lateral tilt while maintaining spinal precautions.
- Consult obstetrical and neonatal specialists (providers and nurses) to evaluate the patient and fetus.
- Evaluate for traumatic injury associated with domestic violence.

Ongoing Care

The ongoing patient care priorities evolve from the initial trauma injury, the patient's diagnosis, and the surgical procedure to reducing the risk of prolonged consequences of injury. In the acute hospital phase, careful attention is given to anticipating potential problems and intervening when actual problems are identified. Perform a comprehensive reassessment every 4 hours to identify changes in the patient's status, prepare for additional diagnostic procedures, and intervene appropriately. Evaluate the patient continuously for alterations in oxygenation, ventilation, acid-base balance, perfusion, metabolic status, and hemodynamic status and for signs and symptoms of infection. Potential complications include infections (e.g., pneumonia, urinary tract infections, and sepsis), ARDS, and VTE. The goal of ongoing care is to prevent these complications.

Optimal nutritional support is considered an integral component of care of the critically injured patient. The nutritional needs of the patient are addressed early in the postoperative phase (within 24 to 48 hours) to assist with healing and meeting the body's needs related to an elevated metabolic demand. The route of administration (oral, enteral, or parenteral), type of nutritional replacement, and rate of administration depend on the severity of illness or injury and the expected recovery period. In critically ill patients who are unable to maintain oral intake, early initiation of enteral nutrition, within 24 to 48 hours, is recommended and associated with a reduction in mortality and morbidity.[81,82] Obtain a nutritional consultation to evaluate the metabolic needs of the patient and determine the optimal feeding formula and rate of administration (see Chapter 7, Nutritional Therapy).

Ensure that the patient has pharmacological prophylaxis for VTE and stress ulceration and an aggressive protocol for mobilization. Immobility places a patient at increased risk of developing VTE, pneumonia, pressure ulcers, urostasis, and delirium. Strategies to prevent complications of immobility include frequent turning, off-loading pressure on bony prominences with pillows, frequent skin assessments, application of moisture barriers to skin to prevent maceration from feces or leaking drainage devices, coughing and deep-breathing exercises, early extubation, urinary catheter care and early removal of the catheter, and early ambulation.

Patients with multisystem injuries are at high risk for myriad complications associated with the overwhelming stressors of the injury, prolonged immobility, and consequences of inadequate tissue perfusion. Even with optimal care, the stressors and overwhelming inflammatory responses to injury influence the risk of secondary complications. These include respiratory impairment (abdominal compartment syndrome, ARDS, pneumonia), infection (catheter infection, sepsis), acute kidney injury, high nutritional demands, and MODS. A full discussion of these secondary complications can be found in other chapters within this text.

SPECIAL CONSIDERATIONS AND POPULATIONS

Alcohol and Drug Use

Many injuries have alcohol and drug use as a contributing factor. Most trauma patients who have a high blood alcohol concentration on admission meet criteria that indicate an alcohol use disorder. Because of the high incidence of traumatic events involving the use of alcohol and drugs, trauma prevention cannot be successful unless these concerns are addressed. Screening and brief intervention for alcohol use is required of all Level I and Level II trauma centers, and the Committee on Trauma recommends all trauma centers incorporate it as part of routine trauma care.[9,83]

Evidence-based programs are available to guide intervention programs and provide tools to address alcohol and drug use disorders in patients during an acute hospital admission. These include the *Screening, Brief Intervention, and Referral to Treatment* (SBIRT) services provided by Medicare and Medicaid.[84] Trauma centers need to have alcohol and drug intervention programs that can be implemented at the time of admission and maintained throughout the hospitalization by appropriately trained staff. Brief interventions initiated during hospitalization affect the high correlation of alcohol and/or illicit drug use and serious traumatic injury by decreasing the incidence of trauma recidivism.[83]

Substance use and misuse impair a patient's cognitive processes and create physiological stress. Multiple categories of drugs may be used by the trauma patient, ranging from inhalant intoxicants to hallucinogens, stimulants, sedatives, dissociatives, cannabinoids, psychedelics, and prescription opioids.

Drug use, especially drug overdose, causes significant physiological stressors. After addressing the traumatic injury, the physiological consequences of the drug and subsequent drug withdrawal must be addressed. Nursing care of the trauma patient with an alcohol or substance use disorder provides both a challenge and an opportunity. Because addiction or misuse is associated with physiological dependence, serious or life-threatening withdrawal may occur when the patient no longer consumes these agents. Closely monitor the patient's physiological status during withdrawal. Implement protocols to address withdrawal by providing preemptive treatment. Common signs and symptoms include increased agitation, anxiety, auditory and visual hallucinations, disorientation, headache, nausea and vomiting, paroxysmal diaphoresis, and tremors (Box 20.3). Assess the time of the patient's last use of the drug or alcohol to plan treatment strategies. As patients experience withdrawal, medications may be ordered to ease the physiological and behavioral symptoms. Assess the patient hourly, especially in the presence of worsening anxiety, hallucinations, and other symptoms, to ensure patient safety. Someone may be designated to sit with the patient at all times during acute drug or alcohol withdrawal. Implement drug and alcohol prevention interventions before discharge from the hospital.

BOX 20.3 Signs and Symptoms of Alcohol Withdrawal

- Irritability, anxiety, agitation, and/or confusion
- Hallucinations and delusions
- Tremors
- Nausea, vomiting, and diarrhea
- Diaphoresis
- Tachycardia and hypertension
- Seizures

Vulnerable Populations and Intimate Partner Violence

Vulnerable populations (i.e., children, mentally and/or physically dysfunctional adults, and older adult patients who cannot care for themselves) are at risk for abuse. Many states have mandatory reporting laws for reported or suspected abuse in these vulnerable populations. When abuse is suspected, the nurse must follow the hospital's reporting processes and provide emotional support to the patient.

Intimate partner violence, also called *domestic* or *dating violence,* can be physical, sexual, stalking, or psychological.[85] Several questionnaires are available to screen for intimate partner violence: *Humiliation, Afraid, Rape, Kick* (HARK); *Hurt/Insult/Threaten/Scream* (HITS); *Extended Hurt/Insult/Threaten/Scream* (E-HITS); *Partner Violence Screen* (PVS); and *Woman Abuse Screening Tool* (WAST). Intimate partner violence is not restricted to heterosexual couples. Individuals who identify as lesbian, gay, bisexual, transgender, and queer or questioning (LGBTQ+) also experience intimate partner violence, as well as other types of violence, and may not seek help or disclose the mechanism of injury. Trauma nurses and teams have a unique opportunity to identify intimate partner violence, care for these patients, and provide resources in a safe environment.[16]

Family and Patient Coping

Traumatic injury is frequently unexpected and is a potentially devastating event, producing physical, psychological, and emotional stress for the patient and family. The event leaves the patient and family feeling overwhelmed, vulnerable, and often ill-prepared to cope with ramifications of the injury. The traumatic event often creates a crisis within the patient's family unit. Critical decisions for the patient frequently must be made in seconds by family members. The trauma team can assist the patient and family in crisis by helping them establish a consistent communication process between the healthcare team and the family. Explore the patient's and family's perception of the event, support systems, and coping mechanisms. Involve the social worker early to assist the patient and family with coping and decision-making. Coordinate a family conference early in the emergency care phase and frequently during the critical care phase to assist with communication and understanding of the patient's and family's expectations for care and to enhance the decision-making and coping skills of the patient and family.

Posttraumatic stress disorder (PTSD) and *acute stress disorder* (ASD) are trauma- and stressor-related psychiatric disorders that can occur after experiencing or witnessing events involving physical injury, death, or other threats to physical integrity.[86] Symptoms of trauma- and stressor-related disorders include reexperiencing the traumatic event and avoidance of trauma-related stimuli. If the patient exhibits symptoms of ASD or PTSD during screening, obtain consultations and provide resources such as the Trauma Survivors Network support group and crisis intervention call-in lines.

REHABILITATION PHASE

The final phase of trauma care encompasses rehabilitation of the patient. The initiation of the rehabilitative process begins the moment the patient is admitted to the trauma center. Prevention of complications that prolong hospitalization and delay rehabilitation is imperative. Early involvement of physical medicine and rehabilitation personnel is vital to achieving positive functional patient outcomes. Early in this phase of trauma care, a case manager or discharge planner evaluates the patient for the need for extensive rehabilitation at a specialty center. An individualized plan is developed for each patient based on physical injuries and rehabilitation potential, patient and family preferences, and insurance coverage.

Nursing interventions in the critical care phase influence the patient's rehabilitative needs. For example, focus on positioning the immobile patient to prevent foot drop. This intervention facilitates ambulation during recovery. Apply splints to injured extremities to improve functionality. Provide emotional support to both the patient and the family as the patient convalesces through the critical care phase and begins more independent activities. Prepare them for the rehabilitation phase of trauma recovery.

Transition of the patient into rehabilitation is both an exciting and a frightening time for the patient and family. The patient has relied on the nursing staff for encouragement and support at a critical time in the patient's life. Transfer to another center brings with it uncertainty in new relationships, as well as excitement, because rehabilitation is the last step before returning to the patient's home.

CLINICAL EXEMPLAR

Quality and Safety

A nurse notices that essential life-saving equipment (e.g., manual resuscitation bag, oxygen flow meter, Lactated Ringer's solution, suture material) are often missing from the trauma room designated for admission of patients with traumatic injury. The lack of essential equipment in the room causes delays in care as team members leave the room to obtain necessary supplies and increases the tension of the team during the acute admission. On exploring the reasons for missing items, the nurse discovers that there is no checklist for what is considered essential equipment for the trauma room. The nurse surveys the trauma team (providers, nurses, technicians, support staff, laboratory personnel) to understand what equipment each healthcare professional deems essential to provide initial care to the trauma patient. After developing the list of items to be stocked in the trauma room, the nurse approaches the unit leadership to ask for a trauma cart so that the equipment needed may be more easily stocked and stored in the trauma room. The list of essential items is attached to the trauma cart, and the technicians agree to use the list to stock the cart as part of daily routines. The nurse agrees to track the efficiency in care (i.e., reduced interruptions in care to retrieve essential equipment and consistency of the trauma cart being fully stocked) resulting from having a trauma cart stocked with essential items. Team huddles are used to review the efficiency of the trauma cart and suggest ongoing improvements for efficiency of care of patients with traumatic injuries.

CASE STUDY

Mr. M., a 27-year-old male, was dropped off in the emergency department (ED) with a gunshot wound to his right chest. He was awake on arrival, but his level of consciousness quickly declined as the trauma team transported him to the resuscitation room. Once in the resuscitation room, Mr. M. became unresponsive with a weak pulse. Vital signs were as follows: heart rate and rhythm, sinus tachycardia at 125 beats/min; blood pressure, 72/48 mm Hg; respiratory rate, 8 breaths/min; oxygen saturation (SpO_2), 75%; and temperature, 35.8°C. The patient was immediately intubated to secure his airway and placed on the ventilator at 100% fraction of inspired oxygen (FiO_2). Two large-bore peripheral IV catheters were placed, the patient's blood was typed and crossmatched, and the massive transfusion protocol was initiated at a ratio of 1:1:1 (packed red blood cells, fresh frozen plasma, and platelets). The focused assessment with sonography for trauma (FAST) examination was positive for free fluid in the abdomen. The patient was transported to the operating room for damage-control surgery. A thoracotomy was performed, and the site of hemorrhage was located; the bullet had lacerated the descending aorta. The aorta was repaired, chest tubes were placed, and the patient was transported to the critical care unit in critical condition.

Upon arrival to the unit, the critical care nurses performed a rapid and systematic primary and secondary survey. The airway remained secure via the endotracheal tube, the patient was tolerating mechanical ventilation, and his bilateral lung sounds were clear. He had equal chest rise and fall, and his oxygen saturation was 95%. Circulation assessment revealed normal pulses, heart rate was sinus tachycardia at 110 beats/min, blood pressure was 95/67 mm Hg, respiratory rate was 18 breaths/min, and temperature was 35.9°C. The patient was not responsive to verbal commands or moving any extremities, and his pupils were 2 mm and reactive to light. During the head-to-toe assessment and inspection of posterior surfaces of the secondary survey, a small wound was discovered in the midline posterior aspect of his cervical spine, consistent with a penetrating injury. No other injuries were discovered. Laboratory results were as follows:

Hemoglobin	7.2 g/dL
Hematocrit	22.3%
White blood cell count	16,000 cells/microliter
Platelet count	200,000/microliter
Potassium	5.5 mEq/L
Other electrolyte levels	Unremarkable
Arterial Blood Gas Results	
pH	7.19
Partial pressure of arterial oxygen (PaO_2)	160 mm Hg
Partial pressure of arterial carbon dioxide ($PaCO_2$)	42 mm Hg
Bicarbonate (HCO_3^-)	18 mEq/L
Base deficit	−14
Lactate	8 mmol/L

The patient was transported for computed tomography to evaluate his head and spine for additional injuries. The ED contacted his family, who were in the waiting room of the critical care unit.

Questions

1. Describe the priority interventions on arrival of the patient in the ED based on his vital signs.
2. Explain additional procedures you anticipate in the emergent evaluation and treatment of this patient, considering his mechanism of injury.
3. Explain why it is important to administer platelets and fresh frozen plasma along with packed red blood cells to a patient who requires a massive blood transfusion.
4. Interpret and describe the laboratory results. Prioritize interventions you anticipate based on these results.
5. Describe how hypothermia affects the care of the postoperative patient. Describe your nursing interventions to address Mr. M.'s postoperative hypothermia.
6. How will you assess the needs of the family and coordinate meeting those needs?

KEY POINTS

- Injury prevention is an overarching goal in trauma care. Nurses are poised to lead injury prevention by identifying patients at risk, educating patients and families, collaborating with injury-prevention specialists, and referring to community resources where available.
- The primary survey is a rapid assessment to simultaneously identify and manage life-threatening injuries in a systematic approach through the pneumonic ABCDEFG.
- The secondary survey is initiated after all actual or potential life-threatening injuries have been addressed and resuscitation has been initiated. It is a methodological approach to obtaining the patient and event history and a complete head-to-toe assessment of the patient.
- Large volumes of crystalloid fluid resuscitation are associated with increased mortality. Resuscitation with blood products is recommended to minimize coagulopathies using a ratio-based transfusion of one part PRBCs to one part thawed plasma to one part platelets (1:1:1 ratio).
- Nursing priorities include minimizing the risk and incidence of hypothermia, coagulopathy, and acidosis, which are associated with the trauma triad of death.
- Knowledge and understanding of the mechanism of injury assist the trauma team in early identification and management of injuries. Ongoing assessment, management of specific organ injuries, and awareness of the patient's response to the injury due to patient factors, comorbidities, or medications are vital during the resuscitative and critical care phase of trauma care.

REFERENCES

1. Merriam-Webster.com Dictionary. Trauma. https://www.merriam-webster.com/dictionary/trauma. Accessed February 19, 2023.
2. Peterson C, Miller GF, Barnett SBL, Florence C. Economic cost of injury—United States, 2019. *MMWR Morb Mortal Wkly Rep*. 2021;70(48):1655–1659. https://doi.org/10.15585/mmwr.mm7048a1.
3. Centers for Disease Control and Prevention. Leading Causes of Death and Injury. https://www.cdc.gov/injury/wisqars/LeadingCauses.html. Updated January 19, 2023. Accessed February 19, 2023.
4. Centers for Disease Control and Prevention. Transportation Safety. https://www.cdc.gov/transportationsafety/index.html. Updated June 29, 2023. Accessed December 19, 2023.
5. Centers for Disease Control and Prevention. Drug Overdose Deaths. https://www.cdc.gov/drugoverdose/deaths/index.html. Updated August 22, 2023. Accessed December 19, 2023.
6. American College of Surgeons. *Advanced Trauma Life Support: Student Course Manual*. 10th ed. Chicago, IL: American College of Surgeons; 2018.
7. Porter A, Karim S, Bowman SM, Recicar J, Bledsoe GH, Maxson RT. Impact of a statewide trauma system on the triage, transfer, and inpatient mortality of injured patients. *J Trauma Acute Care Surg*. 2018;84(5):771–779. https://doi.org/10.1097/ta.0000000000001825.
8. David JS, Bouzat P, Raux M. Evolution and organisation of trauma systems. *Anaesth Crit Care Pain Med*. 2019;38(2):161–167. https://doi.org/10.1016/j.accpm.2018.01.006.
9. American College of Surgeons, Committee on Trauma. Regional trauma systems: optimal elements, integration, and assessment. In: *Resources for Optimal Care of the Injured Patient*. Chicago, IL: American College of Surgeons, Committee on Trauma; 2014.
10. U.S. Department of Health and Human Services. Model Trauma System Planning and Evaluation. https://www.facs.org/media/p0nfw0n0/hrsa-mtspe.pdf. Published 2006.
11. American College of Surgeons, Committee on Trauma. Descriptions of trauma center levels and their roles in a trauma system. In: *Resources for Optimal Care of the Injured Patient*. Chicago, IL: American College of Surgeons Committee on Trauma; 2022.
12. Rauf R, von Matthey F, Croenlein M, et al. Changes in the temporal distribution of in-hospital mortality in severely injured patients—an analysis of the Trauma Register DGU. *PLoS One*. 2019;14(2):e0212095. https://doi.org/10.1371/journal.pone.0212095.
13. American College of Surgeons. Committee on trauma. Prevention. In: *Resources for Optimal Care of the Injured Patient*. Chicago, IL: American College of Surgeons, Committee on Trauma; 2014.
14. U.S. Department of Health and Human Services. StopBullying.gov. https://www.stopbullying.gov. Accessed February 19, 2023.
15. Snow S. ENA position statement: the role of the emergency nurse in injury prevention. *J Emerg Nurs*. 2018;44(6):640–644. https://doi.org/10.1016/j.jen.2018.10.002.
16. Emergency Nurses Association. *Trauma Nurse Core Course Provider Manual*. 8th ed. Sudbury, MA: Jones and Bartlett; 2020.
17. Huis In't Veld MA, Craft CA, Hood RE. Blunt cardiac trauma review. *Cardiol Clin*. 2018;36(1):183–191. https://doi.org/10.1016/j.ccl.2017.08.010.
18. Patel KM, Kumar NS, Desai RG, Mitrev L, Trivedi K, Krishnan S. Blunt trauma to the heart: a review of pathophysiology and current management. *J Cardiothorac Vasc Anesth*. 2022;36(8 Pt A):2707–2718. https://doi.org/10.1053/j.jvca.2021.10.018.
19. Baum GR, Baum JT, Hayward D, MacKay BJ. Gunshot wounds: ballistics, pathology, and treatment recommendations, with a focus on retained bullets. *Orthop Res Rev*. 2022;14:293–317. https://doi.org/10.2147/orr.S378278.
20. Westrol MS, Donovan CM, Kapitanyan R. Blast physics and pathophysiology of explosive injuries. *Ann Emerg Med*. 2017;69(1s):S4–S9. https://doi.org/10.1016/j.annemergmed.2016.09.005.
21. Schenk E, Wijetunge G, Mann NC, Lerner EB, Longthorne A, Dawson D. Epidemiology of mass casualty incidents in the United States. *Prehosp Emerg Care*. 2014;18(3):408–416. https://doi.org/10.3109/10903127.2014.882999.
22. Goolsby C, Schuler K, Krohmer J, et al. Mass shootings in America: consensus recommendations for healthcare response. *J Am Coll Surg*. 2023;236(1):168–175. https://doi.org/10.1097/xcs.0000000000000312.
23. Herstein JJ, Schwedhelm MM, Vasa A, Biddinger PD, Hewlett AL. Emergency preparedness: what is the future? *Antimicrob Steward Healthc Epidemiol*. 2021;1(1):e29.

24. Binkley JM, Kemp KM. Mobilization of resources and EMERGENCY RESPONSE ON THE NATIONAL SCALE. *SURG CLIN NORTH AM*. 2022;102(1):169–180. https://doi.org/10.1016/j.suc.2021.09.014.
25. Melmer P, Carlin M, Castater CA, et al. Mass casualty shootings and emergency preparedness: a multidisciplinary approach for an unpredictable event. *J Multidiscip Healthc*. 2019;12:1013–1021. https://doi.org/10.2147/jmdh.S219021.
26. Cleary M, Kornhaber R, Thapa DK, West S, Visentin D. The effectiveness of interventions to improve resilience among health professionals: a systematic review. *Nurse Educ Today*. 2018;71:247–263. https://doi.org/10.1016/j.nedt.2018.10.002.
27. American College of Surgeons, Committee on Trauma. Prehospital trauma care. In: *Resources for Optimal Care of the Injured Patient*. Chicago, IL: American College of Surgeons, Committee on Trauma; 2014.
28. Holcomb JB, Tilley BC, Baraniuk S, et al. Transfusion of plasma, platelets, and red blood cells in a 1:1:1 vs a 1:1:2 ratio and mortality in patients with severe trauma: the PROPPR randomized clinical trial. *JAMA*. 2015;313(5):471–482. https://doi.org/10.1001/jama.2015.12.
29. Brown J, Sajankila N, Claridge JA. Prehospital assessment of trauma. *Surg Clin North Am*. 2017;97(5):961–983. https://doi.org/10.1016/j.suc.2017.06.007.
30. Ramesh GH, Uma JC, Farhath S. Fluid resuscitation in trauma: what are the best strategies and fluids? *Int J Emerg Med*. 2019;12(1):38. https://doi.org/10.1186/s12245-019-0253-8.
31. Guyette FX, Sperry JL, Peitzman AB, et al. Prehospital blood product and crystalloid resuscitation in the severely injured patient: a secondary analysis of the prehospital air medical plasma trial. *Ann Surg*. 2021;273(2):358–364. https://doi.org/10.1097/sla.0000000000003324.
32. Lecky F, Woodford M, Edwards A, Bouamra O, Coats T. Trauma scoring systems and databases. *Br J Anaesth*. 2014;113(2):286–294. https://doi.org/10.1093/bja/aeu242.
33. Harris T, Davenport R, Mak M, Brohi K. The evolving science of trauma resuscitation. *Emerg Med Clin North Am. Feb*. 2018;36(1):85–106. https://doi.org/10.1016/j.emc.2017.08.009.
34. American College of Surgeons. Hemorrhage Control Devices: Tourniquets and Hemostatic Dressings. https://www.stopthebleed.org/media/xt0hjwmw/hartford-consensus-compendium.pdf. Accessed February 19, 2023.
35. Richards JR, McGahan JP. Focused assessment with sonography in trauma (FAST) in 2017: what radiologists can learn. *Radiology*. 2017;283(1):30–48. https://doi.org/10.1148/radiol.2017160107.
36. Matsushima K, Khor D, Berona K, et al. Double jeopardy in penetrating trauma: get FAST, get it right. *World J Surg*. 2018;42(1):99–106. https://doi.org/10.1007/s00268-017-4162-9.
37. Engles S, Saini NS, Rathore S. Emergency focused assessment with sonography in blunt trauma abdomen. *Int J Appl Basic Med Res*. 2019;9(4):193–196. https://doi.org/10.4103/ijabmr.IJABMR_273_19.
38. Tyler JA, Perkins Z, De'Ath HD. Intraosseous access in the resuscitation of trauma patients: a literature review. *Eur J Trauma Emerg Surg*. 2021;47(1):47–55. https://doi.org/10.1007/s00068-020-01327-y.
39. Gonzalez E, Moore EE, Moore HB, et al. Goal-directed hemostatic resuscitation of trauma-induced coagulopathy: a pragmatic randomized clinical trial comparing a viscoelastic assay to conventional coagulation assays. *Ann Surg*. 2016;263(6):1051–1059. https://doi.org/10.1097/sla.0000000000001608.
40. American College of Surgeons, Committee on Trauma. ACS Trauma Quality Improvement Program: Massive Transfusion in Trauma Guidelines. https://www.facs.org/media/zcjdtrd1/transfusion_guildelines.pdf. Accessed February 19, 2023.
41. Crowe E, DeSantis SM, Bonnette A, et al. Whole blood transfusion versus component therapy in trauma resuscitation: a systematic review and meta-analysis. *J Am Coll Emerg Physicians Open*. 2020;1(4):633–641. https://doi.org/10.1002/emp2.12089.
42. Duchesne J, Smith A, Lawicki S, et al. Single institution trial comparing whole blood vs balanced component therapy: 50 years later. *J Am Coll Surg*. 2021;232(4):433–442. https://doi.org/10.1016/j.jamcollsurg.2020.12.006.
43. Meneses E, Bonova D, McKenney M, Elkbuli A. Massive transfusion protocol in adult trauma population. *Am J Emerg Med*. 2020;38(12):2661–2666. https://doi.org/10.1016/j.ajem.2020.07.041.
44. CRASH-2 Collaborators. Effects of tranexamic acid on death, vascular occlusive events, and blood transfusion in trauma patients with significant haemorrhage (CRASH-2): a randomised, placebo-controlled trial. *Lancet*. 2010;376(9734):23–32. https://doi.org/10.1016/s0140-6736(10)60835-5.
45. The CRASH-2 Collaborators. The importance of early treatment with tranexamic acid in bleeding trauma patients: an exploratory analysis of the CRASH -2 randomised controlled trial. *Lancet*. 2011;377(9771):1096–1101. e1-2. https://doi.org/10.1016/s0140-6736(11)60278-x.
46. Hagebusch P, Faul P, Klug A, Gramlich Y, Hoffmann R, Schweigkofler U. Elevated serum lactate levels and age are associated with an increased risk for severe injury in trauma team activation due to trauma mechanism. *Eur J Trauma Emerg Surg*. 2022;48(4):2717–2723.
47. Rösli D, Schnüriger B, Candinas D, Haltmeier T. The impact of accidental hypothermia on mortality in trauma patients overall and patients with traumatic brain injury specifically: a systematic review and meta-analysis. *World J Surg*. 2020;44(12):4106–4117. https://doi.org/10.1007/s00268-020-05750-5.
48. Family presence during resuscitation and invasive procedures. *Crit Care Nurse*. 2016;36(1):e11–e14. https://doi.org/10.4037/ccn2016980.
49. Vanhoy MA, Horigan A, Stapleton SJ, et al. Clinical practice guideline: family presence. *J Emerg Nurs*. 2019;45(1).e1-76.e29. https://doi.org/10.1016/j.jen.2018.11.012. 76.
50. Vardanjani AE, Golitaleb M, Abdi K, et al. The effect of family presence during resuscitation and invasive procedures on patients and families: an umbrella review. *J Emerg Nurs*. 2021;47(5):752–760. https://doi.org/10.1016/j.jen.2021.04.007.
51. Peck KA, Ley EJ, Brown CV, et al. Early anticoagulant reversal after trauma: a Western Trauma Association critical decisions algorithm. *J Trauma Acute Care Surg*. 2021;90(2):331–336. https://doi.org/10.1097/ta.0000000000002979.
52. Emergency Nurses Association. ENA Topic Brief—Avoiding the Log Roll Maneuver: Alternative Methods for Safe Patient Handling. https://enau.ena.org/Users/LearningActivity/LearningActivityDetail.aspx?LearningActivityID=LJMRSp85WwPew%2BHMK6%2B5YQ%3D%3D&tab=4. Accessed October 2, 2022.
53. Benz D, Balogh ZJ. Damage control surgery: current state and future directions. *Curr Opin Crit Care*. 2017;23(6):491–497. https://doi.org/10.1097/mcc.0000000000000465.
54. Gupta A, Kumar S, Sagar S, et al. Damage control surgery: 6 years of experience at a level I trauma center. *Ulus Travma Acil*

Cerrahi Derg. 2017;23(4):322–327. https://doi.org/10.5505/tjtes.2016.03693.

55. Centers for Disease Control and Prevention. Traumatic brain injury and concussion. https://www.cdc.gov/traumaticbraininjury/. Updated December 15, 2022. Accessed February 19, 2023.
56. Geeraerts T, Velly L, Abdennour L, et al. Management of severe traumatic brain injury (first 24 hours). *Anaesth Crit Care Pain Med.* 2018;37(2):171–186. https://doi.org/10.1016/j.accpm.2017.12.001.
57. Tran J, Haussner W, Shah K. Traumatic pneumothorax: a review of current diagnostic practices and evolving management. *J Emerg Med.* 2021;61(5):517–528. https://doi.org/10.1016/j.jemermed.2021.07.006.
58. Schellenberg M, Inaba K. Critical decisions in the management of thoracic trauma. *Emerg Med Clin North Am.* 2018;36(1):135–147. https://doi.org/10.1016/j.emc.2017.08.008.
59. Požgain Z, Kristek D, Lovrić I, et al. Pulmonary contusions after blunt chest trauma: clinical significance and evaluation of patient management. *Eur J Trauma Emerg Surg.* 2018;44(5):773–777. https://doi.org/10.1007/s00068-017-0876-5.
60. Brasel KJ, Moore EE, Albrecht RA, et al. Western Trauma Association critical decisions in trauma: management of rib fractures. *J Trauma Acute Care Surg.* 2017;82(1):200–203. https://doi.org/10.1097/ta.0000000000001301.
61. Brenner M, Bulger EM, Perina DG, et al. Joint statement from the American College of Surgeons Committee on Trauma (ACS COT) and the American College of Emergency Physicians (ACEP) regarding the clinical use of resuscitative endovascular balloon occlusion of the aorta (REBOA). *Trauma Surg & Acute Care Open.* 2018;3(1):e000154.
62. Brenner M, Hicks C. Major abdominal trauma: critical decisions and new frontiers in management. *Emergency Medicine Clinics.* 2018;36(1):149–160.
63. Tignanelli CJ, Joseph B, Jakubus JL, Iskander GA, Napolitano LM, Hemmila MR. Variability in management of blunt liver trauma and contribution of level of American College of Surgeons Committee on Trauma verification status on mortality. *J Trauma Acute Care Surg.* 2018;84(2):273–279. https://doi.org/10.1097/ta.0000000000001743.
64. Coccolini F, Montori G, Catena F, et al. Splenic trauma: WSES classification and guidelines for adult and pediatric patients. *World J Emerg Surg.* 2017;12:40. https://doi.org/10.1186/s13017-017-0151-4.
65. Cone J, Inaba K. Lower extremity compartment syndrome. *Trauma Surg Acute Care Open.* 2017;2(1):e000094. https://doi.org/10.1136/tsaco-2017-000094.
66. Raza H, Mahapatra A. Acute compartment syndrome in orthopedics: causes, diagnosis, and management. *Adv Orthop.* 2015;2015:543412. https://doi.org/10.1155/2015/543412.
67. American College of Surgeons, Committee on Trauma. ACS Trauma Quality Improvement Program: Best Practices in the Management of Orthopedic Trauma. https://www.facs.org/media/mkbnhqtw/ortho_guidelines.pdf. Accessed February 19, 2023.
68. Prevaldi C, Paolillo C, Locatelli C, et al. Management of traumatic wounds in the emergency department: position paper from the academy of emergency medicine and care (AcEMC) and the world society of emergency surgery (WSES). *World J Emerg Surg.* 2016;11:30. https://doi.org/10.1186/s13017-016-0084-3.
69. Long B, Koyfman A, Gottlieb M. An evidence-based narrative review of the emergency department evaluation and management of rhabdomyolysis. *Am J Emerg Med.* 2019;37(3):518–523. https://doi.org/10.1016/j.ajem.2018.12.061.
70. Yorkgitis BK, Berndtson AE, Cross A, et al. American association for the surgery of trauma/American College of surgeons-committee on trauma clinical protocol for inpatient venous thromboembolism prophylaxis after trauma. *J Trauma Acute Care Surg.* 2022;92(3):597–604. https://doi.org/10.1097/ta.0000000000003475.
71. Brill JB, Badiee J, Zander AL, et al. The rate of deep vein thrombosis doubles in trauma patients with hypercoagulable thromboelastography. *J Trauma Acute Care Surg.* 2017;83(3):413–419. https://doi.org/10.1097/ta.0000000000001618.
72. Rothberg DL, Makarewich CA. Fat embolism and fat embolism syndrome. *J Am Acad Orthop Surg.* 2019;27(8):e346–e355. https://doi.org/10.5435/jaaos-d-17-00571.
73. Wheeler DS, Sheets AM, Ryckman FC. Improving transitions of care between the operating room and intensive care unit. *Transl Pediatr.* 2018;7(4):299–307. https://doi.org/10.21037/tp.2018.09.09.
74. Abraham J, Meng A, Tripathy S, Avidan MS, Kannampallil T. Systematic review and meta-analysis of interventions for operating room to intensive care unit handoffs. *BMJ Qual Saf.* 2021;30(6):513–524. https://doi.org/10.1136/bmjqs-2020-012474.
75. American Society of PeriAnesthesia Nurses. *2021-2022 Perianesthesia Nursing Standards, Practice Recommendations and Interpretive Statements.* Cherry Hill, NJ: American Society of PeriAnesthesia Nurses; 2020.
76. American College of Surgeons, Committee on Trauma. ACS Trauma Quality Improvement Program: Geriatric Trauma Management Guidelines. https://www.facs.org/media/314or1oq/geriatric_guidelines.pdf. Accessed February 19, 2023.
77. American Geriatrics Society 2019 Updated AGS Beers Criteria® for potentially inappropriate medication use in older adults. *J Am Geriatr Soc.* 2019;67(4):674–694. https://doi.org/10.1111/jgs.15767.
78. Karam BS, Patnaik R, Murphy P, et al. Improving mortality in older adult trauma patients: are we doing better? *J Trauma Acute Care Surg.* 2022;92(2):413–421. https://doi.org/10.1097/ta.0000000000003406.
79. Clare D, Zink KL. Geriatric trauma. *Emerg Med Clin North Am.* 2021;39(2):257–271. https://doi.org/10.1016/j.emc.2021.01.002.
80. Huls CK, Detlefs C. Trauma in pregnancy. *Semin Perinatol.* 2018;42(1):13–20. https://doi.org/10.1053/j.semperi.2017.11.004.
81. McClave SA, Taylor BE, Martindale RG, et al. Guidelines for the provision and assessment of nutrition support therapy in the adult critically ill patient: Society of Critical Care Medicine (SCCM) and American Society for Parenteral and Enteral Nutrition (A.S.P.E.N.). *JPEN J Parenter Enteral Nutr.* 2016;40(2):159–211. https://doi.org/10.1177/0148607115621863.
82. Singer P, Blaser AR, Berger MM, et al. ESPEN guideline on clinical nutrition in the intensive care unit. *Clin Nutr.* 2019;38(1):48–79. https://doi.org/10.1016/j.clnu.2018.08.037.
83. American College of Surgeons, Committee on Trauma, US Department of Health and Human Services, Department of Transportation. Alcohol Screening and Brief Intervention (SBI) for Trauma Patients. https://www.facs.org/media/bshd3vaq/sbirtguide.pdf. Accessed February 19, 2023.
84. Centers for Medicare and Medicaid Services. SBIRT Services. https://www.cms.gov/Outreach-and-Education/Medicare-Learning-Network-MLN/MLNProducts/downloads/sbirt_factsheet_icn904084.pd. Accessed February 19, 2023. f.

85. Centers for Disease Control and Prevention. Fast Facts: Preventing Intimate Partner Violence. https://www.cdc.gov/violenceprevention/intimatepartnerviolence/fastfact.html. Updated October 11, 2022. Accessed February 19, 2023.
86. Ophuis RH, Olij BF, Polinder S, Haagsma JA. Prevalence of post-traumatic stress disorder, acute stress disorder and depression following violence related injury treated at the emergency department: a systematic review. *BMC Psychiatry*. 2018;18(1):311. https://doi.org/10.1186/s12888-018-1890-9.

21

Burns

Sarah Taylor, MSN, RN, ACNS-BC, CBRN

INTRODUCTION

There is no greater challenge in critical care nursing than caring for a severely burned patient. Approximately once every minute, someone in the United States (U.S.) sustains a burn injury that is serious enough to require treatment.[1] Burn injuries result in an estimated 486,000 hospital emergency department (ED) visits and 45,000 acute hospital admissions each year in the U.S.[2] Although injury prevention efforts have resulted in a reduction of burn injuries, such injuries constitute a major worldwide health problem, with low-socioeconomic populations being disproportionately at highest risk for injury.[2,3] Initial burn care often occurs in EDs outside of burn centers, so a fundamental knowledge of initial assessment and resuscitation is crucial for the multiprofessional team.

Burn injuries lead to significant economic and social consequences, as well as marked morbidity and mortality. Application of research-based advances in fluid resuscitation, early excision and closure of the wound, tissue healing and engineering, metabolic and respiratory support, microbial surveillance, and infection prevention have dramatically improved survival and recovery from burn injury.[4,5] Morbidity and mortality remain significant in patients with inhalation injuries, burns on greater than 50% of total body surface area (TBSA), and advancing age.[2] Knowledge of the physiological changes and the potential complications associated with burn injuries prepares the critical care nurse to care for these complex patients and optimizes outcomes.

REVIEW OF ANATOMY AND PHYSIOLOGY OF THE SKIN

The skin, also called the *integumentary system,* is the largest organ of the body. It is a vital organ because of its many functions, including provision of a protective barrier against infection and injury, regulation of fluid loss, thermoregulatory (or body heat) control, synthesis of vitamin D, sensory contact with the environment, and determination of identity and cosmetic appearance. The skin is composed of two layers, the *epidermis* and the *dermis,* with an underlying *subcutaneous* fat tissue layer that binds the dermis to organs and tissues of the body (Fig. 21.1). The *epidermis* is the outermost and thinnest skin layer. The *dermis* is considerably thicker and contains collagen and elastic fibers, blood and lymph vessels, sweat glands, hair follicles, sebaceous glands, and sensory fibers for the detection of pain, pressure, touch, and temperature. The underlying subcutaneous tissue is a layer of connective tissue and fat deposits. When an extensive amount or depth of skin is damaged from burn injury, alterations of these multiple physiological functions place the patient at risk for complications.

MECHANISMS AND ETIOLOGY OF INJURY

Burn injuries are classified into three types: *thermal, chemical,* and *electrical.* Approximately 90% of burn injuries are thermally induced (e.g., flame, scald, contact). Chemical and electrical burns account for the remaining 10% of the injuries.[1,6] These types of injuries can also occur with *inhalation injury.* Approximately one-third of patients with burn injuries have concomitant inhalation injury, which may also occur without skin injury.[2,6]

There is a bimodal distribution, with most adult burns occurring between 20 and 60 years of age and in pediatric populations from birth to 16 years of age. The majority of burn injuries occur in the home. Children under 5 years of age are at the greatest risk of home fire death and injury.[2]

Thermal Injury: Flame, Scald, and Contact

Thermal injury is caused when the skin comes in contact with a source of sufficient temperature to cause cell injury. This can occur from flame, scalding liquids, steam, or direct contact with a heat source. Children and the elderly are at greatest risk for thermal injury because of their thinner skin and decreased mobility to avoid harm. The most common mechanisms of thermal injury are flame and scald, accounting for 78% of injuries.[2] The severity of injury is related to the heat intensity and the duration of contact.

Chemical Injury

Chemical burns are caused by contact, inhalation of fumes, and ingestion or injection of particles. Although chemical injuries account for only a small percentage of admissions, they can be severe and have both local and systemic effects. The severity of injury is related to the type, volume, duration of contact, and concentration of the chemical agent. Tissue damage continues until the chemical is completely removed or neutralized. Chemical agents are found in every home and workplace, so the potential for injury from exposure is great. The U.S. Occupational Safety and Health Administration requires that

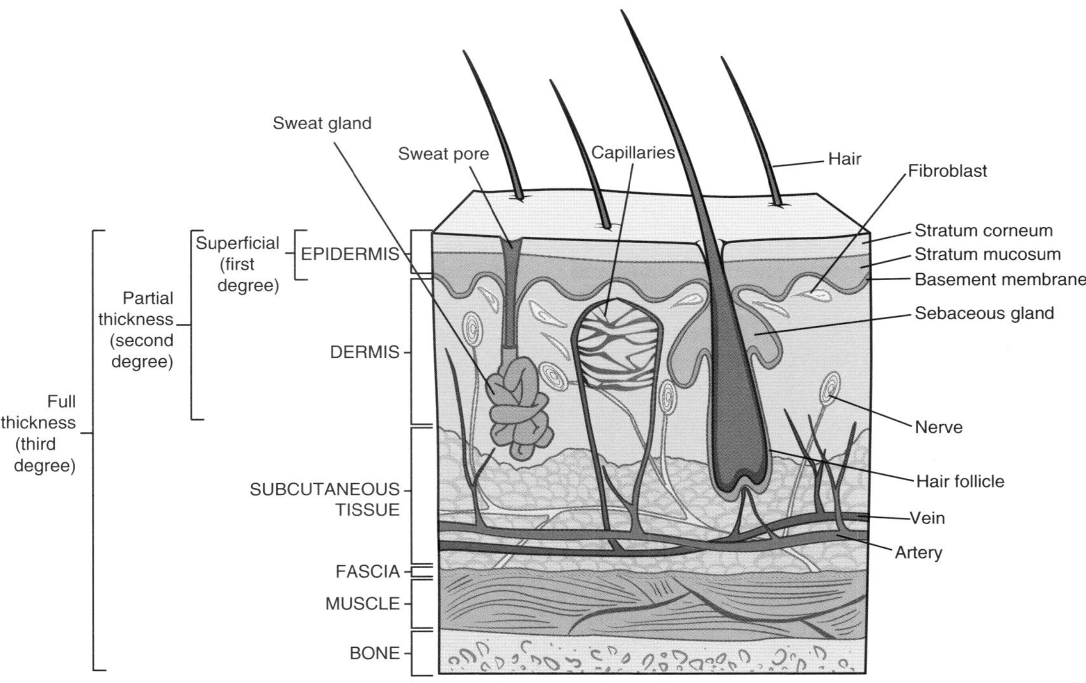

Fig. 21.1 Anatomy of the skin.

employees receive educational training on hazardous materials in the workplace and that Material Safety Data Sheets (MSDSs) be posted in work areas. MSDSs list information on chemicals in the workplace, including composition, side effects, and potential for systemic toxicity.

There are three categories of chemical agents: alkalis, acids, and organic compounds. Alkalis (i.e., bases) commonly encountered in the home and industrial environments include oven cleaners, lye, wet cement, and fertilizers. Burns caused by alkalis are more severe than those caused by acids because alkalis damage tissue through protein denaturation and liquefaction necrosis, allowing the chemical to diffuse deeply into the tissue. Alkalis also bind to tissue proteins and make it more difficult to stop the burning process.

Acids are found in products such as bathroom cleansers, rust removers, and pool chemicals. The depth of burn injury from acids tends to be limited because acids cause tissue coagulation necrosis and protein precipitation. Hydrofluoric acid is especially dangerous because it causes hypocalcemia by rapidly binding to free calcium in the body, increasing the risk of seizures and lethal cardiac arrhythmias.

Organic compounds such as phenols and petroleum hydrocarbon products (e.g., gasoline, kerosene, chemical disinfectants) can produce cutaneous burns and can be absorbed with resulting systemic effects. Chemical pneumonitis and bronchitis may occur from inhalation of toxic fumes. Phenols cause severe coagulation necrosis of dermal proteins and produce a layer of thick, nonviable burn tissue called *eschar*.[6] Petroleum hydrocarbon products such as gasoline promote cell membrane injury and dissolution of lipids with resulting skin necrosis. The systemic effects of petroleum hydrocarbon products can be severe or even fatal and include central nervous system (CNS) depression, hypothermia, hypotension, pulmonary edema, intravascular hemolysis, hepatic and renal failure, and sudden death.[6]

Natural disasters, industrial accidents, warfare, terrorist attacks, mass casualty incidents, and illicit drug manufacturing can produce burn injuries from chemical or thermal exposure.[6] A mass casualty event with significant burn and inhalation injuries can quickly exceed local resources, and critical care nurses must be prepared for such a situation.[6] (See Chapter 20, Trauma and Surgical Management for disaster management.)

Electrical Injury

Electrical injury is caused by contact with varied electrical sources, such as household or industrial current, car batteries, electrosurgical devices, high-tension electrical lines, and lightning. Electrical injuries are frequently work related.[2] Electricity flows by either alternating current (AC), as in most home and commercial applications, or direct current (DC), as in lightning and car batteries. Although AC and DC are both dangerous, AC has a greater probability of producing cardiopulmonary arrest by ventricular fibrillation. The AC causes tetanic muscle contraction that may "lock" the patient to the source of electricity and cause respiratory muscle paralysis. Electrical injuries are classified as high voltage (>1000 V) or low voltage (≤1000 V).[6]

In electrical burns, tissue damage occurs during the process of converting electrical energy to heat. The resulting dissipation of heat energy is often greatest at the points of contact (i.e., entry and exit), which are frequently on the extremities. Several factors affect the extent of injury: type and pathway of the current, duration of contact, environmental conditions, body tissue resistance, and cross-sectional area of the body involved. Electricity follows the path of least resistance; the low resistance of nerve tissue is theorized to pose the highest risk of damage or degeneration. The density and high resistance of bone tissue generate high levels of heat, which directly damages adjacent muscle tissue.[6] The external examination of a patient with electrical conduction injury may underestimate the extent of deep tissue injury related to these processes.

Inhalation Injury

Lung injury caused by inhalation of smoke, chemical toxins, and products of incomplete combustion is associated with increased mortality.[2] Inhalation injury is classified as (1) systemic injury caused by exposure to toxic gases, (2) supraglottic injury, and (3) subglottic injury, or a combination of these.[6,7] Table 21.1 summarizes the pathology of each type of injury. A universally accepted standardized inhalation injury severity scoring system does not currently exist. Diagnosis is based on injury history, clinical signs, and bronchoscopy findings. Inhalation injury stimulates an airway inflammatory response with physiological changes in biochemical mediators and cells, which often results in lung damage.[8]

Carbon Monoxide and Cyanide Poisoning. *Carbon monoxide* and *hydrogen cyanide* are common byproducts of combustion. Carbon monoxide is released when organic compounds, such as wood or coal, are burned. It has an affinity for hemoglobin that is 200 times greater than that of oxygen.[6] When carbon monoxide is inhaled, it binds to hemoglobin to form *carboxyhemoglobin* (COHgb) and prevents red blood cells from transporting oxygen to body tissues, leading to systemic hypoxia. Mild carbon monoxide poisoning is difficult to detect because it may not manifest with significant clinical findings. CNS dysfunction of varying degrees (e.g., restlessness, confusion) manifests at levels of 15% to 40%. Loss of consciousness occurs at COHgb levels of 40% to 60%, and death typically occurs when the COHgb level exceeds 60%. Blood oxygen saturation measured by pulse oximetry and arterial blood gas is usually normal. However, serum laboratory analysis will report an elevated COHgb level as the percentage of hemoglobin molecules that are bound with carbon monoxide.[2] Levels lower than 10% to 15% are found in mild carbon monoxide poisoning and are similar to levels associated with heavy smoking and continual exposure to dense traffic pollution (Table 21.2). The initial management of patients exposed to carbon monoxide includes the following[9]: (1) Remove patient from environment suspected of containing carbon monoxide, and (2) administer high-flow oxygen. The half-life of carbon monoxide is 4 to 5 hours at room air (21% oxygen). Providing high-flow oxygen (100% oxygen) can increase removal and clear carbon monoxide in 30 to 90 minutes. This can be achieved with a non-rebreather oxygen mask in responsive patients but may require bag-valve-mask ventilation or intubation in patients who are unconscious.

Hyperbaric therapy remains controversial for treatment of carbon monoxide poisoning. Recent studies do not demonstrate benefits over standard oxygen therapies, but hyperbaric therapy may be considered when concomitant injuries or burns are not present.[9]

Cyanide poisoning occurs from inhalation of smoke byproducts. Combustion of household synthetics, commonly polyurethane, is the primary source of exposure.[6,10,11] Cyanide impedes cellular respiration and oxygen use by binding with the aa3-type cytochrome *c* oxidase, which is present in high concentrations in the mitochondria. This action inhibits cell metabolism and adenosine triphosphate (ATP) production, resulting in a shift from aerobic to anaerobic metabolism. The state of anaerobic metabolism depletes cellular ATP and leads to lactic acidosis and cell death.[10,11] The clinical symptoms of cyanide poisoning mimic those of carbon monoxide poisoning, and both may be present concomitantly. Patients with suspected cyanide poisoning should be treated presumptively because cyanide levels cannot be obtained in a clinically relevant time frame. The U.S. Food and Drug Administration (FDA) has approved the use of hydroxocobalamin (CyanoKit) for treatment of suspected

TABLE 21.1 Types and Pathology of Inhalation Injury

Type of Injury	Pathology
Systemic: Injury caused by exposure to toxic gas	Carbon monoxide poisoning: Carbon monoxide binds to hemoglobin molecules more rapidly than oxygen molecules do; tissue hypoxia results
	Cyanide poisoning: Cyanide binds to respiratory enzymes in the mitochondria, inhibiting cellular metabolism and use of oxygen
Supraglottic: Inhalation injury above the glottis	Most often a thermal injury; heat absorption and damage occur mostly in the pharynx and larynx; may cause airway obstruction from edema
Subglottic: Inhalation injury below the glottis	Usually a chemical injury that produces impaired ciliary activity, erythema, hypersecretion, edema, ulceration of mucosa, increased blood flow, and spasm of bronchi and/or bronchioles

TABLE 21.2 Carboxyhemoglobin

Carboxyhemoglobin Level[a]	Clinical Presentation
<10%–15%	No symptoms, or minor changes in visual acuity and headache
15%–40%	Central nervous system dysfunction: restlessness, confusion, impaired dexterity, headache, dizziness, nausea and vomiting
40%–60%	Loss of consciousness, tachycardia, tachypnea, seizures, cherry-red or cyanotic skin
>60%	Coma; death generally ensues

[a]Percentage of hemoglobin molecules bound with carbon monoxide.

cyanide exposure. The indications for use include any of the following: hypotension, systolic blood pressure (SBP) < 90 mm Hg, cardiac arrest, Glasgow Coma Scale (GCS) ≤ 9, and profound lactic acidosis > 10 mmol/L.[12] Red discoloration of urine and body fluids is an expected side effect of hydroxocobalamin therapy and may interfere with some clinical laboratory evaluations.

Injury Above the Glottis. Inhalation injury above the glottis, also referred to as *upper airway injury,* is caused by breathing in heat or noxious chemicals that are produced during the burning process. The nose, mouth, and throat dissipate the heat and prevent damage to lower airways, but the patient is still at high risk for airway obstruction due to edema resulting from upper airway thermal injury. Airway obstruction clinically manifests as hoarseness, dry cough, labored or rapid breathing, difficulty swallowing, or stridor.

Injury Below the Glottis. Injury below the glottis may be caused by inhalation of super-heated air, breathing noxious chemical byproducts of combustion, or a combination of both. Extensive damage to alveoli and impaired pulmonary functioning result from the injury (see Table 21.1). Lower airway constriction and spasms characterized by coughing and wheezing occur within minutes to several hours after injury.[6] Acute respiratory failure and acute respiratory distress syndrome (ARDS) are critical complications of this injury. Respiratory tract mucosal sloughing may further complicate ventilation. Chest radiographs may reveal reduced lung expansion, atelectasis, and diffuse lung edema or infiltrates. Fiberoptic bronchoscopy is indicated to provide a definitive diagnosis.[13]

! CLINICAL ALERT

Clinical Indicators of Inhalation Injury

- History of exposure in confined or enclosed space
- Facial burns
- Singed nasal hairs
- Presence of soot around mouth and nose and in sputum (carbonaceous sputum)
- Signs of hypoxemia (e.g., tachycardia, dysrhythmias, agitation, confusion, lethargy, loss of consciousness)
- Abnormal breath sounds
- Signs of respiratory difficulty (e.g., change in respiratory rate, use of accessory muscles, flaring nostrils, intercostal or sternal retractions, stridor, hoarseness, difficulty swallowing)
- Elevated carboxyhemoglobin levels
- Abnormal arterial blood gas values

BURN CLASSIFICATION AND SEVERITY

Burn injury severity is determined by the type of injury, wound characteristics (i.e., depth, extent, body part burned), concomitant injuries, patient age, and preexisting health status. Accurate classification and assessment of injury severity enable appropriate triage and transfer of patients to a burn center.

Depth of Injury

Burn depth predicts wound care treatment requirements and need for skin grafting and affects scarring, cosmetic, and functional outcomes. Burn injuries are often classified as first, second, or third degree. However, the terms *superficial, partial-thickness,* and *full-thickness* burns more closely correlate with the pathophysiology of burn injury and the level of skin layer involvement (see Fig. 21.1). Accurate depth assessment is difficult to determine initially because progressive edema formation and compromised wound blood flow during the first 48 to 72 hours after injury may increase the definitive burn depth.[14]

Superficial burns involve only the first layer of skin or the epidermis, traditionally referred to as *first-degree burns,* and typically heal in 3 to 5 days without treatment. Superficial burn injuries are not included in estimations (i.e., extent of burn injury) or calculations for fluid resuscitation requirements.

Partial-thickness burns involve injury to the second skin layer or dermal layer, traditionally referred to as *second-degree burns,* and are further subdivided into superficial and deep classifications. *Superficial partial-thickness* burn injuries involve the epidermis and a limited portion of the dermis. Injuries typically heal by growth of undamaged basal cells within 7 to 10 days. *Deep partial-thickness* burns involve destruction of the epidermis and most of the dermis. Although such wounds may heal spontaneously within 2 to 4 weeks, they are typically excised and grafted to reduce healing time.

Full-thickness burns, traditionally referred to as *third-degree burns,* involve destruction of all layers of the skin down to or past the subcutaneous fat, fascia, muscles, or bone. When bone or muscle are involved, these wounds may be described as a fourth-degree burn. *Full-thickness burns* create a thick, leathery, nonelastic, coagulated layer of necrotic tissue called *eschar.* The nerves are destroyed, resulting in a painless wound. These injuries always require skin grafting for permanent wound closure. Table 21.3 describes the characteristics of superficial, partial-thickness, and full-thickness burn injuries.

Partial- and full-thickness burns have the potential to progress within the first few days postinjury. The three zones of thermal injury explain this phenomenon (Fig. 21.2) by illustrating the relationship between depth and extent of injury and viability of damaged tissue. The outermost area of minimal cell injury is called the *zone of hyperemia* and has early spontaneous recovery; it is commonly seen in superficial burns. The *zone of coagulation* at the core of the wound contains the greatest area of tissue necrosis and is often irreversible. This is often encountered in full-thickness burns. Surrounding this area is a *zone of stasis,* where vascular damage and reduced blood flow occur. Secondary insults such as inadequate resuscitation, edema, infection, and vasoconstriction caused by hypothermia and vasoactive agents or poor nutrition result in conversion of this potentially salvageable area to full-thickness skin destruction with irreversible tissue *necrosis.*

CHECK YOUR UNDERSTANDING

1. Which would be the priority intervention in the care of a patient with a superficial partial-thickness (second-degree) burn?
   A. Administer 100% oxygen.
   B. Administer prescribed analgesics.
   C. Administer vasoactive agents to support blood pressure.
   D. Encourage nutrition high in protein.

TABLE 21.3 Depth of Burn Injury

Degree of Injury	Morphology	Healing Time	Wound Characteristics
Superficial (first degree)	Destruction of epidermis only	3-5 days	Pink or red, dry, painful
Superficial partial thickness (second degree)	Destruction of epidermis and some dermis	7-10 days	Moist, pink or mottled red; very painful; blisters; blanches briskly with pressure
Deep partial thickness (second degree)	Destruction of epidermis and most of dermis; some skin appendages remain	2-4 weeks	Pale, mottled, pearly red/white; moist or somewhat dry; typically less painful; blanching decreased and prolonged; difficult to distinguish from full-thickness injury
Full thickness (third degree)	Destruction of epidermis, dermis, and underlying subcutaneous tissue	Does not heal; requires skin grafting	Thick, leathery eschar; dry; white, cherry red, or brown-black; painless; does not blanch with pressure; thrombosed blood vessels
Full thickness (fourth degree)	Involves underlying fat, fascia, muscle, tendon, and/or bone	Does not heal; may require amputation or extensive debridement	Black, charred, thick, leathery eschar may be present; bone, tendon, or muscle may be visible

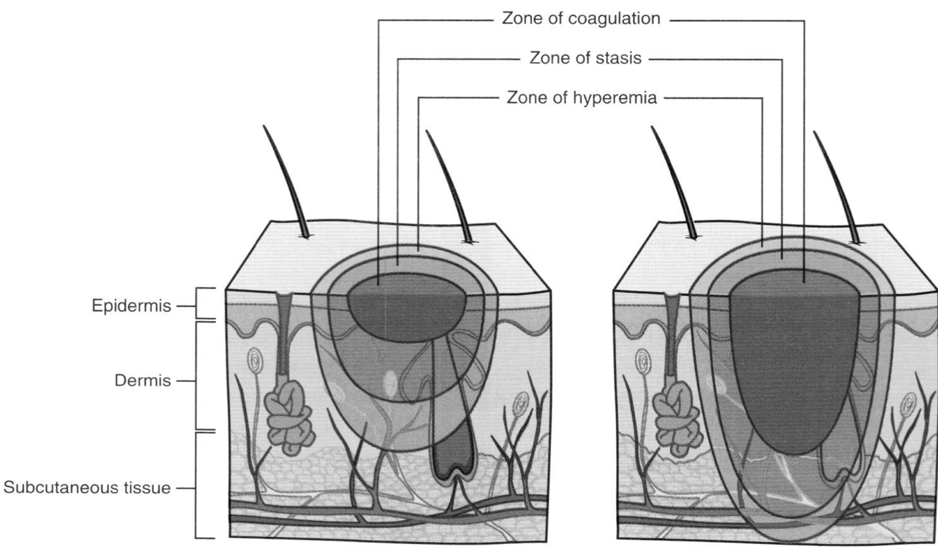

Fig. 21.2 Zones of thermal injury.

Extent of Injury

The extent of injury or size of a burn is expressed as a percentage of *total body surface area* (%TBSA). Accurate calculation of the extent of injury is essential for assessing burn severity and for estimating fluid resuscitation requirements. The %TBSA is calculated by summing all areas of partial- and full-thickness burns (superficial burns are not included because depth of injury involves only the epidermis). The *rule of nines* is the most common method to calculate %TBSA. This technique divides the TBSA into areas representing 9% or multiples of 9% (Fig. 21.3). The rule of nines varies between children and adults because children have a proportionally larger head compared with adults. An alternative method to %TBSA calculation is the palmar method. The nurse can use the size of the patient's palm (including fingers) to calculate injury extent of irregular or scattered small burns; the patient's palm represents 1% of the TBSA.[6]

The *Lund and Browder chart* (Fig. 21.4) provides a more accurate determination of the extent of burn injury by correlating body surface area with age-related proportions. Mobile, three-dimensional computer modeling technology may also facilitate more reliable and accurate %TBSA calculations.[15]

CHECK YOUR UNDERSTANDING

2. The nurse assesses the burn injury to be approximately three palmar surfaces. This would equate to approximately what %TBSA?
   A. 12%
   B. 1%
   C. 3%
   D. 5%

PHYSIOLOGICAL RESPONSES TO MAJOR BURN INJURY

The body responds to major burn injuries (>20% TBSA) with significant hemodynamic, metabolic, and immunological effects that occur locally and systemically because of cellular

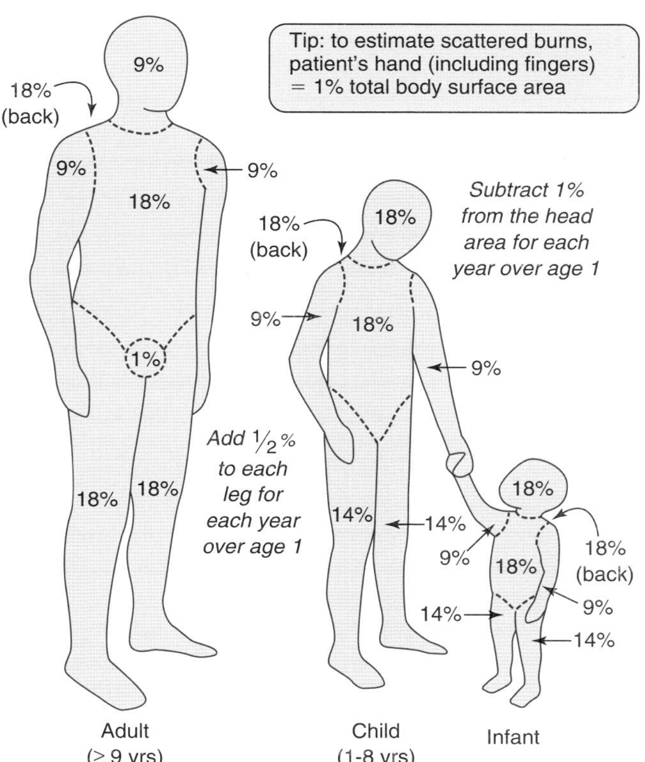

Fig. 21.3 The rule of nines. For example, the calculation for an adult with superficial burns to the face and partial-thickness burns to the lower half of the right arm, entire left arm, and chest is 4.5% (lower right arm) + 9% (entire left arm) + 9% (chest or upper anterior trunk), for a total of 22.5% total body surface area (TBSA). (Superficial burns to the face are not included in the %TBSA calculation.) (Courtesy University of Michigan Trauma Burn Center, Ann Arbor, MI.)

damage (Table 21.4). The magnitude and duration of the systemic response and the degree of physiological changes are proportional to the %TBSA injured. Direct thermal damage to blood vessels causes intravascular coagulation, with arterial and venous blood flow ceasing in the wound injury area. The damaged and ischemic cells release *mediators,* endogenously produced substances that initiate a protective inflammatory response. Mediators such as histamine, prostaglandins, bradykinins, catecholamines, and cytokines are stimulated and released, causing vasoactive, cellular, and cardiovascular effects. Gaps between endothelial cells in vessel wall membranes develop, making vessel walls porous. This *increased capillary membrane permeability* allows a significant shift of protein molecules, fluid, blood components, and electrolytes from the *intravascular space* (inside the blood vessels) into the *interstitium* (the space between cells and the vascular system) in a process also referred to as *third-spacing* (Fig. 21.5). There is rapid and dramatic edema formation. Cellular swelling also occurs as the result of a decrease in cell transmembrane potential and a shift of extracellular sodium and water into the cell.[16] The movement of proteins into the interstitium dramatically lowers the intravascular *oncotic pressure,* which draws additional intravascular fluid into the interstitium. The combination of these processes leads to edema formation and burn shock. Burn shock is a unique combination of distributive and hypovolemic shock, characterized by intravascular volume depletion, increased systemic vascular resistance, and decreased cardiac output. Fluid resuscitation is critical to restore intravascular fluid volume and cardiac output.[6] Edema may be further exacerbated as lymph drainage flow is obstructed due to either direct damage of lymphatic vessels or blockage by serum proteins in the interstitium. Edema is a natural inflammatory response to injury that aids transport of white blood cells to the site of injury for bacterial digestion; however, the extent and rate of edema formation associated with a major burn injury far exceed the intended beneficial inflammatory effect.[17] Following burn injury, edema may occur for up to 24 hours. Reabsorption and resolution begin 1 to 2 days after a burn injury.[17]

In summary, significant burn injuries trigger local and systemic responses involving many complex mechanisms and cascades of physiological events that stress all body systems. The magnitude of the physiological response produces dramatic shifts in intravascular fluid, mediator activation, exaggerated inflammatory cascade reaction, and extensive edema formation. The specific organ system responses are summarized in the following sections and in Table 21.4.

CLINICAL JUDGMENT ACTIVITY

Explain the goals of fluid resuscitation in the patient with a major burn injury.

Cardiovascular Response

Loss of intravascular volume after a major burn injury produces a decrease in cardiac output and oxygen delivery to the body tissues. The sympathetic nervous system activates as a compensatory mechanism, with the release of catecholamines causing tachycardia and vasoconstriction to maintain arterial blood pressure. Alterations in tissue and multiorgan perfusion occur when the blood flow redistributes early in the postburn period to perfuse essential organs such as the heart and brain. Early after a burn injury, cardiac dysfunction may develop, causing a negative inotropic effect on myocardial tissues. The magnitude of myocardial depression exceeds that which would be explained by intravascular fluid volume loss.[18–20] The exact mechanism is unknown; however, secretion of inflammatory cytokine mediators, such as tumor necrosis factor and interleukins, within the myocardium and systemic activation of the complement system with production of anaphylatoxins are implicated as major contributors to contractile dysfunction.[20,21] Cardiac instability in burn patients is further exacerbated by underresuscitation (hypovolemia), overresuscitation (hypervolemia), or increased afterload. Inhalation of cyanide and carbon monoxide may also contribute to cardiac dysfunction. Impaired cardiac function improves approximately 24 to 30 hours after injury.[6,7,9] Initial postburn fluid resuscitation aids in restoring normal cardiac output and perfusion to tissues.

Immune System Response

The loss of skin from a burn injury destroys the body's primary barrier to microorganisms. Tissue damage invokes simultaneous

Burn Estimate and Diagram

Age vs. Area

Area	Birth 1 yr	1–4 yr	5–9 yr	10–14 yr	15 yr	Adult	2°	3°	Total	Donor Areas
Head	19	17	13	11	9	7				
Neck	2	2	2	2	2	2				
Ant. Trunk	13	13	13	13	13	13				
Post. Trunk	13	13	13	13	13	13				
R. Buttock	2 ½	2 ½	2 ½	2 ½	2 ½	2 ½				
L. Buttock	2 ½	2 ½	2 ½	2 ½	2 ½	2 ½				
Genitalia	1	1	1	1	1	1				
R. U. Arm	4	4	4	4	4	4				
L. U. Arm	4	4	4	4	4	4				
R. L. Arm	3	3	3	3	3	3				
L. L. Arm	3	3	3	3	3	3				
R. Hand	2 ½	2 ½	2 ½	2 ½	2 ½	2 ½				
L. Hand	2 ½	2 ½	2 ½	2 ½	2 ½	2 ½				
R. Thigh	5 ½	6 ½	8	8 ½	9	9 ½				
L. Thigh	5 ½	6 ½	8	8 ½	9	9 ½				
R. Leg	5	5	5 ½	6	6 ½	7				
L. Leg	5	5	5 ½	6	6 ½	7				
R. Foot	3 ½	3 ½	3 ½	3 ½	3 ½	3 ½				
L. Foot	3 ½	3 ½	3 ½	3 ½	3 ½	3 ½				
						Total				

Burn Diagram

Age ____________

Sex ____________

Weight __________

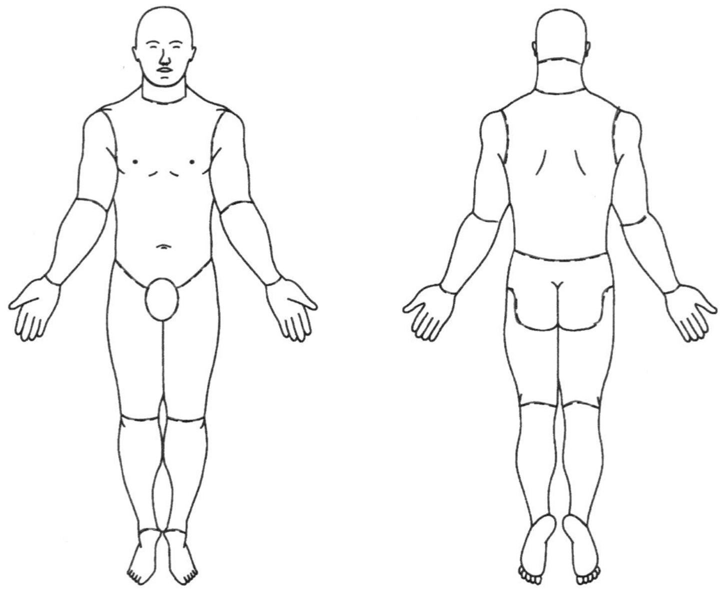

Fig. 21.4 Burn estimate and diagrams. *Ant,* Anterior; *L,* left; *L. L.,* left lower; *L. U.,* left upper; *Post,* posterior; *R,* right; *R. L.,* right lower; *R. U.,* right upper.

TABLE 21.4 Pathophysiology: Local and Systemic Responses to a Major Burn Injury

System	Response
Neurological	↓ LOC from inhalation injury, carbon monoxide or cyanide poisoning, concomitant trauma, polysubstance use, and/or hypoglycemia Massive stress response with activation of sympathetic nervous system ↑ Catecholamine release
Respiratory	↑ O_2 demand from ↑ O_2 consumption Tissue damage from direct heat, edema, or inhaled noxious chemicals Release of vasoconstrictive substances ↓ O_2 tension and lung compliance Transient pulmonary hypertension Hypoxemia If inhalation injury present (see Tables 21.1 and 21.2), ↑ mortality above expected for %TBSA burn Acid-base disturbances
Gastrointestinal	↓ GI blood flow Oral medications and fluids not absorbed Increased risk of ileus Stress or Curling's ulcer (if no prophylaxis)
Integumentary: Skin/tissue/cells	Direct heat-induced tissue damage or ischemia and cell lysis Stimulation of inflammatory response (can be massive) Extensive edema in burned and unburned areas (maximum effect about 18-36 h after burn) ↓ Tissue perfusion and ↑ potential tissue necrosis Cellular dysfunction • ↓ Cell transmembrane potential • Cell edema Loss of skin barrier Loss of thermoregulation (↓ ability to regulate temperature) ↑ Evaporative H_2O loss
Immunological	Release of multiple mediators, cellular enzymes, and vasoactive substances Activation of complement system Overstimulation of suppressor T cells Impaired immune function or response: ↑ risk of opportunistic infections until burn wound closes Leukocyte sequestration
Resuscitation and late effects	With adequate fluid resuscitation, in 24-36 h: • Cell transmembrane potential and capillary wall integrity restored • Cardiac output returns to normal or ↑ • Diuresis • ↓ Edema (cell and tissue) Without adequate resuscitation: • Multiple organ dysfunction due to ↓ perfusion • Reperfusion oxidation injury with returned blood flow Biphasic initial hypofunction, then hyperfunction pattern of all systems Normal cardiac output and organ function returns when burn wounds are closed (healed or are covered) Hypermetabolic state may continue for months to 3 years
Cardiac	↑ Myocardial depressant cytokines (TNF and interleukins) with ↓ cardiac function ↓ Cardiac contractility Tachycardia ↓ Cardiac output (leads to ↑ SVR and resulting ↑ afterload) ↓ Blood pressure ↑ SVR (due to catecholamine-induced peripheral vasoconstriction) leads to redistribution of blood flow to priority organs
Renal	↓ Renal blood flow ↓ Glomerular filtration rate ↓ Urine output or oliguria Hemoglobin or myoglobin in urine (especially with electrical injury from cell lysis or rhabdomyolysis) ↑ Risk of acute kidney injury related to inadequate fluid resuscitation

Continued

TABLE 21.4 Pathophysiology: Local and Systemic Responses to a Major Burn Injury—cont'd

System	Response
Vascular	Heat-induced hemolysis, cell lysis, and endothelial injury ↑ Capillary permeability or "leak" • Shift of protein, fluid, and electrolytes from intravascular to extravascular (interstitial) space • Third-spacing • Oncotic pressure effects • ↑ Edema Serum electrolyte imbalances • Hyperkalemia or hypokalemia • Hyponatremia or hypernatremia ↓ Circulating blood volume (up to 50%) and "burn shock" Hypovolemia ↑ Concentration of red blood cells with ↑ hematocrit and ↑ blood viscosity (hyperviscosity)
Metabolic	Stress response and ↑ catecholamine release triggers adrenal corticoid hormones ↑ Catabolism or hypermetabolism (100%-200% above basal rates) • ↑ Corticosteroid levels, hyperglycemia, and poor wound healing • Protein wasting and weight or muscle mass loss • Bone demineralization • Degree of response depends on %TBSA, age, sex, nutritional status, and preexisting medical conditions Acid-base disturbances

GI, gastrointestinal; *H_2O*, water; *LOC*, level of consciousness; *O_2*, oxygen; *SVR*, systemic vascular resistance; *TBSA*, total body surface area; *TNF*, tumor necrosis factor.

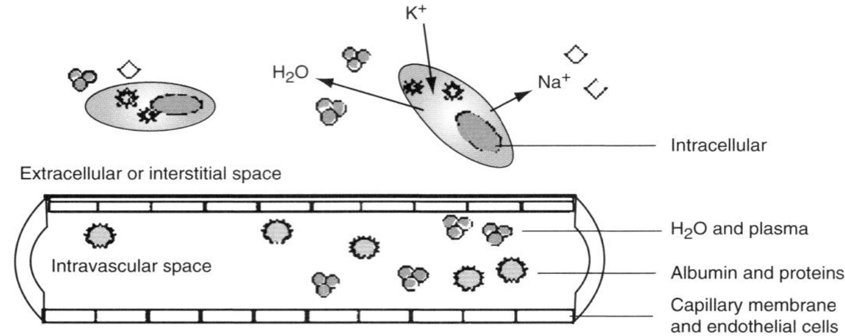

NORMAL PHYSIOLOGY BEFORE BURN INJURY
Intact capillary wall membranes keep large protein molecules within the blood vessels or intravascular space. This maintains normal protein oncotic pressure and retains intravascular fluid volume.

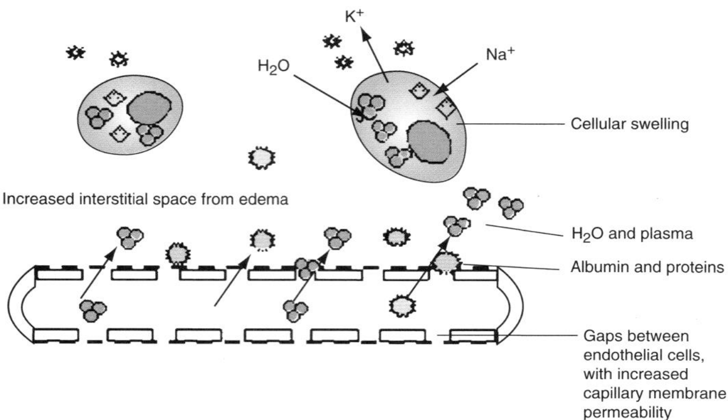

PHYSIOLOGICAL CHANGES FOLLOWING BURN INJURY
Gaps develop between endothelial cells, causing increased capillary membrane permeability. Intravascular proteins and fluids flow into the interstitium in a process called third-spacing and produce tissue edema. Loss of intravascular proteins decreases intravascular oncotic pressure, pulls additional fluid into the interstitium, and reduces intravascular fluid volume. Decreased cell transmembrane potential shifts sodium into the cells, drawing in water and producing cellular swelling and further tissue edema.

Fig. 21.5 Burn edema and shock development. *H_2O*, Water; *K^+*, potassium; *Na^+*, sodium.

activation of all inflammatory response cascades, including the complement, fibrinolytic, clotting, and kinin systems. Immunosuppression interferes with the ability of the patient's host defense mechanisms to fight invading microorganisms, increasing the risk for developing infection and sepsis.

Pulmonary Response

Release of vasoconstrictive mediator substances causes an initial transient pulmonary hypertension associated with decreased oxygen tension and lung compliance. This occurs in the absence of lung injury and edema.[7,22] Inhalation injury complicates the pulmonary response; the pathology of inhalation injury is described in Table 21.1.

Renal Response

The renal circulation is sensitive to decreasing cardiac output and hypovolemia. Hypoperfusion and a decreased glomerular filtration rate signal the nephrons to initiate the renin-angiotensin-aldosterone cascade. Sodium and water are retained to preserve intravascular fluid to increase cardiac preload. Oliguria occurs, and urine becomes more concentrated. If fluid resuscitation is inadequate, acute kidney injury can develop. Fluid resuscitation is aimed at maintaining adequate renal perfusion. Urine output is an easily accessible measurement used to assess the effectiveness of fluid resuscitation interventions.

Gastrointestinal Response

The inflammatory response and hypovolemia after a major burn injury trigger the gastrointestinal (GI) circulation to undergo compensatory vasoconstriction and redistribution of blood flow to preserve perfusion to the brain and heart. Hypoperfusion of the stomach and duodenal mucosa places burn patients at high risk of developing a duodenal ulcer, called a *stress ulcer* or *Curling's ulcer.* Initiation of stress ulcer prophylaxis reduces the risk of gastric bleeding. GI motility is also decreased, which may result in an ileus that clinically manifests as gastric distension, nausea, vomiting, and decreased bowel sounds.

Metabolic Response

Two phases of metabolic dysfunction occur after a major burn injury. First, organ function decreases, followed by a second phase of a hypermetabolic and hyperfunctional response of all systems. Hypermetabolism begins as resuscitation is completed and is one of the most significant and persistent alterations observed after burn injury. The postburn hypermetabolic response is greater than that seen in any other form of trauma.[18] Patients with severe burns have metabolic rates that are 100% to 200% above their basal rates, with some degree of elevation continuing for 1 to 3 years after injury.[18] The rapid metabolic rate is caused by the secretion of inflammatory response mediators or catabolic hormones such as catecholamines, cortisol, and glucagon in an effort to support gluconeogenesis, tissue remodeling, and repair.[10,23] The hypermetabolic state produces a catabolic effect on the body, with skeletal muscle breakdown, decreased protein synthesis, increased glucose use, and rapid depletion of glycogen stores.[10,21,23] The amount of protein wasting and weight loss that occurs is affected by several factors, including %TBSA burned, age, sex, preburn nutritional status, comorbidities, medical conditions, exercise, and nutrient intake.

PHASES OF BURN CARE ASSESSMENT AND COLLABORATIVE INTERVENTIONS

Assessment and management of the burn-injured patient consist of three phases of care: resuscitative, acute, and rehabilitative. The *resuscitative phase* or emergency phase begins at the time of injury and continues until the massive fluid and protein shifts have stabilized. This commonly occurs within 48 hours of burn injury. The primary focus of assessment and intervention is on maintenance of the ABCs (airway, breathing, and circulation) and prevention of burn shock. The resuscitative phase spans care in the prehospital setting, the ED, and the critical care unit, ideally in a burn center.

The *acute phase* begins when resuscitation is complete, which usually occurs between 48 and 72 hours postburn injury. This phase typically lasts for weeks or months. Nursing care focuses on the promotion of wound healing, the prevention of infections and complications, and the provision of psychosocial support. During this phase the multiprofessional team collaborates, addressing nutritional needs, pain management, and physical therapy needs.

Although the critical care nurse is not typically involved in the *rehabilitative phase,* the care given in the first two phases is instrumental in achieving optimal rehabilitative outcomes. The primary goals in the rehabilitative phase are to improve function and range of motion (ROM); minimize scarring and contractures; and restore the patient's ability to return to preburn family, social, and career roles.

In both the resuscitative and acute phases of care, patient assessment and management are prioritized and follow the primary and secondary surveys described in the *Advanced Burn Life Support* course.[6] Pain control, wound management, infection prevention, special considerations for unique burn injuries, and psychosocial concerns are important issues throughout all phases of burn care. See the Plan of Care for Acute Care and Resuscitative Phases of Major Burn Injury for more information. These care plans include only burn-specific interventions not otherwise shown in the Collaborative Plan of Care for the Critically Ill Patient (Chapter 1, Overview of Critical Care Nursing).

Resuscitative Phase: Prehospital

Primary Survey. Prehospital personnel are the first healthcare providers to arrive at the scene of injury. The patient's likelihood of survival is greatly affected by the care rendered during the first few hours after a significant burn injury. The priorities of prehospital care and management are to extricate the patient safely, stop the burning process, identify life-threatening injuries, and minimize time on the scene by rapidly transporting the patient to an appropriate care facility. As with any other type of trauma, the primary survey is used to provide a fast, systematic assessment that prioritizes evaluation of the patient's airway, breathing, and circulatory status (Fig. 21.6).

Stop the burning process. The priority of patient care is to stop the burning process by removing the patient from the source

PLAN OF CARE

Acute Care and Resuscitative Phases of Major Burn Injury

Patient Problem

Potential for Decreased Gas Exchange. Risk factors include tracheal or interstitial edema, inhalation injury, or circumferential torso eschar.

Desired Outcomes

- $PaO_2 > 90$ mm Hg; $PaCO_2 < 45$ mm Hg; $SaO_2 > 95\%$; COHgb < 10%.
- Respiration rate 16 to 20 breaths/min and unlabored; chest wall excursion symmetrical and adequate.
- On teaching, the patient demonstrates an effective cough.
- After interventions, the patient's airway is free of excessive secretions and adventitious breath sounds.

Nursing Assessments/Interventions	Rationales
• Assess respiratory rate, depth, and rhythm every hour; monitor COHgb.	• Assess early warning signs of impending respiratory difficulties.
• Ensure that the patient performs deep-breathing with coughing exercises at least every 2 hours.	• Clear the airway of secretions.
• If patient is not intubated, assess for stridor, hoarseness, use of accessory muscles, and wheezing every hour.	• Identify airway edema and need for immediate intubation or airway control.
• Administer 100% humidified oxygen as ordered.	• Expedite elimination of carbon monoxide to prevent or treat hypoxemia; decrease viscosity of secretions.
• Evaluate need for chest escharotomy during fluid resuscitation.	• Improve ventilation and oxygenation by alleviating constricted chest wall movement.
• Elevate HOB.	• Decrease edema of face, neck, and mouth.
• Alternate periods of increased activity (e.g., wound care, ROM, therapy activities, mobility) with periods of rest to avoid fatigue.	• Prevents atelectasis and promotes oxygenation.

Patient Problem

Potential for Shock, Hypovolemic and Distributive. Risk factors include fluid shifts into the interstitium and evaporative loss of fluids from the injured skin.

Desired Outcomes

- Heart rate 60 to 100 beats/min.
- Blood pressure ≥ 90 mm Hg (adequate in relation to pulse and urine output).
- Pulse pressure variation (PPV) < 12% (if greater than 12%, patient requires fluid resuscitation).
- Hemodynamic parameters at upper ends of normal range.
- Sensorium clear.
- Nonburned skin warm and pink.
- Urine output 0.5 mL/kg/h (1.5 mL/kg/h in electrical injury).
- Serum laboratory values WNL.
- Urine specific gravity normal except during diuresis; urine negative for glucose and ketones.

Nursing Assessments/Interventions	Rationales
• Monitor vital signs and urine output every hour until stable; evaluate mental status every hour for at least 48 hours.	• Assess perfusion and oxygenation status.
• Titrate calculated fluid requirements in first 48 hours to maintain urinary output and hemodynamic stability.	• Restore intravascular volume. • Urine output closely reflects renal perfusion and overall tissue perfusion status.
• Record daily weight and hourly I&O; evaluate trends.	• Evaluate fluid loss and replacement.
• Monitor serum electrolytes, hematocrit, hemoglobin, serum glucose, BUN, and serum creatinine levels at least twice daily for first 48 hours and then as required by patient status.	• Evaluate need for electrolyte and fluid replacement associated with large fluid and protein shifts.

Patient Problem

Hypothermia. Risk factors include loss of skin and/or external cooling.

Desired Outcome

- Rectal or core temperature 37°C to 38°C (98.6°F to 101.3°F).

Nursing Assessments/Interventions	Rationales
• Monitor and document rectal or core temperature every 1 to 2 hours.	• Evaluate body temperature status.
• Assess for shivering.	• After a major thermal injury, routine methods of heat conservation are inadequate.
• Minimize skin exposure; maintain environmental temperatures.	• Prevent evaporative and conductive losses.
• For temperatures <37°C (98.6°F), institute rewarming measures.	• Prevent complications of wound progression related to vasoconstriction.

PLAN OF CARE—cont'd

Acute Care and Resuscitative Phases of Major Burn Injury

Patient Problem

Decreased Peripheral Tissue Perfusion. Risk factors include hypovolemia or impaired vascular circulation in extremities with circumferential deep partial- or full-thickness burns.

Desired Outcomes

- Peripheral pulses present and strong.
- Warm extremities.
- Absence of compartment syndrome.

Nursing Assessments/Interventions	Rationales
• Assess peripheral pulses, color, and temperature every hour for 72 hours; notify provider of changes in pulses, capillary refill, color, temperature, or pain sensation.	• Assess peripheral perfusion and the need for escharotomy.
• Elevate upper extremities with IV poles or on pillows; elevate lower extremities on pillows.	• Decrease edema formation.
• Assist with escharotomy or fasciotomy in circumferential burns to an extremity.	• Escharotomy or fasciotomy allows for edema expansion and permits peripheral perfusion.

Patient Problem

Acute Pain. Risk factors include burn trauma and medical-surgical interventions.

Desired Outcome

- Using the appropriate pain scale, pain is either reduced or at an acceptable level within 1 to 2 hours.
- Patient participates in wound care and ROM and therapy activities.

Nursing Assessments/Interventions	Rationales
• Administer IV analgesic and/or anxiolytic medications during critical care phases.	• Facilitate pain relief and anxiety. • IM and oral medications are not consistently absorbed, especially during early postburn fluid shifts and ileus.
• Medicate patient before wound care, dressing changes, bathing, ROM, therapy, and major procedures as needed.	• Assist patient to perform at higher level of function. • Exposed nerve endings increase pain.
• Explore use of nonpharmacological pain management strategies (e.g., guided imagery, virtual games, music) as adjuncts to pharmacological pain management strategies.	• Provide optimal pain relief and provide the patient with control over pain treatment options.

Patient Problem

Potential for Wound Infection. Risk factors include loss of skin, impaired immune response, and invasive therapies.

Desired Outcomes

- Absence of inflamed burn wound margins.
- No evidence of burn wound, donor site, or invasive catheter site infection.
- Autograft or allograft skin is adherent to healthy tissue.

Nursing Assessments/Interventions	Rationales
• Monitor burn wound healing, including presence of exudate and/or odor.	• Facilitate early detection of developing infection.
• Use appropriate protective isolation; provide meticulous wound care with antimicrobial topical agents as ordered; clip or shave hair (except eyebrows) 1 inch around burn wounds.	• Decrease exposure to pathogens; hair is a medium for microorganism growth; proper hand washing and use of protective barriers decrease contamination. • Reduce scarring.
• Obtain wound cultures as ordered.	• Determine infection source and specific invading microorganism to guide topical or systemic antimicrobial therapy.

Patient Problem

Weight Loss. Risk factors include increased metabolic demands secondary to physiological stress and wound healing.

Desired Outcomes

- Normal intake of food within restrictions, as indicated.
- Evidence of weight maintenance or gain.

Continued

PLAN OF CARE—cont'd

Acute Care and Resuscitative Phases of Major Burn Injury

Nursing Assessments/Interventions	Rationales
• Place nasogastric tube for gastric decompression if burns >20% TBSA.	• Prevent nausea, emesis, and aspiration.
• Administer medications for stress ulcer prophylaxis.	• Prevent stress ulcer development.
• Consult dietitian. Initiate enteral feeding and evaluate tolerance; provide high-calorie or protein supplements; record all oral intake and count calories.	• Caloric or protein intake must be adequate to maintain positive nitrogen balance and promote healing.
• Schedule interventions and activities to avoid interrupting feeding times.	• Pain, fatigue, and sedation interfere with the desire to eat.

Patient Problem

Decreased Mobility. Risk factors include burn injury, therapeutic splinting, immobilization requirements after skin graft, and/or contractures.

Desired Outcomes

- The patient verbalizes understanding of the use of analgesics and adjunctive methods to decrease pain.
- The patient uses mobility aids safely if required.
- Demonstrates ability to care for burn wounds.
- No evidence of permanent decreased joint function.
- Vocation resumed with burn-associated limitation adaptations, or adjustment to new vocation.

Nursing Assessments/Interventions	Rationales
• Perform active and passive ROM of extremities every 2 hours while patient is awake. • Increase activity as tolerated. • Reinforce importance of maintaining proper joint alignment with splints and antideformity positioning.	• Prevent burn wound contractures and loss of joint movement or function.
• Elevate burned extremities.	• Decreases edema and promotes ROM and mobility.
• Provide pain relief measures before self-care activities, ROM therapy, OT/PT therapies.	• Facilitates mobility and assists patient to perform at a higher level of function.

Patient Problem

Decreased Ability to Cope. Risk factors include acute stress of critical burn injury and potential life-threatening crisis.

Desired Outcomes

- Before hospital discharge, the patient verbalizes feelings, identifies strengths and coping behaviors, and does not demonstrate ineffective coping behaviors.
- Patient and family coping is realistic for phase of hospitalization and the family's processes at precrisis level.

Nursing Assessments/Interventions	Rationale
• Consult social worker for assistance in discharge planning and psychosocial assessment issues; consult psychiatric services for inadequate coping skills or substance abuse treatment; promote use of group support sessions.	• Provide expert consultation and intervention; assist patient and family in understanding experiences and reactions after burn injury and methods of dealing with trauma.
• Encourage patient and family to identify previous methods of coping.	• Identify known strategies that promote stress management.

BUN, Blood urea nitrogen; *COHgb,* carboxyhemoglobin; *HOB,* head of bed; *I&O,* intake and output; *IM,* intramuscular; *OT/PT,* occupational therapy/physical therapy; *$PaCO_2$,* partial pressure of carbon dioxide; *PaO_2,* partial pressure of oxygen; *ROM,* range of motion; *SaO_2,* oxygen saturation; *TBSA,* total body surface area; *WNL,* within normal limits.

Adapted from Synder J, Sump C. *Swearingen's All-in-One Nursing Care Planning Resource.* 6th ed. St. Louis, MO: Elsevier; 2024.

while preventing further injury.[6] Extinguish flame burns by rolling the patient on the ground, smothering the flames with a blanket or other cover, or dousing the flames with water. Never apply ice or cold water to the wounds because further tissue damage may occur because of vasoconstriction and hypothermia. Remove jewelry quickly because metal retains heat and can cause continued burning. Treat scald, tar, and asphalt burns by immediately removing saturated clothing, rinsing with cool water if available, or both. Do not attempt to remove adherent tar or clothing (i.e., clothing that is burned into and stuck to the skin) at the scene because this can cause increased tissue damage and bleeding.

Treat electrical injuries with prompt removal of the patient from the electrical source while protecting the rescuer. Ensure that the source of electricity is no longer in contact with the patient or is turned off before attempting rescue.

The burning process of chemical injuries continues for as long as the chemical is in contact with the skin; immediately remove all clothing, brush off any powder chemicals to avoid reaction, and institute water lavage (unless contraindicated) before and during transport. Apply copious amounts of clean water lavage. If the chemical is in or near the eyes, remove contact lenses if present and irrigate the eyes with saline or clean water. Prevent cross-contamination of the opposite eye during

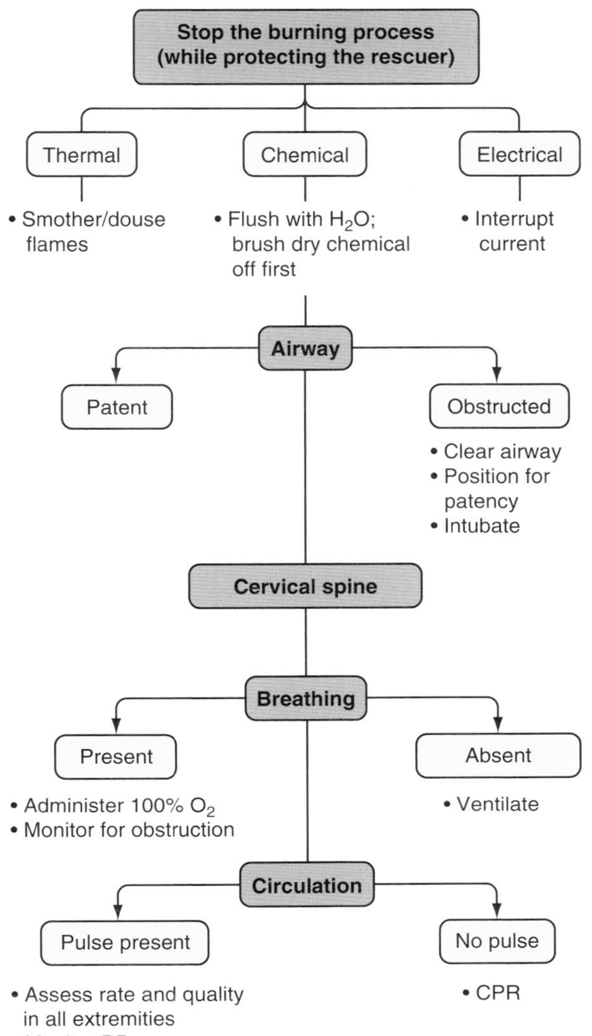

Fig. 21.6 Major burn injury: primary survey. *BP,* Blood pressure; *CPR,* cardiopulmonary resuscitation; *H_2O,* water; *O_2,* oxygen.

lavage by irrigating in the direction from inner to outer canthus. Do not use neutralizing agents, unless indicated, on chemical burns because heat is produced when such agents come into contact with chemicals, further increasing the depth of injury. Chemical decontamination should ideally be performed by providers who are trained in hazardous materials containment. Wear protective barrier garments such as plastic gowns, gloves, goggles, and a face shield to prevent exposure during initial treatment and lavage of chemical injuries.

Airway (with cervical spine precautions). Any suspicion of inhalation injury requires immediate airway assessment. Respiratory stridor, oral swelling, and severe facial burns increase the likelihood that endotracheal intubation is required. Cervical spine immobilization should be maintained if concomitant trauma injury is suspected. Frequent reassessment of the airway during resuscitation is crucial because the development of edema may quickly impair ventilation (Fig. 21.7).

Breathing. All patients with suspected smoke inhalation are treated at the scene with 100% humidified oxygen delivered by nonrebreather mask or endotracheal tube to reduce the half-life of carbon

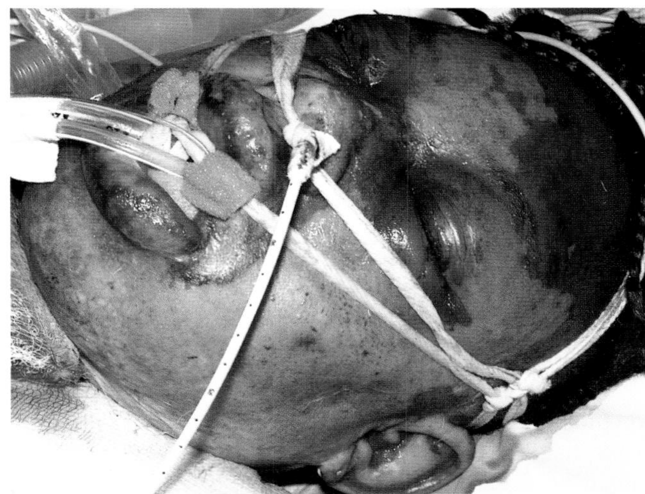

Fig. 21.7 Facial edema. (Courtesy University of Michigan Trauma Burn Center, Ann Arbor, MI.)

monoxide. Monitor for clinical signs of decreasing oxygenation, such as changes in respiratory rate or neurological status. Pulse oximetry may not be accurate in acute inhalation injuries because the pulse oximeter cannot distinguish between carbon monoxide and oxygen attached to the hemoglobin. Consider and treat cyanide poisoning in patients involved in closed-space fires.

! CLINICAL ALERT

Cyanide Toxicity

Clinical indicators of cyanide toxicity:

- Patient involved in a closed-space fire
- Unexplained hypotension
- Unexplained hypoxemia
- Persistent lactic acidosis (>10 mmol/L)
- Cardiac arrest

CHECK YOUR UNDERSTANDING

3. The appropriate priority management of a patient with a documented inhalation injury includes:
   A. Fluid restriction to minimize lung injury
   B. Colloid infusion to decrease extravascular lung water
   C. Prophylactic antibiotics to decrease the incidence of pneumonia
   D. 100% humidified oxygen to decrease carboxyhemoglobin levels

Circulation. Assess central and peripheral pulse quality, particularly in areas with circumferential burn injury. Insert two large-bore (i.e., ≥16-gauge) IV catheters, preferably through nonburned tissue, and initiate volume resuscitation. For burns >20% TBSA, infuse Lactated Ringer's solution (LR) at 500 mL/h for patients 14 years and older, 250 mL/h for children 6 to 13 years old, and 125 mL/h for children 5 years and younger until fluid requirements are met as calculated based on the %TBSA.[6] IV fluids should be administered at a constant rate to maintain perfusion; however, bolus administration of fluids should be avoided to reduce third-spacing. Monitor closely for signs of hypovolemia, such as changes in level of consciousness, rapid or thready pulses, decreased blood pressure, or narrowing pulse pressure. Burn injuries rarely result in hypovolemic shock in the early prehospital phase. Consequently, suspect associated internal or external injuries if evidence of shock is present.

Disability. Assess patient's neurological status. This includes patient's level of consciousness, pupil evaluation, and neurological response.

Exposure and environmental control. Remove contact lenses if present, as well as all nonadherent clothing and jewelry because both may maintain heat. Cover the patient with a clean, dry sheet and blankets to prevent hypothermia because heat loss occurs rapidly and to prevent further wound contamination.

Secondary Survey. Perform a brief secondary survey in the prehospital setting so as not to delay transport to a hospital. A rapid head-to-toe assessment is completed to rule out any additional trauma as part of the secondary survey. In patients with an injury mechanism suggestive of spinal injury, ensure spinal immobilization (e.g., cervical collar, log rolling before transport).

Often the patient is most alert during this initial period. Obtain an accurate history of the events that led to the burn injury, including the time of injury, the source of burns, and events leading to the injury. Also obtain a brief medical history, including allergies; current medical problems; medications taken, to include prescribed, over-the-counter, and herbal agents; past surgical procedures and/or trauma; time of last meal; and history of tetanus immunization.[6]

In preparation for transport, a short-acting IV analgesic, such as morphine sulfate or fentanyl, may be administered for pain relief. Intramuscular medications are not given during the resuscitative phase because perfusion of edematous tissues is poor and produces sporadic absorption and effectiveness. The patient receives nothing by mouth before or during transport to prevent vomiting and aspiration.

Resuscitative Phase: Emergency Department and Critical Care Burn Center

Preferably, the burn patient is transferred from the scene to a burn center, but logistics or patient condition may require initial transport to the closest ED. Patients with a major burn injury require complex care and the expertise of a specially trained multiprofessional team. Burn team members include nurses, providers and surgeons (general, plastic and reconstructive, and critical care), occupational and physical therapists, dietitians, respiratory therapists, infection prevention specialists, pharmacists, social workers, psychiatrists, psychologists, chaplains, injury prevention educators, and provider specialists (rehabilitation, neurosurgeons) as indicated. Burn centers provide a dedicated and trained staff and resources to improve burn patient care and outcome, prehospital and community education, injury prevention, and research. Hospitals without a burn center may not have the personnel or supplies necessary for specialized burn care. The recommendations for referral to a burn center are outlined in the Clinical Alert box.

! CLINICAL ALERT

Guidelines for Burn Center Referral[6]

- Partial-thickness burns 10% of total body surface area (TBSA)
- Full-thickness burns
- Burns involving the face, hands, feet, genitalia, perineum, or major joints
- Chemical injury
- Electrical burns and lightning injury
- Inhalation injury
- Preexisting medical conditions
- Associated trauma
- Hospital without qualified personnel or equipment to care for burn-injured children
- Patients requiring special social, emotional, or rehabilitative intervention

When considering transfer to a burn center, the referring provider directly contacts the burn center provider. The mode of transportation (ground or air) and necessary treatment to stabilize the patient for transport are determined.[6] Transport is optimally completed during the resuscitative phase, based on guidelines provided by the receiving burn center. A standardized transfer form is used to summarize information on a burn patient's status to ensure continuity of care between facilities.[6]

? CLINICAL JUDGMENT

Generate a list of the resources required for management of major burn injuries.

Primary Survey. On arrival at either the ED or the burn center, reassess the patient using a systematic approach such as the ABCDE (airway, breathing, circulation, disability, and exposure) primary survey. Once the patient arrives in the critical care burn unit, perform a thorough primary and secondary assessment.

Airway. Airway management issues related to tracheal edema may occur early or may not be apparent until after fluid resuscitation is initiated. Frequently monitor patients with suspected inhalation injuries for hoarseness, stridor, or wheezing. Massive edema formation is an anticipated response to fluid resuscitation in an extensively burned patient. Anticipate assisting with early intubation of patients with inhalation injuries and/or severe facial burns. A fiberoptic bronchoscopy may be performed to confirm the presence of inhalation injury. If the patient is already intubated, assess for accurate tube position. Securely tie (not tape) the endotracheal tube in place to prevent accidental extubation. Attention should be given to tie placement to prevent pressure injuries to burned ears (see Fig. 21.7). Protecting the artificial airway is critical because it may be difficult to reintubate the patient after massive edema and airway obstruction have developed, necessitating an emergency cricothyroidotomy or tracheostomy. Elevate the head of the patient's bed to reduce facial and airway edema.

Breathing. Assess for impaired gas exchange related to carbon monoxide poisoning, cyanide poisoning, or inhalation injury.

Evaluate breath sounds, characteristics of respirations, work of breathing, sputum color and consistency, and symmetry of chest wall expansion. Measure arterial blood gases and COHgb. Administer humidified 100% oxygen until COHgb levels normalize (<10%), then wean oxygen as tolerated. The goal is a PaO_2 greater than 90 mm Hg and an oxygen saturation (SaO_2) greater than 95%. In suspected cyanide poisoning, continue treatment with 100% oxygen (see Clinical Alert: Cyanide Toxicity).

Patients with circumferential full-thickness burns of the thorax may demonstrate inadequate ventilatory effort due to edema and restrictive eschar inhibiting chest wall expansion. Early signs of inadequate ventilatory effort may include increased peak inspiratory pressure and decreased tidal volumes. Clinically, patients with a pneumothorax, hemothorax, or tension pneumothorax present in similar ways, so these differential diagnoses are ruled out first. In this situation, an immediate chest wall *escharotomy* (Fig. 21.8) may be indicated if the patient continues to show signs of inadequate ventilation from restrictive eschar. An escharotomy is an incision performed at the bedside (or in the operating room) through a full-thickness burn to reduce constriction caused by the tight, nonelastic band of eschar. This relieves pressure, restores ventilation, and improves blood flow.

Perform ongoing assessment of breath sounds, arterial blood gases, and ventilatory status. Provide aggressive pulmonary-focused interventions to patients with inhalation injury. Turn patients at least every 2 hours to promote skin integrity and facilitate secretion movement. In addition, encourage coughing, deep breathing, suctioning as needed, and early mobility to optimize pulmonary function.[8] Continuously monitor pulse oximetry and end-tidal carbon dioxide as appropriate. Lung-protective ventilation strategies are used in intubated patients with inhalation injury, such as lower tidal volumes (6 mL/kg of ideal body weight) and plateau pressures lower than 30 mm Hg.[24,25] Prone positioning may be implemented because this intervention has been shown to increase oxygenation.[24] Research also suggests that administration of nebulization therapy with aerosolized heparin, β_2-adrenergic agonist agents (e.g., albuterol, terbutaline), and *N*-acetylcysteine (Mucomyst) may be beneficial treatment adjuncts to open airways and reduce inflammatory response effects.[8]

Circulation

Fluid resuscitation. Fluid resuscitation is a critical intervention for burn management. To estimate fluid resuscitation requirements, assess the depth and extent of injury. Estimate fluid resuscitation requirements according to body weight in kilograms, the %TBSA burned, time of injury, and the patient's age. IV fluid resuscitation is instituted in patients with burns greater than 20% TBSA. These patients have more diffuse capillary leak and greater intravascular fluid loss. Patients with smaller %TBSA burns may be resuscitated with oral hydration.

Historically, the *Parkland formula* was one of the most widely used burn resuscitation fluid formulas. It approximated fluid replacement requirements by calculating the amount of LR to infuse during the first 24 hours after injury at 4 mL/kg per %TBSA.[7,16] Half of the calculated amount is given over the first 8 hours after injury, and the remaining half is given over the next 16 hours. Based on research, the American Burn Association (ABA) recommends using a modified version of the Parkland formula, called the *Advanced Burn Life Support (ABLS) fluid resuscitation formula*.[6] This formula replaces fluid requirements over the first 24 hours after injury at 2 mL/kg/%TBSA for adult patients and 3 mL/kg/%TBSA for pediatric patients. Half of the calculated amount is given over the first 8 hours after injury, and the remaining half is given over the next 16 hours, as shown in Box 21.1. This calculation is only an estimation of fluid required; titration of fluid should be based on the patient's urine output and blood pressure. Fluid requirements for those with high-voltage electrical injuries are higher during the initial 48 hours after the burn; the ABA recommends resuscitation at 4 mL/kg/%TBSA.

Two large-bore (i.e., ≥ 16-gauge) peripheral IV catheters or intraosseous (IO) devices are inserted. Central venous catheters are commonly inserted in patients with major burns to facilitate large IV fluid infusion requirements and monitor resuscitation

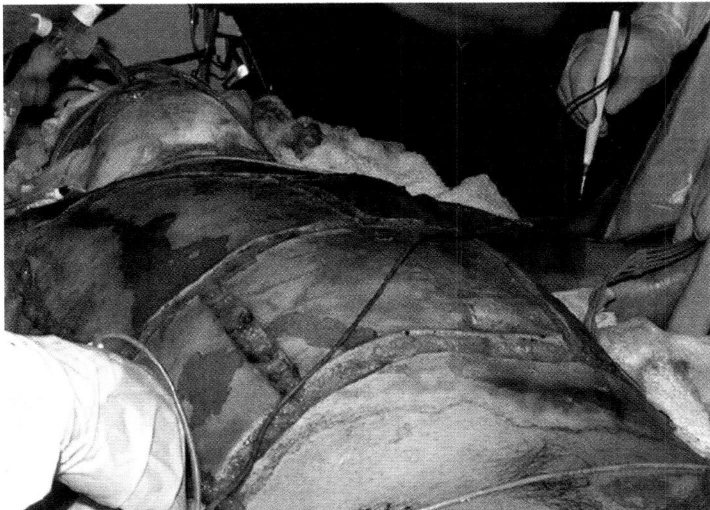

Fig. 21.8 Escharotomy. (Courtesy University of Michigan Trauma Burn Center, Ann Arbor, MI.)

BOX 21.1 Burn Fluid Resuscitation Formulas

During First 24 Hours Administer Fluid According to ABLS Resuscitation Formula[6]

- *Adults:* LR, 2 mL/kg/%TBSA[a]
- *Adults with high-voltage electrical injuries:* LR, 4 mL/kg/%TBSA[a]
- *Children 12 years old and younger and weighing 10 to 30 kg:* LR, 3 mL/kg/%TBSA[a] plus a weight-based maintenance fluid of D5LR.
  - 4 mL/kg/h for the first 10 kg, plus
  - 2 mL/kg for the second 10 kg, plus
  - 1 mL/kg for each remaining kg
- Give half over the first 8 hours after injury and the remaining half over the next 16 hours.
- Titrate fluids to maintain urine output of 0.5 mL/kg/h, or 30 to 50 mL/h in adults, and 1 mL/kg/h in children weighing less than 30 kg.

Example: For an adult weighing 75 kg with a 55% TBSA burn injury:

- 2 mL LR × 75 kg × 55% TBSA = 8250 mL of LR infused over 24 hours
- First 8 hours after burn injury: 4125 mL of LR infused over 8 hours, or 515.6 mL/h
- Next 16 hours after burn injury: 4125 mL of LR infused over 16 hours, or 257.8 mL/h

[a] *%TBSA,* Percentage of TBSA with second- or third-degree burns. *ABLS,* Advanced Burn Life Support; *D5LR,* dextrose in 5% Lactated Ringer's solution; *LR,* Lactated Ringer's solution; *TBSA,* total body surface area.

end points. Lactated Ringer's (LR) solution is the preferred initial IV fluid for burn resuscitation.[6,7] It is a crystalloid solution with an osmolality and electrolyte composition similar to normal body fluids. It does not contain dextrose, which can cause a misleadingly high urine output due to glycosuria and osmotic diuresis. LR does not provide any intravascular protein replacement to increase intravascular oncotic pressure. In the presence of increased capillary membrane permeability, the intravascular retention of LR is only about 25% of the infused volume, necessitating large fluid volume infusions to maintain circulating blood volume.[26] Typically 0.9% normal saline is not used because of its high sodium and chloride concentrations, which can cause hyperchloremic acidosis.

The ABLS fluid resuscitation formula serves as a guide for estimating initial fluid needs. Patients react differently to burn injury and may require varying amounts of IV fluid to support perfusion. Several factors affect fluid requirements: age, depth of burn, concurrent inhalation injury, preexisting disease or comorbidities, delay in treatment of burn injury, use of methamphetamine or other polysubstances, and associated injuries. Patients with inhalation and electrical injuries typically require larger-volume fluid resuscitation. Patients with electrical injuries require larger fluid resuscitation volumes to prevent acute tubular necrosis by clearing the renal tubules from precipitating myoglobin caused by skeletal muscle damage or *rhabdomyolysis* (see Chapter 16, Acute Kidney Injury; Chapter 20, Trauma and Surgical Management).

Increased crystalloid infusion alone is incapable of restoring cardiac preload in burn shock and can cause complications such as compartment syndrome from fluid overload. Colloids, such as albumin, that contain proteins are often used in burn resuscitation to increase intravascular oncotic pressure. The increase in intravascular oncotic pressure pulls fluid from the interstitium into the circulating intravascular volume, reducing edema and ameliorating burn shock. Historically, colloid administration was avoided within the first 12 hours after burn injury, when capillary permeability is at its highest level.[26–28] Current practice supports administering colloids (e.g., albumin or fresh frozen plasma) within the first 12 hours as part of burn shock resuscitation to reduce mortality and compartment syndrome, enhance intravascular volume preservation, decrease overall edema formation, and reduce fluid resuscitation requirements.[7,29,30] Other alternative fluids and augmenting agents, such as high-dose antioxidant vitamin C, are being explored to dampen the inflammatory response, reduce resuscitation fluid requirements, and decrease edema.[30] Additional clinical interventions, including plasma exchange, continuous venovenous hemofiltration, and absorbing membranes, are employed to eliminate proinflammatory cytokines to regulate cytokine homeostasis, modulate inflammatory reactions, and decrease myoglobin during the initial resuscitation.[20] During the second 24 hours after burn injury, as capillary permeability decreases, fluid resuscitation continues incorporating colloids, dextrose, and electrolyte replacement, promoting reabsorption of fluid from the interstitium into the intravascular space supporting the circulatory system.

CHECK YOUR UNDERSTANDING

4. Initial fluid resuscitation requirements are calculated based on which of the following parameters?
   A. Age, total body surface area burned, patient weight, and cause of burn injury
   B. Injury mechanism (flame or nonflame), total body surface area burned, and patient weight
   C. Total body surface area burned, patient weight, and the presence of inhalation injury
   D. Age category (adult or child), patient temperature, and total body surface area burned

End-point monitoring. The goal of burn resuscitation is to maintain tissue perfusion and organ function while preventing the complications of inadequate or excessive fluid therapy.[4,9] Resuscitation fluid infusion rates are titrated to physiological end points, including urine output, blood pressure, and hemodynamic parameters such as cardiac preload, systemic vascular resistance, and stroke volume.[6,29] Insert an indwelling urinary catheter to evaluate resuscitation adequacy. Adjust IV infusion rates to ensure a urinary output of 0.5 mL/kg/h, typically 30 to 50 mL/h in adults.[6] During the resuscitation phase, fluid is administered as a continuous infusion, and adjustments are guided by resuscitation end points. Fluid boluses should be avoided to reduce third-spacing and burn edema.[6]

Peripheral circulation. Special attention is given to full-thickness burns of the extremities that are *circumferential* (completely surrounding a body part). Pressure from areas of eschar or from edema that develops as resuscitation proceeds may impair blood flow to underlying and distal tissue. Elevate extremities to reduce edema. Assess pain, sensation, and peripheral pulses every hour, particularly in circumferential burns of the extremities, to confirm adequate circulation. Use an ultrasonic flowmeter (Doppler) to auscultate radial, palmar, digital, and/or pedal pulses. Closely monitor for signs of developing extremity *compartment syndrome* (see Clinical Alert box). Compartment syndrome occurs when tissue pressure in the extremities increases, compressing and occluding blood vessels and nerves. Absent distal pulses and poor capillary refill are not reliable in diagnosing compartment syndrome because they are often late signs.

If signs and symptoms of extremity compartment syndrome are present, prepare for an escharotomy to relieve pressure and restore circulation. If decreased perfusion is not quickly detected, ischemia and necrosis with loss of the limb may occur. A *fasciotomy* (incision through fascia) may be indicated for deep electrical burns or severe muscle damage to restore blood flow. Escharotomy and fasciotomy sites are treated with a topical antimicrobial agent and closely monitored for bleeding. Cautery, silver nitrate sticks, or sutures may be used to stop continued bleeding.

! CLINICAL ALERT

Clinical Indicators of Extremity Compartment Syndrome

- Presence of circumferential deep partial- or full-thickness extremity burns
- Electrical injury
- Pain: increasing, greater than expected, or out of proportion to the injury
- Increasing edema: muscle compartments tense on palpation or asymmetrical in size
- Altered sensation (e.g., tingling, numbness)
- Late signs (often associated with pending limb necrosis or loss): pallor, poor capillary refill, and absent distal pulses

Secondary Survey. The secondary survey includes a head-to-toe assessment, a complete history and physical examination, reassessment of interventions implemented during the primary survey, and vital signs. If associated trauma is suspected, continue spinal immobilization precautions until spinal injury has been ruled out. Assess indices of essential organ function to evaluate adequacy of burn shock resuscitation and prevent complications. Monitor blood pressure, heart rate, cardiac rhythm, respiration quality and rate, temperature, peripheral pulse presence and quality, and urinary output at least hourly. Weigh the patient on admission and daily thereafter. Closely monitor and manage pain levels. Assessment, early detection, and intervention in the resuscitative phase are essential to prevent complications in the various body systems that are discussed in the following sections.

Cardiovascular system. A mean arterial pressure greater than 70 mm Hg and absence of tachycardia (heart rate < 120 beats/min) have been standard assessments of adequate burn shock resuscitation.[4] However, the cardiovascular response of the patient to burn injury warrants special consideration. Metabolic changes occur hours after burn injury and often cause elevated baseline heart rates of 100 to 120 beats/min. In patients with associated trauma, hemorrhage must be ruled out as a contributor to tachycardia and/or hypotension. Compensatory mechanisms prevent hypotension until significant intravascular volume losses have occurred; therefore decreasing blood pressure is a late sign of inadequate perfusion. Noninvasive cuff pressure readings may be altered by peripheral tissue edema.[6] Arterial line placement may be required for accurate blood pressure assessment. Changes in heart rate and blood pressure may occur secondary to anxiety or fear.

The routine insertion of pulmonary artery catheters is not universally supported; however, patients with significant cardiopulmonary disease, older adults, and those who have unexplained large resuscitation fluid volume requirements may benefit from more intensive monitoring.[6] Hypercoagulability and immobility place the burn patient at risk for developing deep vein thrombosis (DVT) and/or pulmonary embolism (PE), known collectively as *venous thromboembolism* (VTE). Clinical findings of DVT may be obscured by extremity burn wound pain, edema, or erythema. As many as 25% of burn patients develop a VTE, with greater risk in patients with a body mass index (BMI) >30 kg/m^2.[26] Recommendations for VTE prophylaxis vary. Inferior vena cava (IVC) filters are not recommended but may be beneficial in high-risk patient populations.[31] Closely monitor the burn patient for sudden respiratory deterioration, which may indicate PE.

Neurological system. When a burn patient presents with a decreased level of consciousness (LOC), additional injuries or contributing factors must be ruled out. These include head injury, respiratory compromise, metabolic derangement, carbon monoxide or cyanide poisoning, drug overdose, and alcohol intoxication. Perform a neurological examine frequently after admission. Increased agitation, confusion, or a decreased LOC may be an indication of hypovolemia, hypoxemia, or both. Elevate the head of the bed 30 degrees if increased intracranial pressure is suspected or diagnosed from an associated injury.

Renal system. Urine output closely reflects renal perfusion, which is sensitive to decreasing cardiac output and developing shock. Urinary output is the most frequently used indicator of adequate fluid resuscitation. Titrate fluid requirements according to hourly urine output and closely monitor color and concentration because oliguria occurs if fluid resuscitation is inadequate. Polyuria may indicate hyperglycemia and/or overresuscitation and requires clinical intervention.

Gastrointestinal system. The development of ileus and gastric/duodenal ulcers is common following major burn injury. Gastric mucosal atrophy, changes in pH, increased intestinal permeability, and disrupted absorption are all contributing factors to these potential clinical complications.[32] Assess for the presence of abdominal distension, gastric pH, characteristics of gastric secretions, and the presence of GI bleeding. Insert a nasogastric tube and connect it to low suction to prevent vomiting and reduce the risk of aspiration. Most burn patients require nutritional support in the form of nutritional supplements and/or enteral feeding. Provision of stress ulcer prophylaxis is essential.

Intra-abdominal hypertension (IAH) is a serious complication caused by circumferential torso eschar, bowel edema from aggressive fluid resuscitation, and the burn inflammatory response. Overresuscitation during burn care is a major contributor to the development of IAH.[33] IAH is defined as intra-abdominal pressure (IAP) of at least 12 mm Hg; it causes compression of intra-abdominal contents and leads to renal, gut, and hepatic ischemia.[33] If not treated, IAH can progress to abdominal compartment syndrome (ACS). *ACS* is defined as the presence of a sustained IAP greater than 20 mm Hg, with or without abdominal perfusion pressure (APP; APP = mean arterial pressure [MAP] – IAP) less than 60 mm Hg, and associated new organ system dysfunction or failure.[33]

To facilitate early detection of IAH, perform serial IAP measurements using bladder pressure monitoring because physical symptoms are unreliable in diagnosing IAH and ACS. ACS is a life-threatening complication that mandates immediate decompression by laparotomy. Without timely intervention, multiple-organ dysfunction and death may occur.

! CLINICAL ALERT

Clinical Indicators of Abdominal Compartment Syndrome

- Poor abdominal wall compliance (e.g., circumferential full-thickness burns of the torso or trunk, excessive fluid resuscitation)
- Increasing IAH, not resolved by chest or torso escharotomy, repositioning, gastric decompression, sedation, chemical paralysis, or other interventions
- Decreased urine output despite increased fluid administration
- Increasing lactate concentration >2 mmol/L
- Distended abdomen with an IAP greater than 20 mm Hg
- Increased ventilator requirements (e.g., increased FiO_2, increased peak airway pressure, increased PEEP)

FiO_2, Fraction of inspired oxygen; *IAH,* intraabdominal hypertension; *IAP,* intraabdominal pressure; *PEEP,* positive end-expiratory pressure.

Integumentary system. Burn wounds place the patient at risk of tetanus. Administer tetanus toxoid–containing vaccine (e.g., Tdap, Td, or DTaP) if more than 5 years have elapsed since the last dose or if the patient's immunization history is unknown.[6] Monitor the patient's temperature closely to address the hypothermia risk due to loss of the protective skin layer and administration of large amounts of room-temperature fluids. Implement interventions to minimize heat loss, including limiting skin exposure; using fluid or blood warmers for IV fluid infusion; increasing room temperature; closing room doors to prevent air drafts; and using external heat lamps, warming blankets, or radiant heat shields.

Blood and electrolytes. Measure serum electrolyte levels on admission and with changes in the patient's status. Patients receiving large amounts of 0.9% normal saline should be monitored for the development of hyperchloremic acidosis. Monitor serum potassium because values may be elevated from the release of potassium from injured tissue; conversely, values may be low secondary to losses in the urine from fluid resuscitation. Blood urea nitrogen (BUN) levels may increase when excessive protein catabolism occurs. Hyperglycemia develops in response to catecholamine release. Arterial blood gas values and serum lactate levels may be used to diagnose the development of metabolic acidosis resulting from inadequate tissue perfusion (see Laboratory Alert box).

Acute Care Phase: Critical Care Burn Center

With successful resuscitation, burn shock usually stabilizes 48 to 72 hours after injury. At this point, the acute phase of burn care beings. Interventions in this phase focus on promoting wound healing, preventing complications, and improving function of the various body systems.

Respiratory System. Continue assessment for signs of respiratory compromise or the development of pneumonia. Inhalation injury and mechanical ventilation increase the risk for pneumonia.[4,18,34] Tachypnea, abnormal breath sounds, fever, leukocytosis, purulent secretions, and infiltrations on chest radiographs indicate developing pneumonia. Refer to Chapter 10, Ventilatory Assistance and Chapter 15, Acute Respiratory Failure for nursing interventions. Collaborate with respiratory therapy personnel to perform spontaneous awakening and breathing trials to promote early extubation.[35]

CLINICAL EXEMPLAR

Quality and Safety

A nurse in the burn clinic notices that patients returning to the clinic after critical care unit discharge are having a difficult time with activities of daily living. Specifically, the patients cannot tie their shoes or brush their hair if they have sustained hand burns. When exploring the reasons that this may be occurring, the nurse discovers that there is no standard hand range of motion (ROM) exercises for the bedside critical care unit nurse to perform. The clinic nurse collaborates with physical and occupational therapy to understand the role and amount of therapy a patient in the critical care unit requires. The clinic nurse also works with the critical care unit nurses to understand their role in mobility of the burn patient in the critical care unit. With the help of physical and occupational therapy, a list of upper body ROM exercises, including specifics for the hand, is developed for the critical care unit bedside nurses to perform outside of the standard therapy sessions. The clinic nurse agrees to track patients' upper extremity, specifically hand, ROM when they return for clinic visits and share the findings with critical care nurses and the entire burn team at the monthly quality meeting.

! LABORATORY ALERT

Alterations Seen During Acute Care Management of the Adult Burned Patient

Laboratory Test	Normal Range	Critical Value[a]	Significance
Carboxyhemoglobin	Nonsmoker: <3% Smoker: ≤12%	>20%	Present in carbon monoxide poisoning
Hematocrit	Male: 42%-52% Female: 37%-47% Pregnant person: >33%	<15% >60%	↑ In hypovolemia; ↓ as third-spaced fluid reenters the intravascular compartment or with concomitant traumatic injury
Lactic acid (lactate)	Venous blood: 0.6-2.2 mmol/L Arterial blood: 0.3-0.8 mmol/L	>2 mmol/L	↑ In metabolic acidosis; should ↓ if fluid resuscitation is adequate
Potassium	3.5-5.0 mEq/L	<2.5 mEq/L >6.5 mEq/L	↑ Related to tissue damage; assess for cardiac dysrhythmias. Value may ↓ as potassium reenters cells
Sodium	136-145 mEq/L	<120 mEq/L >160 mEq/L	Levels approach the sodium concentration of fluids being administered. May ↑ with inadequate fluid replacement or ↓ with diuresis.
Blood urea nitrogen	10-20 mg/dL	>100 mg/dL	May ↑ from catabolism or hypovolemia; monitor nutrition and volume status. May be higher in older adults.
Platelets	150,000-400,000/mm3	<50,000 or >1 million/mm3	↓ In large %TBSA burns, hypothermia-induced bleeding disorders, or infection
White blood cell count	5000-10,000/mm3	<2,500 or >30,000/mm3	Transient ↓ from use of topical silver sulfadiazine; ↑ with infection

[a]Critical values vary by facility and laboratory.
%TBSA, Percentage of total body surface area.
From Pagana K, Pagana T. *Mosby's Diagnostic and Laboratory Test Reference.* 16th ed. St. Louis, MO: Elsevier; 2023.

Cardiovascular System. As capillary permeability stabilizes, IV fluid requirements decrease. Patients are then transitioned to maintenance IV fluid infusions that match their overall fluid output. Daily weight, intake, and output should continue to be monitored closely. Increased fluid resuscitation requirements after debridement and grafting operations are often required because the inflammatory response is triggered by surgical intervention. Continue frequent monitoring of vital signs to assess ongoing IV replacement needs.

Neurological System. Perform ongoing assessment for changes in neurological status, which may indicate hypoxemia, hypoperfusion, or sepsis.

Renal System. Continue hourly urine output assessment. Postburn diuresis starts approximately 48 to 72 hours after injury. After fluid resuscitation, urinary output should correlate with intake of IV and oral fluids.

Gastrointestinal System. Monitor the patient for the development of a stress ulcer. Assess enteral feeding tolerance. Nutritional considerations are a treatment priority.

Integumentary System. The burn wound becomes the major focus of the acute phase of burn recovery. Continue monitoring for burn wound healing, burn wound depth conversion, and signs of infection. Protective isolation precautions are often implemented as a standard of care (see Evidence-Based Practice box).

Blood and Electrolytes. Although fluid and protein shifts stabilize during the acute care phase, blood and electrolyte abnormalities related to other processes may be observed. Hemodilution with an associated decreased hematocrit may result from reentry of fluid into the intravascular compartment and from loss of red blood cells destroyed at the burn injury site.[16] Hyponatremia from diuresis may occur but commonly resolves within 1 week after onset. Inadequate replacement of evaporative water loss may produce hypernatremia. Electrolyte shifts affect the ability to maintain a proper acid-base balance, and metabolic acidosis may develop. Hypoproteinemia and negative nitrogen balance may occur from an increase in metabolic rate and insufficient nutrition. Leukopenia is a recognized complication from the administration of the topical antimicrobial agent silver sulfadiazine. Hyperglycemia may develop as a result of infection and excessive carbohydrate loading. In addition, infection or sepsis may result in leukocytosis, prolonged coagulation times, and thrombocytopenia.

SPECIAL CONSIDERATIONS AND AREAS OF CONCERN

Burns of the face, ears, eyes, hands, feet, major joints, genitalia, and perineum pose distinct concerns because they contribute to overall burn injury severity and require unique management.

EVIDENCE-BASED PRACTICE

Decreasing the Incidence of Hospital-Acquired Infections in the Burn Unit

Problem

Burn patients are susceptible to various types of infections due to compromised skin integrity. Skin is the body's primary protection against infections. As the size of a wound increases, the immunological function of the patient decreases, which places the patient at a higher risk of infection. Common infections in burn patients include pneumonia, bloodstream infections, urinary tract infections, and wound infections. Many of the infections that develop contain multidrug-resistant organisms due to the patient's long hospital length of stay. Without new antibiotics to treat these infections, patient morbidity and mortality may increase.

Clinical Question

Does the implementation of protective isolation precautions in the burn unit decrease the incidence of hospital-acquired infections?

Evidence

A systematic review and meta-analysis were conducted to understand the relationship between protective isolation precautions and hospital-acquired infections in the burn unit. The literature review focused on articles written in English only, burn patients of all ages, all percentages of total body surface area burn sizes, and only patients in a burn unit. The analysis concluded:

1. Protective isolation includes strict hand hygiene and glove use; the use of masks, gowns, and sterile gloves during wound care; and single-patient isolation rooms.
2. A significant reduction in colonization and infection rates was observed through the implementation of protective precautions.
3. The use of protective isolation precautions for burn patients in daily practice was recommended.

Implications for Nursing

This study remains the most current systematic review and meta-analysis examining the science to guide the use of protective isolation precautions—including strict hand hygiene with glove use; the use of masks, gowns, and sterile gloves during wound care; and the use of single-patient rooms—to decrease the rate of hospital-acquired infections and colonization of bacteria in burn patients. The studies reviewed were lower-quality before/after studies; however, due to the ethical nature of creating a randomized, placebo-controlled, double-blind study for isolation practices in burn patients, higher-level studies for review are not available. Implementation of protective isolation precautions in burn units can reduce the risk of hospital-acquired infections.

Level of Evidence

A—Systematic Review and Meta-analysis

Reference

Raes K, Blot K, Vogelaers D, et al. Protective isolation precautions for the prevention of nosocomial colonization and infection in burn patients: a systematic review and meta-analysis. *Intensive Crit Care Nurs.* 2017;42:22–29.

Burns of the Face

Suspect inhalation injury with any head or neck burns. Associated facial edema may lead to a compromised airway. Closely monitor the patient's respiratory status. Elevate the head of bed to facilitate ventilation and edema reabsorption. Take special care during cleansing of facial burns to prevent excessive bleeding and damage to new tissue growth. The removal of hair may be indicated to decrease bacterial load. Once the wound is cleaned and debrided, apply a topical antimicrobial agent according to unit protocol. Because of the rich blood supply in the face, partial-thickness burns usually heal quickly as long as infection is prevented. Perform regular oral hygiene.

Burns of the Ears

The ears are especially prone to inflammation and infection of the cartilage *(chondritis),* which may lead to complete loss of ear cartilage. Ear burns are treated with a topical antimicrobial agent, mafenide acetate (Sulfamylon), because of its ability to penetrate the cartilage. Prevent mechanical pressure on the ears from dressings or other external sources such as endotracheal tube ties or pillows.

Burns of the Eyes

Immediate examination of the eyes is necessary on arrival to the hospital because eyelid edema forms rapidly. Eyelid edema can cause the cornea to become exposed as the eyelid retracts. Remove contact lenses if present. A thorough examination by an ophthalmologist is mandatory for serious injuries because orbital pressure measurements and potential canthotomy intervention may be warranted. The eyes are stained with fluorescein to rule out corneal injury. Irrigation may be required for chemical exposures. Frequently apply ophthalmic ointment or artificial tears to protect the cornea and conjunctiva from drying. Carefully observe eyelashes because they may invert and cause corneal abrasions.

Burns of the Hands, Feet, or Major Joints

Extensive burns of the hands and feet can cause permanent disability, necessitating a long convalescence. After prioritizing life-sustaining interventions, it is important to preserve limbs and function. Elevate burned hands above the level of the heart on slings or wedges to reduce edema formation. Individually wrap fingers and toes during dressing changes with gauze, bandages, or biological products to keep digits separated to prevent *webbing,* which is the adhesion of skin between burned body parts. Occupational and physical therapists guide the evaluation of function and mobility. Although ROM exercises can be painful or tiring, they should be initiated as soon as possible after injury and frequently performed. Active ROM exercises prevent muscle atrophy, reduce the shortening of ligaments, prevent joint contracture formation, and decrease edema. If patients are unable to move their extremities actively, perform passive ROM exercises.

Burn wounds over joints are prone to scar tissue contractures that limit ROM. The position of comfort often leads to contracture and deformity development. Splinting and positioning are required to maintain function and prevent complications of mobility when healing. When the patient is ambulating or sitting, apply a compression bandage over burn wounds of the lower extremities to prevent venous stasis and pooling of blood. Venous pooling may delay wound healing, contribute to autograft loss, and increase the risk of VTE. Remove the elastic bandage when the feet are elevated. When establishing a plan of care, remember that patients with bilateral burned hands are dependent on others to assist in meeting their physical needs.

 CLINICAL JUDGMENT ACTIVITY

Describe interventions the nurse can implement in the critical care unit to promote early rehabilitation of a patient with a burn injury.

Burns of the Genitalia and Perineum

Patients with perineal burns often require hospitalization for monitoring of urinary tract obstruction. An indwelling urinary catheter is only indicated if strict monitoring of intake and output is required or if there are full-thickness burns of the genitalia. Meticulous wound care is essential because of the high risk of urine or fecal contamination and resulting risk of infection. Clip perineal hair over wound areas. Because scrotal edema is common, elevate the scrotum on towels or foam.

Electrical Injury

Cardiopulmonary arrest is a common complication of high-voltage electrical injury. Other severe complications are summarized in Box 21.2. Hypoxemia may occur secondary to respiratory arrest. Oxygen and endotracheal intubation with mechanical ventilation are implemented as indicated. Evaluate patients for spinal fractures from tetanic contractions or from falls during the injury event. Implement spinal precautions until injury is ruled out. Cardiac monitoring is indicated in all patients with electrical injuries to monitor for cardiac dysrhythmias. When present, cardiac monitoring should continue for 24 hours after injury, and 12-lead electrocardiogram (ECG) and serial serum troponin measurements may be indicated. Rhabdomyolysis commonly occurs because of electrical injury. Clinically, dark or tea-colored urine indicates the presence of myoglobin released as a result of severe deep muscle damage. To prevent kidney injury, large volumes of IV fluid are administered to maintain urine output at 75 to 100 mL/h, and fluid rate is adjusted to patient response until urine pigment clears.[4] Routine alkalization of the urine is not indicated. Closely monitor affected extremities for the development of compartment syndrome. Surgical intervention may be required to manage devitalized tissue from the initial injury.

Chemical Injury

Treatment of chemical injuries focuses on stopping the burning process while maintaining the safety of the burn team. Decontamination is best performed by teams trained in hazardous material management. The burn team must wear protective gear such as plastic gowns, gloves, masks, and goggles during decontamination. Decontamination is also required if the burn injury is suspected to be from illegal drug manufacturing, such as methamphetamine. Illegal production often involves toxic and corrosive chemicals. For all chemical exposures, immediately remove the patient's clothing, brush off dry chemicals, and continuously flush the area with water for at least 30 minutes. Question the patient and significant others to identify the specific chemical agent involved. Some chemicals, such as alkalis, require lengthy lavage, which can be quite uncomfortable for the patient. Control pain and minimize heat loss caused by continual irrigation. Closely monitor the patient for signs of systemic chemical absorption. Consultation of the MSDS and with Poison Control Centers may be instrumental in effective decontamination.

BOX 21.2 Manifestations and Complications of Electrical Injury

- Cardiac dysrhythmias or cardiopulmonary arrest
- Hypoxia secondary to tetanic contractions and paralysis of the respiratory muscles
- Deep tissue necrosis
- Compartment syndrome of extremities
- Long bone or vertebral fractures from tetanic muscle contractions
- Rhabdomyolysis and acute kidney injury
- Acute cataract formation
- Neurological deficits such as spinal cord paralysis, traumatic brain injury, peripheral neuropathy, seizures, deafness, neuropathic pain, and motor and sensory deficits

Current Trends in Burn Injury Epidemiology

Injury resulting from illegal drug manufacturing is a challenging issue in burn care. Examples include methamphetamine (meth) production in clandestine laboratories and extracting butane hash oil to make concentrated marijuana.[6] Legislative changes have been enacted to restrict access to production components. A recent challenge is the use of in-vehicle mobile laboratories to manufacture smaller quantities of methamphetamine while avoiding law enforcement surveillance. When injury occurs, both thermal and chemical burns result. These cases are associated with more extensive %TBSA injury and inhalation injuries, requiring longer mechanical ventilation and longer length of stay.[4] Clinicians caring for these patients are at risk for chemical exposure if patients are not properly decontaminated. In most methamphetamine-related injuries, patients test positive for additional illegal intoxicants, making pain management challenging.[6] Suspect potential drug manufacturing–related injuries when observing burns to the face and hands, signs of agitation and substance withdrawal, lack of social support, and a vague or inconsistent injury history.

A rise in the use of home medical oxygen therapy also poses unique challenges. Despite the high risk, many patients choose to continue smoking while using home oxygen, resulting in flash or flame burns and explosions. The incidence of burns involving home oxygen has quadrupled in the past decade.[36] These patients are three to five times more likely to have respiratory failure requiring mechanical ventilation, leading to increased mortality.[37] To address this challenging issue, multiprofessional team members must collaborate to provide the patient and family safety education as well as smoking cessation treatment for patients on home oxygen therapy. In addition, enhanced equipment safety by medical suppliers, including home safety checks, written safety instructions, and bidirectional thermal fuses in the oxygen tubing, are utilized for injury prevention.

Injuries from electronic cigarettes are also on the rise. Injuries occur from exploding batteries or contact with an overheating device.[34] The burn caused by an electronic cigarette can be particularly concerning because it involves a flame or contact burn from the device exploding as well as a chemical burn from the lithium battery, which produces lithium hydroxide.[34] This is a growing problem, which may necessitate intervention from injury prevention experts.

Abuse and Neglect

Burns are a prevalent form of abuse and can result either from an active intent to injure or from neglect. Vulnerable populations such as children, older adults, disabled persons, persons with cognitive disabilities, and those with substance use disorders are at increased risk of abuse and neglect. Critical care nurses play a key role in recognizing and identifying potential abuse or neglect cases because they spend the most time interfacing with the patient and significant others. Elicit the injury history and circumstances surrounding the event. Accurately document the wound appearance and the pattern of injury, including the use of photographs. Observe and document the interactions between the patient and caregivers or family. When abuse or neglect is suspected, obtain the history from the injured individual separately from the family or caregiver. Discrepancies between reported accounts of the injury event and physical assessment findings indicate a potential abuse or neglect situation. The presence of other injuries, such as associated bruising, fractures, abrasions, or other trauma, and the distribution and characteristics of the burn wound also provide key information on the accurate etiology of the burn injury. For example, a scald burn with clear demarcation or symmetrical wound pattern on the extremities without splash marks raises suspicion for an intentional immersion injury (Fig. 21.9). Lack of witnesses to the injury event, blaming of others, and delay in seeking care are also indicators of potential abuse situations. It is mandatory to report all potential or suspected abuse cases to the appropriate authorities as governed by state laws. The patient may require hospitalization until social workers and protective services have investigated the home environment to determine whether the patient is safe upon discharge.

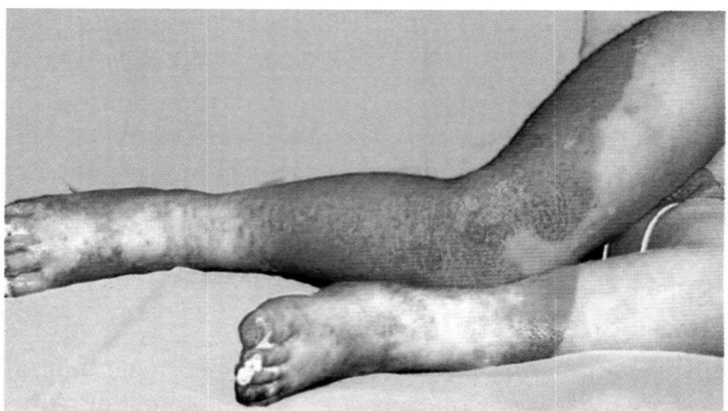

Fig. 21.9 Abuse by hot water immersion. The thigh burn wound edges have a clear demarcation line (are in a straight line), and there are no splash marks. The caregivers delayed seeking medical treatment for the patient's burns until 3 days after injury (notice the dry, crusty appearance of the wounds). The patient also had a forearm fracture and multiple bruises. (Courtesy University of Michigan Trauma Burn Center, Ann Arbor, MI.)

 **CRITICAL JUDGMENT ACTIVITY**

Describe an injury history and physical assessment findings that might lead you to suspect that a burn was caused by abuse.

MANAGEMENT PRIORITIES

Pain Control

Pain is a challenging sequela to burn injury and is present in all phases of burn recovery. Pain is experienced during initial wound care and debridement, dressing changes, following surgical intervention, as a result of splint application, and during both physical and occupational therapies.[24,37,38] Proactive pain management is thus important. Altered pharmacokinetics, frequent dressing changes, positioning, and primary pain from direct thermal injury are all considerations that affect pain control.[38] Burn patients may have histories of mental health and/or substance use disorders that further complicate effective pain management.[39]

The quantities of analgesics required by burn patients often exceed those of standard dosing guidelines.[9,36] Inaccurate assessment of a patient's pain level or concern for addiction may lead to undermedication. Inadequate pain control is associated with long-term negative patient outcomes, such as decreased compliance with care plans and physical and occupational therapies and increased incidence of chronic pain and postinjury stress disorders.[24,37] To successfully manage pain, perform serial pain assessments and involve the patient in creating an individualized treatment plan.[37] Assess pain levels before, during, and after all procedures and treatments. Serve as the patient's advocate by ensuring that the individualized pain management plan is appropriately implemented and updated throughout all phases of burn care.

Opioids are the analgesics most commonly used to treat burn pain. Subcutaneous or intramuscular injections are avoided because absorption is inconsistent, increasing the risk of under- or overmedication. IV medication administration is the route of choice until the patient can be transitioned to oral medications (see Chapter 6, Comfort and Sedation). Itching that occurs during the healing process also contributes to the patient's overall discomfort and may be treated with antihistamine agents.

Burn care and treatment experiences produce anxiety and agitation, which may exacerbate pain.[24,37,38] The ideal pain management regimen incorporates treatment of both pain and anxiety. Fear and a perceived loss of control increase patients' anxiety. Provide frequent and repeated explanations of care plans, interventions, and procedures at a level appropriate for the patient's age and education. Encourage patients to participate as much as possible in their wound care, medication administration, feeding, and exercise therapy. Anxiolytics are commonly administered in the acute care phase as an essential addition to pain management interventions. Virtual reality technology and techniques such as relaxation, music therapy, massage, hypnosis, distraction, and guided imagery also serve as useful adjuncts for reducing anxiety and enhancing pain relief.

Infection Prevention

Prevention of infection is an important nursing intervention in burn patient care. Burn patients have a high risk of infection related to disruption of normal skin integrity and altered immune response. When the skin's natural mechanical barrier protection is lost, susceptibility to infection increases. In addition, other host defense mechanisms are impaired, and immunosuppression develops. Although great strides in management have been made, the incidence of infection is higher in burn patients than in other patient groups and remains a predominant determinant of outcome.[18,29,35] The incidence of infection with multidrug-resistant organisms is an ongoing issue in burn centers worldwide and contributes to an increased risk of sepsis.[7,18] Concomitant inhalation injury places the burn patient at a particularly high risk of developing pneumonia, which further increases the mortality rate.[4] Invasive monitoring and the presence of indwelling urinary catheters, IV catheters, and endotracheal tubes also are potential sources of infection.

Because the inflammatory response is a common mechanism in burns, the ABA consensus panel adapted sepsis definitions that are more applicable to the unique pathophysiological state of patients with burn injury.[18] The hypermetabolic state unique to burn patients can increase baseline temperatures to 38.5°C (101.3°F), thus making the presence of a low-grade fever (without other symptoms) an inaccurate indication of infection.[18]

The goals of infection prevention in burn care include preserving existing immune defenses, preventing transmission of exogenous organisms, and controlling the transfer of endogenous organisms (i.e., normal flora) to sites at increased risk for infection. In addition to Standard Precautions, specific interventions for infection prevention are listed in Box 21.3.

BOX 21.3 Strategies for Infection Prevention for Burn Injuries

- Provide aseptic management of the wound and the environment, including effective decontamination of equipment and hydrotherapy rooms.
- Use topical antibacterial agents.
- Properly care for invasive catheters with special consideration to IV catheters placed through or near burn wounds where occlusive dressings will not adhere.
- Provide aggressive wound management with close monitoring for changes in wound appearance.
- Prevent infection from multidrug-resistant organisms through prudent and microbial-guided use of systemic antibiotics.
- Provide adequate nutrition.
- Closely monitor laboratory values and clinical signs of infection.
- Facilitate early wound closure to restore the protective barrier of skin.
- Prohibit live plants and flowers as they may harbor mold or water-borne organisms.

CRITICAL JUDGMENT ACTIVITY

Specify strategies and interventions the critical care nurse can utilize to reduce the incidence of infection in burn patients.

Wound Management

Although burn wound care protocols and procedures vary among burn centers, the underlying goals of wound care are the same: removal of nonviable tissue to promote epithelialization and prompt coverage via skin grafts or biological dressings when necessary. Perform interventions to attain these goals, such as wound cleansing, debridement, topical antimicrobial and/or biological/biosynthetic dressing therapy, and definitive surgical wound closure.

Wound Care. Meticulous wound care is essential to prevent infection and promote healing of the burn wound. Wound care is typically completed once or twice a day, depending on the healing status of the wound, the dressing or topical agents used, and the number of postoperative days since grafting. Before initiating wound care, explain the procedure and encourage patient participation as appropriate. Administer analgesics (and sedatives or anxiolytic agents if indicated) before starting the procedure. Cleanse all wounds with a mild soap or surgical disinfectant, then rinse with warm tap water. Do not "soak" or tub-bathe the patient in water because immersion creates a significant potential for cross-contamination of wounds, leading to infections. Instead, allow water to flow over the wounds and immediately drain away. This regimen is best accomplished in a shower or hydrotherapy stretcher, but bed baths may be used for hemodynamically unstable patients. Remove all previously applied topical agents, necrotic tissue, exudate, and fibrous debris from the wound to expose healthy tissue, control bacterial proliferation, and promote healing. Debride loose eschar and wound debris with washcloths or gauze sponges, scissors, and forceps. Avoid mechanical trauma and damage from aggressive cleansing of newly formed epithelial skin buds or healing granulation tissue. Facial hair may be clipped in the immediate surroundings associated with the wound bed (except eyebrows) to eliminate a medium for bacterial growth and facilitate wound assessment. Closely inspect all wounds and carefully document wound location, size, color, texture, and drainage. Use standardized language to describe wounds, healing, and signs of infection assessed. During wound care, monitor the patient's temperature and maintain the room temperature at a minimum of 30°C (85°F) to 32°C (90°F) to prevent chilling and excessive body heat loss.

Topical Agents and Dressings. One of the most rapidly changing aspects of burn care is the development of novel tissue engineering techniques for wound treatment. Numerous new topical agents and biosynthetic dressings are available, with many others in development. These new products have broader, longer-lasting antimicrobial actions; interact with wound growth factors and collagen fibers to accelerate healing, stop the zone of stasis from expanding, and help fill in defects; and may reduce scarring. These actions positively affect outcomes by reducing infection, shortening healing time, preventing wound conversion to full-thickness depth, decreasing pain (due to less frequent dressing changes), and improving long-term cosmetic appearance and scarring. After each hydrotherapy session, cover the unhealed or unexcised burn wound with an antimicrobial topical agent, a dressing, or both. Table 21.5 describes various agents that are commonly used in the U.S. and related nursing considerations. The multitude of ever-evolving available agents and dressings precludes a complete listing. Many agents are also used in nonburn, chronic, or surgical wounds. The selection of an agent and dressing is determined by wound depth, anatomical location, frequency of wound visualization desired, and presence and type of microorganisms identified. The ideal antimicrobial agent demonstrates long-lasting, broad-spectrum activity against microorganisms with a low risk of developing resistance, penetrates eschar, and has limited adverse effects. The burn center provider orders the antimicrobial agent, as well as the frequency and method of application.

Advances in wound dressing development and skin substitutes provide many new options in coverage for major burns. Temporary wound coverings or dressings are classified as either *biological* or *biosynthetic* (a combination of biological and synthetic properties). Table 21.6 describes common types and uses for biological and biosynthetic coverings. Biological or biosynthetic wound coverings are used as dressings for partial-thickness burns, meshed autograft skin, or donor sites to promote healing. Temporary wound coverings have the added benefits of controlling heat and fluid loss, decreasing infection risk, stimulating the healing process, and increasing patient comfort.

Enzymatic agents may be used for debridement of smaller necrotic tissue areas on deep partial- and full-thickness burns. Topical enzymatic agents are proteolytic enzyme ointments that act as potent digestants of nonviable protein matter or necrotic tissue. Enzymatic agents do not have antimicrobial properties and do not harm viable tissue.

Burn wounds are treated by either an open or a closed method. The decision of which method to use depends on the location, size, and depth of the burn and on specific burn center protocols. Each method has advantages and disadvantages. With the *open method,* the burn wounds are left open to air after application of the antimicrobial agent. Superficial burns of the face, perineum, and joints are commonly treated with the open method by applying a topical antimicrobial agent. The open method provides increased wound visualization and more opportunities for observation, eliminates dressing supplies, and improves joint mobility that is otherwise limited by the presence of restrictive dressings. The open method has some disadvantages. It allows direct contact between the wound and the environment; the topical antimicrobial agent may rub off on clothing, bedding, or equipment; and wound exposure time and the risk of hypothermia are increased.

With the *closed method,* a gauze dressing is placed over the agent that was applied directly to the wound, or the wound is covered with gauze dressings saturated with a topical antimicrobial agent. The closed method is commonly used on full-thickness and deep partial-thickness burns or newly grafted areas. The closed method reduces heat loss and pain or sensitivity from wound exposure and assists in protecting wounds from external mechanical trauma. The dressings applied may also assist with debridement. The closed method requires a dressing change to assess the wound, and the presence of dressings may impair ROM.

TABLE 21.5 Topical Antimicrobial Agents for Burn Wound Management

Agent	Indications	Nursing Considerations
Clotrimazole cream or nystatin (Mycostatin)	Fungal colonization of wounds	Apply 1-2 times daily. Use with an antibacterial topical agent. May cause skin irritation.
Mafenide acetate (Sulfamylon)	Active against most Gram-positive, Gram-negative, and *Pseudomonas* pathogens; agent of choice for ear burns; penetrates thick eschar and ear cartilage	Apply 1-2 times daily. Strong carbonic anhydrase inhibitor, can cause metabolic acidosis; monitor respiratory rate, electrolyte values, and ABGs. Hydroscopic (draws water out of tissue) and can be painful for 15-60 min after application. Slows eschar separation. Assess for sulfa allergy before use.
Silver-coated dressings	Silver-coated, flexible, nonadhesive wound dressings with or without absorptive layer; as long as dressing is moist, provides continuous release of silver ions for 3-14 days (depending on product); effective broad-spectrum coverage for numerous pathogens (gram-negative/gram-positive bacteria, antibiotic-resistant bacteria, yeast, mold); alternative for patients allergic to sulfa medications	Apply new dressing every 1-7 days to moist open wound with (1) wound exudate maintaining silver activation until drainage stops or wound heals or (2) rewetting with sterile water every 4-6 h to keep dressing moist (not wet). Use sterile water to moisten dressings; saline renders silver ions ineffective. A decrease in number of required dressing changes increases patient comfort and cost-effectiveness. Always reference the dressing instructions as some do not require wetting.
Silver nitrate	Effective against wide spectrum of common wound pathogens; acts on surface microorganisms only; poor eschar penetration; alternative for patients allergic to sulfa medications	Apply 0.5% solution to wet dressing 2-3 times daily; rewet every 2 h to keep moist. Hypotonic solution causes electrolyte leaching; monitor serum electrolyte levels and replace according to protocol. May cause burning sensation and irritation of skin. Assess for methemoglobinemia. Must be kept in light-resistant container. Causes staining; protect equipment and floors with plastic.
Silver sulfadiazine (SSD, Silvadene)	Active against wide spectrum of gram-negative, gram-positive, and *Candida albicans* pathogens; acts only on cell wall and membrane; does not penetrate thick eschar	Apply thin layer, approximately 1/16 inch thick, 1-2 times daily. Wrap wounds or leave as open dressing. Can cause leukopenia; monitor white blood cell count. Assess for sulfa allergy before use.

ABGs, Arterial blood gases.

TABLE 21.6 Biological and Biosynthetic Dressings

Type of Dressing	Definition
Biological Dressings	**Temporary Wound Cover From Human or Animal Tissue**
Allograft (homograft)	Graft of skin transplanted from another human, living or cadaver
Xenograft (heterograft)	Graft of skin (usually pigskin) transplanted between different species
Biological Dressings	**Wound Cover From Biological and Synthetic Materials**
Epidermal Replacements (Epicel, Epidex, MySkin)	Commercially manufactured cultured epidermal autografts (CEAs) from autologous keratinocytes (via skin biopsy) and murine fibroblasts delivered on a silicone or gauze layer.
Dermal Substitutes	
AlloDerm	Transplantable tissue consisting of human cryopreserved allogeneic dermis from which the epidermal cells, fibroblasts, and endothelial cells targeted for immune response have been removed.
Integra	Dressing system composed of two layers: (1) dermal layer of animal collagen and glycosaminoglycan that interfaces with wound and functions as dermal matrix for cellular growth and collagen synthesis; (2) temporary outer synthetic epidermal layer of Silastic that acts as a barrier to water loss and bacteria. Dermal layer biodegrades within months as new wound collagen matrix is synthesized. Silastic layer is removed in 14-21 days and replaced with thin autograft.
TransCyte	Temporary dressing composed of outer polymer membrane and nylon mesh seeded with human neonatal fibroblasts and porcine collagen; matrix contains proteins and growth factors but no viable cells because of cryopreservation.
Bilayer Dermo-Epidermal Substitutes (Apligraf, OrCel)	Consist of an outer epidermal layer of cultured allogeneic (from another human) neonatal keratinocytes and a bottom dermal layer matrix embedded with neonatal fibroblasts and bovine collagen; the matrix's viable or living cells secrete growth factors and cytokines to promote healing.

Negative pressure wound therapy (NPWT) or vacuum-assisted closure (VAC) devices can be used for grafts, partial-thickness burns, and deep surgical wounds. NPWT consists of a sponge and suction tubing placed on the wound bed and covered with an occlusive dressing (Fig. 21.10). The device creates a negative pressure dressing to decompress edematous interstitial spaces and increase local perfusion; helps draw wound edges closed uniformly; removes wound fluid; and provides a closed, moist wound healing environment. NPWT allows the collection and quantification of wound drainage. NPWT has been associated with increased granulation tissue formation, earlier epithelialization, removal of wound exudate, lower wound bacterial counts, a reduction in large wound defects, and a reduction in graft loss due to reduced edema and preservation of blood flow.[39,40]

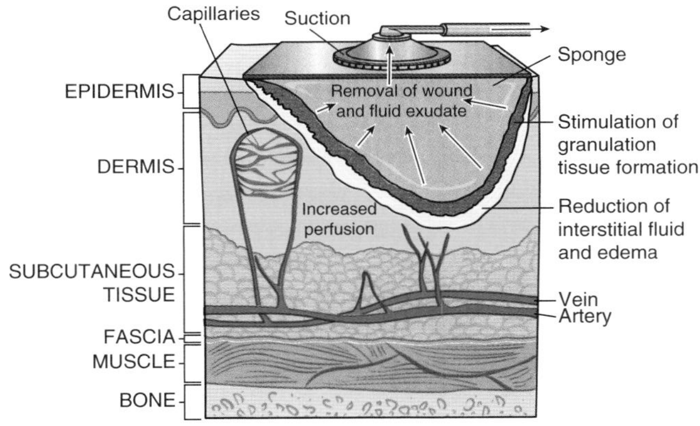

Fig. 21.10 Negative pressure wound therapy (NPWT) consists of a negative pressure dressing to decompress edematous interstitial spaces; increase wound perfusion; remove wound exudate fluid; stimulate granulation tissue growth; and provide a closed, moist wound healing environment.

Surgical Excision and Grafting. The depth of the injury determines whether a burn will require skin grafting. Superficial (first-degree) and partial-thickness (second-degree) burns heal because the necessary elements to generate new skin remain. Full-thickness burns are nonvascular, and all dermal appendages have been destroyed. As a result, full-thickness burns require skin grafting to achieve wound closure. Deep partial-thickness burns are also commonly grafted to decrease the risk of infection by achieving earlier wound closure. This approach may also minimize scarring, promote function, and improve cosmetic appearance. *Excision* is surgical debridement by scalpel or electrocautery to remove necrotic tissue until a layer of healthy, well-vascularized tissue is exposed. *Skin grafting* describes the placement of donor skin on the excised burn wound (Fig. 21.11A). Several types of donor skin can be used for skin grafting. These include *autograft* (the patient's own skin, which is transferred to a new location on the body), *allograft* (skin from another human, such as cadaver skin; also called *homograft*), and *xenograft* (skin from another animal). Autografts are the only permanent type of skin grafting (Table 21.7). Allografts and xenografts are temporary biological dressings (see Table 21.6). With autografts, a partial-thickness wound called a *donor site* is created, where skin is excised (harvested) or removed from the patient with a tool called a *dermatome.* Excision and grafting are performed in the operating room and are typically initiated within the first week after burn injury. Early excision within the first 1 to 3 days has been associated with decreased mortality and morbidity.[7,21] Advantages reported include modulation of the hypermetabolic response, reduced infection and wound colonization rates, increased graft take, and decreased length of hospitalization.[7,21]

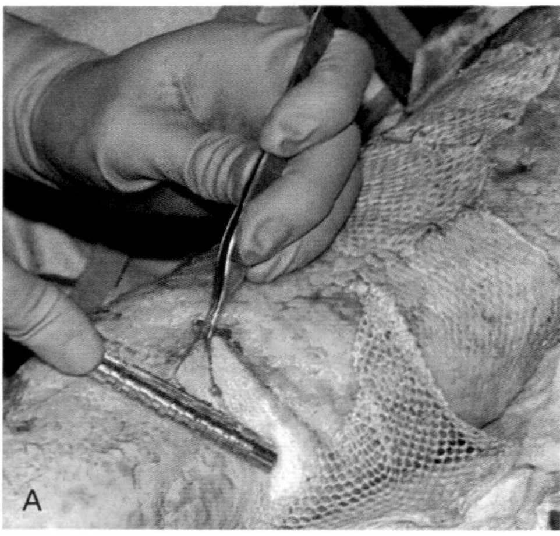

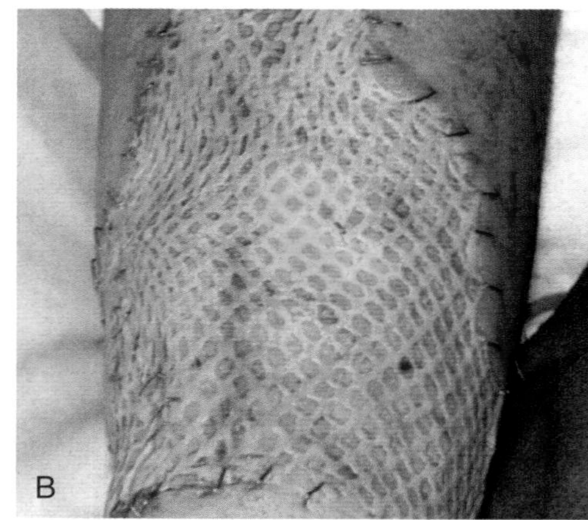

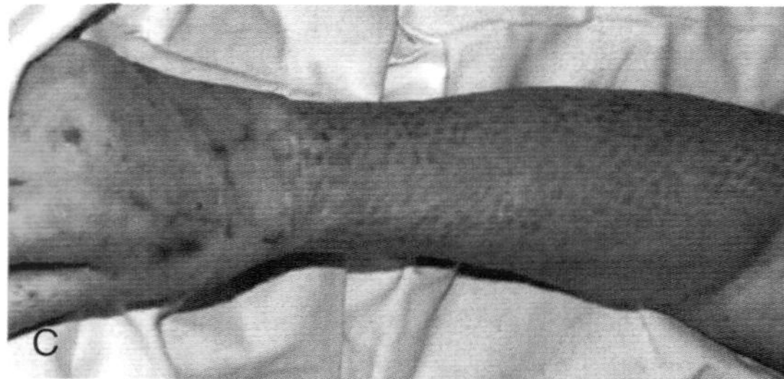

Fig. 21.11 Excision and autografting. **A,** Surgical debridement (excision) with meshed autograft placement in the operating room. **B,** Meshed autograft on postoperative day 2. **C,** Comparison of sheet autograft (on hand) and meshed autograft (on forearm) 3 weeks postoperatively. Use of meshed autograft allows larger body surface area coverage but also typically leads to more scarring and a less cosmetically pleasing appearance. (Courtesy University of Michigan Trauma Burn Center, Ann Arbor, MI.)

Depending on the size of the burn and the presence of infection, sequential or repeated surgical debridement and grafting may be required. In major burns it is often not possible to graft all full-thickness wound areas initially, either because of the patient's hemodynamic instability from the size and severity of burned areas or because of a lack of donor sites to provide adequate coverage. Priority areas for autograft skin application include the face, the hands, the feet, and over joints. In addition, other temporary and permanent biosynthetic products have been developed to substitute for a person's own skin (see Table 21.6). These products allow early burn wound coverage while delaying autografting until previously used donor sites have healed and can be excised again.

Autograft skin is applied as meshed grafts or as sheet grafts. *Sheet* (nonmeshed) grafts are often used on the face and hands for better cosmetic results. Meshed grafts are commonly used elsewhere on the body (see Fig. 21.11B). A meshed graft is created by using a device called a *skin graft mesher,* which places multiple tiny slits or holes in the piece of skin that was harvested from the donor site. The wider the graft's mesh, the larger the area that can be covered with the autograft skin. However, wider-mesh grafts also contribute to more scarring and a less cosmetically pleasing appearance (see Fig. 21.11C). Table 21.7 summarizes the types of skin autografts used, along with nursing care requirements. Graft sites are splinted as indicated to prevent movement and shearing of the grafts until adherence occurs. Elevate extremities to prevent pooling of blood and edema, which can lead to increased pressure and graft loss.

Many types of dressings can be used on donor sites (Table 21.8), but the product chosen must promote healing of the donor site within 7 to 10 days. Donor sites can be reused again once healed. When patient donor sites are limited because of the severity of the burn injury, cultured epidermal autograft (CEA) can be used to provide coverage for a major burn injury. With CEA, a skin biopsy is obtained from the patient and is sent to a laboratory where keratinocytes are cultured and grown. The process takes about 3 weeks and results in small pieces of skin. These fragile pieces of skin are surgically applied to a clean, excised burn wound. The disadvantage of CEA is its extreme fragility, which is partly the result of the lack of a durable dermis. To overcome these shortcomings, researchers are actively investigating novel approaches in tissue engineering, such as developing different types of epidermal substitutes, incorporating CEA with a dermal layer to increase durability, constructing biologically active dermo-epidermal replacements, integrating stem cells, and using topical nanoemulsion technology.[21,41,42]

Burn centers vary in their protocols for treating grafted areas and donor sites. Apply basic wound care principles, with infection prevention always being the primary goal. Although the critical care nurse may not actually develop the wound treatment plan, input from and involvement by all burn team experts are essential for positive patient outcomes. The use of a standard wound treatment documentation method facilitates day-to-day team communication of care requirements.

Inherent in all wound care management is the necessity to improve and maintain function. Consult occupational and physical therapists on the day of admission to develop a treatment plan. Often the position of comfort for the patient is one that leads to dysfunction or deformity. Prevent future complications by using specialized splints, antideformity positioning, and exercises throughout the acute burn care phase. Continually reinforce the need for splinting or positioning and monitor for compliance.

Nutritional Considerations

Adequate nutrition plays an important role in the survival of burned patients. A major burn injury produces a stress-induced hypermetabolic-catabolic response greater than any other disease process or injury. Skeletal muscle is the major protein store in the body. Postburn hypermetabolism is associated with

TABLE 21.7 Autograft Skin: Nursing Implications

Type of Autograft	Definition	Nursing Implications
Split-thickness *sheet* graft	Sheet of skin composed of epidermis and a variable portion of dermis harvested at a predetermined thickness. Sheet is kept intact (not meshed) to improve cosmetic appearance; often used on face and hands.	Immobilize grafted area. Evacuate pockets of serous or serosanguineous fluid by needle aspiration or rolling of the fluid with cotton-tip applicator toward the skin edges; if fluid is not evacuated, graft adherence is compromised.
Split-thickness *meshed* graft	Split-thickness sheet graft that is mesh-cut to expand the graft 1.5 to 9 times its original size before being placed on a recipient bed of granulation tissue; used to cover large surface areas.	Cover graft with layers of fine and coarse mesh gauze to prevent shearing, wrap with absorbent gauze, and splint for immobilization. Keep dressings moist (not saturated) to promote epithelialization of meshed skin interstices. Perform first dressing change within 3-5 days.
Full-thickness graft	Sheet of skin is harvested down to subcutaneous tissue (all layers of skin); typically used for eyelids or later reconstructive procedures.	Requires same care as a split thickness sheet skin graft.
RECELL Autologous Cell Harvesting Device (RECELL System, or RECELL)	Suspension of noncultured, disaggregated, autologous skin cells that uses 1 cm^2 of the patient's skin to treat up to 80 cm^2 of excised burn.	Initial dressing change occurs at 48 hours. Remove all outer and secondary dressings, leave primary dressing in place to not disrupt newly forming skin. Primary dressing stays in place 6-8 days for re-epithelialization. Reapply secondary and outer dressings. Subsequent dressing changes occur every 48 hours.
Cultured epidermal autograft (CEA)	Autologous epidermal keratinocytes derived from skin biopsy of patient are grown in a laboratory using tissue culture techniques (takes <3 weeks). Epidermal layer replacement only. Typically used with extensive percent total body surface area burns when limited donor sites are available.	Perform daily dressing changes of outer gauze for 7-10 days (underlying coarse mesh and petroleum jelly gauze layers are not disturbed); outer dressing must remain dry. Many topical antimicrobial agents are toxic to CEA skin and should not come into contact with graft dressings. Remove petroleum jelly gauze when it becomes loose (7-10 days), and begin gentle range-of-motion exercises. Use moist saline dressings until graft is well adherent (typically 21 days).

TABLE 21.8 Donor Site Dressings

Dressing	Description
BioBrane	Bilaminate dressing composed of nylon mesh embedded with a collagen derivative and an outer silicone membrane; permeable to wound drainage and topical antimicrobial agents; peels away as wound heals
Calcium alginate dressings	Hydrophilic, flexible dressings in which alginate fibers convert to a gel when activated by wound exudates; change dressing within 7 days or more frequently if there is a large amount of drainage.
Hydrocolloid dressing	Hydrocolloid dressing that adheres by interacting and bonding with skin moisture. Creates a moist wound environment facilitating healing.
Fine mesh gauze	Cotton gauze placed directly on wound; a crust or "scab" is formed as gauze dries and wound epithelialization occurs under the dressing; gauze peels away as wound heals.
N-Terface	Translucent, nonabsorbent, and nonreactive surface material used between the burn wound and outer dressing.
Transparent film dressing	Thin, elastic film that is occlusive, waterproof, and permeable to air and moisture vapor; fluid under dressing may need to be evacuated.
Hydrogel dressing	Colloidal suspension on a polyethylene mesh that provides a moist environment; permeable to air and water vapor.
Silver-coated dressings	Silver-coated, flexible dressings (with or without absorptive layer) that provide continuous release of silver ions for 3-14 days while dressing is moist.
Xeroform	Fine mesh gauze containing 3% bismuth tribromophenate in a petrolatum blend; promotes healing as with other mesh gauze dressings.

significant skeletal muscle breakdown and protein degradation, causing deleterious complications such as weight loss, delays in wound healing, skin graft loss, impaired immunological responsiveness, sepsis, and physiological exhaustion or even death.[18,21] Muscle weakness and atrophy also contribute to prolonged mechanical ventilation, delayed ambulation, impaired activities of daily living, and extended acute rehabilitation.

Nutritional therapy should be started immediately after the burn injury, ideally within 4 hours, to meet energy demands, maintain host defense mechanisms, replenish body protein stores, and curtail progressive loss of lean body mass. Collaborate with the patient, the registered dietitian, and the provider to coordinate a nutritional plan. If the patient can tolerate an oral diet, provide a high-calorie, high-protein diet with supplements and perform daily calorie counts to monitor dietary intake. If oral intake is not tolerated or caloric intake is insufficient, enteral nutrition (EN) may be required. Early EN, within the first 24 hours after burn injury, decreases the production of catabolic hormones, improves nitrogen balance, reduces the wound infection rate, maintains gut integrity, lowers the incidence of diarrhea, and decreases hospital stay.[10,21] The small bowel (rather than the stomach) is the preferred location for tube placement so that enteral feedings can be continued during wound care requiring conscious sedation and/or surgical operative procedures.

Ongoing research efforts target the use of anabolic and anticatabolic agents to ameliorate the hypermetabolic-catabolic response to burn injury.[10,21] Most studies have focused on the administration of beta-blockers in the pediatric population, which has been found to reduce the hypermetabolic response and comorbidities from burn injuries; however, there is insufficient evidence to show effects on mortality and length of hospital stay.[43] Further research is needed to show benefit of the use of beta-blockers and impact on metabolism in adults and older adults.[10] Refer to Chapter 7, Nutritional Therapy for additional nutrition information.

CRITICAL JUDGMENT ACTIVITY

Determine nutritional strategies the critical care nurse can employ to meet the high caloric needs of burn patients.

Psychosocial Considerations

As improvements in critical care protocols and technologies have increased survival from burn injury, quality of life and psychosocial considerations become priorities in treatment plans. Burns are one of the most complex and psychologically devastating injuries to patients and their families. There is a threat to survival, psychological and physical pain, fear of disfigurement, and uncertainty of long-term effects of the injury. These factors can precipitate psychosocial stress on both the patient and family. During the acute and rehabilitative phases, the patient may exhibit behaviors described in the stages of psychological adaptation (Box 21.4). A patient may not manifest the behaviors of every stage, but support and therapy should be provided for any patient and family experiencing major burn injury.

To facilitate a person's emotional adjustment to burn injury, consider the complex interaction of preinjury personality, extent of injury, social support systems, cultural factors, and home environment.[6] Burn injuries can result from a variety of etiologies, including poor supervision, abuse, suicide attempts, assaults, illegal activities, safety code violations, arson, or military involvement. Common psychological stressors include the loss of loved ones, injury event flashbacks, loss of home and belongings, job or financial concerns, societal repercussions, or fear of assailants. There may also be potential legal consequences associated with the injury event. Preinjury psychiatric disorders and alcohol and substance use frequently exist in the burn patient population.[37,38] Assess the patient's and family's support systems, coping mechanisms, and potential for developing acute stress disorder (ASD) and posttraumatic stress disorder (PTSD). Inadequate coping may be demonstrated by changes in behavior, anxiety, agitation, manipulation, regression, acting out, psychosis, hallucinations, apathy, sleep disturbances, or depression. The most effective interventions are based on individual assessments and incorporate cultural considerations. Assistance will likely be required from hospital support personnel such as chaplains, clinical nurse specialists, child life specialists, psychiatrists, psychologists, and social workers. As the patient is transferred from the critical care unit, it is important to maintain support mechanisms and continuity of care. The psychosocial recovery after burn injury is lengthy and often requires outpatient support. Several integrative support programs are available to positively facilitate a burn survivor's return to society, family, work, and school (Box 21.5).

If a burn injury is not survivable, support the patient and family members, participate in withdrawal of therapy discussions, and provide compassionate palliative and end-of-life care.

BOX 21.4 Stages of Postburn Psychological Adaptation

Survival Anxiety

Often manifested by anxiety, shock, fear, grieving, anger, mood swings, feelings of helplessness, lack of concentration, easy startle response, tearfulness, social withdrawal, and inappropriate behavior or outbursts. Repeat instructions and give the patient time to verbalize concerns and fears. Increased reports of pain are frequently associated with high levels of anxiety.

Search for Meaning

Patient repeatedly recounts events leading to the injury and tries to determine a logical explanation that is emotionally acceptable. Listen actively, participate in the discussions, provide support, and avoid judging the patient's reasoning.

Investment in Recuperation and Treatment Plan

Patient is cooperative with the treatment plan, is motivated to be independent, and takes pride in small accomplishments. Educate the patient on discharge goals and involve both patient and family in planning an increased self-care program. Provide the patient with much praise and verbal encouragement.

Investment in Rehabilitation

As self-confidence increases, patient is focused on achieving as much preburn function as possible. Depression may occur as new losses in function are realized. This phase usually occurs after hospital discharge, when the patient is undergoing outpatient rehabilitation. Although staff support is typically limited in this phase, provide praise, support, and continued information as possible.

Reintegration of Identity

Patient accepts losses and recognizes that changes have occurred. Adaptation is completed, and staff involvement is terminated.

Modified from Rosenburg L, Rosenburn M, Rimmer RB, Fauerbach JA. Psychosocial recovery and reintegration of patients with burn injuries. In: Herndon DN, ed. *Total Burn Care.* 5th ed. Philadelphia, PA: Saunders Elsevier; 2018.

CRITICAL JUDGMENT ACTIVITY

Many patients with burn injuries are treated at institutions far from home. Determine what approaches can be used to meet the psychosocial needs of these patients and their families.

BOX 21.5 Support Programs for Patients With Burn Injuries and Families

- The Phoenix Society for Burn Survivors, a national organization that provides tools and support networks to assist survivors and families in their journey of healing: http://www.phoenix-society.org
- Peer support, such as Survivors Offering Assistance in Recovery (SOAR): http://www.phoenix-society.org/phoenix-soar
- The Model Systems Knowledge Translation Center, which provides evidence-based resources for those living with burn injuries: http://www.msktc.org/burn
- Burn units at local hospitals
- Burn survivor retreats and camps
- School reintegration programs, such as "The Journey Back" and REACH (Return to Education and Continued Healing)

LIFESPAN CONSIDERATIONS

Many unique pathophysiological, physical, and cognitive changes occur across the lifespan, and their impact affects burn injury, treatment, and outcomes (see Lifespan Considerations box). Regardless of age, a patient's physical and mental health greatly affect critical care management and outcome.[2,6] Despite improved survival rates, advanced age, especially in combination with deeper burns or inhalation injury, is a major determinant of mortality after thermal injury.[2,34] Carefully consider the decision to proceed with resuscitation in older adult patients with large burns and concomitant inhalation injury.[6] Guidance from advance directives, next of kin, and/or the designated healthcare surrogate or proxy is also vital to this decision-making process. Preexisting dementia exacerbated by injury and medications has major implications for an older adult patient's ability to participate in rehabilitation to regain function and independence. Aggressive burn treatment that promotes extension of life must be balanced with quality of life, including comfort, dignity, and patient wishes when known. Poor outcomes after burn injury highlight the importance of prevention of these injuries in the older adult patient.

NONBURN INJURIES

The expertise of the burn team in providing excellent wound and critical care has led to burn center admissions of patients with various other severe exfoliative and necrotizing skin disorders, such as toxic epidermal necrolysis (TEN), staphylococcal scalded skin syndrome (SSSS), and necrotizing fasciitis. These conditions create a clinical wound picture like that of a burn wound and require similar patient management and wound care. Management of these conditions in a burn center is associated with a marked increase in survival.[35,44]

Severe Exfoliative Disorders

Stevens-Johnson syndrome (SJS), TEN, and erythema multiforme (EM) are conditions in which the body sloughs its epidermal layer. The exact pathophysiological mechanism remains unclear, but the sloughing is thought to result from a direct toxic effect, a genetic susceptibility, and/or an immune-mediated response to a causative agent.[42] A common clinical finding is a positive *Nikolsky sign*, elicited by applying lateral pressure to the skin surface with resultant sloughing of the epidermis. Diagnosis of this related continuum of disorders is based on the skin biopsy histopathology (separation at the epidermal-dermal junction) and the extent of involvement of dermal detachment. EM is characterized by less than 10% TBSA affected, with peripheral distribution of lesions. Patients with SJS also have less than 10% TBSA affected, but lesions are widespread. If SJS occurs with TEN, lesions appear on 10% to 30% of TBSA. TEN is characterized by involvement of more than 30% TBSA, and lesions are extensive and widespread.[42]

LIFESPAN CONSIDERATIONS

Older Adults

- Older adults have thinner dermal layers, resulting in deeper burn injuries at lower temperatures or with shorter exposure times.[6]
- Older adults have reduced physiological reserves and capacity to respond to the significant metabolic stressors, hemodynamic demands, and inflammatory challenges after a burn injury. Preexisting cardiovascular, renal, and pulmonary diseases lead to challenges in fluid resuscitation, repeat hospitalizations, and increased morbidity and mortality.[6,29]
- Diminished manual dexterity, reaction time, senses, vision, hearing, balance, mobility, and judgment render older adults more vulnerable to burn injuries. Many older adults live alone, and they are often physically or mentally incapable of responding appropriately to an emergency.
- Advanced hemodynamic monitoring may help guide fluid administration.
- Age-related decline in immune system functioning contributes to increased susceptibility to infection.
- Frail older adults are at higher risk for hypothermia. Small muscle mass decreases the ability to generate heat by shivering.
- Factors contributing to the burn injury (e.g., dangers in the home environment, abuse, supervision or caregiving assistance, syncope, medication side effects) must be addressed before elderly patients are discharged.

Toxic Epidermal Necrolysis. TEN is the most extensive form of severe exfoliative disorder. It is associated with a mortality rate of 25% to 50%, compared with only 1% to 5% for SJS.[42] The most common cause of TEN is a pharmacological reaction, particularly from antibiotics (especially sulfa drugs), phenobarbital, allopurinol, phenytoin, and nonsteroidal anti-inflammatory drugs. In some cases, a definitive etiology is never identified.[42] Patients initially have fever and flu-like symptoms, with erythema and blisters developing within 24 to 96 hours. As large bullae develop, the skin and mucous membranes slough, resulting in a significant and painful partial-thickness injury. TEN is also associated with mucosal wound involvement of conjunctival, oral, GI tract, and/or urogenital areas.[42] Immune suppression occurs and contributes to life-threatening infection-related complications such as sepsis and pneumonia. Primary treatment includes immediate discontinuation of the potential offending drug. Although anticonvulsants and antibiotics are the most common causes, suspect any medication initiated in the past 3 to 4 weeks.[42] Optimal wound treatment consists of early coverage of cutaneous wounds with silver-based or biological dressings. Severe exfoliative disorders typically require intensive critical care management to provide fluid resuscitation and nutritional support. Corticosteroids are not indicated in the management of these patients.[42] Low-sucrose IV immune globulin administration may be beneficial in modulating the causative inflammatory response.[42] Supportive care and infection prevention limit wound progression to full-thickness depth. Long-term follow-up with the burn team is important to monitor for the development of commonly reported ophthalmic, skin, nail, and vulvovaginal complications.[42]

Staphylococcal Scalded Skin Syndrome. SSSS occurs primarily in young children and often manifests with a clinical picture similar to that of TEN. SSSS is caused by a reaction to a staphylococcal toxin, with intraepidermal splitting (unlike the epidermal-dermal separation seen in TEN) resulting in skin sloughing. Differential diagnosis is critical because the treatment for SSSS involves antibiotics, which can exacerbate TEN. Diagnosis is made by microscopic examination of the denuded skin to determine the level of skin separation. SSSS is limited to superficial epidermal involvement and does not affect the mucous membranes. SSSS is best treated with antibiotic therapy and wound care management.

Necrotizing Soft Tissue Infections

Necrotizing soft tissue infections (NSTIs) are a group of rapidly invasive infections that include diagnoses such as necrotizing fasciitis, gas gangrene, hemolytic streptococcal gangrene, Fournier gangrene (NSTI specifically involving the perineum and scrotum), and necrotizing cellulitis. NSTIs occur more frequently in middle-aged adults and are associated with high mortality rates, particularly if treatment is delayed or sepsis develops.[40] NSTIs are caused by polymicrobial organisms, including at least one anaerobic species in combination with one or more facultative anaerobic species. These may be introduced from minor skin disruptions such as insect bites or cuts. Diabetes mellitus, obesity, immune suppression, end-stage renal failure, IV drug use, smoking, recent surgery, and hypertension are common risk factors for NSTI.[40] NSTIs typically have a subtle initial presentation of a localized, painful edematous area with increasing erythema and induration. Crepitus, necrosis, and anesthesia are infrequently seen and are late signs. The pain is severe and out of proportion to cutaneous findings. Because of the rapidly progressive infectious nature of NSTIs, patients can quickly become critically ill, with observed high rates of sepsis and septic shock.[18,40] Early diagnosis, prompt and aggressive surgical excision, appropriate wound care, and empirical broad-spectrum antibiotic therapy are essential for a positive outcome.

Skin Failure

Skin failure should be considered in the care of critically ill patients.[45] Skin failure is a complex problem in which the skin, as the largest organ in the body, fails, similar to processes associated with other organs that fail. Several pathophysiological processes contribute to skin failure. These include hypoperfusion, hypoxia, inflammation, vascular permeability, and edema.[45,46] Hypoperfusion leads to decreased oxygen and nutrient flow to the skin, causing cellular damage and death.

Excessive pressure against the skin can also compromise perfusion, leading to tissue injury and death. It is important to continually assess the patient's skin to include looking under devices to prevent hospital associated pressure injuries (HAPI).

Hypoxia causes changes in cellular metabolism, creating the buildup of lactic acid and further shunting of blood to vital organs, decreasing peripheral perfusion. Skin mottling may be visible with compromised perfusion and hypoxia. Acute and chronic conditions can cause hypoxia, so skin failure can be both an acute and chronic problem often seen in the lower extremities of individuals with diabetes mellitus, heart failure, and renal failure. Inflammation can affect vascular endothelium, creating edema, which impairs the function of the dermal barrier and underlying tissue. With changes in vascular permeability, there is a predisposition for skin failure because of structure compromise that impairs oxygen and nutrient transport and an inability to remove waste. As fluid accumulates in the cells or interstitial space in the form of edema, the space to transport nutrients and oxygen increases. This can cause damage to cells and eventual cell death.

Pharmaceutical agents may also increase the susceptibility of skin to failure. Medications, such as vasopressors, steroids, and chemotherapeutic agents, decrease perfusion, weaken or decreases collagen synthesis, and alter immune function. When assessing the skin and wounds, it is important to ensure that all proper strategies for pressure injury prevention are employed prior to considering skin failure.

DISCHARGE PLANNING

Discharge planning for critically ill burned patients and for those who have sustained a nonburn injury begins on the day of admission. Assessments are made regarding patient survival, the potential or actual short-term or long-term functional disabilities secondary to the injury, the financial resources available, the family roles and expectations, and the psychological support systems. Educate both the patient and the family to prepare for transfer from the critical care unit and eventual discharge from the hospital. Be aware that preexisting learning disabilities or new cognitive deficits caused by the injury can affect a patient's understanding.[38] Patients and families who are returning home must understand how to manage their physical requirements and care for their psychological and social needs. Nurses play an important role in the multiprofessional team discharge planning by providing patient and family education and evaluating the need for additional resources to meet the patient's long-term rehabilitative and home care requirements.

BURN PREVENTION

The majority of burns and fire-related injuries are preventable. Typically, injuries do not occur from random events or "accidents" but rather predominantly from predictable incidents. If people are not aware of potential risks, they do not take appropriate precautions to prevent an injury from occurring. Alcohol and substance use contribute to high-risk behavior. Successful prevention efforts consider the targeted population and focus on interventions involving education, engineering of environment, or enforcement. Critical care nurses have an active and vital role in teaching prevention concepts and in promoting safety legislation to assist in reducing fires and burn injuries.[47] The incidence of burn injuries has been successfully decreased with widespread public safety education and government-mandated regulations such as improved building codes, fire retardant products, and home safety measures. Child-resistant lighters, preset water heater temperature, self-extinguishing cigarettes, fire sprinklers, and mandatory smoke alarms are all examples of successful injury prevention efforts.[1,47] The National Fire Protection Association provides multiple resources for preventing burn injuries (https://www.nfpa.org/Public-Education). Prevention is the best strategy for reducing burn injuries.

CASE STUDY

A 75-year-old female sustained a thermal burn injury in a house fire. She was smoking a cigarette in bed while receiving home medical oxygen therapy. She was trapped in the bedroom for approximately 15 minutes before being rescued by firefighters. No smoke alarms were noted in the home.

Questions

1. Once the patient is removed from the fire, identify priorities that are essential in her initial management.
2. The patient weighs 65 kg. She has burned an estimated 30% of her body. Calculate the estimated fluid requirement during the first 24 hours.
3. Given the patient's age and past medical history, identify assessments that will need to be implemented by the nurse during aggressive fluid resuscitation to evaluate signs of under- and overresuscitation.
4. Circumferential, white, leathery burn wounds are assessed on both arms. Based on this information, what type of burn wound does she have? List and prioritize nursing assessments and interventions that should be performed. What type of surgical treatment and wound care should be expected during the resuscitative phase and later in the acute care phase?
5. Considering the circumstances surrounding the patient's injury, identify discharge needs and resources she may need for successful discharge from the hospital.

KEY POINTS

- Prehospital care of the burn patient can affect long-term clinical outcomes.
- The care of the burn patient involves a multiprofessional team and is ideally delivered at a dedicated burn center.
- Definitive airway management should be considered early in the clinical course of patients with known or suspected inhalation injury, those with facial burns, or those requiring aggressive fluid resuscitation.
- Age-specific formulas are used to calculate fluid needs based on patient weight, percentage and depth of burn areas, and time.
- Adequate urine output guides fluid resuscitation titration.
- Effective pain management is a cornerstone of both acute and rehabilitative burn care.
- Wound care, including debridement and grafting, is a critical intervention for infection prevention.
- Adequate nutrition is essential to wound healing.
- Early physical and occupational therapy are necessary in preventing complications in mobility and preserving preburn functional status.

REFERENCES

1. American Burn Association. *Burn Incident and Treatment in the United States*. Chicago, IL: American Burn Association; 2016.
2. American Burn Association. *Annual Burn Injury Summary Report 2021 Update: Report of Data from 2015–2020*. Chicago, IL: American Burn Association; 2021.
3. Stoddard Jr FJ, Ryan CM, Schneider JC. Physical and psychiatric recovery from burns. *Surg Clin North Am*. 2014;94(4):863–878.
4. Masch JL, Bhutiani N, Bozeman C. Feeding during resuscitation after burn injury. *Nutr Clin Pract*. 2019;34(5):666–671.
5. Daugherty S, Spear M. Skin and skin substitutes—an overview. *Plast Surg Nurs*. 2015;35(2):92–97.
6. American Burn Association. *Advanced Burn Life Support Course: Provider's Manual*. Chicago, IL: American Burn Association; 2022.
7. Legrand M, Barraud D, Constant C, et al. Management of severe thermal burns in the acute phase in adults and children. *Anaesth Crit Care Pain Med*. 2020;39(2):253–267.
8. Deutsch CJ, Tan A, Smailes S, Dziewulski. The diagnosis and management of inhalation injury: an evidence based approach. *Burns*. 2018;44(5):1040–1051.
9. Wolf SJ, Maloney GE, Shih RD, et al. Clinical policy: critical issues in the evaluation and management of adult patients presenting to the emergency department with acute carbon monoxide poisoning. *Ann Emerg Med*. 2017;69(1):98–107.
10. Gus EI, Shahrokhi S, Jeschke MG. Anabolic and anticatabolic agents used in burn care: what is known and what is yet to be learned. *Burns*. 2020;46(1):19–32.
11. Borron S, Baud F, Barriot P, et al. Prospective study of hydroxocobalamin for acute cyanide poisoning in smoke inhalation. *Ann Emerg Med*. 2007;49(6):794–801.
12. *CYANOKIT [package insert]*. BTG International Inc; 2021.
13. Woodson LC, Branski LK, Enkhbaatar P, Talon M. Diagnosis and treatment of inhalation injury. In: Herndon DN, ed. *Total Burn Care*. 5th ed. St. Louis, MO: Elsevier; 2018:184–194.
14. Spectral MD burn image assessment study ("BIAS") results. *Newswire*. 2022. https://www.newswire.com/news/spectral-md-burn-image-assessment-study-bias-results-21839378. Accessed March 28, 2023.

15. Chong HP, Quinn L, Jeeves A, et al. A comparison study of methods for estimation of a burn surface area: Lund and Browder, e-burn and Mersey burns. *Burns*. 2020;46(2):483–489.
16. Cope D, Moore FD. The redistribution of body water in the fluid therapy of the burn patient. *Ann Surg*. 1947;126(6):1010–1045.
17. Demling RH, Mazess RB, Witt RM, et al. The study of burn wound edema using dichromatic absorptiometry. *J Trauma*. 1978;18(2):124–128.
18. Yan J, Hill WF, Rehou S, et al. Sepsis criteria versus clinical diagnosis of sepsis in burn patients: a validation of current sepsis score. *Surgery*. 2018;164(6):1241–1245.
19. Palmieri T. Pediatric burn resuscitation. *Crit Care Clin*. 2016;32(4):547–559.
20. Abraham P, Monard C, Schneider A, Rimmele T. Extracorporeal blood purification in burns: for whom, why, and how? *Blood Purif*. 2023;52(1):17–24.
21. Houschyar M, Borrelli M, Tapking C, et al. Burns: modified metabolism and the nuances of nutrition therapy. *J Wound Care*. 2020;29(3):184–191.
22. Demling RH, Wong C, Jin LJ, et al. Early lung dysfunction after major burns: role of edema and vasoactive mediators. *J Trauma*. 1985;25(10):959–966.
23. Tejiram S, Romanowski KS, Palmieri T. Initial management of severe burn injury. *Curr Opin Crit Care*. 2019;25(6):647–652.
24. Bittner EA, Shank E, Woodson L, et al. Acute and perioperative care of the burn-injured patient. *Anesthesiology*. 2015;122(2):448–464.
25. Gigengack RK, Cleffken BI, Loer SA. Advanced in airway management and mechanical ventilation in inhalation injury. *Curr Opin Anaesthesiol*. 2020;33(6):774–780.
26. Saffle JR. Fluid creep and over-resuscitation. *Crit Care Clin*. 2016;32(4):587–598.
27. Greenhalgh DG, Cartotto R, Taylor SL, et al. Burn resuscitation practices in North America: results of the acute burn resuscitation multicenter prospective trial (ABRUPT). *Ann Surg*. 2023;277(3):512–519.
28. Cartotto R, Greenhalgh D. Colloids in acute burn resuscitation. *Crit Care Clin*. 2016;32(4):507–523.
29. Cartotto R, Greenhalgh DG, Cancio C. Burn state of the science: fluid resuscitation. *J Burn Care Res*. 2017;38(3):e596–e604.
30. Rizzo JA, Rowan MP, Driscoll IR, et al. Vitamin C in burn resuscitation. *Crit Care Clin*. 2016;32(4):539–546.
31. Meizoso JP, Ray JJ, Allen CJ, et al. Hypercoagulability and venous thromboembolism in burn patients. *Semin Thromb Hemost*. 2015;41(1):43–48.
32. Lopez ON, Bohanon FJ, Radhakrishnan RS, Chung DH. Surgical management of complications of burn injury. In: Herdon DH, ed. *Total Burn Care*. Philadelphia, PA: Saunders; 2018:386–395.e3.
33. De Laet IE, Malbrain ML, De Waele JJ. A clinician's guide to management of intra-abdominal hypertension and abdominal compartment syndrome in critically ill patients. *Critical Care*. 2020;24(97):1–9.
34. Jones CD, Ho W, Gunn E, et al. E-cigarette burn injuries: comprehensive review and management guidelines proposal. *Burns*. 2019;45(4):763–771.
35. Palmieri TL. Infection prevention: unique aspects of burn units. *Surg Infect*. 2019;20(2):111–114.
36. Assimacopoulos EM, Heard J, Liao J, et al. The national incidence and resource utilization of burn injuries sustained while smoking on home oxygen therapy (HOT). *J Burn Care Res*. 2016;37(1):25–31.
37. Romanowski KS, Carson J, Pape K, et al. American Burn Association guidelines on the management of acute pain in the adult burn patient: a review of the literature, a compilation of expert opinions, and next steps. *J Burn Care Res*. 2020;41(6):1129–1151.
38. Stoddard Jr FJ, Ryan CM, Schneider JC. Physical and psychiatric recovery from burns. *Psychiatr Clin North Am*. 2015;38(1):105–120.
39. Kantak NA, Mistry R, Halvorson EG. A review of negative-pressure wound therapy in the management of burn wounds. *Burns*. 2016;42(8):1623–1633.
40. Bonne SL, Kadri SS. Evaluation and management of necrotizing soft tissue infections. *Infec Dis Clin N Am*. 2017;31(3):497–511.
41. Dolgachev VA, Ciotti SM, Eisma R, et al. Nanoemulsion therapy for burn wounds is effective as a topical antimicrobial against gram negative and gram positive bacteria. *J Burn Care Res*. 2016;37(2):e104–e114.
42. Woolum JA, Bailey AM, Baum RA, et al. A review of the management of Stevens-Johnson syndrome and toxic epidermal necrolysis. *Adv Emerg Nurs J*. 2019;41(1):56–64.
43. Kopel J, Brower GL, Sorensen G, Griswold J. Application of beta-blockers in burn management. *Proc Bayl Univ Med Center*. 2022;35(1):46–50.
44. Real DS, Reis RP, Piccolo MS, et al. Oxandrolone use in adult burn patients: systematic review and meta-analysis. *Acta Cir Bras*. 2014;29(suppl 3):68–76.
45. Levine JM, Delmore B, Cox J. Skin failure: concept review and proposed model. *Adv Skin Wound Care*. 2022;35(3):139–148.
46. Ayello EA, Levine JM, Langemo D, et al. Reexamining the literature on terminal ulcers, scale, skin failure, and unavoidable pressure injuries. *Adv Skin Wound Care*. 2019;32(3):109–121.
47. Klas KS, Smith SJ, Matherly AF, et al. Multicenter assessment of burn team injury prevention knowledge. *J Burn Care Res*. 2015;36(3):434–439.

ANSWER KEY

CHECK YOUR UNDERSTANDING ANSWERS

CHAPTER 1

1. **A.** The mission of the American Association of Critical Care Nurses is to drive excellence in acute and critical care for nurses, patients and families. AACN supports acute and critical care nurses in practice.
2. **D.** By obtaining certification, nurses are able to demonstrate their skill mastery and knowledge about caring for acutely and critically ill patients. Once certified, nurses must complete ongoing education and professional development to maintain certification.
3. **B.** Crew resource management is psychological training used in the airline industry to assist crew members in avoiding or mitigating threats by developing, communicating, and implementing an action plan after identifying potential and existing threats.
4. **C.** The AACN defines a healthy work environment as integrating the following six standards to achieve improved patient, nurse, and family outcomes: skilled communication, true collaboration, appropriate staffing, meaningful recognition, effective decision-making, and authentic leadership.

CHAPTER 2

1. **A.** Asking questions can help families better understand the patient's condition and the medical interventions being provided. Families who ask questions can be more involved in the patient's care, and this can lead to improved communication and a greater sense of control. When you encourage families to ask questions, it can help build trust in the healthcare team and the medical decisions being made. Overall, encouraging family members to ask questions can help improve communication, involvement, trust, and outcomes for both the patient and the family.
2. **C.** Even if a patient appears to be unresponsive, they may still be able to hear and understand what is happening around them. For this reason, healthcare providers should always use caution when speaking near a sedated patient and ensure the conversations are respectful and appropriate. Music therapy can help reduce stress and anxiety, improve sleep, and promote relaxation in critically ill patients. Hearing familiar voices and sounds can also provide comfort and a sense of security. The likelihood of a patient becoming combative while sedated is minimal, but it may happen due to delirium or confusion.
3. **D.** PICS was defined by the Society of Critical Care Medicine in 2013 as a persistent condition that affects the physical, cognitive, and mental status of survivors of critical illness who have been hospitalized in a critical care unit. This definition recognizes that PICS can have a range of symptoms that include physical weakness, cognitive impairment, depression, anxiety, and posttraumatic stress disorder. Delirium is an acute cognitive impairment occurring in the critical care unit that contributes to the development of PICS. ICU psychosis is not a recognized term.
4. **C.** Though each intervention may alleviate the family's concerns to a degree, the most effective intervention is to coordinate a multiprofessional team meeting with the family. This instills confidence regarding the caliber of care being provided to the patient. In addition, each team member can address questions specific to their specialty.

CHAPTER 3

1. **D.** Options A, B, and C are all examples of nursing actions that are aligned with the ANA Code of Ethics.
2. **C.** Protecting patient confidentiality is a core ethical principle. While you may wish to calm the caller, you cannot provide information about a patient without their consent and, as in this case of the patient being a minor, consent of the parent(s).
3. **C and D.** One of the nurse's roles in the informed consent process is to advocate for the patient by making sure they have been provided the necessary information to give informed consent. The nurse can witness the signature on the consent form. A and B are roles of the nurse; it is the provider's duty to provide the patient with information regarding the risks, benefits, and alternatives of the procedure.
4. **D.** This is an example of the doctrine of double effect. It is ethically acceptable for a nurse to titrate medication to relieve suffering, even if the medication causes the patient to stop breathing.

CHAPTER 4

1. **A.** Multiple factors influence the continuation of aggressive care in the face of a poor prognosis, including cultural and religious beliefs.
2. **D.** All of the above are concepts important to share with the new critical care clinician to facilitate their understanding of the role of palliative care in critical care settings.
3. **D.** Both B and C would ensure the nurse is appropriately advocating for the patient and their wishes while engaging the family and multiprofessional team in the goals of care discussion.

CHAPTER 5

1. **A and B.** Goals of care discussions should occur often, if not daily, to go over the patient's wishes and ensure the treatment plan aligns with the goals of care. Brain death testing is recommended given the absence of reflexes identified on assessment. C and D are not appropriate options. Tracheostomy is

not to be discussed without first identifying the goals of care and whether the patient is legally dead per neurological criteria. Based on the evidence for decoupling, the primary care team should not approach the discussion of organ donation with the family.

2. **D.** Based on the limited number of donation exclusion criteria, all patients listed would be medically suitable for organ donation.
3. **B.** Most OPOs prefer a history negative for smoking, diabetes, dyslipidemia, and hypertension. Low LDL levels are desirable.

CHAPTER 6

1. **A.** The pain type is visceral, characterized by diffuse, poorly localized pain to the epigastrium, which refers to the patient's back.
2. **A.** In nonverbal patients, observe behaviors using either the Behavioral Pain Scale (BPS) or the Critical-Care Pain Observation Tool (CPOT). Both tools demonstrate the greatest validity and reliability for monitoring pain in noncommunicative patients.
3. **B.** Activation of the SNS results in tachycardia and hypertension and may lead to hyperventilation. Drowsiness and vertigo are not related to agitation.
4. **C.** The patient would not be appropriate for CAM-ICU assessment and would be scored as unable to assess. Patients receiving deep sedation should be weaned from sedation as appropriate to allow for CAM-ICU assessment.

CHAPTER 7

1. **A.** Obtain enteral access. Based on the brief assessment, the patient is appropriate for enteral nutrition and could benefit from early initiation of enteral nutrition once access is achieved. The tube can also be used for decompression upon intubation.
2. **B, C, and D.** Stopping the enteral nutrition should be avoided. Critically ill patients are often on medications that decrease motility, such as narcotics and sedatives; therefore, a prokinetic agent may be beneficial. Rarely is EN formula the cause; however, consultation with the dietitian may be helpful to determine opportunities to change the rate or type of formula. Post-pyloric access is preferred in patients with demonstrated gastric EN intolerance.
3. **D.** The patient has experienced a prolonged time to initiation of EN (>7 days), and EN continues to be contraindicated based on high dose vasopressors and GI discontinuity.

CHAPTER 8

1. **C.** The increased heart rate reduces ventricular filling time and coronary artery perfusion (both of which occur during ventricular diastole). Lack of coronary artery perfusion with increased heart rate causes stress on the heart and may lead to angina from excessive oxygen consumption needs.
2. **C.** No visualization of P waves rules out sinus rhythm, sinus arrhythmia, and premature atrial contractions, as all three of these rhythms contain P waves. The term sinus implies there is a P wave. In addition, the term atrial indicates there is likely to be a P wave. Therefore, the answer most likely correct is junctional rhythm.
3. **B.** The patient is symptomatic, evidenced by his complaint of lightheadedness and low blood pressure. Emergency interventions include administering adenosine, so anticipating the need to assist with this intervention is the first priority.
4. **D.** The patient has a symptomatic bradycardia rhythm, as the heart rate is <60 beats/min. The cardiac monitor likely shows a third-degree block, in which there is no relationship between the atria and ventricles. Because the patient is symptomatic, temporary pacing via the transcutaneous method is most appropriate to increase the heart rate.

CHAPTER 9

1. **B.** Elevated RAP is associated with hypervolemia; thus, the treatment is to reduce the circulating blood volume through diuresis. Blood transfusions would further exacerbate hypervolemia. Vasopressors could also further increase RAP. Coughing and deep breathing only transiently reduce intrathoracic pressure and consequently RAP.
2. **A.** The PAC is primarily used to measure pulmonary artery occlusive pressures, providing a measure of left ventricular preload. Pulmonary artery pressures are also provided as a measure of the pulmonary vasculature (but not of the mechanics of the lungs). Right atrial and ventricular function can be assessed with less invasive means.
3. **B.** Expect administration of 500 mL of 0.9% normal saline IV, as the SVV is greater than 10%, indicating hypovolemia. Initiation of dobutamine may improve stroke volume by stimulating beta-1 receptors; however, the stimulation of beta-2 receptors results in vasodilation, exacerbating the hypovolemia. Initiation of norepinephrine results in vasoconstriction, but in the presence of hypovolemia, it may reduce tissue perfusion even more. Epinephrine 0.5 mg IV push is not indicated, as this is an incorrect dose and used only in cardiopulmonary resuscitation.

CHAPTER 10

1. **A.** Color change from purple to yellow on the end-tidal carbon dioxide ($ETCO_2$) detector, providing objective verification of correct placement of the endotracheal tube (ETT) in the trachea (versus incorrect placement in the esophagus), is imperative and is obtained through clinical assessment and confirmation devices. Either a handheld or disposable $ETCO_2$ detector provides immediate objective indication of the presence of CO_2. Clinical assessment includes auscultating the epigastrium and anterior, upper lung fields and observing for bilateral chest expansion. Auscultating the lower, posterior lung fields is not pragmatic and could pick up sounds referred from air in the stomach with an esophageal intubation.

2. **Matching:** Volume-controlled ventilation modes include: volume assist/control and volume intermittent mandatory ventilation. Pressure ventilation modes include: pressure support, pressure-assist/control, and airway pressure release ventilation.
3. **A.** Noninvasive ventilation (NIV) is indicated for the treatment of acute exacerbations of chronic obstructive pulmonary disease (COPD) and respiratory failure associated with pneumonia. The other patients have contraindications for NIV (i.e., hemodynamic instability, high risk for aspiration secondary to copious secretions, active ST elevation myocardial infarction [STEMI]).

CHAPTER 11

1. **D.** Rapid response teams (RRTs) have been implemented to address changes in a patient's clinical condition before a cardiac or respiratory arrest occurs; therefore, it is appropriate for the nurse to call the rapid response team for all of these patients.
2. **C.** Symptomatic bradycardia occurs when the heart rhythm is slow enough to cause hemodynamic compromise and poor perfusion with signs and symptoms such as hypotension, diaphoresis, chest pain, shortness of breath, decreased level of consciousness, and syncope. The cause of these signs and symptoms is related to the decreased cardiac output associated with the decreased heart rate. The appropriate initial intervention for this patient is administration of atropine 1 mg. Though the patient may require temporary pacing, transvenous pacing would not be the initial intervention.
3. **A.** Checking the patient's pulse would be the priority, as the management differs depending on the presence or absence of a pulse. If the patient has a pulse, each of these interventions may be appropriate for the treatment of the patient's rhythm, depending upon the patient's stability.
4. **D.** Both B and C would be appropriate assessments and potential interventions if the water temperature began to decrease. Both shivering and fever generate heat, which would require the water temperature to decrease in an effort to maintain the goal temperature set for targeted temperature management.

CHAPTER 12

1. **B.** The patient's clinical presentation describes the compensatory stage of shock. The patient's neural, endocrine, and chemical compensatory mechanisms are being initiated. His symptoms are becoming apparent, and shock is potentially reversible with minimal morbidity if appropriate interventions are initiated.
2. **A.** The patient is experiencing distributive (septic) shock secondary to the urinary tract infection. The nurse would expect the patient to have elevated lactic acid values as a result of the anaerobic metabolism.
3. **C.** In neurogenic shock, there is an interruption of impulse transmission or a blockage of sympathetic outflow that results in vasodilation, inhibition of baroreceptor response, and impaired thermoregulation. These reactions result in hypotension, bradycardia, and warm, dry skin. Priorities would include stabilizing the spine to reduce the risk of severe neurogenic shock and improving the blood pressure and heart rate through appropriate resuscitation and medication management.

CHAPTER 13

1. **A.** Sleep apnea causes periods of low PaO_2 and elevated $PaCO_2$, which cause vessels to constrict, increasing stress on the heart and the risk of heart disease. Chemoreceptors are sensitive to changes in partial pressure of arterial oxygen (PaO2), partial pressure of arterial carbon dioxide ($PaCO_2$), and pH blood levels. Chemoreceptors stimulate the vasomotor center in the medulla; this center controls vasoconstriction (decreased PaO_2 and/or increased $PaCO_2$ and decreased pH) and vasodilation (increased PaO_2 and/or decreased $PaCO_2$ and increased pH).
2. **D.** P stands for provocation. The fact that the chest pain is associated with strenuous activity suggests it is associated with provocation.
3. **D.** The LVEF is the percentage of blood ejected from the left ventricle during systole, normally 55% to 60%.
4. **B.** Variant, or Prinzmetal's, angina is caused by coronary artery spasms. It often occurs at rest and without other precipitating factors. The electrocardiogram (ECG) shows a marked ST elevation (usually seen only in acute myocardial infarction [AMI]) during the episode.
5. **A.** The patient needs to be informed of contraindications for taking NTG if a phosphodiesterase type 5 inhibitor was taken.
6. **C.** Place the patient in semi-fowlers position and administer a diuretic.

CHAPTER 14

1. **A.** The brainstem controls vital functions, such as the basic rhythm of respiration via the medulla, and is the origin for the cranial nerves responsible for pupillary response (III), cough and gag (IX and X), and hearing (VIII).
2. **B.** The patient's ICPs are sustained, as they have been above 20 mm Hg for more than 5 minutes. Elevating the head of bed to 30 degrees and ensuring the patient's head and neck are midline facilitates venous drainage and decreases the risk of venous obstruction. This would be the first intervention to implement, as there is no sedative or blood pressure side effects. If ineffective, administration of an analgesic or hypertonic saline may be appropriate.
3. **D.** To determine potential eligibility for thrombolytic therapy within 4.5 hours or mechanical thrombectomy within 24 hours, time of symptom onset must be clearly identified.
4. **A.** The patient should be placed on droplet precautions.
5. **C.** Neurogenic shock is characterized by hypotension, bradycardia, and hypothermia.

CHAPTER 15

1. **D.** The patient meets the Berlin definition of ARDS criteria based on the following: acute onset within 1 week after clinical insult, bilateral pulmonary opacities, respiratory failure that does not appear to have a cardiac origin of edema (i.e., cardiac failure, fluid overload), and a PaO_2/FiO_2 ratio of 96.7 (PaO_2 58/FiO_2 0.6 = 96.7). The PaO_2/FiO_2 ratio determines the severity of ARDS, which is severe in this case.
2. **B.** Lower tidal volumes are an evidence-based method for preventing ventilator-induced lung injury and are a part of the lung protective ventilation strategies.
3. **D.** All of the above are methods for treating ARF in COPD. Early treatment with noninvasive ventilation has been found to decrease mortality. Bronchodilators can decrease airway resistance, and corticosteroids can decrease inflammation and edema, improving lung function.
4. **C.** Components of the ventilator bundle to prevent VAP include head of bed elevation to at least 30 degrees, a protocol to guide a daily spontaneous breathing trial with assessment of need for continuing mechanical ventilation, improving physical conditioning, and provision of oral care with toothbrushing without chlorhexidine.
5. **A.** This patient has four risk factors for DVT (i.e., multiple trauma, lower extremity fractures, older than 75 years of age, and immobility expected to last longer than 3 days based on his injuries). The other patients do not have as many risk factors as this patient, who may also be unable to obtain VTE pharmacological prophylaxis in a timely manner depending on the evolution of his traumatic brain injury. All of these are acquired risks for the development of DVT.

CHAPTER 16

1. **A.** Diabetes is a non-modifiable risk factor for the development of AKI.
2. **C.** Patients with renal failure develop metabolic acidosis (pH less than 7.35 and HCO_3 below 22 mEq/L).
3. **D.** Patients with diabetes (as evidenced by an elevated HbA1c) are at risk for the development of AKI.
4. **D.** A low creatinine clearance (i.e., glomerular filtration rate) indicates the presence of AKI to the critical care nurse.
5. **A.** For critically high potassium levels, administration of IV insulin and 50% dextrose rapidly reduces serum potassium levels by shifting the potassium intracellularly. Albuterol (a pure $ß_1$ agonist) may also be used and temporarily pushes potassium back into the cell from the bloodstream. Definitive treatment is required with critical hyperkalemia conditions (e.g., hemodialysis, sodium polystyrene sulfonate [Kayexalate]).
6. **B.** Hypocalcemia is a complication associated with CRRT and is most likely attributed to the use of citrate anticoagulation.

CHAPTER 17

1. **C.** The band neutrophils are referred to as immature neutrophils. A shift to the left happens with an increased number of bands or band neutrophils.
2. **C.** Bleeding precautions are a priority intervention, as the patient may have vitamin B_{12} deficiency anemia associated with age and alcohol use disorder history; RBC suggests anemia, and low platelet count increases the risk for bleeding.
3. **B.** Thrombocytopenia is defined as a quantitative deficiency of platelets, specifically a platelet count less than 150,000/mm^3. The best treatment option for this condition is infusion of platelets.
4. **D.** Gram-negative bacterial infection is one of the listed "infections" to cause DIC. In addition, abruptio placentae is one of the obstetrical causes of DIC. Transfusion reactions are an identified case of hematological disorders that cause DIC. Acute renal failure is not a likely cause of DIC. See Table 17.12 for reference.

CHAPTER 18

1. **D.** All of the above would be appropriate assessments and interventions. The liver is highly vascular, so the nurse can expect to monitor for signs and symptoms of bleeding (i.e. hemoglobin, hematocrit, blood pressure, and heart rate). Serial abdominal assessments assist with identifying changes in the patient's pain, abdominal girth, and distention, which can assist in identifying bleeding, the development of a concomitant injury, or abdominal compartment syndrome.
2. **C.** Assessment of pain assists in identifying potential problems. Assessment of the usual diet provides information on intake that may contribute to constipation, such as low fiber intake.
3. **A.** The patient is most likely experiencing a PUD secondary to *H. pylori* based on ulcer location, positive urea breath test, and concomitant use of NSAIDs. The first-line treatment for *H. pylori* infection consists of triple therapy with a proton pump inhibitor (PPI; e.g., esomeprazole, omeprazole, pantoprazole, rabeprazole) plus use of the antibiotics amoxicillin and clarithromycin.
4. **D.** The patient presents with liver disease. Clinical signs and symptoms are those of heart failure and include jugular vein distension, pulmonary crackles, and decreased perfusion to all organs secondary to portal hypertension. When a patient experiences low blood pressure, dysrhythmias are common. Overtime, esophageal varices can develop, which may have been the cause of the patient's recent upper GI bleed. The patient may be altered secondary to an elevated ammonia level.

CHAPTER 19

1. **C.** With two elevated findings greater than 300 mg/dL in a 12-hour period, it is a priority to ensure that safe and quality care is administered to this patient in a timely manner. Consistently high blood glucose levels require insulin management to establish lower glycemic levels for improved patient outcomes.
2. **C.** With SGLT-2 inhibitor euglycemic DKA, the nurse obtains data about the patient's blood glucose, presence of ketones in the urine, and a full set of vital signs.

3. **D.** Options for the 15/15 rule include the following: 3-4 glucose tablets; one-half cup (4 oz or 120 mL) of fruit juice; 1 tablespoon corn syrup, 8 oz of skim or low-fat milk; 1 tablespoon (15 grams) of sugar. Choosing any one of these appropriate doses of the sugar replacement is acceptable. Once glucose is given, fingerstick glucose is reassessed in 15 minutes to evaluate effectiveness.
4. **B.** Patients may need emergency treatment. Dexamethasone can be given and does not interfere with the results of the test.
5. **A.** Marked tachycardia is commonly noted in thyroid storm secondary to the increase in metabolism and the stimulation of catecholamines produced by excess thyroid hormones.

CHAPTER 20

1. **C.** The primary survey encourages continual evaluation for uncontrolled hemorrhage and life-threatening conditions, which require immediate intervention through the ABCDEFG mnemonic.
2. **A.** The focused assessment with sonography for trauma (FAST) or extended FAST (E-FAST) exams are typically the first-line diagnostic tools used for the emergent evaluation of a patient presenting with traumatic injuries.
3. **A, B, and E.** The "trauma triad of death" is a vicious cycle that occurs in the severely injured patient. The patient can lose the ability to autoregulate temperature as a result of the injuries or hypovolemic shock, which causes hypothermia. Acidosis occurs secondary to hypothermia, lactic acid production during hypovolemic shock, and/or over-resuscitation with unbalanced crystalloids. Coagulopathy occurs secondary to the aforementioned hypothermia and acidosis but is worsened via consumption of coagulation factors and potential dilution from over-resuscitation with crystalloids.
4. **D.** An elevated lactate level indicates the patient's cellular perfusion is poor and anaerobic metabolism is still occurring. Adequate ventilation and successful fluid resuscitation lead to a decrease in lactate levels.
5. **B.** A patient developing compartment syndrome typically complains of an increasing throbbing pain disproportionate to the injury. Attempts to reduce the pain with narcotics do not relieve the pain.

CHAPTER 21

1. **B.** Superficial partial-thickness burns are wounds that are moist, pink or mottled red, and very painful and that blanch briskly with pressure. Addressing the patient's pain with prescribed analgesics is a priority in care.
2. **C.** Using the palmar surface method, the palm, including the fingers, of the patient's hand represents 1% of his or her total body surface area. Thus, three palmar surface areas would equate to approximately 3% TBSA.
3. **D.** Humidified 100% oxygen via face mask or endotracheal tube is administered in the patient with an inhalation injury until carboxyhemoglobin (COHgb) levels are determined. Once COHgb levels normalize (<10%), wean oxygen as tolerated.
4. **A.** During the first 24 hours, age, total body surface area burned, patient weight, and cause of burn injury are used to guide fluid resuscitation.

INDEX

Page numbers followed by *"f"* indicate figures, *"b"* indicate boxes, and *"t"* indicate tables.

F

G

O

P

Q

R

S

T

SPECIAL FEATURES

CASE STUDIES

CLINICAL ALERTS

CLINICAL EXEMPLARS

CLINICAL JUDGMENT ACTIVITIES

EVIDENCE-BASED PRACTICE BOXES